Comprehensive Migraine Management

Teshamae S. Monteith • Nina Riggins
Peter J. Goadsby
Editors

Comprehensive Migraine Management

Springer

Editors
Teshamae S. Monteith
Department of Neurology
Miller School of Medicine, University of Miami
Miami, FL, USA

Nina Riggins
Headache Center of Excellence
VA Palo Alto, CA, USA

Peter J. Goadsby
Department of Neurology
University of California, Los Angeles (UCLA) Health
Los Angeles, CA, USA

ISBN 978-3-031-86922-8 ISBN 978-3-031-86923-5 (eBook)
https://doi.org/10.1007/978-3-031-86923-5

This Springer imprint is published by the registered company Springer Nature Switzerland AG
The registered company address is: Gewerbestrasse 11, 6330 Cham, Switzerland

Foreword

Do we need new books on migraine? Well this one shows that we actually do need them and *Comprehensive Management of Migraine* is such a book. Edited by neurologists with an in-depth knowledge of migraine and experience in the clinical and scientific basis of subject matter makes this book a timely offering. Their stewardship presents us with up-to-date information on migraine in a way that should appeal to new readers of the subject as well as experienced clinicians and all those interested in the burgeoning field of migraine therapeutics.

When I first learned about the development of this new book, I was impressed with the topics showing the remarkable breadth and depth of the subject. Divided into seven parts, this allows one to read the core knowledge necessary to manage migraine or explore multiple other areas of interest. Migraine has been a subject of human observations for centuries. In the last couple decades of the twentieth century and up to the present in this century the knowledge about migraine management has made remarkable strides.

This is a generational book including many new authors, from several continents, in conjunction with senior authors in their fields of interest in migraine. Migraine is one of the leading causes of neurological disabilities in the world, and there is much to learn on the subject when it comes to managing people with migraine. It is all here in this book of 40 chapters. Careful attention to many topics has been outlined by the editors in the Introduction to follow. For example, you need to know how to diagnose migraine to ensure you know exactly what you are treating and not treating, including migraine variants and comorbid disorders. Migraine has to be diagnosed in the presence of less common primary disorders and secondary headache diseases.

You can learn about the history of migraine, its epidemiology, its relations to epilepsy and stroke, along with pediatric migraine and those in the elderly. Also, how to manage migraine when other pain disorders exist and how to manage chronic migraine. It is truly comprehensive as you can see from the table of contents. Most chapters are supported by case histories, questions and answers with brief discussions, allowing context to the subject for the readers. Summaries and key points are added, as are excellent diagrams and tables. The references cover the pertinent literature and are up-to-date.

There have been rapid changes in treatment options in the last few decades. This is where this book stands out. It represents more than a snapshot of the management issues but more of unique story of where we were, how did we get to where we are now, and what is to come in the future. The growth in management options has been punctuated over time by new discoveries in understanding migraine and new medications, such as the triptans and now the calcitonin gene-related peptide antagonists, but also by unique non-pharmacological treatments.

Every once in a while I like to sit down and get a worthwhile pause and update my learning on a subject. A good book which is truly comprehensively and covers the topics succinctly is best for that purpose. One can know too little or too much in medicine about any subject and in migraine and its management this is easy to do. Migraine knowledge has to be disseminated for others to learn. Numerous new papers on migraine come online daily and one cannot always keep up, but a book like this allows a way to keep clinically relevant in migraine. The subject is enormous and important, to people with migraine.

I should note that at the end of the book there is a chapter on teaching migraine around the world. I was a co-writer invited to prepare this chapter, and although it does not deal directly with migraine management, it underlies a big challenge to all who practice and teach about migraine. There are just not enough health professionals in the world to see all those who need assessment and management so it is so important to teach about migraine.

If you want to learn about migraine, use this book as a guide and a source of information to direct you. It covers advocacy efforts, national associations, and organizations that work in this field regularly to help people with migraine. Go to the ample local, regional, and national meetings on migraine in person or online. Learn and teach others about migraine, as it plays a huge role in the practice of medicine. No matter what you do in medicine, you will benefit from learning more about migraine and neurology. Migraine is a great teacher of neurology.

So, enjoy this new book, read it and learn and teach from it. It provides a wide range of useful, pragmatic information and would be of value to anyone who sees, studies, or does research regarding people with migraine. It should pique your curiosity about the brain and migraine, and provide the "tools to optimize treatment plans" as the Editors suggest. I congratulate them on preparing this essential and valuable book.

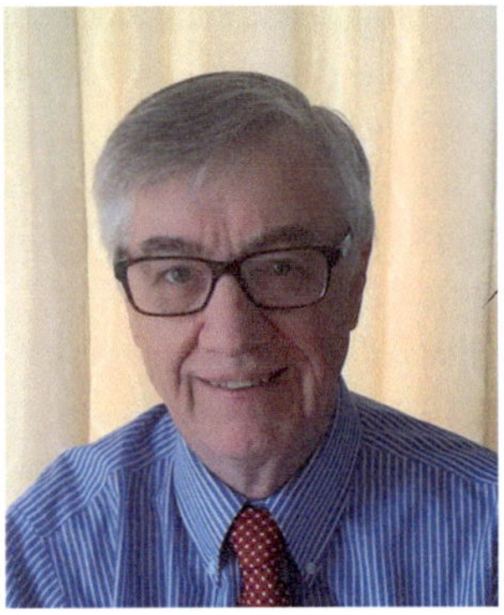

R. Allan Purdy
Professor of Medicine (Neurology)
Dalhousie University
Halifax, NS, Canada
July 22, 2024

Preface

While as an undergraduate student at Florida International University, I was lucky to learn about neuroscience and receive mentorship as a recipient of a program funded by the National Institutes of Health. I soon became committed to become a doctor, the perfect opportunity to provide service to humanity and public health, engage in science, and help people. Along my journey, I had great opportunities to learn about medicine and clinical research from brilliant and passionate doctors who inspired me. While I considered several subspecialities, it was neurology that I loved the most and headache medicine that seemed to be the best fit. I loved the idea of caring for and empowering many different types of people across the lifespan, as well as the overlap with women's health.

I was fascinated by the potential impact of headache medicine (given the huge prevalence) and the modifiable nature of disorders such as migraine that impact quality of life. After completing my neurology residency at the New York University School of Medicine, I completed a headache fellowship at the Thomas Jefferson University Jefferson Headache Center in Pennsylvania under the direction of Stephen Silberstein, MD. This experience was fundamental for developing a comprehensive and systematic approach to headache management. I met Peter J. Goadsby, MD, PhD, DSc, FRS, at the American Headache Society and learned about his research vision and the opportunities to advance headache disorders. It was not long before I chose to do a second fellowship at the University of California, San Francisco, where he worked. It has been a great honor to co-edit this book with both Peter J. Goadsby, MD, PhD, and Nina Riggins, MD, PhD.

I have dedicated my professional career to people living with headache disorders. As a busy professor of clinical neurology, chief of a headache division, and fellowship program director, I understand the highly rewarding yet challenging nature of what we do. For me, it was critical to develop a comprehensive book on migraine that can help provide knowledge and insights to advance migraine care. I believe this book will be both enjoyable and contribute to the competence necessary to provide high quality migraine care. I am grateful for my family, friends, colleagues, mentors, and patients that both support and inspire me. I would especially like to thank Nedra Kalish her wisdom and generous support over the years. We have an amazing collection of leading authors for which I am also grateful. I hope you will enjoy learning from this book as much as we enjoyed developing it.

Miami, FL, USA Teshamae S. Monteith

Preface

From a very young age, I was intrigued by the wonders and untapped potential of the human brain. I was determined to make this my life's work. After earning my medical degree, I remained driven to improve our knowledge, insights, and research into the brain, and strove to learn to find ways to keep it healthy. In addition, my clinical work, in both practice and research, provided me with continuous motivation to determine the causes and seek remedies to fight pain.

Upon continuing my extensive training and fellowship in headache medicine, I felt hopeful that breakthroughs could be made in the near future. I would like to dedicate this work to our headache community, patients living with migraine, and to the outstanding teacher and mentor, Dr. Goadsby, whose work revolutionized the field of headache medicine and who is the Senior Editor of this book.

In time I was able to discern how the unfolding complexity of pain mechanisms can help to develop new ways to enable patients and their doctors to manage migraine. The opportunity to embrace this field practically and philosophically from my outstanding mentor empowered me to keep moving forward in my research and personal learning. I am also fortunate enough to have become a mentor myself, and have developed multiple learning materials for those who are working tirelessly on our united goal of helping patients with migraine and other headache disorders.

I am confident that this book will connect many leaders in the field of headache, as well as their mentees and students. This book will be an auspicious starting point for fruitful conversations aimed toward providing the foundation to meet any clinical issues arising in this field. I believe it will also highlight what we love about working in the field of headache, and that it will invite more brilliant minds to work with us in our journey to provide our patients with treatments they need. The book will be a comprehensive guide, providing a complete understanding of our present knowledge, and help to diagnose and treat our patients in a timely and helpful manner. This book includes a chapter on advocacy and can be viewed as an Advocacy for our patients through the knowledge, research, education, and strengthening of the Migraine and all Headache medicine community.

VA Palo Alto, CA, USA — Nina Riggins

Preface

When my two previous students, Drs. Monteith and Riggins, asked me to be involved in this endeavor, I felt one of those apogees of pleasure that can only come from mentoring and promoting colleagues. I co-authored a book with my mentor, Prof. James W Lance, so there is a particular pride in this project. Headache disorders, once not even the Cinderella, and certainly not invited, have evolved in a truly exciting manner such that a jeremiad on the past serves no purpose. Headache science has pursed the anatomy, physiology, and pharmacology of our disorders at the bench, which has offered understanding and therapeutic direction. Translational medicine has been promethean in its latitude, while clinical trials with mellifluous and precise activity have delivered us new therapies, effective, well-tolerated treatments that are transformational for many patients. While not wishing to sound unnecessarily Panglossian, sedulous efforts have transformed headache medicine, and thus reduced our patients' burden. I am sure they will continue to do so. I hope the breadth, expertise, and experience of our writers imparts much that is useful and certainly a measure of the simply fascinating.

Los Angeles, CA, USA Peter J. Goadsby

Introduction

Migraine is a chronic, debilitating neurological disorder of the brain, which has a significant impact on the individual, family, and society. Migraine is more than just a headache: it is a multiphasic disorder that includes a plethora of neurological and systemic symptoms. Migraine has always been a fascinating area of study; perhaps not so realized by all in neurology. More recently, there have been tremendous strides in the basic and clinical understanding of migraine, leading to advances in therapies. The goal of this book is to prepare clinicians with the knowledge to provide excellent care for people living with migraine. The aim is to provide a comprehensive overview of migraine management.

Each chapter has a summary abstract and then goes on to elaborate key points of the chapter's focus. We also envision the book could be useful for additional purposes. For example, this could include preparation about migraine for medical examinations or assisting a clinical provider in providing care for challenging cases. We hope the book will stimulate the curiosity of both medical educators and students alike and will become part of future educational activities and curriculums in the teaching of migraine pathophysiology, diagnosis, and treatment. We believe this book provides deeper learning going beyond the mere memorization of answers; it calls for changes in practices and critical thinking. It is sensitive to the diverse approach to migraine treatment around the world and mirrors the International Headache Society's curriculum that states that headache management should be one that "allows for flexibility, and the exact content should be further defined by local headache specialists in the country in which it is used" [1, 2].

We are thankful for the extraordinary contributions of our authors, who are leading researchers, clinicians, educators, and advocates in the field of headache medicine. Our authors strive to include many timeless concepts in the management of the migraine. They have provided new clinical insights in advances in migraine and the best practices, both pharmacological and non-pharmacological interventions. Clinical guidance available is based on new knowledge, and the hope is that this will build confidence and provide the reader with the tools to optimize treatment plans.

Overview of the Book This volume is composed of seven major topics in the area of migraine, and includes 40 chapters.

1. Migraine History, Epidemiology, and Diagnosis
Key learning objectives covered in this part include:

- Describing significant milestones in the historical development of migraine research and scientific understanding of the disease
- Recognizing the impact and epidemiology of migraine
- Identifying criteria for migraine and other headache disorders, and recognizing the differential diagnosis and factors that distinguish migraine from other primary and secondary headache disorders

2. Migraine Brain: From Bench to Bedside

This part offers the reader a vertical integration of topics, such as pathophysiology, biology of migraine, and development of targeted therapeutic options.

- Identifying advances in genetics and pathophysiology of migraine and future directions of research
- Recognizing what is known about migraine biomarkers, triggering experiments, and novel targets
- Describing migraine with aura, the underlying pathophysiology, and its best management

3. Migraine Comorbidities

This part deals with the following topics that are important to recognize when managing a patient with migraine:

- Recognizing overlapping pain conditions and impact on psychosocial functioning in patients living with migraine
- Becoming familiar with psychiatric, neurological, and systemic disorders comorbid with migraine
- Gaining expertise in the management of migraine, which may be complicated by comorbidities

4. Lifestyle Factors and Wellness

This part explores the role of lifestyle and lifestyle changes in the management of the migraine patient and will include:

- Listing of important lifestyle modifications in the management of migraine
- Recognizing the role of triggers for migraine attacks
- Describing non-pharmaceutical and behavioral therapy options in the treatment of patients with migraine

5. Migraine Management

Topics covered in this part include:

- Listing of acute and preventive options of therapy available for patents living with migraine
- Recognition of the different mechanism of actions and targeted treatments for migraine
- Understanding emerging treatments for migraine and how they compare to traditional, non-specific therapies
- Description of medication overuse headache as a common complication of migraine

6. Special Patient Populations

This part explores more individualized treatment regimens for patients with other medical issues, including:

- Identifying special populations which require specific management strategies while treating migraine
- Describing vestibular migraine diagnostic criteria and treatment
- Recognizing headache associated with traumatic brain injury
- Understanding the care of migraine in women, including during menstruation, pregnancy, lactation, and perimenopause
- Gaining knowledge of how to treat migraine across the lifespan, including in children and older adults

7. Practice of Headache Medicine: Systems of Care, Underserved Populations, Healthcare Administration, Advocacy, and Education

The final part of the book covers a number of "big picture" issues importantly involved in migraine medicine and includes:

- Defining the role, structure of systems of care, and ways of healthcare administration for management of migraine
- Recognizing the impact of health disparity, inequity, and social determinants of health and migraine
- Illustrating how advocacy can be an essential part of every treatment plan for patients living with migraine
- Listing the main components of education for clinicians and patients while learning about migraine

We are also grateful to our patients, mentors, and readers. We are hopeful that this book will contribute to patient-centered approach to migraine and strengthen care for people living with migraine. We would also like to acknowledge Drs. Allan Purdy and Aarno Palotie for contributing to chapter reviews.

Teshamae S. Monteith
Nina Riggins
Peter J. Goadsby

References

1. The International Headache Society's Core Curriculum on Headache for Neurologists. Br J Pain. 2012;6(3):103–5.
2. The International Headache Society. IHS Core Curriculum [Learning Center]. 2024. Available from: https://ihs-headache.org/en/learning-centre/ihs-core-curriculum/.

Patient Perspective

My Migraine Journey: Insights for Healthcare Workers

I've been affected by migraine since birth, growing up with a debilitated mother who spent countless days in bed. While growing up, I shouldered the burden of the entire family as the primary caregiver, since I was the eldest child. I made dinner, cleaned the kitchen, cared for my mom and siblings, and pacified my dad, who did not understand the disability of migraine while being a loving husband. Furthermore, because she couldn't keep down medications due to prolonged vomiting, I learned to give her intramuscular injections when I was 16 years old.

I developed chronic migraine at 23, but I went undiagnosed by my primary care doctor. Eventually, a family friend suggested I see a neurologist, who diagnosed me. Over the course of a year, I saw him every six weeks, and he adjusted my medication as needed. During that time, I tried over 20 preventive medications and many abortives, but nothing worked. I felt discouraged and overwhelmed, and looking back, I wish I had received more information and education about this disabling disease. No one ever explained that migraine is a lifelong condition and that its invisibility causes stigma. I felt isolated because I didn't know anyone else with this disease, and at that time, resources were limited. I didn't realize that the medications he prescribed were often borrowed from other disease classes, as migraine is under-researched and often dismissed as "only a headache." I also didn't understand the range of symptoms migraine can cause; I thought I was just having bad headaches.

If I could go back to that time, given what I now know, I would ask my caring doctor for a toolkit, not just medications. He was well-meaning, but he couldn't offer the resources I needed, as they simply didn't exist then. I needed education, support, advocacy training, community, and other non-medical options beyond just biofeedback.

There are multitude of resources for patients now, and because your time is limited, you may want to consider directing your patients to vetted advocacy organizations. Here is a wish list from 105 patients I surveyed, asking, "What do you want your healthcare provider to understand about people living with migraine?" Here are the top three:

1. *Make advocacy part of the treatment plan.* Tell us that you are prescribing advocacy because this is a complicated disease requiring multiple levels of education, knowledge, and support. Guide us to websites such as CHAMP (Coalition for Headache and Migraine Patients), where we can find vetted nonprofits to fill our toolkit. Miles for Migraine offers numerous free programs and services, and is part of this valuable coalition.
2. Tell us, "*I will never give up on you.*" Many medications have failed us, so please reassure us that you will stay with us for the long haul. Too many healthcare providers have said, "I don't have anything else to offer you."
3. *Validate our journey.* We face stigma and disbelief from friends, family, coworkers, and bosses. Remind us, "It's not your fault. Migraine is disabling, and you deserve support."

Whenever I meet someone pursuing a career in headache medicine, I always express my gratitude because there are too few of you. To all healthcare providers reading this book, thank you for taking the time to better serve your patients.

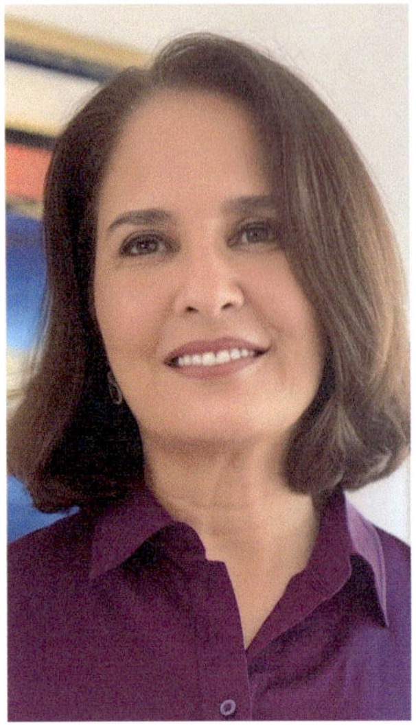

Shirley Kessel

Contents

Part VI Migraine Across the Lifespan and Special Populations

Part VII The Practice of Headache Medicine

About the Editors

Teshamae S. Monteith MD, FAHS, FAAN, graduated from medical school at the University of Miami. While training, she developed an appreciation for the brain and an enthusiasm for the potential of clinical advances to reduce suffering. She went on to complete her neurology residency at the New York University School of Medicine. During her subsequent fellowship at the Thomas Jefferson University, Jefferson Headache Center, she developed a comprehensive approach to headache management under the guidance of Stephen Silberstein, MD. Dr. Monteith pursued a second fellowship at the University of California, San Francisco, where she was involved in research studies involving migraine and other headache disorders under the direction of Peter James Goadsby, MBBS, MD, PhD.

Currently, she is a professor of clinical neurology, chief of the Headache Division, and the headache medicine fellowship director at the University of Miami's Miller School of Medicine. As a result of her passion for training the next generation of specialists, Dr. Monteith became the founding chair of the New Investigator and Trainee Section of the American Headache Society and is currently co-chair of the American Headache Society Leadership Committee. Dr. Monteith is on the Board of Directors for the American Migraine Foundation, is co-chair of the International Headache Society's (IHS) Membership Committee, and was a former member of the IHS Board of Trustees. Her research interest is in migraine, including therapeutics; she was a co-investigator for the Northern Manhattan Study under the mentorship of the late Ralph Sacco, MD, MS, and Tatjana Rundek, MD, PhD. She is involved in editorial work for the American Migraine Foundation, the journal *Cephalalgia* and *Neurology*, and for the American Academy of Neurology's *Brain and Life Magazine*. She also serves as an associate editor of the Continuum Audio and is the deputy editor for the Neurology Minute. Dr. Monteith has been a guest editor for the New England Journal of Medicine Group and was featured in the Lancet Neurology's Lifeline. She has been awarded the American Headache Society's Women's Health Science Award and is a recipient of the American Academy of Neurology's Palatucci Advocacy Leadership Forum co-advocate of the year.

Nina Riggins MD, PhD, FAAN, FAHS, FANA, is a Board-certified Neurologist at the Headache Center of Excellence (HCoE), VA Palo Alto, California. She is a UCNS-certified Headache Specialist. Dr. Riggins is a member of UCNS Headache Medicine examination committee and VA National HCoE Education Committee. Dr. Riggins completed her Internal Medicine internship at Texas Tech University, and her neurology residency at Penn State Medical Center. She completed her clinical neurophysiology fellowship at the State University of New York, Buffalo, and headache medicine fellowship at the University of California, San Francisco. She then progressed in her professional career to the associate professor at the University of California, San Fransisco (UCSF) and then at the University of California, San Diego (UCSD). She led Headache center at the UCSD and Headache Center at The Neuron Clinic in San Diego. Her research and publications are centered around new treatment options for patients with primary and secondary headache disorders. She is a Social Media editor of the International Headache Society Journals, *Cephalalgia* and *Cephalalgia Reports*.

Dr. Riggins is a Vice Chair of the American Academy of Neurology Headache & Facial pain section and Co-Chair of the First Contact Program of American Headache Society. She is a

Chair of the Women's Health Special Interest Group at the American Headache Society and a Vice Chair of the BrainPAC of the American Academy of Neurology. She is devoted to advocacy and is a board member of the "Miles for Migraine." Dr. Riggins is a Director of Women in Neurology (WNG) CME Education.

Peter J. Goadsby FRS, is Director, NIHR King's Clinical Research Facility, Professor of Neurology, King's College London, an Honorary Consultant Neurologist at King's College Hospital and the Hospital for Sick Children, Great Ormond St, London, UK. He is a National Institute for Health and Care Research Senior Investigator. He is Professor Emeritus of Neurology, University of California, Los Angeles. His major research interests are in the basic mechanisms of primary headache disorders, such as migraine and trigeminal autonomic cephalalgias, in both experimental and clinical settings, and translating mechanistic insights into better management.

Peter J. Goadsby obtained his medical degree and training at the University of New South Wales (UNSW), Australia, and neurology training with James W. Lance and clinical neurophysiology with David Burke. He did post-doctoral work in New York with Don Reis at Cornell, and Jacques Seylaz, Paris, and post-graduate neurology training at Queen Square, London, with C. David Marsden, Andrew Lees, Anita Harding, and W. Ian McDonald. He returned to UNSW, and the Prince of Wales Hospital, Sydney, as a consultant neurologist and became an Associate Professor of Neurology. He was appointed Wellcome Senior Research Fellow at the Institute of Neurology, University College London and was Professor of Clinical Neurology and Honorary Consultant Neurologist at the National Hospital for Neurology and Neurosurgery, Queen Square, London. He was Professor of Neurology, at University of California, San Francisco.

Peter J. Goadsby is considered one of the most prolific neurologists of the twenty-first century and was elected a Fellow the Royal Society in 2022. His career spans three continents; he is the past president of the International Headache Society (IHS), the American Headache Society, and the British Association for the Study of Headache. He is the chair of the Scientific Committee of the Migraine Trust (in the UK) and the Classification Committee of the IHS. He has been a lead investigator for many clinical trials. Peter J. Goadsby was a co-recipient of the 2021 Brain prize for decades-long work unraveling the cause of migraine, including the role of calcitonin gene-related peptide. His findings have led to effective treatments that are giving new hope to people suffering from migraine.

Part I

Migraine History, Epidemiology, and Diagnosis

History of Migraine in Medicine and Society

1

Janice Zehentbauer

Introduction

Migraine appears first among the primary headaches identified by the International Classification of Headache Disorders-3 (ICHD-3) [1]. This 2018 document, published 30 years after its first edition, divides migraine into six categories, including migraine without aura (formerly common migraine) and migraine with aura (formerly classical migraine), among others. In the preface, the Classification Committee alludes to past difficulty in classifying headaches [1, 2], and certainly, historical accounts of migraine substantiate that statement. Depending upon cultural contexts, the disorder's complexity was reflected in differing terminology, constellation of symptoms, and treatment. Western medical archives reveal that physicians did generally recognize a specific type of head pain that differed from a common headache or head injury, with one often-cited symptom: recurring unilateral head pain. Discussion of such head pain surfaces in ancient Egyptian papyri and Greco-Roman *materia medica*, the latter of which influenced Western medicine for millennia. Beginning with these early documents, this chapter provides a brief history of migraine, highlighting physicians' accounts of the disorder as well as narratives circulating among medical and social texts.

Questions

1. Physicians focused upon the visual disturbances preceding migraine in which century?
   A. Eighteenth century
   B. Nineteenth century
   C. Twentieth century
   D. Twenty-first century
2. The concept of a "migraine personality" was espoused by which neurologist?
   A. Sigmund Freud
   B. Samuel Auguste André David Tissot
   C. William Richard Gowers
   D. Harold Wolff

Etymology

The word "migraine" entered English via the French in the fifteenth century, diversely spelled "megrim" or "meagrim"; sometimes it materialized among analyses of other conditions such as "bilious headache" or "sick headache." "Megrim" not only indicated a severe headache but also encompassed general malaise, low spirits, and more disparagingly, a whim, fancy, or fad [3]. Eighteenth-century British literature is rife with examples of the latter meaning; in Fanny Burney's novel *Evelina* (1778), a patriarch roars, "There are fools enough in your world, without you adding to their number. I'll have no daughter of mine affect them sort of megrims" [4]. According to scholar Esther Lardreau, medieval French adopted the terms "hemigrania" and "migrania" from the Latin "hemicrania" [5, 6]. World languages have similar terms; for example, in medieval Persia, physicians referred to half-head pain as "shaqhiqheh" [7], while past and present Spanish refer to "migraña" and, from the Arabic, "jaqueca."

J. Zehentbauer (✉)
Faculty of Humanities and Social Sciences, Sheridan College, Trafalgar Campus, Oakville, ON, Canada

T. S. Monteith et al. (eds.), *Comprehensive Migraine Management*, https://doi.org/10.1007/978-3-031-86923-5_1

Ancient Egypt

Egyptologist Lutz Popko suggests that the Greek term for "disease of half of the skull" may have originated from an Egyptian one: "(mhr.t m) gs-dp," translated as "(pain/ disease in) half-of-the-head." The Papyrus Ebers (sixteenth century BCE) contains a remedy for such pain, specifically in recipe no. EB 250, lines 47.14–15: anneal a catfish skull with fat or oil, and place the mixture on the sufferer's head for 4 days. The treatment's efficacy remains unknown, and Popko emphasizes that this is the only reference to half-head pain in the Papyrus Ebers. However, he does point to another remedy—rather, incantation—against pain in half of the head, on the Papyrus Chester Beatty V (1292–1190 BCE), verso, lines 4.1–9. Healers invoked a group of nine Egyptian gods (an ennead) including Re, Shu, Anubis, among others, and recited an incantation over a clay figure of a crocodile with a grain in its mouth (the type of grain is unknown, as the word is missing) (Fig. 1.1). Then, a strip of linen with the gods' images was wrapped around the patient's head (or perhaps the crocodile's). A second recital was then performed over another image of the gods. Pain was considered a demonic adversary, and the ritual was supposed to drive it into the crocodile figure, which was then discarded or perhaps broken. According to Popko, the linen strip was a special amulet, tied only briefly around the sufferer's head, and not a compress that might relieve headaches, as some modern reports have speculated [8].

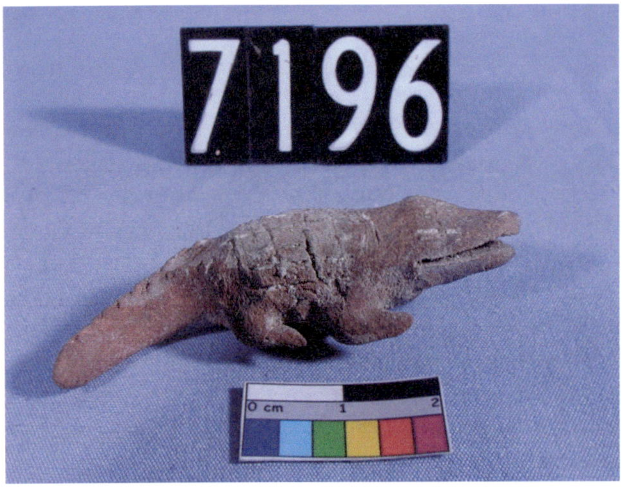

Fig. 1.1 Clay crocodile that may have been used in Egyptian rituals to drive away migraine, UC7196. (Courtesy of The Petrie Museum of Egyptian and Sudanese Archeology, UCL)

The Greco-Roman Era

A nineteenth-century doctoral thesis suggests that a description of migraine appeared in Mesopotamian poems dating to 3000 BCE [9, 10]. In ancient Greece, head pain in general, and what might be diagnosed as today's migraine with aura, also appears in the Hippocratic corpus circa 200 BCE. Neurologist Mervyn J. Eadie draws attention to Phoenix's case, a man who saw flashing lights in his right eye with intense pain arriving in his right temple shortly thereafter. Phoenix could not move his head or open his mouth, and the half-headache eased or ceased only after vomiting. The case describes Phoenix's symptoms only, without theorizing its genesis or treatment [11, 12].

Histories of migraine recognize Aretæus of Cappadocia (c. first century to second-century CE) for his clear distinction of three types of head pain [13–15]. His extant writings, written in Greek and influenced by Hippocrates, devote a section to "On Cephalæa." After distinguishing between "cephalalgia" (temporary headache) and "cephalæa," (headaches more severe, protracted, and recurrent), Aretæus identifies a third type: "heterocrania." This pain occurs on either the right or left half of the head, remaining only in the affected half; additional symptoms include facial spasms, deep eye pain, dizziness, nausea, and vomiting of bilious matters. He adds that sufferers cannot bear light, are averse to certain sounds and smells, and may experience vertigo [16].

Galen of Pergamon was active in the second century CE a little after Aretæus, and his extensive medical writing influenced European thought well into the early modern era. He propounded the Grecian theory of the humors, in which four fluids circulated throughout the human body governing health, personality, and behavior. The humors included black and yellow bile, blood, and phlegm, and corresponded to the elements of earth, fire, air, and water [17]. Healthy bodies maintained the humors in equilibrium, while excess resulted in physical or mental illness. Galen's work also differentiates head pain, but he calls unilateral head pain "hemicrania" and asserts that is incited by yellow bile, or hot or cold vapors, ascending from the stomach to the head [10, 11]. Medieval and early modern texts reflect Galen's unabating authority among medical practitioners. For example, history of medicine scholar Katherine Foxhall points to Bald's *Leechbook*, a collection of health remedies written c. 950 in Old English. Identifying unilateral head pain as "healfes heafdes ece" caused by "evil vapors," the text recommends phlebotomy (via leeches), in addition to various mixtures like vinegar and rue seeds applied to the back of the neck. Foxhall notes that such herbal ingredients were deemed hot and dry, thus counteracting the half-headache caused by an imbalance of cold and moist humors [15]. As late as the eighteenth century, an English medical text rehearses Aretæus' headache categories and asserts that headaches are the result of obstructed blood flow in the head; remedies based on the humoral theory feature rhubarb purges for hemicrania, and cupping, leeches, and blistering plasters to combat the blood excess of other headaches [15, 18].

The Early Modern Era

Throughout the seventeenth century, Western physicians gradually abandoned the humor model for more scientific inquiry. For nascent neurology, studies by English anatomist and physician Thomas Willis (1621–1675) advanced knowledge of the brain and nerves. He explicitly refers to "meagrim" in "The Second Part, Pathological" of *Two Discourses Concerning the Soul of Brutes* (1683), proposing a vasodilation theory as migraine's etiology [10, 11]. Willis distinguishes between pain outside of the skull or within its cavity; the latter, he contends, is more severe due to the brain's membrane sensitivity to intense blood flow. The pressure of the blood coursing through the arteries "bring hurt to the *Meninges*, hence the pain is caused that is interior… and sometimes produces a Meagrim on the side, sometimes in the forepart, and sometimes in the hinderpart of the Head" [19]. He details a now-famous case of a lady of "quality" whose prolonged headache attacks left her prostrate in a darkened room for days, unable to endure sound or light, but without symptoms like vertigo or "scotomia." Treatments included phlebotomy, salivation by mercury ointment, hot baths, spa waters, and other ultimately unavailing interventions [20]. Willis does not explicitly diagnose her with "meagrim," but this case history anticipates late-eighteenth century social representations of chronic pain and the ineffectuality of then-current treatments.

The Eighteenth Century

Other foundational neurological studies appeared in late eighteenth-century Europe, including the work by famed Swiss physician Samuel Auguste André David Tissot (1728–1797), whose case histories in *Traité des nerfs et leurs maladies* (1789) provide extensive evidence regarding migraine. He too discusses unilateral head pain, "principally in the forehead, eye, and temple," which he regards as particularly violent. Noting that migraine is hereditary, he emphasizes its debilitating nature; like other physicians, he writes that vomiting or sleep may help relieve attacks. Tissot promotes a sympathetic theory of migraine, involving a tight neural coupling between the stomach and the head [21]. Elsewhere, describing migraines and vapors among people of "fashion," Tissot criticizes sufferers' sedentary living and unhealthy diet [22].

In England, Tissot's near-contemporary John Fothergill (1712–1780) produced a short essay about sick-headache in 1778. Fothergill too qualifies cases according to social position, observing that sick headache predominantly affects people in the middle and upper classes. Rather than treating it as a nervous disorder, the physician argued that sick headache was the consequence of diet, a surfeit of fatty meat, pepper, tea, bread, and butter (he had a horror of butter). He does not refer to "hemicrania" but does discuss unilateral head pain accompanied by giddiness, nausea, and vomiting. Fothergill's paper links sick headache with a detailed account of transient vision loss; his own experience includes glimmers with "objects swiftly changing their apparent position, surrounded with luminous angles, like those of a fortification" [23]. Ophthalmologists and neurologists of the next century would become obsessed with this symptom as they pursued their studies of vision, light, and migraine.

In aligning migraine, sick headaches, and vapors with class and lifestyle, Tissot and Fothergill's work reflected some physicians' increasing tendency to subsume disorders within the amorphous category of "nerves." Literary critic Peter Melville Logan argues that long-existing conditions such as spleen, melancholia, vapors, and hysteria assumed new meanings in eighteenth-century medicine and society. "Nerves," "vapors," and "sensibility" started to signify overly sensitive people who were susceptible to external impressions; sensory impressions that accumulated and remained too long in the nervous system would dangerously agitate distempers. Logan examines the work of naval physician Thomas Trotter (1760–1832), who was influenced by George Cheyne's *The English Malady* (1733) (Cheyne famously diagnosed melancholia as the disease of wealthy aristocrats). According to Trotter, such nervous conditions were infecting the middle class as it too became more prosperous [24]. In *A View of the Nervous Temperament* (1807), he blames bilious attacks on over-eating and drinking; other socio-economic circumstances complicated conditions, like sedentary labor in banks and offices. For Trotter, women, historically classified as "emotional," were (not surprisingly) prone to nervous conditions; yet he also frets that British culture was promoting supposedly "effeminate" manners among men. In discussing hemicrania, he mentions with some surprise that men too suffer from this hysterical headache [25]. As such medical thought infiltrated popular consciousness, migraine was sometimes deemed an affectation (as evinced by Burney's novel). Later novels featured young women with overwrought nerves and perennial ennui using migraines as "excuses" to escape society, as in Émile Zola's *La Curée* (1872; *The Kill*). In Spain, Benito Pérez Galdós's *Fortunata y Jacinta* (1886–7) follows a young man whose severe migraine ("jaqueca") episodes are compounded by hysteria, leading him to eventual confinement in an "insane" asylum. Cultural devaluation of migraine pain and sensational representations carried alarming consequences. Indeed, by the fin-de-siècle, migraine was connected to mental illness, particularly hysteria. Neurologist and migraine-sufferer and person-with-migraine Sigmund Freud (1856–1939) noted, in his study of Frau Emmy von N, that women were known to experience coincident migraine attacks and hysterical episodes [26]. Clearly, considerations of class and gender informed migraine discourse in medicine and society well into the nineteenth century and beyond.

The British notion that "megrim" signified a flight of fancy undermined the very real suffering of migraine and chronic headache, as social documents of the era testify. Late eighteenth-century poems by Jane Cave (later Winscom; c. 1754–1813) focus on the patient's headache pain as well as its treatment, bathing in the waters in Teignmouth, England. The 1793 poem "The Head-Ache, Or An Ode to Health" features Winscom herself, the patient, tortured by a chronic headache which leaves her prostrate in bed; moreover, the verse specifically locates the pain in her temple, brain, and eyes [27]. Although she does not use the then-current medical and vernacular terms "megrim" or "sick-headache," the image of a woman pinned to her bed with inescapable pain concentrated in her temple, brain, and eyes is one often associated with migraine sufferers in medicine and society. Winscom designed her work as a literary text [28], and it is problematic to impose today's diagnoses upon a poem; nonetheless, her writing from the patient's view [29] articulates unbearable pain and reflects images of migraine that have circulated between medicine and society.

The Nineteenth Century

The nineteenth century was a period in which technological and scientific innovations enabled further study of the body and its functions. More comprehensive studies regarding migraine, in addition to new understandings about opthalmology, visual disruptions and aura, emerged in mid-century Europe. For example, Pierre Adolphe Piorry (1794–1879) finds that migraine, or "ophthalmic neuralgia," occurs among those with weakened eyesight or those suddenly subject to dazzling lights. This migraine was common to those in sedentary positions, laboring over office work or sewing, or in young women reading late at night. He delineates the visual disruption as darkness yielding to a shimmering arc, with colored zig-zags that oscillate for a few minutes. He suggests that exciting causes like bright light on the retina and iris affect eye nerves, causing oscillating and vibrations [30].

British physicians proved to be especially fascinated by these visual disruptions. Mid-century, personal accounts of hemicrania and hemiopsy (half sight) began to circulate in public forums dedicated to medicine and philosophy. These subjective narratives gained authority as empirical evidence, which somewhat counters the concept of nineteenth-century medicine's clinical, objectifying gaze. Responding to other papers, in 1865 the Royal Astronomer, George B. Airy (1801–1892) addresses his encounter with temporary, partial vision loss in the *Philosophical Magazine*, supplementing his narration with a sketch. He details a series of geometric arcs, like Norman arches, that gradually enlarge, and suggests that the condition's seat was in the brain, a "species of paralysis" with hemiopsy as a secondary symptom [31].

In 1870, Airy's son, Hubert, developed his father's observations in "On a Distinct Form of Transient Hemiopsia." Hubert Airy (1838–1903), himself a Cambridge-graduated physician, contributed to neurology a rich description of scintillating scotoma, accompanied by visually stunning colored plates. According to Hubert, the drawings offer a "veritable 'Photograph' of a morbid process going on in the brain" [32], and indeed they were used as an authoritative model by physicians thereafter to help diagnose migraine with aura, reproduced in work by contemporaries like Latham (below) and Jean-Martin Charcot (1825–1893) [33]. Acknowledging debts to previous scientists' study of the visual phenomena, the younger Airy describes his own experiences of visual disturbances before unilateral head pain; "cloud spots" emerged in the center of his vision, which then developed into shapes like serrated horseshoes. The shapes, tinged with color—the plates show blues, reds, and yellows—expanded and flickered, at five vibrations per second. He employs the neologism "teichopsia" (Greek: teichos, town-wall; opsis, vision) to indicate the shapes' similarity to a walled town (reminiscent of Fothergill's "fortifications"). Airy inclines to agree with Wollaston that the visual disturbance is seated in the brain. In addition to narrative and art, Airy quotes from Tennyson's poem "Œnone" to enhance his description [32], one of several examples of nineteenth-century physicians drawing upon literature to lend authority to their own work.

In 1873 two monographs were published by Cambridge-educated physicians, one by Peter Wallwork Latham (1832–1923) and the other by Edward Liveing (1832–1919). Latham's text, based upon case histories and studies of galvanism, proffers a vasodilation theory as a cause of sick headache. Of migraine sufferers themselves, he contends, "their brains are excitable, their senses acute, and their imaginations free"; intense brain work, and mental or emotional excitement or strain triggered attacks, as did women's menstrual cycles [34]. Liveing's more copious study, *On Megrim, Sick-headache, and Some Allied Disorders: A Contribution to the Pathology of Nerve-Storms* proved more influential. Liveing uses the English vernacular "megrim" in preference to "hemicrania," arguing that the meaning of the latter is too restrictive when considering migraine's myriad of relatives, including sick, blind, and bilious headache. Liveing's case histories reflect people of varying genders, ages, and social statuses. He attributes males' migraine attacks to excessive intellectual labor, and females' to menstruation, or to domestic occupational hazards, like eye strain when sewing. He agrees with other physicians that migraine is hereditary, diet could ease or elicit attacks, and environmental factors like barometrical pressure change could wreak havoc on those susceptible to the disorder. Liveing also focuses upon the role that fast-paced nineteenth-century modernity played: sensory overload due to glaring lights, noise, and foul air, as well as stuffy spaces like factories and railway cars, could provoke episodes. While he considers the vascular theory, Liveing's central thesis is that migraine (like epilepsy) is caused by "a hereditary vice or the morbid disposition of the nervous system," in which nervous centers irregularly accumulate and discharge their nerve force, disrupting the functionality of the nervous system. He likens these paroxysms to "nerve storms," and after their eruption, the nervous system regains its equilibrium [35].

Nineteenth-century migraine studies adopted the term "aura" from long-established thought regarding epilepsy [36]. A Greek word indicating "breeze" or "wind," something invisible yet felt, aura came to signify the premonitory symptoms of migraine. These premonitions were discussed by Liveing and some before him, and confirmed by eminent Victorian neurologists. Although his primary interests were epilepsy and Parkinson's disease, William Richard Gowers (1845–1914) reviews migraine in *A Manual of Diseases of the Nervous System* (1888). He concurs with Liveing that migraine is a paroxysmal disturbance of the nervous system with headache as its most constant symptom, though he theorizes that nerves are disturbed in the cerebral cortex rather than the thalamus [10]. He catalogues migraine aura, particularly disruptions to the visual field, and includes symptoms like transient aphasia, paresthesia, stupor, and a sensation of "double consciousness" before head pain. Ultimately, Gowers asserts skepticism of Latham's vasodilation theory because he does not see evidence for spasms in the cranial arteries [37].

The Twentieth and Twenty-First Centuries

Entering the twentieth century, debates about migraine's pathogenesis generally volleyed between vasodilation and neural explanations. During Gowers' era, physician Edmund Woakes (1837–1912) discovered that a liquid extract of ergot proved successful in treating a case of hemicrania [38, 39]; this discovery lent weight to the vasodilation theory, and ergotamine derivatives proved popular in migraine treatment throughout the twentieth century. A proponent for the vasodilation theory, American neurologist Harold Wolff (1898–1962) published influential studies throughout the 1940s to the 1960s regarding migraine, with evidence accrued through empirical study and clinical observation. His seminal *Headache and Other Pain* (1948), contends that the narrowing of cerebral arteries produces the aura, and then the pulsating headache begins when the vessels dilate [40]. As Foxhall observes, Wolff's work also developed the concept of a "migraine personality," shifting from nineteenth-century' assumptions about class (though, as seen above, Wallwork attributes character traits to his patients). People with migraine were thought to be driven perfectionists; the migraine-personality hypothesis seeped into social consciousness, perpetuating the perception that migraine was psychosomatic [15].

The cortical spreading depression phenomenon and the discovery of serotonin also contributed to twentieth-century advances in migraine treatment [10]. Aristides A. P. Leão, while studying epilepsy in the 1940s, observed that an electrical stimulation of the cerebral cortex produced a gradual wave of lowered electrical activity [41]. It is now generally accepted that the cortical spreading depression generates migraine aura, originating in the cerebral cortex [11, 42]. Also in the 1940s, while researching elements of serum released during blood clotting, biochemists isolated a substance that they named "serotonin;" one research member determined its structure to be 5-hydroxytryptamine (5-HT) [11, 15]. Additional study revealed serotonin's role in the nervous system, helping regulate mood, sleep, and other functions, leading neurologists to wonder how 5-HT functioned as a neurotransmitter in migraine. Toward the end of the century, Patrick Humphrey and his research team identified a serotonin receptor type (5-HT_{1B}), located in cranial blood vessels, and developed the drug treatment sumatriptan [43]. Sumatriptan successfully curbed oncoming migraine episodes once they started; however, in some cases, the drug negatively affected those with underlying heart conditions [13].

For Peter J. Goadsby and other contemporary neurologists, the vasodilation theory alone does not adequately account for all the neurophysiological symptoms that occur during a migraine; vasodilation is indeed a factor, but not a cause. Ergot-based medicine helped stop a migraine episode in some cases, but not others, while some triptans had negative side effects. Goadsby contends that Liveing and Gowers were correct to suspect that migraine is primarily neural [44]. To this point, lasmiditan, a serotonin receptor type (5-HT_{1F}) agonist, has not been shown to vasoconstrict blood vessels vessels, yet has been established as effective for acute migraine attacks. Moreover, research shows a link between migraine and calcitonin-gene related peptide (CGRP) [45]. The clinical usage of the new CGRP monoclonal antibodies can help prevent migraine in many patients [46], marking a new era of personalized medicine. Moreover, gepants, nonvasoconstrictive agents which are directed as antagonists to CGRP receptors, are showing benefit for migraine prevention and for treating acute attacks. Certainly, this migraine sufferer can attest to life-changing efficacy of CGRP inhibitors; however, as with any medication, it may not work for everyone. New targets are greatly needed to further accelerate therapeutic treatment for migraine.

Conclusion

Migraine ranks as the second-highest cause of global disability in the *Global Burden of Disease Study* of 2016 [47]. Physicians, people with migraine, and their support networks recognize that it entails more than a common headache. Migraine is a disability, an invisible disability, and it can be difficult to articulate the violence of its pain, although many do so during doctor appointments, and in novels, journals, poetry, and art. As evinced in Western medical and social documents, migraine's nomenclature and nosology have changed, but it has long been identified as "more" than a headache. Egyptian papyri recorded a remedy and incantations for half-head pain; Greek writings of the Hippocratic school also indicate a case of migraine with aura. Greco-Roman thought divided headache into three distinct categories, with hemicrania signaling recurrent, unilateral pain with attendant symptoms like photophobia and nausea. Though eschewing the humoral theory, physicians of the early modern era continued the tripartite division of headaches while developing a greater comprehension of the brain and nervous system. Though hypotheses for migraine pathophysiology had been proposed earlier, nineteenth-century neurologists solidified the competition between the vascular and the neuronal theories. The former theory dominated twentieth-century medical thought and treatment, but toward the end of the century and into the new millennium, a clearer understanding of biochemistry shifted support to the neuronal. Historical knowledge combined with modern scientific research and new technology has greatly advanced our understanding of migraine's complexities and potential treatments. Medical studies read alongside cultural representations of migraine reflect the variability and complexity of the migraine experience, while today's treatments hold optimism for the future.

Teaching Points

1. The Papyrus Chester Beatty V cites an incantation against demonic spirits thought to cause half-head pain; the ritual was supposed to drive the spirits into a crocodile figure made of clay.
2. The history of migraine includes many biases and assumptions of the female gender, presumably because women were thought to be more "emotional" than men and prone to nervous conditions.
3. Historically, the English term "megrim" indicated both unilateral head pain and a whim or fancy.
4. Hubert Airy's illustrations of teichopsia were ground-breaking for aiding a migraine diagnosis.
5. Competition between the vascular and the neuronal theories of migraine pathogenesis was solidified in the mid-to-late nineteenth century.
6. Late twentieth and early twenty-first centuries research demonstrates the efficacy of medication that directly or indirectly affects calcitonin-gene-related peptides (CGRP) can effectively treat migraine.

Acknowledgment I would like to thank Dr. Lutz Popko for his kind correspondence with me regarding my questions about the Papyrus Chester Beatty V.

Questions and Answers

1. Physicians focused upon the visual disturbances preceding migraine in which century?
   A. Eighteenth century
   B. Nineteenth century
   C. Twentieth century
   D. Twenty-first century

The correct answer is B. The Nineteenth century. Although prior physicians like John Fothergill recognized and wrote about visual disturbances, Hubert Airy's drawings of his experience of "teichopsia" (scintillating scotoma) became a definitive diagnostic tool for physicians working with migraine.

2. The concept of a "migraine personality" was espoused by which neurologist?
   A. Sigmund Freud
   B. Samuel Auguste André David Tissot
   C. William Richard Gowers
   D. Harold Wolff

The correct answer is D. Harold Wolff.

References

1. Headache Classification Committee of the International Headache Society (IHS). The international classification of headache disorders, 3rd edition. Cephalalgia. 2018;38(1):1–211. https://doi.org/10.1177/0333102417738202.
2. Olesen J. The International Classification of Headache Disorders: history and future perspectives. Cephalalgia. 2024;41(1). https://doi.org/10.1177/03331024231214731.
3. OED. Megrim. In: Oxford English Dictionary; 2013. http://www.oed.com.proxy2.lib.uwo.ca/view/Entry/115933. Accessed 01 May 2013.
4. Burney F. Evelina. In: Bloom EA, editor. Oxford, UK: Oxford University Press; 1991.
5. Lardreau E. La migraine: biographie d'une maladie. Paris: Les Belles Lettres; 2014.
6. Lardreau E. A curiosity in the history of sciences: the words "megrim" and "migraine". J Hist Neurosci. 2012;21:31–40.
7. Gorji A, Khaleghi GM. History of headache in medieval Persian medicine. Lancet Neurol. 2002;1:510–5.
8. Popko L. Some notes on papyrus Ebers, ancient Egyptian treatments of migraine, and a crocodile on the patient's head. Bull Hist Med. 2018;92:352–67.
9. Allory AL. Concerning migraine. Thesis. Paris; 1879.
10. Pearce JMS. Historical aspects of migraine. J Neurol Neurosurg Psychiatry. 1986;49:1097–103.
11. Eadie MJ. A history of migraine. In: Borsook D, May A, Goadsby PJ, editors. The migraine brain: imaging structure and functions. Oxford: Oxford University Press; 2012. p. 3–16.
12. Eadie MJ. Headache through the centuries. Oxford: Oxford University Press; 2012.
13. Sacks O. Migraine. New York: Vintage; 1999.
14. Koehler PJ, van de Wiel TWM. Aretæus on migraine and headache. J Hist Neurosci. 2001;10(3):253–61.
15. Foxhall K. Migraine: a history. Baltimore: Johns Hopkins University Press; 2019.
16. Aretæus. On cephalæa. In: Adams F, editor and translator. The extant works of Aretæus the Cappadocian. London: Syndeham Society; 1856. p. 294–5.
17. Duffin J. History of medicine: a scandalously short introduction. 2nd ed. Toronto: University of Toronto Press; 2010.
18. Buchan W. Of the headache (sic). Domestic medicine; 1785. AmericanRevolution.org. https://www.americanrevolution.org/medicine/med34.php. Accessed 08 Feb 2022.
19. Willis T. Of the headache (sic). In: Pordage S, translator. Two discourses concerning the soul of brutes. London: Thomas Dring; 1683. p. 105–25.
20. Willis T. Instructions and prescripts for the cure of headache (sic). In: Eugenius, editor and translator. The London practice of physick: or the whole practical part of physick contained in the works of Dr. Willis. London: Thomas Bassett and William Crooke; 1685. p. 370–89.
21. Tissot SAAD. De la migraine. In : Traité des nerfs et leurs maladies, de la catalepsie, de'extase, de anoesthésie, de la migraine, et des maladies du cerveau. Lausanne: F. R. Grasset and Co; 1789. p. 90–173. archive.org/details/traitdesnerfse00tisse. Accessed 02 Apr 2021.
22. Tissot SAAD. Megrims or vapours. In: Lee FB, translator. An essay on the disorders of people of fashion. London: Richardson and Urquhart; 1771. ECCO. 02 Nov 2013.
23. Fothergill J. Remarks on that complaint commonly known under the name of the sick head-ach. In: Medical observations and inquiries, by a society of physicians in London, vol 6. London; 1757–84. p. 103–37. ECCO. 03 May 2013.
24. Logan PM. Nerves and narratives: a cultural history of hysteria in 19th-century British prose. Berkeley: University of California Press; 1997.
25. Trotter T. A view of the nervous temperament: being a practical enquiry into the increasing prevalence, prevention, and treatment of those diseases commonly called nervous, bilious, stomach and liver complaints; indigestion; low spirits; gout, etc. London: Printed by Edw. Walker, for Longman, Hurst, Rees, and Orme; 1807.
26. Freud S, Breuer J. In: Philips A, Bowlby R, editors. Luckhurst N, translator. Studies in hysteria. New York: Penguin; 2004.
27. Winscom JC. The head-ache: or, an ode to health. In: Lonsdale R, editor. Eighteenth-century women poets. Oxford: Oxford University Press; 1989. p. 378.
28. McKim AE. Making poetry of pain: the headache poems of Jane Cave Winscom. Lit Med. 2005;24(1):93–108. https://doi.org/10.1353/lm.2005.0030.
29. Porter R. The patient's view: doing medical history from below. Theory Soc. 1985;14(2):175–98. https://doi.org/10.1007/BF00157532.
30. Piorry PA. Mémoire: Sur l'une des affections désignées sous le nom de migraine ou hémicrânie. In: Du procédé opératoire à suivre dans l'exploration des organes par la percussion médiate, accompagné de mémoires sur la circulation. Paris: Germer-Bailliere; 1835. p. 405–25.
31. Airy GB. The astronomer royal on hemiopsy. Philos Mag. 1865;30(200):19–21. Microfilm.
32. Airy H. On a distinct form of transient hemiopsia. Philos Trans R Soc Lond. 1870;160:247–64.
33. Charcot JM, Cinquième leçon. Leçons sur les maladies du système nerveux : œuvres complètes. Tome III. Paris: Bureaux du Progrès Médical; 1890. p. 60–79.
34. Latham PW. On nervous or sick-headache, its varieties and treatment: two lectures. Cambridge: Deighton, Bell, and Co; 1873.
35. Liveing E. On megrim, sick-headache, and some allied disorders: a contribution to the pathology of nerve-storms. London: J. & A. Churchill; 1873.
36. Lardeau E. The difference between epileptic auras and migrainous auras in the 19th century. Cephalalgia. 2007;27(12):1378–85.
37. Gowers WR. Migraine: paroxysmal headache. In: A manual of diseases of the nervous system. London: J. & A. Churchill; 1888. p. 776–95.
38. Koehler PH, Isler H. The early use of ergotamine in migraine: Edward Woakes' report of 1868, its theoretical and practical background and its international reception. Cephalalgia. 2002;22:686–91.

39. Woakes E. On ergot of rye in the treatment of neuralgia. Br Med J. 1861;2:360–1.
40. Wolff HG. Headache and other pain. Oxford: Oxford University; 1948.
41. Charles AC, Baca SM. Cortical spreading depression and migraine. Nat Rev Neurol. 2013;9:637–44. https://doi.org/10.1038/nrneurol.2013.192.
42. Lauritzen M. Pathophysiology of the migraine aura: the spreading depression theory. Brain. 1994;117:199–210.
43. Humphrey PPA. The discovery and development of triptans, a major breakthrough. Headache. 2008;48(5):685–7.
44. Goadsby PJ. The vascular theory of migraine—a great story wrecked by the facts. Brain J Neurol. 2009;132:6–7. https://doi.org/10.1093/brain/awn321.
45. Tajti J, Szok D, Nyári A, Vécsei L. CGRP and CGRP-Receptor as Targets of Migraine Therapy: Brain Prize-2021. CNS Neurol Disord Drug Targets. 2022;21(6):460–78. https://doi.org/10.2174/1871527320666211011110307. PMID: 34635045.
46. Russo AF, Hay DL. CGRP physiology, pharmacology, and therapeutic targets: migraine and beyond. Physiol Rev. 2023;103(2):1565–644. https://doi.org/10.1152/physrev.00059.2021. Epub 2022 Dec 1. PMID: 36454715; PMCID: PMC9988538.
47. GBD 2016 Neurology Collaborators. Global, regional, and national burden of neurological disorders, 1990–2016: a systematic analysis for the Global Burden of Disease Study 2016. Lancet Neurol. 2019;18(5):459–80. https://doi.org/10.1016/S1474-4422(18)30499-X.

Epidemiology, Impact, and Disability

2

Luis Idrovo, María Dolores Villar-Martínez, David Moreno-Ajona, and Jan Hoffmann

Introduction

Migraine is a major public health problem that has an impact on both the individual sufferer and on society [1]. Migraine is a primary headache disorder characterized by unilateral or bilateral, moderate to severe pain that lasts 4–72 hours and is associated with symptoms that can include aura (visual, somatosensory, speech or motor), photophobia, phonophobia, nausea with or without vomiting, and intolerance to physical activity [2, 3]. Recent data estimates more than 1.33 billion individuals are affected worldwide and a global prevalence of 11.6% [4]. Migraine ranks as the second most common cause of disability (all sexes, all ages) as measured by years lived with disability (YLDs), and it continues to be ranked as the leading cause of disability in women aged 15–50 years [4, 5].

Questions

1. What is the earliest manifestation of migraine in prepubertal ages?
   A. Infantile colic
   B. Cyclical vomiting
   C. Abdominal migraine
   D. Benign paroxysmal vertigo
2. What proportion of the people with migraine develop chronic migraine in their lifetime?
   A. 65–68%
   B. 45–48%
   C. 25–28%
   D. 5–8%

Migraine Incidence

The occurrence of new cases over a specified period of time is scarce due to its challenging methodological aspects. Consequently, little is known about the definite incidence of migraine worldwide [6–8]. Based on a prevalence study of the Turkish general population in 2008, an incidence study was designed using a two-step approach: a telephone-based screening followed by a headache specialist survey. This 5-year longitudinal study revealed an incidence of 23.8 per 1000 person-years overall, with a higher proportion in women [5, 7]. In a similar fashion, a Danish study found an overall incidence of 8.1 per 1000 person-years. People under the age of 35 years of age reported the highest incidence rates with higher rates in women (23 vs 10 per 1000 person-years). Unsurprisingly, the incidence rates declined with age [5]. In the classic American Migraine Prevalence and Prevention (AMPP) study, the incidence was investigated using the age of migraine onset. Using this methodology, Lipton et al. found peak incidence rates at age 20–24 years in women (18.2 per 1000 person-years) and 15–19 years in men (6.2 per 1000 person-years).

Migraine Prevalence

Precise estimates of migraine prevalence have shown variable results, probably because of differences in study methodology [6]. Migraine is ubiquitous and the prevalence—the proportion of the population found to be affected by a specific medical condition at a specific time—of those fulfilling ICHD-3 criteria who have had at least one attack in the previous year ranges between 10% and 15% worldwide. However, its epidemiology and prevalence vary according

L. Idrovo · M. D. Villar-Martínez · D. Moreno-Ajona
J. Hoffmann (✉)
Wolfson Sensory, Pain and Regeneration Centre,
Institute of Psychiatry, Psychology & Neuroscience,
King's College London, London, UK

T. S. Monteith et al. (eds.), *Comprehensive Migraine Management*, https://doi.org/10.1007/978-3-031-86923-5_2

to age, sex, race, geographical distribution, socioeconomic status, genetics, and migraine subtype, among other factors. Overall, the 1-year and lifetime prevalence are 18% and 33% in women, respectively, and 6% and 13% in men. Migraine is most frequent between the ages of 25 and 55 years of age, and the prevalence increases through early adult life and then falls thereafter [9]. The AMPP study estimated that approximately 35 million US residents had migraine, meaning that nearly 25% of households had someone with this disorder [10]. One of every four women who had migraine experienced 4 or more monthly migraine days and more than a third experienced less than four migraine days. Similar frequency patterns were observed for men [10].

Geographical Distribution

Migraine prevalence varies across geographical areas [11–24]. In a European cross-sectional study—The Eurolight project—a survey was conducted on the basis of a structured questionnaire, including diagnostic questions based on ICHD-II and various measures of impact. Data collected from 9 European countries revealed an overall 1-year prevalence of 35% after sex adjustment [13]. By contrast, US-based estimates have reported a 1-year prevalence of 13%, remaining stable over time. Estimates from Europe and the United States are not consistent, and this could be explained by methodological inclusion criteria. In addition, the European project considered both definite and probable migraine patients after first excluding the differential diagnosis of tension-type headache. Studies from the United States included only definite migraine, whereas probable migraine accounted for approximately 40% of ascertained cases in the Eurolight project [10, 11]. Based on the 2016 Global Burden of Diseases study, Nepal ranks at the top of the list and China was reported to have the lowest prevalence [5, 25].

The 'Lifting the Burden: The Global Campaign to Reduce the Burden Worldwide', developed with the World Health Organization(WHO), aimed to assess migraine prevalence and the headache burden globally, to raise awareness among local agencies, and to test regionally appropriate health-care solutions [26]. The results of this comprehensive project showed a migraine prevalence of 35% in the European Union, 20% in Russia, 19% in Lithuania, 16.7% in Turkey, 16% in Georgia, and 14.3% in England. Middle Eastern countries such as Kuwait, UAE, and Saudi Arabia showed a migraine prevalence of 11.7%, 13.7%, and 22%, respectively. In Africa, studies revealed a migraine prevalence of 18% in Ethiopia and 23% in Zambia, and in the Western Pacific, studies have consistently found the lowest migraine prevalence, particularly in Japan with 8.4%, China with 9%, and South Korea with 9.2% [5, 11, 23, 27]. Regional variations were small, although China, with a relatively low headache frequency in a population of 1.3 billion, reduced regional estimates in the Western Pacific. In contrast, individuals affected by more than 15 monthly headache days appear to be a particular problem in eastern European countries [1].

Ethnicity and Migraine

Epidemiological studies suggest variations in migraine prevalence in different ethnic groups. The AMPP study found differences according to race with a high migraine prevalence in white women, intermediate in African Americans, and the lowest in Asian Americans (20.4%, 16.2%, and 9.2% respectively) [27]. The prevalence of migraine is highest in whites compared with Blacks or Hispanics. American Indians and Alaska Natives (19.2%) were found to have the highest 3-month prevalence in the 2014 National Health Interview Survey (NHIS), an important source of information on the health of the civilian noninstitutionalized population of the United States among other ethnic backgrounds. This survey focused on a broad spectrum of people from underrepresented minority groups which also found Native Hawaiian or Pacific Islanders (13.2%) and Asians as the least affected by migraine [27].

Childhood and Adolescence

Migraine affects approximately 10% of school-aged children (5–18 years) and at prepubertal ages infantile colic (abdominal pain with no other gastrointestinal disorder) has emerged as one of the earliest manifestations of migraine [9]. Classic migraine attacks typically begin during puberty and adolescence. The prevalence of migraine rises during puberty, more frequently in girls [6, 10, 28, 29]. After puberty, the prevalence of migraine increases gradually in men but much more rapidly in women. In the United States, the AMPP study estimates the prevalence of migraine in people aged 12–19 years to be 6.3% (boys 5.0%, girls 7.7%). Throughout adolescence, the prevalence in boys (adjusted for socioeconomic status) increases by 2.9–4.1%. The adjusted prevalence in girls peaks at age 17 years at 9.8% [27].

Gender and Age-Related Epidemiology

There is evidence suggesting sex hormone-related differences in brain physiology may alter pain perception and processing [29]. Functional brain MRI studies found that female study participants with a history of migraine show altered processing functions at a resting state compared to the brains of male study participants with migraine. Furthermore, there is evidence that oestrogen can lower the threshold for cortical spreading depression (CSD), while testosterone raises it [29].

Menstrual migraine is a common term for two subtypes of migraine associated with menstruation included in ICHD-3: pure menstrual migraine and menstrually related migraine with and without aura [28, 30]. The "oestrogen withdrawal" concept, proposed in 1972, is still widely used to explain the mechanism through which migraine is triggered by the sudden decline in oestrogen levels [31]. In the general population, menstrual migraine can affect more than 50% of females with migraine. However, observational studies with stricter criteria show that up to 25% of females with migraine have menstrual migraine without aura. In contrast, the overall prevalence of menstrual migraine with aura is estimated to be less than 10%. The discrepancy in prevalence data between clinic and population-based studies is likely to be the result of differing diagnostic criteria and selection biases [30].

The natural history of migraine during pregnancy shows that up to 80% of pregnant women will continue having migraine attacks at some time during pregnancy. From observational studies and clinical practice, migraine attacks are most active during the first trimester and tend to improve as pregnancy progresses. Half of women report an improvement in their migraine burden just before week 12th of pregnancy, and more than 75% see an improvement by the second trimester [29, 32]. There is a sudden drop in oestrogen levels following delivery, leading to several symptoms, including migraine attacks. During the peripartum period, about 30% of women will experience the reappearance of migraine within 1 week postdelivery, and almost 75% will have an attack within a month [33]. During the perimenopausal period, oestrogen and progesterone levels can fluctuate potentially triggering migraine attacks. On the other hand, menopause is characterized by hormonal stability due to the decline of hormonal production by the ovaries [28, 31, 34, 35].

There are very few prospective cohort studies that determine the impact of menopause on migraine. Considering methodological limitations, the prevalence of migraine in perimenopausal women attending menopause and headache clinics reports a point prevalence between 10% and 30%. In a cross-sectional study of 1436 menopausal women aged ≥40 years, almost 70% reported having at least one headache in the previous year, and 16.5% were diagnosed with migraine according to International Headache Society criteria [36]. Conversely, another cross-sectional study looking at middle-aged women attending a headache clinic found a comparable prevalence of migraine among women in the peri- and postmenopausal periods [37]. Of note, the prevalence of postmenopausal women with migraine without aura declines with time in contrast to migraine with aura which does not seem to be directly affected by menopause [28, 35, 38].

Migraine tends to improve after spontaneous menopause compared to induced menopause [35]. In one study, migraine improvement occurred in 67% of women after spontaneous menopause compared to 33% after surgical menopause [39]. Wang et al. analysed the impact of menopause in more detail and found a higher prevalence of migraine in patients with surgical menopause compared to patients that experienced spontaneous menopause, particularly among patients with a history of premenstrual syndrome (44% vs 7%; $P = 0.0001$), while surgical menopause did not significantly affect prevalence if no history of premenstrual syndrome was reported [36]. In summary, current data suggests that compared to the reproductive years, migraine prevalence tends to remain stable or increases in perimenopause and declines after menopause [40].

Older Adults

In individuals over the age of 50, the prevalence of migraine declines to roughly 5% in both men and women [38, 41–43]. Accurate lifetime prevalence figures are generally difficult to estimate as the general population does not easily recognize early attacks and, particularly older adults, do not recall they have had migraine attacks [38].

Acephalgic migraine (typical aura without headache) attacks can occur at any age, but it is more commonly described in the elderly. Miller Fisher described late-life migraine accompaniments and elegantly summarized the clinical characteristics of 205 cases with suspected transient ischaemic attacks [44, 45]. Headache was present in only 40% of these attacks and 65% of patients had a history of recurrent migraine headache in the past. A more recent prospective French study recruited more than 3700 migraine older adult patients and found that migraine with aura was reported in 26% of the cases [46]. Of these, 6% were aged at least 50 years. About 30% of patients experienced migraine aura for the first time after age 50 and men had more migraine attacks than women.

Population studies conducted in headache patients from Italy, Denmark, and the United States revealed a prevalence of acephalgic migraine ranging from 1% to 6% and a prevalence of first-time migraine aura after age 50 of 1.8% [12, 38, 47, 48]. In a subset of the Framingham cohort which included 2110 individuals, almost 9% reported first-ever episodes of sudden visual defect and 15% of these corresponded to visual aura in migraine. The age of onset was greater than

50 years in 77%, and 58% of those with visual symptoms never had a headache [49].

Epidemiology of Migraine Subtypes and Episodic Syndromes That May Be Associated with Migraine

Episodic and Chronic Migraine

Most patients have the episodic form of migraine, with clearly defined attacks and attack-free periods [50]. However, between 5% and 8% of patients develop chronic migraine in their lifetime. Even though an increment of the attack frequency can occur spontaneously, certain modifiable factors can increase the risk of developing chronic migraine, including increased caffeine consumption, high baseline attack frequency, snoring, obesity, and medication overuse [9]. The annual incidence of chronic migraine among people with episodic migraine is less than 3% and the population prevalence of chronic migraine is <2%. Persons with chronic migraine are more likely to suffer from severe disability, such as the inability to work, attend social functions, and perform routine chores. The American Migraine Prevalence and Prevention (AMPP) Study demonstrated the burden of chronic migraine: compared with those with episodic migraine, chronic migraine patients miss nearly three times as many family activities due to headaches. Nearly 60% of chronic migraineurs report reduced household work productivity, missed more days of work, and had more days where their productivity was reduced due to headaches. As a result, chronic migraine has an enormous socio-economic impact [10, 51]. The Chronic Migraine Epidemiology and Outcomes (CaMEO) Study, a large Internet survey of the US population designed to identify individuals with EM and CM and analyse their prospective course with assessments every 3 months over 1 year found that chronic migraineurs were 52% more likely to be female, 41% more likely to be white, 34% more likely to be obese, 205% more likely to have depression, and 140% more likely to have anxiety than episodic migraineurs [52]. A few epidemiological studies have also investigated the differences in the socio-economic impact between episodic and chronic migraine in the population. The CaMEO Study demonstrated that socioeconomic status was decreased in those with CM compared with those with EM. This study showed that chronic migraine sufferers have less education and less full- or part-time employment and are more likely to have lower annual incomes [50, 52–54]. Moreover, the International Burden of Migraine study (IBMS) showed that chronic migraine patients in the United States visit primary care physicians two times more often than episodic migraine patients and are more likely to visit emergency rooms and their primary care physicians than patients with episodic migraine. This has definite implications and higher costs for the healthcare system [55].

Hemiplegic Migraine, Childhood Episodic Syndromes, and Vestibular Migraine

Hemiplegic migraine (HM) is an uncommon subtype of migraine with aura that is clinically and genetically heterogeneous. It can present as sporadic, or familial (FHM) forms and it may well be a diagnostic challenge for the clinician because of the aggressive nature resembling other serious acute neurological disorders, for example, an ischaemic stroke [56] (Table 2.1).

An episodic syndrome that may be associated with migraine (previously known as paediatric migraine variants or childhood periodic syndromes) is a group of paroxysmal disorders occurring in individuals who might also have migraine with or without aura, or who have an increased risk of developing it [57–59]. Cyclic vomiting syndrome (CVS) and abdominal migraine are the two most common entities under this group of disorders with a high prevalence of developing classic migraine attacks in later life [57–61]. Benign Paroxysmal torticollis of infancy and alternating hemiplegia of childhood (AHC) are less common disorders that paediatricians may encounter in their routine clinical practice (Table 2.1) [62, 63].

Patients with migraine and vestibular symptoms are frequently seen in our headache clinics [3, 64–66]. Considering that vestibular migraine ranks as the second most common cause of dizziness after benign paroxysmal positional vertigo (BPPV), in the outpatient setting current epidemiological aspects of VM are scarce (Table 2.1) [64–66].

Table 2.1 Epidemiology of migraine subtypes and episodic syndromes that may be associated with migraine

	Chronic migraine	Vestibular migraine	Familial hemiplegic migraine	Cyclic vomiting	Abdominal migraine	Benign paroxysmal torticollis	Alternating hemiplegia of childhood
Demographics	Peaks—late teens and early 40s Female 3:1 male	Female preponderance 64% and mean age 40.9 years	Female preponderance Onset ages 12–17	Paediatric patients were significantly more likely to be female compared to adult patients (86 vs 57%)	Female predominance in ages 4.2–7 years of age	First attack mean age 7 month (1–30 months of age) Female predominance 71% prevalence	First symptoms before the age of 6 months in more than 50% of patients
Diagnostic features ICHD3	A. Headache (migraine-like or tension-type-likes) on ≥15 days/month for >3 months, fulfilling criteria B and C B. Occurring in a patient who has had at least five attacks fulfilling criteria B-D for 1.1 *Migraine without aura* and/or criteria B and C for 1.2 *Migraine with aura* C. On ≥8 days/month for >3 months, fulfilling any of the following: 1. Criteria C and D for 1.1 *Migraine without aura* 2. Criteria B and C for 1.2 *Migraine with aura* 3. Believed by the patient to be migraine at onset and relieved by a triptan or ergot derivative D. Not better accounted for by another ICHD-3 diagnosis	A. At least five episodes fulfilling criteria C and D B. A current or past history of 1.1 *Migraine without aura* or 1.2 *Migraine with aura* C. Vestibular symptoms of moderate or severe intensity, lasting between 5 minutes and 72 hours D. At least half of episodes are associated with at least one of the following three migrainous features: 1. Headache with at least two of the following four characteristics: (a) Unilateral location (b) Pulsating quality (c) Moderate or severe intensity (d) Aggravation by routine physical activity 2. Photophobia and phonophobia 3. Visual aura E. Not better accounted for by another ICHD-3 diagnosis or by another vestibular disorder.	A. Attacks fulfilling criteria for 1.2.3 *Hemiplegic migraine* B. At least one first- or second-degree relative has had attacks fulfilling criteria for 1.2.3 *Hemiplegic migraine*.	A. At least five attacks of intense nausea and vomiting, fulfilling criteria B and C B. Stereotypical in the individual patient and recurring with predictable periodicity C. All of the following: 1. Nausea and vomiting occur at least four times per hour 2. Attacks last for ≥1 hour, up to 10 days 3. Attacks occur ≥1 week apart D. Complete freedom from symptoms between attacks E. Not attributed to another disorder	A. At least five attacks of abdominal pain, fulfilling criteria B–D B. Pain has at least two of the following three characteristics: 1. Midline location, periumbilical or poorly localized 2. Dull or "just sore" quality 3. Moderate or severe intensity C. At least two of the following four associated symptoms or signs: 1. Anorexia 2. Nausea 3. Vomiting 4. Pallor D. Attacks last 2–72 hours when untreated or unsuccessfully treated E. Complete freedom from symptoms between attacks F. Not attributed to another disorder	1. Recurrent attacks in a young child, fulfilling criteria B and C 2. Tilt of the head to either side, with or without slight rotation, remitting spontaneously after minutes to days 3. At least one of the following five associated symptoms or signs: 1. Pallor 2. Irritability 3. Malaise 4. Vomiting 5. Ataxia 4. Normal neurological examination between attacks 5. Not attributed to another disorder.	A. Recurrent attacks of hemiplegia alternating between the two sides of the body and fulfilling criterion B B. Onset before the age of 18 months C. At least one other paroxysmal phenomenon associated with the bouts of hemiplegia or occurring independently D. Evidence of mental and/or neurological deficit(s) E. Not attributed to another disorder.

(continued)

Table 2.1 (continued)

	Chronic migraine	Vestibular migraine	Familial hemiplegic migraine	Cyclic vomiting	Abdominal migraine	Benign paroxysmal torticollis	Alternating hemiplegia of childhood
Prevalence and incidence	P: <2% of the migraine population I: Annual <3% from those with episodic migraine	P: Point prevalence 0.89–2.7%	Prevalence 0.01%	P: 2% among school aged children 1.9–2.3% I: Annual 3.5/100,000	P: 1.7–4.1% most common episodic syndrome of childhood	Unknown	I: 1: 1 million individuals P: unknown
Prognosis	Variable	Variable	Attack frequency and severity decrease with increasing age		Interferes with daily life activities in about 72% of the affected Can occur up to 17 times a year	Most patients will develop benign paroxysmal vertigo, abdominal pain and eventually migraine attacks	Usually, diagnosis delayed up to the age of 3 years
Genetics	Multiple genes/loci involved in recent GWAS studies	No genetic studies	At least 7–14% of patients with FHM will have Specific mutations CACNA1A ATP1A SCN1A	82% of children affected have a positive family history of migraine	Unknown	Unknown	CACNA1A, ATP1A, SCN1A genes involved Translocation chromosome 9:13

Disability of Migraine

Migraine disability can be challenging to quantify. This difficulty relies mainly on the interindividual bio-psycho-social differences, as well as in the intrapersonal migraine changes, that can even follow a circannual pattern [67, 68]. Therefore, calibrating a totally subjective experience requires the clinician to follow an objective and holistic approach.

A simple way of 'quantifying' disability is through the use of validated questionnaires that assess the magnitude in which migraine affects patients' quality of life. The Headache Impact Test Six (HIT-6) and the migraine disability assessment questionnaire (MIDAS) are the two most frequently used in clinical and research settings to assess the burden of a particular migraine patient [69, 70]. Other measures of disability including quality of life and health-related issues can be assessed by the use of the Migraine Specific Quality of Life questionnaire (MSQ), the World Health Organization Disability Assessment Schedule (WHO DAS II), and the SF-36 (Medical Outcome survey 36 items short-form health survey) [77–82].

The disability derived from migraine does not depend on the painful experience alone. Migraine has been associated with other health problems, and, unsurprisingly, health-related quality of life can be detrimental in patients with a higher headache frequency [71]. Other comorbidities, such as epilepsy [72], are more frequent in people with migraine than in healthy controls. The rate of psychiatric comorbidities can be particularly high in patients with migraine [73] including major depressive, bipolar, and panic disorders, as well as social phobias [74]. Depression, anxiety, and generalized chronic pain rates can be double in those with the chronic form [75], therefore, it has been recommended to systematically screen for psychiatric comorbidities in patients consulting for migraine [76]. Individuals with chronic migraine not only have a higher risk of developing other psychiatric disorders but also other pathological conditions such as vascular risk factors or respiratory disorders [75]. Patients with asthma, chronic bronchitis, and hay fever have a risk of 1.5 higher to having headaches in comparison with controls [77]. Associated musculoskeletal complaints and chronic pain syndromes are not uncommon [78, 79], and might have a bidirectional relationship [80].

Drivers of disability include the avoidance of light, sounds, smells, touch, or movement, which could be translated into the associated symptoms of photophobia, photic allodynia and oculodynia, phonophobia, osmophobia, cutaneous allodynia, and movement sensitivity or vertigo symptoms, respectively [81]. These associated symptoms can represent one of the leading causes of disability and even the main reason for requesting medical assessment. Research focused on the disability related to associated symptoms has mainly looked into the main canonical symptoms [3] associated with migraine, although these might not necessarily be the most prevalent or the most incapacitating.

Photophobia is a marker of migraine disability and is related with psychiatric, and other medical co-morbidities [89] have a higher discomfort in performing daily tasks [90], anxiety and depression scores [91, 92], and worst sleep quality [91].

Similar to photophobia, using close-ended questions can [87] occur in more than 80% of patients with migraine [93]. Discomfort with certain sounds has been assessed in several studies. Hearing discomfort is worse during the ictal [94, 95] and interictal phases of a migraine attack and have a lower threshold [95–97], which might worsen with age [96] and be more marked in female patients [98]. The disability of phonophobia might, however, not only be related to finding annoying certain sounds at normal frequency or intensity but also involving a higher risk of hearing loss, as demonstrated in a recent meta-analysis [99].

Nausea is a canonically associated symptom of migraine, the second most bothersome migraine symptom, reported in almost one-third of migraineurs [100] and might be present in up to fifty per cent of episodes. Nausea also bears a higher risk for migraine chronification at 24 months [101] and has a high economic impact and detrimental influence on the quality of life [102, 103]. The presence of nausea can correlate with a more florid ictal headache phenotype, especially in women [104].

The prevalence of cutaneous allodynia can be up to 80% when measured specifically [105], which can also be quantified from a subjective point of view, by questionnaires [106, 107] or objectively [108, 109]. Hypersensitivity to touch can also depict a manifestation of central sensitization. Ictal and interictal thresholds for auditory stimuli can be lower in episodic migraineurs with cranial and extracranial cutaneous allodynia [110].

The disabling symptoms of migraine are not limited to the migraine phase. Premonitory-like symptoms such as neck stiffness, lethargy, altered frequency of toilet visits, or changes in eating habits are frequently encountered in migraine patients [111]. Similarly, the postdrome phase of migraine can be highly disabling [112]. Moreover, patients with the chronic form of migraine have a higher likelihood of having occupational disability or not being able to sustain a full-time job, as well as lower incomes in the household [80] as described below.

Impact of Migraine

Socioeconomic Aspects in Migraine Epidemiology

There have been discrepancies of the influence of socioeconomic factors in migraine across North American and European studies. American studies have been able to demonstrate an inverse relationship between migraine frequency and socioeconomic condition, as measured by income or level of education. European studies, on the contrary, have not been able to replicate these findings. The NHIS studies found that the prevalence of migraine was highest in those with an annual family income less than $35,000, and an association between increasing annual income and decreasing headache and migraine prevalence has been established [5].

In contrast, studies from Denmark and the Netherlands did not reproduce this inverse relationship. This may be due to less socioeconomic disparities and better access to healthcare services in the European countries compared to the United States. However, the social causation hypothesis could explain that factors associated with low income, such as a stressful lifestyle or poor diet, could increase the rate of migraine. Another possibility is the social selection hypothesis, which states that illness itself interferes with social or occupational function and causes low income [27, 40, 83].

Economic Burden of Migraine

Migraine is highly prevalent and tends to affect patients in the most productive years of life [5]. This translates to a more prominent economic cost of this disorder in contrast with other neurological disorders which are far less common and tend to affect elderly patients [84]. The economic cost of migraine has only been studied recently and we can only access some estimates of the real cost of some factors implicated leading to an underestimated burden. The distinction between different sources of economical cost has helped us understand the real cost of diseases. The latest reviews have taken into consideration the direct, indirect, and intangible costs of migraine [5].

The direct cost of migraine considers the medical care dedicated to the disorder such as tests that may be required for its diagnosis. The diagnosis of migraine is clinical; however, symptoms should 'not be better accounted for by another ICHD-3 diagnosis' [3]. This can require the completion of neuroimaging studies or blood tests to exclude other causes of headaches when red flags are present. Migraine treatment also accounts a direct cost. Both acute and preventive medications are included [85] and, within the latter, the latest migraine treatments which, albeit efficacious, are more expensive [86, 87].

Some studies showing data on direct costs have had different methodologies and hence obtained different results. The Eurolight study, completed in 2012, estimated €1222 of direct health-related costs per person in 2011 in Europe [88]. Combining the United States and Canada, the International Burden of Migraine Study (IBMS) estimated a cost of $1036 for chronic migraine over 3 months and $383 for episodic migraine. Although chronic migraine patients require more of both acute and preventive medications, especially refractory patients [89], episodic migraine patients constituted the main source of direct costs given the higher prevalence of episodic migraine [90]. More recently, following a web-based survey study in the United States, the mean total cost per in people with chronic migraine was more than three times that of episodic migraine ($8243 vs. $2649, $P < 0.001$) [91]. Nevertheless, the direct cost of headache treatment is probably not the main source of cost. Especially when compared to other neurological disorders such as neuromuscular disorders that may cost up to €30,000 per person [84].

The main source of economic cost in migraine is most likely its indirect cost. The loss of productivity is understandable and even more so given that concentration difficulties, word-finding difficulties, or the so-called 'brain-fog' are typically reported by patients. Wisely, a distinction between absenteeism from presenteeism has been postulated. The former cost is derived from the absence of the worker due to migraine-related sick leave. Presenteeism, however, relates to reduced productivity at work [5]. Given the high prevalence of migraine and the pressure to be at work, it is likely that presenteeism is underreported.

Data shows that in the United States, migraine patients missed 9 more workdays than individuals without migraine leading to a cost of $2350 per person in 2018 [92]. The most complete study to date, which used a comprehensive sum of individual cost estimates taking into account different items from patient surveys, calculated an estimated total cost of 50–111 billion euros in Europe only in 2011. Indirect costs were 93% of the total in contrast with 7% for direct costs [13, 93, 94]. A previous study in the United States estimated 12 billion dollars as indirect costs and 11 billion dollars as direct costs which reflects how different methodologies can dramatically affect the outcome [95, 96]. In Japan, the yearly indirect estimated cost of migraine is more than $10,700, and this is around 90% due to presenteeism and 10% to absenteeism [97]. Intangible costs involving the patient's colleagues, family, and caregivers are not easy to measure but are undoubtedly paramount. The CaMEO [98, 99] and Eurolight [13] studies took these aspects into account but with no economic cost estimate.

Conclusion

Migraine is a major public health problem that has an impact on both the individual and the society. Migraine is common and treatable, and it is the most debilitating condition in middle-aged women. Migraine prevalence varies according to age, sex, race, geographical distribution, socioeconomic status, genetics, and migraine subtype. Overall, the accepted prevalence of migraine ranges between 10% and 15% worldwide. Women tend to have fluctuations of their migraine attacks during their lifetime with an onset in their teens, increasing in their adult life, fluctuating in perimenopause, and with a tendency to decline after menopause. Episodic migraine is more common and has a higher risk of transforming into chronic migraine particularly if certain factors such as medication overuse and obesity are present. Various subtypes of migraine have different demographics and epidemiological aspects. Migraine disability depends on the pain experience, the associated symptoms, and debilitating medical and psychiatric comorbidities. The impact and economic burden of migraine have recently drawn more attention as well as strategies to address this chronic, modifiable disorder.

Teaching Points

1. Migraine prevalence ranges between 10% and 15% worldwide, it varies by age, geographical distribution, ethnicity, genetic background, and it may be influenced by socioeconomic factors.
2. Episodic migraine is more common, and certain preventable factors can increase the likelihood of chronification in patients.
3. Episodic syndromes of childhood that can be associated with migraine are common and debilitating and may be underreported.
4. Epidemiological data suggests that compared to the reproductive years, migraine prevalence tends to remain stable or increases in perimenopause and declines after menopause.
5. Migraine disability is multifactorial, and it is likely related to the pain burden and associated symptoms, the interictal burden of the disease, and the frequent association with medical and psychiatric comorbidities.
6. The economic impact of migraine remains understudy due to its complexity in assessing true indirect and direct costs.

Disclosures *Luis Idrovo* reports honoraria for consulting activities and/or serving on advisory boards from Allergan, Abbvie, Novartis, and Eli Lilly. He also reports research support from Eli Lilly.

Maria Dolores Villar-Martinez reports no financial disclosures.

David Moreno-Ajona reports no financial disclosures.

Jan Hoffmann is currently a full-time employee of H. Lundbeck A/S. Prior to this employment he received honoraria for consulting activities and/or serving on advisory boards and/or as a speaker from Allergan, Abbvie, Autonomic Technologies Inc., Cannovex BV, Chordate Medical AB, Eli Lilly, Hormosan Pharma, H. Lundbeck A/S, Novartis, Pfizer, Sanofi, and Teva. He holds stock options from Chordate Medical AB. He received personal fees for Medico-Legal work as well as from NEJM Journal Watch Neurology, Oxford University Press, Quintessence Publishing, Sage Publishing, and Springer Healthcare. He also reports a research grant from Bristol Myers Squibb, the National Institute for Health and Care Research (NIHR), the Medical Research Council (MRC), the International Headache Society (IHS), and the Migraine Trust. Jan Hoffmann serves or has served as Associate Editor for Cephalalgia, Cephalalgia Reports, The Journal of Headache and Pain, Journal of Oral & Facial Pain and Headache, and for Frontiers in Pain Research. He served as an elected member of the Board of Trustees of the International Headache Society (IHS) and as a Council Member and Treasurer of the British Association for the Study of Headache (BASH). All these activities are unrelated to the submitted work.

Questions and Answers

1. What is the earliest manifestation of migraine in prepubertal ages?
   A. Infantile colic
   B. Cyclical vomiting
   C. Abdominal migraine
   D. Benign paroxysmal vertigo

The correct answer is A. Migraine affects approximately 10% of school-aged children (5–18 years) and at prepubertal ages infantile colic (abdominal pain with no other gastrointestinal disorder) has emerged as one of the earliest manifestations of migraine. Answers B, C, D are not the earliest manifestations of migraine and therefore are not correct.

2. What proportion of the people with migraine develop chronic migraine in their lifetime?
   A. 65–68%
   B. 45–48%
   C. 25–28%
   D. 5–8%

The correct answer is D. Most patients have an episodic form of migraine. However, between 5–8% of patients develop chronic migraine in their lifetime. Answers A, B, C are not reflecting data and therefore are not correct.

References

1. Stovner L, Hagen K, Jensen R, Katsarava Z, Lipton R, Scher A, et al. The global burden of headache: a documentation of headache prevalence and disability worldwide. Cephalalgia. 2007;27(3):193–210.
2. Göbel CH, Karstedt SC, Münte TF, Göbel H, Wolfrum S, Lebedeva ER, et al. ICHD-3 is significantly more specific than ICHD-3 beta for diagnosis of migraine with aura and with typical aura. J Headache Pain. 2020;21(1):2.
3. Headache Classification Committee of the International Headache Society (IHS). The International Classification of Headache Disorders, 3rd edition. Cephalalgia. 2018;38(1):1–211.

4. Gendolla A, Rauer N, Kraemer S, Schwerdtner I, Straube A. Epidemiology, demographics, triptan contraindications, and prescription patterns of patients with migraine: a German claims database study. Neurol Ther. 2022;11(1):167–83.
5. Ashina M, Katsarava Z, Do TP, Buse DC, Pozo-Rosich P, Ozge A, et al. Migraine: epidemiology and systems of care. Lancet. 2021;397(10283):1485–95.
6. Bigal ME, Lipton RB. The epidemiology, burden, and comorbidities of migraine. Neurol Clin. 2009;27(2):321–34.
7. Baykan B, Ertas M, Karlı N, Uluduz D, Uygunoglu U, Ekizoglu E, et al. Migraine incidence in 5 years: a population-based prospective longitudinal study in Turkey. J Headache Pain. 2015;16:103.
8. Stewart WF, Wood C, Reed ML, Roy J, Lipton RB. Cumulative lifetime migraine incidence in women and men. Cephalalgia. 2008;28(11):1170–8.
9. Dodick DW. Migraine. Lancet. 2018;391(10127):1315–30.
10. Lipton RB, Bigal ME, Diamond M, Freitag F, Reed ML, Stewart WF. Migraine prevalence, disease burden, and the need for preventive therapy. Neurology. 2007;68(5):343–9.
11. Saylor D, Steiner TJ. The global burden of headache. Semin Neurol. 2018;38(2):182–90.
12. Stang PE, Yanagihara PA, Swanson JW, Beard CM, O'Fallon WM, Guess HA, et al. Incidence of migraine headache: a population-based study in Olmsted County, Minnesota. Neurology. 1992;42(9):1657–62.
13. Steiner TJ, Stovner LJ, Katsarava Z, Lainez JM, Lampl C, Lantéri-Minet M, et al. The impact of headache in Europe: principal results of the Eurolight project. J Headache Pain. 2014;15(1):31.
14. Takeshima T, Wan Q, Zhang Y, Komori M, Stretton S, Rajan N, et al. Prevalence, burden, and clinical management of migraine in China, Japan, and South Korea: a comprehensive review of the literature. J Headache Pain. 2019;20(1):111.
15. El-Metwally A, Toivola P, AlAhmary K, Bahkali S, AlKhathaami A, Al Ammar SA, et al. The epidemiology of migraine headache in Arab countries: a systematic review. ScientificWorldJournal. 2020;2020:4790254.
16. Huang GB, Yao LT, Hou JX, Zhang ZJ, Xin YT, Wu XY, et al. Epidemiology of migraine in the She ethnic minority group in Fujian province, China. Neurol Res. 2013;35(7):684–92.
17. Kandil MR, Hamed SA, Fadel KA, Khalifa HE, Ghanem MK, Mohamed KO. Migraine in Assiut Governorate, Egypt: epidemiology, risk factors, comorbid conditions and predictors of change from episodic to chronic migraine. Neurol Res. 2016;38(3):232–41.
18. Lanteri-Minet M, Geraud G. Epidemiology of migraine: French key descriptive data. Rev Neurol (Paris). 2016;172(1):56–8.
19. Matsumori Y, Ueda K, Komori M, Zagar AJ, Kim Y, Jaffe DH, et al. Burden of migraine in Japan: results of the ObserVational Survey of the Epidemiology, tReatment, and Care Of MigrainE (OVERCOME [Japan]) study. Neurol Ther. 2022;11(1):205–22.
20. Navarro-Pérez MP, Marín-Gracia M, Bellosta-Diago E, Santos-Lasaosa S. Epidemiology of migraine in Spain and Latin America. Rev Neurol. 2020;71(3):110–8.
21. Pozo-Rosich P. Chronic migraine: its epidemiology and impact. Rev Neurol. 2012;54(Suppl 2):S3–11.
22. Rabiee B, Zeinoddini A, Kordi R, Yunesian M, Mohammadinejad P, Mansournia MA. The epidemiology of migraine headache in general population of Tehran, Iran. Neuroepidemiology. 2016;46(1):9–13.
23. Sakai F, Igarashi H. Prevalence of migraine in Japan: a nationwide survey. Cephalalgia. 1997;17(1):15–22.
24. Steiner TJ, Scher AI, Stewart WF, Kolodner K, Liberman J, Lipton RB. The prevalence and disability burden of adult migraine in England and their relationships to age, gender and ethnicity. Cephalalgia. 2003;23(7):519–27.
25. Global, regional, and national burden of migraine and tension-type headache, 1990–2016: a systematic analysis for the Global Burden of Disease Study 2016. Lancet Neurol. 2018;17(11):954–76.
26. Steiner TJ. Lifting the burden: the global campaign to reduce the burden of headache worldwide. J Headache Pain. 2005;6(5):373–7.
27. Burch RC, Buse DC, Lipton RB. Migraine: epidemiology, burden, and comorbidity. Neurol Clin. 2019;37(4):631–49.
28. MacGregor EA. Menstrual and perimenopausal migraine: a narrative review. Maturitas. 2020;142:24–30.
29. Burch R. Epidemiology and treatment of menstrual migraine and migraine during pregnancy and lactation: a narrative review. Headache. 2020;60(1):200–16.
30. Vetvik KG, MacGregor EA. Menstrual migraine: a distinct disorder needing greater recognition. Lancet Neurol. 2021;20(4):304–15.
31. Somerville BW. The role of estradiol withdrawal in the etiology of menstrual migraine. Neurology. 1972;22(4):355–65.
32. Sacco S, Ripa P. Migraine in pregnancy. J Headache Pain. 2015;16(Suppl 1):A24.
33. Pavlović JM. Headache in women. Continuum (Minneap Minn). 2021;27(3):686–702.
34. Shifren JL, Gass ML. The North American Menopause Society recommendations for clinical care of midlife women. Menopause. 2014;21(10):1038–62.
35. Ripa P, Ornello R, Degan D, Tiseo C, Stewart J, Pistoia F, et al. Migraine in menopausal women: a systematic review. Int J Women's Health. 2015;7:773–82.
36. Wang SJ, Fuh JL, Lu SR, Juang KD, Wang PH. Migraine prevalence during menopausal transition. Headache. 2003;43(5):470–8.
37. Oh K, Jung KY, Choi JY, Seo WK, Park KW. Headaches in middle-aged women during menopausal transition: a headache clinic-based study. Eur Neurol. 2012;68(2):79–83.
38. Vongvaivanich K, Lertakyamanee P, Silberstein SD, Dodick DW. Late-life migraine accompaniments: a narrative review. Cephalalgia. 2015;35(10):894–911.
39. Neri I, Granella F, Nappi R, Manzoni GC, Facchinetti F, Genazzani AR. Characteristics of headache at menopause: a clinico-epidemiologic study. Maturitas. 1993;17(1):31–7.
40. Launer LJ, Terwindt GM, Ferrari MD. The prevalence and characteristics of migraine in a population-based cohort: the GEM study. Neurology. 1999;53(3):537–42.
41. Soni PP, Lee M, Shadbehr N, Ahmed ZA. Recent advances in the management of migraine in older patients. Drugs Aging. 2020;37(7):463–8.
42. Dees B, Coleman-Jackson R, Hershey LA. Managing migraine and other headache syndromes in those over 50. Maturitas. 2013;76(3):243–6.
43. Riggins N, Ehrlich A. Episodic migraine and older adults. Curr Pain Headache Rep. 2022;26(4):331–5.
44. Fisher CM. Late-life migraine accompaniments as a cause of unexplained transient ischemic attacks. Can J Neurol Sci. 1980;7(1):9–17.
45. Fisher CM. Late-life migraine accompaniments--further experience. Stroke. 1986;17(5):1033–42.
46. Donnet A, Daniel C, Milandre L, Berbis J, Auquier P. Migraine with aura in patients over 50 years of age: the Marseille's registry. J Neurol. 2012;259(9):1868–73.
47. Schwaiger J, Kiechl S, Seppi K, Sawires M, Stockner H, Erlacher T, et al. Prevalence of primary headaches and cranial neuralgias in men and women aged 55–94 years (Bruneck Study). Cephalalgia. 2009;29(2):179–87.
48. Rasmussen BK, Jensen R, Olesen J. A population-based analysis of the diagnostic criteria of the International Headache Society. Cephalalgia. 1991;11(3):129–34.

49. Wijman CA, Wolf PA, Kase CS, Kelly-Hayes M, Beiser AS. Migrainous visual accompaniments are not rare in late life: the Framingham Study. Stroke. 1998;29(8):1539–43.
50. Diener HC, Solbach K, Holle D, Gaul C. Integrated care for chronic migraine patients: epidemiology, burden, diagnosis and treatment options. Clin Med (Lond). 2015;15(4):344–50.
51. Lipton RB, Manack Adams A, Buse DC, Fanning KM, Reed ML. A comparison of the Chronic Migraine Epidemiology and Outcomes (CaMEO) Study and American Migraine Prevalence and Prevention (AMPP) Study: demographics and headache-related disability. Headache. 2016;56(8):1280–9.
52. Adams AM, Serrano D, Buse DC, Reed ML, Marske V, Fanning KM, et al. The impact of chronic migraine: the Chronic Migraine Epidemiology and Outcomes (CaMEO) Study methods and baseline results. Cephalalgia. 2015;35(7):563–78.
53. Katsarava Z, Buse DC, Manack AN, Lipton RB. Defining the differences between episodic migraine and chronic migraine. Curr Pain Headache Rep. 2012;16(1):86–92.
54. Ferrari A, Leone S, Vergoni AV, Bertolini A, Sances G, Coccia CP, et al. Similarities and differences between chronic migraine and episodic migraine. Headache. 2007;47(1):65–72.
55. Blumenfeld AM, Varon SF, Wilcox TK, Buse DC, Kawata AK, Manack A, et al. Disability, HRQoL and resource use among chronic and episodic migraineurs: results from the International Burden of Migraine Study (IBMS). Cephalalgia. 2011;31(3):301–15.
56. Di Stefano V, Rispoli MG, Pellegrino N, Graziosi A, Rotondo E, Napoli C, et al. Diagnostic and therapeutic aspects of hemiplegic migraine. J Neurol Neurosurg Psychiatry. 2020;91(7):764–71.
57. Lagman-Bartolome AM, Lay C. Pediatric migraine variants: a review of epidemiology, diagnosis, treatment, and outcome. Curr Neurol Neurosci Rep. 2015;15(6):34.
58. Lipton RB. Diagnosis and epidemiology of pediatric migraine. Curr Opin Neurol. 1997;10(3):231–6.
59. Bhandari S, Jha P, Thakur A, Kar A, Gerdes H, Venkatesan T. Cyclic vomiting syndrome: epidemiology, diagnosis, and treatment. Clin Auton Res. 2018;28(2):203–9.
60. Al-Twaijri WA, Shevell MI. Pediatric migraine equivalents: occurrence and clinical features in practice. Pediatr Neurol. 2002;26(5):365–8.
61. Thiessen PN. Recurrent abdominal pain. Pediatr Rev. 2002;23(2):39–46.
62. Verret S, Steele JC. Alternating hemiplegia in childhood: a report of eight patients with complicated migraine beginning in infancy. Pediatrics. 1971;47(4):675–80.
63. Mikati MA, Kramer U, Zupanc ML, Shanahan RJ. Alternating hemiplegia of childhood: clinical manifestations and long-term outcome. Pediatr Neurol. 2000;23(2):134–41.
64. Morganti LO, Salmito MC, Duarte JA, Bezerra KC, Simões JC, Ganança FF. Vestibular migraine: clinical and epidemiological aspects. Braz J Otorhinolaryngol. 2016;82(4):397–402.
65. Formeister EJ, Rizk HG, Kohn MA, Sharon JD. The epidemiology of vestibular migraine: a population-based survey study. Otol Neurotol. 2018;39(8):1037–44.
66. Neuhauser HK, Radtke A, von Brevern M, Feldmann M, Lezius F, Ziese T, et al. Migrainous vertigo: prevalence and impact on quality of life. Neurology. 2006;67(6):1028–33.
67. Radziwon J, Waszak P. Seasonal changes of internet searching suggest circannual rhythmicity of primary headache disorders. Headache. 2022;7(10):14329.
68. Alstadhaug KB, Bekkelund S, Salvesen R. Circannual periodicity of migraine? Eur J Neurol. 2007;14(9):983–8.
69. Bigal ME, Rapoport AM, Lipton RB, Tepper SJ, Sheftell FD. Assessment of migraine disability using the migraine disability assessment (MIDAS) questionnaire: a comparison of chronic migraine with episodic migraine. Headache. 2003;43(4):336–42.
70. Kosinski M, Bayliss MS, Bjorner JB, Ware JE Jr, Garber WH, Batenhorst A, et al. A six-item short-form survey for measuring headache impact: the HIT-6. Qual Life Res. 2003;12(8):963–74.
71. Meletiche DM, Lofland JH, Young WB. Quality-of-life differences between patients with episodic and transformed migraine. Headache. 2001;41(6):573–8.
72. Lipton RB, Ottman R, Ehrenberg BL, Hauser WA. Comorbidity of migraine: the connection between migraine and epilepsy. Neurology. 1994;44(10 Suppl 7):S28–32.
73. Breslau N, Davis GC. Migraine, major depression and panic disorder: a prospective epidemiologic study of young adults. Cephalalgia. 1992;12(2):85–90.
74. Jette N, Patten S, Williams J, Becker W, Wiebe S. Comorbidity of migraine and psychiatric disorders--a national population-based study. Headache. 2008;48(4):501–16.
75. Buse DC, Manack A, Serrano D, Turkel C, Lipton RB. Sociodemographic and comorbidity profiles of chronic migraine and episodic migraine sufferers. J Neurol Neurosurg Psychiatry. 2010;81(4):428–32.
76. Lanteri-Minet M, Radat F, Chautard MH, Lucas C. Anxiety and depression associated with migraine: influence on migraine subjects' disability and quality of life, and acute migraine management. Pain. 2005;118(3):319–26.
77. Aamodt AH, Stovner LJ, Langhammer A, Hagen K, Zwart JA. Is headache related to asthma, hay fever, and chronic bronchitis? The Head-HUNT Study. Headache. 2007;47(2):204–12.
78. Von Korff M, Crane P, Lane M, Miglioretti DL, Simon G, Saunders K, et al. Chronic spinal pain and physical-mental comorbidity in the United States: results from the national comorbidity survey replication. Pain. 2005;113(3):331–9.
79. Hestbaek L, Leboeuf-Yde C, Kyvik KO, Vach W, Russell MB, Skadhauge L, et al. Comorbidity with low back pain: a cross-sectional population-based survey of 12- to 22-year-olds. Spine (Phila Pa 1976). 2004;29(13):1483–91; discussion 92.
80. Hagen K, Linde M, Steiner TJ, Zwart JA, Stovner LJ. The bidirectional relationship between headache and chronic musculoskeletal complaints: an 11-year follow-up in the Nord-Trondelag Health Study (HUNT). Eur J Neurol. 2012;19(11):1447–54.
81. Goadsby PJ, Holland PR, Martins-Oliveira M, Hoffmann J, Schankin C, Akerman S. Pathophysiology of migraine: a disorder of sensory processing. Physiol Rev. 2017;97(2):553–622.
82. Suzuki K, Suzuki S, Shiina T, Okamura M, Haruyama Y, Tatsumoto M, et al. Investigating the relationships between the burden of multiple sensory hypersensitivity symptoms and headache-related disability in patents with migraine. J Headache Pain. 2021;22(1):021–01294.
83. Rasmussen BK. Migraine and tension-type headache in a general population: psychosocial factors. Int J Epidemiol. 1992;21(6):1138–43.
84. Gustavsson A, Svensson M, Jacobi F, Allgulander C, Alonso J, Beghi E, et al. Cost of disorders of the brain in Europe 2010. Eur Neuropsychopharmacol. 2011;21(10):718–79.
85. Goadsby PJ, Lipton RB, Ferrari MD. Migraine--current understanding and treatment. N Engl J Med. 2002;346(4):257–70.
86. Moreno-Ajona D, Chan C, Villar-Martínez MD, Goadsby PJ. Targeting CGRP and 5-HT. Headache. 2019;59(Suppl 2):3–19.
87. Dodick DW, Turkel CC, DeGryse RE, Aurora SK, Silberstein SD, Lipton RB, et al. OnabotulinumtoxinA for treatment of chronic migraine: pooled results from the double-blind, randomized, placebo-controlled phases of the PREEMPT clinical program. Headache. 2010;50(6):921–36.
88. Linde M, Gustavsson A, Stovner LJ, Steiner TJ, Barré J, Katsarava Z, et al. The cost of headache disorders in Europe: the Eurolight project. Eur J Neurol. 2012;19(5):703–11.
89. Pozo-Rosich P, Lucas C, Watson DPB, Gaul C, Ramsden E, Ritter S, et al. Burden of migraine in patients with preventive

treatment failure attending European headache specialist centers: real-world evidence from the BECOME study. Pain Ther. 2021;10(2):1691–708.
90. Stokes M, Becker WJ, Lipton RB, Sullivan SD, Wilcox TK, Wells L, et al. Cost of health care among patients with chronic and episodic migraine in Canada and the USA: results from the International Burden of Migraine Study (IBMS). Headache. 2011;51(7):1058–77.
91. Messali A, Sanderson JC, Blumenfeld AM, Goadsby PJ, Buse DC, Varon SF, et al. Direct and indirect costs of chronic and episodic migraine in the United States: a web-based survey. Headache. 2016;56(2):306–22.
92. Bonafede M, Sapra S, Shah N, Tepper S, Cappell K, Desai P. Direct and indirect healthcare resource utilization and costs among migraine patients in the United States. Headache. 2018;58(5):700–14.
93. Stovner LJ, Andrée C, Committee ES. Impact of headache in Europe: a review for the Eurolight project. J Headache Pain. 2008;9(3):139–46.
94. Andrée C, Stovner LJ, Steiner TJ, Barré J, Katsarava Z, Lainez JM, et al. The Eurolight project: the impact of primary headache disorders in Europe. Description of methods. J Headache Pain. 2011;12(5):541–9.
95. Hawkins K, Wang S, Rupnow M. Direct cost burden among insured US employees with migraine. Headache. 2008;48(4):553–63.
96. Hawkins K, Wang S, Rupnow MF. Indirect cost burden of migraine in the United States. J Occup Environ Med. 2007;49(4):368–74.
97. Kikui S, Chen Y, Todaka H, Asao K, Adachi K, Takeshima T. Burden of migraine among Japanese patients: a cross-sectional National Health and Wellness Survey. J Headache Pain. 2020;21(1):110.
98. Buse DC, Scher AI, Dodick DW, Reed ML, Fanning KM, Manack Adams A, et al. Impact of migraine on the family: perspectives of people with migraine and their spouse/domestic partner in the CaMEO study. Mayo Clin Proc. 2016;91:596.
99. Buse DC, Powers SW, Gelfand AA, VanderPluym JH, Fanning KM, Reed ML, et al. Adolescent perspectives on the burden of a parent's migraine: results from the CaMEO study. Headache. 2018;58(4):512–24.
100. Munjal S, Singh P, Reed ML, Fanning K, Schwedt TJ, Dodick DW, et al. Most Bothersome Symptom in Persons With Migraine: Results From the Migraine in America Symptoms and Treatment (MAST) Study. Headache. 2020;60(2):416–29.
101. Reed ML, Fanning KM, Serrano D, Buse DC, Lipton RB. Persistent frequent nausea is associated with progression to chronic migraine: AMPP study results. Headache. 2015;55(1):76–87.
102. Lipton RB, Buse DC, Saiers J, Serrano D, Reed ML. Healthcare resource utilization and direct costs associated with frequent nausea in episodic migraine: results from the American Migraine Prevalence and Prevention (AMPP) Study. J Med Econ. 2013;16(4):490–9.
103. Gajria K, Lee LK, Flores NM, Aycardi E, Gandhi SK. Humanistic and economic burden of nausea and vomiting among migraine sufferers. J Pain Res. 2017;10:689–98.
104. Lipton RB, Buse DC, Saiers J, Fanning KM, Serrano D, Reed ML. Frequency and burden of headache-related nausea: results from the American Migraine Prevalence and Prevention (AMPP) study. Headache. 2013;53(1):93–103.
105. Burstein R, Yarnitsky D, Goor-Aryeh I, Ransil BJ, Bajwa ZH. An association between migraine and cutaneous allodynia. Ann Neurol. 2000;47(5):614–24.
106. Ashkenazi A, Silberstein S, Jakubowski M, Burstein R. Improved identification of allodynic migraine patients using a questionnaire. Cephalalgia. 2007;27(4):325–9.
107. Lipton RB, Bigal ME, Ashina S, Burstein R, Silberstein S, Reed ML, et al. Cutaneous allodynia in the migraine population. Ann Neurol. 2008;63(2):148–58.
108. Ashkenazi A, Sholtzow M, Shaw JW, Burstein R, Young WB. Identifying cutaneous allodynia in chronic migraine using a practical clinical method. Cephalalgia. 2007;27(2):111–7.
109. Nahman-Averbuch H, Shefi T, Schneider VJ, 2nd, Li D, Ding L, King CD, et al. Quantitative sensory testing in patients with migraine: a systematic review and meta-analysis. Pain. 2018;159(7):1202–23.
110. Ashkenazi A, Yang I, Mushtaq A, Oshinsky ML. Is phonophobia associated with cutaneous allodynia in migraine? J Neurol Neurosurg Psychiatry. 2010;81(11):1256–60.
111. Karsan N, Bose P, Goadsby PJ. The Migraine Premonitory Phase. Continuum (Minneap Minn). 2018;24(4, Headache):996–1008.
112. Karsan N, Perez-Rodriguez A, Nagaraj K, Bose PR, Goadsby PJ. The migraine postdrome: Spontaneous and triggered phenotypes. Cephalalgia. 2021;41(6):721–30.

Migraine Diagnosis and Classification

3

Claire E. J. Ceriani and Stephen D. Silberstein

Introduction

Migraine is a disabling neurologic disorder that causes attacks of headache accompanied by a constellation of neurologic and gastrointestinal symptoms. The headache of migraine is typically of moderate to severe intensity, unilateral, throbbing in quality, and aggravated by routine physical activity. Associated symptoms include photophobia, phonophobia, and nausea. It should be noted that migraine symptoms vary from person to person and attack to attack, and not all of these features are required for diagnosis. The International Classification of Headache Disorders (ICHD) provides specific diagnostic criteria to facilitate the diagnosis of migraine and its subtypes [1]. Additional symptoms of migraine, such as osmophobia, allodynia, neck pain, sinus pain, and mood changes, are not included in these diagnostic criteria but are seen in many patients [2].

Migraine is a primary headache, meaning there is no other underlying cause of the headache. Primary headache disorder diagnoses are based on clinical symptoms. Without specific examination or imaging findings or biomarkers to define a diagnosis, clinicians and researchers have had to rely on patterns in the clinical presentation of headache disorders to diagnose primary headaches. As headache medicine grew as a field, it became essential to have a standardized classification system for headache disorders to ensure that clinicians and researchers were applying diagnostic criteria in a consistent way. This was first attempted in 1962 by an ad hoc committee formed by the National Institutes of Health [3]. This classification listed headache types with brief definitions rather than specific diagnostic criteria, leaving them somewhat open to the interpretation of the user. Headache diagnoses were listed in groups, with the first group being "vascular headache of migraine type," which included classic migraine, common migraine, cluster headache, hemiplegic and ophthalmoplegic migraine, and lower-half headache [3]. This classification system was utilized worldwide, but was eventually seen as unhelpful for advancing headache understanding due to the lack of evidence used to support its headache classes [4].

Questions

1. A 32-year-old woman presents to clinic with severe right sided headaches which respond to sumatriptan in 45 minutes. The attacks are associated with vomiting and can debilitating. They occur several times per year for the past 10 years. What characteristic is most indicative of a primary headache disorder?
   A. Recurrent and remitting
   B. Unilateral location
   C. Presence of vomiting
   D. Response to sumatriptan
2. A 64-year-old man presents with chronic headaches, occurring every day for the past 6 months. She has a history of mild bilateral headache that was non-disabling in her 40s, but nothing since. These headache are throbbing, and worsen with activity. She recalls this started the day before Thanksgiving and has not stopped since it started. She also reports mild nausea but no sensitivity to light or sound. She is unable to identify any triggers and has a normal examination. What is the most likely diagnosis?
   A. Chronic cluster headache
   B. Cervicogenic headache
   C. Chronic tension-type headache
   D. Chronic migraine
   E. New daily persistent headache

C. E. J. Ceriani (✉) · S. D. Silberstein
Jefferson Headache Center, Department of Neurology, Thomas Jefferson University, Philadelphia, PA, USA

T. S. Monteith et al. (eds.), *Comprehensive Migraine Management*, https://doi.org/10.1007/978-3-031-86923-5_3

The History of the Headache Classification

In 1985, the International Headache Society (IHS) formed the Classification Committee, chaired by Dr. Jes Olesen. Their purpose was to devise a headache classification system with consistent diagnostic criteria, drawing on the expertise of headache clinicians and researchers from around the world. The ICHD was published in 1988 [5], with a second edition in 2004 [6] and a third edition in 2018 [1]. The third edition was subjected to field testing by first publishing a beta version in 2013 [7]. Many field-testing studies were published evaluating the proposed diagnostic criteria for various diagnoses, and the findings were taken into consideration when revising the criteria for the third edition. For example, one such study compared the diagnostic criteria for migraine with aura in the main body of the ICHD-3 beta to the criteria contained in the appendix and found that the appendix criteria were better at distinguishing migraine with aura from transient ischemic attack [8]. This allowed for a more evidence-based revision of the ICHD with the publication of the third edition. This edition also included cross-specialty criteria developed with other specialty societies. The criteria for vestibular migraine were developed in collaboration with the Bárány Society [9], and the criteria for trigeminal neuralgia were developed by a joint committee with members of the IHS and members of the International Association for the Study of Pain [10].

The ICHD-3 uses a hierarchical classification system (Table 3.1). Headache diagnoses are classified into three major groups ("primary headaches", "secondary headaches," and "neuropathies, facial pains, and other headaches") with further subdivisions for specific headache types and subforms. Each diagnosis is given a numeric code of up to five digits, with each digit adding additional detail to the diagnosis. The level of detail can therefore be chosen to suit the needs of the clinician or researcher making the diagnosis. The group "migraine" (code 1) contains six subgroups, some of which are further broken down into additional subdivisions with each subdivision adding another digit to the code (Table 3.2). A two-digit code may be adequate for the primary care physician, whereas a researcher may wish to use the maximally detailed five-digit code. This flexibility makes the ICHD-3 useful in primary care, subspecialty care, and research.

Table 3.1 ICHD-3 classification

Part I: The primary headaches
1. Migraine
2. Tension-type headache
3. Trigeminal autonomic cephalalgias
4. Other primary headache disorders
Part II: The secondary headaches
5 . Headache attributed to trauma or injury to the head and/or neck
6. Headache attributed to a cranial or cervical vascular disorder
7. Headache attributed to nonvascular intracranial disorder
8. Headache attributed to a substance or its withdrawal
9. Headache attributed to infection
10. Headache attributed to disorder of homeostasis
11. Headache or facial pain attributed to a disorder of the cranium, neck, eyes, ears, nose, sinuses, teeth, mouth, or other facial or cervical structure
12. Headache attributed to psychiatric disorder
Part III: Neuropathies and facial pains and other headaches
13. Painful lesions of the cranial nerves and other facial pain
14. Other headache disorders
Part IV: Appendix

Table 3.2 ICHD-3 migraine classification

1. *Migraine*
1.1 *Migraine without aura*
1.2 *Migraine with aura*
1.2.1 Migraine with typical aura
1.2.1.1 Typical aura with headache
1.2.1.2 Typical aura without headache
1.2.2 Migraine with brainstem aura
1.2.3 Hemiplegic migraine
1.2.3.1 Familial hemiplegic migraine (FHM)
1.2.3.1.1 FHM type 1
1.2.3.1.2 FHM type 2
1.2.3.1.3 FHM type 3
1.2.3.1.4 FHM, other loci
1.2.3.2 Sporadic hemiplegic migraine
1.2.4 Retinal migraine
1.3 *Chronic migraine*
1.4 *Complications of migraine*
1.4.1 Status migrainosus
1.4.2 Persistent aura without infarction
1.4.3 Migrainous infarction
1.4.4 Migraine aura-triggered seizure
1.5 *Probable migraine*
1.5.1 Probable migraine without aura
1.5.2 Probable migraine with aura
1.6 *Episodic syndromes that may be associated with migraine*
1.6.1 Recurrent gastrointestinal disturbance
1.6.1.1 Cyclic vomiting syndrome
1.6.1.2 Abdominal migraine
1.6.2 Benign paroxysmal vertigo
1.6.3 Benign paroxysmal torticollis

ICHD-3 Criteria for Migraine

The main diagnostic criteria for migraine are listed under "1.1 Migraine without aura" in the ICHD 3rd edition [1]. Most importantly for the diagnosis, the presentation should not be accounted for by another ICHD-3 diagnosis which may be challenging due to phenotypic overlap with primary and secondary disorders.

Though not listed as a diagnosis in the ICHD, the term episodic migraine (EM) is often used to describe migraine that occurs on fewer than 15 days per month [11]. Migraine without aura is diagnosed clinically, if a patient has experienced at least five attacks. Headache attacks should last 4–72 hours, if untreated or unsuccessfully treated. In addition, the headache has at least two of the following four characteristics: unilateral location, pulsating quality, moderate or severe pain intensity, aggravation by or causing avoidance of routine physical activity (e.g., climbing, walking, etc.). Other criteria during headache must include at least one of the following: nausea and/or vomiting, or alternatively photophobia and phonophobia.

Chronic migraine (CM) is listed in the ICHD-3 with the numeric code 1.3 and describes migraine that occurs 15 days or more per month (migraine-like or tension-type-like) for >3 months [1]. For CM, patients should meet the criteria for migraine without aura and/or migraine with aura. On ≥8 days/month for >3 months, attacks should be fulfilling any of the following: migraine without aura, migraine with aura, and the attack should be perceived as migraine at the onset and be relieved by a migraine-specific treatment (e.g., triptan or ergot derivative).

CM is discussed in further detail later in this chapter. Migraine may also be diagnosed as "with" or "without aura." Migraine with aura and its subtypes are discussed elsewhere in this book. When patients meet all but one of the criteria for migraine without aura or migraine with aura, the diagnosis is probable migraine [1]. Patients with probable migraine may experience a decrease in health-related quality of life and significant disability, just as patients with migraine [12]. Recognition of this diagnosis is therefore essential to ensure that these patients are offered appropriate migraine treatment.

Complications of Migraine

Complications of migraine are included in Sect. 1.4. Status migrainosus is defined as a debilitating migraine attack lasting more than 72 hours, though remissions of up to 12 hours due to medications or sleep are accepted [1]. The reported prevalence of status migrainous varies widely in the medical literature but is thought to be more common in patients with EM [13]. Nondebilitating attacks lasting >72 hours are coded as probable migraine without aura, and headache persisting for 3 months or more should be diagnosed as chronic migraine or new daily persistent headache [2].

Persistent aura without infarction is defined as aura symptoms lasting for at least 1 week with no evidence of infarction on neuroimaging [1]. The aura should be typical of the patient's previous auras, except for the duration. This is a rare but well-documented phenomenon, the pathophysiology of which is still poorly understood [14]. Aura persisting for more than 1 hour, but less than 1 week should be diagnosed as probable migraine with aura [1]. When an aura symptom persists for more than 1 hour and there is an ischemic infarction on neuroimaging in a relevant area, this is diagnosed as migrainous infarction. Ischemic stroke of other causes may coexist with migraine or may present with symptoms resembling migraine, but in order to diagnose migrainous infarction, the infarction must occur during the course of a typical attack of migraine with aura. Migrainous infarction is most common in younger women and typically occurs in the posterior circulation [1].

Migraine-aura-triggered seizure is a seizure that fulfills diagnostic criteria of an epileptic attack and occurs during or within 1 hour after an attack of a migraine aura [1]. This is sometimes termed migralepsy. Migraine and epilepsy are comorbid disorders. Post-ictal headache is common, occurring in nearly half of patients with epilepsy [15]. This should be distinguished from a migraine-aura-triggered seizure, which is rare and must occur during or following the migraine with an aura attack. There is little evidence for an association with migraine without aura [1].

Episodic Syndromes That May Be Associated with Migraine

These disorders occur in patients with migraine with or without aura, or in those with an increased risk of developing migraine. They were previously termed "periodic syndromes of childhood," but they occur in adults as well. Though not included in the criteria for these disorders, the ICHD does note that these patients may also experience motion sickness and periodic sleep disorders, such as sleepwalking, sleep talking, night terrors, and bruxism [1].

Recurrent gastrointestinal disturbance is defined as recurrent episodic attacks of abdominal pain/discomfort and/or nausea and/or vomiting. This includes the diagnoses of cyclic vomiting syndrome and abdominal migraine. Cyclic vomiting syndrome consists of attacks of intense nausea and vomiting that occur with predictable timing of the episodes. Abdominal migraine is characterized by episodic attacks of moderate to severe midline abdominal pain associated with nausea and vomiting and lasting 2–72 hours. These attacks occur without a headache, and the diagnosis of migraine should be considered if the headache is present. Many children with abdominal migraine will develop more typical migraine later in life. Other causes of gastrointestinal symptoms must be ruled out in these disorders [1].

Benign paroxysmal vertigo is defined as brief attacks of vertigo that occur without warning and resolve after minutes to hours. Attacks are associated with nystagmus, ataxia, vomiting, pallor, and/or fearfulness. The neurologic and vestibular exam must be normal in between attacks, and it is essential to rule out posterior fossa tumors, seizures, and vestibular disorders. Benign paroxysmal torticollis is defined as recurrent attacks of head tilt that resolve after minutes to days and are associated with pallor, irritability, malaise, vomiting, and/or ataxia. Onset is in the first year of life, and may evolve into benign paroxysmal vertigo or migraine with aura [1].

Chronic Migraine: Evolution of a Diagnosis

It is particularly interesting to trace the history of chronic migraine as a diagnosis, in order to see how our understanding of this disorder has evolved and improved. The term "transformed migraine" was first introduced by Mathew in 1987 to describe patients with episodic migraine that progressed in frequency to daily or near-daily occurrence [16]. These patients had features of both migraine and tension-type headache, and most had migraine without aura. They were also more likely to report gastrointestinal symptoms and were more likely to have a positive family history of migraine [17]. Patients with headaches occurring as many days as not (i.e., 15 or more days per month) for at least 3 months may be said to have a chronic daily headache (CDH) [2]. The original ICHD did not include transformed or chronic migraine, but instead placed CDH in the chronic tension-type headache (CTTH) group [5]. In a study of 100 patients with CDH, 30% did not meet the criteria for tension-type headaches because they had more than one migrainous feature [18]. Multiple studies had found an association between the overuse of acute medications for headaches and the development of CDH [19–21]. It had also been observed that the majority of patients with CDH had previously had episodic migraine [22]. For patients with CDH with migrainous features and frequent acute medication use, three ICHD-1 diagnoses were required: CTTH, migraine, and medication overuse headache. The classification system intended to improve and simplify headache diagnosis was not capable of easily diagnosing the transformed or chronic migraine patient.

As the ICHD-1 criteria were subjected to more scrutiny, many researchers found that patients with CDH were difficult to classify accurately. Sanin et al. [23] classified 400 randomly selected patients and found that more than half met the criteria for more than one diagnosis. Of the patients diagnosed with migraine, 75% also had CTTH, medication-induced headache, or both. More than a third of patients had CDH, 86.6% of whom had migraine as one of their diagnoses. Pure CTTH alone was seen in a small minority of patients. Sanin et al. concluded that the ICHD-1 could classify individual attacks of headache, but did not consider the natural history of migraine as a disorder, impeding the progress of studying CDH [23]. A study by Silberstein et al. [24] evaluated 300 patients admitted to an inpatient headache unit with CDH. More than two-thirds were overusing acute medications, and a subset of 50 of these patients were followed for 2 years. The majority (74%) had chronic migraine, some (24%) had new daily persistent headache, and only a few (2%) had CTTH. Following the discontinuation of overused medication, 80% returned to an episodic headache pattern, suggesting that acute medication overuse is associated with progression from episodic to chronic migraine [24]. Sandrini et al. [25] classified 90 consecutive patients with CDH seen at a clinic and found that 75% had evolved from migraine, while only 7.7% had evolved from episodic tension-type headache. The findings of these studies illustrate that CDH is much more likely to emerge in patients with migraine than tension-type headache, and that the role of overused acute medications should be considered in these patients. Simply classifying these patients as CTTH according to the ICHD-1 criteria was therefore inaccurate and ignored the impact of medication overuse.

In 1994, Silberstein and Lipton proposed new criteria for transformed migraine that would address the limitations of the ICHD-1 [26]. CDH was subdivided into transformed migraine, CTTH evolved from episodic tension-type headache, new daily persistent headache, and hemicrania continua. The criteria for transformed migraine required a history of episodic migraine, headache at least 15 days per month with an average duration of 4 hours per day, and a history of increasing headache frequency with decreasing severity of migrainous features over at least 3 months. Transformed migraine could be further subclassified as "with medication overuse" or "without medication overuse." Silberstein and Lipton chose not to include specific headache characteristics in the criteria due to the pleiomorphic nature of daily headaches, with many patients experiencing headaches that would not meet ICHD-1 migraine criteria on all days [2]. This was an effort to move away from diagnosing individual headache attacks and instead consider the history and progression of a primary headache disorder. After field testing found that 40% of patients with CDH could not be classified, often due to patients' poor recall of characteristics of their prior headaches, the criteria were revised to require only one of the following: history of episodic migraine, history of increasing headache frequency with decreasing severity of migrainous features over at least 3 months, or headache at some time meets the IHS criteria for migraine other than duration [27].

The IHS released the second edition of the ICHD in 2004 with the inclusion of chronic migraine as a diagnosis. The criteria required headaches that fulfilled migraine criteria on 15 or more days per month for more than 3 months without medication overuse [6]. Field studies found that most patients who met the Silberstein-Lipton criteria for TM did not meet the ICHD-2 criteria for CM [28–30]. The criteria were too restrictive, not allowing for patients with varying headache phenotypes and requiring that medication overuse be ruled out. With so many studies demonstrating that the majority of CDH patients did not meet these criteria, the IHS released revised CM criteria in 2006. These criteria required 15 or more headache days per month but with a minimum of 8 days on which the headache meets migraine criteria or is relieved by a triptan or an ergot [31]. After multiple studies validated the revised criteria [32, 33], they were incorporated into the third edition of the ICHD (Table 3.1) [1].

Diagnosing Chronic Migraine

The current IHS criteria for CM are more evidence-based and easier to use than the original criteria included in the ICHD-2, but the diagnosis of CM can still be challenging. Some patients may have difficulty recalling how many days their headaches met migraine criteria or responded to triptans or ergot derivatives, and some patients may not be able to take these acute medicines due to side effects or other medical problems. The use of a headache diary can provide a more accurate history, but this may not be available at an initial office visit. CM must also be differentiated from other primary and secondary headache disorders that can cause daily or near-daily headaches.

The possibility of secondary headache should always be considered in the patient presenting with CDH. Intracranial hypertension may cause daily headaches and may be missed if papilledema is absent. Intracranial hypertension may be idiopathic, or secondary to an underlying etiology, including dural venous sinus thrombosis, head trauma, brain mass, meningitis, middle ear or mastoid infection, sleep apnea, endocrine disorders (Addison, hypoparathyroidism), central venous hypertension, renal failure, hypervitaminosis A, or medications (tetracycline, doxycycline, sulfa, lithium, steroid withdrawal) [34]. Spontaneous intracranial hypotension may also cause CDH, typically with a positional component and often worsening throughout the day [35]. Daily headaches that are present upon awakening may be caused by obstructive sleep apnea, which should be considered in patients with a snoring history, large neck size, or obesity [36]. Occipital neuralgia and cervicogenic headache should be considered when there is significant occipital or nuchal pain [37]. Sphenoid rhinosinusitis may present as an intractable headache with poor response to analgesics and interference with sleep [38]. Other infectious causes should be considered in high-risk patients.

If secondary headache is suspected, MRI is generally the imaging modality of choice. Gadolinium should be used if there is suspicion of spontaneous intracranial hypotension, neoplasm, or abscess. Magnetic resonance venography (MRV) should be performed as well if there is a concern for increased intracranial pressure. CT may be a better choice for patients in whom sinus disease is suspected [38]. Spinal MRI may also be helpful in suspected spontaneous intracranial hypotension [35]. If intracranial hypertension is suspected, a lumbar puncture with measurement of the opening pressure is an essential part of the workup.

When secondary headache has been ruled out, other primary headache disorders may be considered. Headaches in CM will typically last at least 4 hours unless successfully treated. Other headache disorders lasting longer than 4 hours include CTTH, NDPH, nummular headache, and hemicrania continue (HC). These disorders may have clinical overlap with CM and are discussed in further detail below. Headache disorders with shorter duration include cluster headaches, chronic paroxysmal hemicrania, short-lasting unilateral neuralgiform headaches, primary stabbing headaches, and hypnic headaches. These disorders may all present as daily or near-daily headaches, but their shorter attacks make them more clinically distinct from CM.

CTTH is defined by the ICHD-3 as a headache occurring on 15 or more days per month for at least 3 months. The headaches must meet the TTH criteria with only one migrainous feature permitted (photophobia, phonophobia, or mild nausea) [1]. Patients with CM may have headaches with TTH phenotype, but the diagnosis requires the presence of 8 or more migraine days per month. Technically a patient could have 15 headache days per month meeting TTH criteria, plus an additional 8 headache days per month meeting migraine criteria, which would seem to satisfy diagnostic criteria for both CTTH and CM. In these cases, the presence of 8 migraine days makes the diagnosis CM, and CTTH should not be diagnosed.

NDPH is an unremitting headache that occurs daily from its onset and may have features of migraine, TTH, or both [39]. It does not evolve from a history of worsening EM or ETTH. To meet the ICHD-3 criteria, it must become continuous within 24 hours of onset [1]. Though patients with NDPH may meet the criteria for CM or CTTH, the diagnosis of NDPH takes precedence over both.

A nummular headache, also known as "coin-shaped headache," occurs in a small circumscribed area of the scalp in the absence of an underlying structural lesion. To meet the ICHD-3 criteria, the headache can be continuous or intermittent and must occur in an area of the scalp that is sharply contoured, fixed in size and shape, round or elliptical, and 1–6 cm in diameter [1]. It is most often parietal in location and may be multifocal in some patients [40]. Allodynia and sensory disturbances over the area may be seen. Migrainous features and autonomic symptoms are rare but have been reported [40]. Duration of headache attacks may vary, and there is no required duration in the ICHD-3 criteria, but patients with continuous pain or longer-lasting attacks may be misdiagnosed with CM.

HC is characterized by a strictly unilateral, persistent headache associated with either autonomic symptoms unilateral to the headache or a sense of restlessness or agitation, and responding absolutely to indomethacin [1]. Because HC may also have migrainous features, there may be clinical overlap with CM. Any patient with a strictly unilateral persistent headache should be given an indomethacin trial.

The presence of acute medication overuse should always be considered in patients with CM. Medication overuse headache (MOH) is diagnosed when there is a headache occurring on 15 or more days per month in a patient with a pre-existing headache disorder who is overusing one or more acute headache medications for more than 3 months [1]. The ICHD-3 defines medication overuse as using nonopioid analgesics on 15 or more days per month or using triptans, ergot derivatives, opioids, combination analgesics, or multiple classes of medications on 10 or more days per month. Unlike in prior diagnostic criteria where MOH had to be ruled out before diagnosing CM, the ICHD-3 allows for MOH to be diagnosed in addition to other headache disorders. Patients should be given the diagnosis for their pre-existing headache disorder as well as MOH. Patients who meet criteria for CM and MOH should be given both diagnoses [1]. MOH is more common in women and in those with comorbid anxiety, depression, or other pain disorders. All patients presenting with frequent headaches should be evaluated for possible MOH, as MOH may be exacerbating the pre-existing headache disorder and may interfere with the effectiveness of preventive medications [41]. Many patients with CM and MOH will revert back to EM once the overused medication is withdrawn, with additional benefit seen when preventive medication is also initiated [41].

Migraine Chronification

CM rarely begins de novo but rather evolves from pre-existing EM. Understanding the epidemiology of and risk factors for CM aids the clinician in recognizing EM patients who may be at higher risk of migraine chronification. Modification of risk factors, initiation of preventive medication, and patient education regarding medical overuse may help patients avoid progression to daily or near-daily headaches.

The global prevalence of CM is estimated at 1.4–2.2%, with the prevalence highest in Europe, followed by the Western Pacific and then the Americas [42]. The American Migraine Prevalence and Prevention (AMPP) Study [43] mailed surveys to 120,000 US households to collect data on headache frequency, demographics, and disability. The study found that CM is more common in women than men (sex prevalence ratio of 4.57), in midlife, and in households with the lowest annual income. CM represented 7.7% of migraine cases overall, with the proportion increasing with age. The analysis also showed that 2.5–3% of people with EM in 1 year meet criteria for CM the following year [43].

Granella et al. [44] found that head trauma, analgesic use with every attack, and long duration of oral contraceptive use were all risk factors for chronification in patients with migraine without aura. Scher et al. [45] interviewed patients 2 times over an average of 11 months apart to determine factors that predicted CDH onset and remission. CDH at baseline was more common in women, Caucasians, those previously married, those with BMI >30, those with a lower level of education, and those with a diagnosis of diabetes or arthritis. New-onset CDH was associated with obesity, high baseline headache frequency, snoring, and stressful life events. The remission rate of CDH back to less than 1 headache per week was 14% and associated with higher education, non-white race, and being married. Other studies have found an association between obesity and CM, but obesity does not appear to be a significant risk factor for CTTH [46]. Patients with high-frequency EM (8–14 headache days/month) have a higher risk of progressing to CM than those with low-frequency EM (4–7 headache days/month) [47, 48]. Other reported risk factors for CDH include head or neck trauma, high caffeine consumption, depression, and sleep disorders [49–51].

In a longitudinal population-based cohort study, Hagen et al. [52] evaluated risk factors for both CDH and MOH. Subjects were sent surveys at baseline and approximately 11 years later. Of the subjects who did not report CDH at baseline, 1.0% had CDH without medication overuse and 0.8% had MOH 11 years later. Risk factors for developing MOH were regular use of tranquilizers, chronic musculoskeletal complaints, gastrointestinal complaints, elevated Hospital Anxiety and Depression Scale score, smoking, and physical inactivity. These factors did not increase the risk of developing CDH without medication overuse [52].

Multiple comorbidities have been identified in CM. Peres et al. [53] enrolled 101 consecutive TM patients (as diagnosed by the Silberstein-Lipton criteria) and found that 35.6% also met diagnostic criteria for fibromyalgia. The patients with fibromyalgia also had more insomnia, were older, and found their headaches more incapacitating. The majority (87.7%) had at least mild depression, and Beck Depression Inventory scores correlated with pain intensity [53]. In a separate study, Peres et al. [54] evaluated TM patients for fatigue and found that 66.7% met the criteria for chronic fatigue syndrome established by the Centers for Disease Control [54]. Buse et al. [55] analyzed the data from the AMPP survey and found that chronic pain disorders such as arthritis were more common in CM than in EM. They also found higher incidences of allergies/hay fever, asthma, sinusitis, bronchitis, COPD, heart disease, stroke, hypertension, and hyperlipidemia.

The pathophysiological mechanisms of CM and its progression from EM remain poorly understood. Dysfunction of the descending pain modulatory pathway, enhanced cortical hyperexcitability, central sensitization, and structural brain changes have been proposed as important considerations in the development of chronic migraine [56]. It is conceivable that patients with CM are in a constant premonitory phase which may perpetuate abnormalities in the descending pain modulatory pathway, cortical hyperexcitability, and central sensitization.

Patients with CM have increased cortical excitability, demonstrated by lower phosphene thresholds on magnetic visual evoked responses, decreased cortical inhibition, and persistent inter-ictal excitability of the visual cortex between migraine attacks, which is suggestive of central inhibitory dysfunction [57]. Coppola et al. [58] found that the response pattern of the somatosensory cortex to repeated somatosensory evoked potentials in CM is similar to that seen during migraine attacks in EM: an initial sensitization response followed by habituation. They hypothesized that this sensory sensitization may be explained by an increase in the strength of connections between the thalamus and cortex. CM patients have also been shown to have lower pain thresholds than EM patients [59]. Whether these observed differences between CM and EM are the cause or result of migraine chronification is not clear. The mechanisms that lead to chronification likely include increased peripheral nociception activation and sensitization, altered sensory neuron excitability, central sensitization, changes in the expression of receptors/transmitters/ion channels, synaptic reorganization caused by cell death or sprouting, and decreased pain modulation due to loss of local and descending input [2]. More research is needed to fully understand the process of migraine chronification and the role that medication overuse may play.

Conclusion

This chapter provides a broad overview of the approach to headaches, the diagnosis of migraine, episodic syndromes that may be associated with migraine, and the approach to chronic headache. For optimal care of migraine, the first step is to provide a correct diagnosis. The classification of headache disorders has evolved over the years to equip clinicians with criteria to distinguish between primary and secondary headache disorders as well as different types of migraine. It is important to take a historical account of chronic headache, as symptoms may evolve over time. Until biomarkers come to be available, history taking skills, understanding the classification, and knowledge of the criteria is essential to prevent misdiagnoses and optimal migraine management.

Teaching Points

1. The ICHD is a classification system that has undergone extensive revision over three decades to be comprehensive, evidence-based, and flexible enough to be used in clinical practice and research.
2. The ICHD includes diagnostic criteria for migraine with and without aura, chronic migraine, probable migraine, complications of migraine, and episodic syndromes associated with migraine.
3. The diagnosis of chronic migraine has changed as our understanding of this disorder has improved. The third edition of the ICHD defines chronic migraine as a >3 month history of 15 or more headache days per month with at least 8 days meeting migraine criteria or relieved by a triptan or ergot derivative.
4. The differential for chronic daily headache is broad and should include consideration of secondary causes of headache and other primary headache disorders.
5. Medication overuse is a risk factor for migraine chronification. Patients may be diagnosed with both chronic migraine and medication overuse headaches simultaneously.
6. The pathophysiology of migraine chronification is poorly understood but likely involves dysfunction of the descending pain modulatory pathway, enhanced cortical hyperexcitability, central sensitization, and structural brain changes.

Questions and Answers

1. A 32-year-old woman presents to clinic with severe right sided headaches which respond to sumatriptan in 45 minutes. The attacks are associated with vomiting and can debilitating. They occur several times per year for the past 10 years. What characteristic is most indicative of a primary headache disorder?
   A. Recurrent and remitting
   B. Unilateral location
   C. Presence of vomiting
   D. Response to sumatriptan

The correct answer is A. The patient has a long standing history of recurrent and remitting unilateral headache with vomiting. While further history is needed, the longstanding nature of the headache is a green flag, suggesting this is a primary headache disorder such as migraine and possibly cluster headache. Choices B–D can all be seen with both primary and secondary headache.

2. A 64-year-old man presents with chronic headaches, occurring every day for the past 6 months. She has a history of mild bilateral headache that was non-disabling in her 40s, but nothing since. These headache are throbbing, and worsen with activity. She recalls this started the day before Thanksgiving and has been constant since it started. She also reports mild nausea but no sensitivity to light or sound. She is unable to identify any triggers and has a normal examination. What is the most likely diagnosis?
   A. Chronic cluster headache
   B. Cervicogenic headache
   C. Chronic tension-type headache
   D. Chronic migraine
   E. New daily persistent headache

The correct answer is E. The patient has continuous headache for over 3 months that began one day, and since then has not gone way. This history is concerning for new daily persistent headache (NDPH) as a primary diagnosis, once secondary causes are ruled out. The condition may have migraine or tension type like headache. Both chronic migraine and tension type headache evolve over time.

References

1. Headache Classification Committee of the International Headache Society. The International Classification of Headache Disorders, 3rd edition. Cephalalgia. 2018;38(1):1–211.
2. Dodick DW, Silberstein SD. Migraine. 3rd ed. New York: Oxford University Press; 2016.
3. Ad Hoc Committee on Classification of Headache of the National Institute of Health. Classification of headache. JAMA. 1962;179:717–8.
4. Levin M. International classification of headache disorders and classification and diagnosis of migraine. In: Levin M, editor. Comprehensive review of headache medicine. New York: Oxford University Press, Inc; 2008. p. 59–72.
5. International Headache Society Classification Committee. Classification and diagnostic criteria for headache disorders, cranial neuralgias and facial pain. Cephalalgia. 1988;8:1–96.
6. Headache Classification Committee of the International Headache Society. The International Classification of Headache Disorders, 2nd edition. Cephalalgia. 2004;24:9–160.
7. Headache Classification Committee of the International Headache Society. The International Classification of Headache Disorders, 3rd edition (beta version). Cephalalgia. 2013;33(9):629–808.
8. Li D, Christensen AF, Olesen J. Field-testing of the ICHD-3 beta/proposed ICD-11 diagnostic criteria for migraine with aura. Cephalalgia. 2015;35(9):748–56.
9. Lempert T, Olesen J, Furman J, Waterston J, Seemungal B, Carey J, et al. Vestibular migraine: diagnostic critera: consensus document of the Bárány Society and the International Headache Society. J Vest Res. 2012;22:167–72.
10. Olesen J. Problem areas in the International Classification of Headache Disorders, 3rd edition (beta). Cephalalgia. 2014;34:1193–9.
11. Bigal ME, Serrano D, Buse D, Scher A, Stewart WF, Lipton RB. Acute migraine medications and evolution from episodic to chronic migraine: a longitudinal population-based study. Headache. 2008;48:1157–68.
12. Patel NV, Bigal ME, Kolodner KB, Leotta C, Lafata JE, Lipton RB. Prevalence and impact of migraine and probable migraine in a health plan. Neurology. 2004;63(8):1432–8.
13. Chua A, Grosberg B, Evans R. Status migrainosus in children and adults. Headache. 2019;59(9):1611–23.
14. Thissen S, Vos I, Schreuder T, Schreurs W, Postma L, Koehler P. Persistent migraine aura: new cases, a literature review, and ideas about pathophysiology. Headache. 2014;54(8):1290–309.
15. Caprara F, Letícia A, Rissardo J, Leite M, Silveira J, Jauris P, et al. Characteristics of post-ictal headaches in patients with epilepsy: a longitudinal study. Seizure. 2020;81:244–9.
16. Mathew NT, Reuveni U, Perez F. Transformed or evolutive migraine. Headache. 1987;27(2):102–6.
17. Mathew NT. Transformed migraine. Cephalalgia. 1993;13:78–83.
18. Solomon S, Lipton RB, Newman LC. Evaluation of chronic daily headache: comparison to criteria for chronic tension-type headache. Cephalalgia. 1992;12(16):365–8.
19. Mathew NT, Stubits E, Nigam MP. Transformation of episodic migraine into daily headache: analysis of factors. Headache. 1982;22(2):66–8.
20. Mathew NT, Kurman R, Perez F. Drug induced refractory headache: clinical features and management. Headache. 1990;30(10):634–8.
21. Bigal ME, Sheftell FD, Rapoport AM, Lipton RB, Tepper SJ. Chronic daily headache in a tertiary care population: correlation between the International Headache Society diagnostic criteria and proposed revisions of criteria for chronic daily headache. Cephalalgia. 2002;22(6):432–8.
22. Saper JR. Headache disorders: current concepts in treatment strategies. Littleton: Wright-PSG; 1983.
23. Sanin LC, Mathew NT, Bellmeyer LR, Ali S. The International Headache Society (IHS) headache classification as applied to a headache clinic population. Cephalalgia. 1994;14(6):443–6.
24. Silberstein SD, Schulman EA, Hopkins MM. Repetitive intravenous DHE in the treatment of refractory headache. Headache. 1990;30(6):334–49.
25. Sandrini G, Manzoni GC, Zanferrari C, Nappi G. An epidemiological approach to the nosography of chronic daily headache. Cephalalgia. 1993;13:72–7.
26. Silberstein SD, Lipton RB, Solomon S, Mathew NT. Classification of daily and near-daily headaches: proposed revisions to the IHS criteria. Headache. 1994;34(1):1–7.
27. Silberstein SD, Lipton RB, Sliwinski M. Classification of daily and near-daily headaches: field trial of revised IHS criteria. Neurology. 1996;47(4):871–5.
28. Lipton RB. Chronic migraine, classification, differential diagnosis, and epidemiology. Headache. 2011;51:77–83.
29. Manack AN, Buse DC, Lipton RB. Chronic migraine: epidemiology and disease burden. Curr Pain Headache Rep. 2011;15:70–8.
30. Bigal ME, Tepper SJ, Sheftell FD, Rapoport AM, Lipton RB. Chronic daily headache: Correlation between the 2004 and the 1988 International Headache Society diagnostic criteria. Headache. 2004;44(7):684–91.
31. Headache Classification Committee. New appendix criteria open for a broader concept of chronic migraine. Cephalalgia. 2006;26(6):742–6.
32. Zeeberg P, Olesen J, Jensen R. Medication overuse headache and chronic migraine in a specialized headache centre: field-testing proposed new appendix criteria. Cephalalgia. 2009;29(2):214–20.
33. Bigal ME, Rapoport AM, Sheftell FD, Tepper SJ, Lipton RB. The International Classification of Headache Disorders revised criteria for chronic migraine: field testing in a headache specialty clinic. Cephalalgia. 2007;27(3):230–4.

34. Toscano S, Fermo SL, Reggio E, Chisari CG, Patti F, Zappia M. An update on idiopathic intracranial hypertension in adults: a look at pathophysiology, diagnostic approach and management. J Neurol. 2021;268(9):3249–68.
35. Upadhyaya P, Ailani J. A review of spontaneous intracranial hypotension. Curr Neurol Neurosci Rep. 2019;19(5):1–6.
36. Russell MB, Kristiansen HA, Kværner KJ. Headache in sleep apnea syndrome: epidemiology and pathophysiology. Cephalalgia. 2014;34:752–5.
37. Barmherzig R, Kingston W. Occipital neuralgia and cervicogenic headache: diagnosis and management. Curr Neurol Neurosci Rep. 2019;19(5):20.
38. Ceriani CEJ, Silberstein SD. Headache and rhinosinusitis: a review. Cephalalgia. 2021;41(4):453–63.
39. Yamani N, Olesen J. New daily persistent headache: a systematic review on an enigmatic disorder. J Headache Pain. 2019;20(1):80.
40. Wilhour D, Ceriani CEJ, Nahas SJ. Nummular headache. Curr Neurol Neurosci Rep. 2019;19(6):1–7.
41. Diener H-C, Dodick D, Evers S, Holle D, Jensen RH, Lipton RB, et al. Pathophysiology, prevention, and treatment of medication overuse headache. Lancet Neurol. 2019;18(9):891–902.
42. Burch RC, Buse DC, Lipton RB. Migraine: epidemiology, burden, and comorbidity. Neurol Clin. 2019;37(4):631–49.
43. Buse DC, Manack AN, Fanning KM, Serrano D, Reed ML, Turkel CC, et al. Chronic migraine prevalence, disability, and sociodemographic factors: results from the American Migraine Prevalence and Prevention Study. Headache. 2012;52(10):1456–70.
44. Granella F, Cavallini A, Sandrini G, Manzoni GC, Nappi G. Long-term outcome of migraine. Cephalalgia. 1998;18(Suppl 21):30–3.
45. Scher AI, Stewart WF, Ricci JA, Lipton RB. Factors associated with the onset and remission of chronic daily headache in a population-based study. Pain. 2003;106:81–9.
46. Bigal ME, Lipton RB. Obesity is a risk factor for transformed migraine but not chronic tension-type headache. Neurology. 2006;67(2):252–7.
47. Ford JH, Jackson J, Milligan G, Cotton S, Ahl J, Aurora SK. A real-world analysis of migraine: a cross-sectional study of disease burden and treatment patterns. Headache. 2017;57(10):1532–44.
48. Silberstein SD, Stauffer VL, Day KA, Lipsius S, Wilson M-C. Galcanezumab in episodic migraine: subgroup analyses of efficacy by high versus low frequency of migraine headaches in phase 3 studies (EVOLVE-1 & EVOLVE-2). J Headache Pain. 2019;20(1):1–11.
49. Wang SJ, Fuh JL, Lu SR, Liu CY, Hsu LC, Wang PN, et al. Chronic daily headache in Chinese elderly: prevalence, risk factors, and biannual follow-up. Neurology. 2000;54(2):314–9.
50. Wiendels NJ, Neven AK, Rosendaal FR, Spinhoven P, Zitman FG, Assendelft WJJ, et al. Chronic frequent headache in the general population: prevalence and associated factors. Cephalalgia. 2006;26(12):1434–42.
51. Couch JR, Lipton RB, Stewart WF, Scher AI. Head or neck injury increases the risk of chronic daily headache: a population-based study. Neurology. 2007;69(11):1169–77.
52. Hagen K, Linde M, Steiner TJ, Stovner LJ, Zwart J-A. Risk factors for medication-overuse headache: an 11-year follow-up study. Pain. 2012;153(1):56–61.
53. Peres MF, Young WB, Kaup AO, Zukerman E, Silberstein SD. Fibromyalgia is common in patients with transformed migraine. Neurology. 2001;57(7):1326–8.
54. Peres MFP, Zukerman E, Young WB, Silberstein SD. Fatigue in chronic migraine patients. Cephalalgia. 2002;22(9):720–4.
55. Buse DC, Manack A, Serrano D, Turkel C, Lipton RB. Sociodemographic and comorbidity profiles of chronic migraine and episodic migraine sufferers. J Neurol Neurosurg Psychiatry. 2010;81(4):428–32.
56. Mungoven TJ, Henderson LA. Meylakh N, vol. 2. Chronic migraine pathophysiology and treatment: a review of current perspectives: Front Pain Res; 2021. p. 705276.
57. Torres-Ferrús M, Ursitti F, Alpuente A, Brunello F, Chiappino D, Vries T, et al. From transformation to chronification of migraine: pathophysiological and clinical aspects. J Headache Pain. 2020;21(1):42.
58. Coppola G, Iacovelli E, Bracaglia M, Serrao M, Lorenzo CD, Pierelli F. Electrophysiological correlates of episodic migraine chronification: evidence for thalamic involvement. J Headache Pain. 2013;14(1):1–8.
59. Kitaj MB, Klink M. Pain thresholds in daily transformed migraine versus episodic migraine headache patients. Headache. 2005;45(8):992–8.

Headache History and Examination

4

Seniha Nur Ozudogru and Kathleen Digre

Introduction

Despite the new advancements in neuroimaging and diagnostic modalities, we still rely mostly on history and physical examination in headache diagnosis. Diagnostic testing is mainly used to rule out secondary causes or confirm our clinical diagnosis. A complete headache history can take time, but it is the most important part of the evaluation in headache diagnosis. It should include open- and close-ended questions to help us understand the characteristics of the headache and its impact on patients' lives. Because of its importance, a structured headache history will cover important key elements of the history in a focused manner. A structured headache history comprises five main categories: family history, life history, attack history, past medical and psychiatric history, and treatment history (Table 4.1). In this chapter, clinical pearls for a detailed evaluation of migraine will be discussed.

Questions

1. A 28-year-old woman presents to the clinic with right-sided headache. She never had headaches until 4 years ago. It started as an intermittent attack and became daily last 15 months. She describes her headache as a continuous right-sided headache, associated with ipsilateral photophobia and rhinorrhea, red eye. She also has periods of nausea. There is no prior family history of headache. Her MRI is normal. What is the best diagnosis?
   - A. Chronic migraine
   - B. Cluster headache
   - C. Hemicrania continua
   - D. Idiopathic stabbing headache
2. In which clinical scenario, would ordering neuroimaging be appropriate?
   - A. Headache started at age 12
   - B. Side-locked headache with autonomic symptoms
   - C. Patient with chronic migraine who did not respond to topiramate treatment
   - D. Thirty-year-old male with chronic tension headache and normal neurological exam

Table 4.1 Five history of headaches

1. Family history
2. Life history
3. Attack history:
A. Location of the headache
B. Duration and frequency of attacks
C. Characteristic and severity of the pain
D. Associated symptoms (light and sound sensitivity, nausea or vomiting) and autonomic
Symptoms: red eye, nasal congestion, rhinorrhea, tearing, ptosis
E. Onset and end of the attack (prodrome and postdrome)
F. Precipitating and relieving factors
4. Past medical and psychiatric history
5. Medication and treatment history

Dr. Digre is supported in part by an Unrestricted Grant from Research to Prevent Blindness, Inc., New York, NY, to the Department of Ophthalmology & Visual Sciences, University of Utah.

S. N. Ozudogru (✉)
Division of Headache and Facial Pain, Department of Neurology, University of Pennsylvania School of Medicine, Philadelphia, PA, USA

K. Digre
Division of Headache and Neuro-Ophthalmology, Department of Neurology, University of Utah School of Medicine, Salt Lake City, UT, USA

T. S. Monteith et al. (eds.), *Comprehensive Migraine Management*, https://doi.org/10.1007/978-3-031-86923-5_4

Family History

The family history often identifies if the patient is genetically prone to migraine and other comorbidities. There is a high percentage of undiagnosed migraine that is self-diagnosed as tension or sinus headache [1]. That is why when we ask this question, we should make sure patients also think about family members with sinus and tension and "hormonal" headaches. Sometimes we ask "you mean no one in your family has ever had a headache?" Out of this may come more information. Searching the family history for other neurological, rheumatological, and psychiatric diseases can be helpful. Untreated autoimmune disorder can be the reason for the intractability of chronic migraine. We should also ask about a family history of cerebral aneurysm, intracranial bleed, and hemorrhagic stroke to help decide if a patient requires magnetic resonance imaging (MRI) or computed tomography (CT) angiogram.

Life History

The life history determines early signs of migraine attacks and life-changing events which can explain the progression of headaches. Car sickness, night terrors, recurrent abdominal pain, and colic as a child are frequent precursors of migraine [2]. Episodic nausea or abdominal pain as a child can be a presentation of migraine in children. Age of onset and progression in years are very important to determine primary versus secondary headache disorders. For example, headaches starting at puberty are more likely primary headache disorders, where a new headache starting in middle or older age, should be a red flag for a secondary headache. It is important to ask when and how the headaches became daily from chronic or episodic headaches; headache onset may be abrupt, progressive, or relapsing and remitting. If a patient's history of headache onset fits the criteria for primary migraine, but we cannot explain acute exacerbation of episodic migraine to chronic migraine, we should consider underlying systemic or structural etiology (Table 4.2).

The impact of social determinants of health (SDH) on neurological disorders, including migraine, is increasingly recognized. According to Healthy People 2030, five domains include economic stability, access and quality to education and healthcare, environmental factors, and social and community context [3]. Moreover, life stressors like the death of relatives, marriage, divorce, and moving to another city can be important triggers for the chronification of migraine that need to be elicited specifically.

Table 4.2 SNOOP pneumonic for clues to secondary headaches

*S*ystemic symptoms and risk factors	Fever, high blood pressure, cancer, immunocompromised state, weight loss
*N*eurological signs and symptoms	Change in mental status, abnormal neurological exam
*O*nset, Older	Thunderclap headache, acute onset, new headache after age 50
*O*ther associated conditions	Prolonged aura, postural headache
*P*rior headaches, postural, precipitated by exertion, pulsatile tinnitus, pregnancy	Change in the characteristics, frequency, and severity of headaches, symptoms of high or low intracranial pressure, pregnancy

Attack History

Since many people have more than one type of headache [4], it is important to confirm how many types of headaches the patient has. Then we ask about the details of each headache type. The important associated factors are light, smell and sound sensitivity, allodynia, nausea and/or vomiting, and worsening with activity for migraine. To distinguish from the trigeminal autonomic cephalalgias (TAC), we focus on laterality, duration, and lacrimation, rhinorrhea, ptosis, and nasal stuffiness as cranial autonomic features, along with agitation. See Table 4.3 for a summary of headache characteristics for migraine without aura and TACs. It is important to note that cranial autonomic symptoms also occur in migraine, although symptoms are generally less common and severe.

Location of the Headache

Headache can be unilateral or bilateral. Unilateral headaches should be differentiated as side-locked and shifting headaches. Unilateral shifting headache is a common presentation of primary migraine disease. The frontotemporal area is the common location for migraine when presented as bilateral pain [5]. However, unilateral side-locked headache can be secondary to an underlying structural disease like a tumor, cervical disease, or venous sinus thrombosis. Or it can be a type of TAC-like cluster headache or paroxysmal hemicrania. When we discover that a patient has a unilateral side-

Table 4.3 Differentiating migraine from trigeminal autonomic cephalalgias

Migraine without aura	Trigeminal autonomic cephalalgia
Unilateral shifting headache	Unilateral side-locked headache
Associated with; (a) Photophobia (b) Phonophobia (c) Nausea and vomiting (d) Aggravation with activity (e) Relieves with rest	Associated with ipsilateral autonomic symptoms; (a) Erythema (b) Lacrimation (c) Rhinorrhea (d) Ptosis and/or Miosis (e) Restlessness and agitation Also look for Indomethacin response for Hemicrania, seasonal attacks for Cluster headache, short lasting attacks for SUNCT/SUNA

locked headache, we should ask about the associated autonomic symptoms such as erythema and lacrimation of the eye, ptosis, and rhinorrhea.

Duration and Frequency of Attacks

Information about the duration and frequency of attacks is not only important to make the diagnosis but also help us to understand the treatment response to rescue and preventive therapy. If the rescue medication can stop the attack in 2 hours but the patient continues to suffer from more than 4 monthly headache days, or the attacks significantly affect the patient's daily activities, preventive therapy should be recommended [6]. Whereas the patient who suffers from 2 attacks a month, each attack lasting 3 days needs a change in their rescue medication. Monthly migraine days, mild-moderate-severe headache days, and the number of days rescue medication was taken can give important additional information. One of the most helpful questions that can be asked is "How many total headache-free days do you have excluding any mild ones"? Individuals may have migraine or migraine-like attacks and only mention the worst headache, but the individual is having many more headache days than reported. In addition to diurnal and *seasonal* rhythmicity, duration and frequency of attacks are also important to differentiate from TAC subtypes. Shorter attacks are more likely to be TACs.

Characteristic and Severity of the Pain

Throbbing, pulsating, or pounding is the common description of migraine, whereas electric, shooting pain from the occipital area with a history of trauma is an indicator of occipital neuralgia. Tension-type headaches usually present as mild to moderate intensity and migraine moderate to severe. Thunderclap headache is the most severe headache, reaching its maximum intensity within 60 seconds and often signals a secondary headache (hemorrhage, vasoconstriction syndrome) so neuroimaging must be done for thunderclap headache even if the neurological exam is normal.

Associated Symptoms

Migraine may be accompanied by many associated symptoms besides the usual light and sound and smell sensitivity, nausea, and vomiting; these symptoms may be easy to miss if mild or infrequent. Commonly, vertigo and visual blurring can occur. Sometimes the diagnosis of migraine is missed because patients do not report light sensitivity but when they are asked about what helps or what you do when you have a headache, they sometimes report being in a dark, quiet room alleviates the pain.

Migraine attacks may have autonomic symptoms, but TACs are classified by having some autonomic symptoms (or agitation) and can occasionally have migraine features. Ipsilateral autonomic symptoms are most likely signs of TACs. Insomnia, cognitive decline, and mood swings along with headache after trauma are signs of post-concussion syndrome [7].

Onset and End of the Attack

Prodrome and aura are the phases of migraine that mostly occur prior to the headache. Common premonitory symptoms are stiff neck, fatigue, and yawning. It may help to encourage patients to identify their prodromal symptoms, which may have treatment implications and better help them plan their day. Some prodrome symptoms may be hunger, yawning, and even feeling elated. It is also important to ask about the end of the attack, known as the postdrome, which may occur for days after the headache resolves. The postdrome is often described as a hangover feeling, and is associated with fatigue, and changes in mood, concentration, and other cognitive complaints.

Aura is a discrete, transient neurological event—usually visual, but occasional language, motor, sensory, or brainstem symptoms. Migraine aura occurs for 5–60 minutes and can occur before, during, or after a headache. The aura can be followed by a headache or not. Multiple aura symptoms can happen in succession (e.g., 3 × 10) and motor aura can last up to 72 hours. Aura can sometimes last longer than 60 minutes. If a person has prolonged aura, workup should be completed for systemic and/or structural diseases. Blurred vision is frequently mistaken for aura, so specific questions are important. Visual auras are characteristically zig-zag lines (teichopsias) starting centrally or peripherally and then moving across the visual field. Individuals often claim that the aura is in one eye, but to help demonstrate the aura is in both eyes, ask the patient to read a page with each eye individually and if the letters are obscured in both eyes, the aura is coming from the occipital lobe. Based on the duration and frequency of the aura, we might change the treatment to target the aura specifically with medications like aspirin and lamotrigine. It is important to note that not all visual disturbances are due to aura, as orthostatic phosphenes, sparkles are common and benign, and transient visual obscurations or dimming occurs in the presence of increased intracranial pressure.

Precipitating and Relieving Factors

A variety of triggers can initiate migraine attacks. Stress, stress letdown, menstrual cycle, weather changes, sleep disturbances, and fasting are some very well-known examples. Premonitory symptoms like neck tightness, light sensitivity, and food cravings can mimic triggers. That is why triggers can be so difficult to determine.

A rigorous evaluation of factors that may be associated with migraine attacks is important for distinguishing between primary versus secondary headaches and for identification of triggers. Headache worsening upon sitting and standing up, improving with lying down should raise suspicion for low-pressure headache. Cough may aggravate migraine, but if cough produces headache secondary causes should be considered. One of the most important differences between migraine and tension type headache is that activity aggravates the headaches in migraine but can be helpful for tension type headache.

Past Medical and Psychiatric History

Other medical and surgical diseases are very important to know for the treatment options. This is true to prevent possible complications from the therapy like using triptans if a patient has a history of coronary artery disease or prescribing topiramate to a patient who suffers from glaucoma. Moreover, it can also help to choose the treatment that might help comorbid illnesses like tricyclic antidepressants for insomnia or serotonin-norepinephrine reuptake inhibitors (SNRIs) for depression [8]. When a patient suffers from obesity, diabetes, and chronic migraine, topiramate can be chosen to help weight loss and chronic migraine at the same time. Table 4.4 consists of a list of medical and psychiatric conditions that may complicate migraine and headache diagnoses.

Table 4.4 Common medical and psychiatric comorbidities with chronic migraine [7]

Common medical comorbidities with chronic migraine	Common psychiatric comorbidities with chronic migraine
1. Insomnia or sleep apnea 2. Cervical spine disease 3. Irritable bowel syndrome 4. Thyroid disease 5. Fibromyalgia 6. Hypertension 7. Asthma 8. Head injury 9. Obesity	1. Depression 2. Anxiety 3. PTSD with or without nightmares 4. Early childhood maltreatment 5. Adult ADHD 6. Bipolar Disease

A detailed history of other pain conditions like cervical spine disease can guide us to understand the etiology of the headache like cervicogenic headaches or what other diseases might be precipitating to the headache. Untreated mental health illnesses can be the reason for the intractability of chronic headache [9]. Childhood maltreatment and a history of physical, sexual, and emotional abuse are known contributors to intractable chronic migraine [10].

In this section, sleep should be assessed. The diagnosis and management of insomnia, sleep apnea, and post-traumatic stress disorder (PTSD) with nightmares can be the key to successfully treating chronic primary headaches.

Treatment History

Current and past treatments should be listed carefully. When we ask about past treatments, we should note the dose, duration, and response of the treatment. If a patient took amitriptyline with minimal response only for 3 weeks and stopped due to side effects, prescribing a less potent tricyclic antidepressant can be a good option. Treatments should be divided into preventive interventions (medication and nonmedication or devices) and acute interventions (medication and nonmedication or devices). Encouraging a patient to keep a list of what was tried for the length of time and if appropriate the dose. This is so important for further treatment. Medication adherence should also be assessed; persistence of oral preventive medication is poor at 6 months and declines further by 12 months according to claim analyses [11].

Medication or caffeine overuse should be evaluated since both can cause chronic daily headaches [12]. When assessing acute medication use, it is important to find out how many days in a month a person uses the rescue medication—since medication overuse is a common cause of chronic migraine and medication overuse headaches. Be sure to ask about herbal products and vitamins, since many will not consider these medications.

Physical and Neurological Examination

The clinical examination should include a general physical exam and a neurological exam. Vital signs can show evidence for infectious etiology like fever and hypertension. Even if hypertension may not change the diagnosis of chronic migraine, a patient with uncontrolled hypertension should not be placed on triptans and this fact may guide a choice for a preventive medication. Obesity or notable weight gain may alert us to consider idiopathic intracranial hypertension which is a risk factor for chronic migraine.

General examination should include a thorough examination of the head and neck areas including tenderness in response to pressure along the temporal arteries, occipital nerves, supraorbital, supratrochlear, and auriculotemporal nerves. The temporomandibular joint, cervical paraspinal, and trapezius muscles should be checked for focal tenderness. The fundoscopic exam is a very important part of the exam for the evaluation of headache disorders; look for signs of papilledema that may signal high pressure, or spontaneous venous pulsations that will signal normal intracranial pressure (Fig. 4.1). A neurological examination should be complete and cranial nerve examination should be done properly. Abnormalities on the neurological exam should prompt the physician to consider appropriate testing (Table 4.5) when exam findings are suggestive of secondary headache syndromes.

Diaries and Questionnaires

Diaries provide more objective data on the number of headaches and headache days patients are having. A diary can include information about the headache days, severity of the headache, and use of rescue medication. There are many free apps available for this purpose. Diaries not only help us to make the diagnosis of acute versus chronic headache and/or menstrual migraine but also show the response to the treatment.

The impact of the headache on the patient's life is another important part of the evaluation. Some patients might have one or two migraine attacks a month but if the headache makes them miss a day at work or school, proper treatment changes should be reviewed. For this purpose, questionnaires assessing the impact of headaches can be used at the initial and follow-up visit. The Migraine Disability Assessment Test (MIDAS) [13] and the Headache Impact Test (HIT-6) [14] are short and adequate tools. Other tools that can be useful are readily available depression and anxiety screening tools such as the Patient Health Questionnaire (PHQ) 9, 5, or 2 and the Generalized Anxiety Disorder (GAD) 7 or 2 [15].

At the end of the structured headache history and examination, the provider should have a primary or secondary headache diagnosis, a list of comorbidities, and a list of previous preventive and acute treatments. Red flags should signal a reason for further evaluation to exclude a secondary headache disorder. The provider will want to write out the diagnosis for the patient as well as the treatment plan at the end of the visit.

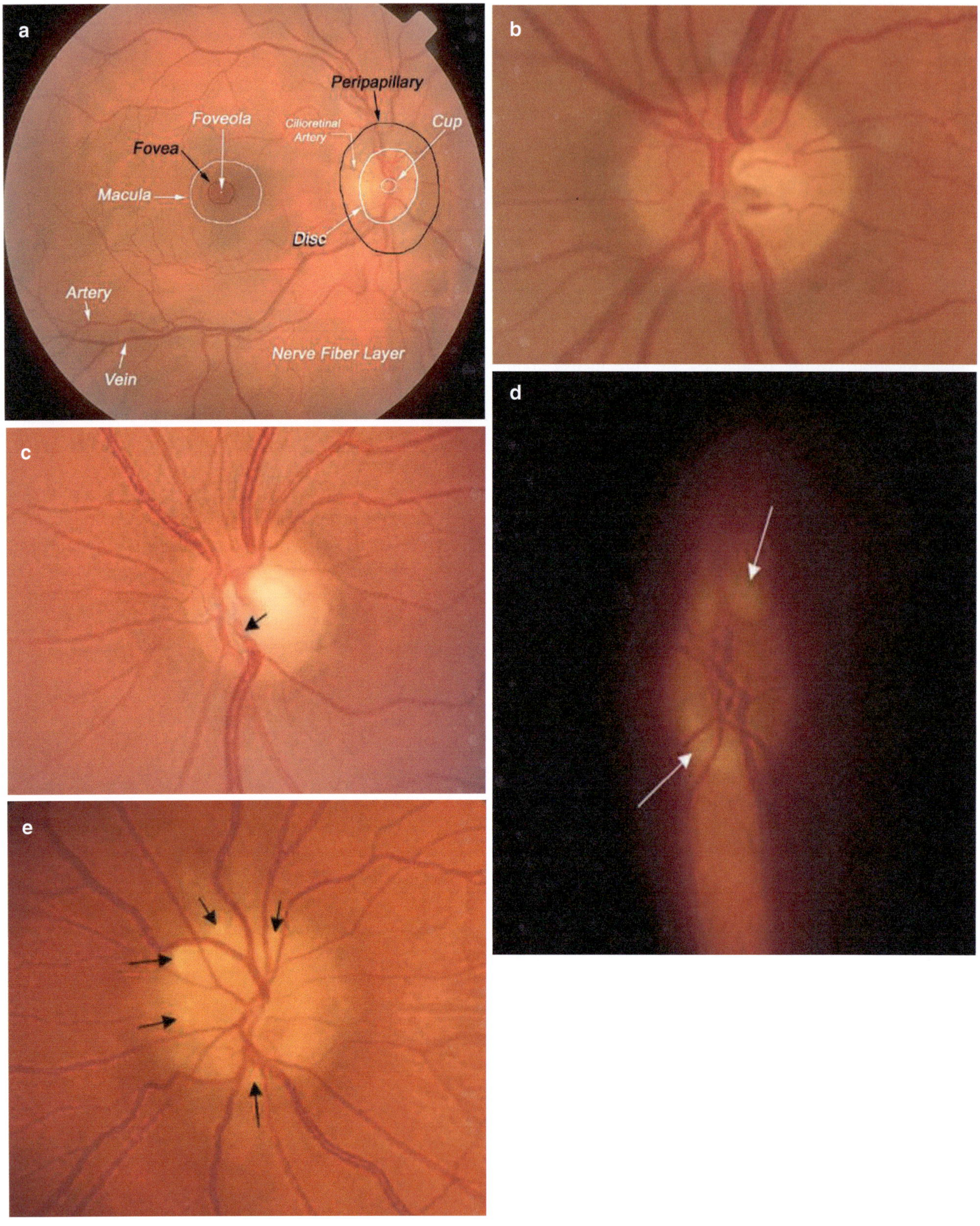

Fig. 4.1 Funduscopic findings from practical viewing of the optic disc [17]. (**a**) What to look for in a fundus examination. (**b**) Optic disc normal; Look at the cup/disc ratio; normal vasculature. (**c**) Venous pulsations; Look on the edges of the disc to see. (**d**) Elevation; Use your slit beam to determine if it is elevated. (**e-f**) Pseudo edema from Disc drusen; These can be buried (right) or visible (left); use the green light on the ophthalmoscope to see. (**g**) Pseudo edema from crowded or cupless disc; When there is a cupless disc—look carefully; these are frequently anomalous and often mistaken for papilledema. (**h**) True papilledema; Should obscure the disc margin and first appear superiorly and inferiorly. (**i**) Mild; Only c-shaped swelling. (**j**) Moderate; 360 degree elevation but major vessels not obscured. (**k**) Severe; 360 degree elevation and major vessels are obscured

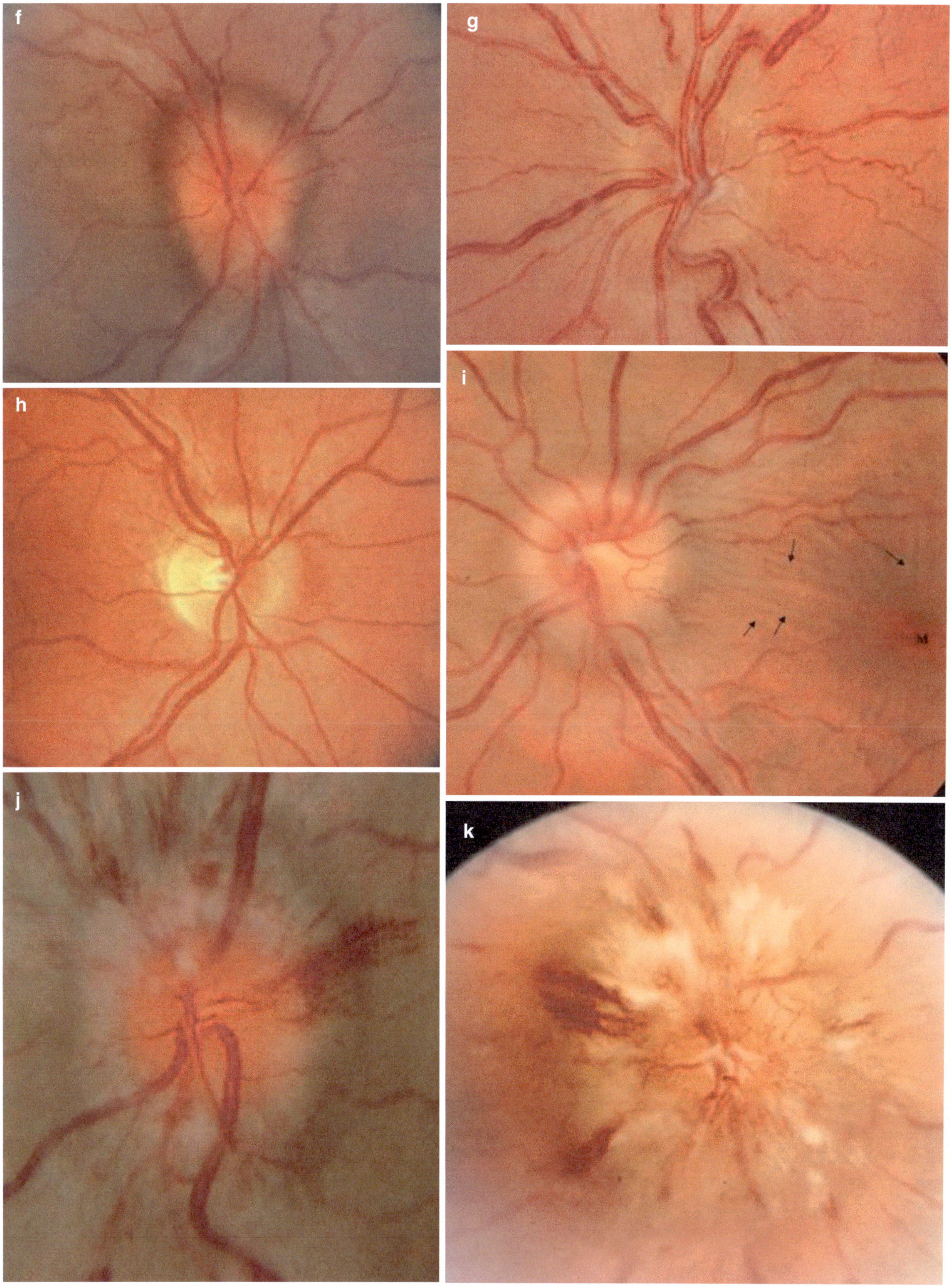

Fig. 4.1 (continued)

Table 4.5 Exam findings indicative of secondary cause of headache

Finding	Rule out
Vital signs	
Elevated temperature	Infectious causes, GCA
Elevated blood pressure	PRES, CVD
Tachycardia	Orthostatic hypotension, POTS
Bradycardia	Hypothyroidism
Body mass index >25	Idiopathic intracranial hypotension
General	
Wasted appearance	HIV, Malignancy, GCA
Joint hypermobility Skin laxity	Intracranial hypotension Intracranial aneurysm Cervical artery dissection
Hair loss, dry skin, edema, hoarse voice	Hypothyroidism
Diaphoresis, rhinorrhea, mydriasis, restlessness, yawning, tremor	Opioid withdrawal
Cardiac	
Temporal artery tendersness/ induration Diminished/asymmetric pulse Aortic regurgitation	GCA
Neurologic	
Papilledema	Intracranial hypertension
Horner's sign	Carotid artery dissection
Trigeminal sensation loss	Trigeminal neuropathy
Abducens paresis	Intracranial hypertension Other focal lesion
Oculomotor paresis and/or mydriasis	Intracranial aneurysm, ION, Other focal lesion
Head and Neck	
Trochlear tenderness aggravated by vertical duction	Trochlear headache
Tympanic vesicles	Herpes zoster
Hard papule near frenulum or adjacent to second upper molar	Sialolithiasis
Restricted neck rotation	C2/3 facet arthropathy
Pericranial and/or occipital nerve tenderness	Trigeminal branch or occipital neuralgia
Limited TMJ range of motion	TMJ syndrome

Reproduced with permission from Smith [16]

Conclusion

A complete history and examination are essential for the diagnosis and treatment of headache disorder. First, we should differentiate if this is a primary or a secondary headache. Then determine what specific headache disorder the patient has. If there is a concern for a secondary headache disease, appropriate workup should be completed. Treatment choices should be decided considering the comorbid illnesses and symptoms the patient suffers from.

Teaching Points

1. Ask how many headache-FREE days the patient has.
2. If the patient says there is no light or sound sensitivity, ask if they prefer a dark quiet room.
3. Always think of the red flags that signal a secondary headache type.
4. On examination, always look at the disc to determine if there is swelling or spontaneous venous pulsations.
5. If the patient does not respond to treatments, recheck your headache diagnosis and possible underlying systemic or structural disease to cause intractability.

Case

A 31-year-old female presented to the clinic with a 2-year history of daily headaches. Her mother and 2 other siblings suffer from headaches. Headaches began at age 12 around the time she had her first period. Until 2 years ago she would get a headache once or twice a month. But for the last 2 years, she has been having daily severe headaches. She did not have any life-changing events that could be a trigger. She has one type of headache which is holocephalic, associated with light and sound sensitivity along with severe nausea and vomiting. She can fall asleep easily but wakes up multiple times at night with pounding headaches. She reported no other medical disease or history of surgery. Her family history was also negative for aneurysm, stroke, or rheumatological diseases. She used to be able to treat headaches with over-the-counter painkillers in her teenage years. She tried amitriptyline 50 mg at night for 2 months without any benefit.

The patient's examination showed normal vital signs and a normal neurological exam. Due to unexplained significant change in the frequency and severity of the headaches, MRI brain with contrast was obtained. On the MRI brain, she was found to have a nonenhancing expansile lesion within the medial right frontal lobe which was diagnosed as diffuse astrocytoma WHO grade 2 with an IDH 1 mutation. After the surgical treatment, the headache frequency returned to her usual frequency of a couple a month.

Case Discussion

In this case, the change in her headache frequency, nocturnal awakening triggered further evaluation. See Table 4.2—for red flags of secondary headache, use the SNOOP pneumonic—for features of headaches that should suggest a secondary headache. However, most patients that present for evaluation of headache will have a primary headache disorder. Reassuring signs include a history of long duration before the age of 50, stable disease, recurrent symptoms of a similar nature, an association with typical migraine triggers (e.g., menses, changes in sleep, and sensory stimulation), and a normal examination.

Questions and Answers

1. A 28-year-old woman presents to the clinic with right sided headache. She never had headaches until 4 years ago. It started as an intermittent attack and became daily last 15 months. She describes her headache as continuous right sided headache, associated with ipsilateral photophobia and rhinorrhea, red eye. She also has periods of nausea. There is no prior family history of headache. Her MRI is normal. What is the best diagnosis to consider?
   A. Chronic migraine
   B. Cluster headache
   C. Hemicrania continua
   D. Idiopathic stabbing headache

The correct answer is C. The patient has a strictly unilateral headache that is continuous and associated with cranial autonomic symptoms. Given this presentation, hemicrania continua should be strongly considered. Cluster headaches occur up to 8 times per day but lasts 15 minutes to 3 hours. A positive indomethacin test is needed to confirm the diagnosis of hemicrania continua, although chronic migraine can be considered if there is a negative indomethacin response. Stabbing pain may co-occur both with migraine and TACs, but other symptoms go against idiopathic stabbing headache.

2. In which clinical scenario ordering neuroimaging would be appropriate?
   A. Headache started at age 12
   B. Side locked headache with autonomic symptoms
   C. Patient with chronic migraine who failed Topiramate treatment
   D. 30 years old male with chronic tension headache and normal neurological exam

The correct answer is B. Headache that does not switch sides, and only localizes to one side of the head raises the concern for underlying structural disease. Side locked headache with autonomic symptoms leads to diagnosis of trigeminal autonomic cephalalgia headaches. These are rare headache syndromes and that must be evaluated for secondary causes. A long history of recurrent headache of pediatric onset is reassuring. A lack of response to treatment is not a red flag and is not uncommon in clinical practice.

References

1. Eross E, Dodick D, Eross M. The sinus, allergy and migraine study (SAMS). Headache. 2007;47(2):213–24.
2. Lagman-Bartolome AM, Lay C. Pediatric migraine variants: a review of epidemiology, diagnosis, treatment, and outcome. Curr Neurol Neurosci Rep. 2015;15(6):34.
3. Gomez CA, et al. Addressing health equity and social determinants of health through healthy people 2030. J Public Health Manag Pract. 2021;27(Suppl 6):S249–57.
4. Blumenfeld A, Schim J, Brower J. Pure tension-type headache versus tension-type headache in the migraineur. Curr Pain Headache Rep. 2010;14:465–9.
5. Turkdogan D, Cagrici S, Soylemez D, Sur H, Bilge C, Turk U. Characteristic and overlapping features of migraine and tension-type headache. Headache. 2006;46(3):461–8.
6. American Headache Society. The American Headache Society position statement on integrating new migraine treatments into clinical practice. Headache. 2019;59(1):1–18.
7. Elliott JE, et al. Different methods for traumatic brain injury diagnosis influence presence and symptoms of post-concussive syndrome in United States veterans. J Neurotrauma. 2021;38:3126–36.
8. Yin J-H, et al. Prevalence and association of lifestyle and medical-, psychiatric-, and pain-related comorbidities in patients with migraine: a cross-sectional study. Headache. 2021;61(5):715–26.
9. Lipton RB, Silberstein SD, Saper JR, Bigal ME, Goadsby PJ. Why headache treatment fails. Neurology. 2003;60(7):1064–70.
10. Tietjen GE, et al. History of childhood maltreatment is associated with comorbid depression in women with migraine. Neurology. 2007;69(10):959–68.
11. Hepp Z, Dodick DW, Varon SF, Chia J, Matthew N, Gillard P, Hansen RN, Devine EB. Persistence and switching patterns of oral migraine prophylactic medications among patients with chronic migraine: a retrospective claims analysis. Cephalalgia. 2017;37(5):470–85. https://doi.org/10.1177/0333102416678382. Epub 2016 Nov 12. PMID: 27837173; PMCID: PMC5405847.
12. Chen X, Chen Z, Dong Z, Liu M, Shengyuan Y. Morphometric changes over the whole brain in caffeine-containing combination-analgesic-overuse headache. Mol Pain. 2018;14:1744806918778641.
13. Stewart WF, Lipton RB, Dowson AJ, Sawyer J. Development and testing of the Migraine Disability Assessment (MIDAS) questionnaire to assess headache-related disability. Neurology. 2001;56(6 Suppl. 1):S20–8.
14. Yang M, Rendas-Baum R, Varon SF, Kosinski M. Validation of the Headache Impact Test (HIT-6™) across episodic and chronic migraine. Cephalalgia. 2011;31(3):357–67.
15. Baldacci F, et al. Migraine features in migraineurs with and without anxiety-depression symptoms: a hospital-based study. Clin Neurol Neurosurg. 2015;132:74–8.
16. Smith JR. Ruling out secondary headache. Pract Neurol (US). 2018;18(3):41–9.
17. Digre KB, Corbett JJ. Practical viewing of the optic disc. Boston: Butterworth-Heineman; 2003.

Diagnostic Approach to Headache and Secondary Disorders

5

Jacob Van Orman and Robert Cowan

Introduction

Headache is a common clinical complaint. Its causes range from benign syndromes to more sinister presentations of head pain associated with life-threatening pathologies. In the clinical literature, headache is divided into two broad categories: primary headache and secondary headaches.

A primary headache is a head pain syndrome without an apparent pathologic cause. A secondary headache is a head pain syndrome attributed to some separate pathology or process known to produce a symptomatic headache and whose clinical course corresponds to the natural history of the underlying cause. A secondary headache is also present when a primary headache syndrome is substantially worsened or changed in correlation with the discovery of a secondary pathology. The clinic entities included within each of these categories are well laid out in the International Classification of Headache Disorders published by the International Headache Society [1].

In this chapter, we review the pathophysiology and clinical features of secondary headaches to help guide work-up and diagnosis.

Questions

1. Which headache symptom should raise concern for a secondary pathology?
   A. Photophobia and phonophobia are extremely severe
   B. Throbbing quality is bilateral
   C. Pain peaks in less than 60 seconds from onset
   D. Pain is rated as severe and behind one eye
2. A 30-year-old obese female is complaining of headaches that are worse with lying flat, transient visual obscurations, and pulsatile tinnitus. Head imaging shows an empty sella sign and venous sinus stenosis but is otherwise normal. A lumbar puncture will likely show
   A. An opening pressure of less than 6 cm H_2O
   B. Xanthochromia
   C. A high red blood cell count that does not clear from tubes 1 to 4
   D. An opening pressure of greater than 25 cm H_2O

Pathophysiology of Secondary Headache

The parenchyma of the brain lacks nociceptive afferents [2]. However, the supportive architecture of the brain, face, and neck have sensory afferents in abundance and relay increased signals to the trigeminal nucleus caudalis (TNC) when sufficiently stimulated [3, 4]. Second-order sensory neurons ascend from the brainstem to the diencephalon, brainstem, limbic system, and cerebral cortex [5].

At the same time, nuclei in the periaqueductal gray (PAG) and rostral ventral medulla (RVM) receive inputs from forebrain structures and muster a descending modulatory effect on pain signaling in the trigeminal system [3]. Thus, the patient's pain experience is a complex of sensory and modulatory signals that drive a combination of autonomic, affec-

J. Van Orman (✉) · R. Cowan
Department of Neurology, Stanford University, Palo Alto, CA, USA

T. S. Monteith et al. (eds.), *Comprehensive Migraine Management*, https://doi.org/10.1007/978-3-031-86923-5_5

tive, and behavioral responses. Any process that disturbs the pain-sensitive architecture of the head and neck can manifest as headaches.

Because the differential for secondary headaches is broad, identifying the causative pathology can be a significant diagnostic and management challenge. In 1988, The International Headache Society released the first version of the International Classification on Headache Disorders (ICHD) to create an operational diagnostic framework. Subsequent editions in 2004 and 2018 added significant revisions and additions to the secondary headache category, the product of new knowledge ascertained through research-driven classification [6].

This begs the question: will all headaches eventually become secondary? Migraine is currently considered a primary headache disorder, though evidence supports the role of familial transmission and receptor mutation as part of its pathophysiology [7]. New Daily Persistent Headache (NDPH) is a treatment refractory primary headache disorder often accompanied by migraine or tension-type features. The pathophysiology of this condition is poorly understood. Rozen et al. reviewed 97 cases of NDPH where 47% of patients reported precipitating factors, including flu-like illness, stressful life events, and surgical intubation [8]. Another study screened 12 NDPH patients and found that the majority had cervical spine and widespread joint hypermobility [9]. Connective tissue disorders that lead to altered states of CSF pressure and post-infectious CNS inflammation are among the proposed mechanisms that contribute to NDPH [10, 11].

Cluster headache is a primary headache disorder in the family of Trigeminal Autonomic Cephalalgias (TAC). Epidemiologic data support the genetic basis of this condition with several hypothalamic gene variants under investigation as a pathologic mechanism [12–14]. Though the precise pathologic mechanism(s) in migraine, tension headache, and the trigeminal autonomic cephalalgias remain uncertain, future editions of the ICHD may struggle to ascribe the title of "primary headache" as it is currently understood should those mechanisms be identified, whether acquired or inherited.

Clinical Features of Secondary Headache

Headache characterization requires a review of the location, quality, severity, and time course. But other clinically meaningful features of the patient's history should be explored so that a secondary cause is not missed. This is especially relevant in the emergency setting where nontraumatic headache is a common presentation.

Most nontraumatic headache cases are benign, though an estimated 3% are the presenting feature of a serious secondary cause [15]. A 2006, single-center study of 558 patients with nontraumatic headaches in the emergency setting identified three historical features that were independent predictors of a serious secondary cause: patient age over 50 years old, sudden onset headache, and an abnormal neurologic examination [16].

Dodick, in 2010, published a review article in Seminars in Neurology that popularized a mnemonic to screen for "red flags" that should prompt a secondary evaluation [17]. The SNOOP4 screen is designed to be a 2-minute interview added to the initial evaluation. A study of 90 patients in a single tertiary center demonstrated a negative predictive value of 96% for secondary nontraumatic headache and a negative SNOOP4 screen. The positive predictive value was low at 26% [18].

More recently, the mnemonic has been expanded to SNOOP10, including many additional features of nonemergent secondary headaches [19]. An effective and easy-to-use tool like the SNOOP screen can be a helpful guide to the neurologist, emergency physician, primary care physician, or headache specialist while performing their due diligence in addressing secondary causes in their history taking. Should there be one or more responses on the screen that raise suspicion for secondary pathology, an appropriate diagnostic evaluation should be considered.

In the following section, we will address several "red-flag symptoms" with corresponding diseases. We will focus on clinical features and diagnosis rather than treatment. It is our hope that familiarity with these patterns can provide the clinician some degree of confidence when approaching headaches in the clinical setting.

Positional Headache

Pathophysiology

A headache that worsens while in a vertical or horizontal body position should raise concern for a pathological alteration to intracranial pressure (ICP). Normal physiologic variations to blood and cerebrospinal fluid (CSF) flow dynamics with changes in body position have been demonstrated on MRI flow studies of healthy patients. In the vertical position, total blood flow in the cranium is 12% of the flow rate in the spinal canal and cranial CSF flow is 58% of the spinal canal flow rate [20]. The relationship between CSF volume and pressure is exponential, with experimental human modeling of low-pressure states demonstrating that a 10% removal of CSF volume corresponds to a 40% reduction in vertex pressure in the upright position [21–22]. Small alterations to CSF volume can induce large changes to intracranial pressure leading to the development of headache and other symptoms.

Intracranial CSF travels in the ventricles and subarachnoid space surrounded by meningeal layering, venous sinuses, and pial arteries. Increased pressure may compress these pain-sensitive structures [23]. Reduced CSF pressure will cause the brain to sink and apply traction, distortion, or compression to the surrounding dura and vasculature [24]. Headache that awakens from sleep happens in the morning after waking, or worsens with Valsalva raises concern for high ICP. A headache that persists during the second half of the day and improves with recumbency suggests low ICP.

Idiopathic Intracranial Hypertension

Idiopathic intracranial hypertension (IIH) is a condition of pathologically elevated CSF pressure. Childbearing age, female gender, obesity, use of tetracycline antibiotics, glucocorticoids, vitamin A derivatives, and co-morbid endocrinopathies are risk factors with an incidence of 0.5 to 2 per 100,000 per year in the general population [25]. Headache is the most frequently reported symptom and, though the phenotype is variable, a constant bilateral frontal headache with a pressing or pulsing quality is the most often seen [26, 27].

Sensory sensitivity and nausea can accompany the headache. Positionally provoked transient visual obscuration, or distortion of vision that lasts less than 60 seconds, is seen in about 68% of patients [26, 28]. Pulsatile tinnitus, or a swooshing sound in the ear(s), may be related to turbulent blood flow in the transverse sinuses and is seen in about 52% of patients [26]. Nasal field defects, an enlarged blind spot, and generalized field constriction are the most reported visual complaints [29].

The 2013 update of the Modified Dandy Criteria guides work-up [30]. Fundoscopic eye examination may reveal loss of spontaneous venous pulsations and papilledema. Optic Coherence Tomography (OCT) can measure papilledema, with retinal nerve fiber layer (RNFL) thickness found to be significantly higher in IIH patients compared to controls [31].

Neurologic examination should be normal except for potential oculomotility dysfunction which can be a sign of high intracranial pressure. Brain imaging with contrasted MRI and MR Venogram are recommended to rule out structural lesions, masses, hydrocephalus, meningeal enhancement, or venous sinus thrombosis. An empty sella, optic nerve sheath distention, or posterior globe flattening are found in 70%, 45%, and 80% of IIH patients, respectively [32]. Finally, lumbar puncture in the lateral decubitus position with leg extension will reveal an opening pressure of 25 cm H_2O or greater with normal composition (Fig. 5.1).

Headache Attributed to Low Intracranial Pressure

Low intracranial pressure headache is a condition of low CSF volume and pressure related to CSF leakage from the spinal column. Leaks are commonly found in the cervicothoracic and thoracic spine and result from dural rents, meningeal diverticula, CSF-venous fistulas, or uncertain sources. These are referred to as Type 1–4 leaks, respectively. Annual incidence is reported at 5 per 100,000, affecting women in the 4th and 5th decade of life disproportionately [33, 34]. Isolated joint hypermobility and marfanoid skeletal features are found in one-fifth and two-fifth of patients, respectively [35, 36]. Evidence supports the role of connective tissue disorders in the pathogenesis of the condition in many cases [37].

Headache phenotype is variable though bilateral occipital pain with a throbbing or nonthrobbing quality is most often reported. Pain occurs or worsens within 15 minutes of being upright, though some patients report hours for pain to manifest. Headache more reliably improves with recumbency within 15–30 minutes [38]. Rarely, it can present suddenly like a thunderclap headache. The postural component can dampen or even disappear with chronic CSF leaks [39]. Additional symptoms include neck stiffness, tinnitus, hyperacusis, nausea, photophobia, and vertigo that may mirror headaches by improving with recumbency [38]. Examination may demonstrate a rare constellation of findings including galactorrhea, bulbar dysfunction, and cognitive impairments [40–42].

Diagnosis is established through radiographic or physiologic evidence of low CSF pressure and leak localization. Cranial MRI may demonstrate a combination of subdural fluid collection, enhancement of the pachymeninges, engorgement of venous structures, pituitary hyperemia, and sagging of the brain (SEEPS). In 2019, The University of Bern quantified the 6 most relevant MRI brain findings into a 3-tier scoring system that ascribes a likelihood of positive spinal imaging, which may help triage invasive localization procedures to high-yield cases [43]. About 20% of patients will not have abnormalities on cranial MRI [44]. Lumbar puncture less than 6 cm H_2O is another line of evidence to support the diagnosis though patients can have normal values. CSF fluid composition may show elevated protein, xanthochromia, or lymphocytic pleocytosis [37–38]. An initial noninvasive spinal MRI can assess for signs of leak (dural enhancement, vein engorgement, diverticula, fluid collections). If this is nonrevealing, procession to conventional CT or MR myelogram is most appropriate. Delayed or hyperdynamic variations of the technique may be applied depending on the size and rate of the leak. Lateral Decubitus Digital Subtraction Myelogram (LDDSM) has

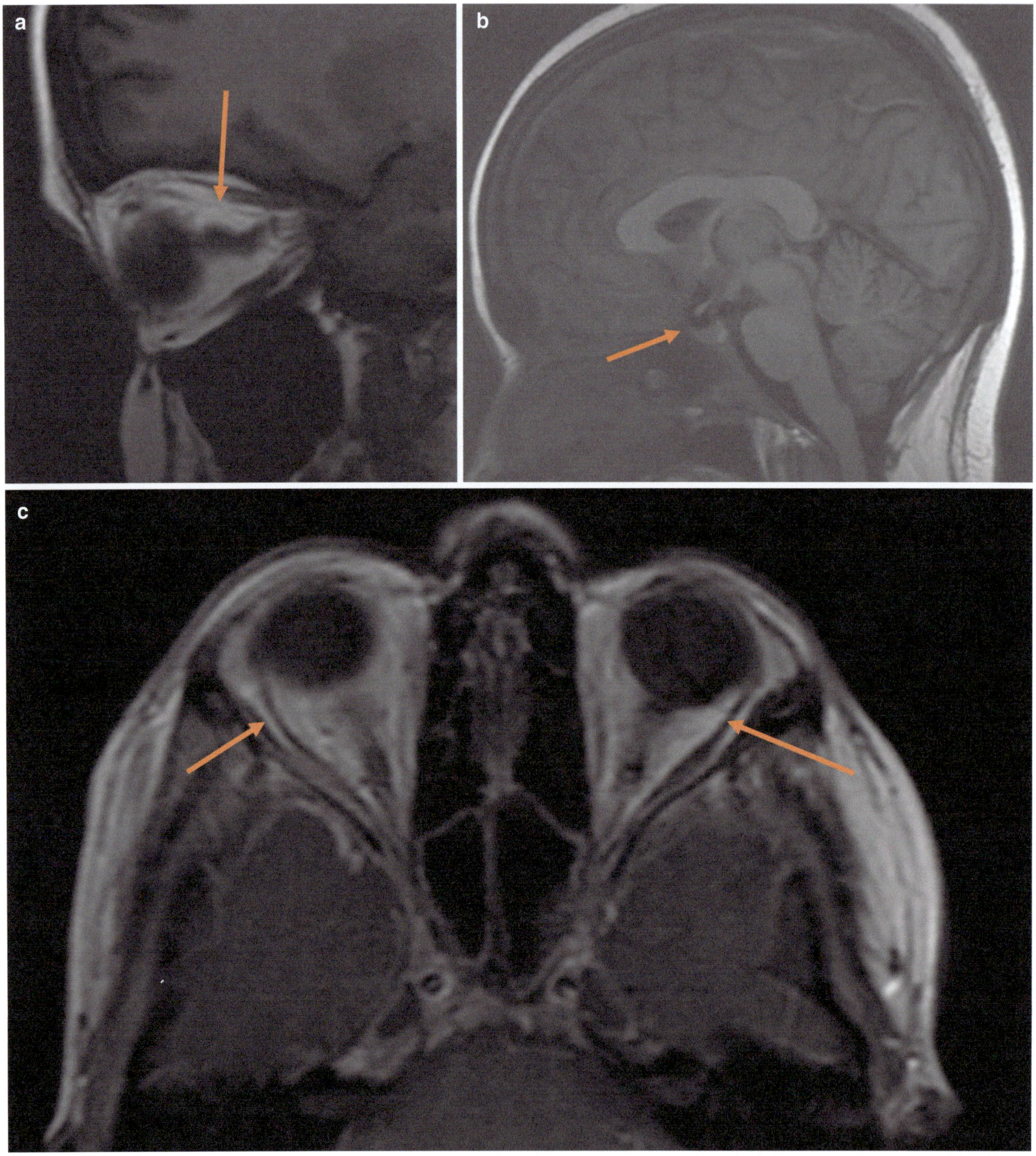

Fig. 5.1 Idiopathic intracranial hypertension. (**a**) Sagittal MRI brain T1 Flair: Tortuous optic nerves with distention. (**b**) Saggital MRI brain T2 Flair: Partially empty sella. (**c**) Axial MRI brain T1 + C: Posterior orbital globe flattening

shown the ability to identify type 2–4 CSF leaks with higher sensitivity than MRI or conventional CT and should be considered in patients with high Bern Scores and negative conventional spinal imaging [45]. Procession to image-guided Epidural Blood Patching (EBP) with whole blood or fibrin glue products can be considered, ideally after the leak location has been established, and close observation of clinical response should follow. If the leak location is uncertain, a blinded lumber EBP can be attempted (Figs. 5.2 and 5.3).

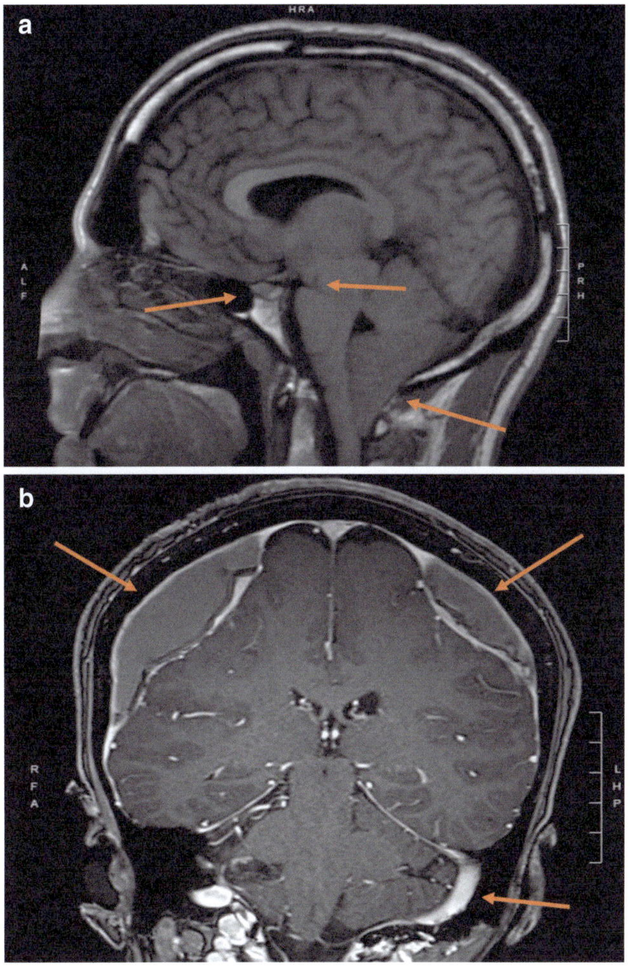

Fig. 5.2 Intracranial hypotension. (**a**) Sagittal MRI brain T1 Flair: Pituitary hyperemia, ton-sillar descent, narrowed mamillo-pontine distance. (**b**) Coronal MRI brain T1 + C: Bilateral subdural fluid collections, venous engorgement

Thunderclap Headache

Pathophysiology

A severe, abrupt-onset headache that reaches peak severity within one minute should raise concern for a differential of intracranial conditions with high morbidity and mortality [46]. Day and Raskin described the phenotype in 1986, coining the term "thunderclap headache" as a sudden, severe headache in a patient with an unruptured cerebral aneurysm [47]. The pain was like a "clap of thunder" with patients frequently using the description "worst headache of my life" to describe their pain experience [48].

The most common "thunderclap" etiologies have a vascular origin: aneurysmal subarachnoid hemorrhage (aSAH), reversible cerebrovascular vasoconstrictive syndrome (RCVS), central venous thrombosis (CVT), arterial dissection, ischemic or hemorrhagic stroke, and reversible posterior leukoencephalopathy (RPLE). Pituitary apoplexy and low CSF pressure headaches are rarer. The primary form according to the ICHD-3 is diagnosed when secondary sources have been ruled out with imaging and lumbar puncture and no clear triggers are identified [49].

The unifying feature of the various diseases that induce the thunderclap phenotype is the sudden nature of their pathology. A 2008 study evaluating human exposure to conditioned gradual vs sudden pain stimulation under adaptive conditions found that the gradual exposure group had 4 times the level of pain reduction with repeat pain testing [50]. This suggests that descending inhibitory pathways require greater time of signal exposure to modulate ascending pain signals. Abrupt tissue damage to sensitive brain structures may lack this modulation leading to a severe, abrupt form of head pain.

Aneurysmal Subarachnoid Hemorrhage

Aneurysmal subarachnoid hemorrhage results from a rupture to a weakened arterial outpouching with subsequent hemorrhage into the subarachnoid space. These most commonly occur at proximal branch points of the great intracranial arteries. Modifiable risk factors include cigarette smoking, hypertension, and moderate to heavy alcohol consumption [51]. Annual global incidence was 6.1 per 100,000 persons in 2010 [52].

Headache phenotype can have several distinguishing features including occipital location, sharp character, peaks within 1 second of onset, and is accompanied by meningismus [53]. Rarely, altered levels of consciousness and seizure can accompany the syndrome and neurologic deficits corresponding to the site of the bleed may be present on physical examination. The use of a clinical decision-making tool like the Ottawa SAH rule can help risk stratify patients based on clinical features and avoid unnecessary testing. The absence of seven high-risk features, including questions about meningismus, patient age, provoking factors, and rapidity of onset, was able to rule out SAH with 100% sensitivity and negative predictive value [54].

Patients with high-risk features should proceed to head imaging with a noncontrasted computer tomography. This is 100% sensitive and specific for SAH detection at 6 hours, 93% sensitive at 24 hours, and 58% sensitive at day 5 [55]. If there is ongoing uncertainty a lumbar puncture should be performed, which is most sensitive between 2 to 12 hours from the onset of symptoms [56]. The presence of xanthochromia, elevated opening pressure, and raised red blood cell counts without clearing from CSF tubes 1 to 4 are supportive of an SAH diagnosis. Use of CT angiogram after or with initial noncontrast head CT has shown some benefit with aneurysm localization, showing a sensitivity and specificity of 91 and 85 percent compared to catheter angiography [57].

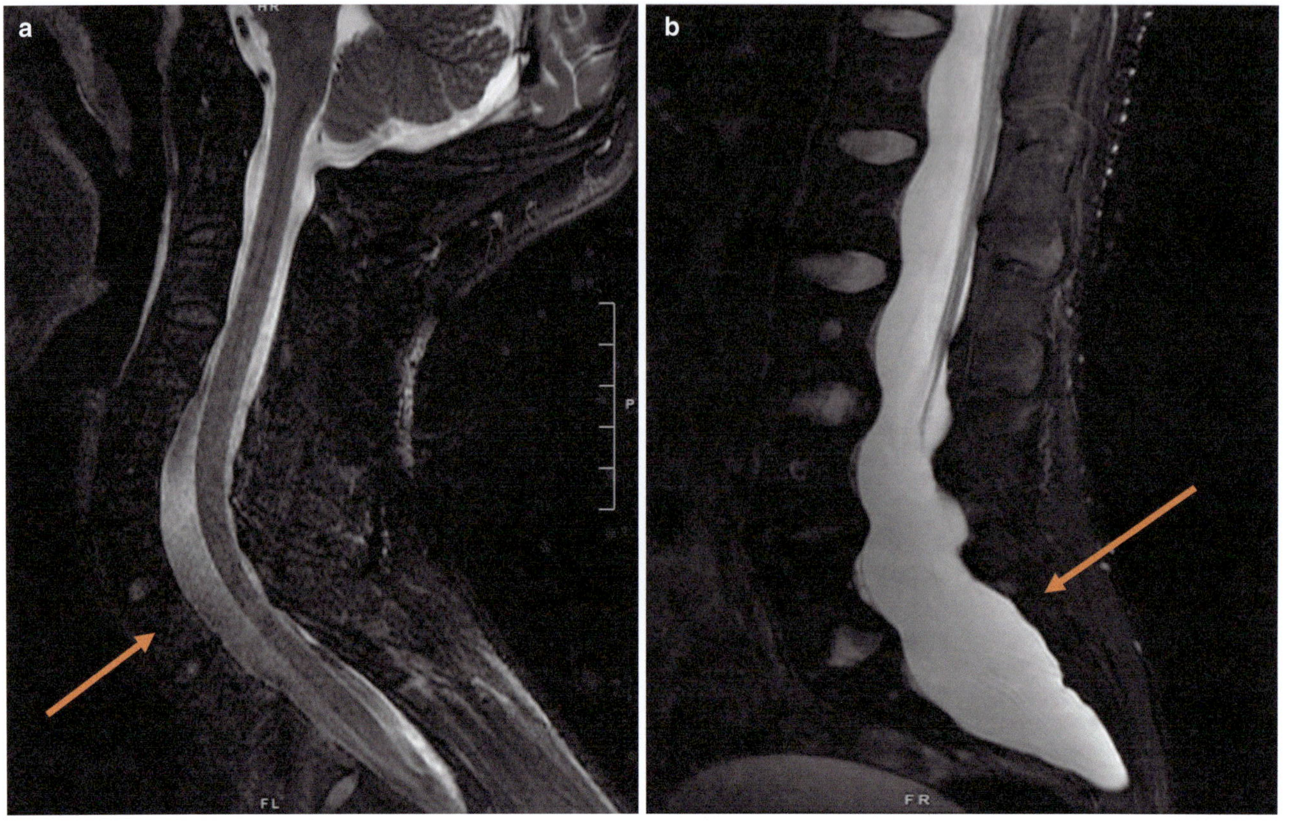

Fig. 5.3 Intracranial hypotension. (**a**) Sagittal C-Spine MRI T2 Fat Saturated: Cervical dural ectasia with bal-looning. (**b**) Sagittal L-Spine MRI T2 Fat Saturated: Lumbar dural ectasia with balloon-ing

This does not preclude the need for lumbar puncture if initial head CT remains equivocal. If an unsecured aSAH is diagnosed, emergent catheter angiography is indicated for lesion characterization and stabilization (Fig. 5.4).

Reversible Cerebral Vasoconstrictive Syndrome

Reversible cerebral vasoconstrictive syndrome is a condition affecting one or multiple segments of the intracranial arteries. It is considered a transient abnormality of vascular tone triggered by sympathetic hyperactivity and endothelial dysfunction. It is affiliated with conditions including pregnancy, use of vasoactive drugs and medications, cerebrovascular injury, and migraine [58, 59] The 2016 national incidence was 4.62 per million population and 4 times as likely in women [60].

The classic headache phenotype is a severe, bilateral, occipitally located headache with diffuse spread lasting an average of one to three hours and reaching peak severity within seconds. Sensory sensitivities and nausea can be seen [61]. Eighty percent of cases have a trigger involving Valsalva, physical exertion, or activities that affect sympathetic tone [62]. The disease course is progressive with recurrent headache attacks occurring over 1–4 weeks and many patients endorse low grade pain between attacks [63]. Stroke, hemorrhage, seizure, and RPLE are possible complications [64].

The diagnostic evaluation balances clinical and radiographic evidence gathering to support RVCS while ruling out other causes of thunderclap headache and cerebral arteriopathy. Brain imaging in three-fourth of cases will demonstrate a lesion (RPLE, edema, infarction, or hemorrhage) though 55% of initial scans are normal [64]. Noninvasive angiography with CT or MRI of the head and neck may demonstrate smooth, proximal narrowing of the cerebral arteries, like "beads on a string." Twenty percent of initial angiography will be normal [65]. A lumbar puncture is used to rule out aSAH, CNS infection, and inflammation and should have a normal composition. Serum labs can screen for vasoactive drug intoxication, electrolytes, and catecholamine levels. The RCVS2 score is a helpful screen looking at clinical and radiographic factors with high sensitivity and specificity for ruling in and ruling out RCVS in the high and low score groups, respectively [66] (Fig. 5.5).

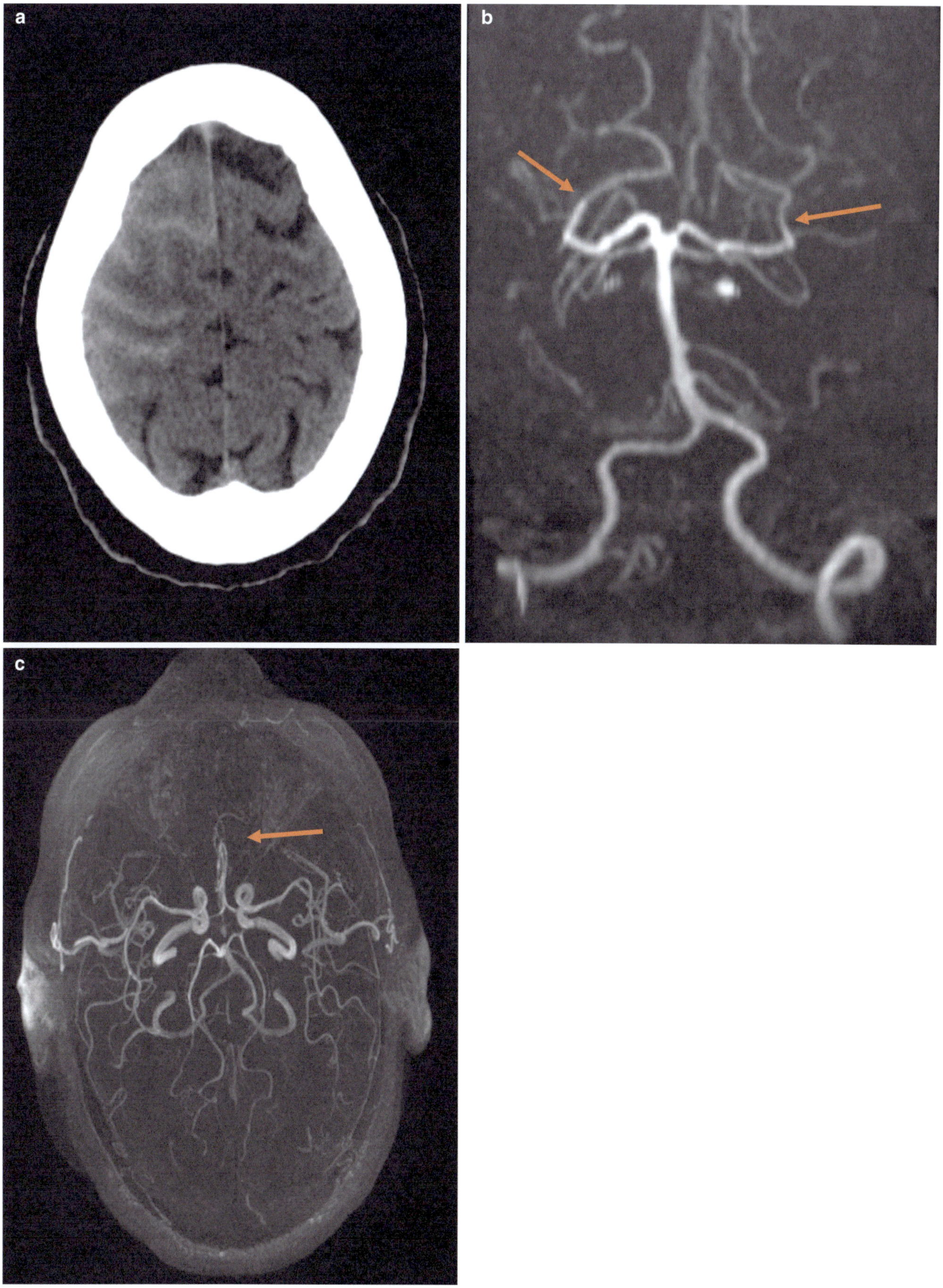

Fig. 5.4 Aneurysmal non-traumatic subarachnoid hemorrhage (SAH). (**a**) Axial CT head without contrast: Right sylvian and frontal SAH. (**b**) Axial CT Angiogram head: Saccular anterior communicating aneurysm. (**c**) Sagittal CT Angiogram head: Saccular anterior communicating aneurysm

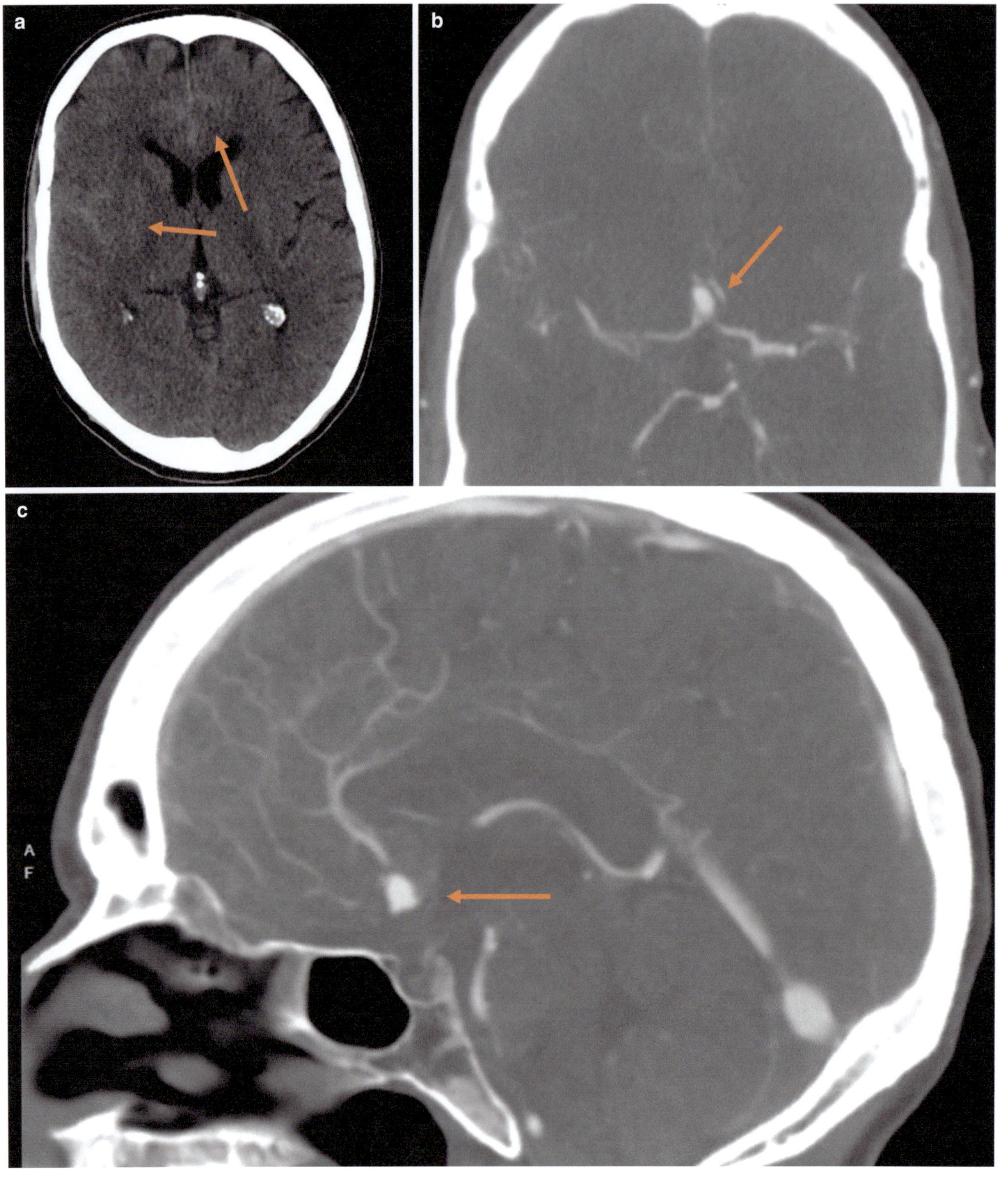

Fig. 5.5 Reversible cerebral vasocon-strictive syndrome. (**a**) Axial CT head without contrast: Right frontal subarachnoid hemorrhage on initial imaging. (**b**) MR Angiogram head Circle of Willis (COW): Bilateral posterior cerebral artery narrowing. (**c**) MR Angiogram head COW: Bilateral proximal anterior cerebral artery spasm with poor distal flow

Headache with Neurologic Deficits

Pathophysiology

An abnormality on neurologic examination is an independent predictor of serious secondary pathology during a headache evaluation in the emergency department [16]. An altered level of consciousness suggests dysfunction of the ascending reticular activating system and when combined with headache, meningismus, and fever there should be concern for infective, inflammatory, or neoplastic meningoencephalitides.

Focal deficits of motor, complex motor, sensory, bulbar, or cortical function suggest discrete lesions like stroke or tumor with progressive neurologic deterioration raising concern for more rapid processes like hemorrhage or infection. Headache can be seen with any pathology that affects pain-sensitive brain structures including dura, meninges, and vasculature.

Acute Spontaneous Intracerebral Hemorrhage

Acute spontaneous intracerebral hemorrhage accounts for 10–20% of stroke with the incidence varying by race and increasing with age [67]. Modifiable risk factors include cholesterol levels, hypertension, cigarette smoking, excessive ethanol consumption, and the use of anti-thrombotic medications.

About 33–50% of ICH patients who are able to report symptoms complain of headache [68, 69]. Headache onset can be sudden or gradual, mild or severe, and lobar hemorrhages produce more headache than deep hemorrhages. Occipital lesions tend to produce ipsilateral periorbital/orbital pain, whereas anterior lesions cause ipsilateral temporal or frontal headaches [70]. Cerebellar ICH tends to produce occipital headaches with rare frontal radiation [71, 72]. Nausea is more prevalent than in aSAH.

Focal neurologic deficits with progressive neurologic deterioration and acute hypertension may accompany the syndrome. Emergent noncontrast CT of the head will show hyperdense parenchyma lesions consistent with acute blood. MRI brain or LP should be considered in CT negative patients to look for other etiologies.

Brain Tumor

CNS tumors are estimated to account for 1.4% of new cancer diagnoses and 2.6% of cancer deaths in 2015, with tumor type varying by age [73]. Headache is present in 48 to 71% of undifferentiated intracranial tumors with higher prevalence in patients younger than 45 years and a history of primary headache disorder [74–76]. Intraventricular or infratentorial tumor location, glioblastomas, and secreting pituitary tumors have higher rates of headache compared to supratentorial non-gliomas [74, 77].

Up to 55% of patients with known malignancy and isolated new or changed headaches will have intracranial metastasis [78]. The headache phenotype is variable though an initially intermittent bilateral pain that is moderate to severe in intensity and progressive is the most reported [79]. Focal neurologic deficits, signs of altered ICP, meningismus, or fever may accompany the headache syndrome. The majority of headaches do not fit the criteria for a primary headache disorder with approximately 15% and 30% reporting migraine and tension-type phenotypes, respectively [74].

Pituitary tumors may produce symptomatic TAC syndromes with SUNCT, paroxysmal hemicrania, and cluster headache being the most common [80]. Skull-based tumors have a variety of classic syndromes with regional pain and neurologic deficits depending on lesion location [81]. Diagnosis is made with imaging, using MRI with contrast, though internal auditory canal, skull base, or FIESTA special sequences can increase image resolution and rate of tumor detection. A neoplastic work-up should follow MRI findings using a combination of serum and CSF labs, body scans, SPECT or functional brain imaging, and brain biopsy.

Headache Attributed to Substance and Systemic Infection

Pathophysiology

Headache is a frequent complaint with systemic infection, substance usage, and withdrawal. In infection, the body's inflammatory response drives the production of pyrogens, such as interleukin, a-interferon, and cyclooxygenase products like prostaglandin that interact with neurovascular endothelium and the trigeminal vascular system to induce headache [82]. Medications like nitric oxide donors can cause headaches through vasoactive properties and direct nociceptive receptor activation [83]. Medication overuse or substance withdrawal is related to pain promoting changes in the endogenous pain system from chronic exposure to substances with analgesic properties. This happens by central sensitization and impaired pain inhibition via several mechanisms including depletion of 5-HT, overexpression of 5-HT_{2A} receptors, and increased expression of CGRP [84].

Systemic Infection

Several systemic infections can have headache associated with the acute febrile phase of the illness including influenza, adenovirus, legionella, and mycoplasma pneumonia [85–88]. SARS-CoV-2 infection has a strong association with headache and is frequently an early symptom of the disease [89]. Herpes Simplex Virus and Epstein Barr Virus are implicated in the development of chronic or delayed headaches and affiliated with conditions like chronic fatigue syndrome and new daily persistent headaches [90, 91].

The headache phenotype with systemic infection is typically moderate to severe, diffuse, or bilateral pain, though focal pain over the frontal or retro-orbital areas has been reported. Sensory sensitivity, meningismus, nausea with vomiting, and exacerbation by Valsalva or head movements can be seen. The headache mirrors the natural history of the infection, though chronic forms of the syndrome are diagnosed if headaches persist for longer than 3 months.

Medication Overuse

Medication Overuse Headache (MOH) is the clinical deterioration of a primary headache syndrome with regular overuse of acute headache medication for more than 3 months. Its 1-year prevalence is 1–2% and is most common in women in their 4th and 5th decade of life [92]. A pre-existing primary headache disorder is required for the diagnosis as chronic analgesic use in headache free patients rarely produces MOH [93]. The most common primary disorder complicated with MOH is migraine [94].

Overuse is defined as greater than 15 days per month with simple analgesics (NSAIDs, acetaminophen, aspirin) and greater than 10 days per month with triptans, ergots, opiates, barbiturates, and combination formulations [1]. Headache phenotype can persist or change from the initial primary syndrome, depending on the class of overused medication. People with migraine overusing triptans tend to have preserved phenotype compared to migraineurs overusing simple analgesics where phenotype can shift to a continuous tension pattern [95]. Diagnosis is clinical and requires verification of an initial primary headache disorder, quantification of acute medication usage, and review of changes to headache burden.

Conclusion

Headache remains a common and challenging problem, affecting nearly half of the world population and ranking as a top contributor to global disability. Though the majority of headaches are primary disorders, a wide array of secondary causes for headaches has been and will continue to be identified. Conditions with life-threatening morbidity and mortality often present with headache as their most noxious symptom. Once diagnosed, a timely condition-specific treatment should be offered to the patient. For example, catheter angiography or craniotomy to secure intracerebral aneurysm rupture in nontraumatic SAH can be lifesaving. In IIH, treatment includes the management of obesity or other precipitants when present, diuretics, VP shunt placement, and optic fenestration for severe cases, as well as treatment of any comorbid migraine. CSF spinal leaks can require several blood or fibrin glue patches or surgery to correct dural rents. Identifying these conditions can be a high-risk diagnostic challenge to providers across a broad collection of specialties. These challenges demand a logical and effective approach to evaluation that will coalesce into an often-simultaneous combination of accurate diagnosis and appropriate intervention. Tools like the SNOOP screen have been helpful to this end, though a familiarity with the ICHD-3 general diagnostic criteria for secondary headache can also guide providers as they thoughtfully explore the unique features of a patient's headache syndrome.

Teaching Points

1. Secondary headache is a head pain syndrome with a close temporal relationship to the natural history of another pathology known to produce headache.
2. Condition that disturbs the supportive vascular, meningeal, and osseous architecture around the brain or the adjacent bones and soft tissues of the face and neck can produce headaches.
3. Screens like the SNOOP4 or SNOOP10 can be helpful for remembering red-flag symptoms of common secondary headache syndromes.
   Positional headaches refer to syndromes with symptoms worsening in either the vertical or horizontal position and suggest pathologic alterations to ICP.
4. Thunderclap headaches are sudden headaches that reach severe levels of pain within 60 seconds of onset. This type of headache is affiliated with intracranial vascular conditions with high mortality and morbidity.
5. Overuse of acute analgesic medications more than 10 days per month for more than 3 months can make primary headache syndromes like migraine and tension-type headaches more frequent and severe.

Clinical Case

A 24-year-old female presented to the emergency department (ED) with a severe, sudden-onset headache triggered while lifting her kids or coughing. She does not have a prior history of recurrent headaches. She has a history of generalized anxiety disorder and has been using THC/CBD gummies for sleep. She recently started a combination of buspirone and escitalopram. With coughing she would experience a sudden onset bilateral occipital throbbing cephalgia with rapid holocephalic spread, rated as a 10/10 or the worst pain she's ever experienced in her life. She also has a sensitivity to lights and sounds with nausea and neck tension. Pain will resolve completely over the course of 2–3 hours. There have been a total of 3 episodes over the course of a week prior to seeking medical evaluation. In the ED, neurologic and physical examination plus screening serum labs were unremarkable. CT head w/o contrast and MRI brain w/o contrast were unremarkable. CT angiogram of the head revealed a short segment of moderate narrowing of the midportion of the basilar artery which was reconfirmed on MRA of the head. No aneurysm was seen. Lumbar puncture CSF analysis was unremarkable.

Case Discussion

A neurology consultation to the ED resulted in a diagnosis of reversible cerebrovascular vasoconstrictive syndrome (RCVS) secondary to selective serotonin reuptake inhibitor and CBD/THC usage. Offending agents were stopped and she was started on verapamil ER 120 mg daily. At outpatient follow-up, she reported full resolution of symptoms immediately after starting the calcium channel blocker. Follow-up MR angiogram of the brain demonstrated resolution of basilar artery narrowing 3 months after stopping SSRI and CBD/THC.

The presentation demonstrates features of a thunderclap headache, a red flag symptom whereby a severe headache reaches peak intensity in less than 60 seconds as well as triggering by exertion. An appropriate work-up was completed in the ED consisting of brain and vascular imaging which revealed large arterial narrowing supportive of a diagnosis of RCVS. Antecedent usage of serotonergic agents like SSRIs and recreational drugs should be screened and discontinued. The use of calcium channel blockers can help stabilize vascular tone and prevent recurrent episodes. Re-imaging 3 to 6 months after initial diagnosis and management to look for resolution of arterial narrowing is recommended.

Questions and Answers

1. Which headache symptom should raise concern for a secondary pathology?
   A. Photophobia and phonophobia are extremely severe
   B. Throbbing quality is bilateral
   C. Pain peaks in less than 60 seconds from onset
   D. Pain is rated as severe and behind one eye

The correct answer is C. A severe headache that reaches peak intensity within 60 seconds is considered a thunderclap headache, a red flag for potential secondary intracranial conditions that require prompt medical attention.

A. B. C. Photophobia and phobia, nausea and severe headache pain alone are non-specific findings that are described both in secondary headaches and common primary headaches such as migraine.

2. A 30-year-old obese female is complaining of headaches that are worse with lying flat, transient visual obscurations and pulsatile tinnitus. Head imaging shows an empty sella sign and venous sinus stenosis but is otherwise normal. Lumbar puncture will likely show?
   A. An opening pressure of less than 6 cm H_2O
   B. Xanthochromia
   C. A high red blood cell count that doesn't clear from tube 1 to 4
   D. An opening pressure of greater than 25 cm H_2O

The correct answer is D. The patient is a young, obese, reproductive-age female describing a positional quality to her headache with visual and auditory phenomenon plus head imaging findings that suggest a secondary condition like idiopathic intracranial hypertension (IIH). To meet Modified Dandy Criteria for a diagnosis of IIH the CSF composition must be normal and pressure greater than 25 cm H_2O.

A. An opening pressure of less than 6 cm H_2O is described in headache attributed to low CSF pressure patients.

B. C. Xanthochromia and an elevated RBC count that does clear from tube 1–4 is described in cases of aneurysmal subarachnoid hemorrhage.

References

1. Headache classification committee of the international headache society (IHS). The international classification of headache disorders, 3rd edition. Cephalalgia. 2018;38(1):1–211.
2. Marino MH, Watanabe TK. Posttraumatic pain management. In: Rehabilitation after traumatic brain injury. Elsevier; 2019. p. 165–77.
3. Özge A, Uludüz D, Karadaş Ö, Bolay H. Peripheral interventional management in headache. New York: Springer Berlin Heidelberg; 2019. p. 7–16.
4. Ray BS, Wolff HG. Experimental studies on headache: pain-sensitive structures of the head and their significance in headache. Arch Surg. 1940;41(4):813–56.

5. Ashina M, Geppetti P, editors. Pathophysiology of headaches: from molecule to man. 1st ed. Cham: Springer International Publishing: Imprint: Springer; 2015. p. 1–29. 1 p. (Headache)
6. Gobel H. Introduction to the secondary headaches [Internet]. ICHD-3. [cited 2021 Nov 14]. Available from: https://ichd-3.org/introduction-secondary-headaches/
7. Sutherland HG, Albury CL, Griffiths LR. Advances in genetics of migraine. J Headache Pain. 2019;20(1):72.
8. Rozen TD. Triggering events and new daily persistent headache: age and gender differences and insights on pathogenesis-a clinic-based study. Headache. 2016;56(1):164–73.
9. Rozen TD, Roth JM, Denenberg N. Cervical spine joint hypermobility: a possible predisposing factor for new daily persistent headache. Cephalalgia. 2006;26(10):1182–5.
10. Rozen T, Swidan SZ. Elevation of CSF tumor necrosis factor alpha levels in new daily persistent headache and treatment refractory chronic migraine. Headache. 2007;47(7):1050–5.
11. Peng KP, Robbins MS, Wang SJ. New daily persistent headache. In: Oxford textbook of headache syndromes; 2020. p. 267.
12. Russell MB, Andersson PG. Clinical intra- and interfamilial variability of cluster headache. Eur J Neurol. 1995;1(3):253–7.
13. El Amrani M, Ducros A, Boulan P, Aidi S, Crassard I, Visy JM, et al. Familial cluster headache: a series of 186 index patients. Headache. 2002;42(10):974–7.
14. Costa M, Squassina A, Piras IS, Pisanu C, Congiu D, Niola P, et al. Preliminary transcriptome analysis in lymphoblasts from cluster headache and bipolar disorder patients implicates dysregulation of circadian and serotonergic genes. J Mol Neurosci. 2015;56(3):688–95.
15. Chu KH, Howell TE, Keijzers G, Furyk JS, Eley RM, Kinnear FB, et al. Acute headache presentations to the emergency department: a statewide cross-sectional study. Acad Emerg Med. 2017;24(1):53–62.
16. Locker TE, Thompson C, Rylance J, Mason SM. The utility of clinical features in patients presenting with nontraumatic headache: an investigation of adult patients attending an emergency department. Headache. 2006;46(6):954–61.
17. Dodick DW. Pearls: headache. Semin Neurol. 2010;30(1):74–81.
18. Wongtanasarasin W, Wittayachamnankul B. Clinical availability of SNOOP4 in acute non-traumatic headache patients admitted to the emergency department. Hong Kong J Emerg Med. 2020;29:102490792092868.
19. Do TP, Remmers A, Schytz HW, Schankin C, Nelson SE, Obermann M, et al. Red and orange flags for secondary headaches in clinical practice: SNNOOP10 list. Neurology. 2019;92(3):134–44.
20. Alperin N, Hushek SG, Lee SH, Sivaramakrishnan A, Lichtor T. MRI study of cerebral blood flow and CSF flow dynamics in an upright posture: the effect of posture on the intracranial compliance and pressure. Acta Neurochir Suppl. 2005;95:177–81.
21. Miller JD. Volume and pressure in the craniospinal axis. Clin Neurosurg. 1975;22:76–105.
22. Kunkle EC, Ray BS, Wolff HG. Experimental studies on headache: analysis of the headache associated with changes in intracranial pressure. Arch Neurol Psychiatr. 1943;49(3):323–58.
23. King JO, Mitchell PJ, Thomson KR, Tress BM. Manometry combined with cervical puncture in idiopathic intracranial hypertension. Neurology. 2002;58(1):26–30.
24. Mokri B. Headache associated with abnormalities in intracranial structure or function: low cerebrospinal-fluid-pressure headache. In: Wolff's headache; 2007. p. 513–31.
25. Raoof N, Sharrack B, Pepper IM, Hickman SJ. The incidence and prevalence of idiopathic intracranial hypertension in Sheffield, UK. Eur J Neurol. 2011;18(10):1266–8.
26. Wall M, Kupersmith MJ, Kieburtz KD, Corbett JJ, Feldon SE, Friedman DI, et al. The idiopathic intracranial hypertension treatment trial: clinical profile at baseline. JAMA Neurol. 2014;71(6):693–701.
27. Amico D, Curone M, Ciasca P, Cammarata G, Melzi L, Bussone G, et al. Headache prevalence and clinical features in patients with idiopathic intracranial hypertension (Iih). Neurol Sci. 2013;34(Suppl 1):S147–9.
28. Sadun AA, Currie JN, Lessell S. Transient visual obscurations with elevated optic discs. Ann Neurol. 1984;16(4):489–94.
29. Pollak L, Zohar E, Glovinsky Y, Huna-Baron R. Reevaluation of presentation and course of idiopathic intracranial hypertension--a large cohort comprehensive study. Acta Neurol Scand. 2013;127(6):406–12.
30. Friedman DI, Liu GT, Digre KB. Revised diagnostic criteria for the pseudotumor cerebri syndrome in adults and children. Neurology. 2013;81(13):1159–65.
31. Savini G, Bellusci C, Carbonelli M, Zanini M, Carelli V, Sadun AA, et al. Detection and quantification of retinal nerve fiber layer thickness in optic disc edema using stratus OCT. Arch Ophthalmol. 2006;124(8):1111–7.
32. Brodsky MC, Vaphiades M. Magnetic resonance imaging in pseudotumor cerebri. Ophthalmology. 1998;105(9):1686–93.
33. Schievink W, Roiter V. Epidemiology of cervical artery dissection. In: Handbook on cerebral artery dissection, vol. 20; 2005. p. 12–5.
34. Miyazawa K, Shiga Y, Hasegawa T, Endoh M, Okita N, Higano S, Takahashi S, Itoyama Y. CSF hypovolemia vs intracranial hypotension in "spontaneous intracranial hypotension syndrome". Neurology. 2003;60(6):941–7.
35. Schievink WI, Gordon OK, Tourje J. Connective tissue disorders with spontaneous spinal cerebrospinal fluid leaks and intracranial hypotension: a prospective study. Neurosurgery. 2004;54(1):65–71.
36. Schievink WI, Reimer R, Folger WN. Surgical treatment of spontaneous intracranial hypotension associated with a spinal arachnoid diverticulum: case report. J Neurosurg. 1994;80(4):736–9.
37. Schievink WI, Meyer FB, Atkinson JL, Mokri B. Spontaneous spinal cerebrospinal fluid leaks and intracranial hypotension. J Neurosurg. 1996;84(4):598–605.
38. Schievink WI. Spontaneous spinal cerebrospinal fluid leaks and intracranial hypotension. JAMA. 2006;295(19):2286–96.
39. Mokri B. Spontaneous CSF leaks: low CSF volume syndromes. Neurol Clin. 2014;32(2):397–422.
40. Yamamoto M, Suehiro T, Nakata H, Nishioka T, Itoh H, Nakamura T, Hashimoto K. Primary low cerebrospinal fluid pressure syndrome associated with galactorrhea. Intern Med. 1993;32(3):228–31.
41. Mokri B, Piepgras DG, Miller GM. Syndrome of orthostatic headaches and diffuse pachymeningeal gadolinium enhancement. Mayo Clin Proc. 1997;72(5):400–13. Elsevier.
42. Whiteley W, Al-Shahi R, Myles L, Lueck CJ. Spontaneous intracranial hypotension causing confusion and coma: a headache for the neurologist and the neurosurgeon. Br J Neurosurg. 2003;17(5):456–8.
43. Dobrocky T, Grunder L, Breiding PS, Branca M, Limacher A, Mosimann PJ, Mordasini P, Zibold F, Haeni L, Jesse CM, Fung C. Assessing spinal cerebrospinal fluid leaks in spontaneous intracranial hypotension with a scoring system based on brain magnetic resonance imaging findings. JAMA Neurol. 2019;76(5):580–7.
44. Schoffer KL, Benstead TJ, Grant I. Spontaneous intracranial hypotension in the absence of magnetic resonance imaging abnormalities. Can J Neurol Sci. 2002;29(3):253–7.

45. Kim DK, Carr CM, Benson JC, Diehn FE, Lehman VT, Liebo GB, Morris JM, Morris PP, Verdoorn JT, Cutsforth-Gregory JK, Atkinson JL. Diagnostic yield of lateral decubitus digital subtraction myelogram stratified by brain MRI findings. Neurology. 2021;96(9):e1312–8.
46. Ravishankar K. Looking at "thunderclap headache" differently? Circa 2016. Ann Indian Acad Neurol. 2016;19(3):295.
47. Day JW, Raskin N. Thunderclap headache: symptom of unruptured cerebral aneurysm. Lancet. 1986;328(8518):1247–8.
48. Ferrante E, Tassorelli C, Rossi P, Lisotto C, Nappi G. Focus on the management of thunderclap headache: from nosography to treatment. J Headache Pain. 2011;12(2):251–8.
49. Gobel H. 4.4 Primary thunderclap headache [Internet]. ICHD-3. [cited 2021 Nov 16]. Available from: https://ichd-3.org/other-primary-headache-disorders/4-4-primary-thunderclap-headache/
50. Fornabia C. Resistance to gradual versus sudden exposure to pain with visual stimulation. Hofstra University; 2008.
51. Feigin VL, Rinkel GJE, Lawes CMM, Algra A, Bennett DA, van Gijn J, et al. Risk factors for subarachnoid hemorrhage: an updated systematic review of epidemiological studies. Stroke. 2005;36(12):2773–80.
52. Etminan N, Chang HS, Hackenberg K, De Rooij NK, Vergouwen MD, Rinkel GJ, Algra A. Worldwide incidence of aneurysmal subarachnoid hemorrhage according to region, time period, blood pressure, and smoking prevalence in the population: a systematic review and meta-analysis. JAMA Neurol. 2019;76(5):588–97.
53. Mac Grory B, Vu L, Cutting S, Marcolini E, Gottschalk C, Greer D. Distinguishing characteristics of headache in nontraumatic subarachnoid hemorrhage. Headache. 2018;58(3):364–70.
54. Bellolio MF, Hess EP, Gilani WI, VanDyck TJ, Ostby SA, Schwarz JA, Lohse CM, Rabinstein AA. External validation of the Ottawa subarachnoid hemorrhage clinical decision rule in patients with acute headache. Am J Emerg Med. 2015;33(2):244–9.
55. Dubosh NM, Bellolio MF, Rabinstein AA, Edlow JA. Sensitivity of early brain computed tomography to exclude aneurysmal subarachnoid hemorrhage: a systematic review and meta-analysis. Stroke. 2016;47(3):750–5.
56. Edlow JA, Wyer PC. Evidence-based emergency medicine/clinical question. How good is a negative cranial computed tomographic scan result in excluding subarachnoid hemorrhage? Ann Emerg Med. 2000;36(5):507–16.
57. Pedersen HK, Bakke SJ, Hald JK, Skalpe IO, Anke IM, Sagsveen R, et al. CTA in patients with acute subarachnoid haemorrhage. A comparative study with selective, digital angiography and blinded, independent review. Acta Radiol. 2001;42(1):43–9.
58. Dodick DW, Brown RD Jr, Britton JW, Huston J III. Nonaneurysmal thunderclap headache with diffuse, multifocal, segmental, and reversible vasospasm. Cephalalgia. 1999;19(2):118–23.
59. Singhal AB, Bernstein RA. Postpartum angiopathy and other cerebral vasoconstriction syndromes. Neurocrit Care. 2005;3(1):91–7.
60. Patel SD, Oliver Otite F, Lima J, Khandelwal P, Ollenschleger M. Abstract WP207: current incidence, epidemiological and clinical characteristics of reversible cerebral vasoconstriction in the United States. Stroke. 2020;51(Suppl_1):AWP207.
61. Ducros A, Wolff V. The typical thunderclap headache of reversible cerebral vasoconstriction syndrome and its various triggers. Headache. 2016;56(4):657–73.
62. Chen SP, Fuh JL, Lirng JF, Chang FC, Wang SJ. Recurrent primary thunderclap headache and benign CNS angiopathy: spectra of the same disorder? Neurology. 2006;67(12):2164–9.
63. Ducros A, Boukobza M, Porcher R, Sarov M, Valade D, Bousser MG. The clinical and radiological spectrum of reversible cerebral vasoconstriction syndrome. A prospective series of 67 patients. Brain. 2007;130(12):3091–101.
64. Singhal AB, Hajj-Ali RA, Topcuoglu MA, Fok J, Bena J, Yang D, Calabrese LH. Reversible cerebral vasoconstriction syndromes: analysis of 139 cases. Arch Neurol. 2011;68(8):1005–12.
65. Marder CP, Donohue MM, Weinstein JR, Fink KR. Multimodal imaging of reversible cerebral vasoconstriction syndrome: a series of 6 cases. Am J Neuroradiol. 2012;33(7):1403–11.
66. Rocha EA, Topcuoglu MA, Silva GS, Singhal AB. RCVS2 score and diagnostic approach for reversible cerebral vasoconstriction syndrome. Neurology. 2019;92(7):e639–47.
67. An SJ, Kim TJ, Yoon BW. Epidemiology, risk factors, and clinical features of intracerebral hemorrhage: an update. J Stroke. 2017;19(1):3.
68. Mohr JP, Caplan LR, Melski JW, Goldstein RJ, Duncan GW, Kistler JP, Pessin MS, Bleich HL. The Harvard cooperative stroke registry: a prospective registry. Neurology. 1978;28(8):754.
69. Gorelick PB, Hier DB, Caplan LR, Langenberg P. Headache in acute cerebrovascular disease. Neurology. 1986;36(11):1445.
70. Ropper AH, Davis KR. Lobar cerebral hemorrhages: acute clinical syndromes in 26 cases. Ann Neurol. 1980;8(2):141–7.
71. Ott KH, Kase CS, Ojemann RG, Mohr JP. Cerebellar hemorrhage: diagnosis and treatment: a review of 56 cases. Arch Neurol. 1974;31(3):160–7.
72. Rothrock JF. Headaches due to vascular disorders. Neurol Clin. 2004;22(1):21–37.
73. McNeill KA. Epidemiology of brain tumors. Neurol Clin. 2016;34(4):981–98.
74. Valentinis L, Tuniz F, Valent F, Mucchiut M, Little D, Skrap M, Bergonzi P, Zanchin G. Headache attributed to intracranial tumours: a prospective cohort study. Cephalalgia. 2009;
75. Suwanwela N, Phanthumchinda K, Kaoropthum S. Headache in brain tumor: a cross-sectional study. Headache. 1994;34(7):435–8.
76. Lowry JK, Snyder JJ, Lowry PW. Brain tumors in the elderly: recent trends in a Minnesota cohort study. Arch Neurol. 1998;55(7):922–8.
77. Wilne S, Collier J, Kennedy C, Koller K, Grundy R, Walker D. Presentation of childhood CNS tumours: a systematic review and meta-analysis. Lancet Oncol. 2007;8(8):685–95.
78. Argyriou AA, Chroni E, Polychronopoulos P, Argyriou K, Papapetropoulos S, Corcondilas M, Lepoura N, Heras P. Headache characteristics and brain metastases prediction in cancer patients. Eur J Cancer Care. 2006;15(1):90–5.
79. Kirby S, Purdy RA. Headaches and brain tumors. Neurol Clin. 2014;32(2):423–32.
80. Cittadini E, Matharu MS. Symptomatic trigeminal autonomic cephalalgias. Neurologist. 2009;15(6):305–12.
81. Greenberg HS, Deck MD, Vikram B, Chu FC, Posner JB. Metastasis to the base of the skulk clinical findings in 43 patients. Neurology. 1981;31(5):530.
82. Marinis MD, Welch KM. Headache associated with non-cephalic infections: classification and mechanisms. Cephalalgia. 1992;12(4):197–201.
83. Ashina M, Bendtsen L, Jensen R, Olesen J. Nitric oxide-induced headache in patients with chronic tension-type headache. Brain. 2000;123(9):1830–7.
84. Srikiatkhachorn A, le Grand SM, Supornsilpchai W, Storer RJ. Pathophysiology of medication overuse headache—an update. Headache. 2014;54(1):204–10.
85. Mohammad S, Korn K, Schellhaas B, Neurath MF, Goertz RS. Clinical characteristics of influenza in season 2017/2018 in a German Emergency Department: a retrospective analysis. Microbiol Insights. 2019;12:1178636119890302.

86. Turner MA, Istre GR, Beauchamp HE, Baum MA, Arnold SA. Community outbreak of adenovirus type 7a infections associated with a swimming pool. South Med J. 1987;80(6):712–5.
87. Helms CM, Viner JP, Renner ED, Chiu LC, Weisenburger DD. Legionnaires disease among pneumonias in Iowa (FY 1972-1978) II. Epidemiologic and clinical features of 30 sporadic cases of L. pneumophila infection. Am J Med Sci. 1981;281(1):2–13.
88. Atmar RL, Greenberg SB. Pneumonia caused by Mycoplasma pneumoniae and the TWAR agent. Semin Respir Infect. 1989;4(1):19–31.
89. Caronna E, Ballvé A, Llauradó A, Gallardo VJ, Ariton DM, Lallana S, López Maza S, Olivé Gadea M, Quibus L, Restrepo JL, Rodrigo-Gisbert M. Headache: a striking prodromal and persistent symptom, predictive of COVID-19 clinical evolution. Cephalalgia. 2020;40(13):1410–21.
90. Holmes GP, Kaplan JE, Gantz NM, Komaroff AL, Schonberger LB, Straus SE, Jones JF, Dubois RE, Cunningham-Rundles C, Pahwa S, Tosato G. Chronic fatigue syndrome: a working case definition. Ann Intern Med. 1988;108(3):387–9.
91. Diaz-Mitoma F, Vanast W, Tyrrell DJ. Increased frequency of Epstein-Barr virus excretion in patients with new daily persistent headaches. Lancet. 1987;329(8530):411–5.
92. Evers S, Marziniak M. Clinical features, pathophysiology, and treatment of medication-overuse headache. Lancet Neurol. 2010;9(4):391–401.
93. Lance F, Parkes C, Wilkinson M. Does analgesic abuse cause headaches de novo? Headache. 1988;28(1):61–2.
94. Limmroth V, Katsarava Z, Fritsche G, Przywara S, Diener HC. Features of medication overuse headache following overuse of different acute headache drugs. Neurology. 2002;59(7):1011–4.
95. Colas R, Munoz P, Temprano R, Gomez C, Pascual J. Chronic daily headache with analgesic overuse: epidemiology and impact on quality of life. Neurology. 2004;62(8):1338–42.

Part II

The Migraine Brain: Advances from Bench to Bedside

Migraine Genetics

6

Marta Vila-Pueyo and Patricia Pozo-Rosich

Introduction

Migraine is a complex neurological disorder that aggregates in families, an observation that was done by clinicians after many patients reported family members with migraine [1]. This observation prompted the study of the potential genetic factors underlying migraine to determine whether migraine is a genetic disorder. The focus of this chapter will highlight the major advances in migraine genetics through the evolution of the studies over time, depending on the technological capabilities of studying genetics.

Initially, studies were focused on understanding hemiplegic migraine, a rare subtype of migraine with aura, which is a monogenic disorder where a pathogenic variant in a single gene (*CACNA1A*, *ATP1A2* or *SCN1A*) leads to the disorder with nearly complete penetrance [2]. Later on, thanks to technological improvements and their cost-reduction, we have been able to study the genetic basis of common migraine. Migraine is considered one of the most heritable disorders among the neurological and psychiatric diseases after generalized epilepsy and obsessive–compulsive disorder. In fact, its estimated single nucleotide polymorphism (SNP)-heritability is 15% [3]. Previous studies estimated the heritability of migraine from twin data, not genotype data, with a percentage that ranged from 36% to 74% [4–6]. The heritability of migraine could be explained by two non-excluding main hypotheses: the presence of rare, penetrant variants that follow a Mendelian inheritance and/or the accumulation of several polygenic common variants, each carrying a small individual effect. Over the past decades, several approaches have been used to study the genetics of common migraine which point to the latter hypothesis, suggesting that migraine is a complex polygenic disorder.

M. Vila-Pueyo
Headache and Neurological Pain Research Group, Vall d'Hebron Research Institute, Departament de Medicina, Universitat Autònoma de Barcelona, Barcelona, Spain

P. Pozo-Rosich (✉)
Headache and Neurological Pain Research Group, Vall d'Hebron Research Institute, Departament de Medicina, Universitat Autònoma de Barcelona, Barcelona, Spain

Headache Unit, Neurology Department, Vall d'Hebron University Hospital, Barcelona, Spain

Questions

1. What is the main genetic difference between hemiplegic migraine and common migraine?
   (a) Hemiplegic migraine is a rare disorder, in contrast to common migraine.
   (b) Hemiplegic migraine is a monogenic disorder, whereas common migraine is a polygenic disorder.
   (c) In common migraine, a pathogenic variant in a single gene leads to the disorder, but in hemiplegic migraine, it does not.
   (d) There are no genetic differences between hemiplegic migraine and common migraine.
2. Several approaches have been used to study the genetic basis of migraine. The approach that has contributed the most to a better understanding of the genetic basis of migraine is
   (a) Genetic linkage studies.
   (b) Candidate-gene sequencing.
   (c) Candidate-gene association studies.
   (d) Genome-wide association studies (GWAS).

Genetic Studies in Common Migraine

This section will review the different approaches that have been used in the past decades to study the genetic basis of migraine and their most relevant outcomes, following a chronological order, including genetic linkage studies,

T. S. Monteith et al. (eds.), *Comprehensive Migraine Management*, https://doi.org/10.1007/978-3-031-86923-5_6

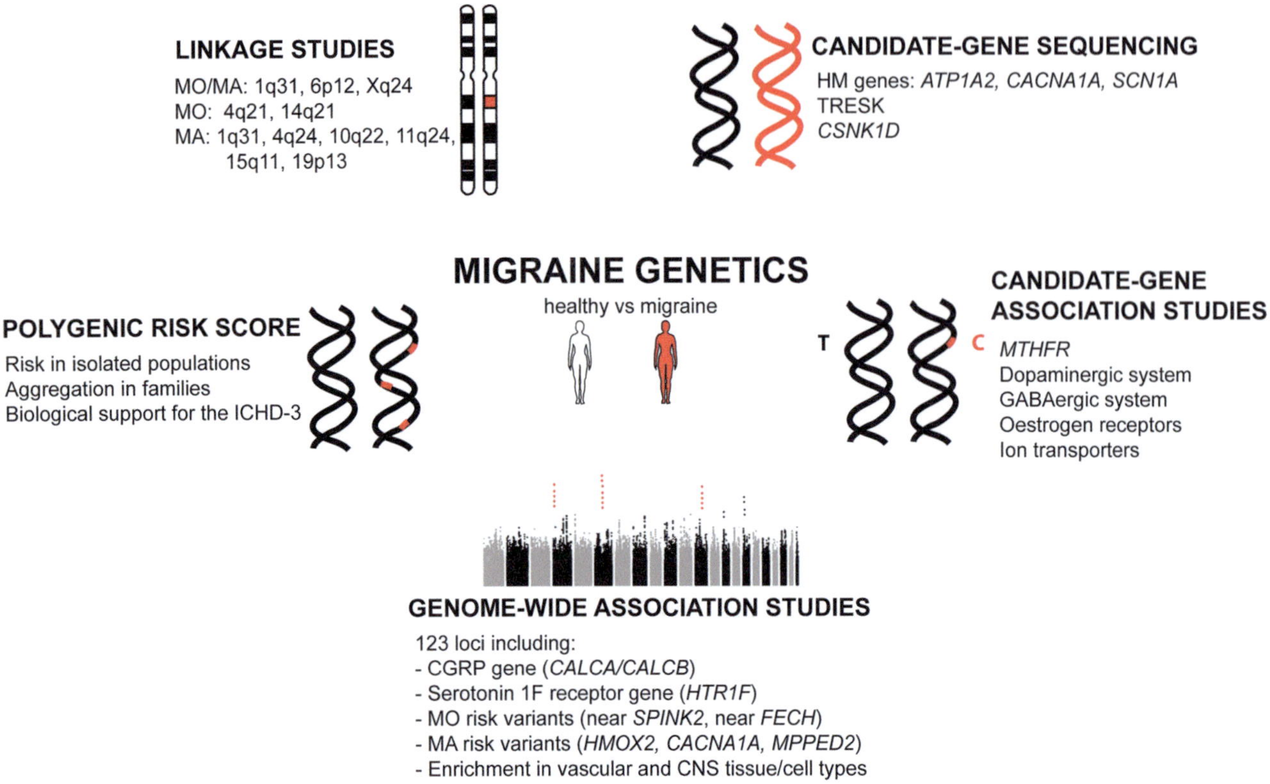

Fig. 6.1 Summary of the most relevant approaches that have been used to study migraine genetics and their key outcomes

candidate-gene sequencing, candidate-gene association studies, genome-wide association studies and the analysis of the polygenic risk score (Fig. 6.1).

Genetic Linkage Studies

Initially, the most commonly used strategy to identify migraine susceptibility genes was genetic linkage analysis. This type of analysis uses a family-based approach to localize chromosomal loci that are genetically linked to the disorder of interest and hence may contain the causative genetic variant. Although some of the studies linked several genomic loci to an increased susceptibility to develop common migraine, including loci 1q31, 4q21, 4q24, 6p12.2–p21.1, 10q22–q23, 11q24, 14q21.2–q22.3, 15q11–q13, 19p13 and Xq24–q28, none of them successfully identified the causative gene variant [7]. The lack of robust findings in linkage studies is likely a reflection of the polygenic nature of migraine and the fact that there are no high penetrant variants associated with it; hence, the linkage method has been proven inappropriate to study the genetic basis of migraine.

Candidate-Gene Sequencing

Hemiplegic Migraine Genes: Are They Relevant for Common Migraine?

Candidate-genes sequencing is another approach that has also been used to determine the genetic basis of common migraine. The first studies that used this approach focused on sequencing the causative genes of the monogenic, rare form of migraine with aura, hemiplegic migraine (HM), including *CACNA1A*, *ATP1A2* and *SCN1A*, which encode ion channel and transport proteins [8]. Although these studies were not able to find a causative genetic variant underlying common migraine, a recent GWAS has identified the SNP rs10405121, located in an intron of *CACNA1A*, as a risk variant for migraine with aura [9]. This provides the first support for the presence of common variants between hemiplegic and common migraine. The most plausible explanation for the lack of positive outcomes in the candidate-genes strategy is that their samples are too small to identify small effect variants and that their methodological approach was mainly based on sequencing only the exons of the genes [10].

TRESK: A Role in Neuronal Excitability

Another gene-candidate study was focused on sequencing *KCNK18*, which encodes the potassium channel TRESK. TRESK is abundantly expressed in the dorsal root and trigeminal ganglia and is involved in the adjustment of neuronal excitability; hence, the authors considered it to be a potential candidate for conferring susceptibility to migraine [11]. The initial study sequenced this gene in a cohort of 110 migraine patients and found a frameshift mutation (F139Wfsx24) in a large multigenerational pedigree where it fully segregated with migraine with aura [12]. Subsequent functional characterization revealed that this mutation causes a complete loss of the TRESK function and that the mutant subunit suppresses the wild-type channel function through a dominant-negative effect. Although the results of this study supported a role for TRESK in the pathogenesis of migraine with aura, a more recent study from the same group found a different loss-of-function mutation in the same gene both in migraine patients and in healthy individuals [13], undermining the importance of TRESK in migraine.

CSNK1D: Sleep and Migraine

The link between the pathophysiology of migraine and sleep disorders has been established in several studies that have analysed different parameters of sleep quality in migraine patients [14, 15]. However, to date, there exists only one genetic link between both entities and it refers to the familial advanced sleep phase syndrome (FASPS) [16]. Patients with FASPS exhibit specific circadian patterns in which they go to sleep unusually early in the evening and wake unusually early in the morning. In the study conducted by Brennan and colleagues, they identified two families, each with a distinct missense mutation in *CSNK1D*, in which the mutation co-segregated with the presence of both migraine and FASPS. *CSNK1D* encodes the protein casein kinase Iδ which regulates the circadian protein PER2 and allows for a correct functioning of the circadian rhythms. Interestingly, this regulation is truncated with the mutation found in these two families. Moreover, functional studies in transgenic mice harbouring the human mutation in *CSNK1D* have indicated that it confers a higher susceptibility to cortical spreading depression and to migraine-like pain only [17], suggesting that decreases in casein kinase Iδ can contribute to the pathogenesis of migraine. This link, though, has some controversy as one of the families has one patient with the mutation in *CSNK1D* who was diagnosed with FASPS but not migraine and one patient with migraine who did not have the mutation. These inconsistencies could be easily explained by the fact that migraine could have not been expressed yet in the former patient and that migraine has a high prevalence in the population and could be developed by other factors in the latter.

Candidate-Gene Association Studies

Before the next-generation sequencing (NGS) era started, several studies analysed the genetic basis of common migraine by performing case–control association studies in patients with migraine without and with aura in preselected candidate genes. These studies were the most commonly used strategy to study the genetic basis of complex disorders and they tested for significant differences in allele frequencies between cases and controls. In the case of common migraine, some of the candidate–gene association studies include candidate genes such as *MTHFR* [18–22]; genes from the dopaminergic system, including *DRD2* and *SLC6A3* [23]; genes from the serotonergic system, including *HTR2C* [24]; genes from the GABAergic system, including *GABRA5* and *GABRB3* [25]; genes that encode the oestrogen receptors *ESR1* and *ESR2* [26]; and other relevant genes, such as ion transporters [27].

Although these studies found numerous significant associations between particular polymorphisms and migraine with or without aura, none of them presented a robust genetic association and the majority of them could not be replicated in independent cohorts [7]. These inconsistencies may be due to several methodological reasons, including small sample sizes, not taking into account linkage disequilibrium blocks when choosing polymorphisms, inadequate correction for multiple testing and phenotyping issues [28].

Genome-Wide Association Studies (GWAS)

The emergence of improved technology and cost-effective genotyping platforms allowed overcoming some of the methodological issues found on the hypothesis-driven candidate-gene approaches with the development of hypothesis-free genome-wide association studies (GWAS). GWAS are a more unbiased method designed to identify genetic variants involved in complex disorders, such as migraine. They enable the simultaneous analysis of millions of single nucleotide polymorphisms (SNPs), by sequencing approximately 800,000 SNPs that are almost equally distributed over the whole genome, in a single experiment [29]. The genotyped SNPs are used as a proxy for any SNPs that are in strong linkage disequilibrium (LD) and are tested for association with the trait of interest, for example, migraine, by assessing differences in allele frequencies between patients and controls. GWAS require the use of large cohorts of patients and controls and the genetic variants identified undergo rigorous statistical multiple testing correction [30]. In GWAS, SNPs must possess genome-wide significance (GWS) to be reported as being associated with the trait of interest, which is commonly considered as a *P*-value threshold of $\leq 5 \times 10^{-8}$ [31].

Several migraine GWAS have been performed to date and their outcomes have been crucial to advance the understanding of the genetic basis of common migraine [9, 32–39]. The first GWAS was conducted by several groups from the International Headache Genetics Consortium in 2010 and included a discovery sample of 2731 migraine with aura patients and 10,747 controls [33]. This study found an association between migraine and the SNP rs1835740, which is located between two genes implicated in glutamate homeostasis: *MTDH*, encoding a regulator of the glutamate transporter SLC1A2; and *PGCP*, encoding a protein involved in the accumulation of glutamate in the synaptic cleft. Following this initial study, Chasman et al. performed a GWAS in 5122 migraine patients and 18,108 controls [35]. Although none of the SNPs was significantly associated with migraine, a subsequent meta-analysis studied the top three SNPs from the GWAS in an extended sample that included three extra cohorts of patients and controls. This allowed the identification of three intronic SNPs that survived the statistical corrections, including rs2651899, located within *PRDM16*, which encodes a protein involved in the differentiation of brown adipose tissue; rs10166942, located close to the transcription start site of *TRPM8*, encoding the cold and menthol receptor 1; and rs11172113, located within *LRP1*, encoding a lipoprotein receptor that interacts with glutamate receptors [40]. A posterior meta-analysis that analysed 2523 migraine patients and 38,170 controls, studied the top SNPs from this GWAS and concluded that the SNPs located within *TRPM8* and *LRP1* were significantly associated with migraine [41].

Later, a GWAS by Freilinger et al. [32] was performed in a clinic-based cohort of 2326 migraine without aura patients and 4580 controls. Subsequently, the 12 loci that included two or more SNPs associated with migraine with a $P < 1 \times 10^{-5}$ were analysed in an independent cohort of 2508 migraine without aura patients and 2652 controls. This analysis allowed the replication of two of the SNPs: rs3790455 located within *MEF2D*, involved in the control of muscle and neuronal cell differentiation and development, and rs7640543, closely located to *TGFBR2*, encoding a transcription factor that modulates several genes. Moreover, part of the results from the previous GWAS were replicated, indicating again an association between the genes *TRPM8* and *LRP1* and migraine susceptibility. This GWAS allowed, for the first time, the identification of risk variants associated with migraine without aura only and revealed that migraine susceptibility seems to be modulated both by genes involved in synapse and neuronal function and differentiation (*MEF2D* and *ASTN2*) and by genes with vascular functions (*TGFBR2* and *PHCTR1*).

The results from posterior genome-wide studies that included larger sample sizes also confirmed this implication of both neuronal and vascular functions, supporting that neurovascular mechanisms underlie the pathophysiology of migraine [9, 34, 39]. The genome-wide meta-analysis by Anttila et al. analysed 29 GWAS, which included 23,285 migraine patients and 95,425 controls, and allowed the identification of 12 risk loci for migraine [34]. Among them, five new loci were identified: near *AJAP1* at 1p36, near *TSPAN2* at 1p13, within *FHL5* at 6q16, within *C7orf10* at 7p14 and near *MMP16* at 8q21. Gormley et al. carried out a GWAS that included 59,674 migraine patients and 316,078 controls from 22 GWAS [39]. Thirty-eight genomic loci associated with migraine were identified, which included 28 loci not previously reported and, for the first time, a locus located on chromosome X. Subsequent analyses revealed enrichment for genes expressed in vascular and smooth muscle tissues.

The most recent and largest GWAS meta-analysis included a sample of 102,084 cases and 771,257 controls and identified 123 loci of which 86 were novel [9] (Table 6.1). Interestingly, among the new loci there were two genes encoding migraine-specific drug targets: rs1003194, within the calcitonin gene-related peptide gene (*CALCA/CALCB*); and rs6795209, within the serotonin 5-HT_{1F} receptor (*HTR1F*). A subsequent stratification of the risk loci that used 29,679 cases with subtype information (MO or MA) increased the evidence supporting defining both migraine subtypes as separate disease entities. Specifically, this analysis revealed three risk variants that were specific for migraine with aura (in *HMOX2*, *CACNA1A* and *MPPED2*), two variants that were specific for migraine without aura (near *SPINK2* and near *FECH*) and nine variants that increased the susceptibility for migraine in general (near *TRPM8*, near *FGF6* and in *FHL5, LRP1, MRVI1, DLST, SUGCT, PRDM16 and PLCE1*).

Some studies have used GWAS data to analyse the shared heritability between migraine and other disorders, including some of its comorbidities. The biggest study performed to date has sought to understand the genetic underpinnings and categorical distinctions for brain disorders and related phenotypes and the shared heritability between neurological and psychiatric disorders [3]. In this study, genome-wide association data for 265,218 patients and 784,643 controls were used, as well as 17 phenotypes from a total of 1,191,588 individuals, to quantify the degree of overlap for genetic risk factors of 25 common brain disorders (including migraine). The results show a significant correlation in common variant risk for psychiatric disorders, especially among attention deficit hyperactivity disorder (ADHD), bipolar disorder, major depressive disorder (MDD) and schizophrenia. Interestingly, common genetic risk sharing among neurological disorders

Table 6.1 List of the 123 genome-wide significant loci from the latest GWAS, including the closest gene (Locus ID), the RSID and the *P* value of each risk variant

Locus ID	RSID	*P* value	Locus ID	RSID	*P* value	Locus ID	RSID	*P* value
PRDM16	rs10218452	7.26E-71	NSD1	rs10866704	2.10E-08	PDZRN4	rs1458170	5.75E-09
CAMTA1	rs10128028	7.66E-09	PHACTR1	rs9349379	1.41E-47	LRP1	rs11172113	1.38E-90
TMEM51	rs12057629	9.38E-14	Near PRL	rs9295536	7.75E-12	ATP2B1	rs4842676	2.26E-09
INPP5B	rs28739509	2.64E-10	Near IER3	rs9468830	2.38E-08	Near RP11-690J15.1	rs10777902	1.25E-10
MACF1	rs1472662	1.75E-08	EHMT2	rs74434374	4.52E-09	NCOR2	rs1271309	3.74E-08
C1orf87	rs11578492	6.25E-09	KCNK5	rs10456100	9.16E-19	LRCH1	rs7335684	1.05E-08
Near LEPR	rs7511672	1.43E-09	Near KRT19P1	rs34273564	1.00E-10	RNF219-AS1	rs7996252	4.11E-08
Near RP4-598G3.1	rs56019088	7.32E-13	FHL5	rs11153082	7.26E-54	Near COL4A1	rs2000660	4.95E-08
TGFBR3	rs11165300	4.72E-08	REV3L	rs6568677	2.09E-08	Near RP11-384J4.2	rs1245463	5.72E-14
Near TSPAN2	rs2078371	5.87E-42	Near GJA1	rs28455731	8.82E-23	Near LRFN5	rs1542668	2.53E-08
Near ADAMTSL4	rs6693567	1.25E-13	Near PCMT1	rs9383843	1.35E-09	Near ARID4A	rs28756401	6.40E-09
MEF2D	rs2274319	2.74E-41	SUGCT	rs10234636	4.43E-28	DLST	rs55707505	2.48E-08
RABGAP1L	rs11487328	1.70E-08	MLXIPL	rs13235543	3.06E-13	IFT43	rs75002882	9.22E-09
PLA2G4A	rs6668908	2.22E-08	TSPAN12	rs56067931	4.83E-08	Near ITPK1	rs11624776	9.75E-19
Near MAPKAPK2	rs56140113	7.76E-09	PTK2B	rs11782789	3.03E-09	SERPINA1	rs28929474	2.54E-09
KIF26B	rs72764846	5.41E-09	Near RP11-573J24.1	rs4739105	2.85E-08	ABHD17C	rs12708529	8.11E-10
THADA	rs12712881	3.50E-10	NFIB	rs580845	4.30E-08	HMOX2	rs12598836	2.21E-10
ANKRD36C	rs4907224	1.63E-09	Near RP11-373A6.1	rs10156578	3.34E-12	CFDP1	rs8046696	4.76E-14
ZEB2	rs7564469	5.06E-09	TJP2	rs7034179	1.60E-16	Near ZCCHC14	rs8052831	8.25E-15
Near AC064865.1	rs895219	3.74E-11	ZNF462	rs17723637	8.63E-09	SMG6	rs9894634	9.64E-11
Near RNU6-546P	rs843215	2.61E-08	ASTN2	rs3891689	2.28E-21	ZBTB4	rs34914463	2.41E-09
MYO3B	rs4668251	7.58E-09	Near EHMT1	rs4278223	6.24E-10	HOXB3	rs11652860	1.07E-08
Near HOXD10	rs72923449	4.66E-08	Near RNA5SP299	rs7916911	3.18E-12	RP11-81K2.1	rs2119930	6.69E-15
CARF	rs138556413	4.15E-16	Near MLLT10	rs10828247	7.51E-09	MRC2	rs12452590	2.03E-10
Near TRPM8	rs10166942	9.35E-51	PLCE1	rs2274224	3.28E-26	TBC1D16	rs1285294	4.32E-08
Near TGFBR2	rs7371912	1.06E-14	HPSE2	rs12260159	7.33E-16	RNF213	rs8077768	9.32E-13
ATRIP	rs7618883	4.16E-08	CNNM2	rs12260436	7.29E-10	Near RBBP8	rs7506921	1.17E-11
Near HNRNPA3P8	rs950570	1.30E-08	RBM20	rs869432	3.54E-08	Near SKOR2	rs1019990	1.00E-11
Near CADM2	rs73138150	1.95E-08	HTRA1	rs2672592	1.22E-12	Near FECH	rs8087942	9.71E-13
Near C3orf38	rs6795209	1.23E-08	Near GPR26	rs11248546	1.59E-12	CACNA1A	rs10405121	4.74E-10
ITGB5	rs1499963	7.48E-09	INPP5A	rs200314499	6.92E-12	SUGP1	rs74182632	1.43E-08
Near GPR149	rs13078967	2.16E-16	MRGPRE	rs12295710	2.86E-16	B9D2|TMEM91	rs1982072	4.22E-11
Near SEC63P2	rs73805934	1.11E-09	MRVI1	rs4910165	1.09E-24	Near JAG1	rs111404218	2.04E-10
Near SPINK2	rs7684253	4.21E-14	Near INSC	rs1003194	2.43E-10	SLC24A3	rs4814864	1.44E-28
ANKDD1B	rs42854	9.40E-13	MPPED2	rs11031122	6.91E-10	C20orf112	rs6057599	8.73E-14
Near SSBP2	rs12653216	8.08E-09	AMBRA1	rs7932866	2.38E-09	ZMYND8	rs910187	1.14E-10
Near ZNF474	rs11957829	1.58E-09	Near RAB3IL1	rs12787928	6.85E-09	Near MRPS6	rs28451064	3.52E-15
SNX24	rs246326	6.80E-10	RBM14-RBM4|RBM4	rs566673	9.07E-09	RUNX1	rs764508	3.28E-09
Near POU4F3	rs10038882	1.33E-12	YAP1	rs12226331	1.92E-13	Near AC006547.14	rs625686	8.26E-09
TIGD6|HMGXB3	rs4705403	1.18E-08	Near SPATA19	rs10894756	2.83E-08	Near FAM47A	rs1507220	2.67E-08
Near NKX2-5	rs6556059	8.16E-10	Near FGF6	rs2160875	2.72E-36	Near MED14	rs4403550	3.07E-09

Modified from Hautakangas et al. [9]

Remarkably, the list of loci includes genes that encode the recent migraine-specific drug targets calcitonin gene-related peptide (*CALCA/CALCB*) and serotonin 1F receptor (*HTR1F*). Genomic annotations among the 123 risk variants are enriched in vascular and central nervous system tissue and cell types, highlighting the relevance of neurovascular mechanisms in migraine

or across neurological and psychiatric disorders was much lower, except for migraine, which was significantly correlated to ADHD, MDD and Tourette syndrome (TS). These results reflect the comorbidity of migraine with ADHD, MDD and TS that had been previously reported in epidemiological studies [42–45].

The outcomes from the migraine GWAS have greatly contributed to a better understanding of the genetic basis underlying common migraine. The analyses of the genes located near the GWAS loci have revealed the types of gene functions and pathways that may be involved in migraine susceptibility. However, the majority of the risk loci identified to date remain uncharacterized and their contribution towards an increase in the susceptibility to develop migraine is not understood yet, partly because the gene that is influenced by the SNP remains unknown [29]. Future studies will need to focus on unravelling the molecular processes by which this genetic variation influences migraine susceptibility [30].

Polygenic Risk Score: Calculating the Genetic Risk in Migraine

Although the genetic variants that come from GWAS have improved our understanding of the genetic underpinnings of complex disorders, single variants cannot assess the disease risk of an individual. However, there are approaches that combine the genetic load conferred by a set of risk variants to measure a score that provides enough information to potentially identify those at higher risk [46]. This can be calculated with the polygenic risk score (PRS) , which is the weighted sum of the number of risk alleles that an individual carries, so it reflects a person's inherited susceptibility to a certain disease. To date, several studies have shown the validity of PRS in both research- and population-based studies, suggesting a potential use as a clinical diagnostic tool [46–48]. The utility of PRS in migraine has been discussed and analysed in three major studies [49].

A study by Rodriguez-Acevedo et al. tested the contribution of PRS in the Norfolk Island population by using migraine GWAS data [50]. Their results showed that there exists a polygenic contribution to migraine risk in this isolated population. Later on, a study by Gormley et al. calculated the PRS based on GWAS information to assess whether the genetic load of these variants contributes to the aggregation of migraine in families by comparing familial and population cases [51, 52]. They included 8319 individuals across 1589 migraine families and found that the PRS was able to explain 1.6% of the phenotypic variance in the population cases and 3.5% of the familial cases, indicating a higher genetic load in the latter ones. These results demonstrate that the aggregation of migraine in families is partly due to the contribution of common polygenic variation as initially hypothesized. Another study used the PRS to evaluate the consensus criteria included in the International Classification of Headache Disorders (ICHD-3) [52, 53] in a Finnish cohort [54]. Their results showed that all the symptoms of common migraine included in the ICHD-3 criteria correlated with the PRS and that on the PRS scale the complex migraine phenotype shows a continuum from individuals with no headache, to non-migrainous headache up to patients with migraine attacks. This allowed the authors to conclude that there is biological support for the ICHD-3 diagnostic criteria. Another study used the PRS, along with other methodologies, with the aim to elucidate whether chronic migraine (CM) is caused by genetic or environmental factors [55]. The analysis did not retrieve any difference between the PRS of chronic migraine versus episodic migraine patients.

Future studies using PRS in migraine, and other subtypes such as chronic migraine and medication overuse headache, will allow for a better analysis of its utility in the field, although the current results seem promising.

Epigenetic Studies in Common Migraine

While there is a clear genetic component underlying migraine susceptibility, this may also be modulated by internal and external non-genetic factors, such as sex hormones, lifestyle and environmental changes [56–58], which could have an impact through epigenetic mechanisms. Among these, changes in DNA methylation and in the expression of microRNAs have gained some interest as potential players implicated in the modulation of the susceptibility to migraine. Both mechanisms are implicated in the repression of gene expression, the former by inhibiting the binding of transcription factors to the DNA and by recruiting proteins involved in gene repression and the latter by targeting and binding to mRNA [59].

To better understand the role of DNA methylation in migraine, a study by Gerring et al. performed an epigenome-wide association analysis where they quantified genome-wide patterns of DNA methylation in 67 migraine patients and compared them to 67 controls [60]. Their results did not reveal any loci that were significantly associated with migraine, which is probably due to the low number of samples included in the study. However, they identified differentially methylated regions that were enriched in regulatory elements of the genome and were in close proximity to genes involved in solute transportation and haemostasis and suggested that these regions could be relevant for the pathogenesis of migraine.

To study the role of microRNAs in migraine, a pilot study analysed the expression profile of circulating microRNAs in 15 female MO patients compared to 13 controls [61]. Although the small cohort did not allow for the identification of statistically significant differences, they subsequently validated four of the top-ten microRNAs and used them to perform a logistic regression model which showed a high accuracy to identify migraine. This led the authors to conclude that there seemed to be a specific circulating microRNA profile in migraine without aura which should be confirmed in future analysis. A study by Andersen et al. looked for changes in microRNA expression in 24 migraine patients during attacks and in pain-free periods and compared them to healthy controls [62]. Interestingly, they found an aberrant expression of microRNAs both during migraine attacks and in pain-free periods, pointing to an upregulation in miR-34a-5p and miR-382-5p expression. Their subsequent in silico analysis revealed that these microRNAs' targets are involved in GABAergic and anti-inflammatory signalling.

Although these results seem very promising, independent, bigger cohorts should be used to replicate their findings. An independent exploratory study focused on the increased evidence of vascular dysfunction in migraine to analyse whether circulating levels of microRNAs associated with endothelial function were differentially expressed in migraine patients [63]. They compared the expression of four microRNAs that modulate endothelial function (miR-155, miR-126, miR-21 and Let-7g) in 30 migraine patients without overt vascular risk actors with healthy controls. Compared to controls, three of the microRNAs were found to be upregulated in migraine patients (miR-155, miR-126 and Let-7g) and two of them (miR-155 and miR-126) were associated with syncope frequency. This pilot study also points towards a dysregulation of serum microRNAs' expression in migraine patients, although again further replication studies are needed to validate their results.

Future studies including bigger cohorts will certainly increase our understanding regarding the role that epigenetic factors may play in migraine susceptibility. However, there will still remain an important limitation: the tissue used in these analyses. On one hand, the analysis that studies epigenetic mechanisms involved in migraine in blood samples may allow for the identification of biomarkers that could be extremely valuable for patient stratification, diagnosis and precision medicine [64]. But, on the other hand, the uncertainty of the concordance of the epigenetic state between brain tissue and blood [65] suggests that this tissue may not be the best approach to better understand the underlying mechanisms of migraine pathophysiology.

Conclusion

The high heritability of migraine has stimulated the development of multiple genetic studies over the years to unravel its genetic basis. Early research focused on genetic linkage studies, candidate-gene sequencing studies and candidate-gene association studies which highlighted the existence of potential gene candidates associated with migraine susceptibility. However, the lack of robust findings in these early studies is likely a reflection of the polygenic nature of migraine. More recently, genome-wide association studies (GWAS) have allowed the identification of 123 migraine risk variants; although future studies will need to focus on unravelling the molecular processes by which this genetic variation influences migraine susceptibility. Polygenic risk score analysis and epigenetic studies will also improve the understanding of the genetic basis of migraine. Individual genetic profiles of migraine patients will also be able to be used in future pharmacogenetic studies, which are promising tools to develop personalized medicine.

Teaching Points

1. Migraine is a complex neurological disorder with an SNP-heritability of 15%.
2. The study of migraine genetics has evolved over time, according to the development of better and more cost-effective technologies.
3. Initial studies were focused on understanding hemiplegic migraine, which is a monogenic disorder where a pathogenic variant in a single gene (*CACNA1A*, *ATP1A2* or *SCN1A*) leads to the disorder with nearly complete penetrance, in contrast with common migraine, which is a polygenic disorder significantly associated with both vascular and neuronal genes.
4. A lack of robust findings, especially in linkage studies, candidate-gene sequencing and candidate–gene association studies, is mostly due to methodological limitations, including small sample sizes, inadequate correction for multiple testing and phenotyping issues.
5. The genome-wide association studies (GWAS) performed to date have contributed to a better understanding of the genetic basis of migraine and have identified 123 risk variants associated with migraine susceptibility.
6. The epigenetic studies have focused on analysing differences in DNA methylation and microRNA expression.
7. Future studies will need to unravel the molecular processes by which the genetic variation associated with migraine influences its susceptibility and will allow for the use of personalized medicine in migraine through the development of pharmacogenetics in the field.

Case

A 44-year-old woman suffers from severe headaches that are accompanied by photophobia and fatigue and has been diagnosed with migraine without aura. She has been prescribed several treatments over the years, including NSAIDS, triptans and anti-CGRP monoclonal antibodies, without having a substantial effect on the frequency and severity of her attacks. Her 6-year-old twins have been diagnosed with cyclic vomiting syndrome and she wants to know if there is any genetic approach to determine whether they will develop migraine or not and to understand what could be the best treatments for them.

Case Discussion

The doctor explains to the patient that currently there are no genetic tests to determine whether a person will develop migraine or not. They have a consultation with the geneticist who informs the patient of the existence of genetic studies in migraine that have found genetic variants associated with an increased risk of developing migraine, but that these studies are still being developed and cannot be used as diagnostic tools.

Questions and Answers

1. What is the main genetic difference between hemiplegic migraine and common migraine?
   A. Hemiplegic migraine is a rare disorder, in contrast to common migraine.
   B. Hemiplegic migraine is a monogenic disorder, whereas common migraine is a polygenic disorder.
   C. In common migraine, a pathogenic variant in a single gene leads to the disorder, but in hemiplegic migraine, it does not.
   D. There are no genetic differences between hemiplegic migraine and common migraine.

The correct answer is B. Hemiplegic migraine is a monogenic disorder where a pathogenic variant in a single gene (*CACNA1A*, *ATP1A2* or *SCN1A*) leads to the disorder with nearly complete penetrance. Common migraine, instead, is a complex polygenic disorder where several genetic variants contribute to its genetic risk. Answer A can be misleading because the sentence is true, but it does not explain the genetic difference between hemiplegic and common migraine.

2. Several approaches have been used to study the genetic basis of migraine. The approach that has contributed the most to a better understanding of the genetic basis of migraine is.
   A. Genetic linkage studies.
   B. Candidate-gene sequencing.
   C. Candidate-gene association studies.
   D. Genome-wide association studies (GWAS).

The correct answer is D. To date, GWAS have identified 123 risk loci for migraine, whereas the results from genetic linkage studies, candidate-gene sequencing and candidate–gene association studies are not robust and have not been replicated.

References

1. Stewart WF, Staffa J, Lipton RB, Ottman R. Familial risk of migraine: a population-based study. Ann Neurol. 1997;41:166. https://doi.org/10.1002/ana.410410207.
2. Ferrari MD, Klever RR, Terwindt GM, Ayata C, van den Maagdenberg AMJM. Migraine pathophysiology: lessons from mouse models and human genetics. Lancet Neurol. 2015;14:65. https://doi.org/10.1016/S1474-4422(14)70220-0.
3. Anttila V, Bulik-Sullivan B, Finucane HK, et al. Analysis of shared heritability in common disorders of the brain. Science. 2018;360:eaap8757. https://doi.org/10.1126/science.aap8757.
4. Ziegler DK, Hur Y-M, Bouchard TJ, Hassanein RS, Barter R. Migraine in twins raised together and apart. Headache. 1998;38:417. https://doi.org/10.1046/j.1526-4610.1998.3806417.x.
5. Lucas RN. Migraine in twins. J Psychosom Res. 1977;21:147. https://doi.org/10.1016/0022-3999(77)90082-4.
6. Polderman TJC, Benyamin B, de Leeuw CA, Sullivan PF, van Bochoven A, Visscher PM, Posthuma D. Meta-analysis of the heritability of human traits based on fifty years of twin studies. Nat Genet. 2015;47:702. https://doi.org/10.1038/ng.3285.
7. de Vries B, Frants RR, Ferrari MD, van den Maagdenberg AMJM. Molecular genetics of migraine. Hum Genet. 2009;126:115. https://doi.org/10.1007/s00439-009-0684-z.
8. Barrett CF, van den Maagdenberg AMJM, Frants RR, Ferrari MD. Familial hemiplegic migraine. Adv Genet. 2008;63:57–83. https://doi.org/10.1016/S0065-2660(08)01003-1.
9. Hautakangas H, Winsvold BS, Ruotsalainen SE, et al. Genome-wide analysis of 102,084 migraine cases identifies 123 risk loci and subtype-specific risk alleles. Nat Genet. 2022;54:152. https://doi.org/10.1038/s41588-021-00990-0.
10. Brugnoni R, Leone M, Rigamonti A, Moranduzzo E, Cornelio F, Mantegazza R, Bussone G. Is the CACNA1A gene involved in familial migraine with aura? Neurol Sci. 2002;23:1. https://doi.org/10.1007/s100720200015.
11. Enyedi P, Braun G, Czirják G. TRESK: the lone ranger of two-pore domain potassium channels. Mol Cell Endocrinol. 2012;353:75. https://doi.org/10.1016/j.mce.2011.11.009.
12. Lafreniere RG, Cader MZ, Poulin JF, et al. A dominant-negative mutation in the TRESK potassium channel is linked to familial migraine with aura. Nat Med. 2010;16:1157–60.
13. Andres-Enguix I, Shang L, Stansfeld PJ, et al. Functional analysis of missense variants in the TRESK (KCNK18) K channel. Sci Rep. 2012;2:237.
14. Stanyer EC, Creeney H, Nesbitt AD, Robert Holland PR, Hoffmann J. Subjective sleep quality and sleep architecture in patients with migraine: a meta-analysis. Neurology. 2021;97:e1620. https://doi.org/10.1212/WNL.0000000000012701.
15. Holland PR. Headache and sleep: shared pathophysiological mechanisms. Cephalalgia. 2014;34:725. https://doi.org/10.1177/0333102414541687.
16. Brennan KC, Bates EA, Shapiro RE, et al. Casein kinase idelta mutations in familial migraine and advanced sleep phase. Sci Transl Med. 2013;5:1–11. 183ra56
17. Schor LI. IHC Electronic Posters-Saturday and Sunday: cluster headache: investigating severity of pain, suicidality, personal burden, access to effective treatment, and demographics among a large International survey sample. Cephalalgia. 2017;37:172–208. https://doi.org/10.1177/0333102417719574.

18. Lea RA, Ovcaric M, Sundholm J, MacMillan J, Griffiths LR. The methylenetetrahydrofolate reductase gene variant C677T influences susceptibility to migraine with aura. BMC Med. 2004;2:3.
19. Kaunisto MA, Kallela M, Hamalainen E, et al. Testing of variants of the MTHFR and ESR1 genes in 1798 Finnish individuals fails to confirm the association with migraine with aura. Cephalalgia. 2006;26:1462–72.
20. Scher AI, Terwindt GM, Verschuren WM, et al. Migraine and MTHFR C677T genotype in a population-based sample. Ann Neurol. 2006;59:372–5.
21. Schurks M, Zee RY, Buring JE, Kurth T. Interrelationships among the MTHFR 677C>T polymorphism, migraine, and cardiovascular disease. Neurology. 2008;71:505–13.
22. Rubino E, Ferrero M, Rainero I, Binello E, Vaula G, Pinessi L. Association of the C677T polymorphism in the MTHFR gene with migraine: a meta-analysis. Cephalalgia. 2009;29:818–25.
23. Todt U, Netzer C, Toliat M, Heinze A, Goebel I, Nurnberg P, Gobel H, Freudenberg J, Kubisch C. New genetic evidence for involvement of the dopamine system in migraine with aura. Hum Genet. 2009;125:265–79.
24. Johnson MP, Lea RA, Curtain RP, MacMillan JC, Griffiths LR. An investigation of the 5-HT2C receptor gene as a migraine candidate gene. Am J Med Genet B Neuropsychiatr Genet. 2003;117B:86–9.
25. Oswell G, Kaunisto MA, Kallela M, Hamalainen E, Anttila V, Kaprio J, Farkkila M, Wessman M, Palotie A. No association of migraine to the GABA-A receptor complex on chromosome 15. Am J Med Genet B Neuropsychiatr Genet. 2008;147B:33–6.
26. Oterino A, Toriello M, Cayon A, et al. Multilocus analyses reveal involvement of the ESR1, ESR2, and FSHR genes in migraine. Headache. 2008;48:1438–50.
27. Nyholt DR, LaForge KS, Kallela M, et al. A high-density association screen of 155 ion transport genes for involvement with common migraine. Hum Mol Genet. 2008;17:3318–31.
28. Eising E, de Vries B, Ferrari MD, Terwindt GM, van den Maagdenberg AM. Pearls and pitfalls in genetic studies of migraine. Cephalalgia. 2013;33:614–25.
29. Sutherland HG, Albury CL, Griffiths LR. Advances in genetics of migraine. J Headache Pain. 2019;20:72. https://doi.org/10.1186/s10194-019-1017-9.
30. Lappalainen T, MacArthur DG. From variant to function in human disease genetics. Science. 2021;373:1464. https://doi.org/10.1126/science.abi8207.
31. Fadista J, Manning AK, Florez JC, Groop L. The (in)famous GWAS P-value threshold revisited and updated for low-frequency variants. Eur J Hum Genet. 2016;24:1202. https://doi.org/10.1038/ejhg.2015.269.
32. Freilinger T, Anttila V, de Vries B, et al. Genome-wide association analysis identifies susceptibility loci for migraine without aura. Nat Genet. 2012;44:777–82.
33. Anttila V, Stefansson H, Kallela M, et al. Genome-wide association study of migraine implicates a common susceptibility variant on 8q22.1. Nat Genet. 2010;42:869–73.
34. Anttila V, Winsvold BS, Gormley P, et al. Genome-wide meta-analysis identifies new susceptibility loci for migraine. Nat Genet. 2013;45:912–7.
35. Chasman DI, Schurks M, Anttila V, et al. Genome-wide association study reveals three susceptibility loci for common migraine in the general population. Nat Genet. 2011;43:695–8.
36. Chang X, Pellegrino R, Garifallou J, et al. Common variants at 5q33.1 predispose to migraine in African-American children. J Med Genet. 2018;55:831. https://doi.org/10.1136/jmedgenet-2018-105359.
37. Chen S-P, Fuh J-L, Chung M-Y, et al. Genome-wide association study identifies novel susceptibility loci for migraine in Han Chinese resided in Taiwan. Cephalalgia. 2018;38:466. https://doi.org/10.1177/0333102417695105.
38. Pickrell JK, Berisa T, Liu JZ, Ségurel L, Tung JY, Hinds DA. Detection and interpretation of shared genetic influences on 42 human traits. Nat Genet. 2016;48:709. https://doi.org/10.1038/ng.3570.
39. Gormley P, Anttila V, Winsvold BS, et al. Meta-analysis of 375,000 individuals identifies 38 susceptibility loci for migraine. Nat Genet. 2016;48:856. https://doi.org/10.1038/ng.3598.
40. Schurks M. Genetics of migraine in the age of genome-wide association studies. J Headache Pain. 2012;13:1–9.
41. Esserlind AL, Christensen AF, Le H, et al. Replication and meta-analysis of common variants identifies a genome-wide significant locus in migraine. Eur J Neurol. 2013;20:765–72.
42. Barabas G, Matthews WS, Ferrari M. Tourette's syndrome and migraine. Arch Neurol. 1984;41:871–2.
43. Merikangas KR. Migraine and psychopathology. Arch Gen Psychiatry. 1990;47:849.
44. Breslau N, Lipton RB, Stewart WF, Schultz LR, Welch KMA. Comorbidity of migraine and depression: investigating potential etiology and prognosis. Neurology. 2003;60:1308–12.
45. Fasmer OB, Halmøy A, Oedegaard KJ, Haavik J. Adult attention deficit hyperactivity disorder is associated with migraine headaches. Eur Arch Psychiatry Clin Neurosci. 2011;261:595–602.
46. Lewis CM, Vassos E. Polygenic risk scores: from research tools to clinical instruments. Genome Med. 2020;12:44. https://doi.org/10.1186/s13073-020-00742-5.
47. Musliner KL, Mortensen PB, McGrath JJ, et al. Association of polygenic liabilities for major depression, bipolar disorder, and schizophrenia with risk for depression in the Danish population. JAMA Psychiatry. 2019;76:516. https://doi.org/10.1001/jamapsychiatry.2018.4166.
48. Khera AV, Chaffin M, Aragam KG, et al. Genome-wide polygenic scores for common diseases identify individuals with risk equivalent to monogenic mutations. Nat Genet. 2018;50:1219. https://doi.org/10.1038/s41588-018-0183-z.
49. Chalmer MA, Esserlind A-L, Olesen J, Hansen TF. Polygenic risk score: use in migraine research. J Headache Pain. 2018;19:29. https://doi.org/10.1186/s10194-018-0856-0.
50. Rodriguez-Acevedo AJ, Ferreira MA, Benton MC, Carless MA, Goring HH, Curran JE, Blangero J, Lea RA, Griffiths LR. Common polygenic variation contributes to risk of migraine in the Norfolk Island population. Hum Genet. 2015;134:1079. https://doi.org/10.1007/s00439-015-1587-9.
51. Gormley P, Kurki MI, Hiekkala ME, et al. Common variant burden contributes to the familial aggregation of migraine in 1,589 families. Neuron. 2018;98:743. https://doi.org/10.1016/j.neuron.2018.04.014.
52. Chalmer MA, Rasmussen AH, Kogelman LJA, Olesen J, Hansen TF. Chronic migraine: genetics or environment? Eur J Neurol. 2021;28:1726–36.
53. Headache Classification Committee of the International Headache Society (IHS). The international classification of headache disorders, (beta version). Cephalalgia. 2013;33(9):629–808. https://doi.org/10.1177/0333102413485658.
54. Häppölä P, Gormley P, Nuottamo ME, et al. Polygenic risk provides biological validity for the ICHD-3 criteria among Finnish migraine families. Cephalalgia. 2021;42:345. https://doi.org/10.1177/03331024211045651.
55. Le H, Tfelt-Hansen P, Skytthe A, Kyvik KO, Olesen J. Association between migraine, lifestyle and socioeconomic factors: a population-based cross-sectional study. J Headache Pain. 2011;12:157–72.
56. Dzoljic E, Vlajinac H, Sipetic S, Marinkovic J, Grbatinic I, Kostic V. A survey of female students with migraine: what is the influence of family history and lifestyle? Int J Neurosci. 2013;124:82.

57. Macgregor EA, Rosenberg JD, Kurth T. Sex-related differences in epidemiological and clinic-based headache studies. Headache. 2011;51:843–59.
58. Moore LD, Le T, Fan G. DNA methylation and its basic function. Neuropsychopharmacology. 2013;38:23. https://doi.org/10.1038/npp.2012.112.
59. Gerring ZF, McRae AF, Montgomery GW, Nyholt DR. Genome-wide DNA methylation profiling in whole blood reveals epigenetic signatures associated with migraine. BMC Genomics. 2018;19:69. https://doi.org/10.1186/s12864-018-4450-2.
60. Tafuri E, Santovito D, de Nardis V, Marcantonio P, Paganelli C, Affaitati G, Bucci M, Mezzetti A, Giamberardino MA, Cipollone F. MicroRNA profiling in migraine without aura: pilot study. Ann Med. 2015;47:468. https://doi.org/10.3109/07853890.2015.1071871.
61. Andersen HH, Duroux M, Gazerani P. Serum MicroRNA signatures in migraineurs during attacks and in pain-free periods. Mol Neurobiol. 2016;53:1494. https://doi.org/10.1007/s12035-015-9106-5.
62. Cheng C-Y, Chen S-P, Liao Y-C, Fuh J-L, Wang Y-F, Wang S-J. Elevated circulating endothelial-specific microRNAs in migraine patients: a pilot study. Cephalalgia. 2018;38:1585. https://doi.org/10.1177/0333102417742375.
63. Gazerani P. Current evidence on potential uses of MicroRNA biomarkers for migraine: from diagnosis to treatment. Mol Diagn Ther. 2019;23:681. https://doi.org/10.1007/s40291-019-00428-8.
64. Berdasco M, Esteller M. Clinical epigenetics: seizing opportunities for translation. Nat Rev Genet. 2019;20:109. https://doi.org/10.1038/s41576-018-0074-2.
65. Lea RA, Shepherd AG, Curtain RP, Nyholt DR, Quinlan S, Brimage PJ, Griffiths LR. A typical migraine susceptibility region localizes to chromosome 1q31. Neurogenetics. 2002;4:17–22.

7 Migraine Pathophysiology: Structure and Function for Comprehensive Migraine Management

Oyindamola Ogunlaja, Lauren C. Strother, and Peter J. Goadsby

Introduction

Migraine presents with a diverse clinical phenotype with four phases being described that can occur over days [1]. The most common, recognizable, and reasonably well-understood phase of the attack is the headache caused by the activation of the trigeminovascular system. The aura is the least common and probably the best understood. The premonitory and postdromal phases are less understood and are likely underreported owing to the lack of patient and physician recognition. A better understanding and awareness of the entire attack, from the premonitory phase through to the postdrome, will help to improve migraine treatment and management.

Questions

1. With regard to migraine, areas or structures important in is phenotypic expression in all but one of
   A. The trigeminocervical complex in the caudal brainstem and upper cervical spinal cord
   B. Brainstem regions in the dorsal pons and dorsal midbrain
   C. Large cranial arteries
   D. The hypothalamus
   E. Cortical regions, such as the visual cortex in migraine aura
2. Neurotransmitters, neuropeptides or their receptors involved in migraine include the following except
   A. Calcitonin gene-related peptide (CGRP)
   B. Serotonin—5-HT$_{1B/1D}$ receptors
   C. Substance P
   D. Serotonin—5-HT$_{1F}$ receptors
   E. Amines, such as noradrenaline

Premonitory Phase

Most migraine patients experience a range of non-painful symptoms up to 72 h prior to the onset of head pain [2, 3]. These premonitory (prodromal) symptoms vary between patients and can be grouped into broad categories: homeostatic or hormonal alterations, mood and fatigue symptoms, migrainous symptoms and sensory sensitivities, and cranial autonomic symptoms [4]. The most consistent symptoms seem to be cognitive effects, tiredness and mood changes [3, 5]. A full list of commonly reported symptoms can be found in Table 7.1.

O. Ogunlaja
NIHR King's Clinical Research Facility, London, UK

Department of Neurology, Stanford University, Stanford, CA, USA

L. C. Strother
Wolfson Sensory, Pain and Regeneration Research Centre, King's College London, London, UK

P. J. Goadsby (✉)
NIHR King's Clinical Research Facility, London, UK

Wolfson Sensory, Pain and Regeneration Research Centre, King's College London, London, UK

Department of Neurology, University of California, Los Angeles, CA, USA

Wellcome Foundation Building, King's College Hospital, London, UK

T. S. Monteith et al. (eds.), *Comprehensive Migraine Management*, https://doi.org/10.1007/978-3-031-86923-5_7

Table 7.1 Commonly reported premonitory symptoms

Symptomatic category	Symptoms
Homeostatic or hormonal changes	Food cravings Change in appetite Thirst Polyuria Yawning Altered sleep–wake cycle Changes in alertness
Cognitive and fatigue symptoms	Difficulties concentrating Difficulties reading Memory complaints Confusion Disorientation Mood changes (depression, anxiety, irritability, elation) Fatigue
Migrainous symptoms and sensory sensitivities	Mild head discomfort Photophobia Phonophobia Osmophobia Neck stiffness Allodynia Nausea
Cranial autonomic symptoms	Lacrimation Nasal stuffiness Rhinorrhoea Aural fullness Abnormal taste Sensation of throat swelling

Adapted from Karsan and Goadsby [4]

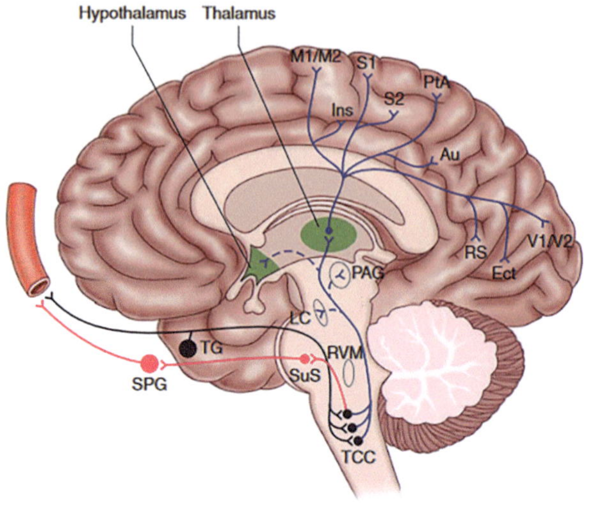

Fig. 7.1 Anatomy of the trigeminovascular system–ascending projections. The trigeminal ganglion (TG) gives rise to pseudo-unipolar trigeminal primary afferents which synapse on intra- and extracranial structures (blood vessels) as well as the spinal cord trigeminocervical complex (TCC). Second-order neurons from the TCC ascend in the quintothalamic (trigeminothalamic) tract synapsing on third-order thalamocortical neurons. Direct and indirect ascending projections also exist to the locus coeruleus (LC), periaqueductal grey (PAG), and hypothalamus. The third-order thalamocortical neurons in turn synapse on a diffuse network of cortical regions including the primary and secondary motor (M1/M2), somatosensory (S1/S2), and visual (V1/V2) cortices. A reflex connection from the TCC to the superior salivatory nucleus (SuS) exists, which projects via the sphenopalatine ganglion (SPG) providing parasympathetic innervation to the extra- and intracranial structures. Ins insula, PtA parietal association, RS retrosplenial, Au auditory, Ect ectorhinal, RVM rostral ventromedial medulla

Pathophysiology of the Premonitory Phase

Based on their manifestation, premonitory symptoms are largely thought to involve the hypothalamus, brainstem, limbic system and cortical brain regions, supported by functional neuroimaging changes in these areas [6–8]. There are many neurotransmitters and neuropeptide systems corresponding to the activated brain areas that likely contribute to the manifestation of premonitory symptoms and migraine pathogenesis. Neuropeptide Y, found in migraine-relevant areas such as the hypothalamus, basal ganglia and limbic system, is associated with appetite changes and food craving [9, 10]; dopaminergic alterations are assumed to underly yawning [11], and also contribute to nausea, together with histaminergic, serotonergic and cholinergic systems [12]. While alterations in hypothalamic orexin signalling and noradrenergic signalling from the locus coeruleus are thought to contribute to changes in the sleep/wake cycle and arousal and fatigue [13, 14] (Fig. 7.1).

Premonitory symptoms are also reliably provoked experimentally with migraine-triggering agents such as nitroglycerin [15], CGRP or PACAP38 [16], suggesting a role for nitric oxide, CGRP and PACAP38 in mediating these symptoms.

In addition to contributing to premonitory symptomatology, these individual neurotransmitters and neuropeptides are known to be involved in pain processing. Specifically, evidence from preclinical investigations has shown neuropeptide Y, dopamine, orexin and noradrenergic mechanisms to modulate trigeminovascular pain processing [10, 13, 17, 18], providing a causal link between premonitory symptoms and the development of pain.

There is particular emphasis on hypothalamic dysfunction as a possible origin for attack initiation where disruption to homeostatic mechanisms through circadian rhythm disruption, sleep disturbances or changes in the appetite may initiate hypothalamic dysfunction and migraine pathogenesis [8, 14, 19]. In support of this, in spontaneous attacks, functional fMRI has revealed early hypothalamic activation and then altered functional connectivity with the spinal trigeminal nuclei and dorsal pons immediately prior to the imitation of migraine [8], suggesting the hypothalamus may modulate the onset of headache (Fig. 7.2).

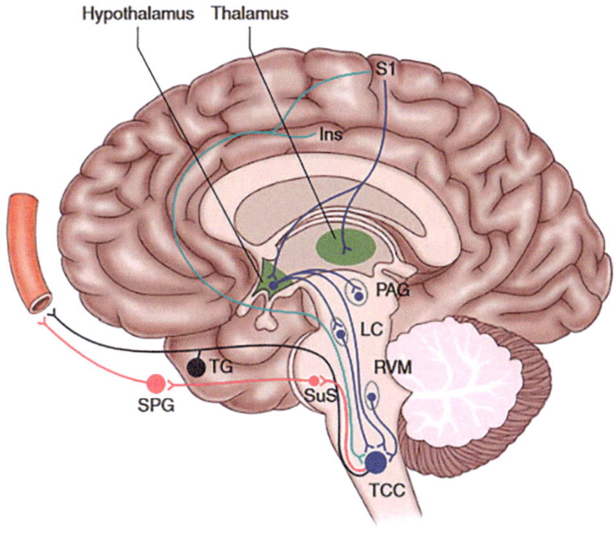

Fig. 7.2 Modulation of trigeminovascular nociceptive transmission–descending projections. The trigeminocervical complex (TCC) is subject to direct and indirect descending pain modulatory pathways arising in the cortex. Direct projections exist from primary somatosensory (S1) and insular (Ins) cortices, while indirect projections arising in S1 that projects via the hypothalamus. A local corticothalamic circuit also exists, which can modulate trigeminothalamic processing. Hypothalamic projections again form direct TCC modulatory projections as well as indirect projections via the locus coeruleus (LC) and periaqueductal gray (PAG), which can further pass via the rostral ventromedial medulla (RVM). This complex network of direct and indirect pathways provides potent anti- and pro-nociceptive modulation of incoming trigeminal nociceptive signaling, the dysfunction of which is thought to contribute to triggering migraine attacks. SPG sphenopalatine ganglion, SuS superior salivatory nucleus, TG trigeminal ganglion

Therapeutic Implications

Premonitory symptoms have been found to predict reliably and reproducibly impending headaches, identifying this phase as a key therapeutic window. Reportedly, 72% of patients can correctly predict headache onset within 72 h [2], with yawning, tiredness, cognitive and mood changes the most consistent and reproducible symptoms [5]. The development of novel treatments for administration during this non-painful phase has the potential to inhibit the initiation of pain. So far, only a few small ones have shown promising results with naratriptan [20] and domperidone [21, 22]. There is a great need for larger studies, some of which are underway (NCT04492020), in order to increase the understanding of this phase and potentially halt attack progression before the onset of headache. Patient and physician education about premonitory symptoms and their heterogenous phenotypes and their ability to predict impending headaches is also required as part of an effective treatment strategy.

Migraine Aura

Up to 30% of migraine patients experience migraine aura: a parallel transient neurological phenomenon that commonly lasts 20–30 min [23]. Aura usually precedes the headache, but can also overlap with headache (typical aura with headache) or can occur in the absence of headache altogether (typical aura without headache) [24]. Aura most commonly manifests as visual disturbance, and can also display as other sensory, motor, speech, brainstem or retinal disturbances [25, 26]. It is widely accepted that the neurological event underlying migraine aura is the human homologue of cortical spreading depression (CSD) [27, 28]. For more details on migraine aura, see Chap. 8.

Headache Phase

Head pain is the key and often most disabling clinical feature of migraine. This head pain is typically unilateral, of moderate or severe intensity, throbbing or pulsating, aggravated by routine physical activity. During this phase, other canonical symptoms are reported, such as nausea, photophobia or phonophobia [1]. Migraine attacks can also be associated with allodynia and cranial autonomic symptoms.

It is widely accepted that head pain is a result of activation, or the perception, of the trigeminovascular system [29–31].

Anatomy and Physiology of the Trigeminovascular System

Activation

The exact events that lead to the activation of the trigeminovascular system remain unknown. Some believe that CSD is the initiating event [32], while others have proposed that physiological events during the premonitory phase may be pivotal [6, 33].

Regardless, migraine pain is perceived when the pathway for nociceptive innervation of the meninges is activated [30]. This leads to the release of neuropeptides such as CGRP [34] and PACAP [35], but not substance P and neurokinin A [36]. It has been argued neuropeptide release triggers an inflammatory response that changes the environment in which these meningeal nociceptors exist [30]. The components of this sterile inflammatory response include vasodilation, plasma protein extravasation, platelet aggregation and mast cell degranulation [37, 38]. Importantly, none of these components has been proven to exist in migraine. Moreover, treatments aimed directly at the proposed sterile inflammatory response failed randomized controlled trials [39, 40]. Preclinical evidence also suggests that the pain of migraine may not arise because of peripheral sensory stimulation alone [41] but that CSD may also produce the pain of migraine via mechanisms intrinsic to the central nervous system (CNS) [41]. Experiments conducted in rats showed that the anaesthetic blockade of the trigeminal ganglion prior to the induction of CSD (by cortical injection of KCl) failed to prevent the development of CSD-induced increases in discharge rates of second-order trigeminovascular neurons [41].

Anatomical Description

Nociceptive nerve fibres consisting of non-myelinated (C-fibers) and thinly myelinated (A delta fibres) originating from the trigeminal ganglion innervate the meninges and intracranial vessels [42–44]. Much of this innervation is through the ophthalmic division of the trigeminal nerve but also to a lesser extent, the maxillary and mandibular divisions [29]. These trigeminal afferents then converge with pain inputs from adjacent skin, paraspinal muscles and other tissues innervated by C1–C2 before synapsing on second-order neurons in the trigeminocervical complex (TCC). The TCC encompasses the trigeminal nucleus caudalis (TNC) and the dorsal horn of C1–C2 [29, 31, 45–48]. Notably, the activation of trigeminovascular nociceptive afferents in primate [49] and cat [50] results in the activation of neurons in the medial caudal nucleus of the tractus solitarius, which are emesis neurons. This is paralleled in humans in the premonitory phase, when nausea is present by activations shown by PET in the rostral dorsal medulla [51].

Ascending pathways from the TCC send signals to several key areas of the brain stem and diencephalon involved in the processing of pain and other sensory information [29]. Functional physiological studies have allowed the mapping of these connections. The activation of these structures is thought to not only be responsible for pain but also the associated autonomic, cognitive and sensory aversive symptoms present throughout a migraine attack [29]. These structures include the rostral ventromedial medulla, nucleus raphe magnus, parabrachial nucleus, locus coeruleus, the cuneiform nucleus, periaqueductal grey and hypothalamic nuclei [29, 52, 53]. Functional nociceptive inputs have been shown from the dura mater to these nuclei [46, 49, 54, 55].

Evidence suggests that the thalamus represents an important first stage for multimodal sensory modulation in migraine [56]. Dural nociceptive projections carrying sensory information from the TCC project primarily to the ventroposteromedial thalamic nuclei [46, 57–59], while spinal dorsal horn neurons primarily target the ventroposterolateral nuclei. In addition, a minority of trigeminal neurons also project to the posterior and intralaminar thalamic nuclei [56].

It has been discovered recently [60] that in addition to the established indirect projections from the TCC to the lateral parabrachial nucleus, there also exist direct projections from the trigeminal ganglion to the parabrachial nucleus in mice. This dual innervation may partially explain heightened craniofacial affective pain in comparison to body pain [61–63].

Sensory information is then relayed from the various brainstem, hypothalamic and thalamic nuclei to the somatosensory, motor, insular, auditory, visual and olfactory cortex [30, 64]. These projections likely account for symptoms including photophobia, phonophobia and osmophobia which are experienced in addition to pain.

Peripheral and Central Sensitization

Once peripheral trigeminovascular neurons are activated, they become sensitized to dural stimuli, i.e. their response threshold decreases and response magnitude increases [65]. Peripheral sensitization is thought, by some, to be responsible for certain clinical manifestations in migraine including the throbbing pain of migraine and the transient worsening of pain with coughing, bending or other activities that temporarily increase intracranial pressure [30]. An alternative view would be that hypothalamic, such as A11 [18], or brainstem, such as locus coeruleus [13], structures through dysmodulation may be responsible for these clinical manifestations.

The clinical manifestation of sensitization of central trigeminovascular neurons in the spinal trigeminal nucleus is the development of cephalic allodynia (includes scalp, muscle tenderness and hypersensitivity to touch). This has been shown to take 30–60 min to develop and 120 min to reach its full extent [30, 66], and has been well described in the literature for many decades [67]. Extracephalic allodynia is because of thalamic sensitization during migraine, and this takes 2–4 h to develop [30, 66].

Pharmacology of Headache/Notable Molecular Mediators with Treatment Implications

Neuropeptides involved in the pain phase include calcitonin gene-related peptide (CGRP), pituitary adenylate cyclase activating polypeptide (PACAP), nitric oxide synthase, vasoactive intestinal peptide (VIP) and orexin [68, 69]. The neurotransmitters, serotonin, dopamine, GABA and noradrenaline are also involved in signalling [25] during this phase.

CGRP and CGRP receptor elements are expressed in trigeminal nerve fibres both peripheral and central branches [70] and levels of CGRP were found to be significantly elevated during migraine attacks in humans [71]. These elevated levels were found to normalize after successful treatment of the attack with triptans [72]. In addition, an intravenous infusion of CGRP was shown to trigger a migraine attack in 57% of patients with migraine [73]. Research into CGRP and its receptors has led to the development of new migraine drugs targeting this pathway including the CGRP monoclonal antibodies (erenumab, fremanezumab, galcanezumab and eptinezumab) as well as the gepants, such as rimegepant, ubrogepant and zavegepant. These are covered in detail in other chapters of this book.

PACAP and its receptor PAC1 have been found in key areas implicated in migraine pathophysiology, specifically the paraventricular nucleus of the hypothalamus, locus coeruleus, ventrolateral periaqueductal grey, solitary nucleus, trigeminal nucleus caudalis and the trigeminal ganglion [53, 74–78]. In addition, trigeminocervical neurons responding to a trigeminovascular nociceptive stimulus are modulated by PACAP-based mechanisms [79].

Like CGRP, plasma levels of PACAP have also been found to be elevated during a migraine attack in patients with migraine in comparison to during the interictal period [35, 80] with a reduction in PACAP levels found 1 h after treatment with sumatriptan [35]. The infusion of PACAP-38 was found to cause a migraine-like attack in 7 out of 12 migraine patients (58%), while none who received placebo experienced this [81]. PACAP has emerged as a promising therapeutic target in migraine, although the PAC-1 receptor alone may not be a useful target [82]. There is ongoing research into developing drugs against the molecule and its receptors [83].

The serotonergic system has been convincingly implicated in the pathophysiology of migraine for a long time [84–86]. Triptans, serotonin $5H_{1B/1D}$ receptor agonists, are successfully used as acute treatment for migraine. Their efficacy was initially thought to be because of the vasoconstrictive effect on meningeal vessels [87]. However, in animal models, triptans have been shown to interrupt nociceptive signalling in the TNC, periaqueductal grey and thalamus [88–90]. In addition, the newly developed ditans—selective serotonin $5HT_{1F}$ receptor agonists—do not have a vasoconstrictive effect [91] but do have clinical efficacy in aborting migraine attacks [92, 93] suggesting a central mechanism of action.

Postdrome

The migraine attack can also include a postdrome phase, where patients are left feeling tired and unwell after headache resolution [94, 95]. These non-painful symptoms typically resolve within 24 h but can last up to 48 h, greatly prolonging the disability of the attack [96]. The least is known about this phase, as patients may fail to recognize these non-painful symptoms as a continuation of the attack, but rather may assume the symptoms are expected following the resolution of pain or a side effect of abortive headache therapy [97].

The postdrome phase is symptomatically similar to the premonitory phase, although less heterogenous, with the most common symptoms being fatigue, mood and cognitive changes [2, 5, 96].

There is some suggestion that the premonitory and postdrome symptoms are consistent within the same individual suggesting a persistence of symptoms throughout the entire attack (a symptom continuum) [97]; however, it is unclear if these symptoms initiate in the prodrome and persist, or if they separately initiate during the headache, or even after headache resolution. In support of a symptom continuum, there is a similarity in brain systems involved in both arousal, cognition and homeostasis [97]; however, there is also support for differential mechanisms where the premonitory phase is associated with significant areas of increased regional blood flow [98], while the postdrome sees a near global hypoperfusion [99]. More work needs to be done to understand further this final stage of the migraine.

Conclusion

The mechanisms underlying migraine are complex and likely vary among individuals given the significant heterogeneity of clinical symptoms in patients with this disorder. Although the phases of migraine are presented here sequentially, they likely overlap and occur in parallel. Our understanding of the pathophysiology of migraine remains incomplete but there is hope that advances in functional imaging and neurophysiology will continue to increase our knowledge of the underlying mechanisms.

Teaching Points

1. Premonitory symptoms are largely thought to involve the hypothalamus, brainstem, limbic system and cortical brain regions.
2. It is widely accepted that a neurological event underlying migraine aura is cortical spreading depression (CSD).
3. Head pain is the key and often most disabling clinical feature of migraine. It is widely accepted that head pain is a result of activation, or perceived activation, of the trigeminovascular system.
4. Ascending pathways from the TCC send signals to the brainstem, hypothalamic, thalamic and basal ganglia nuclei which then project to the somatosensory, motor, insular, auditory, visual and olfactory cortex. These projections likely account for symptoms including photophobia, phonophobia and osmophobia, which are experienced in addition to pain.
5. Multiple neuropeptides and neurotransmitters play a role in the pathophysiology of migraine. Among the most well studied include serotonin, dopamine, CGRP and PACAP.

Questions and Answers

1. With regard to migraine, areas or structures important in its phenotypic expression in all but one of:
   A. The trigeminocervical complex in the caudal brainstem and upper cervical spinal cord
   B. Brainstem regions in the dorsal pons and dorsal midbrain
   C. Large cranial arteries
   D. The hypothalamus
   E. Cortical regions, such as the visual cortex in migraine aura

The correct answer is C. Choice C is incorrect since vascular mechanisms are now thought to be neither sufficient nor necessary for the symptomatic manifestations of migraine.

2. Neurotransmitters, neuropeptides or their receptors involved in migraine include the following except:
   A. Calcitonin gene-related peptide (CGRP)
   B. Serotonin—5-HT$_{1B/1D}$ receptors
   C. Substance P
   D. Serotonin—5-HT$_{1F}$ receptors
   E. Amines, such as noradrenaline

The correct answer is C. Choice C is incorrect because substance P levels are not altered in the cranial circulation during migraine and substance P/neurokinin-1 receptor antagonists are not effective in either the acute or preventive treatment of migraine.

References

1. Headache Classification Committee of the International Headache Society (IHS). The international classification of headache disorders, 3rd edition. Cephalalgia. 2018;38(1):1–211.
2. Giffin NJ, Ruggiero L, Lipton RB, Silberstein SD, Tvedskov JF, Olesen J, et al. Premonitory symptoms in migraine: an electronic diary study. Neurology. 2003;60(6):935–40.
3. Schoonman GG, Evers DJ, Terwindt GM, van Dijk JG, Ferrari MD. The prevalence of premonitory symptoms in migraine: a questionnaire study in 461 patients. Cephalalgia. 2006;26(10):1209–13.
4. Karsan N, Goadsby PJ. Biological insights from the premonitory symptoms of migraine. Nat Rev Neurol. 2018;14(12):699–710.
5. Quintela E, Castillo J, Muñoz P, Pascual J. Premonitory and resolution symptoms in migraine: a prospective study in 100 unselected patients. Cephalalgia. 2006;26(9):1051–60.
6. Maniyar FH, Sprenger T, Monteith T, Schankin C, Goadsby PJ. Brain activations in the premonitory phase of nitroglycerin-triggered migraine attacks. Brain. 2014;137(Pt 1):232–41.
7. Schulte LH, Allers A, May A. Hypothalamus as a mediator of chronic migraine: evidence from high-resolution fMRI. Neurology. 2017;88(21):2011–6.
8. Schulte LH, May A. The migraine generator revisited: continuous scanning of the migraine cycle over 30 days and three spontaneous attacks. Brain. 2016;139(Pt 7):1987–93.
9. Martins-Oliveira M, Akerman S, Holland PR, Hoffmann JR, Tavares I, Goadsby PJ. Neuroendocrine signaling modulates specific neural networks relevant to migraine. Neurobiol Dis. 2017;101:16–26.
10. Martins-Oliveira M, Akerman S, Tavares I, Goadsby PJ. Neuropeptide Y inhibits the trigeminovascular pathway through NPY Y1 receptor: implications for migraine. Pain. 2016;157(8):1666–73.
11. Sanna F, Succu S, Melis MR, Argiolas A. Dopamine agonist-induced penile erection and yawning: differential role of D_2-like receptor subtypes and correlation with nitric oxide production in the paraventricular nucleus of the hypothalamus of male rats. Behav Brain Res. 2012;230(2):355–64.
12. Andrews PL, Sanger GJ. Nausea and the quest for the perfect anti-emetic. Eur J Pharmacol. 2014;722:108–21.
13. Vila-Pueyo M, Strother LC, Kefel M, Goadsby PJ, Holland PR. Divergent influences of the locus coeruleus on migraine pathophysiology. Pain. 2019;160(2):385–94.
14. Holland PR. Headache and sleep: shared pathophysiological mechanisms. Cephalalgia. 2014;34(10):725–44.
15. Karsan N, Bose P, Lowe J, Goadsby P. The phenotype of premonitory symptoms and migraine headache triggered with nitroglycerin. BMJ Publishing Group Ltd; 2016.
16. Guo S, Vollesen ALH, Olesen J, Ashina M. Premonitory and non-headache symptoms induced by CGRP and PACAP38 in patients with migraine. Pain. 2016;157(12):2773–81.
17. Bartsch T, Levy MJ, Knight YE, Goadsby PJ. Differential modulation of nociceptive dural input to [hypocretin] orexin A and B receptor activation in the posterior hypothalamic area. Pain. 2004;109(3):367–78.

18. Charbit AR, Akerman S, Holland PR, Goadsby PJ. Neurons of the dopaminergic/calcitonin gene-related peptide A11 cell group modulate neuronal firing in the trigeminocervical complex: an electrophysiological and immunohistochemical study. J Neurosci. 2009;29(40):12532–41.
19. van Oosterhout W, van Someren E, Schoonman GG, Louter MA, Lammers GJ, Ferrari MD, et al. Chronotypes and circadian timing in migraine. Cephalalgia. 2018;38(4):617–25.
20. Luciani R, Carter D, Mannix L, Hemphill M, Diamond M, Cady R. Prevention of migraine during prodrome with naratriptan. Cephalalgia. 2000;20(2):122–6.
21. Waelkens J. Domperidone in the prevention of complete classical migraine. Br Med J (Clin Res Ed). 1982;284(6320):944.
22. Waelkens J. Dopamine blockade with domperidone: bridge between prophylactic and abortive treatment of migraine? A dose-finding study. Cephalalgia. 1984;4(2):85–90.
23. Viana M, Linde M, Sances G, Ghiotto N, Guaschino E, Allena M, et al. Migraine aura symptoms: duration, succession and temporal relationship to headache. Cephalalgia. 2016;36(5):413–21.
24. Shah DR, Dilwali S, Friedman DI. Migraine Aura without headache [corrected]. Curr Pain Headache Rep. 2018;22(11):77.
25. Akerman S, Holland PR, Goadsby PJ. Diencephalic and brainstem mechanisms in migraine. Nat Rev Neurosci. 2011;12(10):570–84.
26. Russell MB, Rasmussen BK, Fenger K, Olesen J. Migraine without aura and migraine with aura are distinct clinical entities: a study of four hundred and eighty-four male and female migraineurs from the general population. Cephalalgia. 1996;16(4):239–45.
27. Leao AAP. Spreading depression of activity in cerebral cortex. J Neurophysiol. 1944;7:359–90.
28. Migraine CA. Puntos clínicos clave. N Engl J Med. 2017;377(6):553–61.
29. Goadsby PJ, Holland PR, Martins-Oliveira M, Hoffmann J, Schankin C, Akerman S. Pathophysiology of migraine: a disorder of sensory processing. Physiol Rev. 2017;97(2):553–622.
30. Burstein R, Noseda R, Borsook D. Migraine: multiple processes, complex pathophysiology. J Neurosci. 2015;35(17):6619–29.
31. Dodick DW. A phase-by-phase review of migraine pathophysiology. Headache. 2018;58(Suppl 1):4–16.
32. Pietrobon D, Moskowitz MA. Pathophysiology of migraine. Annu Rev Physiol. 2013;75:365–91.
33. Charles A, Hansen JM. Migraine aura: new ideas about cause, classification, and clinical significance. Curr Opin Neurol. 2015;28(3):255–60.
34. Goadsby PJ, Edvinsson L, Ekman R. Release of vasoactive peptides in the extracerebral circulation of humans and the cat during activation of the trigeminovascular system. Ann Neurol. 1988;23(2):193–6.
35. Zagami AS, Edvinsson L, Goadsby PJ. Pituitary adenylate cyclase activating polypeptide and migraine. Ann Clin Transl Neurol. 2014;1(12):1036–40.
36. May A, Goadsby PJ. Substance P receptor antagonists in the therapy of migraine. Expert Opin Investig Drugs. 2001;10(4):673–8.
37. Moskowitz MA, Macfarlane R. Neurovascular and molecular mechanisms in migraine headaches. Cerebrovasc Brain Metab Rev. 1993;5(3):159–77.
38. Moskowitz MA. Neurogenic inflammation in the pathophysiology and treatment of migraine. Neurology. 1993;43(6 Suppl 3):S16–20.
39. Roon KI, Olesen J, Diener HC, Ellis P, Hettiarachchi J, Poole PH, et al. No acute antimigraine efficacy of CP-122,288, a highly potent inhibitor of neurogenic inflammation: results of two randomized, double-blind, placebo-controlled clinical trials. Ann Neurol. 2000;47(2):238–41.
40. Earl N, McDonald S, Lowy M. Efficacy and tolerability of the neurogenic inflammation inhibitor, 4991W93, in the acute treatment of migraine. Cephalalgia. 1999; SCANDINAVIAN UNIVERSITY PRESS PO BOX 2959 TOYEN, JOURNAL DIVISION CUSTOMER ....
41. Lambert GA, Truong L, Zagami AS. Effect of cortical spreading depression on basal and evoked traffic in the trigeminovascular sensory system. Cephalalgia. 2011;31(14):1439–51.
42. McNaughton FL, Feindel WH. Innervation of intracranial structures: a reappraisal. In: Rose FC, editor. Physiological aspects of clinical neurology. Oxford: Blackwell Scientific; 1977. p. 279–93.
43. Penfield W, McNaughton F. Dural headache and innervation of the dura mater. Arch Neurol Psychiatr. 1940;44(1):43–75.
44. Ray BS, Wolff HG. Experimental studies on headache: pain-sensitive structures of the head and their significance in headache. Arch Surg. 1940;41(4):813–56.
45. Noseda R, Burstein R. Migraine pathophysiology: anatomy of the trigeminovascular pathway and associated neurological symptoms, CSD, sensitization and modulation of pain. Pain. 2013;154(Suppl 1):S44. https://doi.org/10.1016/j.pain.2013.07.021.
46. Burstein R, Yamamura H, Malick A, Strassman AM. Chemical stimulation of the intracranial dura induces enhanced responses to facial stimulation in brain stem trigeminal neurons. J Neurophysiol. 1998;79(2):964–82.
47. Bartsch TGP. Anatomy and physiology of pain referral in primary and cervicogenic headache disorders. Headache Curr. 2005;2:42–8.
48. Bartsch T, Goadsby PJ. The trigeminocervical complex and migraine: current concepts and synthesis. Curr Pain Headache Rep. 2003;7(5):371–6.
49. Goadsby PJ, Hoskin KL. The distribution of trigeminovascular afferents in the nonhuman primate brain Macaca nemestrina: a c-fos immunocytochemical study. J Anat. 1997;190(Pt 3):367–75.
50. Kaube H, Keay KA, Hoskin KL, Bandler R, Goadsby PJ. Expression of c-Fos-like immunoreactivity in the caudal medulla and upper cervical spinal cord following stimulation of the superior sagittal sinus in the cat. Brain Res. 1993;629(1):95–102.
51. Maniyar FH, Sprenger T, Schankin C, Goadsby PJ. The origin of nausea in migraine-a PET study. J Headache Pain. 2014;15(1):84.
52. Liu Y, Broman J, Zhang M, Edvinsson L. Brainstem and thalamic projections from a craniovascular sensory nervous centre in the rostral cervical spinal dorsal horn of rats. Cephalalgia. 2009;29(9):935–48.
53. Robert C, Bourgeais L, Arreto CD, Condes-Lara M, Noseda R, Jay T, et al. Paraventricular hypothalamic regulation of trigeminovascular mechanisms involved in headaches. J Neurosci. 2013;33(20):8827–40.
54. Edelmayer RM, Vanderah TW, Majuta L, Zhang ET, Fioravanti B, De Felice M, et al. Medullary pain facilitating neurons mediate allodynia in headache-related pain. Ann Neurol. 2009;65(2):184–93.
55. Hoskin KLBD, Lasalandra M, Jonkman A, Goadsby PJ. Fos expression in the midbrain periaqueductal grey after trigeminovascular stimulation. J Anat. 2001;198:29–35.
56. Goadsby PJ, Holland PR. An update: pathophysiology of migraine. Neurol Clin. 2019;37(4):651–71.
57. Zagami ASLG. Stimulation of cranial vessels excites nociceptive neurones in several thalamic nuclei of the cat. Exp Brain Res. 1990;81:552–66.
58. Zagami AS, Lambert GA. Craniovascular application of capsaicin activates nociceptive thalamic neurones in the cat. Neurosci Lett. 1991;121(1–2):187–90.
59. Burstein R, Jakubowski M, Garcia-Nicas E, Kainz V, Bajwa Z, Hargreaves R, et al. Thalamic sensitization transforms localized pain into widespread allodynia. Ann Neurol. 2010;68(1):81–91.

60. Rodriguez E, Sakurai K, Xu J, Chen Y, Toda K, Zhao S, et al. A craniofacial-specific monosynaptic circuit enables heightened affective pain. Nat Neurosci. 2017;20(12):1734–43.
61. Schmidt K, Schunke O, Forkmann K, Bingel U. Enhanced short-term sensitization of facial compared with limb heat pain. J Pain. 2015;16(8):781–90.
62. Schmidt K, Forkmann K, Sinke C, Gratz M, Bitz A, Bingel U. The differential effect of trigeminal vs. peripheral pain stimulation on visual processing and memory encoding is influenced by pain-related fear. NeuroImage. 2016;134:386–95.
63. Moulton EA, Pendse G, Morris S, Strassman A, Aiello-Lammens M, Becerra L, et al. Capsaicin-induced thermal hyperalgesia and sensitization in the human trigeminal nociceptive pathway: an fMRI study. NeuroImage. 2007;35(4):1586–600.
64. Noseda R, Jakubowski M, Kainz V, Borsook D, Burstein R. Cortical projections of functionally identified thalamic trigeminovascular neurons: implications for migraine headache and its associated symptoms. J Neurosci. 2011;31(40):14204–17.
65. Strassman AM, Raymond SA, Burstein R. Sensitization of meningeal sensory neurons and the origin of headaches. Nature. 1996;384(6609):560–4.
66. Burstein R, Yarnitsky D, Goor-Aryeh I, Ransil BJ, Bajwa ZH. An association between migraine and cutaneous allodynia. Ann Neurol. 2000;47(5):614–24.
67. Selby G, Lance JW. Observations on 500 cases of migraine and allied vascular headache. J Neurol Neurosurg Psychiatry. 1960;23(1):23–32.
68. Edvinsson L, Goadsby PJ. Neuropeptides in the cerebral circulation: relevance to headache. Cephalalgia. 1995;15(4):272–6.
69. Goadsby PJ, Charbit AR, Andreou AP, Akerman S, Holland PR. Neurobiology of migraine. Neuroscience. 2009;161(2):327–41.
70. Edvinsson L. The trigeminovascular pathway: role of CGRP and CGRP receptors in migraine. Headache. 2017;57(Suppl 2):47–55.
71. Goadsby PJ, Edvinsson L, Ekman R. Vasoactive peptide release in the extracerebral circulation of humans during migraine headache. Ann Neurol. 1990;28(2):183–7.
72. Goadsby PJ, Edvinsson L. The trigeminovascular system and migraine: studies characterizing cerebrovascular and neuropeptide changes seen in humans and cats. Ann Neurol. 1993;33(1):48–56.
73. Hansen JM, Hauge AW, Olesen J, Ashina M. Calcitonin gene-related peptide triggers migraine-like attacks in patients with migraine with aura. Cephalalgia. 2010;30(10):1179–86.
74. Vaudry D, Falluel-Morel A, Bourgault S, Basille M, Burel D, Wurtz O, et al. Pituitary adenylate cyclase-activating polypeptide and its receptors: 20 years after the discovery. Pharmacol Rev. 2009;61(3):283–357.
75. Tajti J, Uddman R, Edvinsson L. Neuropeptide localization in the "migraine generator" region of the human brainstem. Cephalalgia. 2001;21(2):96–101.
76. Knutsson M, Edvinsson L. Distribution of mRNA for VIP and PACAP receptors in human cerebral arteries and cranial ganglia. Neuroreport. 2002;13(4):507–9.
77. Eftekhari S, Salvatore CA, Johansson S, Chen TB, Zeng Z, Edvinsson L. Localization of CGRP, CGRP receptor, PACAP and glutamate in trigeminal ganglion. Relation to the blood-brain barrier. Brain Res. 2015;1600:93–109.
78. Rubio-Beltrán E, Correnti E, Deen M, Kamm K, Kelderman T, Papetti L, et al. PACAP38 and PAC1 receptor blockade: a new target for headache? J Headache Pain. 2018;19(1):64.
79. Akerman S, Goadsby PJ. Neuronal PAC1 receptors mediate delayed activation and sensitization of trigeminocervical neurons: relevance to migraine. Sci Transl Med. 2015;7(308):308ra157.
80. Tuka B, Helyes Z, Markovics A, Bagoly T, Szolcsányi J, Szabó N, et al. Alterations in PACAP-38-like immunoreactivity in the plasma during ictal and interictal periods of migraine patients. Cephalalgia. 2013;33(13):1085–95.
81. Schytz HW, Birk S, Wienecke T, Kruuse C, Olesen J, Ashina M. PACAP38 induces migraine-like attacks in patients with migraine without aura. Brain. 2009;132(Pt 1):16–25.
82. Ashina M, Doležil D, Bonner JH, Zhou L, Klatt J, Picard H, et al. A phase 2, randomized, double-blind, placebo-controlled trial of AMG 301, a pituitary adenylate cyclase-activating polypeptide PAC1 receptor monoclonal antibody for migraine prevention. Cephalalgia. 2021;41(1):33–44.
83. Ogunlaja O, Karsan N, Goadsby P. Emerging drugs for the prevention of migraine. Expert Opin Emerg Drugs. 2021;26(3):271–80.
84. Hamel E. Serotonin and migraine: biology and clinical implications. Cephalalgia. 2007;27(11):1293–300.
85. Kimball RW, Friedman AP, Vallejo E. Effect of serotonin in migraine patients. Neurology. 1960;10:107–11.
86. Anthony M, Hinterberger H, Lance JW. Plasma serotonin in migraine and stress. Arch Neurol. 1967;16(5):544–52.
87. Humphrey PP, Feniuk W. Mode of action of the anti-migraine drug sumatriptan. Trends Pharmacol Sci. 1991;12(12):444–6.
88. Bartsch T, Knight YE, Goadsby PJ. Activation of 5-HT(1B/1D) receptor in the periaqueductal gray inhibits nociception. Ann Neurol. 2004;56(3):371–81.
89. Levy D, Jakubowski M, Burstein R. Disruption of communication between peripheral and central trigeminovascular neurons mediates the antimigraine action of 5HT 1B/1D receptor agonists. Proc Natl Acad Sci USA. 2004;101(12):4274–9.
90. Shields KG, Goadsby PJ. Serotonin receptors modulate trigeminovascular responses in ventroposteromedial nucleus of thalamus: a migraine target? Neurobiol Dis. 2006;23(3):491–501.
91. Nelson DL, Phebus LA, Johnson KW, Wainscott DB, Cohen ML, Calligaro DO, et al. Preclinical pharmacological profile of the selective 5-HT1F receptor agonist lasmiditan. Cephalalgia. 2010;30(10):1159–69.
92. Kuca B, Silberstein SD, Wietecha L, Berg PH, Dozier G, Lipton RB. Lasmiditan is an effective acute treatment for migraine: a phase 3 randomized study. Neurology. 2018;91(24):e2222–e32.
93. Goadsby PJ, Wietecha LA, Dennehy EB, Kuca B, Case MG, Aurora SK, et al. Phase 3 randomized, placebo-controlled, double-blind study of lasmiditan for acute treatment of migraine. Brain. 2019;142(7):1894–904.
94. Blau JN. Migraine postdromes: symptoms after attacks. Cephalalgia. 1991;11(5):229–31.
95. Kelman L. The postdrome of the acute migraine attack. Cephalalgia. 2006;26(2):214–20.
96. Giffin NJ, Lipton RB, Silberstein SD, Olesen J, Goadsby PJ. The migraine postdrome: an electronic diary study. Neurology. 2016;87(3):309–13.
97. Karsan N, Peréz-Rodríguez A, Nagaraj K, Bose PR, Goadsby PJ. The migraine postdrome: spontaneous and triggered phenotypes. Cephalalgia. 2021;41(6):721–30.
98. Karsan N, Bose P, Zelaya FO, Goadsby PJ. Alterations in regional cerebral blood (rCBF) during nitroglycerin (NTG) triggered migraine headache assessed using arterial spin-labelled (ASL) functional magnetic resonance imaging (fMRI). Cephalalgia. 2017;37:52–171.
99. Bose P, Karsan N, O'Daly O, Zelaya FO, Goadsby PJ. Alterations in cerebral blood flow during the postdrome phase of a migraine attack captured with arterial spin labelled (ASL) MRI. Cephalalgia. 2017;37:1–24.

Insights into Migraine with Aura

8

Anders Hougaard and Andreas Vinther Thomsen

Introduction

The migraine aura is one of the most fascinating and complex phenomena of clinical neurology and neuroscience. While the earliest known accounts of migraine with aura were provided by Hippocrates [1], the disorder continues to puzzle clinicians and scientists today. Our understanding of migraine with aura, its underlying mechanisms, and relation to the headache phase of migraine and to other neurological conditions is rapidly evolving. In this chapter, we will describe the clinical presentation of the different subtypes of migraine with aura and summarize what is currently known about its pathophysiology, association with other disorders, and treatment. Migraine with aura is characterized by recurrent episodes of fully reversible central nervous system symptoms. The symptoms are most often visual or sensory, usually develop gradually, and are usually followed by headache and other migraine symptoms.

The current definition, according to the third version of the International Classification of Headache Disorders (ICHD) published by the International Headache Society [2], is shown in Table 8.1. In the present chapter, we will use the term "migraine aura" for the transient neurological symptoms per se, not including headache or premonitory symptoms of migraine, while "migraine with aura" refers to the entity defined by the ICHD.

Questions

1. Which of the following symptoms is not a feature of migraine with typical aura?
   A. Speech or language disturbances
   B. Motor weakness
   C. Visual disturbances
   D. Sensory disturbances
2. A diagnosis of migraine with aura may be supported by the following imaging findings:
   A. Increased visual cortical thickness
   B. White matter hyperintensities
   C. Brain atrophy
   D. None of the above

Table 8.1 Diagnostic criteria of migraine with aura

A. At least two attacks fulfilling criteria B and C
B. One or more of the following fully reversible aura symptoms:
1. Visual
2. Sensory
3. Speech and/or language
4. Motor
5. Brainstem
6. Retinal
C. At least three of the following six characteristics:
1. At least one aura symptom spreads gradually over ≥5 min
2. Two or more aura symptoms occur in succession
3. Each individual aura symptom lasts 5–60 min
4. At least one aura symptom is unilateral
5. At least one aura symptom is positive
6. The aura is accompanied, or followed within 60 min, by headache
D. Not better accounted for by another ICHD-3 diagnosis.

A. Hougaard (✉)
Department of Neurology, Copenhagen University Hospital – Herlev and Gentofte, Herlev, Denmark

Department of Clinical Medicine, Faculty of Health and Medical Sciences, University of Copenhagen, Copenhagen, Denmark

A. V. Thomsen
Danish Headache Center, Department of Neurology, Rigshospitalet Glostrup, Faculty of Health and Medical Sciences, University of Copenhagen, Copenhagen, Denmark

T. S. Monteith et al. (eds.), *Comprehensive Migraine Management*, https://doi.org/10.1007/978-3-031-86923-5_8

Classification of Migraine Aura

Some aspects relating to the classification are particularly worth noticing: (1) there are four subtypes of migraine with aura (migraine with typical aura, migraine with brainstem aura, hemiplegic migraine, and retinal migraine), (2) the classification does not include details about the perceived appearance (visual symptoms) or localization (sensory and motor symptoms) of migraine aura symptoms although these are valuable for making the diagnosis in clinical practice, (3) the characteristics that best distinguish migraine with aura from transient ischemic attacks (TIAs) are the gradual spread over 5 min or more and the presence of positive symptoms (see below) [3], and (4) migraine with aura is not necessarily accompanied by headache, and if it is, the headache does not necessarily have the features of migraine without aura. In most cases, the aura symptoms occur before the onset of a headache. It is not uncommon for the headache to begin during the aura [4]. Only a few studies have documented the prevalence of headache onset before aura, which ranges from 3% to 9% of patients [5, 6].

Migraine with aura is a very common condition with an estimated prevalence of 8% in the general population [7]. Interestingly, the true prevalence of migraine aura without headache is unknown. Epidemiological studies to determine migraine prevalence have used initial questions of either "have you ever had a headache?", "have you ever had migraine?", or "have you ever had visual disturbances lasting from 5 to 60 minutes, which were followed by a headache?" These will not capture patients exclusively experiencing migraine aura symptoms. In a survey among Norwegian neurologists, 83 out of 245 responders (34%) reported having experienced migraine aura without headache at least once, suggesting that this condition may be underdiagnosed.

Importantly, the subtype known as *migraine with typical aura*, defined by aura symptoms in the forms of visual and/or sensory and/or language symptoms, is by far the most common. The second most common subtype, hemiplegic migraine, has a prevalence of only 0.01% [8]. The remaining two subtypes are considered very rare, and their existence is even controversial. In migraine with brainstem aura, the aura consists of brainstem symptoms (dysarthria, vertigo, tinnitus, hypacusis, diplopia, ataxia). The previous term for this condition, basilar migraine, is no longer used since the involvement of the basilar artery is considered unlikely [2]. Some experts have suggested that the symptoms reported by patients with so-called brainstem aura actually originate from the cerebral cortex [9], while others disagree [10].

Likewise, the existence of retinal migraine, i.e., monocular visual aura symptoms, is controversial. Even though visual auras generally occur in a hemifield rather than a single eye, many patients erroneously perceive them as monocular at first. While retinal spreading depression has been demonstrated in animals [11], this phenomenon would be expected to cause visual disturbances that are different from visual auras arising from the cortex in terms of speed of progression and appearance. It has been suggested that most cases of retinal migraine are more likely explained by retinal vasospasms [12].

Clinical Features of Migraine with Aura

The most characteristic clinical property of the migraine aura is the gradual spread of symptoms, usually over 5–20 min for each symptom. In contrast, the symptoms of transient ischaemic attacks occur instantaneously, and Jacksonian focal epileptic seizures spread over seconds. Visual symptoms are by far the most common and occur in more than 90% of attacks, followed by sensory symptoms (reported by roughly one-third of patients) and speech and/or language symptoms (10–20% of patients) [5, 13].

If patients experience more than one type of aura symptoms, the symptoms usually follow one another in succession, typically beginning with visual, then sensory, and then language/speech disturbances, but other orders and overlapping symptoms occur as well.

Visual and sensory auras are usually unilateral, but bilateral symptoms are not rarely reported by patients. As a rule, auras are not perceived on the same side in every attack. Consistently side-locked aura symptoms should raise concern about structural brain pathology as a cause of the symptoms [14].

As a clinician, it is important to bear in mind that patients often find it very hard to describe their aura symptoms in a level of detail that is sufficient to make the diagnosis. In these cases, it can be very useful to instruct patients to prospectively record the symptoms using an aura diary.

Visual Symptoms

A classical visual aura will start as a flickering, colorless zigzag line near the center on one side of the visual field, gradually spreading toward the periphery over a course of minutes, leaving a scotoma in its wake. However, visual aura symptoms are extremely multifaceted in terms of perceived appearance and behavior. They may vary tremendously from patient to patient and even from attack to attack in the individual patient, unlike focal epileptic seizures that are usually identical in every attack.

Commonly, visual auras have *positive* features such as flickering, scintillations, and colors, i.e., perception that does not reflect sensory input from the surrounding environment but rather is generated by the brain. Patients will be able to "see" these positive features with their eyes closed. People who are blind due to disorders of the eye or optic nerve may experience visual auras as well [15]. Most visual auras also have *negative* features, i.e., scotomas or blurred, dark, or gray areas. A scotoma, i.e., a blind spot, is usually described by patients as a "missing" area in the visual field. Patients are often unaware of such blind spots and only notice these when actively looking at something in the environment, such as the face of a person.

It has previously been stated that the color of visual disturbances is a main feature in distinguishing visual aura from occipital epileptic seizures, with only the latter being colorful [16], but systematic studies of visual migraine auras have demonstrated that while most auras are black/white or black/silver, more than one-third of patients report colorful auras, often in all colors of the rainbow [5, 17].

Visual auras are most often unilateral and homonymous, reflecting a functional disturbance in one cerebral hemisphere. However, many patients initially report that they experience visual disturbances in one eye. This is likely because patients often attend only to the visual phenomena seen in the temporal field, which is relatively larger than the nasal field.

The appearance of the visual symptoms may take many forms. The classical zigzag lines are considered pathognomonic of migraine with aura [18]. This type of visual disturbance is referred to as a fortification spectrum or teichopsia (*teichos* meaning wall) because it resembles the fortifications of a walled medieval town seen from above (see Fig. 8.1). The zigzag lines possibly reflect the firing of orientation-tuned neurons in the primary visual cortex [19].

Other commonly reported visual aura symptoms include small bright spots that increase in size or number, a growing lateral convex crescent-shaped figure, or the perception of looking through heat waves or water. More rare forms include macropsia/micropsia (objects appearing larger/smaller than they really are), autokinesis (stationary objects appearing to be moving), or even complex hallucinations. For a detailed review of visual aura symptoms, see Viana et al. [20].

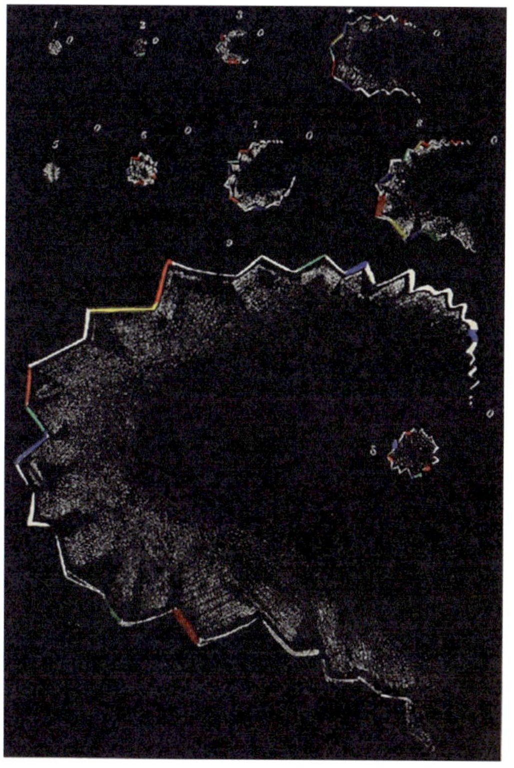

Fig. 8.1 Illustration of a classical visual migraine aura: a gradually expanding visual disturbances with a zigzag-shaped edge. The drawing was made in 1870 by Hubert Airy, a British physician, and is one of the first renderings of a migraine aura

Sensory and Language/Speech Symptoms

Like the visual aura symptoms, sensory aura symptoms may be positive (described by patients as a tingling or "pins and needles" sensation), or negative (hypesthesia or anesthesia) and are often a combination of both. Patients who report sensory auras often do not experience these in every attack, and the localization of sensory symptoms may vary.

The typical sensory aura is unilateral, starting in the hand, gradually spreading to the arm, and then affecting the face and tongue on the ipsilateral side. Nearly all patients with sensory auras experience symptoms in the hand and face (so-called cheiro-oral symptoms), while the trunk and legs are less commonly involved. Approximately 15% of patients report bilateral sensory symptoms [5, 13].

The language or speech disturbances during aura episodes are less well characterized. The typical symptoms are impaired production of language and paraphasia (substitution of words with wrong words or nonwords), usually with preserved comprehension. Some patients may exhibit dysarthria as well [5]. Language production in writing is likely affected in the same way as spoken language, and agraphia may even be the only symptom of migraine aura [21].

In addition, other deficits of higher cortical function, including amnesia and déjà vu phenomena, have been proposed as possible aura symptoms [22].

Hemiplegic Migraine

True motor aura symptoms are extremely rare. An important clinical caveat is that patients often experience decreased function, typically of one hand, during sensory auras due to loss of tactile or proprioceptive input. They will tend to describe their symptoms in terms that may lead physicians to suspect motor weakness. It is important to ask specific questions relating to motor tasks during aura episodes, such as "are you able to lift a cup from a table?" or "are you able to turn a doorknob?". Patients with genuine paresis will report severe difficulties in performing such tasks. Hemiplegic migraine may be either familial (in which at least one first- or second-degree relative has the same phenotype) or sporadic. The two forms are equally prevalent [23].

Interestingly, motor aura symptoms are always negative, i.e., they manifest as motor weakness and never involuntary movement. The motor symptoms typically involve the same areas that are affected during sensory aura, and the severity may vary from clumsiness to paralysis. The weakness is nearly always unilateral but commonly does not affect the same side in every attack. Motor aura symptoms typically last markedly longer than symptoms of typical aura, with a mean duration of 6 h and frequently 2–3 days in patients with familial hemiplegic migraine type 1.

Other features distinguish hemiplegic migraine from migraine with typical aura. Patients with hemiplegic migraine generally tend to have rare attacks. In some hemiplegic migraine patients, attacks can be triggered by a light head trauma. Attacks of hemiplegic migraine may have other, more severe, clinical features that are not seen in typical aura attacks. Attacks with impaired consciousness, leading to coma, fever, or meningism have been reported in one-third of familial hemiplegic migraine type 1 patients [24]. Severe attacks can also include seizures, agitation, and delusions. Clinical investigations in these severe cases will commonly show CSF pleocytosis and cerebral edema. Patients will nearly always recover fully, but symptoms may last for days to several weeks, and cases of fatal brain edema as a result of severe hemiplegic migraine attacks have been reported [25].

A minority of hemiplegic migraine (up to 20% of familial cases) patients have permanent, often progressive, neurological deficits, most often cerebellar signs in the form of nystagmus or ataxia. Less frequently reported is the co-occurrence of epilepsy and cognitive impairment.

Pathophysiology of Migraine Aura

Judged by their clinical presentation, the typical migraine aura symptoms clearly stem from the cerebral cortex. One of the first major clues to the understanding of the underlying mechanism came from Lashley, an American psychologist, in the mid-twentieth century. Lashley meticulously drew his own visual auras and, based on their homonymous presentation and slow spread in the visual field, concluded that they represented a dysfunction of the visual cortex spreading at a rate of approximately 3 mm/min [26]. Around the same time, Leão, a Brazilian physiologist, made his breakthrough discovery of cortical spreading depression (CSD), an electrophysiological phenomenon involving a wave of neuronal and glial depolarization spreading across the cerebral cortex at an approximate rate of 3 mm/min (see Fig. 8.2) (Redrawn) [27]. Since its discovery, the complex mechanisms of CSD, also known as spreading depolariza-

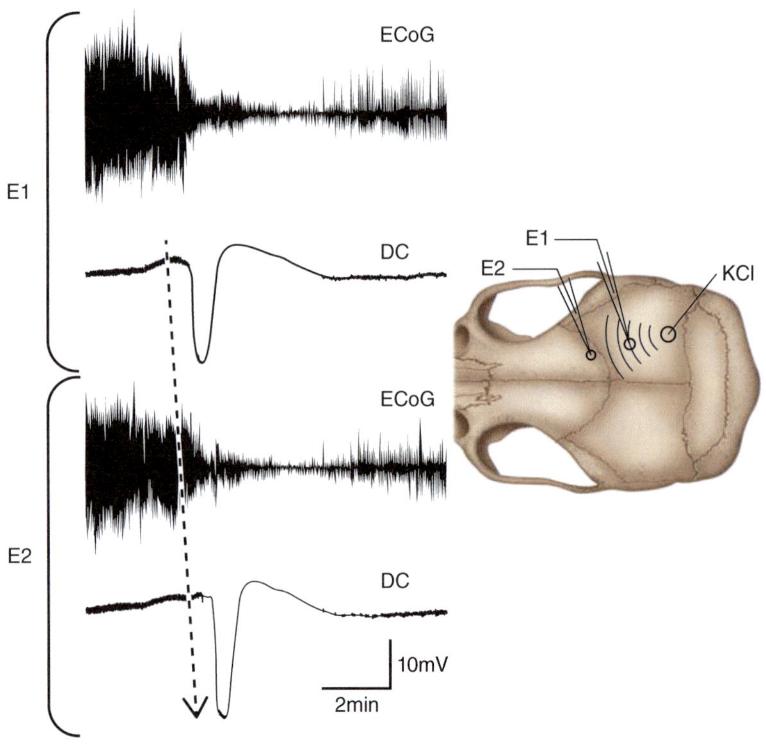

Fig. 8.2 Typical electrophysiological tracings showing electrocorticogram (ECoG) depression spatiotemporally coincident with a large negative extracellular direct coupled (DC) potential shift that lasts up to a minute when recorded by two serial intracortical microelectrodes in the rat as shown in the inset. (From Ayata et al., Cephalalgia 2009)

tion, have been extensively investigated. The wave of CSD is typically associated with a wave of hyperemia, followed by a prolonged phase of oligemia, i.e., reduced cerebral blood flow above the ischemic threshold, but the cerebral hemodynamic response to CSD varies depending on physiological conditions and species [28]. The intense depolarization of neurons and glia cells leads to substantial changes in the extracellular environment in terms of ion and neurotransmitter concentrations and metabolism, including the release of glutamate, potassium ions, hydrogen ions, and nitric oxide. These changes likely lead to depolarization of neighboring cells, thereby causing CSD propagation, but the exact mechanisms behind the spreading behavior are not completely understood [29].

Although Leão suggested that CSD could be the substrate of migraine aura symptoms, this relation was not widely recognized until the 1980s after a series of cerebral perfusion studies performed in patients during migraine aura symptoms, which showed gradually spreading perfusion changes resembling the propagation of CSD (see Fig. 8.3) (Redrawn) [30]. Subsequently, functional MRI data obtained during visual auras have further corroborated that migraine aura is a result of CSD occurring in the human brain [31].

In experimental animals, CSD can be triggered by a wide range of stimuli, mostly noxious, that cause tissue depolarization, including electrical stimulation, depolarizing chemicals, and mechanical cortical damage (usually simply by sticking a pin into the cortex) [32]. CSD may also be triggered noninvasively through neuronal depolarization by the opening of unspecific cation channels using optogenetics [33].

CSD has been directly demonstrated using cortical electrode recordings in damaged human cortex in the context of stroke, subarachnoid hemorrhage, and traumatic brain injury [34, 35]. In most of these cases, patients were unconscious, but electrocorticographic demonstration of CSD during migraine aura-like symptoms following subarachnoid hemorrhage has been reported (see Sect. 5 below) [36].

It is puzzling what could trigger CSD episodes to occur in the otherwise healthy cerebral cortex of migraine patients. Potentially, these patients are susceptible to CSD initiation due to ion channel dysfunction or changes in the extracellular environment leading to neuronal depolarization. In the special case of familial hemiplegic migraine, mutations in genes coding for ion channels and a Na/K-ATPase have been identified [23], but similar pathology has not been demonstrated for migraine with typical aura.

Three genes are known to be involved in familial hemiplegic migraine. In familial hemiplegic migraine type 1, mutations in CACNA1A, encoding the α1 subunit of the voltage-gated channel CaV2.1 calcium, lead to a gain of channel function. Familial hemiplegic migraine type 2 muta-

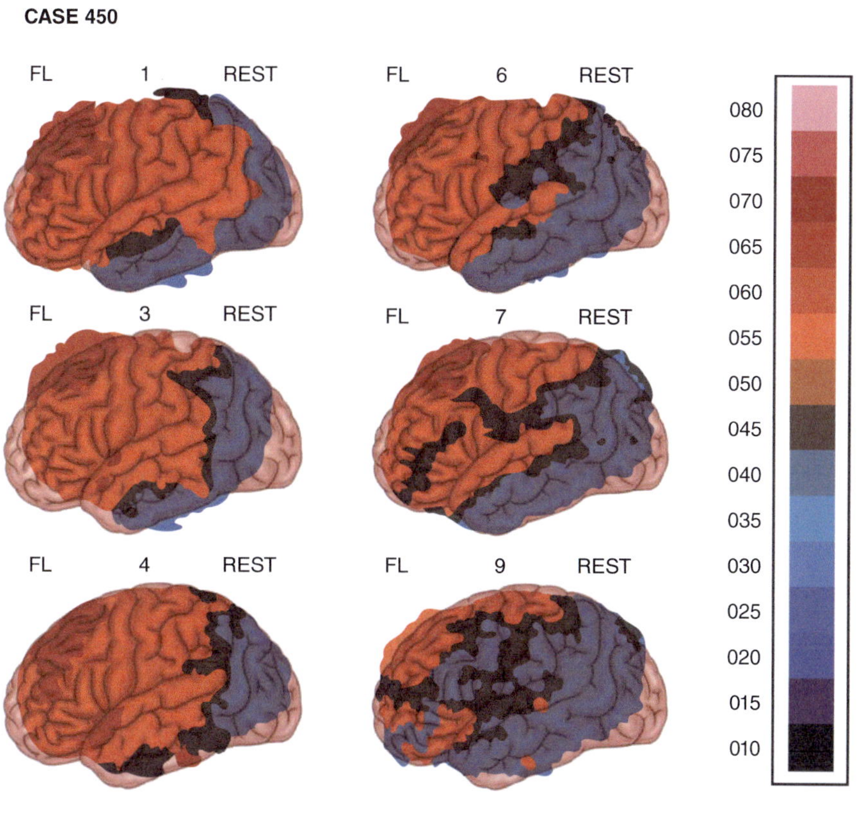

Fig. 8.3 Regional cerebral blood flow (rCBF) in a patient with migraine with aura examined with carotid injection of xenon-133 and 254 detectors in a study by Olesen et al. from 1981. Oligemia starts in the posterior part of the brain and slowly spreads over the hemisphere

tions in the ATP1A2 gene encoding the α2 subunit of Na/K--ATPases result in a loss of function in glial cells. In familial hemiplegic migraine type 3, mutations in the SCN1A gene lead to a gain of function of NaV1.1 sodium channels. These mutations likely facilitate neuronal depolarization. Knock-in mouse models have been developed for all three types of familial hemiplegic migraine, and in these models, an enhanced susceptibility to experimental CSD elicitation has been demonstrated [37].

It is currently not understood how the existence of bilateral aura symptoms can be explained. Possible mechanisms include the spreading of CSD from one hemisphere to the other via the corpus callosum, multiple waves of CSD, and bilateral representation in some cortical areas [38].

While numerous neuroimaging studies, including different modalities of structural and functional MRI investigations, have been performed in migraine with aura patients outside of attacks [39], no robust interictal neuroimaging biomarkers have yet been identified, and the diagnosis of migraine with aura remains purely based on the clinical presentation.

Relation Between Aura and Headache

The mechanisms responsible for the connection between the migraine aura and the headache phase are not clear. One hypothesis holds that CSD leads to the release of pro-inflammatory mediators that, in turn, activate nociceptors of the dura mater and thereby trigger migraine headaches. Indeed, activation of trigeminal nociceptive neurons in the brainstem and thalamus has been demonstrated following CSD [40]. It has also been suggested that CSD may lead to headache by disrupting pain modulatory centers in the brainstem [41] but evidence in support of this hypothesis is limited.

An alternative hypothesis posits that a common mechanism initiates both the aura symptoms and the headache phase of migraine. Observations in support of this relation include that a headache may occur before the onset of aura symptoms during migraine attacks with aura (see above) and that migraine headache is often not located on the contralateral side of perceived aura symptoms as would be expected in CSD-induced activation of ipsilateral nociceptors. Further, erenumab, an anti-calcitonin gene-related peptide monoclonal antibody that likely exhibits its effects outside of the central nervous system appears to be effective in the prevention of both migraine with and without aura [42], suggesting that CSD may not be the primary, initiating event in migraine attacks.

Interestingly, when pharmacological agents that reliably trigger attacks of migraine *without* aura in patients are administered to migraine patients *with* aura, they will commonly trigger the headache phase of migraine and much less frequently trigger migraine aura symptoms, even in patients who always experience aura in their spontaneous migraine attacks. This pattern was observed in provocation studies of migraine patients with aura using calcitonin gene-related peptide [43, 44], glyceryl trinitrate [45, 46], cilostazol [47], sildenafil [48], and levcromakalim [49], which are all vasodilating agents, and a similar effect was observed following exposure of migraine patients with aura to normobaric hypoxia [50]. Intravenous infusion of the vasoconstrictor peptide endothelin-1 did not provoke aura in any patients [51].

Symptomatic Migraine Aura-Like Episodes

Although migraine is, by current definition, a primary headache disorder, meaning that it cannot be attributed to another underlying disorder, it has been consistently reported that conditions including arteriovenous malformations, neoplasms, and stenosis or aneurysm of the carotid artery can cause symptoms that are clinically indistinguishable from migraine with aura. Complete cessation of migraine with aura attacks following treatment of the suspected underlying condition strongly supports a causal relation. These disorders are either of a nature to cause microembolization to the cerebral cortex or to directly irritate the cortex, which could lead to the triggering of CSD and thereby aura, corresponding to CSD experimentally induced by direct cortical irritation or microembolization [52]. Interestingly, no clear-cut cases of migraine *without* aura due to underlying pathology have been published.

Based on these observations, cortical pathology may, in some cases, give rise to migraine aura-like symptoms in patients in the same way that such pathology may cause symptomatic epilepsy. Since these clinical episodes are highly characteristic and, in all likelihood, represent episodes of CSD, perhaps a better term for them would be "symptomatic CSD," when they occur due to cortical pathology entirely outside the context of a migraine attack.

The prevalence of migraine aura-like symptoms caused by underlying conditions is unknown, but the phenomenon seems to be observed frequently in clinical practice [53].

Based on a recent review, patients presenting with migraine aura-like symptoms and the following clinical features should undergo investigation for underlying pathology: (a) side-locked migraine aura, (b) atypical aura (i.e., aura not strictly fulfilling ICHD criteria for migraine with typical aura), (c) increasing aura frequency, or (d) onset of migraine aura after the age of 50 years [54].

Relation to Stroke

Historically, a relation between migraine and stroke has been suspected since the late nineteenth century when the first accounts of supposed "migrainous strokes," e.g., severe migraine attacks leading to permanent neurological deficits or death, were published [55].

As of today, the diagnostic entity of "migrainous infarction," defined as the co-occurrence of migraine aura symptoms and a neuroimaging-verified ischemic brain lesion, is included in the ICHD. Migrainous infarction is considered to be a rare complication of migraine with aura, in which migraine aura causes brain ischemia, potentially via a more severe degree of hypoperfusion following CSD. However, ischemia following CSD has not been demonstrated in healthy cortical tissue, and neuroimaging studies of patients diagnosed with migrainous infarctions did not show ischemic lesions overlapping different vascular territories as would have been expected from ischemia caused by a wave of CSD [56]. Thus, the existence of migraine aura-induced infarctions remains controversial. The reverse causal relation, migraine aura caused by cortical ischemia, on the other hand, is well documented by clinical and preclinical evidence [14].

Longitudinal epidemiological studies have shown that having a diagnosis of migraine *with* aura (not *without* aura) is associated with an increased risk of subsequently obtaining a diagnosis of ischemic or hemorrhagic stroke (hazard ratio of 1.56 in a recent meta-analysis) [57]. Importantly, the diagnostic accuracy of migraine and stroke diagnoses in these studies is generally unknown, and misdiagnosis of migraine as stroke, and vice versa, could falsely strengthen this statistical relation. Currently, no mechanisms that would explain how migraine with aura generally increases the risk of stroke have been firmly established, but some have been suggested. An increased prevalence of patent foramen ovale has been reported in migraine with aura patients [58] and migraine with aura seems to be associated with an increased risk of atrial fibrillation [59] and cervical artery dissection [60]. Such co-morbid conditions could potentially explain an increased risk of ischemic stroke related to migraine with aura.

Pharmacology of Migraine with Aura and CSD Blockade

There are currently no well-established treatment options for migraine with aura specifically. Animal models have demonstrated that the threshold for CSD initiation and CSD propagation can be modulated chemically. CSD-inhibiting drugs could, therefore, be useful for acute or preventive therapy directly targeting migraine aura.

Chronic daily administration of commonly used migraine prophylactic drugs, including topiramate, valproate, propranolol, amitriptyline, and methysergide, increases the threshold for CSD elicitation in rats [61]. However, these drugs are effective for the prevention of migraine with aura as well as migraine without aura, and it is not clear if their effect on CSD is clinically relevant. Interestingly, erenumab, a monoclonal antibody against the calcitonin gene-related peptide receptor, a drug that would be expected to exert its action outside of the central nervous system, is effective for the prevention of migraine with and without aura [42]. Unfortunately, no clinical trials of migraine prophylactics directly compared drug effects between patients with and without aura [62].

NMDA receptor antagonists, including ketamine, have been reported to inhibit CSD initiation and propagation in animal and human cortex [63]. In an open-label trial, intranasal ketamine reduced the duration and severity of aura symptoms in 5/11 patients with familial hemiplegic migraine type 1 [64]. A subsequent randomized, double-blind study of intranasal ketamine, with midazolam as an active control, reduced the severity but not the duration of aura symptoms in patients with prolonged typical migraine aura (i.e., symptoms lasting between 1 h and 7 days).

Tonabersat, a gap junction modulator that blocks CSD in animal models, was not effective for migraine prophylaxis in initial trials, including primarily migraine patients without aura [65]. A subsequent randomized clinical trial of migraine with aura patients exclusively reported a decrease in aura attacks, but no change in monthly days with migraine headache in patients treated with tonabersat compared to placebo, suggesting that tonabersat could have a specific effect on the migraine aura [66]. The drug is currently not marketed.

Lamotrigine, a voltage-sensitive sodium channel blocker that is commonly used for the treatment of epilepsy, is a potent inhibitor of CSD in rats [67]. Randomized clinical trials did not demonstrate efficacy in migraine prophylaxis [68] but emerging evidence from open-label studies suggests that the drug may have a specific effect on migraine aura [69]. In the authors' experience, lamotrigine is widely used for off-label preventive treatment of migraine with aura in clinical practice.

Low-dose aspirin has been proposed as a prophylactic treatment of migraine with aura, although current evidence is limited. In an observational case series of 42 migraine with aura patients aged 34–70 years who were prescribed aspirin 80 mg daily, 39 patients reported a reduction of aura frequency, and 20 reported complete aura cessation [70]. A study of patients undergoing transcatheter closure of an atrial shunt reported that those who were treated with a combination of clopidogrel and aspirin experienced fewer and less severe episodes of migraine with aura compared to patients on aspirin monotherapy [71]. Theoretically, platelet inhibitors may be effective in a subgroup of patients who develop migraine aura-like episodes due to microembolic events.

Conclusion

The pathophysiology underlying migraine aura symptoms is relatively well understood, but future studies are needed to better understand how dysfunction leading to aura arises in the otherwise healthy cortex of migraine patients and by what mechanisms aura is related to headache. The relation between cortical damage or irritation, including stroke, and migraine with aura needs to be further elucidated. Experimental methods for provocation of migraine aura in patients could prove valuable for increasing the understanding of the mechanisms of migraine with aura in patients and for identifying potential new drug targets for the treatment of this highly prevalent disorder.

Teaching Points

1. Migraine with *typical aura* is a very common condition, while hemiplegic migraine and other migraine with aura subtypes are very rare.
2. Cortical spreading depression is the most likely underlying pathophysiology of the migraine aura.
3. Migraine with aura is distinguished from transient ischemic attacks by a gradual spread of symptoms (over minutes) and the presence of positive symptoms.
4. In rare cases, symptoms indistinguishable from migraine aura can result as a symptom of cortical damage or pathology, including ischemic stroke and arteriovenous malformations.

Case

A 33-year-old, previously healthy, currently 12 weeks pregnant woman, presents to the emergency department with a first episode of transient visual disturbances. She describes the visual disturbance as a "flickering zig-zag line on the right side" that starts in the center of the visual field and gradually grows larger and moves toward the periphery. After 20 min, her vision is normal, and she has no headache or other complaints. A neurological exam, including fundoscopy, is within normal limits.

Case Discussion

The prevalence of migraine aura without headache in the general population is unknown, but observational studies suggest that this condition is common. New-onset aura without headache may occur during pregnancy. The vast majority of these episodes are benign. A single episode with typical features, as in this case, generally does not require further workup.

In rare cases, aura-like symptoms may occur due to intracranial disease. The increased risk of cerebrovascular events during pregnancy should be considered. Red flags of underlying disease include side-locked aura symptoms, visual or sensory symptoms without positive features or gradual spread, frequent auras (several episodes per week), atypical aura (i.e., aura not fulfilling ICHD criteria for migraine with typical aura), and an unfavorable cardiovascular risk profile.

Questions and Answers

1. Which of the following symptoms is not a feature of migraine with typical aura?
   A. Speech or language disturbances
   B. Motor weakness
   C. Visual disturbances
   D. Sensory disturbances

The correct answer is B. Migraine with typical aura, as defined by the International Classification of Headache Disorders, involves visual and/or sensory and/or speech/language symptoms.

While migraine with typical aura is a very common condition with a prevalence of around 10% in the general population, migraine with aura involving motor weakness (i.e., hemiplegic migraine) is rare with a prevalence of 0.01%. Migraine with brainstem aura and retinal migraine, the other two subtypes of migraine with aura, are considered extremely rare, and their existence is even controversial.

2. A diagnosis of migraine with aura may be supported by the following imaging finding:
   A. Increased visual cortical thickness
   B. White matter hyperintensities
   C. Brain atrophy
   D. None of the above

The correct answer is D. Currently, no structural neuroimaging findings are useful for diagnosing migraine with aura. An increased prevalence of white matter hyperintensities in migraine patients has been reported. However, this finding has been challenged by large population-based MRI studies and remains controversial. While MRI studies have reported increased visual cortical thickness in groups of patients, this feature is too subtle and too variable to be useful for individual evaluation. Functional neuroimaging may reveal characteristic findings *during* aura symptoms only and are, therefore, not useful in clinical practice.

References

1. Rose FC. The history of migraine from Mesopotamian to Medieval times. Cephalalgia. 1995;15(Suppl 15):1–3.
2. Headache Classification Committee of the International Headache Society. The international classification of headache disorders, 3rd edition. Cephalalgia. 2018;38(1):1–211.
3. Lebedeva ER, Gurary NM, Gilev DV, Christensen AF, Olesen J. Explicit diagnostic criteria for transient ischemic attacks to differentiate it from migraine with aura. Cephalalgia. 2018;38(8):1463–70.
4. Hansen JM, Lipton RB, Dodick DW, Silberstein SD, Saper JR, Aurora SK, et al. Migraine headache is present in the aura phase: a prospective study. Neurology. 2012;79(20):2044–9.
5. Russell MB, Olesen J. A nosographic analysis of the migraine aura in a general population. Brain. 1996;119(Pt 2):355–61.
6. Viana M, Linde M, Sances G, Ghiotto N, Guaschino E, Allena M, et al. Migraine aura symptoms: duration, succession and temporal relationship to headache. Cephalalgia. 2016;36(5):413–21.
7. Russell MB, Rasmussen BK, Thorvaldsen P, Olesen JES. Prevalence and sex-ratio of the subtypes of migraine. Int J Epidemiol. 1995;24(3):612–8.
8. Lykke Thomsen L, Kirchmann Eriksen M, Faerch Romer S, Andersen I, Ostergaard E, Keiding N, et al. An epidemiological survey of hemiplegic migraine. Cephalalgia. 2002;22(5):361–75.
9. Demarquay G, Ducros A, Montavont A, Mauguiere F. Migraine with brainstem aura: why not a cortical origin? Cephalalgia. 2017;38(10):1687–95.
10. Yamani N, Chalmer MA, Olesen J. Migraine with brainstem aura: defining the core syndrome. Brain. 2019;142(12):3868–75.
11. Martins-Ferreira H, Nedergaard M, Nicholson C. Perspectives on spreading depression. Brain Res Rev. 2000;32(1):215–34.
12. Hill DL, Daroff RB, Ducros A, Newman NJ, Biousse V. Most cases labeled as "'retinal migraine"' are not migraine. J Neuroophthalmol. 2007;27(1):6.
13. Viana M, Sances G, Linde M, Ghiotto N, Guaschino E, Allena M, et al. Clinical features of migraine aura: results from a prospective diary-aided study. Cephalalgia. 2016;37(10):979–89.
14. Thomsen AV, Sørensen MT, Ashina M, Hougaard A. Symptomatic migraine: a systematic review to establish a clinically important diagnostic entity. Headache. 2021;61(8):1180–93.
15. Noseda R, Kainz V, Jakubowski M, Gooley JJ, Saper CB, Digre K, et al. A neural mechanism for exacerbation of headache by light. Nat Publ Group. 2010;13(2):239–45.
16. Panayiotopoulos CP. Elementary visual hallucinations in migraine and epilepsy. J Neurol Neurosurg Psychiatry. 1994;57(11):1371–4.
17. Queiroz LP, Friedman DI, Rapoport AM, Purdy RA. Characteristics of migraine visual aura in Southern Brazil and Northern USA. Cephalalgia. 2011;31(16):1652–8.
18. Goadsby P. Migraine, aura, and cortical spreading depression: why are we still talking about it? Ann Neurol. 2001;49(1):4–6.
19. Ohki K, Chung S, Kara P, Hübener M, Bonhoeffer T, Reid RC. Highly ordered arrangement of single neurons in orientation pinwheels. Nature. 2006;442(7105):925–8.
20. Viana M, Tronvik EA, Do TP, Zecca C, Hougaard A. Clinical features of visual migraine aura: a systematic review. J Headache Pain. 2019;20(1):64.
21. Evers S, Homann B, Vollmer J. Agraphia as the only symptom of migraine aura: a case report. Cephalalgia. 1996;16(8):562–3.
22. Petrusic I, Zidverc-Trajkovic J, Podgorac A, Sternic N. Underestimated phenomena: higher cortical dysfunctions during migraine aura. Cephalalgia [Internet] 2013 Feb. Available from: http://cep.sagepub.com/cgi/doi/10.1177/0333102413476373.
23. Russell MB, Ducros A. Sporadic and familial hemiplegic migraine: pathophysiological mechanisms, clinical characteristics, diagnosis, and management. Lancet Neurol. 2011;10(5):457–70.
24. Ducros A, Denier C, Joutel A, Cecillon M, Lescoat C, Vahedi K, et al. The clinical spectrum of familial hemiplegic migraine associated with mutations in a neuronal calcium channel. N Engl J Med. 2001;345(1):17–24.
25. Kors EE, Terwindt GM, Vermeulen FLMG, Fitzsimons RB, Jardine PE, Heywood P, et al. Delayed cerebral edema and fatal coma after minor head trauma: role of the CACNA1A calcium channel subunit gene and relationship with familial hemiplegic migraine. Ann Neurol. 2001;49(6):753–60.
26. Lashley KS. Patterns of cerebral integration indicated by the scotomas of migraine. Arch Neurol Psychiatry [Internet] 1941. Available from: http://archneurpsyc.jamanetwork.com/article.aspx?articleid=648953&ijkey=b2755a90c50502e14885f447afa1f26e3dd2f223&keytype2=tf_ipsecsha.
27. Leao AAP. Spreading depression of activity in the cerebral cortex. J Neurophysiol. 1944;7:359–90.
28. Ayata C, Lauritzen M. Spreading depression, spreading depolarizations, and the cerebral vasculature. Physiol Rev. 2015;95(3):953–93.
29. Somjen GG. Mechanisms of spreading depression and hypoxic spreading depression-like depolarization. Physiol Rev. 2001;81(3):1065–96.
30. Olesen J, Friberg L, Olsen TS, Iversen HK, Lassen NA, Andersen AR, et al. Timing and topography of cerebral blood flow, aura, and headache during migraine attacks. Ann Neurol. 1990;28(6):791–8.
31. Hadjikhani N, Sanchez del Rio M, Wu O, Schwartz D, Bakker D, Fischl B, et al. Mechanisms of migraine aura revealed by functional MRI in human visual cortex. Proc Natl Acad Sci USA. 2001;98(8):4687–92.
32. Ayata C. Pearls and pitfalls in experimental models of spreading depression. Cephalalgia. 2013;33(8):604–13.
33. Houben T, Loonen ICM, Baca SM, Schenke M, Meijer JH, Ferrari MD, et al. Optogenetic induction of cortical spreading depression in anesthetized and freely behaving mice. J Cereb Blood Flow Metab. 2017;37(5):1641–55.
34. Fabricius M, Fuhr S, Bhatia R, Boutelle M, Hashemi P, Strong AJ, et al. Cortical spreading depression and peri-infarct depolarization in acutely injured human cerebral cortex. Brain. 2006;129(3):778–90.
35. Dreier JP, Woitzik J, Fabricius M, Bhatia R, Major S, Drenckhahn C, et al. Delayed ischaemic neurological deficits after subarachnoid haemorrhage are associated with clusters of spreading depolarizations. Brain. 2006;129(12):3224–37.
36. Major S, Huo S, Lemale CL, Siebert E, Milakara D, Woitzik J, et al. Direct electrophysiological evidence that spreading depolarization-induced spreading depression is the pathophysiological correlate of the migraine aura and a review of the spreading depolarization continuum of acute neuronal mass injury. GeroScience. 2020;42(1):57–80.
37. de Boer I, Terwindt GM, van den Maagdenberg AMJM. Genetics of migraine aura: an update. J Headache Pain. 2020;21(1):64.
38. Wilkinson F. Aura mapping: where vision and Somatosensation meet. Vision. 2021;5(4):52.
39. Arca KN, VanderPluym JH, Halker Singh RB. Narrative review of neuroimaging in migraine with aura. Headache. 2021;61(9):1324–33.

40. Zhang X, Levy D, Kainz V, Noseda R, Jakubowski M, Burstein R. Activation of central trigeminovascular neurons by cortical spreading depression. Ann Neurol. 2011;69(5):855–65.
41. Lambert G, Hoskin K, Zagami A. Cortico-NRM influences on trigeminal neuronal sensation. Cephalalgia. 2008;28(6):640–52.
42. Ashina M, Goadsby PJ, Dodick DW, Tepper SJ, Xue F, Zhang F, et al. Assessment of Erenumab safety and efficacy in patients with migraine with and without aura: a secondary analysis of randomized clinical trials. JAMA Neurol [Internet]. 2021 [cited 2022 Feb 3]. Available from: https://doi.org/10.1001/jamaneurol.2021.4678.
43. Al-Khazali HM, Ashina H, Wiggers A, Rose K, Iljazi A, Christensen RH, et al. Calcitonin gene-related peptide causes migraine aura. J Headache Pain. 2023;24(1):124.
44. Hansen JM, Hauge AW, Olesen J, Ashina M. Calcitonin gene-related peptide triggers migraine-like attacks in patients with migraine with aura. Cephalalgia. 2010;30(10):1179–86.
45. Christiansen I, Thomsen LL, Daugaard D, Ulrich V, JJ O. Glyceryl trinitrate induces attacks of migraine without aura in sufferers of migraine with aura. Cephalalgia. 1999;19(7):660–7. discussion 626
46. Sances G, Tassorelli C, Pucci E, Ghiotto N, Sandrini G, Nappi G. Reliability of the nitroglycerin provocative test in the diagnosis of neurovascular headaches. Cephalalgia. 2004;24(2):110–9.
47. Butt JH, Rostrup E, Hansen AS, Lambertsen KL, Kruuse C. Induction of migraine-like headache, but not aura, by cilostazol in patients with migraine with aura. Brain. 2018;141(10):2943–51.
48. Butt JH, Eddelien S, H, Kruuse C. The headache and aura-inducing effects of sildenafil in patients with migraine with aura. Cephalalgia. 2022;42(10):984–92.
49. Al-Karagholi MAM, Ghanizada H, Nielsen CAW, Hougaard A, Ashina M. Opening of ATP sensitive potassium channels causes migraine attacks with aura. Brain. 2021;144(8):2322–32.
50. Arngrim N, Schytz HW, Britze J, Amin FM, Vestergaard MB, Hougaard A, et al. Migraine induced by hypoxia: an MRI spectroscopy and angiography study. Brain. 2016;139(3):723–37.
51. Hougaard A, Younis S, Iljazi A, Sugimoto K, Ayata C, Ashina M. Intravenous endothelin-1 infusion does not induce aura or headache in migraine patients with aura. Headache. 2020;60(4):724–34.
52. Nozari A, Dilekoz E, Sukhotinsky I, Stein T, Eikermann-Haerter K, Liu C, et al. Microemboli may link spreading depression, migraine aura, and patent foramen ovale. Ann Neurol. 2010;67(2):221–9.
53. Scutelnic A, Kreis LA, Beyeler M, Heldner MR, Meinel TR, Kaesmacher J, et al. Migraine aura-like symptoms at onset of stroke and stroke-like symptoms in migraine with aura. Front Neurol. 2022;13:1004058.
54. Rasmussen BK, Jensen R, Schroll M, Olesen J. Epidemiology of headache in a general population-a prevalence study. J Clin Epidemiol. 1991;44(11):1147–57.
55. Fere C. Note sur un cas de migraine opthalmique. Rev Med (Paris). 1883;3:194–201.
56. Wolf ME, Szabo K, Griebe M, Forster A, Gass A, Hennerici MG, et al. Clinical and MRI characteristics of acute migrainous infarction. Neurology. 2011;76(22):1911–7.
57. Mahmoud AN, Mentias A, Elgendy AY, Qazi A, Barakat AF, Saad M, et al. Migraine and the risk of cardiovascular and cerebrovascular events: a meta-analysis of 16 cohort studies including 1 152 407 subjects. BMJ Open. 2018;8(3):e020498.
58. Schwedt TJ, Demaerschalk BM, Dodick DW. Patent foramen ovale and migraine: a quantitative systematic review. Cephalalgia. 2008;28(5):531–40.
59. Sen S, Michelle Androulakis X, Duda V, Alonso A, Chen LY, Soliman EZ, et al. Migraine with visual aura is a risk factor for incident atrial fibrillation: a cohort study. Neurology. 2018;91(24):E2202–10.
60. Rist PM, Diener HC, Kurth T, Schürks M. Migraine, migraine aura, and cervical artery dissection: a systematic review and meta-analysis. Cephalalgia. 2011;31(8):886–96.
61. Ayata C, Jin H, Kudo C, Dalkara T, Moskowitz MA. Suppression of cortical spreading depression in migraine prophylaxis. Ann Neurol. 2006;59(4):652–61.
62. Hansen JM, Charles A. Differences in treatment response between migraine with aura and migraine without aura: lessons from clinical practice and RCTs. J Headache Pain. 2019;20(1):96.
63. Hoffmann J, Charles A. Glutamate and its receptors as therapeutic targets for migraine. Neurotherapeutics. 2018;15(2):361–70.
64. Kaube H, Herzog J, Käufer T, Dichgans M, Diener HC. Aura in some patients with familial hemiplegic migraine can be stopped by intranasal ketamine. Neurology. 2000;55(1):139–41.
65. Silberstein S, Schoenen J, Göbel H, Diener H, Elkind A, Klapper J, et al. Tonabersat, a gap-junction modulator: efficacy and safety in two randomized, placebo-controlled, dose-ranging studies of acute migraine. Cephalalgia. 2009;29(s2):17–27.
66. Hauge AW, Asghar MS, Schytz HW, Christensen K, Olesen J. Effects of tonabersat on migraine with aura: a randomised, double-blind, placebo-controlled crossover study. Lancet Neurol. 2009;8(8):718–23.
67. Bogdanov VB, Multon S, Chauvel V, Bogdanova OV, Prodanov D, Makarchuk MY, et al. Migraine preventive drugs differentially affect cortical spreading depression in rat. Neurobiol Dis. 2011;41(2):430–5.
68. Steiner T, Findley L, Yuen A. Lamotrigine versus placebo in the prophylaxis of migraine with and without aura. Cephalalgia. 1997;17(2):109–12.
69. Buch D, Chabriat H. Lamotrigine in the prevention of migraine with Aura: a narrative review. Headache. 2019;59(8):1187–97.
70. Turk WE, Uiterwijk A, Pasmans R, Meys V, Ayata C, Koehler PJ. Aspirin prophylaxis for migraine with aura: an observational case series. Eur Neurol. 2017;78:287–9.
71. Wilmshurst PT. Clopidogrel reduces migraine with aura after transcatheter closure of persistent foramen ovale and atrial septal defects. Heart. 2005;91(9):1173–5.

Human Migraine Laboratories: Validating Phenotypes, Biomarkers, and Precision Medicine

9

Lanfranco Pellesi and Messoud Ashina

Introduction

Over the past decade, research has made significant progress in unraveling the complex mechanisms underlying migraine [1, 2]. In vitro studies have played a pivotal role in identifying the specific receptors expressed by peripheral sensory afferents and blood vessels within the cranium [3]. Animal models, specifically designed to investigate migraine-related pain, have been essential in uncovering the intricate mechanisms of the trigeminovascular system, the phenomenon of cortical spreading depression, and the transmission of pain through both peripheral and central neural pathways [4, 5]. The activation of C- and Aδ-fibers innervating the intracranial arteries triggers the release of several neurotransmitters, including the calcitonin gene-related peptide (CGRP) and the pituitary adenylate cyclase activating polypeptide-38 (PACAP38) [6, 7]. This mechanism evokes a head pain that closely resembles a migraine headache in terms of localization and quality [8, 9]. Despite the invaluable insights gained from preclinical studies, they inherently fall short of encapsulating the full spectrum of the migraine experience. Migraine is a unique human disorder, and its multifaceted nature is more accurately and richly understood within the human context. Investigating spontaneous migraine attacks presents a logistical challenge as the accompanying pain and disability often preclude people with migraine from seeking immediate medical attention at a hospital. Therefore, experimental models of migraine have emerged as a vital tool, offering a controlled environment to explore the clinical correlates of a migraine attack in depth [10]. In these models, the provocation of an attack in individuals with migraine, but not in people without migraine, suggests the role of specific triggering molecules in the pathogenesis of the condition. If an endogenous compound is found to provoke migraine, neutralizing its effect could pave the way for therapeutic interventions. The origins of this approach date back to 1949, when the administration of nitroglycerin and histamine to individuals experiencing headaches was first employed as a diagnostic tool to identify specific types of the condition [11]. In this chapter, we provide a concise and comprehensive review of the human models of migraine, outlining the main steps involved in their development. In addition, we will discuss the most recent human studies to elucidate the relevant findings and to illustrate future prospects and directions for novel targeted treatments.

Questions

1. Which of the following is not a peptide?
   A. CGRP
   B. Erenumab
   C. VIP
   D. PACAP38
2. Migraine provocation studies typically are
   A. Case-control studies
   B. Observational studies
   C. Double-blind, cross-over studies
   D. Cross-sectional studies

L. Pellesi
Department of Neurology, Danish Headache Center, Copenhagen University Hospital – Rigshospitalet, Copenhagen, Denmark

Clinical Pharmacology, Pharmacy and Environmental Medicine, Department of Public Health, University of Southern Denmark, Odense, Denmark

M. Ashina (✉)
Department of Neurology, Danish Headache Center, Copenhagen University Hospital – Rigshospitalet, Copenhagen, Denmark

Department of Clinical Medicine, Faculty of Health and Medical Sciences, University of Copenhagen, Copenhagen, Denmark

T. S. Monteith et al. (eds.), *Comprehensive Migraine Management*, https://doi.org/10.1007/978-3-031-86923-5_9

Human- Model of Migraine

Provocation studies, often conducted as double-blind crossover trials, randomly assigned participants to receive either an intravenous infusion, an oral tablet of the triggering molecule, or a placebo. These studies allow for the evaluation of various aspects, ranging from discovering of signaling pathways involved in migraine pathogenesis to the identification of imaging or biochemical markers [12]. During these experiments, different recording techniques can be employed, such as transcranial Doppler ultrasonography [13] or magnetic resonance imaging angiography [14, 15], to investigate vascular biomarkers. Functional magnetic resonance imaging is also utilized to explore the activation of deep brain structures [16, 17]. To assess headache intensity, an 11-point pain numbered rating scale (NRS-11) is used, with 0 representing no headache, 1 indicating a very mild headache (including a feeling of throbbing or pressing), 5 representing a moderate headache, and 10 marking the worst imaginable headache. Features of the headache and accompanying symptoms are meticulously recorded during the experiments and subsequently in a headache diary. Typically, only participants with migraine develop experimentally induced migraine, while healthy participants report only mild headaches [10]. Provocations in healthy volunteers are valuable for examining headaches and certain physiological responses, such as vascular responses. Generally, healthy volunteers with first-degree family members suffering from migraine are excluded from the research. The most promising compounds are subsequently tested in people with migraine, who must be headache-free for at least 5 days before the experiment. Preferably, participants with a mild or moderate frequency of migraine days, and without preventive medication, are selected for recruitment. The phenotype of experimentally induced migraine closely resembles that of spontaneous migraine. However, there are distinctions; experimentally induced migraines are not spontaneous, symptoms develop gradually, and they may not meet the International Headache Society criteria [18]. Participants may be asked to abstain from abortive therapy until they meet the criteria, but treatment cannot be withheld indefinitely. Therefore, different criteria are utilized in these studies (Table 9.1) [12].

Table 9.1 The criteria for migraine attacks in human provocation models described in Ashina et al. [12]

	Migraine after experimental provocation
Diagnostic criteria	Migraine must fulfill either 1 or 2: 1. Headache fulfilling criteria A and B. A. Headache with at least two of the following characteristics: (a). Unilateral location (b). Pulsating quality (c). Moderate to severe pain intensity (d). Aggravation or avoidance of routine physical activity B. Headache must be accompanied by at least one of the following symptoms: (a). Nausea and/or vomiting (b). Photophobia and phonophobia 2. Headache that mimics the patient's usual migraine attacks and is treated with a rescue medication.

Calcitonin Gene-Related Peptide (CGRP) and Migraine Provocation

Human provocation models using CGRP have been instrumental in advancing the development of migraine treatments that target the CGRP or its receptor [19]. CGRP, a sensory peptide, is widely expressed within the trigeminovascular system, including locations such as perivascular sensory afferents, trigeminal ganglion, and trigeminal nucleus caudalis [20]. The potential mechanisms associated with CGRP-induced migraine are multifaceted, including vasodilation through cyclic adenosine monophosphate (cAMP), activation of perivascular sensory afferents, and modulation of specific brain centers. The initial evidence of CGRP-induced migraine was reported in a double-blind, placebo-controlled crossover study involving 12 individuals with migraine without aura [21]. Subsequent research, including two provocation studies, confirmed that CGRP could induce migraine-like attacks in the majority of participants [22, 23]. Similar results were observed in individuals exclusively experiencing migraine with aura. One provocation study revealed that CGRP induced migraine-like attacks in 8 out of 14 participants (57%) and aura symptoms in 4 out of 14 participants (28%) [24]. Two other provocation studies investigated the effects of CGRP infusion in people with familial hemiplegic migraine, an autosomal dominant type of migraine with aura

[25, 26]. Both studies reported that CGRP infusion failed to induce migraine-like attacks in participants with known and unknown mutations. This finding suggests that biological pathways underlying migraine without aura may be distinct from those responsible for familial hemiplegic migraine. The CGRP provocation studies further demonstrated that the response to CGRP is heterogeneous; some individuals developed migraine attacks without aura, while others did not. This variability opens the possibility of using the CGRP provocation model to theoretically stratify people with migraine into responders and nonresponders. If CGRP-induced migraine could be repeatedly demonstrated in selected individuals, it would reinforce the value of CGRP as a migraine-specific biomarker.

Pituitary Adenylate Cyclase-Activating Peptide (PACAP) and Vasoactive Intestinal Polypeptide (VIP) Signaling in Migraine

The initiation of migraine may be associated with the release of potent vasoactive peptides from both afferent and efferent perivascular nerve fibers [2, 27, 28]. Historically, vascular changes in migraine were often regarded more as secondary occurrences rather than causative factors [29]. A compelling argument supporting this view emerged from a single study, demonstrating that a short-lasting infusion of vasoactive intestinal polypeptide (VIP) markedly dilated extracranial arteries without provoking migraine [30]. VIP, a potent human vasodilator, plays a role in vasodilatory, parasympathetic, and secretory functions [31]. It shares a close relationship with PACAP38 and primarily acts on two G-protein coupled receptors located on the endothelium and the media arterial wall: the vasoactive intestinal polypeptide receptor 1 ($VPAC_1$) and the vasoactive intestinal polypeptide receptor 2 ($VPAC_2$) [32]. In a head-to-head study comparing the migraine-inducing properties of a 20-min infusion of PACAP38 and VIP, 16 out of 22 (73%) participants with migraine reported migraine after PACAP38, but only 4 (18%) after VIP [33]. Unlike other vasoactive peptides, VIP caused only transient dilation of cranial arteries, leading to the hypothesis that the absence of migraine provocation might be attributed to the short-lasting vasodilation [30, 33]. Recently, a 2-h infusion model with VIP was developed to further explore the relationship between the prolonged dilation of cranial arteries and headaches [34]. In healthy volunteers, infused VIP over 2 h induced a prolonged extracranial vasodilation and a mild and delayed headache, with three individuals even reporting migraine attacks [34]. When applied in people with migraine, 15 participants with episodic migraine without aura (71%) out of 21 reported migraine attacks and a sustained expansion of the superficial temporal artery for more than 2 h [35]. The incidence of nausea (93%), photophobia (67%), and phonophobia (53%) was

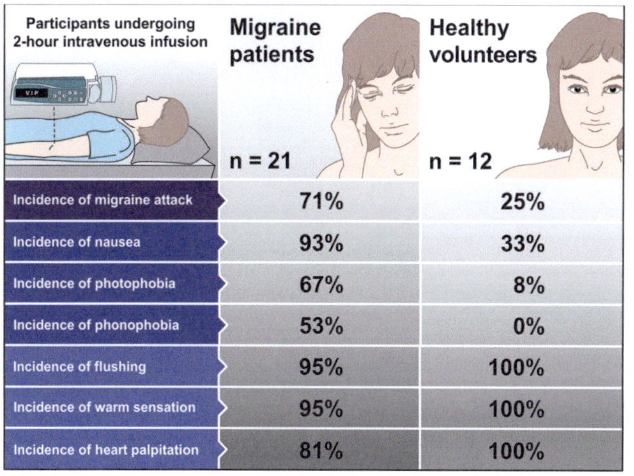

Fig. 9.1 Migraine characteristics and physiological effects after 2-h infusion of vasoactive intestinal polypeptide (VIP) in individuals with migraine and healthy volunteers [26, 27]

consistent with previously described migraine triggers [33, 36, 37]. Interestingly, the high incidence of migraine-associated symptoms was not observed when VIP was administered to healthy volunteers, indicating that such symptoms are not merely side effects of VIP administration [34]. Among healthy individuals, infused VIP over 2 h induced nausea and photophobia in 33% and 8% of cases, respectively, but not phonophobia [34]. Side effects specific to VIP administration, such as heart palpitations, warm sensations, and flushing, were observed in both migraine participants and healthy volunteers (Fig. 9.1) [34, 35]. These findings revive the role of pericranial arteries in migraine, suggesting that sustained dilation of arteries may be a critical factor in migraine initiation. A proposed mechanism involves the activation of $VPAC_1$ and $VPAC_2$ on arterial smooth muscle cells, leading to the upregulation of intracellular cAMP and the opening of ion channels [1]. This process could result in the accumulation of positively charged ions in the perivascular space, culminating in the depolarization of trigeminal perivascular sensory fibers [1].

Intracellular Signaling Pathways

A range of signaling neuropeptides have been used for studying migraine and their underlying pathophysiological mechanisms [10]. A unifying characteristic among all triggering peptides relates to their intracellular effects through either cAMP or cGMP (Fig. 9.2). The pathway mediated via cAMP can be activated by CGRP, which binds to its G-protein coupled receptor, leading to an intracellular increase of cAMP and the subsequent activation of protein kinase A [38]. When cilostazol, a type 3 phosphodiesterase inhibitor that upregulates cAMP, was used as the triggering compound, nearly 90% of migraine participants reported an attack [39].

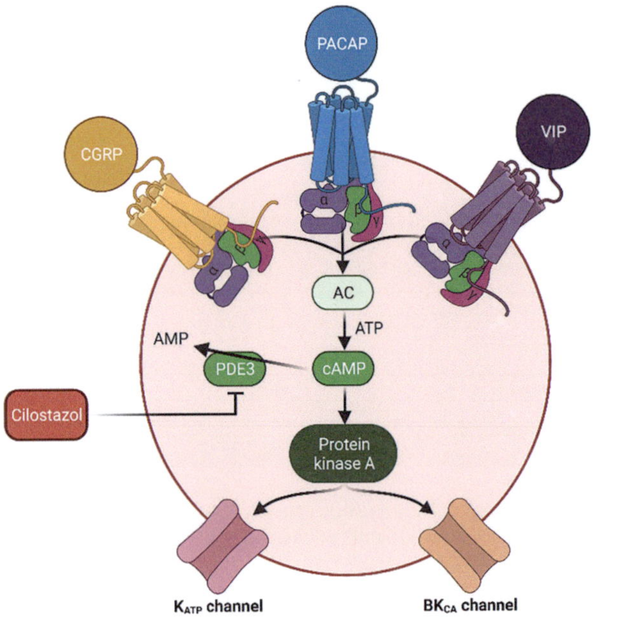

Fig. 9.2 Provocation models of migraine have implicated the cyclic adenosine monophosphate (cAMP) signaling pathway in migraine attack initiation, suggesting a downstream mechanism resulting in the opening of ATP-sensitive potassium (K_{ATP}) channels and the "big" calcium-activated potassium (BKCa) channels. The site of action of the triggering molecules, such as calcitonin gene-related peptide (CGRP), pituitary adenylate cyclase-activating peptide (PACAP), and vasoactive intestinal polypeptide (VIP), is presumably the smooth muscle cell of intracranial arteries

A common and more downstream component of the cyclic nucleotide signaling system is the potassium channels, representing the most widely distributed class of ion channels. Their activation, along with the elevation of extracellular positively charged ions, can activate and sensitize the perivascular fibers, generating nociceptive impulses that culminate in migraine pain [1]. Among these, the ATP-sensitive potassium (K_{ATP}) channels and the "big" calcium-activated potassium (BK_{Ca}) channels are currently considered the most promising ion channels involved in the migraine-signaling cascade. Both the K_{ATP} channels [40–42] and the BK_{Ca} channels [43, 44] are expressed throughout the trigeminovascular system. Interestingly, various migraine-triggering compounds induce vasodilation by opening K_{ATP} and BK_{Ca} channels [45–49]. The role of K_{ATP} channels in migraine was explored through pharmacological provocation with levcromakalim, a K_{ATP} channel opener. When infused for 20 min, levcromakalim provoked migraine in all individuals with migraine without aura, establishing itself as one of the most potent migraine-provoking compounds [50]. Most attacks were localized in the temporal and frontal regions, with a median onset of approximately 3 h [50]. The involvement of BK_{Ca} channels in the pathogenesis of migraine was similarly investigated through a 20-min infusion of MaxiPost, a BK_{Ca} channel opener. The administration led to migraine in 21 out of 22 (95%) participants, accompanied by prolonged dilation of cranial arteries [51]. The median onset of migraine was around 3 h [39] with nausea, photophobia, and phonophobia reported significantly more frequently after MaxiPost compared to placebo [51]. Since levcromakalim can cross the blood–brain barrier and cortical spreading depression could be triggered by an increase of extracellular K^+, the migraine-inducing abilities of levcromakalim were also tested in migraine with aura, resulting in migraine attacks with aura in 59% of participants [52]. These data suggest that levcromakalim could be a valuable tool for investigating migraine aura through experimental protocol. Collectively, these studies underscore the crucial role of the K_{ATP} and BK_{Ca} channels in migraine pathophysiology, highlighting their potential as targets for the development of novel migraine therapeutics.

Methodological Considerations

Migraine remains a complex disorder. Identifying a migraine trigger does not necessarily translate into an effective drug target. For instance, the nitric oxide donor glyceryl trinitrate has been shown to provoke migraine attacks through the nitric oxide-cGMP signaling pathway [53, 54]. The findings initially pointed to the inhibition of a nitric oxide synthase (NOS) isoform—endothelial (eNOS), neuronal (nNOS), or inducible (iNOS)—as a potential target for migraine [55, 56]. However, this promising direction faced setbacks when two different inhibitors of iNOS failed in randomized trials for both acute and preventative treatment of migraine [57, 58]. Similarly, provocation studies using PACAP38 suggested that inhibiting the pituitary adenylate cyclase-activating polypeptide type I (PAC_1) receptor might offer a new therapeutic avenue. Yet, a recent phase 2 study employing a human monoclonal antibody antagonizing PAC_1 did not show any significant benefits [59]. However, a recently initiated phase 2 study is investigating a monoclonal antibody specifically designed to bind and inhibit signaling mediated by PACAP38, which has reported positive results in a proof-of-concept study [60]. Selective nNOS and eNOS inhibitors remain relevant and are still being actively explored in the context of migraine. Despite these challenges, the pursuit of effective treatments continues.

Conclusion

The systematic investigation of signaling neuropeptides in human subjects has substantially augmented our understanding of the pathophysiological mechanisms underlying migraine. This has catalyzed the development of targeted pharmacological agents and initiated a significant shift in migraine translational research. Recent investigations have elucidated that migraine-signaling pathways may be integrated through the modulation of potassium channels, a finding that could have far-reaching implications for therapeutic interventions [1]. In the future, the refinement of current human models, along with the application of innovative laboratory methodologies, will likely address outstanding questions and foster a more nuanced understanding of this prevalent neurological disorder. These advancements are set to enhance the precision and specificity of investigative approaches, potentially paving the way for tailored therapeutic strategies that could revolutionize the treatment of migraine.

Teaching Points

1. Provocation studies, utilizing double-blind cross-over trials, have been instrumental in identifying molecular pathways in migraine, including the role of downstream potassium channels.
2. The integration of animal and human models with cutting-edge laboratory techniques is advancing the understanding of the underlying biology of migraine.
3. Refinement of human models and innovative methodologies is paving the way for the development of tailored therapeutic strategies in migraine treatment.

Questions and Answers

1. Which of the following is not a peptide?
   A. CGRP
   B. Erenumab
   C. VIP
   D. PACAP38

The correct answer is B. Erenumab is an antibody

2. Migraine provocation studies typically are
   A. Case-control studies
   B. Observational studies
   C. Double-blind, cross-over studies
   D. Cross-sectional studies

The correct answer is C. The vast majority of published provocation studies are double-blind, cross-over studies.

References

1. Ashina M. Migraine. N Engl J Med. 2020;383(19):1866–76.
2. Ashina M, Hansen JM, Do TP, Melo-Carrillo A, Burstein R, Moskowitz MA. Migraine and the trigeminovascular system-40 years and counting. Lancet Neurol. 2019;18(8):795–804.
3. Labruijere S, Ibrahimi K, Chan KY, MaassenVanDenBrink A. Discovery techniques for calcitonin gene-related peptide receptor antagonists for potential antimigraine therapies. Expert Opin Drug Discov. 2013;8(11):1309–23.
4. Vuralli D, Wattiez AS, Russo AF, Bolay H. Behavioral and cognitive animal models in headache research. J Headache Pain. 2019;20(1):11.
5. Harriott AM, Strother LC, Vila-Pueyo M, Holland PR. Animal models of migraine and experimental techniques used to examine trigeminal sensory processing. J Headache Pain. 2019;20(1):91.
6. Olesen J, Burstein R, Ashina M, Tfelt-Hansen P. Origin of pain in migraine: evidence for peripheral sensitisation. Lancet Neurol. 2009;8(7):679–90.
7. Tajti J, Szok D, Majláth Z, Tuka B, Csáti A, Vécsei L. Migraine and neuropeptides. Neuropeptides. 2015;52:19–30.
8. Ray BW, Wolff HG. Experimental studies on headache. Pain sensitive structures of the head and their significance in headache. Arch Surg. 1940;41:813–56.
9. Fontaine D, Almairac F, Santucci S, Fernandez C, Dallel R, Pallud J, Lanteri-Minet M. Dural and pial pain-sensitive structures in humans: new inputs from awake craniotomies. Brain. 2018;141(4):1040–8.
10. Ashina M, Hansen JM, Á Dunga BO, Olesen J. Human models of migraine—short-term pain for long-term gain. Nat Rev Neurol. 2017;13(12):713–24.
11. Dalsgaard-Nielsen T. Results of some diagnostic tests in different forms of headache. Acta Psychiatr Neurol. 1949;24(3–4):391–402.
12. Ashina M, Terwindt GM, Al-Karagholi MA, et al. Migraine: disease characterisation, biomarkers, and precision medicine. Lancet. 2021;397(10283):1496–504.
13. Lassen LH, Jacobsen VB, Haderslev PA, et al. Involvement of calcitonin gene-related peptide in migraine: regional cerebral blood flow and blood flow velocity in migraine patients. J Headache Pain. 2008;9(3):151–7.
14. Asghar MS, Hansen AE, Kapijimpanga T, et al. Dilation by CGRP of middle meningeal artery and reversal by sumatriptan in normal volunteers. Neurology. 2010;75(17):1520–6.
15. Asghar MS, Hansen AE, Amin FM, et al. Evidence for a vascular factor in migraine. Ann Neurol. 2011;69(4):635–45.
16. Asghar MS, Hansen AE, Larsson HB, Olesen J, Ashina M. Effect of CGRP and sumatriptan on the BOLD response in visual cortex. J Headache Pain. 2012;13(2):159–66.
17. Asghar MS, Becerra L, Larsson HB, Borsook D, Ashina M. Calcitonin gene-related peptide modulates heat nociception in the human brain-an fMRI study in healthy volunteers. PLoS One. 2016;11(3):e0150334.
18. Headache Classification Committee of the International Headache Society (IHS). The international classification of headache disorders, 3rd edition. Cephalalgia. 2018;38(1):1–211.
19. Ashina H, Schytz HW, Ashina M. CGRP in human models of migraine. Handb Exp Pharmacol. 2019;255:109–20.

20. Russo AF, Hay DL. CGRP physiology, pharmacology, and therapeutic targets: migraine and beyond. Physiol Rev. 2023;103(2):1565–644.
21. Lassen LH, Haderslev PA, Jacobsen VB, Iversen HK, Sperling B, Olesen J. CGRP may play a causative role in migraine. Cephalalgia. 2002;22(1):54–61.
22. Asghar MS, Hansen AE, Amin FM, van der Geest RJ, Koning PV, Larsson HB, Olesen J, Ashina M. Evidence for a vascular factor in migraine. Ann Neurol. 2011;69(4):635–45.
23. Guo S, Vollesen AL, Olesen J, Ashina M. Premonitory and nonheadache symptoms induced by CGRP and PACAP38 in patients with migraine. Pain. 2016;157(12):2773–81.
24. Hansen JM, Hauge AW, Olesen J, Ashina M. Calcitonin gene-related peptide triggers migraine-like attacks in patients with migraine with aura. Cephalalgia. 2010;30(10):1179–86.
25. Hansen JM, Thomsen LL, Olesen J, Ashina M. Calcitonin gene-related peptide does not cause the familial hemiplegic migraine phenotype. Neurology. 2008;71(11):841–7.
26. Hansen JM, Thomsen LL, Olesen J, Ashina M. Calcitonin gene-related peptide does not cause migraine attacks in patients with familial hemiplegic migraine. Headache. 2011;51(4):544–53.
27. Goadsby PJ, Edvinsson L, Ekman R. Release of vasoactive peptides in the extracerebral circulation of humans and the cat during activation of the trigeminovascular system. Ann Neurol. 1988;23(2):193–6.
28. Goadsby PJ, Edvinsson L. The trigeminovascular system and migraine: studies characterizing cerebrovascular and neuropeptide changes in humans and cats. Ann Neurol. 1993;33(1):48–56.
29. Mason BN, Russo AF. Vascular contributions to migraine: time to revisit? Front Cell Neurosci. 2018;12:233.
30. Rahmann A, Wienecke T, Hansen JM, et al. Vasoactive intestinal peptide causes marked cephalic vasodilation, but does not induce migraine. Cephalalgia. 2008;28:226–36.
31. Fahrenkrug J. Transmitter role of vasoactive intestinal peptide. Pharmacol Toxicol. 1993;72:354–63.
32. Couvineau A, Laburthe M. VPAC receptors: structure, molecular pharmacology and interaction with accessory proteins. Br J Pharmacol. 2012;166:42–50.
33. Amin FM, Hougaard A, Schytz HW, et al. Investigation of the pathophysiological mechanisms of migraine attacks induced by pituitary adenylate cyclase-activating polypeptide-38. Brain. 2014;137:779–94.
34. Pellesi L, Al-Karagholi MA, Chaudhry BA, et al. Two-hour infusion of vasoactive intestinal polypeptide induces delayed headache and extracranial vasodilation in healthy volunteers. Cephalalgia. 2020;40(11):1212–23.
35. Pellesi L, Al-Karagholi MA, De Icco R, et al. Effect of vasoactive intestinal polypeptide on development of migraine headaches: a randomized clinical trial. JAMA Netw Open. 2021;4(8):e2118543.
36. Schytz HW, Birk S, Wienecke T, Kruuse C, Olesen J, Ashina M. PACAP38 induces migraine-like attacks in patients with migraine without aura. Brain. 2009;132(1):16–25.
37. Ghanizada H, Al-Karagholi MA, Arngrim N, Olesen J, Ashina M. PACAP27 induces migraine-like attacks in migraine patients. Cephalalgia. 2020;40(1):57–67.
38. Jansen-Olesen I, Mortensen A, Edvinsson L. Calcitonin gene-related peptide is released from capsaicin-sensitive nerve fibres and induces vasodilatation of human cerebral arteries concomitant with activation of adenylyl cyclase. Cephalalgia. 1996;16(5):310–6.
39. Guo S, Olesen J, Ashina M. Phosphodiesterase 3 inhibitor cilostazol induces migraine-like attacks via cyclic AMP increase. Brain. 2014;137(Pt 11):2951–9.
40. Plough KB, Sørensen MA, Strøbech L, et al. KATP channels in pig and human intracranial arteries. Eur J Pharmacol. 2008;601:43–9.
41. Plough KB, Baun M, Hay-Schmidt A, Olesen J, Jansen-Olesen I. Presence and vascular pharmacology of KATP channel subtypes in rat central and peripheral tissues. Eur J Pharmacol. 2010;637:109–17.
42. Plough KB, Amrutkar DV, Baun M, et al. K(ATP) channel openers in the trigeminovascular system. Cephalalgia. 2012;32:55–65.
43. Adelman JP, Shen KZ, Kavanaugh MP, et al. Calcium-activated potassium channels expressed from cloned complementary DNAs. Neuron. 1992;9:209–16.
44. Wulf-Johansson H, Amrutkar DV, Hay-Schmidt A, Poulsen AN, Klaerke DA, Olesen J, Jansen-Olesen I. Localization of large conductance calcium-activated potassium channels and their effect on calcitonin gene-related peptide release in the rat trigemino-neuronal pathway. Neuroscience. 2010;167:1091–102.
45. Armstead WM. Role of ATP-sensitive K+ channels in cGMP-mediated pial artery vasodilation. Am J Phys. 1996;270:H423–6.
46. Wellman GC, Quayle JM, Standen NB. ATP-sensitive K+ channel activation by calcitonin gene-related peptide and protein kinase A in pig coronary arterial smooth muscle. J Physiol. 1998;506:117–29.
47. Hu XQ, Zhang L. Function and regulation of large conductance Ca(2+)-activated K+ channel in vascular smooth muscle cells. Drug Discov Today. 2012;17(17–18):974–87.
48. Syed AU, Koide M, Brayden JE, Wellman GC. Tonic regulation of middle meningeal artery diameter by ATP-sensitive potassium channels. J Cereb Blood Flow Metab. 2017;39:670–9.
49. Tykocki NR, Boerman EM, Jackson WF. Smooth muscle ion channels and regulation of vascular tone in resistance arteries and arterioles. Compr Physiol. 2017;7(2):485–581.
50. Al-Karagholi MA, Hansen JM, Guo S, Olesen J, Ashina M. Opening of ATP-sensitive potassium channels causes migraine attacks: a new target for the treatment of migraine. Brain. 2019;142(9):2644–54.
51. Al-Karagholi MA, Ghanizada H, Waldorff Nielsen CA, et al. Opening of BKCa channels causes migraine attacks: a new downstream target for the treatment of migraine. Pain. 2021;162(10):2512–20.
52. Al-Karagholi MA, Ghanizada H, Nielsen CAW, Hougaard A, Ashina M. Opening of ATP sensitive potassium channels causes migraine attacks with aura. Brain. 2021;144(8):2322–32.
53. Iversen HK, Olesen J, Tfelt-Hansen P. Intravenous nitroglycerin as an experimental model of vascular headache. Basic characteristics. Pain. 1989;38:17–24.
54. Thomsen LL, Kruuse C, Iversen HK, Olesen J. A nitric oxide donor (nitroglycerin) triggers genuine migraine attacks. Eur J Neurol. 1994;1:73–80.
55. Reuter U, Bolay H, Jansen-Olesen I, et al. Delayed inflammation in rat meninges: implications for migraine pathophysiology. Brain. 2001;124(Pt 12):2490–502.
56. Dieterle A, Fischer MJ, Link AS, Neuhuber WL, Messlinger K. Increase in CGRP- and nNOS-immunoreactive neurons in the rat trigeminal ganglion after infusion of an NO donor. Cephalalgia. 2011;31(1):31–42.
57. Van der Schueren BJ, Lunnon MW, Laurijssens BE, et al. Does the unfavorable pharmacokinetic and pharmacodynamic profile of the iNOS inhibitor GW273629 lead to inefficacy in acute migraine? J Clin Pharmacol. 2009;49(3):281–90.
58. Høivik HO, Laurijssens BE, Harnisch LO, et al. Lack of efficacy of the selective iNOS inhibitor GW274150 in prophylaxis of migraine headache. Cephalalgia. 2010;30(12):1458–67.
59. Ashina M, Doležil D, Bonner JH, et al. A phase 2, randomized, double-blind, placebo-controlled trial of AMG 301, a pituitary adenylate cyclase-activating polypeptide PAC1 receptor monoclonal antibody for migraine prevention. Cephalalgia. 2021;41(1):33–44.
60. Ashina M, Phul R, Khodaie M, Löf E, Florea I. A monoclonal antibody to PACAP for migraine prevention. N Engl J Med. 2024;391(9):800–9. https://doi.org/10.1056/NEJMoa2314577.

Part III

Migraine Comorbidities

Migraine and Pain Disorders

10

Tigran Kesayan, Michael P. Flannery, and Nathaniel M. Schuster

Introduction

Over 100 million people in the United States may be affected by chronic pain disorders [1]. The World Health Organization's Global Burden of Disease data suggest that among the world's most disabling disorders, migraine and low back pain rank among the top for socioeconomic impact in terms of years lived with disability [2]. Migraine is often present with comorbid noncephalic pain disorders. While chronic migraine accounts for only a small percentage of the tens of millions who have migraine, it is chronic migraine that is responsible for extraordinary and disproportionate direct and indirect healthcare and societal costs. Thus, the identification of those patients with episodic migraine who have a greater risk of chronification is prudent not only for reducing the disease burden but also mitigating its negative socioeconomic impact.

This chapter discusses migraine and chronic pain conditions and their pathophysiologic similarities, cervicogenic contribution to migraine chronification, interventional treatment options, and an approach to the patient using opioids.

Opioids continue to be excessively used to treat migraine, and this contributes to migraine chronification through mechanisms similar to opioid-induced hyperalgesia. Safe tapering and discontinuation of opioids has been shown to improve disability scores, depression and anxiety, and headache frequency in those with migraine [3, 4]. Awareness and consideration of these concomitant pain disorders and opioids may lead to a coordinated approach to decrease polypharmacy, improve outcomes, and reduce healthcare utilization.

T. Kesayan (✉)
Department of Anesthesiology and Neurology, Vanderbilt University Medical Center, Nashville, TN, USA

M. P. Flannery
Department of Neurology, Division of Headache Medicine, University of California San Francisco, San Francisco, CA, USA

N. M. Schuster
Department of Anesthesiology, Center for Pain Medicine, UC San Diego Health, La Jolla, CA, USA

Questions

1. Which treatment for cervical facet joint pain has the strongest evidence?
   A. Cervical epidural steroid injection
   B. Cervical intra-articular facet injection
   C. Cervical medial branch blocks as prelude to radiofrequency ablation
   D. Trigger point injections
2. A patient on 100 morphine milligram equivalents daily is interested in tapering off opioids. Which is the most appropriate initial percentage reduction per visit?
   A. 10%
   B. 20%
   C. 25%
   D. 50%

Prevalence of Comorbid Noncephalic Pain Disorders in Those with Migraine

Comorbid pain disorders are reported in up to 64% of patients who have migraine [3, 5]. Latent class analysis of the Chronic Migraine Epidemiology and Outcomes (CaMEO) study demonstrated hazard ratios between 1.4 and 3.4 for migraine chronification in those with comorbid pain [6]. Migraine may clinically overlap with numerous noncephalic pain disorders, such as temporomandibular joint disease, neck pain, musculoskeletal pain, fibromyalgia, irritable bowel syndrome, and chronic regional pain syndrome. The

T. S. Monteith et al. (eds.), *Comprehensive Migraine Management*, https://doi.org/10.1007/978-3-031-86923-5_10

CaMEO study identified particular disorders that occur with migraine more often than by chance alone; the former suggests comorbid or multimorbid disease states, and the latter suggests disease co-occurrence.

Neck pain is highly prevalent in patients with migraine and may even be more common than nausea, a cardinal feature of migraine. One study found that even when accounting for and excluding cervicogenic headaches, neck pain was reported by 43–73% of patients with migraine, versus nausea being reported by 18–48% of patients with migraine [7].

Patients with irritable bowel syndrome are 40–80% more likely than the general population to have migraine and/or fibromyalgia. Migraine is twice as likely in those with irritable bowel syndrome than those without (54 vs. 28%) [8]. A retrospective cohort study noted a fibromyalgia and migraine comorbidity rate between 18 and 35% [9].

Those with chronic regional pain syndrome (CRPS) are 3.6 times more likely to have migraine and 2 times more likely to have chronic daily headache compared to the general population [10]. In a study of 124 consecutive pain clinic patients with CRPS, 63% of participants had a diagnosis of migraine, and 82% of those with migraine and CRPS developed onset of headaches prior to developing CRPS symptoms [10]. Furthermore, allodynia, the perception of pain despite non-noxious stimulation, is endorsed more commonly by patients with CRPS and comorbid migraine (72.2%) than by patients with CRPS without a migraine diagnosis (46.2%) [10].

The clinical overlap in comorbid disease states may suggest that there are pathophysiological similarities among migraine, noncephalic pain, and other disorders. For example, abnormality of the serotonin transport receptor 2A gene has been demonstrated in both migraine and irritable bowel syndrome [11]. Chronic migraine and comorbid noncephalic pain disorders are associated with worse physical function, psychosocial function, healthcare utilization, and adverse life experiences when compared to chronic migraine in isolation [13]. Recognition of the coprevalence of these pain conditions carries implications for current and future treatment targets and outcomes research [14].

Shared Pain Mechanisms

Central sensitization is a complex process involving nociceptive pathway hyperexcitability via neuroplastic kindling. It is considered the common pathophysiological substrate in the chronification of migraine and comorbid pain disorders. Release of inflammatory neuropeptides such as calcitonin gene-related peptide (CGRP) increases cellular gain of central nociceptors [13]. The result is cutaneous allodynia.

Allodynia is seen in migraine progression, as well as comorbid noncephalic pain disorders such as CRPS. Cutaneous allodynia in the setting of sensitization and hyperexcitability of trigeminal nociceptive neurons likely increases the risk of developing chronic migraine [14, 15]. As such, central sensitization is likely a shared pathophysiological mechanism of both migraine and noncephalic pain disorders.

Similarly, photophobia is thought to result from the hyperexcitability of retinal photoreceptors in patients with migraine, resulting in hyperexcitability and sensitization [16]. Abnormality of photoreception in these patients leads to a perseverative cycle of retino-thalamo-cortical sensitization, subsequent photoreceptor hyperexcitability and light aversion, and resultant dark adaptation and further sensitivity to light upon re-exposure [16].

Abnormal resting-state cellular hypersensitivity thus has a bidirectional influence, which provides a basis for trigeminocervical complex contribution to migraine pathogenesis. Neck stiffness can be a prodromal migraine symptom, but migraine can also be triggered by upper cervical spinal pathology. Sensory input from the cranium and the cervical spine is involved in the pathophysiology of migraine, and allodynia in the distribution of these nerves can occur with prolonged and frequent migraine [17, 18]. The occipital nerves and peripheral nerves, which innervate cervical spine facet (zygapophyseal) joints, are targets for percutaneous interventions for migraine treatment. This bidirectional communication is evidenced by preclinical evidence showing that cephalic nociceptive afferents sensitize dural afferents, as well as that dural afferents sensitize cephalic neurons [17, 18].

This maladaptive process ultimately results in a reduction in the threshold of pain perception. However, there still remains discordance between headache intensity and disability level. Dysfunctional descending nociception may occur in the thalamus, cingulate gyrus, insula, and other brain structures. Further neuroplastic changes of the limbic-cortical circuitry may provide a basis for these perceptual differences and provide insight into the cognitive and affective contributions to pain [19].

Multidisciplinary Care

Multidisciplinary care is of particular importance for this often difficult-to-treat patient population. Not only does multidisciplinary care among a team of providers increase the likelihood of finding efficacious treatment, but it also reduces individual provider burnout. Multidisciplinary care involving providers in primary care, headache neurology, psychology, psychiatry, and pain management can improve patient reported outcomes as demonstrated by changes in validated outcome measures, such as Neuro-QoL and PROMIS [12].

Cognitive behavioral therapy performed by a psychologist can have a significant impact on the level of function experienced during pain exacerbation. A systemic review on nonpharmacological self-management of headaches suggested that cognitive behavioral therapy not only reduces perceived pain intensity but also disability [18].

Despite multiple attempted pharmacological, nonpharmacological, and interventional treatment options, this patient population may still be difficult to treat. Those with comorbid psychiatric disorders can pose additional barriers to improvement. In the latter group, where pain conditions can "sensitize" psychiatric conditions and vice versa, psychiatry consultation is recommended.

Manual therapies have demonstrated efficacy for the reduction of medication use in pain conditions. In a single study, physical therapy and yoga were demonstrated to be similarly effective in reducing medication use by over 20% [19]. Physical activity alone is known to improve outcomes in this population of patients. Manual treatment options may be of particular benefit for patients with migraine and overlapping craniofacial or craniocervical pain conditions, such as temporomandibular joint disease or chronic cervicalgia.

Evaluation of patients with migraine by a pain management specialist may provide further insight into the treatment of headache disorders, especially in those with overlapping comorbid pain conditions. This can be of particular utility in the patient with comorbid cervicalgia, given the inclusion of further treatment modalities. Information regarding the evaluation and management of this population is discussed in the following section.

Interventional Treatment Options

Migraine and cervicogenic headaches can overlap, and clinicians treating patients with migraine should be vigilant for possible cervicogenic contributors. Those with headache characteristics that meet the diagnostic criteria for migraine may also have imaging, examination, and diagnostic blockade findings that would qualify their headache as cervicogenic (Table 10.1).

With the prevalence of neck pain in migraine ranging as high as 73%, it can be challenging to untangle whether a patient's neck pain is a migraine symptom or whether the neck pain is a migraine trigger and the cause of migraine chronification in a given patient. Furthermore, the location of pain in both migraine and cervicogenic head pain can overlap. Unilateral pain in migraine is common but not necessary. Pain in cervicogenic headaches is often in the neck and posterior head but can also be seen in the temples, forehead, and the top of the head (Fig. 10.1).

Table 10.1 Diagnostic criteria for migraine without aura and cervicogenic headache

Migraine without aura	Cervicogenic headache
Pain that lasts 4–72 h when not treated or incompletely treated	Must have at least two of the following four characteristics:
One or both of the following:	Headache starts at the onset of a cervical disorder or lesion
Nausea or vomiting	Headache improves or resolves when cervical disorder improves or resolves
Light and sound sensitivity	Cervical range of motion is decreased, and provocative testing exacerbated headache
Two of the following four characteristics:	Headache significantly improves or resolves when the cervical structure in question, or its nerve supply, is blocked
Pain is worse with physical activity	
Pain has moderate to severe intensity	
Pain has a pulsating quality	
Pain is unilateral	

History and exam alone in some cases can be strongly suggestive that the neck pain is a symptom of the migraine, such as patients who report neck pain only during migraine attacks, which resolves after the migraine attack, and patients with a reassuring cervical musculoskeletal exam. However, in other patients, history and exam may suggest that cervical pathology may be a migraine trigger or underlie the migraine chronification. The cervical spine, which is comprised of seven cervical vertebrae and their accompanying neural and musculoskeletal structures, contains numerous pain generators that can be identified and treated in patients where clinicians suspect cervicogenic contributors to migraine chronification.

The atlanto-occipital joints, as well as the atlanto-axial joints (sometimes referred to as the C0/C1 and C1/C2 joints, respectively) and cervical facet joints, refer pain to a much larger area than the joint itself. The atlanto-occipital joints and atlanto-axial joints have been shown to refer pain to the occipital region, and this often overlaps with the pain referral pattern of the C2/C3 joint. A placebo-controlled prevalence study has shown that cervical facet pain at the C2/C3 level was prevalent in 50% of those with headaches after whiplash injury. The C2/C3 joint is one of the two most common clinically suspected levels leading to neck pain, as well as one of the most frequent levels to be radiologically affected [20–22].

Several percutaneous treatment options are currently used in clinical practice for suspected cervicogenic contributors to migraine chronification, including trigger point injections, occipital nerve blocks, atlanto-occipital and atlanto-axial joint intraarticular corticosteroid injections, and cervical medial branch blocks and radiofrequency ablation for facet joint-mediated pain. Procedures treating the atlanto-occipital

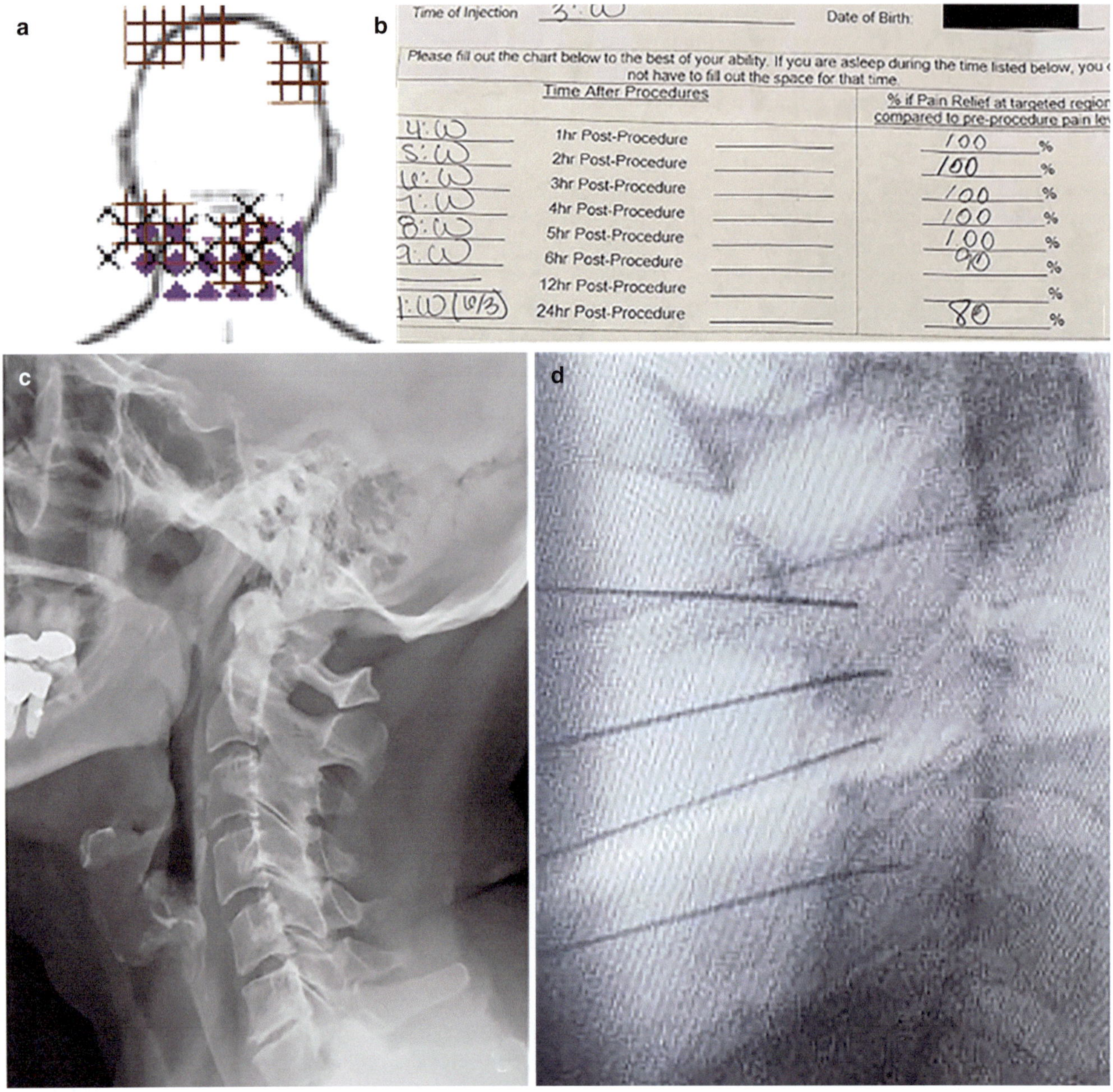

Fig. 10.1 (**a**). Location of pain as marked by the patient on a diagram. (**b**). Pain diary depicting 100% improvement in her head pain after diagnostic medial branch nerve blocks. (**c**). Lateral X-ray of the patient's cervical spine demonstrating cervical facet arthropathy as well as degenerative disc disease. (**d**). Fluoroscopy-guided radiofrequency needle positioning for the C2–4 medial branch ablation

joints, atlanto-axial joints, and cervical facet joints have predominantly been studied by pain and spine researchers, and as such, the presence of migraine in the studied patients is often not described. Cervical facet joint interventions have been predominantly studied in patients with whiplash injuries. Nonetheless, in our experience, such procedures can be effective in carefully selected patients with migraine refractory to standard-of-care treatments with suspected chronification due to cervicogenic contributors.

Trigger Point Injection

Trigger point injections can be used to treat cranial and cervical myofascial pain, and when located in the musculature of the cervico-occipital region, they can radiate pain to the cranium in those with chronic tension-type headache and migraine [23, 24]. While there are no prospective randomized controlled trials at this time that show the efficacy of trigger point injections for those with chronic migraine like there are in chronic tension-type headaches, up to 75% of American Headache Society members utilize this treatment option in the treatment of headaches, including migraine [23, 25].

Occipital Nerve Block

Occipital nerve blocks (ONBs) can be used in the treatment of acute migraine in the clinic or the emergency department, as well as for chronic migraine prevention. The occipital nerves include the greater, lesser, and third occipital nerves. Greater and lesser occipital nerve blocks can be performed either unilaterally, ipsilateral to the pain, or bilaterally, and can be performed with or without imaging guidance [26, 27]. The clinical significance of the third occipital nerve (TON) is chiefly that it innervates the C2–3 joint, and blocking or ablating it can abolish pain coming from the C2–3 joint; TON blocks and ablations require fluoroscopic or ultrasound guidance to perform. In the emergency department, greater occipital nerve blocks (GONBs) are superior to placebo as well as intravenous (IV) nonsteroidal anti-inflammatory drugs (NSAIDs), and are as effective as a combination of IV NSAIDS + IV dopamine receptor antagonist but were less effective than IV metoclopramide in one study in which 71% of GONBs were performed by inexperienced injectors [26–28]. Several studies have evaluated the efficacy of GONBs in chronic migraine with positive results, with a decrease in pain lasting from 2 days to 3 months [29–32]. However, these studies have methodological limitations, and as a result, the American Academy of Pain Medicine has given greater occipital nerve blocks a weak recommendation for chronic migraine prevention [33]. Blockade of the occipital nerves may reduce migraine pain through a reduction of nociceptive neuronal activity of the trigeminocervical complex [34].

Cervical Medial Branch Blocks and Radiofrequency Neurotomy (Ablation)

The C3–4 through L5-S1 facet joints are innervated by the medial branch of the dorsal rami that innervate the joints above and below, while the C2-C3 joint is innervated primarily by the C3 medial branch, also known as the third occipital nerve [22]. For pain that may arise from a specific cervical facet joint, or set of joints, an anesthetic block of the nerves innervating said joints can be helpful for diagnosis. If, for example, the C3-C4 joint is thought to be the pain generator for a predominantly occipital headache, then blocks of the C3 and C4 medial branches will be diagnostic if there is either resolution of pain or significant reduction of pain with this injection.

Those who have a successful diagnostic cervical medial branch block will likely have a successful response to radiofrequency neurotomy, or ablation, of those medical branch nerves. During this procedure, high-frequency current is transmitted through a radiofrequency (RF) probe, which is placed inside an RF cannula positioned in proximity to the desired nerve. The current flowing through the probe's active tip raises the temperature in a small area around the active tip to 80–85 °C for 90 s, leading to a lesion that interrupts unwanted neural signals [35]. Sham-controlled and well-performed prospective studies have demonstrated the efficacy of cervical medial branch neurotomy for the treatment of cervicogenic headache and neck pain [36–38]. Radiofrequency neurotomy of the third occipital nerve at the level of the C2–3 cervical facet has shown a significant reduction in pain, with 88% of those treated with radiofrequency neurotomy experiencing a successful outcome with a median duration of pain relief for 297 days [36]. However, patients in these studies were not studied for the presence of migraine.

Pulsed radiofrequency is a nonablative percutaneous treatment where pulsed stimulation typically at 42 °C—at a temperature below 45 °C, the minimum temperature for irreversible tissue destruction—achieves neuromodulation by proposed mechanisms, including increasing the level of endogenous opioid precursor mRNA, regulating proinflammatory gene expression at the injury site, and possibly by causing microstructure damage [39–41]. In a randomized clinical trial of patients with chronic migraine, 20 patients were treated with pulsed radiofrequency of the third occipital nerve and C3 medial branch (C2–3) joint innervation, and 20 patients were treated with a sham procedure. There was a significant decrease in headache days and disability scores in the pulsed radiofrequency group at 1 month, 2 months, and 6 months after the ablation [42]. Similarly, another randomized, double-blind study of patients with migraine and occipital nerve tenderness or occipital neuralgia found that pulsed radiofrequency of the occipital nerves provided greater and longer-lasting pain relief, sustainable through a 6-month follow-up, compared to anesthetic and deposteroid blockade of the occipital nerves along with a sham ablation [43].

Cervical Joint Steroid Injection

Atlanto-occipital joint injections have been less studied and are rarely performed due to significant risk, especially related to the proximity of the vertebral artery to the needle trajectory. In a study of patients with upper neck pain and headache, careful examination of the atlanto-occipital joint had a decreased range of motion and reproduction of their usual pain, and there was a > 50% pain reduction in 83% of participants [44]. Patients in this study were not evaluated for the presence of migraine.

Atlanto-axial joint injections can be performed safely but carry significant risk and should only be performed by experienced interventionalists. The interventionalist must take care not to let the needle tip stray medial (risking dural puncture and spinal cord injury) or lateral (risking injury to the vertebral artery) during the performance of the procedure. The best evidence for its efficacy is in patients with rheumatoid arthritis, with a randomized, double-blind, double-dummy, comparative effectiveness study showing that atlanto-axial joint injections with steroids and oral placebo pills outperformed atlanto-axial joint injections without steroids and oral steroid pills [45]. While headaches stemming from atlantoaxial (C1-C2) and atlantooccipital (C0-C1) joints have been described and have responded to interventions aimed at these joints, there have been no studies evaluating the role of interventions at these levels in patients with migraine [44, 46, 47].

Pharmaceutical Interventions and Use of Opioids

There are several categories of medications used in the treatment of chronic pain conditions that have also shown benefits as prophylactic treatment for migraine. Antidepressants such as tricyclic antidepressants (TCAs), serotonin norepinephrine reuptake inhibitors (SNRIs), antiepileptics such as topiramate, valproate, and gabapentin, and other medications and supplements such as memantine and magnesium are used as preventative therapies for the treatment of migraine and these can also be helpful for the treatment of chronic noncephalic pain [48]. Clinicians can reduce polypharmacy and help patients avoid the use of analgesics, which may cause medication overuse headaches, by selecting migraine preventives that can also treat the patient's comorbid pain disorders. For example, the TCAs amitriptyline and nortriptyline, SNRIs duloxetine and venlafaxine, and antiepileptic gabapentin are first-line therapies for the treatment of neuropathic pain [49, 50]. Other antileptics such as valproate have also shown benefits in the treatment of neuropathic pain [49]. TCAs, SNRIs, and gabapentin are also used to treat pain in those with fibromyalgia and phantom limb pain [51, 52]. In addition to being a treatment option for chronic migraine prevention, memantine has also been shown to be beneficial in CRPS, fibromyalgia, and phantom limb pain [53, 54]. Although not specifically studied in CRPS, the authors frequently use TCAs and SNRIs in the treatment of neuropathic pain in CRPS. Gabapentin may also have some beneficial role in the treatment of chronic pelvic pain in women [55]. Intravenous magnesium can be an effective adjuvant therapy in postoperative abdominal pain, low back pain with a neuropathic component, fibromyalgia, CRPS, and neuropathic pain [56, 57]. Nonsteroidal anti-inflammatory drugs (NSAIDS), which is used as an acute/abortive therapy for migraine, are also often used as an anti-inflammatory agent and an analgesic in myofascial pain, painful arthritic conditions, and soft tissue injuries [58]. While some studies have suggested topiramate may be useful in the treatment of neuropathic pain, others have not shown benefit [59–61].

However, some pharmaceutical approaches for migraine have not been proven effective for noncephalic chronic pain syndromes to date. Calcitonin genre-related peptide (CGRP) has been shown to play a role in our current understanding of the pathophysiology of migraine, and CGRP antagonists, discussed elsewhere in this book, are effective for migraine prevention. CGRP has been shown in animal models to cause peripheral nociceptive sensitization, is found in abundance in the trigeminal ganglion neurons that innervate meningeal structures, and is also found in posterior gray columns of the spinal cord, as well as nerves innervating these lamina [62, 63]. Despite its potential, CGRP inhibitors have not yet been shown to be effective for noncephalic chronic pain conditions. In the only RCT studying a CGRP inhibitor for a noncephalic pain disorder, galcanezumab, an anti-CGRP blocker, failed to show a reduction in symptoms or signs associated with knee osteoarthritis [64].

Opioids

The use of opioids for the treatment of migraine is not recommended but given their widespread use, clinicians will encounter patients with migraine who are using opioids either for migraine or for other painful conditions. Opioids share key properties with naturally occurring alkaloids derived from the opium poppy, which react with mu, delta, and kappa opioid receptors and can be in the naturally occurring form (opiate) or a semisynthetic or a fully synthetic form (opioids) [65]. Opioid use for noncancer pain increased in the 1990s and 2000s [65, 66]. In the early 2000s, opioids were the most widely used class of medication for treating acute migraine in emergency rooms in North America, with rates up to 60% of those with an acute migraine receiving an opioid, with the majority of these patients being treated without any other nonopioid parenteral medications [67, 68].

Of the 2388 patients with migraine who used prescription medications from 2012 to 2013 in the CaMEO study, 36.3% used opioids [69]. Those in the CaMEO study who used opioids for the treatment of acute migraine had a worse quality of life, more headache-related burden, and more comorbidities than those who did not use opioids [69]. The use of opioids increases the risk of the progression of migraine from episodic to chronic. Longitudinal population studies, case-control studies, and clinic-based studies have shown that exposure to opioids is consistently associated with the development of chronic daily headaches, and around 8 days per month is the critical exposure dose [3, 4, 70–72]. Of the 5796 persons with migraine surveyed in the AMPP study from 2005 to 2009, 30% were either current or previous opioid users [3]. This study found that those who had used opioids in the past, or were currently using opioids, had higher headache-related disability scores, higher monthly headache frequency, and a higher prevalence of depression and anxiety compared to those who were not opioid users [3].

Daily use of opioids for the treatment of chronic migraine or refractory chronic daily headaches carries significant concerns. In a large group of patients with chronic headaches treated with daily opioids, about a quarter had improvement initially; however, in those who showed initial improvement in headache severity, there was no improvement in disability scores [65, 73]. Furthermore, about half of the participants had reported dose violations, lost prescriptions, obtaining opioids from multiple sources, required dose escalations, etc., which raise concerns for aberrancy, misuse and abuse, addiction, and increased risk of overdose [73].

There are several reasons why opioids may lead to the above poor outcomes. Even brief periods of exposure to opioids can lead to opioid-induced hyperalgesia, a paradoxical phenomenon where those who are exposed to opioids develop a greater sensitivity to pain and an increase in pain intensity with a decrease in pain perception threshold [74–76]. Cholecystokinin upregulation exposure in the rostral ventromedial medulla due to opioids may lead to hyperalgesia and increased pain transmission seen in opioid-induced hyperalgesia by activating descending medullary pain facilitation [66, 77]. Chronic opioid exposure may also upregulate CGRP in primary afferent neurons and activate N-methyl-D-aspartate glutamic receptors, which can lead to opioid tolerance and increase spinal cord dynorphin level, which acts as a pro-nociceptive factor and may induce a neuroexcitatory state via activation of toll-like receptors [66, 78].

Tapering and discontinuation of opioid therapy for the treatment of migraine, especially when there is a clinical concern for medication overuse headache and/or opioid-induced hyperalgesia, are necessary for successful treatment. Headache-related disability scores, depression and anxiety, and headache frequency are lower in those who were previously treated with opioids for migraine and have since discontinued this class of medication compared with those who are actively taking opioids [3, 79]. Discontinuation of the overused medication in medication overuse headaches has also been shown to decrease monthly headache days and revert chronic migraine to episodic migraine [80, 81].

There is a clear benefit to tapering and discontinuing opioids in the treatment of the vast majority of people with migraine. However, opioid tapering must be done with caution, as this process can lead to adverse events for the patient in addition to the opioid withdrawal symptoms of hypertension, tachycardia, restlessness, diaphoresis, tremor, abdominal pain and diarrhea, and myalgia and arthralgia. A retrospective cohort study examined 113,618 patients who were on long-term (greater than 12 months) stable doses of opioids ≥50 morphine milligram equivalents per day and measured drug overdose or withdrawal and mental health crises such as depression, anxiety, or suicide attempts. Tapering events were associated with a higher risk of opioid overdose and mental health crisis [82]. Monthly dose reduction velocities higher than 10% per month of morphine milligram equivalents were associated with a higher risk of overdose and mental health crisis [82] cephalic pain disorder, galcanezumab, an anti-CGRP blocker, failed to show a reduction in symptoms or signs associated with knee osteoarthritis [64] (Table 10.2).

Currently, there are no steadfast guidelines for tapering rate/velocity for opioid doses. The Centers for Disease Control suggests that a decrease of 10% of the opioid dose per month is reasonable, and a decrease of 10% per week may be appropriate for patients who have been treated with opioids for a shorter term, i.e., weeks to months [83]. The United States Department of Health and Human Services has put forth a guide to aid clinicians with opioid dose reduction for those who are treated with long-term opioids, which highlights that a taper should be slow enough to minimize opioid withdrawal symptoms and suggests that a 10% or slower taper per month may be better

Table 10.2 Therapeutic roles of common medications used in the treatment of migraine for other pain disorders

	TCA	SNRI	Gabapentin	Valproate	Memantine	Magnesium	NSAIDs
Neuropathic pain	+	+	+	+		+	
Fibromyalgia	+	+			+	+	
CRPS			+		+	+	
Phantom limb pain	+		+		+		
Chronic pelvic pain	+		+				
Myofascial pain							+
Arthritis pain							+

TCA Tricyclic antidepressant, *SNRI* Serotonin norepinephrine reuptake inhibitor, *NSAIDs* Nonsteroidal anti-inflammatory drugs. *CRPS* complex regional pain syndrome tolerated than a more rapid taper [84]. Other strategies have also been suggested, including a recommendation to decrease the dose by 10% of the original dose every 5 to 7 days until 30% of the original dose is reached, followed by a weekly decrease by 10% of the remaining dose [85]. There are also suggested protocols with faster tapers. For example, the Department of Veterans Affairs and the Department of Defense recommend a dose decrease of 5–20% per month in most but do also recommend a taper by 20% to 50% of the starting dose per week, or a daily decrease by 20% to 50% of the initial dose down to a 30–45 mg of morphine equivalents per day followed by decreases every 2–5 days in several special situations such as diversion, illegal activities, or when the risk of a slow taper or continuing the opioid outweigh the risks associated with rapid tapers [86, 87].

We recommend reducing the morphine milligram equivalents by ≤10% per month, with close clinical follow-up to evaluate for withdrawal symptoms, which can be treated supportively with medications such as clonidine, baclofen, diphenhydramine, and other medications as indicated, as well as evaluate for psychiatric and psychological disturbances that may arise or become exacerbated during the opioid dose tapering process [87].

An equianalgesic table (Table 10.3) can be used to assist with doing calculations for performing a wean/taper by ≤10% per month in patients on multiple opioids.

In patients with medication overuse headaches as a result of opioid use in addition to migraine, providers should consider an approach utilizing concomitant weaning of opioids by ≤10% or less per month, optimizing migraine preventative medications and/or percutaneous interventions, and adding nonopioid acute migraine treatments. A course of corticosteroids may also be considered [80]. Some patients may warrant an elective admission for parental therapies such as intravenous dihydroergotamine.

Table 10.3 Equianalgesic doses for commonly prescribed doses

Opioid	Conversion factor
Codeine	0.15
Fentanyl transdermal (in mcg/hr)	2.4
Hydrocodone	1
Hydromorphone	4
Methadone: 1–20 mg/day	4
Methadone: 21–40 mg/day	8
Methadone: 41–60 mg/day	10
Methadone: ≥61–80 mg/day	12
Morphine	1
Oxycodone	1.5
Oxymorphone	3
Tapentadol	0.4

Adapted from https://www.cdc.gov/opioids/providers/prescribing/guideline.html

Conclusion

Many patients with migraine have other chronic pain disorders, and people with chronic pain disorders are more likely to have chronic migraine. People who have chronic migraine as well as other pain conditions appear to have worse physical and psychological functioning, more adverse live experiences, and higher healthcare utilization compared to those with chronic migraine without co-occurring pain conditions. For some patients with migraine and a comorbid chronic pain disorder, such as the aforementioned case of a patient with cervical facet arthropathy, which responded to radiofrequency ablation, the correct percutaneous intervention may be all the patient needs. However, in cases of patients with migraine and multiple chronic overlapping pain conditions, multidisciplinary care, including pharmacologic and nonpharmacologic treatments, is typically the best approach.

Recognition of chronic overlapping pain conditions is essential for the identification of patients with acute and subacute pain conditions who are at higher risk for transitioning to chronic pain states. Current gaps in knowledge that must be addressed to improve outcomes for this population include genetic and epigenetic studies, the identification of novel biomarkers, integrative studies to evaluate the impact of comorbidity, randomized controlled trials for interventional treatments in migraine, and improving pain education across multiple disciplines. Development of the best practice for this population is ongoing.

Central sensitization to pain, a complex process leading to pain pathway hyperexcitability and a reduced pain perception threshold, may lead to the chronification of migraine and other chronic pain conditions. Sensory and nociceptive inputs from peripheral nerves that innervate the head or upper cervical structures are involved in the pathophysiology of migraine and likely contribute to the central sensitization of pain associated with chronic migraine. These peripheral structures offer a target for percutaneous interventions for the treatment of suspected cervicogenic contributors to migraine chronification, and further research studying such interventions as occipital nerve blocks and cervical medical branch radiofrequency neurotomy is warranted.

Opioids are associated with greater headache-related burden, more comorbidities, and worse quality of life and can lead to migraine chronification. We recommend against initiating opioids for the treatment of migraine in the vast majority of patients. In patients already on chronic opioid therapy, caution should be used when tapering opioid doses to avoid adverse physiological and psychological outcomes, and a dose reduction of ≤10% of total morphine milligram equivalents per month typically prevents undesired outcomes associated with opioid tapering, such as precipitating opioid withdrawal or mental health crises.

Teaching Points

1. Comorbid pain disorders are reported in up to 64% of patients who have migraine. Some of these comorbid conditions include temporomandibular joint disease, neck pain, musculoskeletal pain, fibromyalgia, irritable bowel syndrome, and chronic regional pain syndrome.
2. Chronic migraine and comorbid noncephalic pain disorders are associated with worse physical function, psychosocial function, healthcare utilization, and adverse life experiences when compared to chronic migraine in isolation.
3. Central sensitization is likely a shared pathophysiological mechanism of both migraine and noncephalic pain disorders.
4. Migraine and cervicogenic headache can have overlap, and clinicians treating patients with migraine should be vigilant for possible cervicogenic contributors.
5. Several percutaneous treatment options for migraine and other painful conditions involving the head and neck are currently used in clinical practice, including trigger point injections, occipital nerve blocks, atlanto-occipital and atlantoaxial joint intraarticular corticosteroid injections, and cervical medial branch blocks and radiofrequency ablation for facet joint mediated pain which can refer to the head and may be accompanied by migrainous symptoms.
6. There is a clear benefit to tapering and discontinuing opioids in the treatment of the vast majority of people with migraine. However, opioid tapering must be done with caution, as this process can lead to adverse events for the patient, including symptoms of physiological withdrawal and psychological distress.
7. We recommend reducing the morphine milligram equivalents by ≤10% per month, with close clinical follow-up to evaluate for withdrawal symptoms, which can be treated supportively with medications, as well as to evaluate for psychiatric and psychological disturbances which may arise or become exacerbated during the opioid dose tapering process.

Case

A 63-year-old woman with a diagnosis of chronic migraine without aura, diagnosed by a general neurologist, is referred to the pain medicine clinic for further evaluation and treatment. A review of general neurology records shows that she has pain with exacerbations rated at 8/10–10/10 intensity on a 0–10 numeric rating scale, which can last 10–24 h. The pain is located in the upper neck and back of the head (Fig. 10.2a), and radiates to her left more than right temple. Her pain is made worse with physical exertion and is accompanied by nausea, and it meets the diagnostic criteria for migraine if no other diagnosis is evident to the clinician.

She did not respond to treatments with propranolol, topiramate, nortriptyline, and onabotulinumtoxinA for migraine prevention, as well as NSAIDs, acetaminophen, sumatriptan, and eletriptan for exacerbations of her migraine. Upon further evaluation in the pain clinic, it becomes evident that her pain nearly always starts in her upper neck and radiates up to the back of her head. For several years, turning her head to either side led to excruciating pain without any radiation to her arms or down her spine. Examination revealed the reproduction of her headache with palpation over the cervical facet joints and with cervical facet loading maneuvers. Strength, reflexes, and sensory examination were without deficit. X-ray of her cervical spine revealed facet arthropathy (Fig. 10.2c). Based on the clinical history, physical examination findings, and review of diagnostic imaging, there was a suspicion that the cervical spine facet joints may be a significant contributor to her headaches (Fig. 10.2).

Case Discussion

The patient was diagnosed with a cervicogenic headache. Diagnostic cervical medial branch blocks of the C2–4 medial branches were performed with 0.3 ml of 2% lidocaine at each nerve. The diagnostic injection gave her 100% headache relief for 5 h. A diagnosis of the cervicogenic headache in the setting of cervical facet arthropathy was confirmed (Fig. 10.2b).

A radiofrequency ablation of these nerves was carried out at 80C for 90 s (Fig. 10.2d). At the two-month follow-up after the procedure, she denies having any headache exacerbations since the radiofrequency ablation. Six months after the procedure, she continues to have a greater than 75% reduction in the frequency and intensity of her head and neck pain.

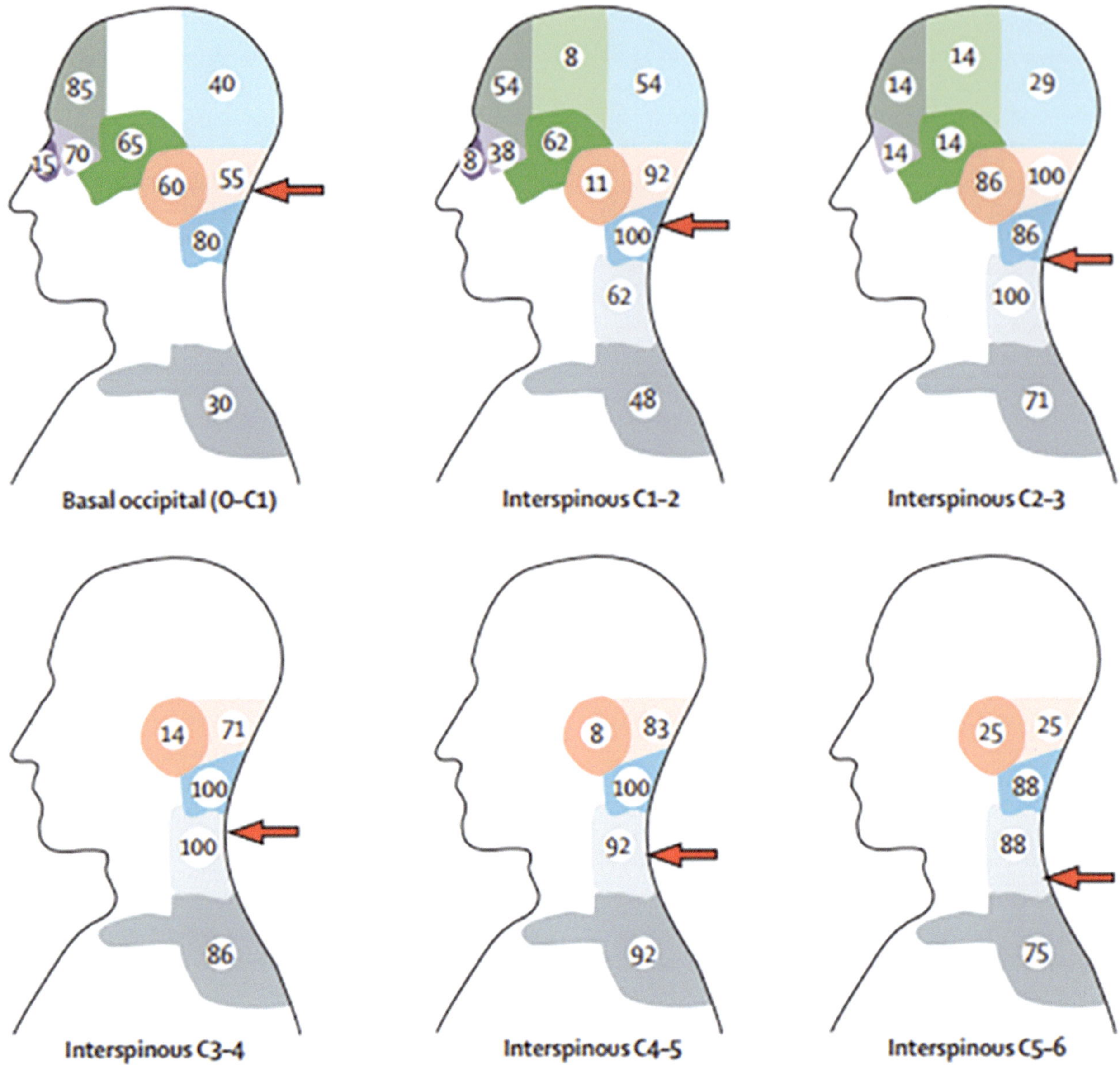

Fig. 10.2 Referred pain patterns after noxious stimulation of the basal occipital periosteum and interspinous muscles at C1–2, C2–3, C3–4, C4–5, and C5–6. The more cephalad the site of stimulation, the more likely it is that pain will be referred to distant regions of the head. The numbers indicate the percentage of individuals who reported pain in the area shown after stimulation at each segmental level. The arrows indicate the approximate site of stimulation. (Adapted from Campbell and Parsons, with permission from Lippincott Williams & Wilkins (J Nerv Ment Dis, 99 (1944), pp. 544–551). Bogduk N, Govind J. Cervicogenic headache: an assessment of the evidence on clinical diagnosis, invasive tests, and treatment. Lancet Neurol. 2009 Oct;8 (10):959–68. doi: 10.1016/S1474-4422(09)70209-1. PMID: 19747657)

Questions and Answers

1. Which treatment for cervical facet joint pain has the strongest evidence?
   A. Cervical epidural steroid injection
   B. Cervical intra-articular facet injection
   C. Cervical medial branch blocks as prelude to radiofrequency ablation
   D. Trigger point injections

The correct answer is C. Multiple studies have shown efficacy of this intervention for cervicogenic headaches and cervical facet joint pain. Furthermore, in those with chronic migraine, pulsed radiofrequency ablation was shown to decrease headache days and disability scores at 1 month, 2 months, and 6 months after the ablation [39] and provides longer lasting pain relief, sustainable through a 6-month follow up, compared to anesthetic and deposteroid blockade of the occipital nerves [43]

2. A patient on 100 morphine milligram equivalents daily is interested in tapering off of opioids. Which is the most appropriate initial percentage reduction per visit?
   A. 10%
   B. 20%
   C. 25%
   D. 50%

The correct answer is A. Tapering chronic opioid doses by greater than 10 morphine milligram equivalents per month is associated with risk of overdose and mental health crisis

References

1. Nahin RL. Estimates of pain prevalence and severity in adults: United States, 2012. J Pain [Internet] 2015 Aug 1 [cited 2022 Aug 28];16(8):769–780. Available from: https://pubmed.ncbi.nlm.nih.gov/26028573/
2. Vos T, Allen C, Arora M, Barber RM, Bhutta ZA, Brown A, et al. Global, regional, and national incidence, prevalence, and years lived with disability for 310 diseases and injuries, 1990–2015: a systematic analysis for the Global Burden of Disease Study 2015. The Lancet [Internet]. 2016 [cited 2022 Aug 28];388:1545–1602. Available from: www.thelancet.com
3. Buse DC, Pearlman SH, Reed ML, Serrano D, Ng-Mak DS, Lipton RB. Opioid use and dependence among persons with migraine: results of the ampp study. Headache. 2012;52(1):18–36.
4. Bigal ME, Lipton RB. Overuse of acute migraine medications and migraine chronification. Curr Pain Headache Rep [Internet]. 2009 [cited 2021 Nov 14];13(4):301–307. Available from: https://pubmed-ncbi-nlm-nih-gov.proxy.library.vanderbilt.edu/19586594/
5. Plesh O, Adams SH, Gansky SA. Self-reported comorbid pains in severe headaches or migraines in a US national sample. Headache [Internet]. 2012 [cited 2021 Dec 6];52(6):946–956. Available from: https://pubmed.ncbi.nlm.nih.gov/22553936/
6. Lipton RB, Fanning KM, Buse DC, Martin VT, Reed ML, Manack Adams A, et al. Identifying natural subgroups of migraine based on comorbidity and concomitant condition profiles: results of the chronic migraine epidemiology and outcomes (CaMEO) study. Headache [Internet]. 2018 Jul 1 [cited 2021 Dec 6];58(7):933–947. Available from: https://pubmed.ncbi.nlm.nih.gov/30024028/
7. Calhoun AH, Ford S, Millen C, Finkel AG, Truong Y, Nie Y. The prevalence of neck pain in migraine. Headache [Internet] 2010 Sep [cited 2021 Dec 6];50(8):1273–1277. Available from: https://pubmed.ncbi.nlm.nih.gov/20100298/
8. Cole JA, Rothman KJ, Cabral HJ, Zhang Y, Farraye FA. Migraine, fibromyalgia, and depression among people with IBS: a prevalence study. BMC Gastroenterol [Internet] 2006 Sep 28 [cited 2021 Dec 6];6. Available from: https://pubmed.ncbi.nlm.nih.gov/17007634/
9. Whealy M, Nanda S, Vincent A, Mandrekar J, Cutrer FM. Fibromyalgia in migraine: a retrospective cohort study. J Headache Pain [Internet] 2018 Jul 31 [cited 2021 Dec 6];19(1). Available from: https://pubmed.ncbi.nlm.nih.gov/30066109/
10. Peterlin BL, Rosso AL, Nair S, Young WB, Schwartzman RJ. Migraine may be a risk factor for the development of complex regional pain syndrome. Cephalalgia [Internet]. 2010 Feb [cited 2021 Dec 6];30(2):214–223. Available from: https://pubmed.ncbi.nlm.nih.gov/19614690/
11. Uluduz D, Cakmak S, Ozge A, Ucbilek E, Sezgin O, Soylemez F, et al. A link between migraine, tension type headache and irritable bowel syndrome: clinical and genetic indicators (P4.120). Neurology. 2016;86(16 Supplement)
12. Barad MJ, Sturgeon JA, Hong J, Aggarwal AK, Mackey SC. Characterization of chronic overlapping pain conditions in patients with chronic migraine: a CHOIR study. Headache. 2021 June 1;61(6):872–81.
13. Woolf CJ. Central sensitization: implications for the diagnosis and treatment of pain. Pain [Internet] 2011 Mar [cited 2021 Dec 6];152(3 Suppl). Available from: https://pubmed.ncbi.nlm.nih.gov/20961685/
14. Boyer N, Dallel R, Artola A, Monconduit L. General trigeminospinal central sensitization and impaired descending pain inhibitory controls contribute to migraine progression. Pain [Internet]. 2014 [cited 2022 Feb 5];155(7):1196–1205. Available from: https://pubmed-ncbi-nlm-nih-gov.proxy.library.vanderbilt.edu/24631586/
15. Bigal ME, Lipton RB. What predicts the change from episodic to chronic migraine? Curr Opin Neurol [Internet]. 2009 Jun [cited 2022 Feb 5];22(3):269–276. Available from: https://pubmed-ncbi-nlm-nih-gov.proxy.library.vanderbilt.edu/19381087/
16. Bernstein CA, Nir RR, Noseda R, Fulton AB, Huntington S, Lee AJ, et al. The migraine eye: distinct rod-driven retinal pathways' response to dim light challenges the visual cortex hyperexcitability theory. Pain [Internet]. 2019 Mar 1 [cited 2021 Dec 6];160(3):569–578. Available from: https://pubmed.ncbi.nlm.nih.gov/30376534/
17. Bartsch T, Goadsby PJ. The trigeminocervical complex and migraine: current concepts and synthesis. Curr Pain Headache Rep [Internet]. 2003 [cited 2021 Dec 6];7(5):371–376. Available from: https://pubmed.ncbi.nlm.nih.gov/12946290/
18. Bartsch T, Goadsby PJ. Stimulation of the greater occipital nerve induces increased central excitability of dural afferent input. Brain [Internet] 2002 [cited 2021 Dec 6];125(Pt 7):1496–1509. Available from: https://pubmed.ncbi.nlm.nih.gov/12077000/
19. McCarberg B, Peppin J. Pain pathways and nervous system plasticity: learning and memory in pain. Pain Med [Internet] 2019 Dec 1 [cited 2021 Dec 6];20(12):2421–2437. Available from: https://pubmed.ncbi.nlm.nih.gov/30865778/
20. Nevalainen MT, Foran PJ, Roedl JB, Zoga AC, Morrison WB. Cervical facet oedema: prevalence, correlation to symptoms, and follow-up imaging. Clin Radiol [Internet]. 2016 June 1 [cited 2021 Nov 15];71(6):570–575. Available from: https://pubmed-ncbi-nlm-nih-gov.proxy.library.vanderbilt.edu/27055743/
21. Aprill C, Dwyer A, Bogduk N. Cervical zygapophyseal joint pain patterns. II: a clinical evaluation. Spine (Phila Pa 1976) [Internet] 1990 [cited 2021 Nov 15];15(6):458–461. Available from: https://pubmed-ncbi-nlm-nih-gov.proxy.library.vanderbilt.edu/2402683/
22. Hurley RW, Adams MCB, Barad M, Bhaskar A, Bhatia A, Chadwick A, et al. Consensus practice guidelines on interventions for cervical spine (facet) joint pain from a multispecialty international working group. Reg Anesth Pain Med [Internet]. 2021 Nov 11 [cited 2021 Nov 15];rapm-2021-103031. Available from: https://pubmed-ncbi-nlm-nih-gov.proxy.library.vanderbilt.edu/34764220/
23. Robbins MS, Kuruvilla D, Blumenfeld A, Charleston L, Sorrell M, Robertson CE, et al. Trigger point injections for headache disorders: expert consensus methodology and narrative review. Headache. 2014 Oct 1;54(9):1441–59.
24. Fernández-de-las-Peñas C, Ge HY, Alonso-Blanco C, González-Iglesias J, Arendt-Nielsen L. Referred pain areas of active myofascial trigger points in head, neck, and shoulder muscles, in chronic tension type headache. J Bodyw Mov Ther [Internet] 2010 Oct [cited 2022 Aug 21];14(4):391–396. Available from: https://pubmed.ncbi.nlm.nih.gov/20850047/
25. Blumenfeld A, Ashkenazi A, Grosberg B, Napchan U, Narouze S, Nett B, et al. Patterns of use of peripheral nerve blocks and trigger point injections among headache practitioners in the USA: results of the American headache society interventional procedure survey (AHS-IPS). Headache [Internet]. 2010 [cited 2022 Jul 4];50(6):937–942. Available from: https://pubmed-ncbi-nlm-nih-gov.proxy.library.vanderbilt.edu/20618812/

26. Korucu O, Dagar S, Çorbacioglu K, Emektar E, Cevik Y. The effectiveness of greater occipital nerve blockade in treating acute migraine-related headaches in emergency departments. Acta Neurol Scand [Internet]. 2018 Sep 1 [cited 2021 Nov 15];138(3):212–218. Available from: https://pubmed-ncbi-nlm-nih-gov.proxy.library.vanderbilt.edu/29744871/
27. Friedman BW, Mohamed S, Robbins MS, Irizarry E, Tarsia V, Pearlman S, et al. A randomized, sham-controlled trial of bilateral greater occipital nerve blocks with bupivacaine for acute migraine patients refractory to standard emergency department treatment with metoclopramide. Headache [Internet]. 2018 Oct 1 [cited 2021 Nov 14];58(9):1427–1434. Available from: https://pubmed-ncbi-nlm-nih-gov.proxy.library.vanderbilt.edu/30144034/
28. Oswald JC, Schuster NM. A randomized, double-dummy, emergency department-based study of greater occipital nerve block with bupivacaine versus intravenous metoclopramide for treatment of migraine: a comment. Headache. 2021 Jan 1;61(1):218.
29. Gul HL, Ozon AO, Karadas O, Koc G, Inan LE. The efficacy of greater occipital nerve blockade in chronic migraine: a placebo-controlled study. Acta Neurol Scand [Internet]. 2017 Aug 1 [cited 2021 Nov 15];136(2):138–144. Available from: https://pubmed-ncbi-nlm-nih-gov.proxy.library.vanderbilt.edu/27910088/
30. Cuadrado ML, Aledo-Serrano Á, Navarro P, López-Ruiz P, Fernández-De-Las-Peñas C, González-Suárez I, et al. Short-term effects of greater occipital nerve blocks in chronic migraine: a double-blind, randomised, placebo-controlled clinical trial. Cephalalgia [Internet]. 2017 Aug 1 [cited 2021 Nov 15];37(9):864–872. Available from: https://pubmed-ncbi-nlm-nih-gov.proxy.library.vanderbilt.edu/27296456/
31. Palamar D, Uluduz D, Saip S, Erden G, Unalan H, Akarirmak U. Ultrasound-guided greater occipital nerve block: an efficient technique in chronic refractory migraine without aura? – PubMed. Pain Physician [Internet] 2015 Mar [cited 2021 Nov 15];18(2):153–162. Available from: https://pubmed-ncbi-nlm-nih-gov.proxy.library.vanderbilt.edu/25794201/
32. Inan LE, Inan N, Karadaş O, Gül HL, Erdemoğlu AK, Türkel Y, et al. Greater occipital nerve blockade for the treatment of chronic migraine: a randomized, multicenter, double-blind, and placebo-controlled study. Acta Neurol Scand [Internet] 2015 Oct 1 [cited 2021 Nov 15];132(4):270–277. Available from: https://pubmed--ncbi-nlm-nih-gov.proxy.library.vanderbilt.edu/25765043/
33. Barad M, Ailani J, Hakim SM, Kissoon NR, Schuster NM. Percutaneous interventional Strategies for migraine prevention: a systematic review and practice Guideline. Pain Med. 2021;0(August):1–25.
34. Hoffmann J, Mehnert J, Koo EM, May A. Greater occipital nerve block modulates nociceptive signals within the trigeminocervical complex. J Neurol Neurosurg Psychiatry [Internet] 2021 [cited 2021 Nov 20];92(12). Available from: https://pubmed.ncbi.nlm.nih.gov/34312221/
35. Cosman ER, Dolensky JR, Hoffman RA. Factors that affect radiofrequency heat lesion size. Pain Med (United States) [Internet]. 2014 Dec 1 [cited 2022 Feb 5];15(12):2020–2036. Available from: https://academic.oup.com/painmedicine/article/15/12/2020/1817249
36. Govind J, King W, Bailey B, Bogduk N. Radiofrequency neurotomy for the treatment of third occipital headache. J Neurol Neurosurg Psychiatry [Internet]. 2003 Jan 1 [cited 2021 Dec 7];74(1):88. Available from: /pmc/articles/PMC1738184/?report=abstract.
37. Jang BL, Jung YP, Park J, Dong JL, Sang DK, Heung SC. Clinical efficacy of radiofrequency cervical zygapophyseal neurotomy in patients with chronic cervicogenic headache. J Korean Med Sci [Internet] 2007 [cited 2021 Dec 7];22(2):326–329. Available from: https://pubmed.ncbi.nlm.nih.gov/17449944/
38. van Suijlekom HA, van Kleef M, Barendse GA, Sluijter ME, Sjaastad O, Weber WE. Radiofrequency cervical zygapophyseal joint neurotomy for cervicogenic headache: a prospective study of 15 patients. Funct Neurol. 13(4):297–303.
39. Vallejo R, Tilley DM, Williams J, Labak S, Aliaga L, Benyamin RM. Pulsed radiofrequency modulates pain regulatory gene expression along the nociceptive pathway. Pain Physician [Internet]. 2013 [cited 2022 Jan 9];16:E601–E613. Available from: www.painphysicianjournal.comwww.painphysicianjournal.com
40. Moffett J, Fray LM, Kubat NJ. Activation of endogenous opioid gene expression in human keratinocytes and fibroblasts by pulsed radiofrequency energy fields. J Pain Res [Internet]. 2012 [cited 2022 Jan 9];5:347–357. Available from: https://pubmed-ncbi-nlm-nih-gov.proxy.library.vanderbilt.edu/23055776/
41. Erdine S, Bilir A, Cosman ER, Cosman ER. Ultrastructural changes in axons following exposure to pulsed radiofrequency fields. Pain Pract [Internet] 2009 Nov [cited 2022 Jan 9];9(6):407–417. Available from: https://pubmed-ncbi-nlm-nih-gov.proxy.library.vanderbilt.edu/19761513/
42. Yang Y, Huang X, Fan Y, Wang Y, Ma K. Efficacy of pulsed radiofrequency on cervical 2–3 posterior medial branches in treating chronic migraine: a randomized, controlled, and double-blind trial. Evid Based Complement Alternat Med [Internet]. 2015 [cited 2021 Nov 15];2015. Available from: https://pubmed-ncbi-nlm-nih-gov.proxy.library.vanderbilt.edu/26170880/
43. Cohen SP, Lee Peterlin B, Fulton L, Neely ET, Kurihara C, Gupta A, et al. Randomized, double-blind, comparative-effectiveness study comparing pulsed radiofrequency to steroid injections for occipital neuralgia or migraine with occipital nerve tenderness. Pain [Internet]. 2015 [cited 2021 Nov 15];156(12):2585–2594. Available from: https://pubmed-ncbi-nlm-nih-gov.proxy.library.vanderbilt.edu/26447705/
44. Lee DG, Cho YW, Jang SH, Son SM, Kim GJ, Ahn SH. Effectiveness of intra-articular steroid injection for atlanto-occipital joint pain. Pain Med [Internet]. 2015 June 1 [cited 2021 Nov 15];16(6):1077–1082. Available from: https://pubmed-ncbi-nlm-nih-gov.proxy.library.vanderbilt.edu/25105892/
45. Hetta DF, Elawamy AM, Hassanein MM, Aljohi AS, Hasan RAR, Mohammed NAA, et al. Efficacy of atlantoaxial joint glucocorticoid injection in patients with rheumatoid arthritis: a randomized trial. Pain Physician [Internet]. 2019 Jul 1 [cited 2022 Feb 5];22(4):E295–E302. Available from: https://pubmed-ncbi-nlm-nih-gov.proxy.library.vanderbilt.edu/31337171/
46. Aprill C, Axinn MJ, Bogduk N. Occipital headaches stemming from the lateral atlanto-axial (C1-2) joint. Cephalalgia [Internet] 2002 [cited 2021 Nov 15];22(1):15–22. Available from: https://pubmed-ncbi-nlm-nih-gov.proxy.library.vanderbilt.edu/11993608/
47. Zhou L, Hud-Shakoor Z, Hennessey C, Ashkenazi A. Upper cervical facet joint and spinal rami blocks for the treatment of cervicogenic headache. Headache [Internet]. 2010 Apr [cited 2021 Nov 15];50(4):657–663. Available from: https://pubmed-ncbi-nlm-nih-gov.proxy.library.vanderbilt.edu/20132336/
48. Robbins MS, Burch R. Preventive migraine treatment. Continuum (Minneap Minn) [Internet]. 2021 June 1 [cited 2022 Aug 21];27(3):613–632. Available from: https://pubmed.ncbi.nlm.nih.gov/34048395/
49. Baron R, Binder A, Wasner G. Neuropathic pain: diagnosis, pathophysiological mechanisms, and treatment. Lancet Neurol [Internet] 2010 Aug [cited 2022 Aug 21];9(8):807–819. Available from: https://pubmed.ncbi.nlm.nih.gov/20650402/
50. Bates D, Carsten Schultheis B, Hanes MC, Jolly SM, Chakravarthy K V Deer TR, et al. A comprehensive algorithm for management of neuropathic pain. Pain Med: The Official Journal of the American Academy of Pain Medicine [Internet] 2019 June 1 [cited 2022 Aug 21];20(Suppl 1):S2. Available from: /pmc/articles/PMC6544553/

51. Chinn S, Caldwell W, Gritsenko K. Fibromyalgia pathogenesis and treatment options update. Curr Pain Headache Rep [Internet] 2016 Mar 1 [cited 2022 Aug 21];20(4):1–10. Available from: https://pubmed.ncbi.nlm.nih.gov/26922414/
52. Urits I, Seifert D, Seats A, Giacomazzi S, Kipp M, Orhurhu V, et al. Treatment strategies and effective management of phantom limb-associated pain. Curr Pain Headache Rep [Internet]. 2019 Sep 1 [cited 2022 Aug 22];23(9). Available from: https://pubmed.ncbi.nlm.nih.gov/31359171/
53. Loy BM, Britt RB, Brown JN. Memantine for the treatment of phantom limb pain: a systematic review. J Pain Palliat Care Pharmacother [Internet] 2016 Oct 1 [cited 2022 Aug 21];30(4):276–283. Available from: https://pubmed.ncbi.nlm.nih.gov/27813692/
54. Duong S, Bravo D, Todd KJ, Finlayson RJ, Tran DQ. Treatment of complex regional pain syndrome: an updated systematic review and narrative synthesis. Can J Anesth[Internet] 2018;65(6):658–684. Available from: https://doi.org/10.1007/s12630-018-1091-5.
55. Speer LM, Mushkbar S, Erbele T. Chronic pelvic pain in women. Am Fam Physician [Internet] 2016 Mar 1 [cited 2022 Aug 21];93(5):380–387. Available from: https://pubmed.ncbi.nlm.nih.gov/26926975/
56. Urits I, Jung JW, Amgalan A, Fortier L, Anya A, Wesp B, et al. Utilization of magnesium for the treatment of chronic pain. Anesth Pain Med [Internet]. 2021 Feb 1 [cited 2022 Aug 21];11(1):1–10. Available from: /pmc/articles/PMC8236839/.
57. Park R, Ho AMH, Pickering G, Arendt-Nielsen L, Mohiuddin M, Gilron I. Efficacy and safety of magnesium for the management of chronic pain in adults: a systematic review. Anesth Analg [Internet] 2020 Sep 1 [cited 2022 Aug 21];131(3):764–775. Available from: https://pubmed.ncbi.nlm.nih.gov/32049671/
58. Bacchi S, Palumbo P, Sponta A, Coppolino MF. Clinical pharmacology of non-steroidal anti-inflammatory drugs: a review. Antiinflamm Antiallergy Agents Med Chem [Internet]. 2012 Oct 19 [cited 2022 Aug 21];11(1):52–64. Available from: https://pubmed.ncbi.nlm.nih.gov/22934743/
59. Wiffen PJ, Derry S, Lunn MPT, Moore RA. Topiramate for neuropathic pain and fibromyalgia in adults. Cochrane Database Syst Rev [Internet] 2013 May 31 [cited 2022 Aug 21];2013(5). Available from: https://pubmed.ncbi.nlm.nih.gov/23996081/
60. Eisenberg E, River Y, Shifrin A, Krivoy N. Antiepileptic drugs in the treatment of neuropathic pain. Drugs [Internet] 2007 [cited 2022 Aug 21];67(9):1265–1289. Available from: https://pubmed.ncbi.nlm.nih.gov/17547471/
61. Nazarbaghi S, Amiri-Nikpour AN, Foroughi Eghbal A, Valizadeh R. Comparison of the effect of topiramate versus gabapentin on neuropathic pain in patients with polyneuropathy: a randomized clinical trial. Electron Physician [Internet] 2017 Oct 25 [cited 2022 Aug 21];9(10):5617–5622. Available from: https://pubmed.ncbi.nlm.nih.gov/29238506/
62. Iyengar S, Johnson KW, Ossipov MH, Aurora SK. CGRP and the trigeminal system in migraine. Headache [Internet]. 2019 May 14 [cited 2020 Jan 11];59(5):659–681. Available from: https://onlinelibrary.wiley.com/doi/abs/10.1111/head.13529
63. Urits I, Li N, Bahrun E, Hakobyan H, Anantuni L, An D, et al. An evidence-based review of CGRP mechanisms in the propagation of chronic visceral pain. Best Pract Res Clin Anaesthesiol. 2020 Sep 1;34(3):507–16.
64. Jin Y, Smith C, Monteith D, Brown R, Camporeale A, McNearney TA, et al. CGRP blockade by galcanezumab was not associated with reductions in signs and symptoms of knee osteoarthritis in a randomized clinical trial. Osteoarthritis Cartilage [Internet] 2018 Dec 1 [cited 2022 Jul 4];26(12):1609–1618. Available from: https://pubmed-ncbi-nlm-nih-gov.proxy.library.vanderbilt.edu/30240937/
65. Levin M. Opioids in headache. Headache. 2014;54(1):12–21.
66. Tepper SJ. Opioids should not be used in migraine. Headache. 2012 May;52(SUPPL. 1):30–4.
67. Vinson DR. Treatment patterns of isolated benign headache in US emergency departments. Ann Emerg Med [Internet] 2002 [cited 2021 Nov 14];39(3):215–222. Available from: https://pubmed--ncbi-nlm-nih-gov.proxy.library.vanderbilt.edu/11867972/
68. Colman I, Rothney A, Wright SC, Zilkalns B, Rowe BH. Use of narcotic analgesics in the emergency department treatment of migraine headache. Neurol Int 2004 May 25 [cited 2021 Nov 14];62(10):1695–1700. Available from: https://pubmed-ncbi-nlm-nih-gov.proxy.library.vanderbilt.edu/15159464/
69. Lipton RB, Buse DC, Friedman BW, Feder L, Adams AM, Fanning KM, et al. Characterizing opioid use in a US population with migraine: results from the CaMEO study. Neurology. 2020;95(5):e457–68.
70. Bigal ME, Lipton RB. Excessive opioid use and the development of chronic migraine. Pain [Internet]. 2009 Apr [cited 2021 Nov 14];142(3):179–182. Available from: https://pubmed-ncbi-nlm-nih-gov.proxy.library.vanderbilt.edu/19232469/
71. Bahra A, Walsh M, Menon S, Goadsby PJ. Does chronic daily headache arise de novo in association with regular use of analgesics? Headache [Internet]. 2003 Mar [cited 2021 Nov 14];43(3):179–190. Available from: https://pubmed-ncbi-nlm-nih-gov.proxy.library.vanderbilt.edu/12603636/
72. Bigal ME, Serrano D, Buse D, Scher A, Stewart WF, Lipton RB. Acute migraine medications and evolution from episodic to chronic migraine: a longitudinal population-based study. Headache [Internet]. 2008 Sep [cited 2021 Nov 14];48(8):1157–1168. Available from: https://pubmed-ncbi-nlm-nih-gov.proxy.library.vanderbilt.edu/18808500/
73. Saper JR, Lake AE, Hamel RL, Lutz TE, Branca B, Sims DB, et al. Daily scheduled opioids for intractable head pain: long-term observations of a treatment program. Neurol Int 2004 May 25 [cited 2021 Nov 15];62(10):1687–1694. Available from: https://pubmed--ncbi-nlm-nih-gov.proxy.library.vanderbilt.edu/15159463/
74. Mercadante S, Arcuri E, Santoni A. Opioid-induced tolerance and hyperalgesia. CNS Drugs 2019 33:10 [Internet]. 2019 Oct 1 [cited 2022 Jan 9];33(10):943–955. Available from: https://link-springer-com.proxy.library.vanderbilt.edu/article/10.1007/s40263-019-00660-0
75. Tröster A, Sittl R, Singler B, Schmelz M, Schüttler J, Koppert W. Modulation of remifentanil-induced analgesia and postinfusion hyperalgesia by parecoxib in humans. Anesthesiology [Internet] 2006 Nov [cited 2022 Jan 9];105(5):1016–1023. Available from: https://pubmed-ncbi-nlm-nih-gov.proxy.library.vanderbilt.edu/17065897/
76. Lee MO, Lee M, Silverman S, Hansen H, Patel V, Manchikanti L. A comprehensive review of opioid-induced hyperalgesia. Pain Physician [Internet]. 2011 [cited 2022 Jan 9];14:145–161. Available from: www.painphysicianjournal.com
77. Ossipov MH, Lai J, King T, Vanderah TW, Malan TP, Hruby VJ, et al. Antinociceptive and nociceptive actions of opioids. J Neurobiol [Internet] 2004 Oct [cited 2021 Nov 15];61(1):126–148. Available from: https://pubmed-ncbi-nlm-nih-gov.proxy.library.vanderbilt.edu/15362157/
78. Watkins LR, Hutchinson MR, Rice KC, Maier SF. The "toll" of opioid-induced glial activation: improving the clinical efficacy of opioids by targeting glia. Trends Pharmacol Sci [Internet] 2009 Nov [cited 2021 Nov 15];30(11):581–591. Available from: https://pubmed-ncbi-nlm-nih-gov.proxy.library.vanderbilt.edu/19762094/
79. Bendtsen L, Munksgaard SB, Tassorelli C, Nappi G, Katsarava Z, Lainez M, et al. Disability, anxiety and depression associated with medication-overuse headache can be considerably reduced by detoxification and prophylactic treatment. Results from a multicentre, multinational study (COMOESTAS project). Cephalalgia [Internet]. 2014 [cited 2021 Nov 15];34(6):426–433. Available from: https://pubmed-ncbi-nlm-nih-gov.proxy.library.vanderbilt.edu/24322480/

80. Diener HC, Holle D, Solbach K, Gaul C. Medication-overuse headache: risk factors, pathophysiology and management. Nat Rev Neurol [Internet] 2016 Oct 1 [cited 2021 Nov 14];12(10):575–583. Available from: https://pubmed-ncbi-nlm-nih-gov.proxy.library.vanderbilt.edu/27615418/
81. Tassorelli C, Jensen R, Allena M, de Icco R, Sances G, Katsarava Z, et al. A consensus protocol for the management of medication-overuse headache: evaluation in a multicentric, multinational study. Cephalalgia [Internet]. 2014 [cited 2021 Nov 15];34(9):645–655. Available from: https://pubmed-ncbi-nlm-nih-gov.proxy.library.vanderbilt.edu/24558185/
82. Agnoli A, Xing G, Tancredi DJ, Magnan E, Jerant A, Fenton JJ. Association of Dose Tapering with overdose or mental health crisis among patients prescribed long-term opioids. JAMA – J Am Med Assoc [Internet] 2021 Aug 3 [cited 2021 Nov 14];326(5):411–419. Available from: https://pubmed-ncbi-nlm-nih-gov.proxy.library.vanderbilt.edu/34342618/
83. Department of Health U, Services H, for Disease Control C. POCKET GUIDE: TAPERING OPIOIDS FOR CHRONIC PAIN *.
84. CDC. HHS Guide for clinicians on the appropriate dosage reduction or discontinuation of long-term opioid analgesics HHS guide for clinicians on the appropriate dosage reduction or discontinuation of long-term opioid analgesics this HHS guide for clinicians on the appropriate dosage reduction or discontinuation of long-term opioid analgesics. [cited 2021 Nov 15]; Available from: https://www.oregonpainguidance.org/guideline/tapering/.
85. Berna C, Kulich RJ, Rathmell JP. Tapering long-term opioid therapy in chronic noncancer pain: evidence and recommendations for everyday practice. Mayo Clin Proc [Internet]. 2015 June 1 [cited 2021 Nov 15];90(6):828–842. Available from: http://www.mayoclinicproceedings.org/article/S0025619615003031/fulltext
86. VA/DoD CLINICAL PRACTICE GUIDELINE FOR OPIOID THERAPY FOR CHRONIC PAIN The Opioid Therapy for Chronic Pain Work Group With support from. [cited 2021 Nov 15]; Available from: www.tricare.mil
87. Department of Veterans Affairs U, Administration H, academic detailing service P. Opioid Taper Decision Tool. [cited 2021 Dec 7]; Available from: https://vaww.portal2.va.gov/sites/ad/SitePages/Home.aspx

Migraine, Psychiatric Disorders and Psychopharmacology

11

Michelle Bravo, Maria Adelaida Rueda-Lara, and Noah Rosen

Introduction

Migraine is a prevalent neurological condition oftentimes accompanied by psychiatric comorbidities such as major depressive disorder (MDD), generalized anxiety disorder (GAD), bipolar disorder, panic disorder, post-traumatic stress disorder (PTSD), and social phobias [1–3]. Although this association is well known, this link has led to negative stigma and even dismissal of individuals presenting with migraine pain [4]. Proper treatment cannot occur without appropriate diagnosis—migraine is diagnosed in just over half of those who suffer from this condition [5]. In addition, psychiatric illness is often not prioritized in medical visits and may go undiagnosed, misdiagnosed, or inappropriately treated [6]. Patients with mood disorders and migraine are more likely to have higher disability assessment scores (i.e., MIDAS scores), greater functional impairment, and lower quality of life [7].

The purpose of this chapter is to provide an overview of the epidemiology of psychiatric comorbidities and migraine, to understand shared pathophysiological mechanisms, diagnosis, and pharmacological treatment.

Questions

1. Which treatment for episodic migraine prevention has class A evidence?
   A. Divalproex sodium
   B. Amitriptyline
   C. Lamotrigine
   D. OnabotulinumtoxinA
2. Which medication can be used for the co-management of bipolar disorder and cluster headache?
   A. Fremanezumab
   B. Clozapine
   C. Olanzapine
   D. Lithium

Epidemiology

Historically, the association between migraine and psychiatric comorbidities had been noted in 1895 by Dr. Liveing, who reported that patients with chronic headaches often times experienced depressive mood, irritability, anxiety, and attention deficit [8]. Dr. Wolff was the first to conduct a systematic study of these psychiatric comorbidities, coining his term "migraine personality," defined as "feelings of insecurity with tension manifested as inflexibility, conscientiousness, meticulousness, perfectionism, and resentment" [9, 10]. Epidemiological research has demonstrated an association between migraine and psychiatric disorders [11–13].

Major Depressive Disorder

MDD is a common problem. Among people with migraine, the 1-year prevalence of MDD is approxi-

The original version of the chapter has been revised. A correction to this chapter can be found at https://doi.org/10.1007/978-3-031-86923-5_41

M. Bravo (✉)
Department of Neurology, Division of Headache Medicine, University of Miami, Miami, FL, USA

M. A. Rueda-Lara
Department of Psychiatry and Behavioral Sciences, University of Miami, Miami, FL, USA

N. Rosen
Department of Neurology, Zucker School of Medicine, Northwell Health System, Manhasset, NY, USA

T. S. Monteith et al. (eds.), *Comprehensive Migraine Management*, https://doi.org/10.1007/978-3-031-86923-5_11

mately 14.7 per 100 (as compared to 7.3 per 100 in the general population), with a lifetime prevalence of 35% [14–16], and the odds ratio of migraine and MDD between 2.2 to 4.0 [17]. Furthermore, people with migraine with or without MDD have a higher risk of suicide than those without migraine [18]. Breslau et al. demonstrated over a 2-year period that MDD raised the incidence of migraine and the presence of migraine raised the incidence of MDD, demonstrating bi-directionality [19]. A study conducted by Zwart et al. suggested that increased frequency of migraine was predictive of a higher incidence of MDD and GAD [20].

Bipolar Disorder

Among people with migraine, the 1-year prevalence of bipolar disorder is as high as 8.8% [21], with adjusted odds ratio of 2.4 for lifetime risk of Bipolar I disorder in migraine without aura, and 7.3 in migraine with aura (as compared to 0.4 and 1.6 in the general population) [14, 16], with adjusted odds ratio of 2.5 for lifetime risk of Bipolar II disorder in migraine without aura, and 5.2 for migraine with aura [16].

Anxiety Disorders and Obsessive-Compulsive Disorder

Prevalence rates of GAD in the general population are about 5%, social phobia 3–13%, panic disorder 1–3.5%, and obsessive-compulsive disorder (OCD) about 2.5% [14]. In people with migraine, the 1-year prevalence of GAD has been estimated to be 9.8%, and social phobia prevalence about 6.6% [22]. The lifetime prevalence of GAD in people migraine was 54% compared to a control group with 27%, GAD was 10% (versus 2%), panic disorder 11% (versus 2%), and OCD 9% (versus 2%) [16], with a bidirectional association [23].

Relationship Between Psychiatric Disorders and Migraine

It is well established there is a link between migraine and psychiatric disorders from epidemiological and genetic evidence [24]. Studies have shown that psychiatric comorbidity is associated with increased migraine attacks, and psychiatric comorbidities are more commonly present in patients with chronic migraine (CM) [7]; thus, it is important to investigate shared biological mechanisms.

Genetic Factors

Genetic studies involving families and twins suggest there is an interplay between genetic and environmental factors. Twin studies estimate a 44% trait-specific heritability for migraine and 52% for MDD, with shared genetics accounting for 20% of the variance observed in migraine disorders and MDD [25]. Candidate gene association studies identify genetic variations linked with a specific trait or disease [26]. Studies have identified a relationship between gene polymorphisms in the 5-HTT (human serotonin transporter) gene promoter in individuals with anxiety-related personality traits that lead to decreased uptake of serotonin [27]. Lower serotonin levels are thought to facilitate cortical spreading of depression-induced trigeminal nociception in migraine by increasing cortical excitability and sensitivity of the trigeminovascular pathway [28–30]. Tryptophan hydroxylase 2 (TPH2 on chromosome 12) single nucleotide polymorphisms have been implicated in the pathophysiology of migraine due to its importance as a rate-limiting step in serotonin synthesis and may contribute to an increased risk of migraine and depression in Whites [24]. Other theories include dopaminergic system dysfunction caused by multiple polymorphisms, MTHFR gene mutations, genes affecting the GABAergic system, and brain-derived neurotrophic factor single nucleotide polymorphisms, which have been linked to an increased risk of migraine and depression [24].

Shared Pathophysiology

Patients who have CM have been found to have dysregulated HPA axis [31]. Various neurotransmitters-- orexin, melatonin, dopamine, somatostatin, and antidiuretic hormone have been implicated as potential culprits, with studies demonstrating decreased peak nocturnal prolactin levels, increased cortisol levels, and delayed nocturnal melatonin peaks [31, 32]. In patients with MDD, hypersecretion of adrenocorticotrophic hormone and increased cortisol levels have been noted. In transgenic mice models, studies support the hypothesis that malfunctioning glucocorticoid receptors are involved in HPA dysfunction, which can be reversed by upregulating glucocorticoid receptors, sensitizing the HPA to glucocorticoid feedback [33].

Migraine is associated with multiple disturbances in neurotransmitters and neuropeptides, including serotonin deficiency. During a migraine attack, Sicuteri et al. noted increased urinary excretion of 5-HIAA (a serotonin metabolite) and low plasma levels of serotonin [34]. During a migraine attack, PET studies demonstrate increased blood flow near the brainstem raphe nucleus, indicating activation of serotonergic neurons that may be part of a "migraine generator center" [35]. Decreased serotonin levels may promote cortical spreading of depression-induced trigeminal nociception via increased cortical excitability and sensitivity of the trigeminovascular pathway [28–30]. The dysfunction of the serotonin (5-HT) membrane transporter protein and the serotonin 1A (5-HT1A), serotonin 1B (5-HT1B), and serotonin 2A (5-HT2A) receptors in depression has been implicated in the pathogenesis of depression and the target of antidepressant therapies [36].

There are no biomarkers to date that consistently aid in the diagnosis of migraine and depression. However, inflammatory markers such as IL-6, tumor necrosis factor-alpha (TF-α), and C-reactive protein (CRP) are elevated. TF-α and IL-6 are thought to be involved in the stimulation of corticotropin-releasing hormone production, activation of the HPA, and hypercortisolemia in depression. There is a link between elevated CRP levels and a higher risk of depression, but more research is needed. Similarly, elevated CRP levels have been found in patients with migraine with aura and migraine without aura [37–39].

Migraine attacks commonly occur in women during the menstrual cycle due to lower estrogen levels. Estrogen affects serotonin synthesis by modulating gene expression and/or binding potentials of serotonin receptors, as well as serotonin reuptake and degradation. Furthermore, mood disturbances can also occur, particularly during the late luteal phase, due to decreased estrogen levels, increased cortisol levels, upregulation of the sympathetic nervous system, and downregulation of the serotonin and GABA pathways [40].

Central sensitization has been theorized to be an explanation for why migraine and affective disorders can progress to chronic states that are refractory to treatment. Depression, anxiety, stress, irritability, and sleep have been shown to affect the homeostasis of signaling from relaying thalamic neurons to the cerebral cortex [41]. The nociceptive input of thalamic trigeminovascular neurons is thought to be influenced by a variety of neurotransmitters, including glutamate, GABA, dopamine, serotonin, noradrenaline, orexin, and melanin concentrating hormone. These neurotransmitters are further influenced by internal and external circumstances that call for behavioral, physiological, and affective adjustments [42].

The relationship between migraine and depression may also be explained by relevant brain structures and function. The anterior cingulate cortex, anterior insula, prefrontal cortex, hippocampus, and amygdala have been found to have structural abnormalities or dysfunction in migraine. This is significant because many of these brain regions are involved in determining emotional reactions to pain, mood, and affect [41]. In one fMRI study, the migraine group had higher activation of the hippocampus, prefrontal cortex, and anterior cingulate cortex, all of which are involved in the emotional response to pain [43]. However, it is unclear whether these atypical imaging findings are baseline findings that predispose an individual to have stronger emotional reactions to painful stimuli, if they are a result of recurrent migraine attacks that lead to a psychiatric comorbidity, or if the presence of a psychiatric comorbidity leads to changes in these brain structures causing individuals to have stronger emotional reactions to noxious stimuli [41].

Diagnosis of Psychiatric Comorbidities

Diagnosis of psychiatric comorbidities may be time consuming and difficult to access in the everyday office. Limited focused tests, such as the Hamilton Anxiety Scale or Beck Depression Inventory, may have more practical use as screening tools for diagnosis or for evaluating interventions. Additionally, the Patient Health Questionnaire (PHQ-9) has an in-depth depression module which has been shown to be a reliable and valid measure of depression severity [44]. Appropriate utilization of self-screening tools, clinician level of engagement, dedicated time to assess, and strong therapeutic alliance can help more than a diagnosis alone [22, 45]. Appropriate screening of psychiatric conditions has become a priority for Quality processes and Medicare reimbursement in the last several years, even as access to care has remained a challenge (Table 11.1).

Table 11.1 [102]- List of psychiatric disorders associated with migraine

Condition	DSM 5-TR criteria	Screening tools
Major Depressive Disorder	Depressed mood Diminished interest Weight loss or weight gain Insomnia or hypersomnia Psychomotor agitation or retardation Fatigue Feelings of worthlessness or excessive guilt Diminished ability to think/concentrate Recurrent thoughts of death, suicidal ideation, or suicide attempt	PHQ-9 [44] Beck Depression Inventory [103] Center for Epidemiologic Studies Depression Scale (CES-D) [104] Hamilton Depression Rating Scale (HAM-D) [105]
Generalized Anxiety Disorder	Excessive anxiety and worry occurring for at least 6 months Difficulty controlling anxiety Restless or feeling on edge Fatigue Irritability Muscle tension Sleep disturbance	GAD-7 [106] GAD-2 [107] Beck Anxiety Inventory (BAI) [103] Generalized Anxiety Disorder Severity Scale (GADSS) [108] Hamilton Anxiety Rating Scale (HARS) [109]
Obsessive-Compulsive Disorder	Presence of obsessions, compulsions, or both. Obsessions: Recurrent and persistent thoughts Suppression of thoughts with some other action/thought Compulsions: Repetitive behaviors done in response to an obsession Behaviors done to prevent a dreaded event or situation Obsessions are time consuming	The Yale-Brown Obsessive-Compulsive Scale (Y-BOCS) [110]
Bipolar I disorder	At least one manic episode which may have been preceded by a hypomanic or major depressive episode. Manic episode: Elevated and/or irritable mood lasting at least 1 week plus 3 or more symptoms: Inflated self-esteem and grandiosity Decreased need for sleep More talkative or pressured speech Flight of ideas Distractibility Increase in goal directed activity Excessive involvement in risky behavior	Young Mania Rating Scale (YMRS) [111] Bech-Rafaelsen Mania Rating Scale (MAS) [112] The Mood Disorder Questionnaire (MDQ) [113]
Post-traumatic Stress Disorder	Exposure to death, serious injury, or sexually violent event Presence of intrusive symptoms (thoughts, flashbacks) associated with traumatic event Persistent avoidance of stimuli associated with traumatic event Negative alterations in cognition and mood (dissociation, detachment, decreased interest) Marked alterations in arousal and reactivity Symptoms of depersonalization and derealization Inability to remember an important aspect of the traumatic event(s)	Self-report Measures: Primary Care PTSD Screen for *DSM-5* (PC-PTSD-5) [114] SPAN [115] SPRINT [116] Trauma Screening Questionnaire (TSQ) [117] Interviews Clinician-Administered PTSD Scale for DSM-5 (CAPS-5) [118, 119] PTSD Symptom Scale Interview (PSS-I and PSS-I-5) [120–122] Structured Clinical Interview; PTSD Module (SCID PTSD Module) [123] Structured Interview for PTSD (SIP or SI-PTSD) [124]

Table 11.2 Basics of psychopharmacology

1. Be certain of your diagnosis and your target symptoms.
2. Determine the most appropriate and simplest medication regimen.
3. Work collaboratively with the patient.
4. Set reasonable goals for treatment.
5. Start low and increase doses slowly to avoid adverse events.
6. Have a method for measuring treatment outcomes.
7. Foster collaboration with mental health professionals.

Psychopharmacology and Treatment Options

Migraine treatment entails a myriad of medications, including non-specific agents (blood pressure medications, anti-seizure medications, and antidepressants) and more specific therapies targeting calcitonin gene-related peptide (CGRP). Before choosing a medication, the practitioner and patient must weigh the likelihood of therapeutic benefit, the risk of side effects, and the possibility of interactions with other medications or conditions [22, 45, 46] (Table 11.2).

Antidepressants

Antidepressant medications fall into select groups: tricyclic antidepressants (TCAs), selective serotonin reuptake inhibitors (SSRIs), serotonin and norepinephrine reuptake inhibitors (SNRIs), monoamine oxidase inhibitors (MAOIs), and other antidepressants including Norepinephrine Dopamine Reuptake Inhibitors (NDRI), Serotonin-2 Antagonists/Serotonin Reuptake Inhibitors (SARI), Serotonin-1A Partial Agonist/Serotonin Reuptake Inhibitors (SPARI), Serotonin Modulator and Stimulators (SMS), and Noradrenergic/Specific Serotonergic Agents (NaSSA). The efficacy of these medications with regard to both their antidepressant and antinociceptive effects is debated, with few head-to-head studies [47]. Many antidepressants have a risk of serotonin syndrome, which could be a complicating factor with concomitant use of triptans [48]. This safety warning has been contested and further work needs to be done to elucidate this issue [49].

Tricyclic Antidepressants

TCAs are among the best researched migraine preventives. Amitriptyline has Level B evidence for migraine prevention [50]. Studies have demonstrated that amitriptyline is at least as effective as propranolol in decreasing migraine frequency compared to placebo with 60–75% of patients experiencing a 50% reduction in mean monthly headache days [51]. There is limited evidence for imipramine, doxepin, nortriptyline, and desipramine [52]. Protriptyline, which has a very different side effect profile than other TCAs, has yet to be studied.

TCAs reduce serotonin synthesis in the brainstem raphe nuclei, while also influencing norepinephrine levels. Tricyclics are colloquially called "dirty" medications because of their broad effect on various neurotransmitters such as acetylcholine, histamine, serotonin, norepinephrine, and alpha-1- adrenergic receptors. This widespread effect can explain their efficacy, but also explains their significant side effects including sedation, dry mouth, dry eyes, urinary retention, weight gain, sedation, impotence, and orthostatic hypotension. As a result, TCAs are rarely used as primary antidepressants or anxiolytics, and are used in lower dosages in the management of chronic headache and other pain disorders. At the lower doses typically prescribed for migraine prophylaxis, they typically do not act as antidepressants. [53] (Table 11.3)

Selective Serotonin Reuptake Inhibitors

SSRIs are the most commonly prescribed medications for depression and anxiety [54]. SSRIs were investigated for migraine prophylaxis because of the TCA's efficacy in migraine prevention, and possible serotonergic underpinnings. Fluvoxamine, fluoxetine, and citalopram have demonstrated relatively low efficacy [55]. While one study demonstrated the superiority of fluoxetine over placebo, the effect size was small [56]. The same can be said about another study that looked at the positive effects of paroxetine [57]. Their high degree of tolerability suggests they are helpful for individuals who have had difficulty tolerating other headache treatments. Common side effects include nausea, vomiting, headache, insomnia, drowsiness, nervousness and agitation, decreased libido, insomnia, weight loss and/or weight gain, and a small increased risk for suicidal events in adolescents and young adults (Table 11.4).

Serotonin Norepinephrine Reuptake Inhibitors

There are currently four SNRI's --desvenlafaxine, duloxetine, venlafaxine, and milnacipran. The first three mostly affect serotonin, and milnacipran predominantly affects norepinephrine. Venlafaxine has been shown to be effective in treating social anxiety disorder, panic disorder, and GAD. Duloxetine is also approved for use in the treatment of neuropathy and fibromyalgia [58].

Venlafaxine has Level B evidence for migraine prevention [50]. In one study comparing venlafaxine and amitriptyline, venlafaxine demonstrated equivalency in migraine prevention over a 12-week period compared to placebo [59]. Amitriptyline was discontinued more often due to hyper-

Table 11.3 Tricyclic antidepressants

Generic name	Trade name	Available dose size	Reported doses	Blood levels can be obtained
Amitriptyline	Elavil	10, 25, 50, 75, 100, 125, 150 mg	10–300 mg	+
Amoxapine		25, 50, 100, 150 mg	50 mg BID to 600 mg/day	–
Clomipramine	Anafranil	25, 50, 75 mg	25–250 mg	–
Desipramine	Norpramin	10, 25, 50, 75, 100, 150 mg	25–300 mg	+
Doxepin		10, 25, 50, 75, 100, 150 mg; 10 mg/ mL	25–300 mg	–
Imipramine	Tofranil	10, 25, 50, 75, 100, 125, 150 mg	25–300 mg	+
Nortriptyline	Pamelor	10, 25, 50, 75; 10 mg/5 mL solution	25–150 mg	+
Protriptyline	Vivactil	5, 10 mg	2.5–20 mg TID	–
Trimipramine	Surmontil	25, 50, 100 mg	25–300 mg	–

Table 11.4 Selective serotonin reuptake inhibitors

Generic name	Trade name	Available dose size	Reported doses	Notes
Fluoxetine	Prozac, Serafem	10, 20, 40 mg, 20 mg/5 ml solution	10–80 mg qDay	All SSRIs now have a black box warning for possible increase in suicidal behavior in children, adolescents and young adults.
Sertraline	Zoloft	25, 50, 100 mg, 20 mg/ml solution	25–200 mg qDay	
Fluvoxamine	Luvox	25, 50, 100, 150 mg ER	50–150 mg BID	
Paroxetine	Paxil	10, 20, 30, 40; 12.5, 25 ER; 10 mg/5 ml	20–75 mg qDay	
Citalopram	Celexa	10, 20, 40 mg; 10 mg/ 5 ml solution	20–60 mg qDay	
Escitalopram	Lexapro	5, 10, 20 mg; 5 mg/ 5 ml solution	10–20 mg qDay	

Table 11.5 Serotonin Norepinephrine reuptake inhibitors

Generic name	Trade name	Available dose size	Reported doses	Notes
Desvenlafaxine	Pristiq	50, 100 mg ER	50–100 mg	Predominant action on Serotonin
Duloxetine	Cymbalta	30, 60 mg	30–60 mg	
Venlafaxine	Effexor	25, 37.5, 37.5 ER 50, 75, 75ER, 100, 150ER, 225ER	37.5–300 mg	
Milnacipran	Savella	12.5, 25, 50, 100 mg	12.5–100 mg BID	Predominant action on Norepinephrine

somnia, difficulty concentrating, and orthostatic hypotension. Another study compared venlafaxine to placebo in 60 patients over a 2-month period with a dose-dependent positive response [60]. SNRI side effects are similar to SSRI side effects, but withdrawal symptoms are more severe (Table 11.5).

Monoamine Oxidase Inhibitors

MAOIs are older antidepressants that have largely been replaced by SSRIs and SNRIs due to their high rate of side effects and interactions with medications and foods. They include the non-selective Mono amine oxidase (MAO)-A and MAO-B hydrazines and non-hydrazines, and selective MAO-A and MAO-B inhibitors. They are highly effective for atypical depression. These medications had historically been used for migraine prophylaxis, but, there is insufficient evidence to support their use for migraine prophylaxis [61]. There is some historical support for the use of phenelzine, tranylcypromine, and selegeline, but no large double-blind, placebo-controlled studies have been conducted [62]. The most common side effect of MAOI's is orthostatic hypotension. In addition, interaction with tyramine-containing compounds and opioids can lead to acute serotonin syndrome and hypertensive crisis. Because earlier MAO inhibitors were irreversible, their effects could last for weeks. These side effects, combined with a long list of drugs and foods to avoid while taking these medications, make adherence difficult. (Table 11.6)

Table 11.6 Mono Amine Oxidase (MAO) inhibitors

Generic name	Trade name	Available dose size	Reported doses	Notes
Isocarboxazid	Marplan	10 mg	10–30 mg BID	Significant side effects, interactions and medicine and food restriction
Phenelzine	Nardil	15 mg	15–30 mg TID	
Selegiline Transdermal	Emsam	6, 9, 12 mg patch	6–12 mg daily	
Tranylcypromine	Parnate	10 mg	10–20 mg TID	

Table 11.7 Other antidepressants

Generic name	Trade name	Available dose size	Reported doses	Notes
Buproprion HBr	Aplenzin	348, 522 ER	348–522 mg	Norepinephrine Dopamine Reuptake Inhibitors
Buproprion HCl	Wellbutrin, SR, XL Budeprion SR, XL	75, 100, 100 ER, 150 ER, 200 ER (12 h) 150 ER, 300 ER (24 h)	75–450 mg	
Maprotiline		25, 50, 75 mg	25–75 mg TID	Tetracyclic inhibits norepinephrine
Mirtazapine	Remeron, Remeron SolTab	15, 30, 45 mg	15–45 mg qHS	Tetracyclic antagonizes 5-HT2 and alpha2-adrenergic
Nefazodone	Serzone	50, 100, 150, 200, 250 mg	50–300 mg BID	Inhibits norepinephrine and serotonin and antagonizes 5-HT2
Trazodone		50, 100, 150, 300 mg	25–200 mg TID	Inhibits serotonin reuptake

Other Antidepressants

Mirtazapine (a NaSSA) has been shown to be effective in treating migraine in low doses, but data is mostly from case reports [63]. There is also some evidence that mirtazapine can be used to treat chronic tension headaches, but the studies were small [64]. Furthermore, one study discovered that trazodone may be effective for headaches that have characteristics of both tension-type headaches and migraine [65]. There is also some evidence that nefazadone may be useful [66]; however, the brand name medication was discontinued in the United States in 20223 due to rare occurrence of severe liver damage. Trazodone (a SARI) may be beneficial in patients with comorbid insomnia. Interestingly, one of trazodone's breakdown products is meta-chlorophenylpiperazine (mCPP), a psychoactive drug known to cause headaches in humans (Table 11.7).

Mood Stabilizers

Mood stabilizing agents have a role in the treatment of comorbid psychiatric conditions and migraine prophylaxis. Commonly used mood stabilizing agents include anti-seizure medications (divalproex sodium, lamotrigine, and carbamazepine), atypical neuroleptics (olanzapine, risperidone, quetiapine, lurasidone, and aripiprazole), and lithium. Divalproex sodium has class A evidence for the prophylactic treatment of episodic migraine, while carbamazepine has class C evidence [49]. Some atypical antipsychotics have been used to treat bipolar disorder and are used as an adjunctive treatment for refractory depression; however, the risk of extrapyramidal symptoms [67] and the development of metabolic syndrome complicate their use; however, risk of EPS is lower with atypical antipsychotics. There is insufficient evidence to recommend the use of olanzapine, risperidone, and aripiprazole in the prevention of migraine [68–70].

Lithium, an ionic salt, has become the treatment of choice for bipolar disorder and is an adjunct treatment in refractory MDD. To date, no studies have convincingly demonstrated effect in the treatment of migraine or tension-type headache but are effective in treatment of cluster headache [71, 72]. It has been used in other trigeminal autonomic cephalalgias with varying degrees of success [73]. With regard to refractory headaches, lithium should be considered in cases where autonomic symptoms are present. There are no current good double-blinded studies of its use in the refractory population. Side effects include tremor, slurred speech, blurred vision, nausea, weakness, thirst, anorexia, and diarrhea. Confusion, ataxia, tremor, nystagmus, EPS, seizures, and death can occur in patients with toxic levels. Chronic use can result in hypothyroidism, polyuria, abnormal renal function, and polymorphonuclear leukocytosis. Lithium also has direct interactions with NSAIDs, carbamazepine, and diuretics, necessitating close monitoring.

Table 11.8 Mood stabilizers

Generic name	Trade name	Available dose size	Reported doses
Carbamazepine	Tegretol	100 CH, 200 mg 100 mg/ 5 ml soln	200–600 mg BID
Divalproex Sodium	Depakote Depakote ER	125, 250, 500 mg 250, 500 mg ER	125–500 mg BID to TID
Lamotrigine	Lamictal	25, 100, 150, 200 mg 2, 5, 25 CH	25–200 mg qDay
Lithium	Lithobid Eskalith	150, 300, 600 mg 300, 450 mg ER	300–900 mg BID
Oxcarbazepine	Trileptal	150, 300, 600 mg 300 mg/ 5 ml	300–1200 mg BID
Valproic Acid	Depakene Stavzor	125, 250, 500 mg 250 mg/ 5 ml	250–500 mg BID to TID

Valproic acid (VPA) is an intriguing drug with a wide range of effects. It raises GABA levels, enhances postsynaptic GABA response, causes neuronal hyperpolarization, and lowers serotonin levels in the dorsal raphe nuclei. It appears to reduce abnormal neuronal firing, raising the seizure threshold. VPA has demonstrated its efficacy in acute and maintenance treatment of bipolar disorder. Both sodium valproate and divalproex sodium are effective in migraine prevention [74]. For each drug, there are at least two placebo-controlled studies [75]. However, there is little evidence that these medications are more effective than other migraine preventives, such as beta-blockers. Divalproex sodium extended-release appears to have preventive efficacy as well [76].

Regardless of the form utilized, VPA appears to have frequent adverse events including nausea, vomiting, and gastrointestinal discomfort. There is also evidence that VPA may affect liver function levels and, in rare cases, lead to hepatitis or pancreatitis. Other adverse reactions include weight gain, hair loss, bleeding disorders, hyperandrogenism, and polycystic ovarian syndrome. VPA is a well-documented teratogen leading to neural tube defects, and its use in women should be closely monitored. VPA interacts with a wide range of medications, both directly and indirectly, through the inhibition of cytochrome P-450.

Carbamazepine was found to be effective for migraine prevention in one placebo-controlled study [76], but other studies have failed to show efficacy over placebo [77]. There is more evidence for controlling bipolar disorder. Several studies have shown efficacy in maintaining euthymia, particularly during the manic phase [78], and in patients who cycle quickly [79]. This medication can cause leukopenia, necessitating close monitoring.

Lamotrigine is used in the treatment of bipolar disorder and as an adjunct therapy in refractory MDD. It works by blocking voltage-gated sodium channels, resulting in inhibition of glutamate release, and decreasing neuronal excitability. Lamotrigine has been studied as a treatment for CM in several open-label studies. In one study, it was used in combination treatment and had some preventive effect in patients with migraine with aura [80]. However, due to adverse events, there was a high dropout rate. Another study looked at its effect on aura, and it appears that using it reduces the frequency and duration of the aura, even in people who have persistent aura [81]. (Table 11.8).

Anxiolytics

Barbiturates and benzodiazepines have a long history of use in the acute treatment of anxiety disorders. Tolerance, dependence, and abuse complicate usage. Barbiturates are rarely used to treat affective disorders but are still commonly used in migraine treatment [82]. Barbiturates have a high risk of respiratory depression, elevation of liver enzymes, and cardiac arrhythmias. This can be especially problematic due to their low therapeutic index [83]. Butalbital, which is found in many headache medications, has a relatively short half-life, which contributes to the risk of medication overuse and headaches. Some people with migraine and GAD may find these preparations appealing, not only because they are effective for headache, but also some mild relief from anxiety symptoms.

Benzodiazepines are a common treatment for GAD and serve to stabilize patients while longer-term treatments are initiated. However, three benzodiazepines (diazepam, lorazepam, and alprazolam) remain among the most commonly abused drugs in the United States and around the world [84]. Benzodiazepines are classified into three types: short-acting, mid-acting, and long-acting. Their common site of action is the GABA-A receptor complex, which results in a sedative-hypnotic effect. They are also used to treat sleep disorders, panic attacks, OCD, akathisia, phobias, and agitation associated with bipolar disorder. While nearly all of these medications list headaches as a potential side effect, there is very little data on whether they contrib-

Table 11.9 Benzodiazepines

Generic name	Trade name	Available dose size	Reported doses	Length of action
Alprazolam	Niravam, Xanax, Xanax XR	0.25, 0.5, 1, 2 ODT, 0.5, 1, 2, 3ER, 1 mg/mL solution	0.25 BID – 2 mg TID	Short-acting and rapid-onset
Midazolam	Versed	2 mg/mL syrup; IM; IV	1 mg IV q 2–3 min	
Oxazepam		10, 15, 30 mg	10–30 mg TID	
Triazolam	Halcion	0.125, 0.25 mg	0.125–0.5 mg qHS	
Estazolam		1, 2 mg	0.5–2 mg qHS	Mid Length of Action
Lorazepam	Ativan	0.5, 1, 2 mg 2 mg/ml solution IV, IM	0.5 qDay – 3 mg TID	
Temazepam	Restoril	7.5, 15, 22.5, 30 mg	7.5 – 30 mg qHS	
Chlordiazepoxide	Librium	5, 10, 25 mg	5–25 mg QID	Long length of Action
Clonazepam	Klonopin, Klonopin Wafer	0.5, 1, 2 mg; 0.125, 0.25, 0.5, 1, 2 ODT	0.125–6 mg TID	
Clorazepate	Tranxene SD, TranxeneT-tab	3.75, 7.5, 15 mg	3.75 – 20 mg TID	
Diazepam	Valium	2, 5, 10 mg 5 mg/5 mL sol 5 mg/ mL nasal IM, IV	2–10 mg BID – QID	
Flurazepam	Dalmane	15, 30 mg	15–30 mg	

Table 11.10 Non-Benzodiazepine Anxiolytics

Generic name	Trade name	Available dose size	Reported doses	Notes
Buspirone	Buspar	5, 7.5, 10, 15, 30 mg	7.5–30 mg BID	
Butabarbital	Butisol	30, 50 mg 30 mg/5 ml	15–30 mg BID to TID	
Hydroxyzine	Atarax	10, 25, 50, 100 mg 10 mg/5 ml soln	50–100 mg q6H	
Meprobamate		200, 400 mg	400 mg TID – QID	
Pentobarbital	Nembutal	IM, IV	150–200 mg	

ute to, cause, or are effective for treating migraine or intractable headaches [85].

Barbiturates and SSRIs are the most common non-benzodiazepine anxiolytics. Other drugs in this category include buspirone, an azaspirone with no sedative, hypnotic, muscle relaxant, or anti-convulsant properties. It is primarily a partial agonist at the 5-HT1A receptor, with some effects at the 5-HT2A receptor, and as a mixed agonist–antagonist at dopamine type 2 receptors [86]. Side effects include nausea, dizziness, occasional insomnia, and headache (Tables 11.9 and 11.10).

Antipsychotics

Antipsychotic medications (neuroleptics) were primarily derived from phenothiazine compounds. The general action of these drugs is 'neurolepsis,' or the suppression of spontaneous complex behaviors, vigilance, aggression, impulsivity, and overactive response to stimuli. Promethazine, developed in the 1930s, failed to show adequate efficacy in treating agitation; however, it is an effective anti-emetic still used today. Chlorpromazine was invented in 1949 to help with anesthesia. Reserpine was discovered in the 1950s and showed some mild antipsychotic effects. The first butyrophene haloperidol, developed in 1958, paved the way for the development of other 'typical' neuroleptics throughout the 1960s and 1970s. Clozapine, the first 'atypical' neuroleptic, was developed in the 1980s. It is a dibenzepine with a low affinity for dopamine receptors (being somewhat D1 selective) as well as 5HT2, muscarinic, alpha-adrenergic, and H1 effects that set it apart from other neuroleptics. Following that, other atypical neuroleptics demonstrated a reduction in EPS, little effect on prolactin levels, and a greater effect on negative schizophrenia symptoms. The first 'third generation' neuroleptic, aripiprazole, was introduced in the twenty-first century, with a mixed agonist antagonist effect. Different classes of neuroleptics are depicted in Tables 11.11 and 11.12.

Dopamine's role in migraine has been speculated. Dopamine stimulation has been shown to cause migraine-related symptoms such as yawning, mood changes, nausea, vomiting, gastrokinetic changes, and hypotensive autonomic

Table 11.11 Neuroleptics

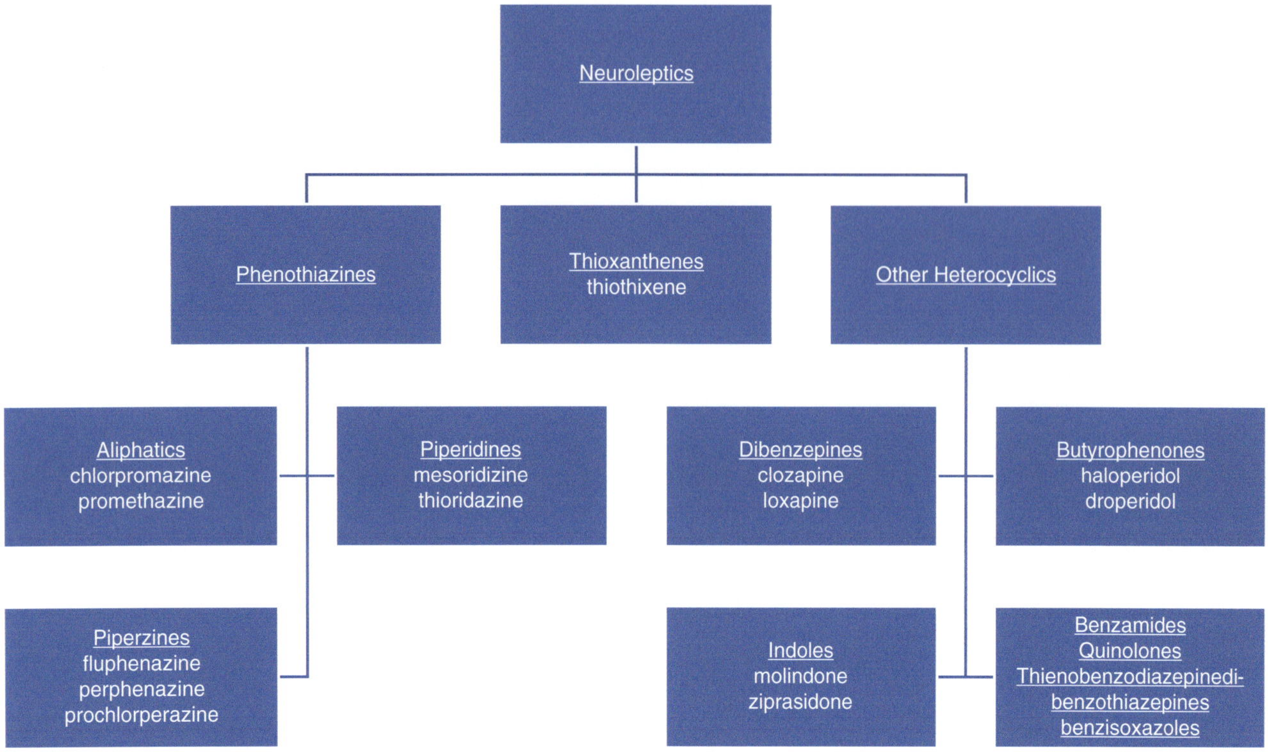

Table 11.12 Dopamine receptors

D1: Thalamus, Superior Chiasmatic Nucleus, Supraoptic nucleus, Arterial walls
D2: Peri Aqueductal Grey, Hypothalamus, Raphe Nuclei, basal Ganglia, Solitary nucleus, Dorsal motor vagal nucleus, sympathetic ganglia
D3: Area postrema, Brainstem
D4: Brainstem
D5: Limbic regions, Basal Ganglia

changes [87]. The dopamine receptor is heterogeneous, with two major receptor families: D1-like (including D1 and D5) and D2-like (including D2, D3 and D4). D1-like receptors stimulate adenylyl cyclase while D2-like inhibits adenylyl cyclase. While most receptors are central, D1 and D2 are also present peripherally. There are four major dopaminergic pathways: the tuberoinfundibular pathway (hypothalamus to the anterior pituitary involved in prolactin release), nigrostriatal pathway (substantia nigra to the striatum involved in movement smoothing), mesocortical pathway (ventral tegmentum to the limbic cortex involved in cognition), and mesolimbic pathway (tegmentum to nucleus accumbens involved in perception).

The neuroleptics have a diverse effect on a range of neurochemical messengers including serotonin, epinephrine, norepinephrine, acetylcholine, and histamine which account for their side effects. These include hyperprolactinemia, dry mouth and eyes, hypotension, weight gain, metabolic syndrome, sedation, QTc prolongation, lowered seizure threshold, and EPS, including tardive dyskinesia [88].

Evidence exists for the use of chlorpromazine, prochlorperazine, haloperidol, droperidol, and metoclopramide in migraine [89–92]. Limited evidence exists for olanzapine, quetiapine, ziprasidone, and aripiprazole [68, 70, 93, 94].Haloperidol prevented migraine in two small open studies in 1995 and 2004, and in a small randomized double blinded study in 2006 [90, 95, 96].One double-blind crossover study of fluphenazine showed benefit with tension-type headache [97]. None of these studies meet Level 1 evidence and further research needs to be done (Tables 11.13 and 11.14).

Table 11.13 1st Generation Antipsychotics

Generic name	Trade name	Available dose size	Reported doses
Chlorpromazine	Thorazine	10, 25, 50, 100, 200 mg IM, IV	10 – 250 mg TID to QID
Fluphenazine	Prolixin	1, 2.5, 5, 10 mg 2.5/ 5 ml elixir	1–10 mg QID
Haloperidol	Haldol	0.5, 1, 2, 5, 10, 20 mg	0.5 – 5 mg TID reports up to 100 mg/ day
Loxapine	Loxitane	5, 10, 25, 50 mg	10 – 50 mg BID
Molindone	Moban	5, 10, 25, 50, 100 mg	5–50 mg TID to QID
Perphenazine	Trilafon	2, 4, 8, 16 mg	4–16 mg BID to QID
Pimozide	Orap	1, 2 mg	1–2 mg qDay to BID
Prochlorperazine	Compazine	5, 10 mg	5 – 10 mg q6-8hr
Thioridazine	Mellaril	10, 15, 25, 50, 100, 150, 200 mg 30; 100 mg / mL	
Thiothixene	Navane	1, 2, 5, 10, 20 mg	
Trifluoperazine	Stelazine	1, 2, 5, 10 mg	

Table 11.14 Second generation antipsychotics

Generic name	Trade name	Available dose size	Reported doses	Notes
Aripiprazole	Abilify	2, 5, 10, 15, 20, 30 mg 1 mg/ mL IM	2–30 mg qDay	D2, 5-HT1A agonist; 5-HT2A antagonist
Clozapine	Clozaril FazaClo ODT Versacolz	12.5, 25, 50, 100, 200 mg	12.5–300 mg BID (max 900 mg/day)	Risk of agranulocytosis
Olanzapine	Zyprexa Zyprexa Zydis Zyprexa IntraMuscular Zyprexa Relpevv Symbyax	2.5, 5, 7.5, 10, 15, 20 mg	2.5–20 mg qDay	
Paliperidone	Invega Invega Sustenna Invega Trinza	3, 6, 9 mg ER	3–12 mg qDay	
Quetiapine	Seroquel Seroquel XR	25, 50, 100, 200, 300, 400 mg 25, 50, 100, 200, 300, 400 mg ER	25–300 mg TID (max 800 mg/day)	
Risperidone	Risperdal Risperidal M-tab Risperidal Consta	0.25, 0.5, 1, 2, 3, 4 mg 1 mg/ ml	0.25–4 mg BID (max 16 mg/ day)	
Ziprasidone	Geodon Zeldox	20, 40, 60, 80 mg	20–80 mg BID	

Attention Deficit and Hyperactivity Disorder

There is little written about the use of stimulant and non-stimulant medications for attention deficit and hyperactivity disorder (ADHD) and their impact on migraine. While headache is listed as a side effect, there is no distinction whether this side effect is medication-induced or acts as a trigger for migraine episodes. Furthermore, some of these medications can cause insomnia and anorexia, which can be migraine triggers (Table 11.15).

Table 11.15 Stimulants and non-stimulants

Generic name	Trade name	Available dose size	Reported doses
Amphetamine/ Dextroamphetamine	Adderall Adderall XR	5, 7.5, 10, 12.5, 15, 20, 30; 5, 10, 15,20, 25, 30 ER	5–60 mg qDay – BID
Atomoxetine	Strattera	10, 18, 25, 40, 60, 80, 100	10–100 mg qDay
Dextroamphetamine	Dexedrine Procentra	5, 10, 15 mg ER	5–60 mg qDay
Dexmethylphenidate	Focalin Focalin XR	2.5, 5, 10 mg; 5, 10, 15, 20 ER	2.5 – 10 mg qDay – BID
Lisdexamfetamine	Vyvanse	20, 30, 40, 50, 60, 70 mg	20–70 mg qDay
Methylphenidate	Ritalin (LA, SR) Metadate (CD,ER) Methylin (ER) Daytrana	2.5, 5, 10, 20 18, 27, 36, 54 ER	2.5–15 mg TID

Table 11.16 CGRP inhibitors

Generic name	Trade name	Available dose size	Reported doses	Notes
Erenumab	Aimovig	70 mg, 140 mg subQ q 30 days	70–140 mg subQ q 30 days	Approved for prevention of migraine
Fremanezumab	Ajovy	225 mg q30 days	225 mg subQ q30 days	Approved for prevention of migraine
Galcanezumab	Emgality	240 mg loading dose, followed by 120 mg subQ q 30 days	240 mg loading dose, followed by 120 mg subQ q 30 days	Approved for prevention of migraine
Eptinezumab	Vyepti	100 mg, 300 mg subQ q 3 months	100 mg or 300 mg subQ q 3 months	Approved for prevention of migraine
Rimegepant	Nurtec	75 mg QOD (preventive) 75 mg daily PRN (abortive)	75 mg QOD (preventive) 75 mg daily PRN (abortive)	Approved for preventive treatment of episodic migraine and abortive treatment of migraine
Atogepant	Qulipta	10 mg, 30 mg, 60 mg daily	10 mg, 30 mg, 60 mg daily	Approved for prevention of migraine
Ubrogepant	Ubrelvy	50 mg, 100 mg daily PRN	50 mg, 100 mg daily PRN	Approved for abortive treatment of migraine
Zavegepant	Zavzpret	10 mg nasal spray daily PRN	10 mg nasal spray daily PRN	Approved for abortive treatment of migraine

Calcitonin Gene-Related Peptide Inhibitors

CGRP inhibitors, which include monoclonal antibodies (that bind to CGRP or CGRP receptor) and gepants (medications that bind to the CGRP receptor) are used for preventive and abortive treatment of migraine with few side effects [98]. Preliminary studies have demonstrated that fremanezumab is associated with a statistically significant reduction in mean monthly migraine days of at least moderate severity in patients with moderate to severe depression [99], suggesting that a decreased migraine burden may positively affect mood. Additionally, they have been shown to be effective in patients with refractory migraine who have failed four medication classes in the past (including TCAs and VPA) [100] (Table 11.16).

OnabotulinumtoxinA

OnabotulinumtoxinA is a neurotoxin that is FDA-approved for the prevention of CM; however, its effect on depression is not understood. A recent meta-analysis shows that onabotulinumtoxinA can have a significant effect on disease severity in patients who have CM and MDD. The mechanism why onabotulinumtoxinA is beneficial in patients with depression is hypothesized to be negative feedback to the brain, which may impact mood by limiting contraction of the procerus and corrugator muscles [101].

Conclusion

Migraine is comorbid with several psychiatric disorders, most commonly anxiety and depression. Patients with migraine and CM have a higher prevalence of MDD, dysthymia, bipolar I and II, GAD, social phobia, and OCD. These comorbidities complicate medical care and necessitate individual evaluation and management.

Many classes of pharmacologic agents are used in the concomitant treatment of headaches and psychiatric disorders. Understanding pharmacological agents is critical because, while their actions can be beneficial, their side effects and interactions can be devastating. Comprehensive management includes evaluation of migraine and the potential impact of psychiatric disorders to improve outcomes. The end goal is the same: to improve function, reduce disability, and do the best we can for our patients.

Teaching Points

1. Psychiatric comorbidities are more common in migraineurs, resulting in higher MIDAS scores, greater functional impairment, and lower quality of life.
2. MDD, GAD, and bipolar disorders are more commonly present in migraineurs than in the general population.
3. Genetic factors, serotonin deficiency, dysregulation of the HPA, central sensitization, and brain abnormalities have been postulated as possible shared pathophysiological mechanisms of both migraine disorders and MDD.
4. The diagnosis of psychiatric comorbidities can be difficult to assess in visits, but screening tools and a multidisciplinary approach can be helpful.
5. Antidepressants, including TCAs and SNRIs, are postulated to work by affecting serotonin levels in the brainstem raphe nuclei and are effective prophylactic agents that can be used in migraine prophylaxis, as well as co-management of MDD. However, caution must be taken since TCAs can have significant side effects.
6. Mood stabilizers such as VPA can be used in the co-management of migraine and MDD. Lamotrigine can be helpful for auras. Lithium is useful for co-management of bipolar disorder and cluster headaches. Caution must be taken as these medications can also have significant side effects.
7. Barbiturates and benzodiazepines have limited evidence for use in management, however benzodiazepines can be used in the acute management of GAD until transitioning to long term management. These medications have a high risk of dependency and are some of the most commonly abused drugs.
8. Neuroleptics such as chlorpromazine, prochlorperazine, haloperidol, droperidol, and metoclopramide are useful in the management of migraine. These medications, particularly droperidol, have a risk of side effects that are significant for EPS and QTc prolongation.
9. There is not much known about the effects of ADHD stimulants and non-stimulants in the management of migraine.
10. Although OnaBot-A and CGRP inhibitors are effective medications in the management of migraine, not much is known about their effects on psychiatric comorbidities.

Case

A 55-year-old woman with a history of chronic migraine (CM) without aura was referred to your headache clinic for management of migraine disorder, which has been refractory to multiple preventive and abortive treatments. Of note, she has a history significant for major depressive disorder (MDD), for which she has seen Psychiatry in the past. She tells you that her headaches have been chronic for the past 10 years. Two years prior to her headaches worsening, you note that your patient was hospitalized for suicidal ideation after her husband of 20 years passed away in a tragic car accident. She has tried tricyclic antidepressants, SSRIs, onabotulinum A, and CGRP inhibitors, which have had limited effect on her migraine frequency. During your neurological examination, she tells you that she has a history of sciatica in her right leg that is exacerbated when sitting for prolonged periods of time, but otherwise, her neurological examination was normal with no focal deficits. What is an appropriate next step in the treatment of this patient?

Case Discussion

The decision is made to start her on duloxetine as a new preventive treatment to co-manage her sciatic pain, depression, and migraine disorder. Nine months later, you have titrated her dose to 90 mg daily, and since then, she has had a 25% reduction in the frequency of her headaches, as well as decreased severity and duration of her migraine attacks. She also appears less distressed and reports that her mood has been improving.

Questions and Answers

1. Which treatment for episodic migraine prevention has class A evidence?
   A. Divalproex sodium
   B. Amitriptyline
   C. Lamotrigine
   D. Onabotulinumtoxin-A

The correct answer is A. Multiple studies have shown that Divalproex sodium has class A evidence for the prevention of episodic migraine. Amitriptyline has class B evidence for the prevention of episodic migraine. Onabotuliniumtoxin A is FDA-approved for the prevention of chronic migraine. Lamotrigine has some evidence for management of auras.

2. Which medication can be used for the co-management of bipolar disorder and cluster headache?
   A. Fremanezumab
   B. Clozapine
   C. Olanzapine
   D. Lithium

The correct answer is D. Lithium can be used for cluster migraine during a bout; however, other medications such as verapamil and galcanezumab are usually preferred initially due to more favorable side effect profiles. Fremanezumab is a fully humanized monoclonal antibody used to prevent episodic migraines. Clozapine and olanzapine are not used for cluster headaches but can be useful mood stabilizers. Olanzapine is useful for the management of bipolar disorder, refractory depression, and schizophrenia. Clozapine is useful for the treatment of schizophrenia that has been refractory to other treatments.

Bibliography

1. Burch R, Rizzoli P, Loder E. The prevalence and impact of migraine and severe headache in the United States: updated age, sex, and socioeconomic-specific estimates from government health surveys. Headache. 2021;61(1):60–8.
2. On behalf of Lifting The Burden: the Global Campaign against Headache, Steiner TJ, Stovner LJ, Jensen R, Uluduz D, Katsarava Z. Migraine remains second among the world's causes of disability, and first among young women: findings from GBD2019. J Headache Pain. 2020;21(1):137. https://doi.org/10.1186/s10194-020-01208-0.
3. Jette N, Patten S, Williams J, Becker W, Wiebe S. Comorbidity of migraine and psychiatric disorders—a national population-based study. Headache. 2008;48(4):501–16.
4. Seng EK, Seng CD. Understanding migraine and psychiatric comorbidity. Curr Opin Neurol. 2016;29(3):309–13.
5. Lipton RB, Serrano D, Buse DC, Pavlovic JM, Blumenfeld AM, Dodick DW, et al. Improving the detection of chronic migraine: development and validation of Identify Chronic Migraine (ID-CM). Cephalalgia. 2016;36(3):203–15.
6. Vermani M, Marcus M, Katzman MA. Rates of detection of mood and anxiety disorders in primary care: a descriptive, cross-sectional study. PCC CNS Disord. 2011;13(2):PCC.10m01013.
7. Radat F. What is the link between migraine and psychiatric disorders? From epidemiology to therapeutics. Rev Neurol. 2021;177(7):821–6.
8. Pompili M, Lamis DA, Andrasik F, Martelletti P. Oxford textbook of headache syndromes. Oxford University Press; 2020.
9. Wolff HG. Personality features and reactions of subjects with migraine. Arch NeurPsych. 1937;37(4):895.
10. Wolff H. Headache and other head pain. New York; 1947.
11. Breslau N, Merikangas K, Bowden CL. Comorbidity of migraine and major affective disorders. Neurology. 1994;44(10 Suppl 7):S17–22.
12. Breslau N. Migraine, suicidal ideation, and suicide attempts. Neurology. 1992;42(2):392–5.
13. Breslau N, Rasmussen BK. The impact of migraine: epidemiology, risk factors, and co-morbidities. Neurology. 2001;56(Supplement 1):S4–S12.
14. Kessler RC. Lifetime and 12-month prevalence of DSM-III-R psychiatric disorders in the United States: results from the national comorbidity survey. Arch Gen Psychiatry. 1994;51(1):8.
15. Merikangas KR, Stevens DE. Comorbidity of migraine and psychiatric disorders. Neurol Clin. 1997;15(1):115–23.
16. Breslau N. Psychiatric comorbidity in migraine. Cephalalgia. 1998;18(22 suppl):56–61.
17. Swartz KL, Pratt LA, Armenian HK, Lee LC, Eaton WW. Mental disorders and the incidence of migraine headaches in a community sample: results from the baltimore epidemiologic catchment area follow-up study. Arch Gen Psychiatry. 2000;57(10):945.
18. Breslau N, Davis GC, Andreski P. Migraine, psychiatric disorders, and suicide attempts: an epidemiologic study of young adults. Psychiatry Res. 1991;37(1):11–23.
19. Breslau N, Lipton RB, Stewart WF, Schultz LR, Welch KMA. Comorbidity of migraine and depression: investigating potential etiology and prognosis. Neurology. 2003;60(8):1308–12.
20. Zwart JA, Dyb G, Hagen K, Ødegård KJ, Dahl AA, Bovim G, et al. Depression and anxiety disorders associated with headache frequency. The Nord-Trøndelag Health Study: The Nord-Trøndelag Health Study (The HUNT Study). Eur J Neurol. 2003;10(2):147–52.
21. Radat F, Swendsen J. Psychiatric comorbidity in migraine: a review. Cephalalgia. 2005;25(3):165–78.
22. Baskin SM, Lipchik GL, Smitherman TA. Mood and anxiety disorders in chronic headache. Headache. 2006;46(s3):S76–87.
23. Guidetti V, Galli F, Fabrizi P, Giannantoni A, Napoli L, Bruni O, et al. Headache and psychiatric comorbidity: clinical aspects and outcome in an 8-year follow-up study. Cephalalgia. 1998;18(7):455–62.
24. Yang Y, Ligthart L, Terwindt GM, Boomsma DI, Rodriguez-Acevedo AJ, Nyholt DR. Genetic epidemiology of migraine and depression. Cephalalgia. 2016;36(7):679–91.
25. Schur EA, Noonan C, Buchwald D, Goldberg J, Afari N. A twin study of depression and migraine: evidence for a shared genetic vulnerability. Headache. 2009;49(10):1493–502.
26. Kwon JM, Goate AM. The candidate gene approach. Alcohol Res Health. 2000;24(3):164–8.
27. Lesch K-P, Bengel D, Heils A, Sabol SZ, Greenberg BD, Petri S, et al. Association of anxiety-related traits with a polymorphism in the serotonin transporter gene regulatory region. Science. 1996;274(5292):1527–31.
28. Cui Y, Kataoka Y, Watanabe Y. Role of cortical spreading depression in the pathophysiology of migraine. Neurosci Bull. 2014;30(5):812–22.
29. Hamel E, Currents H. Serotonin and migraine: biology and clinical implications. Cephalalgia. 2007;27(11):1293–300.
30. Supornsilpchai W, Sanguanrangsirikul S, Maneesri S, Srikiatkhachorn A. Serotonin depletion, cortical spreading depression, and trigeminal nociception. Headache. 2006;46(1):34–9.
31. Peres MFP. Hypothalamic involvement in chronic migraine. J Neurol Neurosurg Psychiatry. 2001;71(6):747–51.
32. Karsan N, Bose P, Goadsby PJ. The migraine premonitory phase. Continuum. 2018;24(4):996–1008.
33. Barden N. Implication of the hypothalamic-pituitary-adrenal axis in the physiopathology of depression. J Psychiatry Neurosci. 2004;29(3):185–93.
34. Sicuteri F, Testi A, Anselmi B. Biochemical investigations in headache: increase in the Hydroxyindoleacetic acid excretion during migraine attacks. Int Arch Allergy Immunol. 1961;19(1):55–8.
35. Weiller C, May A, Limmroth V, Jüptner M, Kaube H, Schayck RV, et al. Brain stem activation in spontaneous human migraine attacks. Nat Med. 1995;1(7):658–60.

36. Fakhoury M. Revisiting the serotonin hypothesis: implications for major depressive disorders. Mol Neurobiol. 2016;53(5):2778–86.
37. Furtado M, Katzman MA. Examining the role of neuroinflammation in major depression. Psychiatry Res. 2015;229(1–2):27–36.
38. Welch KMA, Brandes AW, Salerno L, Brandes JL. C-reactive protein may be increased in migraine patients who present with complex clinical features. Headache. 2006;46(2):197–9.
39. Vanmolkot FH, de Hoon JN. Increased C-reactive protein in young adult patients with migraine. Cephalalgia. 2007;27(7):843–6.
40. Martin VT, Behbehani M. Ovarian hormones and migraine headache: understanding mechanisms and pathogenesis-part I. Headache. 2006;46(1):3–23.
41. Minen MT, Begasse De Dhaem O, Kroon Van Diest A, Powers S, Schwedt TJ, Lipton R, et al. Migraine and its psychiatric comorbidities. J Neurol Neurosurg Psychiatry. 2016;87(7):741–9.
42. Noseda R, Kainz V, Borsook D, Burstein R. Neurochemical pathways that converge on thalamic trigeminovascular neurons: potential substrate for modulation of migraine by sleep, food intake, stress and anxiety. PLoS One. 2014;9(8):e103929.
43. Russo A, Tessitore A, Esposito F, Marcuccio L, Giordano A, Conforti R, et al. Pain processing in patients with migraine: an event-related fMRI study during trigeminal nociceptive stimulation. J Neurol. 2012;259(9):1903–12.
44. Kroenke K, Spitzer RL, Williams JB. The PHQ-9: validity of a brief depression severity measure. J Gen Intern Med. 2001;16(9):606–13.
45. Sheftell FD. Understanding the headache patient with complex psychiatric comorbidities: a headache specialist's perspective. Headache. 2006;46(s3):S165–S7.
46. Hamelsky SW, Lipton RB. Psychiatric comorbidity of migraine. Headache. 2006;46(9):1327–33.
47. Melfi CA, Chawla AJ, Croghan TW, Hanna MP, Kennedy S, Sredl K. The effects of adherence to antidepressant treatment guidelines on relapse and recurrence of depression. Arch Gen Psychiatry. 1998;55(12):1128.
48. Evans RW. The FDA alert on serotonin syndrome with combined use of SSRIs or SNRIs and Triptans: an analysis of the 29 case reports. MedGenMed. 2007;9(3):48.
49. Evans RW, Tepper SJ, Shapiro RE, Sun-Edelstein C, Tietjen GE. The FDA alert on serotonin syndrome with use of Triptans combined with selective serotonin reuptake inhibitors or selective serotonin-norepinephrine reuptake inhibitors: American headache society position Paper: June 2010. Headache. 2010;50(6):1089–99.
50. Silberstein SD, Holland S, Freitag F, Dodick DW, Argoff C, Ashman E. Evidence-based guideline update: pharmacologic treatment for episodic migraine prevention in adults: Table 1: Report of the quality standards subcommittee of the American Academy of neurology and the American Headache Society. Neurology. 2012;78(17):1337–45.
51. Ziegler DK. Migraine prophylaxis: a comparison of propranolol and amitriptyline. Arch Neurol. 1987;44(5):486.
52. Martucci N, Manna V, Agnoli A. Antidepressant drugs and migraine. Cephalalgia. 1985;5(2_suppl):225–8.
53. Feighner JP. Mechanism of action of antidepressant medications. J Clin Psychiatry. 1999;60(Suppl 4):4–11. discussion 2–3
54. Song F, Freemantle N, Sheldon TA, House A, Watson P, Long A, et al. Selective serotonin reuptake inhibitors: meta-analysis of efficacy and acceptability. BMJ. 1993;306(6879):683–7.
55. Saper JR, Silberstein SD, Lake AE, Winters ME. Double-blind trial of fluoxetine: chronic daily headache and migraine. Headache. 1994;34(9):497–502.
56. d'Amato CC, Pizza V, Marmolo T, Giordano E, Alfano V, Nasta A. Fluoxetine for migraine prophylaxis: a double-blind trial. Headache. 1999;39(10):716–9.
57. Park H-J, Lee S-T, Shim J-Y, Kim B, Hwang S-H, Kim S-H, et al. The effect of paroxetine on the reduction of migraine frequency is independent of its anxiolytic effect. J Clin Neurol. 2006;2(4):246.
58. Young WB, Bradley KC, Anjum MW, Gebeline-Myers C. Duloxetine prophylaxis for episodic migraine in persons without depression: a prospective study. Headache. 2013;53(9):1430–7.
59. Bulut S, Berilgen MS, Baran A, Tekatas A, Atmaca M, Mungen B. Venlafaxine versus amitriptyline in the prophylactic treatment of migraine: randomized, double-blind, crossover study. Clin Neurol Neurosurg. 2004;107(1):44–8.
60. Ozyalcin SN, Talu GK, Kiziltan E, Yucel B, Ertas M, Disci R. The efficacy and safety of venlafaxine in the prophylaxis of migraine. Headache. 2005;45(2):144–52.
61. Anthony M, Lance JW. Monoamine Oxidase inhibition in the treatment of migraine. Arch Neurol. 1969;21(3):263–8.
62. Punay NC, Couch JR. Antidepressants in the treatment of migraine headache. Curr Sci. 2003;7(1):51–4.
63. Lévy E, Margolese HC. Migraine headache prophylaxis and treatment with low-dose mirtazapine. Int Clin Psychopharmacol. 2003;18(5):301–3.
64. Bendtsen L, Jensen R. Mirtazapine is effective in the prophylactic treatment of chronic tension-type headache. Neurology. 2004;62(10):1706–11.
65. Pies R. Trazodone and intractable headaches. J Clin Psychiatry. 1983;44(8):317.
66. Saper JR, Lake AE, Tepper SJ. Nefazodone for chronic daily headache prophylaxis: an open-label study. Headache. 2001;41(5):465–74.
67. Beck AT, Epstein N, Brown G, Steer R. Beck anxiety inventory. J Consult Clin Psychol. 1993;
68. Silberstein SD, Peres MFP, Hopkins MM, Shechter AL, Young WB, Rozen TD. Olanzapine in the treatment of refractory migraine and chronic daily headache. Headache. 2002;42(6):515–8.
69. Dusitanond P, Young WB. Neuroleptics and migraine. Cent Nerv Syst Agents Med Chem. 2009;9(1):63–70.
70. LaPorta LD. Relief from migraine headache with aripiprazole treatment. Headache. 2007;47(6):922–6.
71. Peatfield RC. Lithium in Migraine and Cluster Headache: a Review. J R Soc Med. 1981;74(6):432–6.
72. Ekbom K. Lithium for cluster headache: review of the literature and preliminary results of long-term treatment. Headache. 1981;21(4):132–9.
73. Cohen AS, Matharu MS, Goadsby PJ. Trigeminal autonomic cephalalgias: current and future treatments. Headache. 2007;47(6):969–80.
74. Hering R, Kuritzky A. Sodium valproate in the prophylactic treatment of migraine: a double-blind study versus placebo. Cephalalgia. 1992;12(2):81–4.
75. Yoon MS, Savidou I, Diener HC, Limmroth V. Evidence-based medicine in migraine prevention. Expert Rev Neurother. 2005;5(3):333–41.
76. Freitag FG, Collins SD, Carlson HA, Goldstein J, Saper J, Silberstein S, et al. A randomized trial of divalproex sodium extended-release tablets in migraine prophylaxis. Neurology. 2002;58(11):1652–9.
77. Silberstein S, Lipton R, Dodick D. Wolff's headache and other head pain, 8th edn. 2007.
78. Ceron-Litvoc D, Soares BG, Geddes J, Litvoc J, Lima MSD. Comparison of carbamazepine and lithium in treatment of bipolar disorder: a systematic review of randomized controlled trials. Hum Psychopharmacol Clin Exp. 2009;24(1):19–28.
79. Stoner SC, Nelson LA, Lea JW, Marken PA, Sommi RW, Dahmen MM. Historical review of carbamazepine for the treatment of bipolar disorder. Pharmacotherapy. 2007;27(1):68–88.

80. Lampl C. Lamotrigine reduces migraine aura and migraine attacks in patients with migraine with aura. J Neurol Neurosurg Psychiatry. 2005;76(12):1730–2.
81. Chen W-T, Fuh J-L, Lu S-R, Wang S-J. Persistent migrainous visual phenomena might be responsive to lamotrigine. Headache. 2001;41(8):823–5.
82. Evans RW, Baskin SM. Why Do Migraineurs Abuse Butalbital-Containing Combination Analgesics? Headache. 2010;50(7):1194–7.
83. Bigal ME, Serrano D, Buse D, Scher A, Stewart WF, Lipton RB. Acute migraine medications and evolution from episodic to chronic migraine: a longitudinal population-based study. Headache. 2008;48(8):1157–68.
84. Christensen RC, Garces LK. The growing abuse of commonly prescribed psychiatric medications. Am J Emerg Med. 2006;24(1):137–8.
85. Covelli V, Maffione AB, Nacci C, Tatò E, Jirillo E. Stress, Neuropsychiatric Disorders and Immunological Effects Exerted by Benzodiazepines. Immunopharmacol Immunotoxicol. 1998;20(2):199–209.
86. Lee S-T, Park J-H, Kim M. Efficacy of the 5-HT1A agonist, Buspirone hydrochloride, in Migraineurs with anxiety: a randomized, prospective, parallel group, double-blind, placebo-controlled study. Headache. 2005;45(8):1004–11.
87. Fernandez F, Colson N, Quinlan S, MacMillan J, Lea RA, Griffiths LR. Association between migraine and a functional polymorphism at the dopamine β-hydroxylase locus. Neurogenetics. 2009;10(3):199–208.
88. Edlinger M, Hofer A, Rettenbacher MA, Baumgartner S, Widschwendter CG, Kemmler G, et al. Factors influencing the choice of new generation antipsychotic medication in the treatment of patients with schizophrenia. Schizophr Res. 2009;113(2–3):246–51.
89. Miller MA, Levsky ME, Enslow W, Rosin A. Randomized evaluation of octreotide vs prochlorperazine for ED treatment of migraine headache. Am J Emerg Med. 2009;27(2):160–4.
90. Honkaniemi J, Liimatainen S, Rainesalo S, Sulavuori S. Haloperidol in the acute treatment of migraine: a randomized, double-blind, placebo-controlled study. CME. Headache. 2006;46(5):781–7.
91. Silberstein SD, Young WB, Mendizabal JE, Rothrock JF, Alam AS. Acute migraine treatment with droperidol: a randomized, double-blind, placebo-controlled trial. Neurology. 2003;60(2):315–21.
92. Griffith JD, Mycyk MB, Kyriacou DN. Metoclopramide versus hydromorphone for the emergency department treatment of migraine headache. J Pain. 2008;9(1):88–94.
93. Krymchantowski AV, Jevoux C. Quetiapine for the prevention of migraine refractory to the combination of atenolol + nortriptyline + flunarizine: an open pilot study. Arq Neuropsiquiatr. 2008;66(3b):615–8.
94. Boeker T. Ziprasidone and migraine headache. AJP. 2002;159(8):1435-a-6.
95. Fisher H. A new approach to emergency department therapy of migraine headache with intravenous haloperidol: a case series. J Emerg Med. 1995;13(1):119–22.
96. Monzillo PH, Nemoto PH, Costa AR, Sanvito WL. Tratamento agudo da crise de enxaqueca refratária na emergência: estudo comparativo entre dexametasona e haloperidol. Resultados preliminares Arq Neuro-Psiquiatr. 2004;62(2b):513–8.
97. Hakkarainen H. Fluphenazine for Tension Headache; Double-Blind Study. Headache. 1977;17(5):216–8.
98. Levin M, Silberstein SD, Gilbert R, Lucas S, Munsie L, Garrelts A, et al. Basic considerations for the use of monoclonal antibodies in migraine: headache currents. Headache. 2018;58(10):1689–96.
99. Lipton RB. Efficacy of quarterly and monthly Fremanzeumab in patients with migraine and psychiatric comorbidities. MTIS2022.
100. al P-Re. Fremanezumab efficacy in migraine patients with prior inadequate response to ≥ preventive migraine medication classes and depressive symptoms. MTIS2022.
101. Affatato O, Moulin TC, Pisanu C, Babasieva VS, Russo M, Aydinlar EI, et al. High efficacy of onabotulinumtoxinA treatment in patients with comorbid migraine and depression: a meta-analysis. J Transl Med. 2021;19(1):133.
102. American Psychiatric Association. Diagnostic and statistical manual of mental disorders, 5th edn. American Psychiatric Association; 2013 2013/05/22/.
103. Beck AT, Ward CH, Mendelson M, Mock J, Erbaugh J. An inventory for measuring depression. Arch Gen Psychiatry. 1961;4:561–71.
104. Radloff LS. The CES-D scale: a self-report depression scale for research in the general population. Appl Psychol Meas. 1977;1(3):385–401.
105. Hamilton M. A rating scale for depression. J Neurol Neurosurg Psychiatry. 1960;23(1):56–62.
106. Spitzer RL, Kroenke K, Williams JB, Löwe B. A brief measure for assessing generalized anxiety disorder: the GAD-7. Arch Intern Med. 2006;166(10):1092–7.
107. Kroenke K, Spitzer RL, Williams JB, Monahan PO, Löwe B. Anxiety disorders in primary care: prevalence, impairment, comorbidity, and detection. Ann Intern Med. 2007;146(5):317–25.
108. Shear K, Belnap BH, Mazumdar S, Houck P, Rollman BL. Generalized anxiety disorder severity scale (GADSS): a preliminary validation study. Depress Anxiety. 2006;23(2):77–82.
109. Hamilton M. The assessment of anxiety states by rating. Br J Med Psychol. 1959;32(1):50–5.
110. Goodman WK, Price LH, Rasmussen SA, Mazure C, Fleischmann RL, Hill CL, et al. The yale-brown obsessive compulsive scale. I. Development, use, and reliability. Arch Gen Psychiatry. 1989;46(11):1006–11.
111. Young RC, Biggs JT, Ziegler VE, Meyer DA. A rating scale for mania: reliability, validity and sensitivity. Br J Psychiatry. 1978;133:429–35.
112. Bech P, Rafaelsen OJ, Kramp P, Bolwig TG. The mania rating scale: scale construction and inter-observer agreement. Neuropharmacology. 1978;17(6):430–1.
113. Hirschfeld RM, Williams JB, Spitzer RL, Calabrese JR, Flynn L, Keck PE Jr, et al. Development and validation of a screening instrument for bipolar spectrum disorder: the mood disorder questionnaire. Am J Psychiatry. 2000;157(11):1873–5.
114. Prins A, Bovin MJ, Smolenski DJ, Marx BP, Kimerling R, Jenkins-Guarnieri MA, et al. The primary care PTSD screen for DSM-5 (PC-PTSD-5): development and evaluation within a veteran primary care sample. J Gen Intern Med. 2016;31(10):1206–11.
115. Meltzer-Brody S, Churchill E, Davidson JR. Derivation of the SPAN, a brief diagnostic screening test for post-traumatic stress disorder. Psychiatry Res. 1999;88(1):63–70.
116. Connor KM, Davidson JR. SPRINT: a brief global assessment of post-traumatic stress disorder. Int Clin Psychopharmacol. 2001;16(5):279–84.

117. Brewin CR, Rose S, Andrews B, Green J, Tata P, McEvedy C, et al. Brief screening instrument for post-traumatic stress disorder. Br J Psychiatry. 2002;181:158–62.
118. Weathers FW, Blake DD, Schnurr PP, Kaloupek DG, Marx BP, Keane TM. The clinician-administered PTSD scale for DSM-5 (CAPS-5). 2013. Available from: www.ptsd.va.gov
119. Weathers FW, Bovin MJ, Lee DJ, Sloan DM, Schnurr PP, Kaloupek DG, Marx BP. The clinician-administered PTSD scale for DSM-5 (CAPS-5): development and initial evaluation in military veterans. Psychol Assess. 2017;30(3):383–95.
120. Foa EBC, S. Manual for the administration and scoring of the PTSD symptom scale-interview for DSM-5 (PSS-I-5). 2013.
121. Foa E, Riggs DS, Dancu CV, Rothbaum BO. Reliability and validity of a brief instrument for assessing post-traumatic stress disorder. J Trauma Stress. 1993;6(4):459–73.
122. Foa EB, Tolin DF. Comparison of the PTSD symptom scale-interview version and the clinician-administered PTSD scale. J Trauma Stress. 2000;13(2):181–91.
123. First MB WJ, Karg RS, Spitzer RL. Structured clinical interview for DSM-5 disorders, clinician version (SCID-5-CV). 2016.
124. Davidson JRT, Kudler HS, Smith RD Assessment and pharmacotherapy of posttraumatic stress disorder. Giller JEL, editor1990.

Visual Snow Syndrome

12

Francesca Puledda

Introduction

Visual snow (VS) is a brain condition characterized by the presence of a positive visual phenomenon which occupies the entire visual field, is continuous, and is described quite consistently as flickering and moving dots that resemble the static of an old analog television (Fig. 12.1). The static in visual snow can be black and white, transparent, flashing, colored, or a combination of these.

When visual snow was first described in a systematic manner less than ten years ago, it became clear that patients commonly complained of ancillary symptoms in addition to static perception [1]. This notion gave rise to the definition of a specific syndrome, in which the snow is accompanied by at least two additional visual symptoms among palinopsia, photophobia, nyctalopia and exaggerated entoptic phenomena [2, 3]. When these criteria are met, we talk of visual snow syndrome (VSS) [Table 12.1]. Among the additional criteria, after-images, photophobia and floaters are particularly prevalent, constituting a hallmark of the syndrome. VS and VSS do not differ in their main features and seem to represent different degrees of a wide clinical spectrum. Within this continuum, more severe manifestations are characterized by a higher prevalence of additional symptoms and associated comorbidities, such as migraine [4].

This chapter gives an overview of what is currently known about the visual snow phenomenon. The main clinical presentation of visual snow syndrome will be described, as well as its complex relationship with migraine and other comorbid conditions. The most recent advances in the current understanding of the neurobiology of visual snow are then presented, as well as possible management options for affected patients.

Questions

1. Which two are most commonly associated with visual snow syndrome?
   A. aura and depression
   B. migraine and tinnitus
   C. HPPD and migraine
   D. anxiety and depression
2. Which of the following elements is NOT considered suggestive of a common biology between visual snow syndrome and migraine?
   A. high levels of comorbidity between the two conditions
   B. migraine worsens the phenotype of VSS
   C. migraine drugs are used in VSS
   D. both have photophobia

F. Puledda (✉)
Headache Group, Wolfson SPaRC, Institute of Psychiatry, Psychology & Neuroscience, King's College London, London, UK

NIHR-Wellcome Trust King's Clinical Research Facility, SLaM Biomedical Research Centre, King's College Hospital, London, UK

T. S. Monteith et al. (eds.), *Comprehensive Migraine Management*, https://doi.org/10.1007/978-3-031-86923-5_12

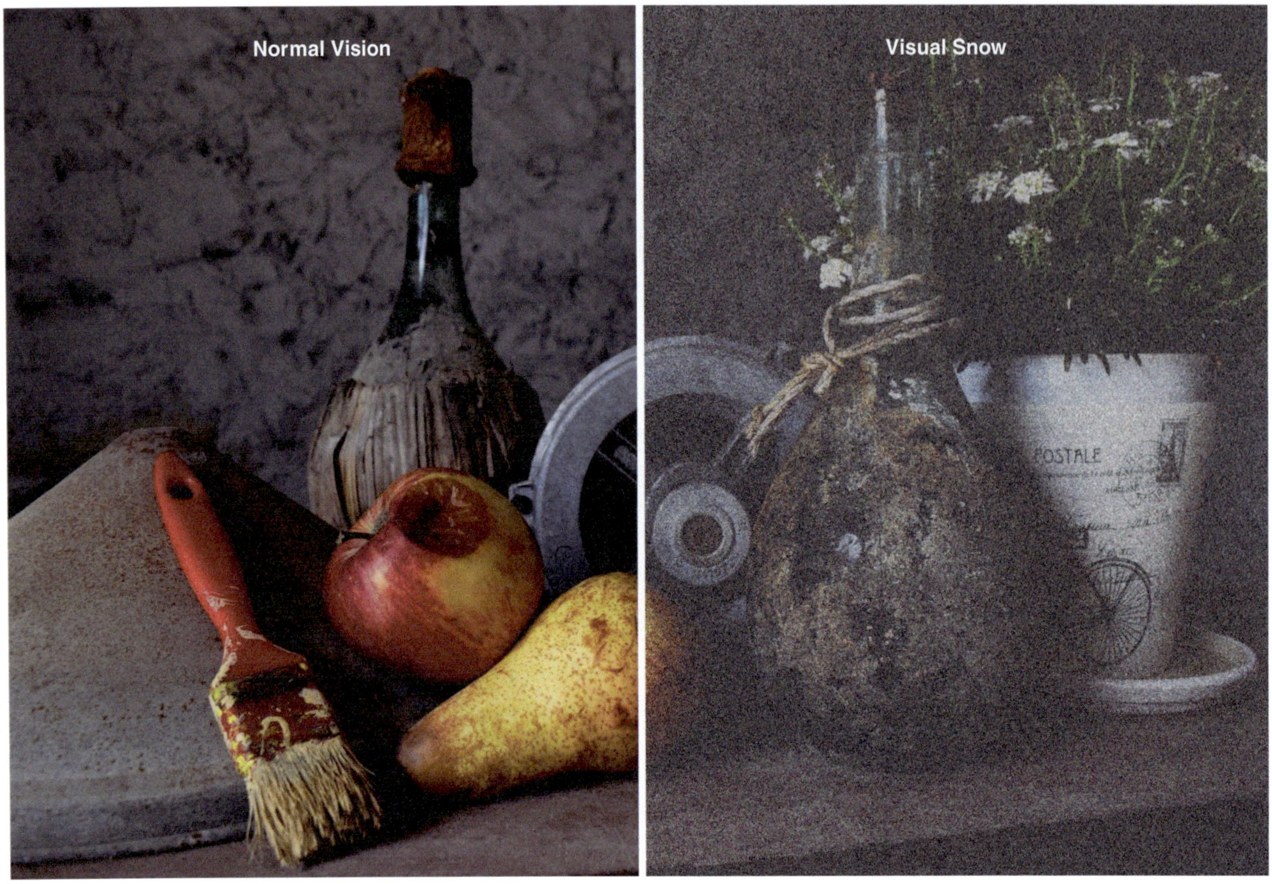

Fig. 12.1 An image of the static typical of visual snow

Table 12.1 Visual snow syndrome criteria from The International Classification of Headache Disorders 3rd edition [2]

A	Dynamic, continuous, tiny dots across the entire visual field[a], persisting for >3 months.
B	Additional visual symptoms of at least two of the following four types: 1. palinopsia[b] 2. enhanced entoptic phenomena[c] 3. photophobia 4. impaired night vision (nyctalopia)
C	Symptoms are not consistent with typical migraine visual aura.[d]
D	Symptoms are not better accounted for by another disorder[e]

[a]Patients compare visual snow to television static. The dots are usually black or gray on a white background and gray or white on a black background, but also reported are transparent dots, white flashing dots and colored dots

[b]Palinopsia may be visual after-images and/or trailing of moving objects. Visual after-images are different from retinal after-images, which occur only after staring at a high-contrast image and are in complementary color

[c]These phenomena, arising from the structure of the visual system itself, include excessive floaters in both eyes, excessive blue field entoptic phenomenon (uncountable little gray/white/black dots or rings shooting over the visual field of both eyes when looking at homogeneous bright surfaces such as the blue sky), self-lighting of the eye (colored waves or clouds perceived when closing the eyes in the dark) and spontaneous photopsia (bright flashes of light)

[d]As described under 1.2.1 of IHCD-3

[e]Normal ophthalmology tests (corrected visual acuity, dilated-pupil fundoscopy, visual field examination and electroretinography) and no intake of psychotropic drugs

The Visual Snow Phenomenon and Its Relationship to Migraine

The relationship between visual snow and migraine is deeply rooted. Before a few seminal papers in the literature marked the clear distinction between the two, visual snow had only been acknowledged in the context of case reports describing individuals with migraine, where typical VSS symptoms were attributed to complex forms of prolonged aura.

The first clear report of visual snow can be traced back to a memorable case series of patients with migraine describing continuous visual disturbances. Of these, three subjects had what we now clearly understand to be visual snow [5]. Several years later, two further descriptions of visual snow were featured in a paper investigating changes of diffusion and perfusion in patients with prolonged visual disturbances [6]. In 2008, a further two subjects with prolonged visual disturbances associated with migraine were described and assessed through the Visual Aura Rating scale [7]. Simpson and colleagues were the first to focus on visual snow as a stand-alone phenomenon through the case report of a teenager describing a sudden onset of visual snow that was clearly distinguishable from her usual migraine symptoms [8].

In 2014, a paper by Schankin and colleagues first defined the criteria for VS and its associated syndrome, presented through the review of 78 patients with self-assessed visual snow performed over the phone [1]. The same research group went on to analyze the relationship between visual snow and migraine, highlighting how the two clearly represent distinct conditions. They were also able to show that not only are VSS and migraine often comorbid, but also that migraine can aggravate the clinical phenotype of visual snow syndrome [9]. This important clinical overlap was later confirmed in a paper that described the clinical features of over one thousand visual snow patients, in which severe cases were significantly more likely to report migraine [4]. The high comorbidity between visual snow and migraine has been described consistently across the larger VSS studies and case series [10–14], although concomitant migraine prevalence seems to be lower if affected subjects are selected from the general population rather than a specialized clinic, and not inquired directly about VSS [15].

Photophobia—where normal light is either perceived as too bright or as painful—is another key element highlighting the strong overlap between VSS and migraine, as it is highly prevalent in both disorders [16]. Photophobia is present in migraineurs during attacks as well as interictally [17] and is reported in up to 80% of VSS individuals [1, 4]. Importantly, photophobia in VSS has shown to be independent of concomitant migraine, with levels of perceived light sensitivity that can reach those present in ictal migraine [18].

Migrainous photophobia is thought to be related to the retino-thalamocortical pathway, notably thalamic dysfunction [19] and possibly visual cortex hyperactivity [20]. The area found to be abnormally active in migraine photophobia anatomically overlaps one that showed hypermetabolism in visual snow subjects [9], possibly suggesting a disturbance in the downstream processing of visual inputs, common to both migraine and VSS.

If the relationship between visual snow and migraine is starting to be understood, its overlap with aura remains slightly more elusive. As described above, visual snow is often mistaken for a persistent or atypical visual aura, due to similar symptomatology and frequent presentation of VS with migraine. Indeed, some of the clinical similarities have suggested a common pathophysiological mechanism between the two phenomena, and some patients even report transient visual snow as part of their common aura experience [13]. While aura seems substantially more prevalent in VSS subjects [4, 15] with respect to the general population [21], it is interesting to find that, unlike migraine, it is not necessarily associated with a more severe phenotype of visual snow [9]. If aura is less likely to drive VSS patients to seek medical attention due to the severity of their symptoms, a true biological link between the conditions, rather than a spurious association due to selection bias, is highly possible. Overall, research studies specifically addressing these important questions are needed in order to understand more about the intricate relationship between visual snow, migraine and aura.

Clinical and Demographic Aspects of Visual Snow Syndrome

Although visual snow syndrome tends to be considered a rare disease [22], evidence from a recent UK web-based epidemiological study places its prevalence in the population at around 2% [15], which is higher than most neurological disorders [23]. This suggests that the visual snow phenomenon has gone largely underestimated, possibly due to the fact that mild manifestations are not necessarily considered troublesome by all of those affected, even though they can range to being extremely disabling in many [24].

The aforementioned population study also showed a very slight prevalence of visual snow in females (female to–male ratio of 1.6:1) and a mean age of patients around 50 years, higher than that of the general population [15]. The association between VSS and older age, however, was not confirmed in other studies [1, 4, 12]. VSS is found to typically start at a young age, with an onset in the first years of life in up to 50% of patients.

Only one study has compared the clinical presentation of VSS in different geographic regions, showing that UK and Italian patients did not largely differ in their main characteristics and had very similar rates of additional visual symptoms [25].

The main comorbidities of visual snow include migraine—thoroughly examined in the previous chapter—tinnitus, and psychiatric disorders.

Tinnitus represents the abnormal sensation of ringing or buzzing in one's year in the absence of an acoustic stimulus and is experienced as a benign symptom by numerous otherwise healthy people. However, around 10–15% of the population reports to have prolonged tinnitus that affects their quality of life [26]. A bilateral, continuous, non-pulsatile tinnitus is reported by up to 75% of visual snow patients [4], making it almost a hallmark feature of the syndrome. This very high association could perhaps be explained by viewing visual snow and tinnitus as intertwined phenomena. It is likely that these disorders represent different manifestations of a similar perceptual anomaly across two sensory modalities. This abnormality, of which the origin is largely unknown, could be leading the brain to perceive phantom sensations even when outside stimuli are absent or subthreshold.

An increased rate of psychiatric disorders, particularly depression and anxiety, has been found in patients with visual snow across several case series. These are also a common report within clinical practice, particularly in subjects who have had an extremely sudden onset of visual snow symptoms, or who report a heavy disease burden. A recent questionnaire-based study involving 125 patients with VSS showed significantly high levels of depression, anxiety, depersonalization, fatigue, and sleep issues [27]. These problems were found to greatly impact the quality of life and were associated with increased visual symptom severity. Although this relationship is certainly concerning, it is relevant to note that appropriate management of psychiatric comorbidities could significantly improve the quality of life of patients affected by VSS, where other treatments have proven useless.

The intake of certain drugs such as hallucinogenics is capable of inducing a persistent visual perception which can sometimes resemble visual static [28, 29], often causing a misattribution of visual snow to the use of recreational substances. This condition, known as hallucinogen persisting perception disorder (HPPD), can present as the delayed effect of psychedelic drugs, such as lysergic acid diethylamide (LSD), ecstasy and psylocibin [30].

The relationship between HPPD and visual snow has been investigated in two studies. A large web-based survey showed that patients with onset of visual snow symptoms following exposure to recreational drugs were more commonly male and had a later onset of symptoms, but did not differ in the main clinical characteristics of the syndrome to VSS patients without prior illicit drug use [4].

A more recent study attempted to compare migraine prevalence in a group of patients complaining of visual snow symptomatology triggered by hallucinogenics to VSS subjects with no prior recreational drug use. Interestingly, no subjects in the HPPD group—most of which were male—reported migraine, whereas over half of the VSS group did [14], suggesting that, even if a form of overlap exists between these two disorders, there are most likely different pathophysiological factors at play in VSS when hallucinogenics are involved.

Although the large majority of cases of visual snow are benign, it is worth to recall that an underlying secondary cause can sometimes bring on a similar symptomatology to the typical static, as recently demonstrated by a large retrospective case series in which over 40% of patients associated visual snow with an inciting event or comorbid illness [13]. The relevance of this finding lies in the fact that when an underlying cause exists, treatment might improve the prognosis of this form of visual snow—defined 'secondary'—with respect to subjects with spontaneous 'primary' VS. Finally, the visual snow phenomenon can sometimes underlie serious ophthalmological [31], brain or systemic disorders [32–34], which should be investigated and excluded through appropriate testing in most patients.

Pathophysiological Hypotheses and Recent Findings

Understanding the pathophysiological brain changes that are at the basis of the visual snow phenomenon has represented a challenge, chiefly because of the lack of recognition of the disorder and its very recent official definition. Several hypotheses have been advanced in order to explain VS, some of which have been corroborated by a growing number of recent studies on the topic.

A well-cited theory puts emphasis on a possible dissociation between sensory thalamic inputs and cortical projections, a mechanism known as thalamocortical dysrhythmia [11]. This dysfunction has also been implicated in migraine pathophysiology [35] and tinnitus [36], which as we know are strongly related to VSS. Other theories include increased cortical excitability [37, 38] and reduced habituation [39, 40], both of which have also been abundantly explored in migraine, and finally stochastic resonance [41] an interesting phenomenon by which the presence of 'noise' in one sensory system is thought to cause altered perception in another [42].

In the last few years studies involving a set of different methodologies, chiefly pertaining to neuroimaging, neurophysiology and neuro-behavioral approaches, have brought to conceptualize visual snow syndrome as a complex network disorder [43]. Within this view, a combination of multiple mechanisms affecting distinct brain systems could be contributing in a variety of different ways to create the altered multi-sensory perception typical of the condition [16]. The most relevant of these studies are summarized below.

Neuroimaging

The first investigation exploring the pathophysiology of visual snow syndrome through the use of neuroimaging was an [18F]-FDG PET study conducted initially on 17 subjects, recently expanded to 20. This study revealed a hypermetabolism of the right secondary visual cortex, specifically the lingual gyrus, in subjects with VSS [44]. Abnormal activation of the lingual gyrus was confirmed by functional magnetic resonance imaging (MRI) and spectroscopy, in a study conducted on 24 patients compared to 24 healthy controls [45]. Results showed increased lactate levels in this associative cortical region, which correlated to a reduced BOLD activation in response to an external visual stimulus mimicking visual snow itself. It was hypothesized that the localized disturbance in extrastriate anaerobic metabolism caused a decreased metabolic reserve in the overly active visual cortex, thus impeding the normal processing of visual stimuli.

An opposing finding was reported in another paper describing three patients with VSS undergoing [123I]-IMP SPECT, one of whom had hypoperfusion in the temporo-occipital area largely corresponding to the ventral visual stream [46].

Increased cortical activation was further found in VSS through the use of arterial spin-labeled MRI. In a recent study [47], patients showed a vast cortical area of increased cerebral blood flow—an indirect measure of neuronal activation—with respect to controls. The affected regions included the bilateral striate and extrastriate visual cortices, motor cortices, the posterior cingulate cortex and the cerebellum; additionally, this activation could be seen both at rest and during a visual task. This suggests that brain networks of cortical hyperactivation in VSS are extensive and not limited to the visual cortex, and that they are present regardless of the underlying brain state.

Two studies have assessed functional brain connectivity of patients with visual snow syndrome. The first, performed on 19 patients and 16 controls during resting state, found increased connectivity between the extrastriate visual cortex and the inferior temporal cortex, as well as between the prefrontal and angular cortices [48]. A second study analyzed VSS brain connectivity both at rest and during a visual task mimicking the snow. Compared to controls, patients showed altered connectivity within the pre-cortical and cortical visual pathways, the visual motion network, as well as the salience and attentional brain networks [49]. Further confirming the involvement of the salience network in VSS biology, the anterior insulae showed reduced BOLD response to an external visual stimulus in an fMRI experiment by the same group [45].

Morphological brain features have also been assessed with neuroimaging in visual snow syndrome. Specifically, increased gray matter volume has been found in multiple areas, both internal to the visual system—V1, visual motion area V5 and the right lingual gyrus [48, 50]—as well as extending beyond it, such as within lobule VI/Crus I of the cerebellum and the temporal and limbic lobes [44, 50]. On the other hand, decreased gray matter volume was found in the superior temporal gyrus, and it was speculated that this could be due to concomitant tinnitus [44].

White matter abnormalities were investigated in two studies: in one, a single VSS patient compared with ten healthy controls presented multiple changes in the dorsal, ventral and integrative visual stream [51]. Similarly, widespread white matter alterations were found in a group of 14 VSS patients within and outside of the visual cortex, in areas involved in visual processing and visual conceptualization [52].

These findings overall confirm that in VSS structural, as well as functional, brain abnormalities involve a large network of neuronal areas including but not limited to the visual system.

Neurophysiology

Non-invasive electrophysiological approaches have attempted to uncover important aspects of the biology of visual snow syndrome, primarily by focusing on cortical excitability and habituation, a phenomenon strongly linked to migraine pathophysiology [53, 54]. Results of these studies, however, have not been completely consistent, and more research is needed in the future to better understand the patterns of neuronal activation in VSS.

Through the use of visual evoked potentials in response to repetitive stimulation, two studies found decreased habituation in VSS, as well as increased cortical excitability over the afferent visual pathways [39, 40]. This abnormal visual habituation was not confirmed in a more recent study by Eren and colleagues [37], who conversely found that patients with VSS presented an increased N145 latency with respect to controls and migraineurs, possibly indicating a dysfunctional processing at the level of the associative visual cortex.

By applying transcranial magnetic stimulation to the occipital cortex, Yildiz et al. found an increased phosphene threshold in VSS patients [40], which they hypothesized to represent a marker of neuronal hyperexcitability in the visual pathway. By contrast, an increased cortical excitability of the primary visual cortex was not confirmed in a later study using TMS to measure magnetic suppression of perceptual accuracy, which was found to be normal in patients [55].

Neuro-behavioral and Neuro-ophthalmologic Evidence

Several types of visual and oculomotor tasks have been used to study changes in neural behavior and visual processing in patients with visual snow syndrome. While the majority of standard ophthalmic examinations appear normal in VSS, one study demonstrated a deficit in spatial contrast sensitivity measured through visual perception thresholds [56].

McKendrick and colleagues applied four different visual tasks specifically targeting visual processing in the striate and extrastriate visual cortex, showing abnormal cortical excitability localized to the primary visual areas, possibly due to an imbalance between excitation and inhibition [57]. A more recent study confirmed these results by assessing visual contrast perception in patients with VSS with and without migraine, healthy controls and migraineurs [58]. Here authors investigated the two competing mechanisms thought to underlie cortical hyperexcitability and attributed these excitatory changes to an increased neural response to external stimuli, rather than to an abnormally elevated neural noise.

In order to assess the integrity of the ocular motor network, Solly et al. used three different types of oculomotor tests, revealing significantly faster eye movements toward new and sudden stimuli and an increased error rate in patients with VSS, regardless of the task difficulty [59]. To further examine visual attentional control, two follow-up studies were performed by the same group, confirming that poor attentional control exists in VSS, regardless of whether attention is directed exogenously or endogenously [60]. Authors also showed that VSS presents a precise saccadic behavioral profile, which might provide a reliable instrument to objectively measure this clinically subjective disorder [61], and hypothesized that these attentional changes might be caused by abnormal communication within intricate thalamocortical processing networks.

Treatment Options for Visual Snow

The direct consequence of our poor understanding of the neurobiology underlying visual snow is the lack of effective treatments for the condition. From the first studies defining the VS syndrome, it has been clear from patient reports that most drugs are not capable of resolving their complex symptoms. Partly, this could be due to the fact that routinely used treatments for VSS include pain medication or migraine preventives [1], even in cases where headache is the least troublesome symptom.

Systematic clinical trials have not been performed in this patient population. Therefore, aside from sporadic empirical evidence, the most reliable data on the pharmacology of visual snow comes from two studies performed respectively in 58 [12] and four hundred cases [62].

In the study by van Dongen et al., the authors retrospectively reviewed the medical charts of VS patients treated in their center, 47 of whom fulfilled the criteria for the syndrome. The most frequently prescribed medication had been lamotrigine, possibly because of a previous single case report in which this drug, given at the dose of 50 mg twice daily, had resulted in remission of symptoms [63]. Some have speculated that this could be due to lamotrigine acting on depersonalization symptoms, which are notably high in VSS [27, 64]. In the van Dongen study, authors found that no patient had complete remission with lamotrigine. However, around a fifth of the 26 subjects who were prescribed this drug had some form of reduction in their visual snow symptomatology. Of the other drugs that were tried—including flunarizine, acetazolamide and valproate—only topiramate brought some improvement in a single patient, albeit at the cost of non-tolerable side effects [12].

The largest effort to evaluate the effect of medication on visual snow syndrome is represented by a recent perspective web-based study [62], in which information on a comprehensive list of commonly used drugs and their effect on VSS was gathered through the use of questionnaires. Medications were divided into categories including but not limited to antidepressants, antiepileptics, benzodiazepines and pain medication. Their effect on VSS symptoms was recorded as either an improvement, a worsening or no modification.

The most common categories of drugs used by patients were antidepressants, followed by antiepileptics, antibiotics and benzodiazepines. It was found that the overwhelming majority of patients reported an absence of effect with any medication, regardless if this was taken for visual snow or for other conditions. In those subjects who detected some form of improvement, the only drug categories in which this was somewhat consistent were vitamins and benzodiazepines.

With regards to lamotrigine, its use was recorded in 34 subjects. Similarly to van Dongen et al., around 20% of these reported some efficacy. However, the drug was found to more often cause a worsening (35%) or no change (44%) in symptoms, and showed comparable efficacy ratios to the broader category of antiepileptics. Importantly, this study also provided evidence on substances that can cause a worsening of VSS symptoms. These often include recreational drugs, alcohol, atypical antidepressants and ADHD medication, which should therefore be avoided as much as possible by patients.

With regards to non-pharmacological and behavioral interventions, there is some sparce evidence for their use in VSS. In the study by Lauschke et al., authors describe improvement of visual snow symptoms in 11 patients who used filtered lenses, particularly within the blue-yellow color spectrum [11]. Given the similarities between VSS and tinnitus, and the positive effect of mindfulness and cognitive behavioral therapy on the latter, it is also possible that these approaches might be beneficial in visual snow, although no study has investigated this to date. Finally, as stated in the previous chapter, treatment of associated conditions such as psychiatric comorbidities [27], as well as the investigation of treatable underlying causes of visual snow [13], can provide important avenues for the management of highly affected patients.

Conclusion

Visual snow syndrome is a neurological disorder characterized by a continuous visual symptomatology resembling static, which often co-occurs with migraine, aura and tinnitus.

The underlying mechanisms causing the phenomenon might be linked to altered cortical excitability and dysfunctional sensory processing in the visual areas of the brain. Pharmacological treatments for visual snow syndrome are not particularly useful and, for this reason, more effort needs to be placed in studying the basic neurobiology of the condition. Diagnostic criteria for VSS appear in the Appendix of the ICHD-3 to raise awareness about the condition and encourage subject homogeneity for future research.

Teaching Points

1. Visual snow syndrome is a relatively novel neurological condition often associated with migraine, aura and tinnitus. It is characterized by a positive and continuous visual symptomatology resembling static, or snow, as well as several additional symptoms such as after-images, photophobia, floaters and nyctalopia.
2. The pathophysiology of visual snow syndrome remains elusive; however, a diffuse alteration of visual and attentional brain networks, as well as cortical disexcitability, are mechanisms likely to be involved.
3. Treatment for visual snow syndrome is complex as most known medication—particularly migraine preventives—have been shown to fail. Focus should be put on non-pharmacological interventions and treatment of comorbidities or secondary causes, when these are present.

Case

A32-year-old woman presents to clinic with a history of migraine with aura, mild depression and anxiety. In the last few months, aside from her typical visual aura characterized by scotoma, colorful zig-zag lines and fortification spectra, she has been noticing a new visual disturbance that never goes away and is very similar to the static of an old, detuned TV. The static is mostly black and white, sometimes flashing; it covers everything she sees.

Aside from the static, she has been getting other bothersome symptoms, such as being more sensitive than usual to bright lights, frequent floaters, and a near to constant ringing in her ears which is most noticeable when there are no sounds. Sometimes when she looks at the sky strange squiggly lines appear, and often when looking at an object and quickly looking away the object stays in her vision. All of these symptoms seem to worsen during an acute migraine attack or when she gets little sleep.

She was seen by her GP and local ophthalmologists, who performed detailed tests and found no eye problems that could explain the disorder. Given her history of migraine, the GP suggests preventive treatment with amitriptyline, which does not improve her symptoms, and requests a brain MRI, which is normal.

The patient is quite distressed by not knowing the nature of her symptoms, which have been dismissed by her GP once all of the tests came back negative, as due to her anxiety. Following a normal neurological examination, a diagnosis of visual snow syndrome is made and a detailed explanation of the disorder is given, reassuring the patient that it is known to be benign.

Case Discussion

The patient is counseled on avoiding recreational drugs, which could potentially worsen her symptoms. Acute migraine therapy can be improved and adjusted to better control the typical VSS worsening during attacks. Other potential avenues of treatment include multivitamins, counseling for management of anxiety related to VSS symptoms, tinted glasses, and improvement of sleep hygiene to avoid symptom worsening.

Questions and Answers

1. Which two are most commonly associated with visual snow syndrome?
   A. aura and depression.
   B. migraine and tinnitus.
   C. HPPD and migraine.
   D. anxiety and depression.

The correct answer is B: Large clinical studies have shown that migraine and tinnitus can co-occur in over 70% of VSS cases. Migraine aura and psychiatric disturbances are certainly more prevalent in VSS than in the general population, but to a lesser degree than migraine and tinnitus. Visual snow syndrome and HPPD can present with overlapping symptomatology; however, their relationship is complex and still under investigation.

2. Which of the following elements is NOT considered suggestive of a common biology between visual snow syndrome and migraine?
   A. high levels of comorbidity between the two conditions
   B. migraine worsens the phenotype of VSS
   C. migraine drugs are used in VSS
   D. both have photophobia

The correct answer is C. Of all the answers, C is false, as recent studies have shown that most preventive migraine drugs are not useful in VSS. A, B and D all describe well-known elements suggesting a shared pathophysiological pathway between migraine and visual snow.

References

1. Schankin CJ, Maniyar FH, Digre KB, Goadsby PJ. 'Visual snow' – a disorder distinct from persistent migraine aura. Brain J Neurol. 2014;137(Pt 5):1419–28.
2. Headache Classification Committee of the International Headache Society (IHS). The International Classification of Headache Disorders, third edition. Cephalalgia. 2018;38(1):1–211.
3. Puledda F, Schankin C, Digre K, Goadsby PJ. Visual snow syndrome: what we know so far. Curr Opin Neurol. 2018;31(1):52–8.
4. Puledda F, Schankin C, Goadsby PJ. Visual snow syndrome. A clinical and phenotypical description of 1,100 cases. Neurology. 2020;94(6):e564–e74.
5. Liu GT, Schatz NJ, Galetta SL, Volpe NJ, Skobieranda F, Kosmorsky GS. Persistent positive visual phenomena in migraine. Neurology. 1995;45(4):664–8.
6. Jager HR, Giffin NJ, Goadsby PJ. Diffusion- and perfusion-weighted MR imaging in persistent migrainous visual disturbances. Cephalalgia. 2005;25(5):323–32.
7. Wang YF, Fuh JL, Chen WT, Wang SJ. The visual aura rating scale as an outcome predictor for persistent visual aura without infarction. Cephalalgia. 2008;28(12):1298–304.
8. Simpson JC, Goadsby PJ, Prabhakar P. Positive persistent visual symptoms (visual snow) presenting as a migraine variant in a 12-year-old girl. Pediatr Neurol. 2013;49(5):361–3.
9. Schankin CJ, Maniyar FH, Sprenger T, Chou DE, Eller M, Goadsby PJ. The relation between migraine, typical migraine aura and "visual snow". Headache. 2014;54(6):957–66.
10. Bessero AC, Plant GT. Should 'visual snow' and persistence of after-images be recognised as a new visual syndrome? J Neurol Neurosurg Psychiatry. 2014;85(9):1057–8.
11. Lauschke JL, Plant GT, Fraser CL. Visual snow: A thalamocortical dysrhythmia of the visual pathway? J Clin Neurosci. 2016;28:123–7.
12. van Dongen RM, Waaijer LC, Onderwater GLJ, Ferrari MD, Terwindt GM. Treatment effects and comorbid diseases in 58 patients with visual snow. Neurology. 2019;93(4):e398–403.
13. Mehta DG, Garza I, Robertson CE. Two hundred and forty-eight cases of visual snow: A review of potential inciting events and contributing comorbidities. Cephalalgia. 2021;41(9):1015–26.
14. van Dongen RM, Alderliefste GJ, Onderwater GLJ, Ferrari MD, Terwindt GM. Migraine prevalence in visual snow with prior illicit drug use (hallucinogen persisting perception disorder) versus without. Eur J Neurol. 2021;28(8):2631–8.
15. Kondziella D, Olsen MH, Dreier JP. Prevalence of visual snow syndrome in the UK. Eur J Neurol. 2020;27(5):764–72.
16. Puledda F, Ffytche DH, O'Daly O, Goadsby PJ. Imaging the visual network in the migraine spectrum. Front Neurol. 2019;10:1325.
17. Main A, Dowson A, Gross M. Photophobia and phonophobia in migraineurs between attacks. Headache. 1997;37(8):492–5.
18. Eren O, Ruscheweyh R, Straube A, Schankin CJ. Quantification of photophobia in visual snow syndrome: a case-control study. Cephalalgia. 2019;40(4):393–8.
19. Noseda R, Copenhagen D, Burstein R. Current understanding of photophobia, visual networks and headaches. Cephalalgia. 2019;39(13):1623–34.
20. Denuelle M, Boulloche N, Payoux P, Fabre N, Trotter Y, Geraud G. A PET study of photophobia during spontaneous migraine attacks. Neurology. 2011;76(3):213–8.
21. Rasmussen BK, Olesen J. Migraine with aura and migraine without aura: an epidemiological study. Cephalalgia. 1992;12(4):221–8.
22. Puledda F, Goadsby PJ. Visual snow syndrome 2018. Available from: https://rarediseases.org/rare-diseases/visual-snow-syndrome/
23. Collaborators GBDN. Global, regional, and national burden of neurological disorders, 1990-2016: a systematic analysis for the Global Burden of Disease Study 2016. Lancet Neurol. 2019;18(5):459–80.
24. Schankin CJ, Puledda F, Goadsby PJ. Visual snow syndrome: is it normal or a disorder – and what to do with patients? Eur J Neurol. 2020;27:2393–5.
25. Viana M, Puledda F, Goadsby PJ. Visual snow syndrome: a comparison between an Italian and British population. Eur J Neurol. 2020;27:2099–101.
26. Heller AJ. Classification and epidemiology of tinnitus. Otolaryngol Clin N Am. 2003;36(2):239–48.
27. Solly EJ, Clough M, Foletta P, White OB, Fielding J. The Psychiatric Symptomology of Visual Snow Syndrome. Front Neurol. 2021;12:703006.
28. Abraham HD. Visual phenomenology of the LSD flashback. Arch Gen Psychiatry. 1983;40(8):884–9.
29. Halpern JH, Lerner AG, Passie T. A Review of Hallucinogen Persisting Perception Disorder (HPPD) and an Exploratory Study of Subjects Claiming Symptoms of HPPD. Curr Top Behav Neurosci. 2018;36:333–60.
30. American Psychiatric Association. Diagnostic and statistical manual of mental disorders. 5th ed. Arlington. 2013.
31. Braceros KK, Asahi MG, Gallemore RP. Visual Snow-Like Symptoms and Posterior Uveitis following COVID-19 Infection. Case Rep Ophthalmol Med. 2021;2021:6668552.
32. Chen BS, Lance S, Lallu B, Anderson NE. Visual snow: Not so benign. J Clin Neurosci. 2019;64:37–9.
33. Catarci T. Occipital ischaemic stroke after visual snow phenomenon – a case report. Cephalalgia. 2021;41(7):871–4.
34. Hang C, Leishangthem L, Yan Y. Not all cases of visual snows are benign: mimics of visual snow syndrome. Neuropsychiatr Dis Treat. 2021;17:3293–300.
35. Coppola G, Di Renzo A, Tinelli E, Lepre C, Di Lorenzo C, Di Lorenzo G, et al. Thalamo-cortical network activity between migraine attacks: insights from MRI-based microstructural and functional resting-state network correlation analysis. J Headache Pain. 2016;17(1):100.
36. Llinas RR, Ribary U, Jeanmonod D, Kronberg E, Mitra PP. Thalamocortical dysrhythmia: a neurological and neuropsychiatric syndrome characterized by magnetoencephalography. Proc Natl Acad Sci USA. 1999;96(26):15222–7.
37. Eren O, Rauschel V, Ruscheweyh R, Straube A, Schankin CJ. Evidence of dysfunction in the visual association cortex in visual snow syndrome. Ann Neurol. 2018;84(6):946–9.
38. Bou Ghannam A, Pelak VS. Visual snow: a potential cortical hyperexcitability syndrome. Curr Treat Options Neurol. 2017;19(3):9.
39. Luna S, Lai D, Harris A. Antagonistic relationship between VEP potentiation and gamma power in visual snow syndrome. Headache. 2018;58(1):138–44.
40. Yildiz FG, Turkyilmaz U, Unal-Cevik I. The clinical characteristics and neurophysiological assessments of the occipital cortex in visual snow syndrome with or without migraine. Headache. 2019;59(4):484–94.
41. Moss F, Ward LM, Sannita WG. Stochastic resonance and sensory information processing: a tutorial and review of application. Clin Neurophysiol. 2004;115(2):267–81.

42. Metzler AI, Robertson CE. Visual snow syndrome: proposed criteria, clinical implications, and pathophysiology. Curr Neurol Neurosci Rep. 2018;18(8):52.
43. Klein A, Schankin C. Visual snow syndrome as a network disorder: a systematic review. Front Neurol. 2021;12:1708.
44. Schankin CJ, Maniyar FH, Chou DE, Eller M, Sprenger T, Goadsby PJ. Structural and functional footprint of visual snow syndrome. Brain J Neurol. 2020;143(4):1106–13.
45. Puledda F, Ffytche D, Lythgoe DJ, O'Daly O, Schankin C, Williams SCR, et al. Insular and occipital changes in visual snow syndrome: a BOLD fMRI and MRS study. Ann Clin Transl Neurol. 2020;7(3):296–306.
46. Shibata M, Tsutsumi K, Iwabuchi Y, Kameyama M, Takizawa T, Nakahara T, et al. [(123)I]-IMP single-photon emission computed tomography imaging in visual snow syndrome: A case series. Cephalalgia. 2020;40(14):1671–5.
47. Puledda F, Schankin CJ, O'Daly O, Ffytche D, Eren O, Karsan N, et al. Localised increase in regional cerebral perfusion in patients with visual snow syndrome: a pseudo-continuous arterial spin labelling study. J Neurol Neurosurg Psychiatry. 2021;92(9):918–26.
48. Aldusary N, Traber GL, Freund P, Fierz FC, Weber KP, Baeshen A, et al. Abnormal connectivity and brain structure in patients with visual snow. Front Hum Neurosci. 2020;14:476.
49. Puledda F, O'Daly O, Schankin C, Ffytche D, Williams SC, Goadsby PJ. Disrupted connectivity within visual, attentional and salience networks in the visual snow syndrome. Hum Brain Mapp. 2021;42(7):2032–44.
50. Puledda F, Bruchhage M, O'Daly O, Ffytche D, Williams SCR, Goadsby PJ. Occipital cortex and cerebellum gray matter changes in visual snow syndrome. Neurology. 2020;95(13):e1792–e9.
51. Latini F, Fahlström M, Marklund N, Feresiadou A. White matter abnormalities in a patient with visual snow syndrome: New evidence from a diffusion tensor imaging study. Eur J Neurol. 2021;28(8):2789–93.
52. Michels L, Stämpfli P, Aldusary N, Piccirelli M, Freund P, Weber KP, et al. Widespread white matter alterations in patients with visual snow syndrome. Front Neurol. 2021;12:723805.
53. Ambrosini A, Schoenen J. The electrophysiology of migraine. Curr Opin Neurol. 2003;16(3):327–31.
54. Coppola G, Di Lorenzo C, Parisi V, Lisicki M, Serrao M, Pierelli F. Clinical neurophysiology of migraine with aura. J Headache Pain. 2019;20(1):42.
55. Eren OE, Ruscheweyh R, Rauschel V, Eggert T, Schankin CJ, Straube A. Magnetic suppression of perceptual accuracy is not reduced in visual snow syndrome. Front Neurol. 2021;12:658857.
56. Yoo YJ, Yang HK, Choi JY, Kim JS, Hwang JM. Neuro-ophthalmologic findings in visual snow syndrome. J Clin Neurol. 2020;16(4):646–52.
57. McKendrick AM, Chan YM, Tien M, Millist L, Clough M, Mack H, et al. Behavioral measures of cortical hyperexcitability assessed in people who experience visual snow. Neurology. 2017;88:1243–9.
58. Brooks CJ, Chan YM, Fielding J, White OB, Badcock DR, McKendrick AM. Visual contrast perception in visual snow syndrome reveals abnormal neural gain but not neural noise. Brain J Neurol. 2021; ahead of print
59. Solly EJ, Clough M, McKendrick AM, Foletta P, White OB, Fielding J. Ocular motor measures of visual processing changes in visual snow syndrome. Neurology. 2020;95(13):e1784–e91.
60. Solly EJ, Clough M, McKendrick AM, Foletta P, White OB, Fielding J. Eye movement characteristics provide an objective measure of visual processing changes in patients with visual snow syndrome. Sci Rep. 2021;11(1):9607.
61. Foletta PJ, Clough M, McKendrick AM, Solly EJ, White OB, Fielding J. Delayed onset of inhibition of return in visual snow syndrome. Front Neurol. 2021;12:738599.
62. Puledda F, Vandenbussche N, Moreno-Ajona D, Eren O, Schankin C, Goadsby PJ. Evaluation of treatment response and symptom progression in 400 patients with visual snow syndrome. Br J Ophthalmol. 2021;106:1318–24. https://doi.org/10.1136/bjophthalmol-2020-318653.
63. Unal-Cevik I, Yildiz FG. Visual snow in migraine with aura: further characterization by brain imaging, electrophysiology, and treatment – case report. Headache. 2015;55(10):1436–41.
64. Naguy A, Al-Enezi N. Lamotrigine uses in psychiatric practice. Am J Ther. 2019;26(1):e96–e102.

Migraine and Epilepsy

13

Ramses Ribot and Andres M. Kanner

Introduction

Migraine and epilepsy are two common neurological disorders characterized by transient paroxysmal episodes resulting from altered brain function [1]. In addition to ranking among the most prevalent neurological disorders affecting millions of patients, both are also among the top five most burdensome neurological conditions in the United States in terms of disability-adjusted life-years (DALYs) rates with 705 [95% UI, 446–1021] per 100,000 population per year for migraine and 124 [95% UI, 75–187] per 100,000 population per year for epilepsy [2].

Numerous studies have highlighted the complex relationship between migraine and epilepsy. Already in the nineteenth century, experts in the field of neurology such as John Hughlings Jackson, Jean-Martin Charcot and Joseph Jules Dejerine had dwelled in the similarities and strong relation between migraine and epilepsy [3]. Sir William Gowers theorizing of this close relationship wrote: "some surprise maybe felt that migraine is given a place in the borderline of epilepsy, but the position is justified by many relations and among them by the fact the two maladies are sometimes mistaken, and more often their distinction is difficult" [4]. The advances in genetics, cellular biology and brain imaging over the last 100 years have allowed for a much deeper understanding of these disorders and their complex relationship, which has therapeutic and diagnostic implications.

In this chapter, we will review the epidemiology of both migraine and epilepsy. We will discuss how common genetic and pathophysiological mechanisms may explain their comorbid occurrence and their possible bidirectional relationship. In addition, we will review the temporal relation of their clinical presentation, highlight common overlaps of their signs and symptoms and consider therapeutic options when they coexist.

R. Ribot (✉) · A. M. Kanner
Epilepsy Division, Department of Neurology, University of Miami Miller School of Medicine, Miami, FL, USA

Questions

1. A 35-year-old man with a history of kidney stones, epilepsy with rare breakthrough seizures on lamotrigine monotherapy and untreated anxiety starts experiencing frequent migraine headaches. Which of the following medications should be considered first as prophylactic treatment for his migraine attacks?
   A. Topiramate
   B. Valproic acid
   C. Gabapentin
   D. Propranolol
   E. Amitriptyline
2. Which of the following migraine subtypes is a good example of the shared genetic susceptibility between seizures and migraine?
   A. Migraine with brainstem aura
   B. Migraine aura-triggered seizure
   C. Familial hemiplegic migraine
   D. Status migrainosus
   E. Retinal Migraine

Epidemiology

As mentioned above, migraine and epilepsy are common neurological disorders that often occur comorbidly in the same patient. In a meta-analysis of population-based studies from 1996 to 2012, there was an overall 52% increase in the prevalence of migraine among persons with epilepsy (PWE) compared to those without epilepsy and an overall 79% increase in the prevalence of epilepsy among individuals with migraine compared to those without migraine [5]. In a more recent systemic review and meta-analysis of studies between 2004 and 2019 that included 5564 subjects, the pooled estimated prevalence among PWE was 48.4% for unspecified headache and 26% for migraine [6].

T. S. Monteith et al. (eds.), *Comprehensive Migraine Management*, https://doi.org/10.1007/978-3-031-86923-5_13

This is much higher than the prevalence of migraine in the general population, which has been reported to occur in 10% [7, 8]. In a review of data from many other studies, Bauer et al. found that 79% of PWE were experiencing headaches, of whom ≤25% were migraine, with no clear relationship between headache type and epileptic focus location, seizure type, seizure frequency or use of antiseizure medication [9]. Although the co-occurrence of epilepsy and migraine in the same patient seems to go beyond their high prevalence, Bauer et al. recognized several methodological limitations in the studies reviewed (e.g., differences in case-ascertainment method, recall bias, misclassification bias), and they call for a cautious interpretation of these data [9].

Migraine and Epilepsy as Comorbidities

The existence of a bidirectional relationship between migraine and epilepsy that goes beyond a strong association has been suggested. This bidirectional relationship would imply the increased likelihood of the occurrence of one disorder if the other is present [10–12]. For example, a retrospective population-based study estimated the adjusted hazard ratio (aHR) of developing epilepsy among 10,016 adults 20 years old or older diagnosed with migraine between 2000 and 2009 when compared to a control cohort of 40,064. In the migraine cohort, the aHR was 1.85 (95% confidence interval [CI] 1.22–2.81). The incidence of developing epilepsy was increased in patients aged 20–44 years, yielding an aHR of 2.14 (95% CI 1.24–3.68); the aHR for developing epilepsy in females with migraine was 2.04 (95% CI 1.20–3.48) and that of males with migraine was 1.53 (95% CI 0.78–3.00) [13]. Another population-based study in Iceland reported a fourfold increased risk for developing epilepsy and a threefold higher risk of developing a first unprovoked seizure in children aged 5 through 15 years old with a history of migraine. Furthermore, migraine with aura was associated with an eightfold risk for developing first unprovoked seizures (95% CI 2.7–24.3) [14]. Conversely, patients with epilepsy were found to have a 2.4-fold increased risk of migraine in a population-based study [15].

This comorbid relationship has clinical significance as it demonstrates a negative impact on the prognosis of epilepsy. For example, in a prospective 5- to 10-year follow-up study comparing patients with epilepsy with and without migraine, those with migraine had a significantly lower cumulative probability of being seizure-free over 10 years compared with patients without migraine (5% vs. 25%) and those patients with migraine also had a seizure disorder of longer duration, a lower early treatment response, a higher incidence of treatment-resistant epilepsy and a lower likelihood of achieving remission with polytherapy for at least the last 2 years of follow-up [16]. The comorbid occurrence of migraine can also worsen the quality of life of PWE [17].

Pathophysiology

Migraine is a complex, multi-phasic, neurovascular disorder of the brain that is associated with abnormal pain processing and sensitivity. The cortical spreading depression (CSD) and trigeminal vascular system (TVS) activation theory are recognized physiopathological mechanisms of migraine. CSD as the substrate of the migraine aura has been reported in multiple studies and is characterized by a self-propagating wave of transient neuronal hyperactivity leading to sustained depolarization and suppression propagating across the cerebral cortex [18–20]. The activation of the TVS involving meningeal nociceptive afferents from trigeminal ganglion sensory neurons causes the headache phase of the migraine. The release of vasoactive mediators such as calcitonin gene-related peptide (CGRP) or substance P, pro-inflammatory mechanisms, and the build-up of extracellular K+ and H+ leading to low pH are among the factors triggering this system [9, 21] Experimental studies in animal models have indicated that the TVS can be activated by CSD, possibly by inflammatory cascades resulting in meningeal inflammation [22–26].

The main pathophysiological mechanism of seizures is cortical hyperexcitability. Events are characterized bisynchronized bursts of action potentials generated by recurrent excitation, which transitions to hypersynchronous electrical activity and recruitment of other neuron populations. The location of these populations and the propagation pattern determine the clinical manifestations of seizures [18–20]. Cortical hyperexcitability has also been proposed as a mechanism to trigger CSD [27] and has been demonstrated in patients with migraine [28, 29], suggesting a pivotal role in migraine.

Clearly, cortical hyperexcitability appears to be a common pathogenic mechanism operant in migraine and epilepsy, which supports their comorbid relationship. In epilepsy, hyperexcitability is turned into hypersynchronous activity while in migraine, hyperexcitability is associated with CSD, as well as photophobia and phonophobia. However, the relationship between CSD and epileptic activity is not completely understood. Depolarization block, the long-lasting depression induced by depolarization that follows the initial hyperexcitability in CSD and migraine, is also observed in dif-

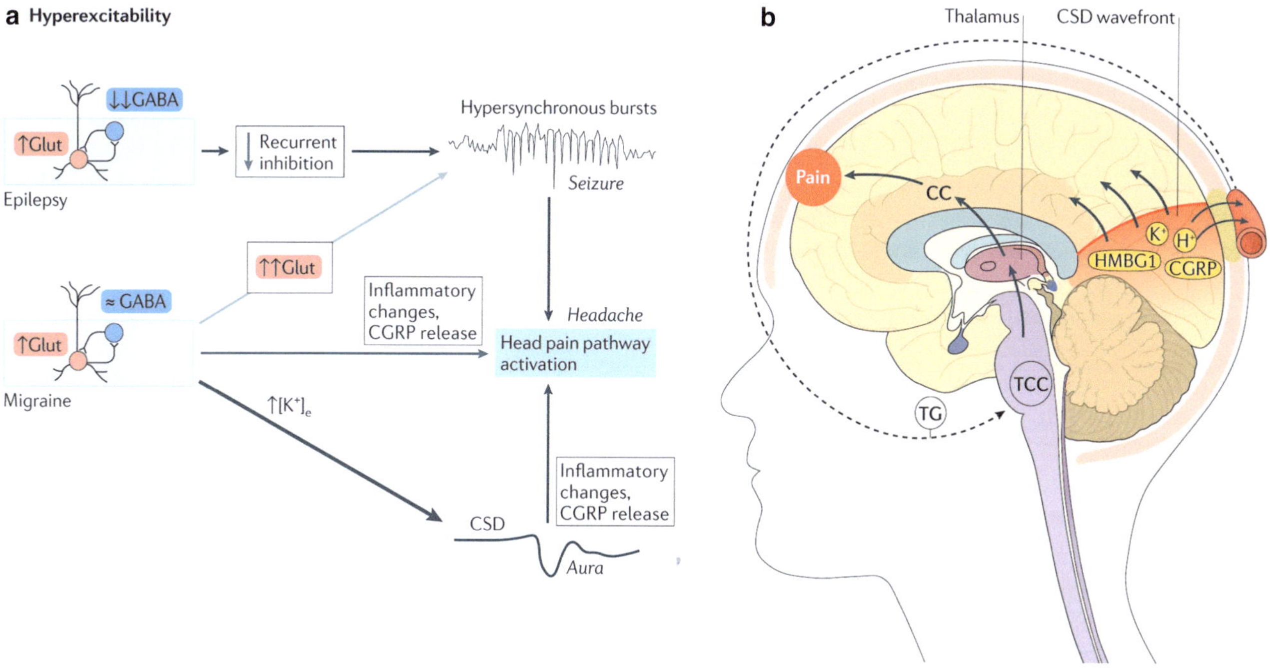

Fig. 13.1 Putative pathophysiological mechanisms linking seizures and headache. (**a**) Hyperexcitability in epilepsy often involves impaired GABAergic transmission, facilitating hypersynchronous seizure bursts. In migraine, hyperexcitability seems to be largely the result of enhanced glutamatergic transmission, which could facilitate pain pathway activation via inflammatory changes and calcitonin gene-related peptide (CGRP) release in the absence or presence of CSD. In migraine, GABAergic transmission seems to be unaltered or could be dynamically enhanced, as indicated by the results of preclinical studies on the effects of mutations associated with familial hemiplegic migraine (FHM) type 3. Strongly enhanced glutamatergic transmission in migraine resulting from pathogenic mutations, as is known to occur in FHM type 1, will increase the likelihood of comorbid epilepsy. (**b**) Cortical spreading depolarization (CSD) is likely to be the neurophysiological mechanism underlying migraine aura. CSD could also trigger migraine headache originating in the trigeminovascular 1178 system. CSD consists of a slowly propagating wave of network depolarization that is presumably caused by cortical hyperexcitability. CSD-associated increases in the concentration of potentially noxious molecules, including K+ and H+ (i.e. low pH), in the extracellular space could reach pial, arachnoid and dural surfaces and activate perivascular sensory afferents from trigeminal ganglion (TG) neurons. Inflammatory changes, involving neuronal release of high mobility group protein 1 (HMBG1) following CSD-induced pannexin channel opening, provide a mechanistic link between CSD and pain pathway activation. Signals from activated meningeal nociceptors are relayed through TG nerve processes to the brainstem trigeminal cervical complex (TCC) and subsequently to thalamic and cortical areas (including cingulate cortex, CC) and produce sensations of pain. (Adapted from Chen et al. Cephalalgia 2019 and Ferrari et al. Lancet Neurology 2015)

ferent types of epileptic activities [18]. Co-occurrence of CSD with epileptic activity was observed in patients with acute brain injury [30] and recurrent CSD appears to increase epileptic activity in experimental studies due to impaired gamma-aminobutyric acid (GABA) inhibitory function [31, 32]. Liao et al. have speculated that both CSD and epilepsy are the result of depolarization and hyper-synchronization, but the threshold of CSD is lower than that of seizures. Consequently, they also suggest that "migraleptic" occurrence (e.g., migraine triggering an epileptic seizure) is very infrequent because the threshold for triggering seizures is higher than the triggering threshold for CSD. Conversely, the trigger of CSD by recurrent seizures may explain the high incidence of peri-ictal migraine-type headaches [33]. Bauer et al. argue the link between hyperexcitability and cortical spreading depression provides a mechanistic framework for some of the clinical observations of headache in epilepsy (Fig. 13.1).

Future studies must investigate the mechanisms responsible for the development of fast, synchronous activity from the common initial cortical hyperexcitability in epilepsy but not in migraine and vice versa.

Genetics in Migraine and Epilepsy

The genetic susceptibility of both migraine and epilepsy is well documented. However, the strength of a genetic association varies among the different epileptic syndromes and migraine subtypes. Symptomatic focal epilepsy and migraine without aura have a less obvious direct genetic linkage and are more likely to relate through complex polygenetic and environmental factors. On the other hand, idiopathic epilepsy and migraine with aura may have a stronger genetic connection [34].

Perhaps the best example of this genetic connection is represented by familial hemiplegic migraine (FHM), an autosomal dominant subtype of migraine with aura characterized by fully reversible motor weakness in addition to the typical presentation of migraine attacks [35]. The three separate genes identified in this condition are CACNA1A (FHM1), ATP1A2 (FHM2) and SCN1A (FHM3), each with different phenotypes and variable manifestations. All three genes are also associated with seizures. Alteration in the genes results in dysfunction of ion channels and imbalance in cortical excitability, a likely central mechanism in both epilepsy and migraine [36–38]. Mutations in another gene, proline-rich transmembrane protein 2 (PRRT2), which leads to altered synaptic neurotransmitter release and dysregulated neuronal excitability, have also been associated with hemiplegic migraine and seizures and are postulated as probably the fourth hemiplegic migraine gene [20, 39–41].

Despite the importance of the genetic findings in FHMH and epilepsy, this monogenetic condition is rare, only accounting for a small number of patients. The genetic linkage between other more common polygenic migraine subtypes and epilepsy is less clear. However, there is evidence of shared genetic susceptibility in both conditions. In a genome-wide association study with the Epilepsy Phenome/Genome Project, 730 participants (probands, siblings or parents) aged 12 or older with either generalized epilepsy or non-acquired focal epilepsy from 501 families were analyzed. The prevalence of migraine with aura increased when two or more additional first-degree relatives were reported to have seizure disorders in the family [34]. As discussed earlier from epidemiologic data, migraine with aura has been associated with an increased risk of developing epilepsy [13, 14], while other studies have reported shared genetic susceptibility evidence for epilepsy and migraine without auras [42, 43].

Structural and metabolic disorders are both associated with an increased risk of migraines and epilepsy. There is evidence of hyperexcitability associated with these conditions and the role this may play in the prevalence of headaches in patients with epilepsy and vice versa [44]. However, it remains unclear whether the susceptibility to seizures is simply due to the structural or metabolic lesion, or whether there is an additional and unique proconvulsant effect resulting from a predisposing genetic component.

Clinical Presentation

An adequate description and accurate classification of headaches that co-occur with epilepsy is pivotal to optimize the diagnosis and treatment of these conditions and an invaluable tool to guide research efforts. Based on their temporal relationship to seizures, headaches are commonly classified as pre-ictal, post-ictal, ictal and interictal headaches. All types may represent migraine as defined by the diagnostic criteria of the International Classification of Headache Disorders, 3rd edition (ICHD-3). The only three specific entities of headache described in association with epilepsy in the ICHD-3 are migraine aura-triggered seizure "migralepsy" (Section 1.4.4), ictal epileptic headache "hemicrania epileptica" (Section 7.6.1) and post-ictal headache (Section 7.6.2) [9, 35].

Pre-ictal headaches typically occur <24 h before a seizure. In one study, the majority of patients reported the headache within 30 min prior to the seizure, and a smaller number had the headache 24 h to 30 min before the seizure onset [45]. Without EEG recording of the headache, it is difficult to distinguish pre-ictal from ictal headaches. For this reason, a classification of pre-ictal headache is not given in the ICHD-3. In a study with video-EEG recording, 3% of individuals with epilepsy reported pre-ictal headaches without epileptic discharges on the EEG [46]. As summarized by Bauer et al., the results of other cohort studies without EEG monitoring suggest pre-ictal headaches occurring in 1–10% of people with epilepsy, with 30–60% reporting migraine-like characteristics [9].

Ictal headache is defined by the ICHD-3 as a headache accompanied by epileptic abnormalities on the EEG [35]. There are several variants within this category. Cianchetti et al. proposed the term epileptic headache as "a headache" (whether migraine or not) with onset, and cessation if isolated, coinciding with an EEG pattern of epileptic seizure (scalp or deep EEG), featuring two variants: "pure" or "isolated" (not followed by other epileptic manifestations) in which the headache/migraine is the sole epileptic semiology and a headache followed by other epileptic manifestations (without discontinuity) thus actually being an epileptic seizure beginning with headache (as an "aura"). Of these two presentations, only the episodes of "pure epileptic headache" have clinical relevance, requiring a diagnostic differentiation from other types of headaches, particularly when no other types of seizures occur, and no epileptic abnormalities are present in the interictal EEG [47]. Some authors have proposed the resolution of the headache and EEG abnormalities after intravenous treatment with antiepileptic drugs as part of the diagnostic criteria [1], but this is not included in the ICHD-3 classification criteria [35]. "Hemicrania epileptica" is a variant of ictal or epileptic headache with unilateral migraine attacks coinciding with ipsilateral EEG epileptic activity. Despite being rare, likely at least in part due to EEG recordings not being common in patients with isolated headaches, several cases have been reported, and it has been accepted in the ICHD-3 [9, 46, 47]. A systematic review of 32 patients with reported ictal headaches summarized the general clinical features of these headaches. They occur at any age and affect both sexes equally. In some patients, they present with features of migraine or tension-type headache, but with no specific correlation between these types and other features or localization. They may last seconds or even days, with the shorter duration associated with temporal and anterior foci. Half the cases had minor accompanying symptoms including phono- and photophobia, nausea, vomiting, pallor, speech difficulty, agitation and irritability. When lesions are present, they may be occipital, parietal, temporal and frontal and may include malformations, dysplasias, dysembryoplastic neuroepithelial tumors (DNET) and neoplasms [47]. There is no unique EEG pattern associated with the ictal epileptic headaches as the ictal activity can be focal, lateralized or generalized and may consist of generalized spike-and-wave or polyspike-and-wave discharges, focal or generalized rhythmic activity, or focal sub-continuous spikes or theta activity that may be intermixed with sharp waves [1]. Ictal headaches are uncommon. Kim et al. reported that only 6 out of 831 patients who underwent EEG monitoring experienced headache as aura, all of whom had focal seizures, making these headaches ictal. For comparison, in the same study the incidence of pre-ictal headache was 6.3% (25/831), and post-ictal headache was 30.9% (257/831) [46]. Fanela et al. identified ictal epileptic headaches in only 5 patients in a retrospective review of 8800 video-EEG recordings of 4800 individuals with epilepsy [48]. However, since most patients with isolated headaches do not undergo EEG monitoring, ictal epileptic headaches are probably underdiagnosed. In addition, scalp EEG recordings may not detect the ictal activity if the headache is the only semiology further exacerbating this underdiagnosis [49]. Ictal epileptic headaches should be suspected with headaches of abrupt onset and ending, and those that do not respond to analgesic treatment warrant an EEG monitoring study [9].

The ICHD-3 refers to seizures that occur during or <1 h after the end of migraine with aura attack as "a seizure triggered by an attack of migraine with aura" or "migraine aura-triggered seizures" and is classified as a complication of migraine. These seizures are sometimes referred to as "migralepsy" [35]. Similar to hemicrania epileptica, migraine aura-triggered seizure is a rare condition with only a few cases reported and in which the evidence of the temporal relation between migraine and epilepsy is unclear, making some experts question this concept altogether [50–52]. The diagnostic challenge lies in the scarcity of EEG recordings for patients with these symptoms since the lack of epileptic EEG abnormalities during the migraine aura phase is essential for diagnosing migraine aura-triggered seizure. Without EEG, it is impossible to establish whether migraine aura symptoms preceded the epileptic seizure (pre-ictal), triggered the seizure (migraine aura-triggered seizures) or is a manifestation of the seizure (ictal). Most studies with EEG recordings of patients with headache and epilepsy have demonstrated that when migraine aura-like symptoms occur <1 h before the obvious ictal phenomena, EEG changes are present during the migraine-aura symptoms phase, confirming an epileptic etiology for such symptoms. The ictal changes on EEG were mostly in the occipital region [50, 52, 53]. Some authors attempting to characterize migraine aura-triggered seizures and occipital lobe seizures mention the duration of symptoms as the most helpful feature for differentiating between migraine-related aura and occipital epilepsy with migraine auras having a median duration of ~25 min, whereas epileptic visual hallucinations typically lasting <1 min [54, 55]. In addition, the progressive centrifugal expansion over minutes of visual symptoms in migraine auras is not described by people with occipital epilepsy in whom visual symptoms are often lateralized [55–57]. Other differentiating features include the description of the visual phenomena, with blurriness, jagged lines, scotomas and flickering lights being more common in migraine aura and visual hallucinations and illusions, palinopsia and oculomotor symptoms more common in occipital epilepsy [56, 57]. Lastly, nausea, vomiting, photophobia and phonophobia occur more often in migraine aura than in occipital epilepsy [55].

A post-ictal headache is defined as a headache that develops within 3 h after the seizure and disappears within 72 h after the seizure [35]. This headache is the most common type of peri-ictal headache, as evidenced in many studies summarized by Bauer et al., and occurs in <45% of patients with epilepsy, with migraine-like characteristics in approximately 50% [9]. A meta-analysis of the post-ictal period in epilepsy reviewed studies up to 2017 and estimated post-ictal headaches in 29% and migraines in 16% of adult patients with epilepsy [58]. Post-ictal headaches are more common in patients with occipital lobe epilepsy and after convulsive seizures than in patients with temporal or frontal lobe epilepsy or non-convulsive seizures [53, 59].

Interictal headaches, including migraine, are those occurring outside of the peri-ictal window, typically <24 h before a seizure and >72 h after the seizure termination. As discussed previously, the shared pathophysiology and genetic overlap between epilepsy and migraine likely make patients with epilepsy particularly susceptible to migraine, as demonstrated in multiple epidemiological studies.

In addition, to the temporal relation of headaches and seizures, there are certain types of migraine and epileptic syndromes that more commonly overlap in the clinical presentation. Migraine with brainstem aura, previously known as basilar migraine, has been associated with EEG abnormalities including diffuse slowing and focal occipital epileptiform activity. Some of its clinical features including dysarthric speech, vertigo, diplopia, paresthesia, ataxia and altered awareness/consciousness are common in epilepsy as well [60–62]. Vestibular migraine can be present in familial hemiplegic migraine. Patients with this syndrome can have, in addition to migraine attacks, vertigo, ataxia and seizures [63]. Migrainous headaches are particularly common in occipital lobe epilepsy syndromes such as benign epilepsy of childhood with occipital paroxysms (Gastaut syndrome), Panayiotopoulos syndrome and lesional occipital lobe epilepsy [64–66]. As discussed above, some of the visual semiology of these syndromes easily overlap with migraine aura symptoms.

Comprehensive management includes screening for catamenial associations and provocations that include disorders of sleep, stress and substance use (i.e., alcohol and sedative). As in most neurological syndromes, a detailed history is essential to aid in establishing the diagnosis of these conditions, especially the myriad of symptoms that present as variants. The role of EEG is also pivotal when a clinical overlap clouds the diagnosis. However, according to the American Academy of Neurology guidelines [67], EEG is typically not useful in the routine management of headaches except in the case of some associated symptoms such as episodic loss of consciousness or atypical migraine aura. Other studies including imaging and genetic tests can aid as well although with less relevance.

Treatment Considerations for Migraine and Epilepsy

Migraine remains underdiagnosed and undertreated in the US [68, 69], including in the pediatric population [70]. Along with disorders of mood and sleep, recognizing migraine as a common comorbidity is a primary concern in the management of patients with epilepsy. Given the pathophysiologic overlap discussed previously, it is not surprising for both migraine and epilepsy to respond to common pharmacological treatments. Among the available antiseizure medications, valproate (VPA) and topiramate (TPM) have the best data supporting effectiveness in migraine prevention, and both are FDA-approved with AAN/AHS Guideline level-A evidence of efficacy. Coincidentally, both drugs have broad spectrum of action and multiple mechanisms of action, although it is unclear if this has any direct relation to their migraine prophylaxis properties.

VPA increases the concentration of gamma-aminobutyric acid (GABA) in the brain, reducing excitatory transmission and blocking voltage-dependent sodium channels, suppressing repetitive neuronal firing. The GABA-ergic action has been postulated to be achieved by the activation of glutamic acid decarboxylase and by inhibition of GABA degradative enzymes. This action is thought to confer the ability to suppress cortical events and neuronal activity in the trigeminal nucleus caudalis, to inhibit ongoing and acute nociceptive activation of central trigeminal neurons, and potentially suppress the cortical spreading depression seen in migraine aura [71–75]. Similar to VPA, TPM increases GABA concentrations in the brain, blocks sodium and calcium channels [76, 77], and, in animal models, has been shown to inhibit CSD [78]; all of which are likely associated with the prevention of migraine attacks. Additional mechanisms of action attributed to TPM include the inhibition of glutamate receptors and carbonic anhydrase. However, the implications of these on the migraine prophylactic effects are not known [71].

The effectiveness of valproate in the prevention of migraine has been demonstrated in five large clinical studies supporting its classification as level-A migraine preventive in the 2000 AAN/AHS Guidelines [79–84]. These studies confirm VPA's ability to reduce the attack rate of migraine, but questions remain on its ability to decrease duration and severity of the residual attacks [85, 86]. Valproic acid is usually started at 250 mg/day with a slow titration to reach 500–1000 mg/day. Common side effects include nausea, weight gain, somnolence, sedation, tremor, alopecia, thrombocytopenia, increased liver function enzyme levels and hyperammonemia [71, 87]. In >95%, hyperammonemia is not clinically relevant and does not call for its discontinuation and/or dose adjustment. These side effects are typically milder given the relatively lower doses used for migraine in comparison with the higher doses used for the treatment of epilepsy [88]. VPA has been associated with an increased risk of severe fetal malformations, autism and cognitive deficits in children exposed in utero [89, 90]. Given this teratogenic profile, the use of VPA is not recommended in women of childbearing potential and is classified as class-X for migraine use and class-D for epilepsy [71]. Lastly, VPA should be used with caution in mitochondrial disorders, which may present with both migraine and epilepsy such as mitochondrial encephalopathy, lactic acidosis and stroke-like episodes (MELAS) [91, 92].

The efficacy of TPM in migraine prophylaxis has been demonstrated in a plethora of clinical studies including four class I studies [93–96] supporting its classification as a level-A migraine preventive treatment. In a meta-analysis by Jackson et al. from 2015, TPM was more effective than placebo at reducing migraine by more than 50%. The study also found evidence that higher doses of topiramate were more effective than lower ones, with a stepwise increment from 50 to 200 mg/day [97]. Typically, the starting dose is 25 mg/day with weekly increments of 25–50 mg/day, as used in clinical trials for migraine prophylaxis [71]. Serious adverse events are rare. Common side effects include paresthesia (dose-dependent), weight loss, cognitive effects (word-finding difficulties), depression, cognitive slowing, renal calculi, acute myopia and angle closure glaucoma [71, 87]. TPM should be avoided or used with caution in patients with glaucoma, severe pulmonary disease, metformin use, hepatic disease, nephrolithiasis, renal failure and depression [87]. TPM has also been shown to increase the risk of severe malformations in fetuses exposed in utero, most commonly cleft palate, especially when used in association with other antiseizure medications [98]. For this reason, it is a pregnancy class-D medication and should be avoided in women of childbearing potential.

Understanding the pharmacokinetic and pharmacodynamic interactions between these two antiseizure medications and other concomitant medications is important to minimize the development of adverse events. VPA is an enzyme inhibitor that can increase levels of other medications used in the treatment of migraine such as amitriptyline and nortriptyline. Accordingly, the doses of these two drugs must be adjusted to avert symptoms associated with their toxicity. Topiramate, on the other hand, has weak inhibiting and inducing actions on hepatic enzymes, minimizing risk of pharmacokinetic interactions.

Many other drugs including lamotrigine, gabapentin, acetazolamide, carbamazepine, oxcarbazepine and zonisamide were suggested to have the preventive role for migraine [71]. However, the evidence supporting their use is weak and often questioned. One of the most recent Cochrane reviews on this topic concluded that at that moment (in 2015), there was no robust evidence to support the use of any of the other antiseizure medications in the preventive management of episodic migraine. The review found some evidence on the efficacy of carbamazepine, gabapentin and levetiracetam, but due to the small sample size and other methodological issues the evidence was considered insufficient [86]. For carbamazepine, a single trial dating from 1970 prevents present-day diagnostic standards from being employed [86]. Two meta-analyses and one randomized double-blind trial concluded that levetiracetam was effective in patients with episodic migraine [97, 99, 100]. But other studies have been less convincing [101]. For gabapentin, four clinical trials have provided some evidence of its efficacy in migraine prophylaxis [102–105], but several other trials demonstrated it was no superior to placebo [97]. Similarly, some small-size trials and a meta-analysis evidenced the effectiveness of lamotrigine in preventing migraine with aura but not for migraine without aura [97, 106]. In other studies, it was no more effective than placebo [95, 107]. Despite some evidence for carbamazepine, a multicenter, double-blind, placebo-controlled trial showed no difference between oxcarbazepine and placebo in the mean change in the number of migraine attacks [108]. Lastly, the efficacy of zonisamide in migraine prevention would seem reasonable, in part due to shared mechanisms of action with topiramate, specifically the inhibition of carbonic anhydrase. Most studies have suggested some benefit in migraine prevention [109–111] including one study from Iran reporting the medications to be equally effective as topiramate in reducing migraine attacks [112]. However, the true effect of zonisamide in migraine prophylaxis remains to be investigated in placebo-controlled trials. Among the third-generation antiseizure medications, perampanel, a non-competitive inhibitor of the glutaminergic AMPA receptor, has been shown to inhibit CGRP release in the rat brainstem, suggesting a potential effect in treating peri-ictal headaches, although this needs further investigation [113].

Paradoxically, headaches are a common (>10%) adverse effect of antiseizure medications and are most often associated with carbamazepine, phenytoin, lamotrigine and levetiracetam [9, 114]. Adverse events are more frequently reported by migraine patients than epileptic patients [115, 116] and people with comorbid epilepsy and migraine are more likely to discontinue medications than those with epilepsy alone [117]. Conversely, medications in the dosage range used for migraine prophylaxis have not been associated with the occurrence of seizures [118] but tramadol, a central opioid agonist used with variable level of evidence for the acute treatment of migraine attacks [119] has been associated with an increased risk of seizures [120], so it should be avoided in patients with epilepsy who have migraine.

Among non-pharmacological treatment options, low-frequency repetitive transcranial magnetic stimulation (TMS) has been associated with reduction in seizure frequency [121] although the evidence of its efficacy in treating seizures has been judged low by other studies [122]. There is also moderate evidence supporting the effectiveness of repetitive TMS in the treatment of headaches including migraine, but with only a few studies reporting changes greater than sham treatment [123]. Single-pulse TMS has been associated with a reduction in headaches in patients with migraine with aura and has been approved by the FDA for the acute treatment of this type of migraine [124–127]. Scarcer data exists for single-pulse TMS and epilepsy. Lastly, transcutaneous vagal nerve stimulation has been shown to be effective in treating migraine acutely [128] and in migraine prevention [129, 130]. This non-invasive stimulation of the vagal nerve was also shown to be effective in drug-resistant epilepsy in three small randomized controlled trials [131–133].

Conclusion

The abundant literature discussed in this chapter has evidenced the complex relationship between migraine and epilepsy. A vast amount of data exists supporting the bidirectional comorbidity, even with a potential causal association in some cases. The diagnostic and treatment challenges that underly their commonalities and differences have been highlighted. However, knowledge of the many factors playing a role in this close relationship remains incomplete. Additional research efforts are needed to elucidate genetics and pathophysiological variables that may increase therapeutic opportunities. Increasing awareness of the many overlaps between migraine and epilepsy among physicians should also translate in increased collaborative research and improvements in the care of the many patients suffering from these conditions.

Teaching Points

1. Migraine and epilepsy are common neurological diseases and often occur as comorbid conditions.
2. There is a strong association between migraine and epilepsy and a bidirectional relationship has often been proposed, negatively impacting the prognosis and quality of life of affected patients.
3. A shared genetic susceptibility as well as pathophysiological mechanisms in which cortical hyperexcitability leads to hypersynchronous activity in epilepsy and cortical spreading depression in migraines have been considered further evidence supporting the comorbid relationship of both conditions.
4. Several signs and symptoms presenting as variants in both migraine and epilepsy and a close temporal relationship at times result in a clinical overlap, often clouding the diagnosis. A detailed history with an adequate description of symptoms and accurate classification of headaches that co-occur with epilepsy is pivotal to optimizing the diagnosis and treatment. Other diagnostic studies including EEG, imaging and genetic tests can aid as well.
5. Migraine and epilepsy respond to common pharmacological treatments. Paradoxically, headaches are a relatively common adverse effect of some antiseizure medications. Recognition of the pharmacokinetic and pharmacodynamic interactions of these medications can minimize the development of side effects.

Case

A 25-year-old woman with a history of focal epilepsy presents with an increased frequency of headaches frequency. The headaches start with auras described as blurred vision, vertigo and difficulty speaking, followed by a pulsating severe unilateral pain associated with nausea and photophobia. These symptoms resolve within 1–2 h, but the headache continues for another 8–12 h. She has had a history of similar headaches since the age of 15, which occurred only a few times per year, particularly after her seizures, which started at the age of 21. Her seizures are described as starting with luminous sparkles and ear buzzing, followed by loss of awareness and hand automatisms. Strangely, in her last two episodes, a seizure occurred within 1 h of her migraine aura. She was initially treated with valproate monotherapy, but after starting to plan for a pregnancy, she was transitioned to lamotrigine monotherapy. Her examination is normal.

Case Discussion

This patient is a good example of the comorbid relationship between migraine and epilepsy. She has focal impaired awareness seizures likely involving posterior head quadrant circuits. She also has a long history of headaches consistent with migraine with aura, which used to follow a post-ictal pattern in association with her seizures. However, there has been a change in both the frequency and the temporal relation between her seizures and migraines. The presence of seizures shortly after the migraine auras suggests migraine-aura-triggered seizures or "migralepsy" and even raises suspicion for ictal migraines. Could the new migraine attacks represent a worsening due to the discontinuation of valproate and the addition of lamotrigine? The former is used as a prophylactic treatment of migraine, and the latter can cause headaches as a side effect. Could the new "migraine attacks" be a manifestation of her seizures due to poor response to lamotrigine? This patient should undergo prolonged EEG monitoring, preferably in an epilepsy monitoring unit to better characterize these events. Treatment considerations include maximizing lamotrigine dose or adding a new migraine prophylactic treatment.

Questions and Answers

1. A 35-year-old man with a history of kidney stones, epilepsy with rare breakthrough seizures on lamotrigine monotherapy, and untreated anxiety starts experiencing frequent migraine headaches. Which of the following medications should be considered first as prophylactic treatment for his migraine attacks?
   A. Topiramate
   B. Valproic acid
   C. Gabapentin
   D. Propranolol
   E. Amitriptyline

The correct answer is B. The patient continues to have seizures on the current dose of lamotrigine, has untreated anxiety and has developed frequent migraine headaches. Valproic acid is a medication that can help with all his symptoms including migraine attacks, seizures and anxiety. Topiramate is less likely to help with anxiety and should be avoided in patients with a history of kidney stones. Gabapentin could help with anxiety, but the anti-seizure efficacy is weak and the data supporting its use for migraine treatment is insufficient. Propranolol and amitriptyline could help with migraine prophylaxis and anxiety but would not address the breakthrough seizures.

2. Which of the following migraine subtypes is a good example of the shared genetic susceptibility between seizures and migraine?
   A. Migraine with brainstem aura
   B. Migraine aura-triggered seizure
   C. Familial hemiplegic migraine
   D. Status migrainosus
   E. Retinal Migraine

The correct answer is C. Familial hemiplegic migraine. Perhaps the best example of the genetic connection between migraine and seizures is familial hemiplegic migraine, an autosomal dominant subtype of migraine with aura characterized by fully reversible motor weakness in addition to typical presentation of migraine attacks. The three separate genes identified in this condition are CACNA1A (FHM1), ATP1A2 (FHM2) and SCN1A (FHM3), each with different phenotypes and variable manifestations. All three genes are also associated with seizures. The genetic linkage between epilepsy and other polygenic migraine subtypes such as migraine with brainstem aura, migraine aura-triggered seizure, status migrainosus and retinal migraine is not clear.

References

1. Parisi P, Paolino MC, Raucci U, et al. Ictal epileptic headache: when terminology is not a moot question. Front Neurol. 2019;10:785.
2. GBD 2017 US Neurological Disorders Collaborators, Feigin VL, Vos T, et al. Burden of neurological disorders across the US from 1990–2017: a global burden of disease study. JAMA Neurol. 2021;78:165–76.
3. Haan J, Terwindt GM, Van den Maagdenberg AMJM, et al. A review of the genetic relation between migraine and epilepsy. Cephalalgia. 2008;28:105–13.
4. Gowers WR. The borderland of epilepsy. In: Arts & Boeve Nijmegen, Chapter V. Philadelphia: P. Blakistons' Son & Co; 1995. p. 76–102.
5. Keezer MR, Bauer PR, Ferrari MD, Sander JW. The comorbid relationship between migraine and epilepsy: a systematic review and meta-analysis. Eur J Neurol. 2014;22:1038–47.
6. Duko B, Ayalew M, Toma A. The epidemiology of headaches among patients with epilepsy: a systematic review and meta-analysis. J Headache Pain. 2020;21:3.
7. Natoli J, Manack A, Dean B, Butler Q, Turkel C, Stovner L, Lipton R. Global prevalence of chronic migraine: a systematic review. Cephalalgia. 2010;30(5):599–609.
8. Woldeamanuel YW, Cowan RP. Migraine affects 1 in 10 people worldwide featuring recent rise: a systematic review and meta-analysis of community-based studies involving 6 million participants. J Neurol Sci. 2017;372:307–15.
9. Bauer PR, Tolner EA, Keezer MR, et al. Headache in people with epilepsy. Nat Rev Neurol. 2021;17:529–44.
10. Kasteleijn-Nolst Trenité DG, Verrotti A, Di Fonzo A, Cantonetti L, Bruschi R, Chiarelli F, et al. Headache, epilepsy, and photosensitivity: how are they connected? J Headache Pain. 2010;11:469–76.
11. Bigal ME, Lipton RB, Cohen J, Silberstein SD. Epilepsy, and migraine. Epilepsy Behav. 2003;4:S13–24.
12. Ottman R, Lipton RB, Ettinger AB, Cramer JA, Reed ML, Morrison A, et al. Comorbidities of epilepsy: results from the Epilepsy Comorbidities and Health (EPIC) survey. Epilepsia. 2011;52:308–15.
13. Harnod T, Wang YC, Kao CH. High risk of developing subsequent epilepsy in young adults with migraine: a nationwide population-based cohort study in Taiwan. QJM. 2015;108:449–55.
14. Ludvigsson P, Hesdorffer D, Olafsson E, Kjartansson O, Hauser WA. Migraine with aura is a risk factor for unprovoked seizures in children. Ann Neurol. 2006;59:210–3.
15. Ottman R, Lipton RB. Comorbidity of migraine and epilepsy. Neurology. 1994;44:2105–10.
16. Velioglu SK, Boz C, Ozmenoglu M. The impact of migraine on epilepsy: a prospective prognosis study. Cephalalgia. 2005;25:528–35.
17. Mameniškienė R, Karmonaitė I, Zagorskis R. The burden of headaches in people with epilepsy. Seizure. 2016;41:120–6.
18. Mantegazza M, Cestèle S. Pathophysiological mechanisms of migraine and epilepsy: similarities and differences. Neurosci Lett. 2018;667:92–102.
19. McCormick DA, Contreras D. On the cellular and network bases of epileptic seizures. Annu Rev Physiol. 2001;63:815–46.
20. Kim DW, Lee SK. Headache and epilepsy. J Epilepsy Res. 2017;7:7–15.
21. Burstein R, Noseda R, Borsook D. Migraine: multiple processes, complex pathophysiology. J Neurosci. 2015;35:6619–29.

22. Bolay H, Reuter U, Dunn AK, Huang Z, Boas DA, Moskowitz MA. Intrinsic brain activity triggers trigeminal meningeal afferents in a migraine model. Nat Med. 2002;8:136–42.
23. Zhang X, et al. Activation of meningeal nociceptors by cortical spreading depression: implications for migraine with aura. J Neurosci. 2010;30:8807–14.
24. Zhang X, et al. Activation of central trigeminovascular neurons by cortical spreading depression. Ann Neurol. 2011;69:855–65.
25. Karatas H, et al. Spreading depression triggers headache by activating neuronal Panx1 channels. Science. 2013;339:1092–5.
26. Schain AJ, et al. Activation of pial and dural macrophages and dendritic cells by cortical spreading depression. Ann Neurol. 2018;83:508–21.
27. Auffenberg E, Hedrich UB, Barbieri R, Miely D, Groschup B, Wuttke TV, Vogel N, Lührs P, Zanardi I, Bertelli S, Spielmann N, Gailus-Durner V, Fuchs H, Hrabě de Angelis M, Pusch M, Dichgans M, Lerche H, Gavazzo P, Plesnila N, Freilinger T. Hyperexcitable interneurons trigger cortical spreading depression in an Scn1a migraine model. J Clin Invest. 2021;1:131.
28. Mulleners WM, Chronicle EP, Palmer JE, et al. Visual cortex excitability in migraine with and without aura. Headache. 2001;41:565–72.
29. Van Der Kamp W, Maassenvandenbrink A, Ferrari MD, Van Dijk G. Interictal cortical excitability to magnetic stimulation in familial hemiplegic migraine. Neurology. 1997;1:1996–8.
30. Fabricius M, Fuhr S, Willumsen L, et al. Association of seizures with cortical spreading depression and peri-infarct depolarisations in the acutely injured human brain. Clin Neurophysiol. 2008;119:1973–84.
31. Gorji A, Speckmann EJ. Spreading depression enhances the spontaneous epileptiform activity in human neocortical tissues. Eur J Neurosci. 2004;19:3371–4.
32. Kruger H, Luhmann HJ, Heinemann U. Repetitive spreading depression causes selective suppression of GABAergic function. Neuroreport. 1996;7:2733–6.
33. Liao J, Tian X, Wang H, Xiao Z. Epilepsy and migraine-Are they comorbidity? Genes Dis. 2018;5:112–8.
34. Winawer, Connors. Evidence of shared genetic susceptibility to migraine and epilepsy. Epilepsia. 2013;54:288–95.
35. Headache Classification Committee of the International Headache Society (IHS): international classification of headache disorders, 3rd edn. Cephalalgia. 2018;38:1–211.
36. Prontera P, Sarchielli P, Caproni S, Bedetti C, Cupini LM, Calabresi P, Costa C. Epilepsy in hemiplegic migraine: genetic mutations and clinical implications. Cephalalgia. 2018;38:361–73.
37. Carreño O, Corominas R, Serra SA, Sintas C, Fernández-Castillo N, Vila-Pueyo M, Toma C, Gené GG, et al. Screening of CACNA1A and ATP1A2 genes in hemiplegic migraine: clinical, genetic, and functional studies. Mol Genet Genomic Med. 2013;1:206–22.
38. Hiekkala ME, Vuola P, Artto V, Häppölä P, Häppölä E, Vepsäläinen S, Cuenca-Leon E, Lal D, et al. The contribution of CACNA1A, ATP1A2 and SCN1A mutations in hemiplegic migraine: a clinical and genetic study in Finnish migraine families. Cephalalgia. 2018;38:1849–63.
39. Marini C, Conti V, Mei D, Battaglia D, Lettori D, Losito E, Bruccini G, Tortorella G, et al. PRRT2 mutations in familial infantile seizures, paroxysmal dyskinesia, and hemiplegic migraine. Neurology. 2012;79:2109–14.
40. Pellacani S, Sicca F, Di Lorenzo C, et al. The revolution in migraine genetics: from aching channels disorders to a next-generation medicine. Front Cell Neurosci. 2016;10:156.
41. Riant F, et al. Hemiplegic migraine associated with PRRT2 variations: a clinical and genetic study. Neurology. 2022;98:e51–61.
42. Clarke T, Baskurt Z, Strug LJ, Pal DK. Evidence of shared genetic risk factors for migraine and rolandic epilepsy. Epilepsia. 2009;50:2428–33.
43. Polvi A, Siren A, Kallela M, Rantala H, Artto V, Sobel EM, Palotie A, Lehesjoki AE, Wessman M. Shared loci for migraine and epilepsy on chromosomes 14q12-q23 and 12q24.2-q24.3. Neurology. 2012;78:202–9.
44. Rogawski MA. Migraine and epilepsy—shared mechanisms within the family of episodic disorders. In: Noebels JL, Avoli M, Rogawski MA, Olsen RW, Delgado-Escueta AV, editors. Jasper's basic mechanisms of the epilepsies [Internet]. 4th ed. Bethesda: National Center for Biotechnology Information (US); 2012.
45. Wang XQ, et al. Comorbidity between headache and epilepsy in a Chinese epileptic center. Epilepsy Res. 2014;108:535–41.
46. Kim DW, Sunwoo JS, Lee SK. Headache as an aura of epilepsy: video-EEG monitoring study. Headache. 2016;56:762–8.
47. Cianchetti C, Dainese F, Ledda MG, Avanzini G. Epileptic headache: a rare form of painful seizure. Seizure. 2017;52:169–75.
48. Fanella M, et al. Ictal epileptic headache in adult life: electroclinical patterns and spectrum of related syndromes. Epilepsy Behav. 2015;53:161–5.
49. Laplante P, Saint-Hilaire JM, Bouvier G. Headache as an epileptic manifestation. Neurology. 1983;33:1493–5.
50. Verrotti A, Coppola G, Di Fonzo A, et al. Should "migralepsy" be considered an obsolete concept? A multicenter retrospective clinical/EEG study and review of the literature. Epilepsy Behav. 2011;21:52–9.
51. Verrotti A, et al. Migralepsy and related conditions: advances in pathophysiology and classification. Seizure. 2011;20:271–5.
52. Hartl E, Rémi J, Noachtar S. Two patients with visual aura – migraine, epilepsy, or migralepsy? Headache. 2015;55:1148–51.
53. Wang XQ, et al. High prevalence of headaches in patients with epilepsy. J Headache Pain. 2014;15:70.
54. Saitowitz Z, Flamini R, Berenson F. Ictal epileptic headache: a review of current literature and differentiation from migralepsy and other epilepsies. Headache. 2014;54:1534–40.
55. Hartl E, Angel J, Rémi J, Schankin CJ, Noachtar S. Visual auras in epilepsy and migraine – an analysis of clinical characteristics. Headache. 2017;57:908–16.
56. Viana M, Tronvik EA, Do TP, Zecca C, Hougaard A. Clinical features of visual migraine aura: a systematic review. J Headache Pain. 2019;20:64.
57. Adcock JE, Panayiotopoulos CP. Occipital lobe seizures and epilepsies. J Clin Neurophysiol. 2012;29:397–407.
58. Subota A, et al. Signs and symptoms of the postictal period in epilepsy: a systematic review and meta-analysis. Epilepsy Behav. 2019;94:243–51.
59. Karaali-Savrun F, Göksan B, Naz Yeni S, Ertan S, Uzun N. Seizure-related headache in patients with epilepsy. Seizure. 2002;11:67–9.
60. De Romanis F, Buzzi MG, Assenza S, et al. Basilar migraine with electroencephalographic findings of occipital spike-wave complexes: a long-term study in seven children. Cephalalgia. 1993;13:192–6.
61. Lapkin ML, French JH, Golden GS, et al. The electroencephalogram in childhood basilar artery migraine. Neurology. 1977;27:580–3.
62. Camfield PR, Metrakos K, Andermann F. Basilar migraine, seizures, and severe epileptiform EE abnormalities. Neurology. 1978;28:584–8.
63. Silberstein SD, Dodick DW. Migraine genetics: part II. Headache. 2013;53:1218–29.
64. Gastaut H. A new type of epilepsy: benign partial epilepsy of childhood with occipital spike-waves. Clin Electroencephalogr. 1982;13:13–22.

65. Panayiotopoulos CP. Benign childhood epilepsy with occipital paroxysms: a 15-year prospective study. Ann Neurol. 1989;26:51–6.
66. Williamson PD, Thadani VM, Darcey TM, et al. Occipital lobe epilepsy: clinical characteristics, seizure spread patterns, and results of surgery. Ann Neurol. 1992;31:3–13.
67. Practice parameter. The electroencephalogram in the evaluation of headache (Summary statement) Report of the Quality Standards Subcommittee of the American Academy of Neurology. Neurology. 1995;45:1411–3.
68. Diamond S, Bigal ME, Silberstein S, Loder E, Reed M, Lipton RB. Patterns of diagnosis and acute and preventive treatment for migraine in the United States: results from the American Migraine Prevalence and Prevention study. Headache. 2007;47:355–63.
69. Lipton R, et al. Diagnosis, consultation, treatment, and impact of migraine in the US: results of the OVERCOME (US) study. Headache. 2022;62:122–40.
70. Kelley SA, Hartman AL, Kossof EH. Comorbidity of migraine in children presenting with epilepsy to a tertiary care center. Neurology. 2012;79:468–73.
71. Bagnato F, Good J. The use of antiepileptics in migraine prophylaxis. Headache. 2016;56:603–15.
72. Johannessen CU. Mechanisms of action of valproate: a commentatory. Neurochem Int. 2000;37:103–10.
73. Galletti F, Cupini LM, Corbelli I, Calabresi P, Sarchielli P. Pathophysiological basis of migraine prophylaxis. Prog Neurobiol. 2009;89:176–92.
74. Cutrer FM, Limnroth V, Moskowitz MA. Possible mechanisms of valproate in migraine prophylaxis. Cephalalgia. 1977;17:93–9.
75. Akerman S, Romero-Reyes M. Targeting the central projection of the dural trigeminovascular system for migraine prophylaxis. J Cereb Blood Flow Metab. 2019;39:704–17.
76. Costa C, Martella G, Picconi B, et al. Multiple mechanisms underlying the neuroprotective effects of antiepileptic drugs against in vitro ischemia. Stroke. 2006;37:1319–26.
77. White HS, Brown SD, Woodhead JH, Skeen GA, Wolf HH. Topiramate modulates GABA-evoked currents in murine cortical neurons by a non-benzodiazepine mechanism. Epilepsia. 2000;41:S 17-20.
78. Akerman S, Goadsby PJ. Topiramate inhibits cortical spreading depression in rat and cat: impact in migraine aura. Neuroreport. 2005;16:1383–7.
79. Silberstein SD for the US Headache Consortium. Practice-parameter: evidence-based guidelines for migraine headache (an evidence-based review): report of the Quality Standards Subcommittee of the American Academy of Neurology. Neurology. 2000;55:754–62.
80. Hering R, Kuritzky A. Sodium valproate in the prophylactic treatment of migraine: a double-blind study versus placebo. Cephalalgia. 1992;12:81–4.
81. Jensen R, Brinck T, Olesen J. Sodium valproate has a prophylactic effect in migraine without aura: a triple-blind, placebo-controlled crossover study. Neurology. 1994;44:647–51.
82. Mathew NT, Saper JR, Silberstein SD, et al. Migraine prophylaxis with divalproex. Arch Neurol. 1995;52:281–186.
83. Klapper J. Divalproex sodium in migraine prophylaxis: a dose-controlled study. Cephalalgia. 1997;17:103–8.
84. Kaniecki RG. A comparison of divalproex with propranolol and placebo for the profilaxis of migraine without aura. Arch Neurol. 1997;54:1141–5.
85. Linde M, Mulleners WM, Chronicle EP, McCrory DC. Valproate (valproic acid or sodium valproate or a combination of the two) for the prophylaxis of episodic migraine in adults. Cochrane Database Syst Rev. 2013;2013(6):CD010611.
86. Mulleners WM, McCrory DC, Linde M. Antiepileptics in migraine pro-phylaxis: an updated Cochrane review. Cephalalgia. 2015;35:51–62.
87. Demarquay G, Rheims S. Relationships between migraine and epilepsy: pathophysiological mechanisms and clinical implications. Rev Neurol. 2021;177:791–800.
88. Nye BL, Thadani VM. Migraine and epilepsy: review of the literature. Headache. 2015;55:359–80.
89. Tomson T, Battino D, Bonizzoni E, Craig J, Lindhout D, Perucca E, et al. Comparative risk of major congenital malformations with eight different antiepileptic drugs: a prospective cohort study of the EURAP registry. Lancet Neurol. 2018;17:530–8.
90. Meador KJ, Baker GA, Browning N, Cohen MJ, Bromley RL, Clayton-Smith J, et al. Fetal antiepileptic drug exposure and cognitive outcomes at age 6 years (NEAD study): a prospective observational study. Lancet Neurol. 2013;12:244–52.
91. Kingston WS, Schwedt TJ. The relationship between headaches with epileptic and non-epileptic seizures: a narrative review. Curr Pain Headache Rep. 2017;21:17.
92. Yorns WR, Hardison HH. Mitochondrial dysfunction in migraine. A review regarding the relationship between mitochondrial and migraine highlighting an important possible etiology. Semin Pediatr Neurol. 2013;20:188–93.
93. Storey JR, Calder CS, Hart DE, Potter DL. Topiramate in migraine prevention: a double-blind, placebo-controlled study. Headache. 2001;41:968–75.
94. Shaygannejad V, Janghorbani M, Ghorbani A, Ashtary F, Zakizade N, Nasr V. Comparison of the effect of topiramate and sodium valproate in migraine prevention: a randomized blinded crossover study. Headache. 2006;46:642–8.
95. Gupta P, Singh S, Goyal V, Shukla G, Behari M. Low-dose topiramate versus lamotrigine in migraine prophylaxis (the Lotolamp study). Headache. 2007;47:402–12.
96. Ashtari F, Shaygannejad V, Akbari M. A double-blind, randomized trial of low dose topiramate vs propranolol in migraine prophylaxis. Acta Neurol Scand. 2008;18:301–5.
97. Jackson JL, Cogbill E, Santana-Davila R, Eldredge C, Collier W, Gradall A, et al. A comparative effectiveness meta-analysis of drugs for the prophylaxis of migraine headache. PLoS One. 2015;10:e0130733.
98. Keni RR, Jose M, Sarma PS, Thomas SV, Kerala Registry of Epilepsy and Pregnancy Study Group. Teratogenicity of antiepileptic dual therapy: dose-dependent, drug-specific, or both? Neurology. 2018;90:790–79.
99. Yen P-H, Kuan Y-C, Tam K-W, Chung C-C, Hong C-T, Huang Y-H. Efficacy of levetiracetam for migraine prophylaxis: a systematic review and meta-analysis. J Formos Med Assoc. 2021;120:755–64.
100. Kashipazha D, Ghadikolaei HS, Siavashi M. Levetiracetam in compared to sodium valproate for prophylaxis in chronic migraine headache: a randomized double-blind clinical trial. Curr Clin Pharmacol. 2017;12:55–9.
101. Verma A, Srivastava D, Kumar A, Singh V. Lecetiracetam in migraine profilaxis: a randomized placebo-controlled study in a rural medical institute in Northen India. Clin Neuropharmacol. 2013;36(6):193–7.
102. Di Trapani G, Mei D, Marra C, Mazza S, Capuano A. Gabapentin in the prophylaxis of migraine: a double-blind randomized placebo-controlled study. Clin Ther. 2000;151:145–8.
103. Mathew NT, Rappapot A, Saper J, et al. Efficacy of gabapentin in migraine prophylaxis. Headache. 2021;41:119–28.
104. Jimenez-Hernandez MD, Torrecillas Narvaez MD, Friera Acebal G. Effectiveness and safety of gabapentin in the preventive treatment of migraine. Rev Neurol. 2002;35:603–6.
105. Silberstein S, Goode-Sellers S, Twomey C, Sajers J, Ascher J. Randomized, double-blind, placebo-controlled, phase II trial of gabapentin enacarbil for migraine prophylaxis. Cephalalgia. 2013;33:101–11.

106. Buch D, Chabriat H. Lamotrigine in the prevention of migraine with aura: a narrative review. Headache. 2019;59:1187–97.
107. Steiner TJ, Findley LJ, Yuen AW. Lamotrigine versus placebo in the prophylaxis of migraine with and without aura. Cephalalgia. 1997;17:109–12.
108. Silberstein SD, Saper J, Berenson F, Somogyi M, McCague MA, D'Souza JD. Oxcarbazepine in migraine headache: a double-blind, randomized, placebo-controlled study. Neurology. 2008;70:548–55.
109. Ashkenazi A, Benlifer A, Korenblit J, Silberstein SD. Zonisamide for migraine prophylaxis in refractory patients. Cephalalgia. 2006;26:1199–202.
110. Bermejo PE, Dorado R. Zonisamide for migraine prophylaxis in patients refractory to topiramate. Clin Neuropharmacol. 2009;32:103–6.
111. Villani V, Ciuffoli A, Prosperini L, Sette G. Zonisamide for migraine prophylaxis in topiramate-intolerant patients: an observational study. Headache. 2011;51:287–91.
112. Mohammadianinejad SE, Abbasi V, Sajedi SA, et al. Zonisamide versus topiramate in migraine prophylaxis: a double-blind randomized clinical trial. Clin Neuropharmacol. 2011;34:174–7.
113. Tringali G, Currò D, Navarra P. Perampanel inhibits calcitonin gene-related peptide release from rat brainstem in vitro. J Headache Pain. 2018;12(19):107.
114. Nevitt S, Sudell M, Weston J, Tudur Smith C, Marson A. Antiepileptic drug monotherapy for epilepsy: a network meta-analysis of individual participant data. Cochrane Database Syst Rev. 2017;6(6):CD011412.
115. Luykx J, Mason M, Ferrari D, Carpay J. Are migraineurs at increased risk of adverse drug responses? A meta-analytic comparison of topiramate-related adverse drug reactions in epilepsy and migraine. Clin Pharmacol Ther. 2009;85:283–8.
116. Romoli M, Costa C, Siliquini S, Corbelli I, Eusebi P, Bedetti C, Caproni S, Cupini LM, Calabresi P, Sarchielli P. Antiepileptic drugs in migraine and epilepsy: who is at increased risk of adverse events? Cephalalgia. 2018;38:274–82.
117. Romoli M, et al. Antiepileptic drugs in migraine and epilepsy: who is at increased risk of adverse events? Cephalalgia. 2018;38:274–82.
118. Kaur A, Selwa L, Fromes G, Ross DA. Persistent headache after supratentorial craniotomy. Neurosurgery. 2000;47:633–6.
119. Marmura MJ, Silberstein SD, Scwedt TJ. The acute treatment of migraines in adults: the American Headache Society evidence assessment of migraine pharmacotherapies. Headache. 2015;55:3–20.
120. Hassamal S, Miotto K, William D, Danovitch I. Tramadol: understanding the risk of serotonin syndrome and seizures. Am J Med. 2018;131:1382.
121. Cooper YA, et al. Repetitive transcranial magnetic stimulation for the treatment of drug-resistant epilepsy: a systematic review and individual participant data meta-analysis of real-world evidence. Epilepsia Open. 2017;3:55–65.
122. Walton D, Spencer DC, Nevitt SJ, Michael BD. Transcranial magnetic stimulation for the treatment of epilepsy. Cochrane Database Syst Rev. 2021;4(4):CD011025.
123. Stilling JM, Monchi O, Amoozegar F, Debert CT. Transcranial magnetic and direct current stimulation (TMS/tDCS) for the treatment of headache: a systematic review. Headache. 2019;59:339–57.
124. Lipton RB, et al. Single-pulse transcranial magnetic stimulation for acute treatment of migraine with aura: a randomised, double-blind, parallel-group, sham-controlled trial. Lancet Neurol. 2010;9:373–80.
125. Starling AJ, et al. A multicenter, prospective, single arm, open label, observational study of sTMS for migraine prevention (ESPOUSE study). Cephalalgia. 2018;38:1038–48.
126. Lan L, Zhang X, Li X, Rong X, Peng Y. The efficacy of transcranial magnetic stimulation on migraine: a meta-analysis of randomized controlled trails. J Headache Pain. 2017;18:86.
127. Food and Drug Administration. Transcranial magnetic stimulator AC adapter. 510(k) Notification K140094. accessdata.fda.gov.
128. Chou DE, et al. Acute migraine therapy with external trigeminal neurostimulation (ACME): a randomized controlled trial. Cephalalgia. 2019;39:3–14.
129. Diener HC, et al. Non-invasive vagus nerve stimulation (nVNS) for the preventive treatment of episodic migraine: the multicentre, double-blind, randomised, sham-controlled PREMIUM trial. Cephalalgia. 2019;39:1475–87.
130. Najib U, et al. Non-invasive vagus nerve stimulation for prevention of migraine: the multicenter, randomized, double-blind, sham-controlled PREMIUM II trial. Cephalalgia. 2022;42:560–9.
131. Aihua L, et al. A controlled trial of transcutaneous vagus nerve stimulation for the treatment of pharmacoresistant epilepsy. Epilepsy Behav. 2014;39:105–10.
132. Rong P, et al. Transcutaneous vagus nerve stimulation for refractory epilepsy: a randomized controlled trial. Clin Sci. 2014;10. https://doi.org/10.1042/CS20130518.
133. Bauer S, et al. Transcutaneous vagus nerve stimulation (tVNS) for treatment of drug-resistant epilepsy: a randomized, double-blind clinical trial (cMPsE02). Brain Stimul. 2016;9:356–63.

Migraine, Vascular Disorders and Complications

14

Alexandra Cocores and Teshamae S. Monteith

Introduction

Historically, the term 'vascular headache' was used to describe migraine given the pulsating and throbbing quality of pain. In the 1940s, it was observed that extracranial blood vessels became distended and pulsated during attacks, leading to the vasogenic theory of migraine. However, migraine is best understood as a neurovascular headache, with a growing body of evidence demonstrating both neuronal and vascular factors [1]. Migraine is associated with cerebral, cardiac, peripheral, and retinal vasculature disorders, according to epidemiological studies. This likely reflects shared biological factors, including endothelial dysfunction and impaired activation and vascular reactivity [2]. Recent genome-wide association studies (GWAS) have revealed multiple independent loci associated with migraine, several of which showed enrichment for genes expressed in vascular and smooth muscle tissues [3]. GWAS studies have also confirmed shared genetic risk loci between migraine and coronary artery disease (CAD) [4], ischemic stroke [5], blood pressure, hyperlipidemia, and heart disease [6]. Given the high prevalence and burden of both migraine and vascular disorders, an understanding of their complex relationships is useful in management of these patients.

Questions

1. Of the following patient scenarios, who might be at the highest risk of ischemic stroke, assuming other risk factors are negative?
   A. A 40-year-old woman with migraine with aura, hypercholesterolemia and obesity.
   B. A 40-year-old woman with migraine with aura who uses combined oral contraceptive and with active tobacco use.
   C. A 40-year-old man with migraine with aura, hypercholesterolemia, and obesity.
   D. A 30-year-old man with migraine with aura, hypercholesterolemia, and with active tobacco use.
   E. A 30-year-old woman with migraine with aura with active tobacco use and physical inactivity.
2. Regarding migraine treatments, which of the following statements is incorrect?
   A. The triptans are generally considered safe even in patients with stable vascular comorbidities but should be used with caution.
   B. The ditans are a class of selective 5-HT_{1F} receptor agonists that do not cause vasoconstriction.
   C. The gepants are a class of calcitonin gene-related peptide receptor antagonists, which are not known to cause vasoconstriction.
   D. Triptan medications carry an FDA contraindication in patients with a history of coronary artery disease (CAD), uncontrolled hypertension, or ischemic stroke.
   E. Gepant medications do not carry FDA contraindications in patients with a history of stroke, CAD, or peripheral vascular disease.

A. Cocores (✉) · T. S. Monteith
Department of Neurology, Miller School of Medicine,
University of Miami, Miami, FL, USA

T. S. Monteith et al. (eds.), *Comprehensive Migraine Management*, https://doi.org/10.1007/978-3-031-86923-5_14

Cerebrovascular Disorders

Ischemic Stroke

Migraine and ischemic stroke, while both neurovascular disorders, have distinct sex preponderance, age of onset, mechanisms, clinical presentation and sequalae, and management [7]. Several meta-analyses indicate that migraine increases the overall risk of cerebrovascular diseases. The relative risk is more than double in migraine with aura but is inconsistent for migraine without aura. Results also suggest increased risk in female sex, age less than 45 years, positive smoking status, and use of oral contraceptive [8–12]. Although the risk of stroke overall increases with age, elderly patients with migraine do not seem to have a substantially greater risk of stroke [13], except if active smokers [14] or in the setting of late-onset migraine with aura, which should be evaluated [15].

In women with migraine with aura in particular, risk is higher in those with certain behavioral factors (smoking, oral contraception use) [16], an attack within the prior year compared to those without recent attack [17] and in those with high attack frequency [18]; though they are more likely to experience stroke with favorable functional outcome (modified Rankin scale 0–1) compared to women without migraine [19].

The precise mechanism behind the migraine-stroke association remains unknown and a history of migraine is associated with a cryptogenic etiology in patients with stroke or transient ischemic attack (TIA) [20]. While migraine patients are more likely to have unfavorable vascular risk factors [21], the increased risk of ischemic stroke has been shown to be even more apparent in people with migraine without conventional cardiovascular risk factors [22]. Migraine was not associated with excess intracranial or extracranial atherosclerosis in patients with acute ischemic stroke [23]. Cortical spreading depression (CSD) may serve as a mechanism for the increased risk in people with migraine aura [24] and there is a shared genetic susceptibility to migraine and ischemic stroke due to large artery and cardioembolic stroke [5]. Analysis of GWAS data revealed that migraine-associated common genetic variants confer a greater risk of posterior than anterior circulation ischemic stroke in patients with unspecified migraine and migraine without aura [25]. Another GWAS revealed concordance between loci for shared genetics of migraine and cervical artery dissection (CeAD) [26] and a population-based study showed that migraine without aura is more common among cervical artery dissection (CeAD) stroke patients compared to non-CeAD stroke patients [27].

Migrainous Infarction

Strokes rarely develop during a migraine attack: One study demonstrated an annual incidence of migrainous infarction to be 0.80 per 100,000 per year, with the incidence in females nearly twofold that of males [28]. A migrainous infarction is defined as an attack in which one or more of the patients' typical migraine aura symptoms persist for greater than 60 minutes and occur in association with an ischemic brain lesion in the appropriate relevant vascular territory (demonstrated by neuroimaging) [29].

A possible explanation is vasoconstriction such as due to large artery vasospasm, persistent oligemia, and decreased blood flow during cortical spreading depression that reaches the ischemic threshold [30]. Though, most commonly during aura and posterior predominant, PET and MRI imaging demonstrate that cerebral blood flow during the oligemic phase of CSD mostly remains above the range associated with ischemic injury [31].

Transient Ischemic Attack

The differentiation between TIA and aura may be challenging even for experienced clinicians. One systematic review concluded that migraine aura is the third most common mimic of acute ischemic in the emergency setting, following seizures and psychiatric disorders [32]. With age, the occurrence of both TIA and atypical aura (without migraine pain) increases [33] and increased aura frequency can be the manifestation of an underlying stroke risk factor including cardioemboli, hemosiderin deposition, or arterial emboli [34].

An update to the diagnostic criteria of migraine with aura in the third edition of the International Classification of Headache disorders (ICHD-3) was made in attempt to improve specificity and distinguish aura from TIA [35]. For example, neurologic symptoms due to migraine aura tend to be accompanied, or followed within 60 minutes, by headache and are typically positive symptoms. In prospective testing of ICHD-3 criteria, a slow spread of symptoms and succession of symptoms were the best features to discriminate between migraine aura and TIA [36]. Interestingly, expert opinion suggests that an ischemic event could also possibly be separated from migraine pathology, considering the involvement of the tongue. Per clinical experience, sensory paresthesia on one side of the tongue may represent migraine aura, unlike stroke [37, 38].

Distinction is necessary clinically as ischemia may trigger migraine, and headache while common following transient neurologic symptoms does not necessarily imply a diagnosis of migraine with aura [39]. Work-up for ischemic events may be implicated, although hemiplegic migraine can involve prolonged hemiparesis and even permanent cerebellar ataxia [40].

Hemorrhagic Stroke

Migraine appears to be associated with an increased risk of hemorrhagic stroke [12, 41, 42], particularly in females and females aged less than 45 years [42, 43]. The influence of migraine type remains unclear [42], but some studies have shown an increased risk in people with migraine with aura, and prevailing theories include possible changes in the vessel wall or associated cardiovascular risk factors [41, 44]. The risk of subarachnoid hemorrhage in particular [45] may be increased in OCP users with a history of migraine. Infratentorial microbleeds were found more commonly on imaging in older patients with migraine without aura than those without migraine, although this migraine population also had increased proportion with hypertension [46].

Genetic Syndromes

Multiple inherited syndromes have been identified which increase the risk of both migraine and cerebral ischemia. These include cerebral autosomal dominant arteriopathy with subcortical infarcts and leukoencephalopathy (CADASIL) (Fig. 14.1), retinal vasculopathy with cerebral leukodystrophy (RVCL), and mitochondrial encephalopathy, lactic acidosis, and stroke-like episodes (MELAS) (Table 14.1). Further work is needed to understand the pathophysiological mechanisms which drive the manifestations of these disease states [47].

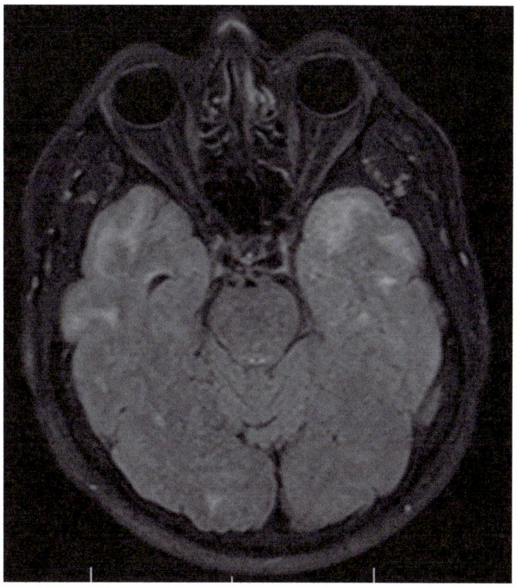

Fig. 14.1 CADASIL: Magnetic resonance imaging of the brain of a 48-year-old male who presented with episodes of transient weakness, cognitive impairment, and depressed mood. T2 FLAIR axial sequences revealed extensive subcortical white matter changes involving the external capsule and the temporal lobe tips. Patient tested positive for the NOTCH3 gene

Table 14.1 Genetic syndromes which include an increased risk for migraine and cerebral ischemia

Genetic syndrome	Cerebral autosomal dominant arteriopathy with subcortical infarcts and leukoencephalopathy (CADASIL)	Retinal vasculopathy with cerebral leukodystrophy (RVCL)	Mitochondrial encephalopathy, lactic acidosis, and stroke-like episodes (MELAS)
Inheritance pattern	Autosomal dominant	Autosomal dominant	Mitochondrial
Chromosome locus	19q12	3p21	Mitochondrial
Gene	NOTCH3	TREX1	Multiple identified: MT-TL1 in 80%
Gene product	Notch3 receptor	3′–5′ exonuclease	tRNALeu in 80%
Clinical features	Migraine with aura Ischemic stroke, TIA Cognitive decline and dementia Psychiatric manifestations	Migraine without aura Progressive visual loss Focal neurological symptoms Cognitive deficit Depression Raynaud's phenomenon Hepatic, renal dysfunction Gastrointestinal bleeding	Stroke-like episodes Encephalopathy Seizures Cognitive impairment: Dementia, learning disabilities Muscle weakness Hearing impairment Peripheral neuropathy Short stature
Neuroimaging findings	White matter hyperintensities in the anterior temporal lobe and external capsule Lacunar infarcts Microhemorrhages	Non-contrast-enhancing T2 hyperintensities or contrast-enhancing mass lesions	Basal ganglia calcifications Focal T2-hyperintensve lesions not clearly related to a vascular territory Brain atrophy

Neuroimaging Studies: White Matter Hyperintensities and Silent Brain Lesions

Many neuroimaging studies have revealed a higher prevalence of asymptomatic (silent) structural brain lesions in people with migraine [48–50], with a more clearly association in patients with aura [49]. Although, some studies have not found any association between migraine with aura and silent brain lesions [51–53]. The mechanisms are not fully understood, although both ischemic and inflammatory mediators have been proposed.

White matter hyperintensities are commonly found in migraine. According to one meta-analysis of 3502 individuals with migraine, the pooled prevalence was 44%, 45%, and 38% in migraine, migraine with aura, and migraine without aura groups, respectively [54]. They are typically small, multiple, punctate high signal lesions seen on T2 weighted images and located in deep or periventricular white matter (Fig. 14.2) [55]. In patients with migraine with aura, the lesion load appears to be independent of the presence of a patent foramen ovale (PFO) and right to left shunt [56].

Silent infarct-like lesions are parenchymal brain signal abnormalities without mass effect, with the same signal as cerebrospinal fluid, and without clinical symptoms [57]; in migraine, they tend to occur in the posterior circulation and especially cerebellar region and are associated with a higher attack frequency, greater or equal to one attack per month [58, 59] (Fig. 14.3). In a recent systematic review and meta-analysis, these lesions were not associated with migraine or migraine aura; however, in a clinic- and population-based exploratory analysis, migraine with aura was significantly associated with silent brain infarction (OR = 1.91 [1.02;3.59], $P = 0.04$), and confirmed the propensity for silent cerebellar infarcts (OR = 2.57 [1.01;6.56], $P = 0.05$) [60].

There does not seem to be a link between progression of white matter abnormalities and frequency, severity, or treatment of migraine [50]. Besides older age, other cardiovascular risk factors do not seem more prevalent in those with silent brain lesions [59, 61]. While data regarding the link between silent brain lesions, clinical features of migraine, and cerebrovascular complications are contradictory, the combination of migraine and white matter hyperintensities may be the earliest manifestation of vascular disorders such as antiphospholipid syndrome, hereditary small vessel disease, and small vessel vasculitis [62].

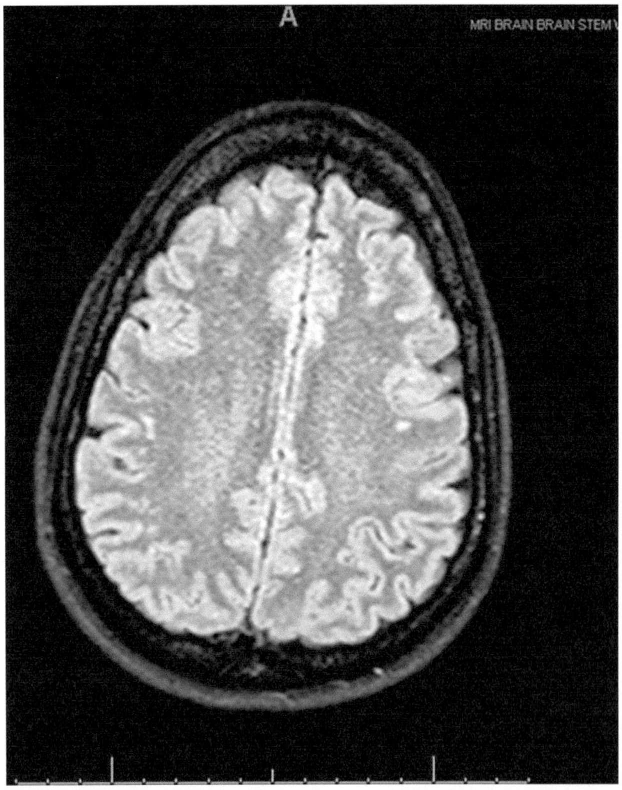

Fig. 14.2 White matter hyperintensities in migraine: Magnetic resonance imaging of the brain of a 48-year-old female with migraine headache disorder who was otherwise healthy and whose neurological examination was normal. T2 FLAIR axial sequences revealed few nonspecific punctate foci of subcortical white matter signal hyperintensity, which are predominately in the frontal and temporal regions

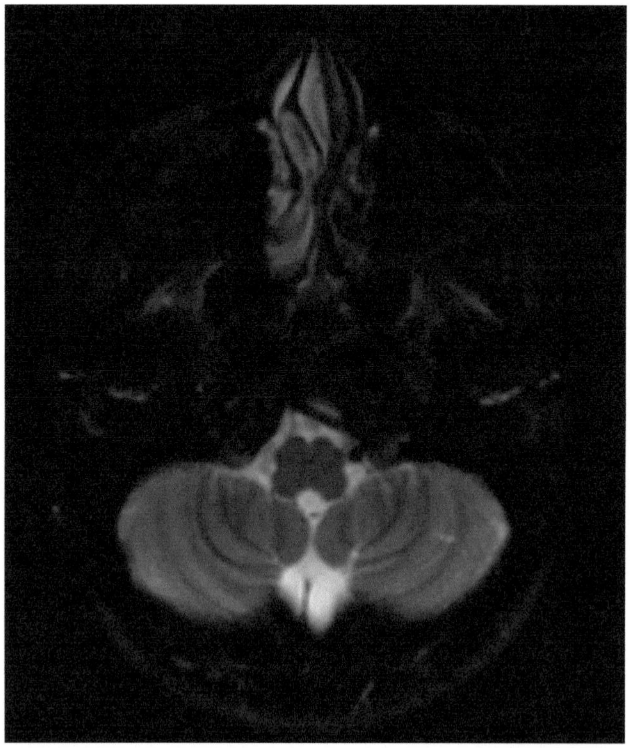

Fig. 14.3 Silent brain infarction: Magnetic resonance imaging of the brain of a 32-year-old female with migraine headache disorder. T2 FSE FS axial sequences revealed ischemic-appearing lesion in the left cerebellar hemisphere which did not correlate to her symptomatology and therefore were considered silent infarct lesion. (Image provided with permission from Sebastian Koch, M.D., University of Miami, Miller School of Medicine)

Cardiovascular Disorders

There is evidence of an association between migraine and cardiovascular disorders including hypertension, myocardial infarction (MI), atrial fibrillation, and venous thromboembolism [41, 63–65]. Migraine, most significantly with aura, is associated with increased risk for cardiovascular disease mortality and coronary heart disease mortality in both males and females [63, 66, 67]. Migraine is now considered a marker of risk in the QRISK3 algorithm validated to predict the 10-year risk of cardiovascular disease in ages 24–84 years [68].

It is unclear whether migraine disorder increases these risks itself or if they share a common underlying pathophysiology. The higher risk of cardiovascular disease in unlikely mediated by any single risk factor. Many studies suggest family history of cardiovascular disease is more frequent in those with migraine compared to those without [69]. Framingham risk score has been shown to be elevated in migraine, most pronounced in migraine with aura, compared to controls and could not be explained by lifestyle factors alone [21, 70].

Observational case studies have observed improvement of aura frequency with antiplatelet therapy [71] and anticoagulation [72]. However, there is no evidence that control of migraine attacks can reduce risk of cardiovascular disease.

Hypertension and Blood Pressure

Chronic hypertensive and hypotensive conditions are highly prevalent worldwide and may occur comorbidly with migraine. Attacks of migraine themselves have been shown to cause transient changes in blood pressure, although data is not consistent [73]. Overall, findings of the relationship between hypertension and migraine have revealed positive, neutral, and inverse associations.

Most large population-based studies report a positive association between migraine and hypertension [21, 74–78]. This is particularly apparent for hypertension of long duration and poor control [79]. Several studies found no association between migraine and hypertension [80–82]. And others reveal a negative association [83–87] between high blood pressure and migraine, in which those with hypertension had a lower risk for migraine or vice versa. The differences in findings are likely attributable to differences in study populations and methodological design. The majority of evidence is derived from cross-sectional data, which limits the ability to draw conclusions on the causal relationship or the directionality of the association.

In investigations of specific blood pressure parameters, migraine is associated with elevated diastolic measurements [80, 81, 88] and lower pulse pressure [84, 87, 89] while associations with elevated systolic measurements are less consistent [80, 88]. Pathophysiologic mechanisms underlying these relationships remain unclear. Potential explanations include endothelial dysfunction, subclinical atherosclerosis, autonomic dysregulation, and increased arterial stiffness [2, 90–93]. In a genome-wide cross-phenotype meta-analysis of the association of migraine and blood pressure, there appears to be an important role for diastolic blood pressure, shared biology, and migraine susceptibility [94].

There is evidence from prospective longitudinal studies that patients with migraine at baseline are at increased risk of developing hypertension [95, 96]. Whether baseline hypertension predicts future migraine remains inconclusive. While patients with hypertension at baseline were at increased risk of having a migraine approximately 10 years later in the NHANES study, a higher SBP at baseline appeared to be protective against the risk of having a migraine 11 years later according to HUNT study data [75, 89].

The identification and management of comorbid hypertension in migraine disorder is paramount. Patients with the two have been shown to have a higher probability of a history of cerebrovascular events compared to those with hypertension alone [97]. In addition, hypertension may act as a risk factor for migraine chronification [98].

Metabolic Syndrome and Obesity

Metabolic syndrome includes a number of abnormalities including hypertension, insulin resistance, atherogenic dyslipidemia, a proinflammatory state, a prothrombotic state, and increased waist circumference or obesity [99]. In a large longitudinal follow-up study, it was found that having migraine with aura was associated with an increased risk for the development of metabolic syndrome [100]. The presence of metabolic syndrome has been associated with a significant risk of cardiovascular disease [101] and stroke [102].

In addition, obesity, both total body and abdominal obesity, is a well-known risk factor for both migraine in both sexes 20–55 years of age [103]. The presence of obesity also has a strong influence on the risk of transformed migraine (a state in which episodic migraine becomes chronic) [104]. This relationship may involve both peripheral and central mechanisms [105], as well as the effects of inflammatory mediators, endogenous and exogenous hormones, neuropeptides, adipokines, in addition to gut microbiota and lifestyle factors (inactivity and dietary patterns) [106].

Cardiac Arrhythmia

Migraine is associated with an increased risk of cardiac arrhythmia, including atrial flutter and fibrillation, in short- and long-term follow-up; the association is stronger for migraine with aura [41]. More specifically, migraine with visual aura was found to be a risk factor for incident atrial fibrillation, more likely to occur in males older than 60 years [107]. Electrocardiogram (EKG) performed during migraine attacks have demonstrated arrhythmia and other conductive changes that were not present on EKG during interictal pain-free periods [108]. It is hypothesized that autonomic dysfunction during attacks may underlie the occurrence of arrhythmia [109]. Interestingly in one study, the frequency and severity of migraine improved after catheter ablation for atrial fibrillation [110].

Ischemic Heart Disease

Multiple population studies have revealed an association between migraine and angina, CAD, MI, coronary revascularization, and ischemic cardiovascular death [17, 111]. One study did reveal an increased risk of angina in migraine with aura, although this did not seem related to increased risk of CAD [112]. Still, other studies found no association between migraine and CAD, MI, or death due to cardiovascular disease [9]. One epidemiologic review concluded that prior literature failed to support an association between migraine and coronary heart disease [113]. The relationship may be explained by shared risk factors and comorbidities including obesity, insulin resistance, dyslipidemia, and proinflammatory state [114].

Congenital Heart Defects

Multiple studies suggest an association between migraine and PFO, a remnant of fetal circulation: the incidence of PFO is significantly higher in those with migraine than in the general population [115], and the incidence of migraine is significantly higher in those with PFO than those without [116]. There is a stronger association with migraine with aura [117] and atypical aura [118]; some studies have shown no association with migraine without aura [119].

It is unclear if this is a causal relationship or rather a coexistence of the two conditions. Proposed pathophysiological mechanisms include shunting of neurochemicals, paradoxical emboli, and sequalae of decreased blood oxygen saturation [120]. In one study, those with frequent aura were found to have a higher degree of right-to-left shunt than those with infrequent aura [121]. Use of antiplatelet medication may reduce attack frequency in migraine patients with PFO [122, 123]. While case series and case–control studies have suggested some benefits for migraine with the PFO closure procedure [120], results in randomized controlled trials are not sufficient to support a recommendation for closure [124–126].

Cardiac Cephalalgia

Headache itself can be a presentation of myocardial ischemia, and the headache may be similar phenotypically to a migraine attack. The ICHD-3 criteria define cardiac cephalalgia as a headache that develops in temporal relation to the onset of acute myocardial ischemia, which must be demonstrated during treadmill or nuclear cardiac stress testing. It is usually but not always aggravated by exercise and is relieved by nitroglycerin [29]. One case series of 30 patients found headache was fully or partially relieved after treatment with drugs or coronary angiogenesis [127].

Cardiac cephalalgia should be considered as a form of atypical angina. The headache of cardiac cephalalgia typically, although not always, occurs along with symptoms of angina pectoris: chest pain, chest tightness, and sweating are most reported [128]. In a prospective study of patients admitted to the hospital with suspected acute coronary syndrome, the prevalence of cardiac cephalalgia was 14.2%. Pain referred to the jaw, concurrent palpitations, and myocardial infarction secondary to disease of the circumflex artery were more frequent in patients with cardiac cephalalgia, while a history of hypertension was less common in these patients [129]. The ability to distinguish between cardiac cephalalgia and an acute migraine attack is crucial, given the potential for worsening ischemia or ischemic complications with triptans and ergot derivatives [29]. On the other hand, nitroglycerin may trigger severe migraine attacks.

Other Female-Specific Considerations

Migraine prevalence is high in females of child-bearing age. The World Health Organization (WHO) medical eligibility criteria fifth edition contraindicates the use of combined oral contraceptives in females with migraine with aura who are over age 35 or under age 35 who also smoke [130]. In 2017, expert consensus found the overall quality of evidence regarding the risk of ischemic stroke associated with the use of hormonal contraceptive in migraine patients is low. Available data suggests that combined hormonal contraceptive may further increase the risk of stroke in migraine, specifically with aura (OR 6.1) compared to those without aura

Table 14.2 Guidelines/Recommendations for combined oral contraception (COC) in females with migraine

Migraine type and patient-related factors		ACOG [182]	IHS [183]	WHO [130]	CDC US MEC [184]
Migraine without aura	Age < 35	No contraindication	No contraindication	Advantages generally outweigh risks	Advantages outweigh risk
	Age ≥ 35	Risk may outweigh benefits; consider progestin-only (or other non-estrogen) methods		Risks usually outweigh benefits	Risk usually outweighs benefit
	Smoker	Risk may outweigh benefits; consider progestin-only (or other non-estrogen) methods	Those with migraine who smoke should stop smoking before starting COCs		Risk usually outweighs benefit
	Additional risk factors[a]	Risk may outweigh benefits; consider progestin-only (or other non-estrogen) methods	There is a potentially increased risk; one must individually assess and evaluate these risks. Risk factors should be treated. Consider non-estrogen methods		Risk usually outweighs benefit
Migraine with aura	Any age	Risk not acceptable; progestin-only (or other non-estrogen) methods. Avoid COC	Low dose COC can be used in cases of simple visual aura. There is a potentially increased risk; COC use may be contraindicated. Consider non-estrogen methods	Unacceptable health risk. Avoid COC	Unacceptable health risk. Avoid COC

ACOG American College of Obstetricians and Gynecologists, *IHS* International Headache Society, *WHO* World Health Organization, *CDC US MEC* Centers for Disease Control and Prevention US Medical Eligibility Criteria
[a]Hypertension, obesity, diabetes, hyperlipidemia

(OR 1.8) [131]. It is therefore recommended to evaluate for migraine (subtype and frequency), vascular risk factors, and type of combined hormonal contraceptive product (Table 14.2). The risk of vascular complication depends mostly on the estrogen compound and is dose-dependent [132]: the risk is greatest for older formations consisting of 50 mcg (2.9–4.8 OR) and lowest for newer 20 mcg of ethinyl estradiol formations (1.7 OR) [133].

During pregnancy and the peripartum period, new-onset or change in migraine should prompt work-up for secondary etiologies including neurovascular disorders. There is an increased risk for reversible cerebral vasoconstriction syndrome (RCVS) and posterior reversible encephalopathy syndrome (PRES), which may present with the headache of migraine phenotype [134]. In migraine patients who are pregnant, there is an increased risk of gestational hypertension, preeclampsia, and thromboembolic events [135].

Migraine Treatment and Vascular Complications/Risk

When formulating a plan for preventive and abortive migraine management, the individual's risk of future vascular events based on prior history and risk factors must be considered. Many of the evidence-based migraine preventive and abortive medications have implications for migraine patients with vascular disease.

Migraine Preventive Medications

Ideally, the migraine preventive agent, in addition to reducing migraine attacks, would prevent a comorbid vascular disease without introducing further risks. Beta-blocker medications show level A (metoprolol, propranolol, and timolol), level B (atenolol and nadolol), and level C (nebivolol and pindolol) evidence for migraine prevention [136, 137] and may be especially useful in migraine prevention for patients with HTN, atrial fibrillation or CAD. They are contraindicated in patients with COPD, asthma, heart failure, severe PVD, or heart block.

Angiotensin-converting enzyme (ACE) inhibitors and angiotensin receptor blockers (ARB) may be particularly suitable for patients with comorbid HTN. Lisinopril and candesartan both have level C evidence for efficacy but are likely to become more strongly recommended in future guidelines [137, 138]. Caution should be taken with cessation in hypertensive patients in order to avoid increases in blood pressure.

Anti-epileptic drugs used for migraine prevention may affect the metabolic status of patients, which can serve to increase or decrease cardiovascular risk. Valproic acid has level A evidence in efficacy but may lead to metabolic syndrome. Topiramate, also with level A evidence, can lead to a reduction in appetite and weight loss, and may be appropriate for patients with obesity or metabolic syndrome.

Anti-depressants of the tricyclic class, including amitriptyline (level B) and nortriptyline, may lead to sinus tachycardia,

QT prolongation, and fluctuations in blood pressure; they should be avoided in patients with orthostatic hypotension. QT prolongation with use of venlafaxine has been demonstrated in case reports and considered clinically insignificant [139].

There is currently no direct evidence to support that a migraine prophylactic treatment can reduce future stroke in people with migraine, although it is sensible to treat frequent migraine aura with prophylactic agents and consider a diagnostic work-up for secondary causes if aura is very frequent or prolonged. Existing comorbid vascular risk factors should be managed adequately in order to reduce risk.

Newer classes of migraine preventive medications act to block the calcitonin gene-related peptide (CGRP) molecule or its receptor. The CGRP small molecule plays a role in migraine production and may have a protective effect in hypertension and ischemia through its vasodilatory function. In theory, its blockage could impact CV health and pose vascular risks. Despite this, efficacy and safety studies for the antibodies have yet to demonstrate any significant cardiovascular adverse events and none carry FDA contraindications in patients with a history of stroke, CAD, or PVD.

Cardiovascular and cerebrovascular adverse events were infrequent and similar to placebo in randomized controlled and open-label studies of erenumab [140–144], fremanezumab [145], galcanezumeb [146], and eptinezumab [147]. These included patients with cardiovascular risk factors but not with active cardiovascular and cerebrovascular disease. Safety analysis of atogepant included patients with risk factors and a history of cardio- and cerebrovascular disease; adverse events between the groups were similar [148]. Rimegepant was also shown to be safe and well-tolerated in subjects with CV risk factors and moderate to high CV risk [149].

In a high cardiovascular-risk population with stable angina, infusion of erenumab did not adversely affect exercise time [150]. With short- and long-term use, there was no significant difference from placebo in blood pressure within 24 hours or over 12 weeks [151], and a pooled analysis also showed no differences in blood pressure changes compared with placebo [152]. Yet, routine post-marketing FDA surveillance identified cases suggesting an association between erenumab and elevated blood pressure, which led to the inclusion of hypertension as a warning and precaution in prescribing information [153]. Long-term safety data of fremanezumab including subjects with cardiovascular risk and disease revealed hypertension in 2% of patients, with the vast majority in patients with a history of hypertension, single findings of elevated measurement, and considered not related to the drug. In addition, in patients with hypertension at baseline, mean and median BP values after 1 year of treatment were lower than baseline [154]. However, the FDA has provided updated warnings of new or worsening hypertension and Raynaud's phenomenon with use of all CGRP monoclonal antibodies and gepants after evaluation of post-marketing data.

Migraine-Specific Abortive Medications

Widely-available and effective first-line abortive treatments include acetaminophen, caffeine, aspirin, and other nonsteroidal anti-inflammatory drugs (NSAIDs). Certain NSAIDs including ibuprofen, aspirin, diclofenac, and naproxen carry an FDA-boxed warning due to their association with increased risk of heart attack and stroke, especially at high doses or duration of use [155]. Therefore, NSAIDs may be contraindicated in patients with CVD and should not be used regularly for frequent attacks in patients with CV risk factors.

Approved in 1992, the triptan class of medication acts as agonist at serotonin receptors $5HT_{1D}$ (where it is shown to exhibit therapeutic relief through the involvement of the trigeminal system and central pain modulating structures) and $5HT_{1B}$ (which may lead to vasoconstriction).

According to FDA-approval terms, triptans are labeled as contraindicated in patients with coronary artery disease or vasospasm, cardiac accessory conduction pathway disorders, uncontrolled hypertension, or history of stroke, transient ischemic attack, or hemiplegic or basilar migraine. Warnings and precautions labels also advise triptan-naïve patients with multiple CVRFs should have CV evaluation prior to receipt of a triptan. After a negative evaluation, it is recommended that patients are closely monitored if prescribed. Although in approval studies, only minimal or no increase in SBP was displayed, it is still advised to avoid triptans in uncontrolled HTN, especially in hypertensive crisis.

In the years following triptan approval, case reports have described acute MI occurring closely after triptan administration. In many, the time of the cardiac event was outside the therapeutic window of the triptan, although many patients did not have a history of MI or angina, and coronary angiography did not show atherosclerotic changes [156]. Two large-scale studies found no evidence of an increased risk of adverse vascular events or death in migraine patients using triptans [157, 158]. An expert panel of headache specialists concluded, based on evidence, including long-term open-label and post-marketing surveillance, that chest symptoms occurring during use of triptans are generally not serious and are not explained by ischemia, and the incidence of serious cardiovascular events with triptans in both clinical trials and clinical practice appears to be extremely low [159].

Initial labeling decisions were likely based on the early assumptions that triptans have vasoconstrictive properties and an early understanding of pathophysiological mechanisms of comorbidities. First, it is now clear that the vast majority of MI occurs secondary to atherosclerotic plaque rupture and not vasospasm. Several studies of patients with CAD have shown triptan use did not produce EKG or troponin level changes [160] nor clinically significant vasoconstriction [161, 162]. Similarly, experts express that the contraindication in cerebrovascular disorders is not clearly justified according to current evidence and understanding of stroke mechanisms, except in cases of subarachnoid hemorrhage or reversible cerebral vasoconstrictive syndrome [163]. Investigations with magnetic resonance angiography during acute treatment of migraine attacks with sumatriptan observed constriction of extracerebral but not intracerebral arteries [164]. Furthermore, hemiplegic migraine is now known to be due to mutations that result in greater susceptibility to cortical spreading depression [165] and previously called 'basilar migraine' is reclassified as migraine with brainstem aura to avoid the implication that basilar artery spasm plays a significant role of this subtype [166]. Several retrospective studies and case reports have suggested the relative safety of triptans and DHE in these patients without a significantly greater risk of ischemic vascular events than in users with more common migraine subtypes [167–170].

A systematic review of three observational studies investigated the CV safety of migraine-specific drugs in clinical practice: the available evidence suggested that there were no strong CV safety issues with triptan use, although no firm conclusions could be drawn, somewhat owing to residual uncontrolled confounding factors. Evidence on stroke risk was deemed conflicting but, if existent, small [171]. A retrospective cohort study found no association between exposure to triptans among migraine patients and an increased risk of cardiovascular events including myocardial infarction, heart failure, and death [172].

Novel agents FDA-approved in late 2019 for the acute management of migraine include the ditan class of selective 5-HT_{1F} receptor agonists and the gepant class of CGRP receptor antagonists. Both classes do not have vasoconstrictive properties [173, 174] and therefore may be more suitable for patients with vascular risk factors or history.

Post-hoc analysis of two phase III trials of lasmiditan, the first ditan approved for use, included subjects with multiple CV risk factors and known CAD, arrhythmia, or uncontrolled HTN. There was no statistical difference in efficacy or frequency of likely CV treatment-emergent adverse events among those with or without risk factors or disease and the only likely treatment-emergent adverse was palpitations [175]. Other post hoc analyses of elderly patients revealed no cardiovascular events during the treatment-emergent or intermediate periods; there were two cases of increased blood pressure during the remote period [176].

First-generation gepants were shown not to effect exercise heart rate or cause ST depression in patients with stable angina [177] and no cardiovascular thrombotic adverse events occurred within 2 weeks of dosing in patients with CAD [178]. The phase IIb study of ubrogepant included subjects with baseline high risk of CVD and observed no significant CV events, although subjects with actual CVD were not included [179]. The phase III studies revealed no increased treatment-emergent or cardiac adverse events in subjects with multiple major CV risk factors [180]. In the phase III trial of rimegepant for acute treatment, there were no serious treatment-attributed adverse events [181]. As previously noted, the FDA has provided updated warnings of new or worsening hypertension and Raynaud's phenomenon with use of CGRP inhibitors after evaluation of post-marketing data.

Non-Pharmacologic Management Strategies

In light of the higher risk of vascular complications in people with migraine with aura, it is important to identify and modify any vascular risk factor. Lifestyle interventions including counseling on cessation of smoking, initiation and maintenance of regular exercise, and proper nutrition may be indicated. The presence of metabolic syndrome significantly increases risk of vascular complications and obesity may be a risk factor for chronic migraine. In those with obstructive sleep apnea, positive airway pressure treatment may improve headache and decrease risk of complications.

Conclusion

The understanding of migraine pathophysiology and the relationship between migraine and vascular disorders and their complications continues to expand and improve. The ability to provide more patient-specific treatments and therapeutic guidance for patients with migraine and vascular disease or risk factors has evolved with the advancement and availability of recent pharmacologic and non-pharmacologic options. Further research is needed to better understand the association between migraine and vascular comorbidities; in addition, clinical investigations to determine personalized approaches to improve the burden of migraine as well as to promote and cardiovascular and cerebrovascular health are warranted.

Teaching Points

1. Association between migraine and vascular comorbidities may be at least in part attributed to endothelial dysfunction; Genome-wide association studies revealed multiple loci associated with both migraine and enrichment for genes expressed in vascular and smooth muscle tissues.
2. The relative risk of ischemic stroke in migraine with aura is more than double that those without migraine and is increased among migraine patients of female sex, age less than 45 years, positive smoking status, and use of combined oral contraception.
3. Neuroimaging studies reveal silent structural brain lesions and white matter hyperintensities to be of increased prevalence in patients with migraine; symptomatic migrainous infarction is a rare complication of migraine.
4. Migraine is considered a marker of risk in the QRISK3 algorithm validated to predict the 10-year risk of cardiovascular disease in ages 24–84 years.
5. When formulating a plan for preventive and abortive migraine management, the individual's risk of future vascular events based on prior history and current risk factors must be considered.
6. Studies on novel migraine preventive and abortive therapies have shown no increased risk of cardiovascular or cerebrovascular adverse events and may be suitable for patients with contraindications to older-generation treatments.

Case

A 53-year-old woman presents to clinic for evaluation of frequently occurring migraine with and without aura. She reports an average of 8 headache days per month with at least three attacks of severe intensity which respond to triptan medication. She has a history of smoking tobacco type II diabetes mellitus, hypertension, and angina; a work-up revealed coronary artery disease, which was treated with percutaneous coronary intervention. Recently, attacks have not responded to adequate prophylactic trials of topiramate, propranolol, and amitriptyline. She treats abortively with acetaminophen as she was advised to avoid triptan medication, but this is insufficiently effective.

Case Discussion

This patient would benefit from improved prophylactic and abortive management. Given her comorbid coronary artery disease, triptan medications are contraindicated and NSAID use should be minimized. She could benefit from gepant or ditan class medication given their favorable safety profile. For preventive measure, a CGRP mAb class medication could be offered, but she should be advised that they have not been studied in combination with gepant treatments (although preliminary real-world studies and clinical experience are reassuring). She should be counseled that migraine can increase the risk of vascular complications, and thus, her vascular comorbidities should be adequately managed with her primary care provider or subspecialists as needed.

Questions and Answers

1. Of the following patient scenarios, who might be at the highest risk of ischemic stroke, assuming other risk factors are negative?
   A. A 40-year-old woman with migraine with aura, hypercholesterolemia and obesity.
   B. A 40-year-old woman with migraine with aura who uses combined oral contraceptive and with active tobacco use.
   C. A 40-year-old man with migraine with aura, hypercholesterolemia, and obesity.
   D. A 30-year-old man with migraine with aura, hypercholesterolemia, and with active tobacco use.
   E. A 30-year-old woman with migraine with aura with active tobacco use and physical inactivity.

The correct answer is B. The use of combined oral contraceptives is contraindicated in women with migraine with aura who are over age 35 or under age 35 who also smoke. The overall quality of evidence regarding the risk of ischemic stroke associated with the use of hormonal contraceptive in migraine patients is low. Available data suggests that combined hormonal contraceptive may further increase the risk of stroke in migraine, specifically with aura. While traditional vascular risk factors may increase the risk of stroke, the risk of stroke in patients with migraine, more often occur in patients with migraine with aura and low cardiovascular risk profiles.

2. Regarding migraine treatments, which of the following statements is incorrect?
   A. The triptans are generally considered safe even in patients with stable vascular comorbidities but should be used with caution.
   B. The ditans are a class of selective 5-HT_{1F} receptor agonists that do no cause vasocontriction.
   C. The gepants are a class of calcitonin gener-related peptide GRP receptor antagonists, which are not known to cause vasoconstriction. .
   D. Triptan medications carry an FDA contraindication in patients with a history of coronary artery disease (CAD), uncontrolled hypertension, or ischemic stroke.
   E. Gepant medications do not carry FDA contraindications in patients with history of stroke, CAD, or peripheral vascular disease.

The correct answer is C. Explanation: All are correct except choice "C" as the gepants are a class of small molecule CGRP receptor antagonists and can be used in patients with comorbid conditions which may prohibit them from use of triptan-class medications.

References

1. Mason BN, Russo AF. Vascular contributions to migraine: time to revisit? Front Cell Neurosci. 2018;12:233. https://doi.org/10.3389/fncel.2018.00233.
2. Tietjen GE. Migraine as a systemic vasculopathy. Cephalalgia. 2009;29(9):987–96. https://doi.org/10.1111/j.1468-2982.2009.01937.x.
3. Gormley P, Anttila V, Winsvold BS, Palta P, Esko T, Pers TH, et al. Meta-analysis of 375,000 individuals identifies 38 susceptibility loci for migraine. Nat Genet. 2016;48(8):856–66. https://doi.org/10.1038/ng.3598.
4. Winsvold BS, Bettella F, Witoelar A, Anttila V, Gormley P, Kurth T, et al. Shared genetic risk between migraine and coronary artery disease: a genome-wide analysis of common variants. PLoS One. 2017;12(9):e0185663. https://doi.org/10.1371/journal.pone.0185663.
5. Malik R, Freilinger T, Winsvold BS, Anttila V, Vander Heiden J, Traylor M, et al. Shared genetic basis for migraine and ischemic stroke: a genome-wide analysis of common variants. Neurology. 2015;84(21):2132–45. https://doi.org/10.1212/WNL.0000000000001606.
6. Siewert KM, Klarin D, Damrauer SM, Chang KM, Tsao PS, Assimes TL, et al. Cross-trait analyses with migraine reveal widespread pleiotropy and suggest a vascular component to migraine headache. Int J Epidemiol. 2020;49(3):1022–31. https://doi.org/10.1093/ije/dyaa050.
7. Donnan GA, Fisher M, Macleod M, Davis SM. Stroke. Lancet. 2008;371(9624):1612–23. https://doi.org/10.1016/S0140-6736(08)60694-7.
8. Etminan M, Takkouche B, Isorna FC, Samii A. Risk of ischaemic stroke in people with migraine: systematic review and meta-analysis of observational studies. BMJ. 2005;330(7482):63. https://doi.org/10.1136/bmj.38302.504063.8F.
9. Schurks M, Rist PM, Bigal ME, Buring JE, Lipton RB, Kurth T. Migraine and cardiovascular disease: systematic review and meta-analysis. BMJ. 2009;339:b3914. https://doi.org/10.1136/bmj.b3914.
10. Spector JT, Kahn SR, Jones MR, Jayakumar M, Dalal D, Nazarian S. Migraine headache and ischemic stroke risk: an updated meta-analysis. Am J Med. 2010;123(7):612–24. https://doi.org/10.1016/j.amjmed.2009.12.021.
11. Hu X, Zhou Y, Zhao H, Peng C. Migraine and the risk of stroke: an updated meta-analysis of prospective cohort studies. Neurol Sci. 2017;38(1):33–40. https://doi.org/10.1007/s10072-016-2746-z.
12. Mahmoud AN, Mentias A, Elgendy AY, Qazi A, Barakat AF, Saad M, et al. Migraine and the risk of cardiovascular and cerebrovascular events: a meta-analysis of 16 cohort studies including 1 152 407 subjects. BMJ Open. 2018;8(3):e020498. https://doi.org/10.1136/bmjopen-2017-020498.
13. Mosek A, Marom R, Korczyn AD, Bornstein N. A history of migraine is not a risk factor to develop an ischemic stroke in the elderly. Headache. 2001;41(4):399–401. https://doi.org/10.1046/j.1526-4610.2001.111006399.x.
14. Monteith TS, Gardener H, Rundek T, Elkind MS, Sacco RL. Migraine and risk of stroke in older adults: Northern Manhattan Study. Neurology. 2015;85(8):715–21. https://doi.org/10.1212/WNL.0000000000001854.
15. Androulakis XM, Sen S, Kodumuri N, Zhang T, Grego J, Rosamond W, et al. Migraine age of onset and association with ischemic stroke in late life: 20 years follow-up in ARIC. Headache. 2019;59(4):556–66. https://doi.org/10.1111/head.13468.
16. MacClellan LR, Giles W, Cole J, Wozniak M, Stern B, Mitchell BD, et al. Probable migraine with visual aura and risk of ischemic stroke: the stroke prevention in young women study. Stroke. 2007;38(9):2438–45. https://doi.org/10.1161/STROKEAHA.107.488395.
17. Kurth T, Gaziano JM, Cook NR, Logroscino G, Diener HC, Buring JE. Migraine and risk of cardiovascular disease in women. JAMA. 2006;296(3):283–91. https://doi.org/10.1001/jama.296.3.283.
18. Kurth T, Schurks M, Logroscino G, Buring JE. Migraine frequency and risk of cardiovascular disease in women. Neurology. 2009;73(8):581–8. https://doi.org/10.1212/WNL.0b013e3181ab2c20.
19. Rist PM, Buring JE, Kase CS, Schurks M, Kurth T. Migraine and functional outcome from ischemic cerebral events in women. Circulation. 2010;122(24):2551–7. https://doi.org/10.1161/CIRCULATIONAHA.110.977306.
20. Li L, Schulz UG, Kuker W, Rothwell PM, Oxford Vascular Study. Age-specific association of migraine with cryptogenic TIA and stroke: population-based study. Neurology. 2015;85(17):1444–51. https://doi.org/10.1212/WNL.0000000000002059.
21. Scher AI, Terwindt GM, Picavet HS, Verschuren WM, Ferrari MD, Launer LJ. Cardiovascular risk factors and migraine: the GEM population-based study. Neurology. 2005;64(4):614–20. https://doi.org/10.1212/01.WNL.0000151857.43225.49.
22. Kurth T, Schurks M, Logroscino G, Gaziano JM, Buring JE. Migraine, vascular risk, and cardiovascular events in women: prospective cohort study. BMJ. 2008;337:a636. https://doi.org/10.1136/bmj.a636.
23. van Os HJA, Mulder IA, Broersen A, Algra A, van der Schaaf IC, Kappelle LJ, et al. Migraine and cerebrovascular atherosclerosis in patients with ischemic stroke. Stroke. 2017;48(7):1973–5. https://doi.org/10.1161/STROKEAHA.116.016133.
24. Eikermann-Haerter K. Spreading depolarization may link migraine and stroke. Headache. 2014;54(7):1146–57. https://doi.org/10.1111/head.12386.
25. Frid P, Xu H, Mitchell BD, Drake M, Wasselius J, Gaynor B, et al. Migraine-associated common genetic variants confer greater risk of posterior vs. anterior circulation ischemic stroke☆. J Stroke Cerebrovasc Dis. 2022;31(8):106546. https://doi.org/10.1016/j.jstrokecerebrovasdis.2022.106546.

26. Daghals I, Sargurupremraj M, Danning R, Gormley P, Malik R, Amouyel P, et al. Migraine, stroke, and cervical arterial dissection: shared genetics for a triad of brain disorders with vascular involvement. Neurol Genet. 2022;8(1):e653. https://doi.org/10.1212/nxg.0000000000000653.
27. Metso TM, Tatlisumak T, Debette S, Dallongeville J, Engelter ST, Lyrer PA, et al. Migraine in cervical artery dissection and ischemic stroke patients. Neurology. 2012;78(16):1221–8. https://doi.org/10.1212/WNL.0b013e318251595f.
28. Sochurkova D, Moreau T, Lemesle M, Menassa M, Giroud M, Dumas R. Migraine history and migraine-induced stroke in the Dijon stroke registry. Neuroepidemiology. 1999;18(2):85–91. https://doi.org/10.1159/000069411.
29. Headache Classification Committee of the International Headache Society (IHS). The international classification of headache disorders, 3rd edition. Cephalalgia. 2018;38(1):1–211. https://doi.org/10.1177/0333102417738202.
30. Kurth T, Chabriat H, Bousser MG. Migraine and stroke: a complex association with clinical implications. Lancet Neurol. 2012;11(1):92–100. https://doi.org/10.1016/S1474-4422(11)70266-6.
31. Cutrer FM, Sorensen AG, Weisskoff RM, Ostergaard L, Sanchez del Rio M, Lee EJ, et al. Perfusion-weighted imaging defects during spontaneous migrainous aura. Ann Neurol. 1998;43(1):25–31. https://doi.org/10.1002/ana.410430108.
32. Terrin A, Toldo G, Ermani M, Mainardi F, Maggioni F. When migraine mimics stroke: a systematic review. Cephalalgia. 2018;38(14):2068–78. https://doi.org/10.1177/0333102418767999.
33. Wijman CA, Wolf PA, Kase CS, Kelly-Hayes M, Beiser AS. Migrainous visual accompaniments are not rare in late life: the Framingham Study. Stroke. 1998;29(8):1539–43. https://doi.org/10.1161/01.str.29.8.1539.
34. Vongvaivanich K, Lertakyamanee P, Silberstein SD, Dodick DW. Late-life migraine accompaniments: a narrative review. Cephalalgia. 2015;35(10):894–911. https://doi.org/10.1177/0333102414560635.
35. Gobel CH, Karstedt SC, Munte TF, Gobel H, Wolfrum S, Lebedeva ER, et al. ICHD-3 is significantly more specific than ICHD-3 beta for diagnosis of migraine with aura and with typical aura. J Headache Pain. 2020;21(1):2. https://doi.org/10.1186/s10194-019-1072-2.
36. Lebedeva ER, Gurary NM, Gilev DV, Olesen J. Prospective testing of ICHD-3 beta diagnostic criteria for migraine with aura and migraine with typical aura in patients with transient ischemic attacks. Cephalalgia. 2018;38(3):561–7. https://doi.org/10.1177/0333102417702121.
37. Evans RW. The clinical features of migraine with and without aura. Pract Neurol. 2014;22:28–32.
38. Purdy RA, Diener HC. Migraine mimicking stroke: what to do? Cephalalgia. 2018;38(14):1995–7. https://doi.org/10.1177/0333102418768087.
39. Olesen J, Friberg L, Olsen TS, Andersen AR, Lassen NA, Hansen PE, et al. Ischaemia-induced (symptomatic) migraine attacks may be more frequent than migraine-induced ischaemic insults. Brain. 1993;116(Pt 1):187–202. https://doi.org/10.1093/brain/116.1.187.
40. Russell MB, Ducros A. Sporadic and familial hemiplegic migraine: pathophysiological mechanisms, clinical characteristics, diagnosis, and management. Lancet Neurol. 2011;10(5):457–70. https://doi.org/10.1016/S1474-4422(11)70048-5.
41. Adelborg K, Szepligeti SK, Holland-Bill L, Ehrenstein V, Horvath-Puho E, Henderson VW, et al. Migraine and risk of cardiovascular diseases: Danish population based matched cohort study. BMJ. 2018;360:k96. https://doi.org/10.1136/bmj.k96.
42. Sacco S, Ornello R, Ripa P, Pistoia F, Carolei A. Migraine and hemorrhagic stroke: a meta-analysis. Stroke. 2013;44(11):3032–8. https://doi.org/10.1161/STROKEAHA.113.002465.
43. Albieri V, Olsen TS, Andersen KK. Risk of stroke in migraineurs using triptans. Associations with age, sex, stroke severity and subtype. EBioMedicine. 2016;6:199–205. https://doi.org/10.1016/j.ebiom.2016.02.039.
44. Kurth T, Kase CS, Schurks M, Tzourio C, Buring JE. Migraine and risk of haemorrhagic stroke in women: prospective cohort study. BMJ. 2010;341:c3659. https://doi.org/10.1136/bmj.c3659.
45. Xu Z, Yue Y, Bai J, Shen C, Yang J, Huang X, et al. Association between oral contraceptives and risk of hemorrhagic stroke: a meta-analysis of observational studies. Arch Gynecol Obstet. 2018;297(5):1181–91. https://doi.org/10.1007/s00404-018-4723-7.
46. Arkink EB, Terwindt GM, de Craen AJ, Konishi J, van der Grond J, van Buchem MA, et al. Infratentorial microbleeds: another sign of microangiopathy in migraine. Stroke. 2015;46(7):1987–9. https://doi.org/10.1161/STROKEAHA.115.009604.
47. Malik R, Winsvold B, Auffenberg E, Dichgans M, Freilinger T. The migraine-stroke connection: a genetic perspective. Cephalalgia. 2016;36(7):658–68. https://doi.org/10.1177/0333102415621055.
48. Bashir A, Lipton RB, Ashina S, Ashina M. Migraine and structural changes in the brain: a systematic review and meta-analysis. Neurology. 2013;81(14):1260–8. https://doi.org/10.1212/WNL.0b013e3182a6cb32.
49. Kurth T, Mohamed S, Maillard P, Zhu YC, Chabriat H, Mazoyer B, et al. Headache, migraine, and structural brain lesions and function: population based epidemiology of vascular ageing-MRI study. BMJ. 2011;342:c7357. https://doi.org/10.1136/bmj.c7357.
50. Palm-Meinders IH, Koppen H, Terwindt GM, Launer LJ, Konishi J, Moonen JM, et al. Structural brain changes in migraine. JAMA. 2012;308(18):1889–97. https://doi.org/10.1001/jama.2012.14276.
51. Gaist D, Garde E, Blaabjerg M, Nielsen HH, Kroigard T, Ostergaard K, et al. Migraine with aura and risk of silent brain infarcts and white matter hyperintensities: an MRI study. Brain. 2016;139(Pt 7):2015–23. https://doi.org/10.1093/brain/aww099.
52. Uggetti C, Squarza S, Longaretti F, Galli A, Di Fiore P, Reganati PF, et al. Migraine with aura and white matter lesions: an MRI study. Neurol Sci. 2017;38(Suppl 1):11–3. https://doi.org/10.1007/s10072-017-2897-6.
53. Monteith T, Gardener H, Rundek T, Dong C, Yoshita M, Elkind MS, et al. Migraine, white matter hyperintensities, and subclinical brain infarction in a diverse community: the Northern Manhattan Study. Stroke. 2014;45(6):1830–2. https://doi.org/10.1161/STROKEAHA.114.005447.
54. Zhang W, Cheng Z, Fu F, Zhan Z. Prevalence and clinical characteristics of white matter hyperintensities in migraine: a meta-analysis. Neuroimage Clin. 2023;37:103312. https://doi.org/10.1016/j.nicl.2023.103312.
55. Colombo B, Dalla Libera D, Comi G. Brain white matter lesions in migraine: what's the meaning? Neurol Sci. 2011;32(Suppl 1):S37–40. https://doi.org/10.1007/s10072-011-0530-7.
56. Adami A, Rossato G, Cerini R, Thijs VN, Pozzi-Mucelli R, Anzola GP, et al. Right-to-left shunt does not increase white matter lesion load in migraine with aura patients. Neurology. 2008;71(2):101–7. https://doi.org/10.1212/01.wnl.0000316798.25510.f2.
57. Zhu YC, Dufouil C, Tzourio C, Chabriat H. Silent brain infarcts: a review of MRI diagnostic criteria. Stroke. 2011;42(4):1140–5. https://doi.org/10.1161/STROKEAHA.110.600114.
58. Scher AI, Gudmundsson LS, Sigurdsson S, Ghambaryan A, Aspelund T, Eiriksdottir G, et al. Migraine headache in middle age and late-life brain infarcts. JAMA. 2009;301(24):2563–70. https://doi.org/10.1001/jama.2009.932.

59. Kruit MC, Launer LJ, Ferrari MD, van Buchem MA. Infarcts in the posterior circulation territory in migraine. The population-based MRI CAMERA study. Brain. 2005;128(Pt 9):2068–77. https://doi.org/10.1093/brain/awh542.
60. Espanol A, Lerebours F, Calviere L, Bonneville F, Ducros A, Larrue V, et al. Silent brain infarct in migraine: systematic review and meta-analysis. Rev Neurol (Paris). 2023;180:486. https://doi.org/10.1016/j.neurol.2023.05.003.
61. Meilan A, Larrosa D, Ramon C, Cernuda-Morollon E, Martinez-Camblor P, Saiz A, et al. No association between migraine frequency, white matter lesions and silent brain infarctions: a study in a series of women with chronic migraine. Eur J Neurol. 2020;27(8):1689–96. https://doi.org/10.1111/ene.14284.
62. Porter A, Gladstone JP, Dodick DW. Migraine and white matter hyperintensities. Curr Pain Headache Rep. 2005;9(4):289–93. https://doi.org/10.1007/s11916-005-0039-y.
63. Hoffman V, Xue F, Ezzy SM, Yusuf A, Green E, Eisele O, et al. Risk of cardiovascular and cerebrovascular events and mortality in patients with migraine receiving prophylactic treatments: an observational cohort study. Cephalalgia. 2019;39(12):1544–59. https://doi.org/10.1177/0333102419856630.
64. Bigal ME, Kurth T, Santanello N, Buse D, Golden W, Robbins M, et al. Migraine and cardiovascular disease: a population-based study. Neurology. 2010;74(8):628–35. https://doi.org/10.1212/WNL.0b013e3181d0cc8b.
65. Sacco S, Ornello R, Ripa P, Tiseo C, Degan D, Pistoia F, et al. Migraine and risk of ischaemic heart disease: a systematic review and meta-analysis of observational studies. Eur J Neurol. 2015;22(6):1001–11. https://doi.org/10.1111/ene.12701.
66. Schurks M, Rist PM, Shapiro RE, Kurth T. Migraine and mortality: a systematic review and meta-analysis. Cephalalgia. 2011;31(12):1301–14. https://doi.org/10.1177/0333102411415879.
67. Kurth T, Winter AC, Eliassen AH, Dushkes R, Mukamal KJ, Rimm EB, et al. Migraine and risk of cardiovascular disease in women: prospective cohort study. BMJ. 2016;353:i2610. https://doi.org/10.1136/bmj.i2610.
68. Hippisley-Cox J, Coupland C, Brindle P. Development and validation of QRISK3 risk prediction algorithms to estimate future risk of cardiovascular disease: prospective cohort study. BMJ. 2017;357:j2099. https://doi.org/10.1136/bmj.j2099.
69. Sacco S, Pistoia F, Degan D, Carolei A. Conventional vascular risk factors: their role in the association between migraine and cardiovascular diseases. Cephalalgia. 2015;35(2):146–64. https://doi.org/10.1177/0333102414559551.
70. Winsvold BS, Hagen K, Aamodt AH, Stovner LJ, Holmen J, Zwart JA. Headache, migraine and cardiovascular risk factors: the HUNT study. Eur J Neurol. 2011;18(3):504–11. https://doi.org/10.1111/j.1468-1331.2010.03199.x.
71. Turk WE, Uiterwijk A, Pasmans R, Meys V, Ayata C, Koehler PJ. Aspirin prophylaxis for migraine with aura: an observational case series. Eur Neurol. 2017;78(5–6):287–9. https://doi.org/10.1159/000481252.
72. Maggioni F, Bruno M, Mainardi F, Lisotto C, Zanchin G. Migraine responsive to warfarin: an update on anticoagulant possible role in migraine prophylaxis. Neurol Sci. 2012;33(6):1447–9. https://doi.org/10.1007/s10072-011-0926-4.
73. Secil Y, Unde C, Beckmann YY, Bozkaya YT, Ozerkan F, Basoglu M. Blood pressure changes in migraine patients before, during and after migraine attacks. Pain Pract. 2010;10(3):222–7. https://doi.org/10.1111/j.1533-2500.2009.00349.x.
74. Lebedeva ER, Kobzeva NR, Gilev DV, Olesen J. Factors associated with primary headache according to diagnosis, sex, and social group. Headache. 2016;56(2):341–56. https://doi.org/10.1111/head.12757.
75. Merikangas KR, Fenton BT, Cheng SH, Stolar MJ, Risch N. Association between migraine and stroke in a large-scale epidemiological study of the United States. Arch Neurol. 1997;54(4):362–8. https://doi.org/10.1001/archneur.1997.00550160012009.
76. Schwaiger J, Kiechl S, Stockner H, Knoflach M, Werner P, Rungger G, et al. Burden of atherosclerosis and risk of venous thromboembolism in patients with migraine. Neurology. 2008;71(12):937–43. https://doi.org/10.1212/01.wnl.0000325918.48056.75.
77. Kuo CY, Yen MF, Chen LS, Fann CY, Chiu YH, Chen HH, et al. Increased risk of hemorrhagic stroke in patients with migraine: a population-based cohort study. PLoS One. 2013;8(1):e55253. https://doi.org/10.1371/journal.pone.0055253.
78. Entonen AH, Suominen SB, Sillanmäki LH, Rautava PT, Kauniskangas K, Mäntyselkä PT, et al. Prevalent migraine as a predictor of incident hypertension. Eur J Pub Health. 2022;32(2):297–301. https://doi.org/10.1093/eurpub/ckab219.
79. Gardener H, Monteith T, Rundek T, Wright CB, Elkind MS, Sacco RL. Hypertension and migraine in the Northern Manhattan Study. Ethn Dis. 2016;26(3):323–30. https://doi.org/10.18865/ed.26.3.323.
80. Gudmundsson LS, Thorgeirsson G, Sigfusson N, Sigvaldason H, Johannsson M. Migraine patients have lower systolic but higher diastolic blood pressure compared with controls in a population-based study of 21,537 subjects. The Reykjavik Study. Cephalalgia. 2006;26(4):436–44. https://doi.org/10.1111/j.1468-2982.2005.01057.x.
81. Hagen K, Stovner LJ, Vatten L, Holmen J, Zwart JA, Bovim G. Blood pressure and risk of headache: a prospective study of 22 685 adults in Norway. J Neurol Neurosurg Psychiatry. 2002;72(4):463–6. https://doi.org/10.1136/jnnp.72.4.463.
82. He M, Yu S, Liu R, Yang X, Zhao G, Qiao X, et al. Elevated blood pressure and headache disorders in China--associations, undertreatment and implications for public health. J Headache Pain. 2015;16:86. https://doi.org/10.1186/s10194-015-0570-0.
83. Wiehe M, Fuchs SC, Moreira LB, Moraes RS, Fuchs FD. Migraine is more frequent in individuals with optimal and normal blood pressure: a population-based study. J Hypertens. 2002;20(7):1303–6. https://doi.org/10.1097/00004872-200207000-00016.
84. Tzourio C, Gagniere B, El Amrani M, Alperovitch A, Bousser MG. Relationship between migraine, blood pressure and carotid thickness. A population-based study in the elderly. Cephalalgia. 2003;23(9):914–20. https://doi.org/10.1046/j.1468-2982.2003.00613.x.
85. Muiesan ML, Padovani A, Salvetti M, Monteduro C, Poisa P, Bonzi B, et al. Headache: prevalence and relationship with office or ambulatory blood pressure in a general population sample (the Vobarno Study). Blood Press. 2006;15(1):14–9. https://doi.org/10.1080/08037050500436089.
86. Bensenor IM, Goulart AC, Lotufo PA, Menezes PR, Scazufca M. Cardiovascular risk factors associated with migraine among the elderly with a low income: the Sao Paulo Ageing & Health Study (SPAH). Cephalalgia. 2011;31(3):331–7. https://doi.org/10.1177/0333102410380754.
87. Tronvik E, Stovner LJ, Hagen K, Holmen J, Zwart JA. High pulse pressure protects against headache: prospective and cross-sectional data (HUNT study). Neurology. 2008;70(16):1329–36. https://doi.org/10.1212/01.wnl.0000309222.79376.57.
88. Courand PY, Serraille M, Girerd N, Demarquay G, Milon H, Lantelme P, et al. The paradoxical significance of headache in hypertension. Am J Hypertens. 2016;29(9):1109–16. https://doi.org/10.1093/ajh/hpw041.
89. Fagernaes CF, Heuch I, Zwart JA, Winsvold BS, Linde M, Hagen K. Blood pressure as a risk factor for headache and

migraine: a prospective population-based study. Eur J Neurol. 2015;22(1):156–62, e10–1. https://doi.org/10.1111/ene.12547.
90. Lee ST, Chu K, Jung KH, Kim DH, Kim EH, Choe VN, et al. Decreased number and function of endothelial progenitor cells in patients with migraine. Neurology. 2008;70(17):1510–7. https://doi.org/10.1212/01.wnl.0000294329.93565.94.
91. Schillaci G, Sarchielli P, Corbelli I, Pucci G, Settimi L, Mannarino MR, et al. Aortic stiffness and pulse wave reflection in young subjects with migraine: a case-control study. Neurology. 2010;75(11):960–6. https://doi.org/10.1212/WNL.0b013e3181f25ecd.
92. Matei D, Constantinescu V, Corciova C, Ignat B, Matei R, Popescu CD. Autonomic impairment in patients with migraine. Eur Rev Med Pharmacol Sci. 2015;19(20):3922–7.
93. Yilmaz Avci A, Akkucuk MH, Torun E, Arikan S, Can U, Tekindal MA. Migraine and subclinical atherosclerosis: endothelial dysfunction biomarkers and carotid intima-media thickness: a case-control study. Neurol Sci. 2019;40(4):703–11. https://doi.org/10.1007/s10072-019-3710-5.
94. Guo Y, Rist PM, Daghlas I, Giulianini F, Kurth T, Chasman DI. A genome-wide cross-phenotype meta-analysis of the association of blood pressure with migraine. Nat Commun. 2020;11(1):3368. https://doi.org/10.1038/s41467-020-17002-0.
95. Entonen AH, Suominen SB, Korkeila K, Mantyselka PT, Sillanmaki LH, Ojanlatva A, et al. Migraine predicts hypertension--a cohort study of the Finnish working-age population. Eur J Pub Health. 2014;24(2):244–8. https://doi.org/10.1093/eurpub/ckt141.
96. Rist PM, Winter AC, Buring JE, Sesso HD, Kurth T. Migraine and the risk of incident hypertension among women. Cephalalgia. 2018;38(12):1817–24. https://doi.org/10.1177/0333102418756865.
97. Mancia G, Rosei EA, Ambrosioni E, Avino F, Carolei A, Dacco M, et al. Hypertension and migraine comorbidity: prevalence and risk of cerebrovascular events: evidence from a large, multicenter, cross-sectional survey in Italy (MIRACLES study). J Hypertens. 2011;29(2):309–18. https://doi.org/10.1097/HJH.0b013e3283410404.
98. Barbanti P, Aurilia C, Egeo G, Fofi L. Hypertension as a risk factor for migraine chronification. Neurol Sci. 2010;31(Suppl 1):S41–3. https://doi.org/10.1007/s10072-010-0269-6.
99. Alberti KG, Zimmet P, Shaw J. Metabolic syndrome--a new worldwide definition. A Consensus Statement from the International Diabetes Federation. Diabet Med. 2006;23(5):469–80. https://doi.org/10.1111/j.1464-5491.2006.01858.x.
100. Winsvold BS, Sandven I, Hagen K, Linde M, Midthjell K, Zwart J-A. Migraine, headache and development of metabolic syndrome: an 11-year follow-up in the Nord-Trφndelag Health Study (HUNT). Pain. 2013;154(8):1305–11. https://doi.org/10.1016/j.pain.2013.04.007.
101. Mottillo S, Filion KB, Genest J, Joseph L, Pilote L, Poirier P, et al. The metabolic syndrome and cardiovascular risk a systematic review and meta-analysis. J Am Coll Cardiol. 2010;56(14):1113–32. https://doi.org/10.1016/j.jacc.2010.05.034.
102. Gupta AK, Dahlof B, Sever PS, Poulter NR. Metabolic syndrome, independent of its components, is a risk factor for stroke and death but not for coronary heart disease among hypertensive patients in the ASCOT-BPLA. Diabetes Care. 2010;33(7):1647–51. https://doi.org/10.2337/dc09-2208.
103. Peterlin BL, Rosso AL, Rapoport AM, Scher AI. Obesity and migraine: the effect of age, gender and adipose tissue distribution. Headache. 2010;50(1):52–62. https://doi.org/10.1111/j.1526-4610.2009.01459.x.
104. Bigal ME, Lipton RB. Obesity is a risk factor for transformed migraine but not chronic tension-type headache. Neurology. 2006;67(2):252–7. https://doi.org/10.1212/01.wnl.0000225052.35019.f9.
105. Farello G, Ferrara P, Antenucci A, Basti C, Verrotti A. The link between obesity and migraine in childhood: a systematic review. Ital J Pediatr. 2017;43(1):27. https://doi.org/10.1186/s13052-017-0344-1.
106. Jahromi SR, Martami F, Morad Soltani K, Togha M. Migraine and obesity: what is the real direction of their association? Expert Rev Neurother. 2023;23(1):75–84. https://doi.org/10.1080/14737175.2023.2173575.
107. Sen S, Androulakis XM, Duda V, Alonso A, Chen LY, Soliman EZ, et al. Migraine with visual aura is a risk factor for incident atrial fibrillation: a cohort study. Neurology. 2018;91(24):e2202–e10. https://doi.org/10.1212/WNL.0000000000006650.
108. Aygun D, Altintop L, Doganay Z, Guven H, Baydin A. Electrocardiographic changes during migraine attacks. Headache. 2003;43(8):861–6. https://doi.org/10.1046/j.1526-4610.2003.03164.x.
109. Melek IM, Seyfeli E, Duru M, Duman T, Akgul F, Yalcin F. Autonomic dysfunction and cardiac repolarization abnormalities in patients with migraine attacks. Med Sci Monit. 2007;13(3):RA47–9.
110. Mohanty S, Mohanty P, Rutledge JN, Di Biase L, Yan RX, Trivedi C, et al. Effect of catheter ablation and periprocedural anticoagulation regimen on the clinical course of migraine in atrial fibrillation patients with or without pre-existent migraine: results from a prospective study. Circ Arrhythm Electrophysiol. 2015;8(2):279–87. https://doi.org/10.1161/CIRCEP.114.002285.
111. Kurth T, Gaziano JM, Cook NR, Bubes V, Logroscino G, Diener HC, et al. Migraine and risk of cardiovascular disease in men. Arch Intern Med. 2007;167(8):795–801. https://doi.org/10.1001/archinte.167.8.795.
112. Rose KM, Carson AP, Sanford CP, Stang PE, Brown CA, Folsom AR, et al. Migraine and other headaches: associations with Rose angina and coronary heart disease. Neurology. 2004;63(12):2233–9. https://doi.org/10.1212/01.wnl.0000147289.50605.dc.
113. Rosamond W. Are migraine and coronary heart disease associated? An epidemiologic review. Headache. 2004;44(Suppl 1):S5–12. https://doi.org/10.1111/j.1526-4610.2004.04103.x.
114. Bigal ME, Kurth T, Hu H, Santanello N, Lipton RB. Migraine and cardiovascular disease: possible mechanisms of interaction. Neurology. 2009;72(21):1864–71. https://doi.org/10.1212/WNL.0b013e3181a71220.
115. Lip PZ, Lip GY. Patent foramen ovale and migraine attacks: a systematic review. Am J Med. 2014;127(5):411–20. https://doi.org/10.1016/j.amjmed.2013.12.006.
116. Truong T, Slavin L, Kashani R, Higgins J, Puri A, Chowdhry M, et al. Prevalence of migraine headaches in patients with congenital heart disease. Am J Cardiol. 2008;101(3):396–400. https://doi.org/10.1016/j.amjcard.2007.08.047.
117. Schwedt TJ, Demaerschalk BM, Dodick DW. Patent foramen ovale and migraine: a quantitative systematic review. Cephalalgia. 2008;28(5):531–40. https://doi.org/10.1111/j.1468-2982.2008.01554.x.
118. Anzola GP, Magoni M, Guindani M, Rozzini L, Volta GD. Potential source of cerebral embolism in migraine with aura: a transcranial Doppler study. Neurology. 1999;52(8):1622–5. https://doi.org/10.1212/wnl.52.8.1622.
119. Dalla Volta G, Guindani M, Zavarise P, Griffini S, Pezzini A, Padovani A. Prevalence of patent foramen ovale in a large series of patients with migraine with aura, migraine without aura and cluster headache, and relationship with clinical phenotype. J Headache Pain. 2005;6(4):328–30. https://doi.org/10.1007/s10194-005-0223-9.

120. Liu K, Wang BZ, Hao Y, Song S, Pan M. The correlation between migraine and patent foramen ovale. Front Neurol. 2020;11:543485. https://doi.org/10.3389/fneur.2020.543485.
121. Yasufumi Kijima NM, Noureddin N, Gevorgyan R, Tobis J. The degree of right-to-left shunt is associated with visual aura due to migraine. J Am Coll Cardiol. 2015;66(15):B301.
122. Reisman AM, Robbins BT, Chou DE, Yugrakh MS, Gross GJ, Privitera L, et al. Ticagrelor for Refractory Migraine/Patent Foramen Ovale (TRACTOR): an open-label pilot study. Neurology. 2018;91(22):1010–7. https://doi.org/10.1212/WNL.0000000000006573.
123. Spencer BT, Qureshi Y, Sommer RJ. A retrospective review of clopidogrel as primary therapy for migraineurs with right to left shunt lesions. Cephalalgia. 2014;34(11):933–7. https://doi.org/10.1177/0333102414523845.
124. Dowson A, Mullen MJ, Peatfield R, Muir K, Khan AA, Wells C, et al. Migraine Intervention With STARFlex Technology (MIST) trial: a prospective, multicenter, double-blind, sham-controlled trial to evaluate the effectiveness of patent foramen ovale closure with STARFlex septal repair implant to resolve refractory migraine headache. Circulation. 2008;117(11):1397–404. https://doi.org/10.1161/CIRCULATIONAHA.107.727271.
125. Mattle HP, Evers S, Hildick-Smith D, Becker WJ, Baumgartner H, Chataway J, et al. Percutaneous closure of patent foramen ovale in migraine with aura, a randomized controlled trial. Eur Heart J. 2016;37(26):2029–36. https://doi.org/10.1093/eurheartj/ehw027.
126. Tobis JM, Charles A, Silberstein SD, Sorensen S, Maini B, Horwitz PA, et al. Percutaneous closure of patent foramen ovale in patients with migraine: the PREMIUM trial. J Am Coll Cardiol. 2017;70(22):2766–74. https://doi.org/10.1016/j.jacc.2017.09.1105.
127. Xu J, Mao N, Wang C, Feng J, Lian Y. Clinical analysis of 30 cases of cardiac cephalalgia. Cephalalgia. 2022;42(9):926–32. https://doi.org/10.1177/03331024221088993.
128. Navarro-Pérez MP, Bellosta-Diago E, Olesen J, Santos-Lasaosa S. Cardiac cephalalgia: a narrative review and ICHD-3 criteria evaluation. J Headache Pain. 2022;23(1):136. https://doi.org/10.1186/s10194-022-01508-7.
129. Navarro-Pérez MP, Espinosa-Rueda J, Ballesta-Martínez S, Revilla-Martí P, Olesen J, Bellosta-Diago E, et al. Prevalence, clinical characteristics and associated factors of cardiac cephalalgia: a prospective study. Cephalalgia. 2023;43(4):3331024231160743. https://doi.org/10.1177/03331024231160743.
130. WHO Guidelines Approved by the Guidelines Review Committee. Medical eligibility criteria for contraceptive use. Geneva: World Health Organization. Copyright © World Health Organization 2015; 2015.
131. Champaloux SW, Tepper NK, Monsour M, Curtis KM, Whiteman MK, Marchbanks PA, et al. Use of combined hormonal contraceptives among women with migraines and risk of ischemic stroke. Am J Obstet Gynecol. 2017;216(5):489.e1–7. https://doi.org/10.1016/j.ajog.2016.12.019.
132. Sacco S, Merki-Feld GS, Ægidius KL, Bitzer J, Canonico M, Kurth T, et al. Hormonal contraceptives and risk of ischemic stroke in women with migraine: a consensus statement from the European Headache Federation (EHF) and the European Society of Contraception and Reproductive Health (ESC). J Headache Pain. 2017;18(1):108. https://doi.org/10.1186/s10194-017-0815-1.
133. Sheikh HU, Pavlovic J, Loder E, Burch R. Risk of stroke associated with use of estrogen containing contraceptives in women with migraine: a systematic review. Headache. 2018;58(1):5–21. https://doi.org/10.1111/head.13229.
134. Pilato F, Distefano M, Calandrelli R. Posterior reversible encephalopathy syndrome and reversible cerebral vasoconstriction syndrome: clinical and radiological considerations. Front Neurol. 2020;11:34. https://doi.org/10.3389/fneur.2020.00034.
135. Wabnitz A, Bushnell C. Migraine, cardiovascular disease, and stroke during pregnancy: systematic review of the literature. Cephalalgia. 2015;35(2):132–9. https://doi.org/10.1177/0333102414554113.
136. Jackson JL, Kuriyama A, Kuwatsuka Y, Nickoloff S, Storch D, Jackson W, et al. Beta-blockers for the prevention of headache in adults, a systematic review and meta-analysis. PLoS One. 2019;14(3):e0212785. https://doi.org/10.1371/journal.pone.0212785.
137. Silberstein SD, Holland S, Freitag F, Dodick DW, Argoff C, Ashman E, et al. Evidence-based guideline update: pharmacologic treatment for episodic migraine prevention in adults: report of the Quality Standards Subcommittee of the American Academy of Neurology and the American Headache Society. Neurology. 2012;78(17):1337–45. https://doi.org/10.1212/WNL.0b013e3182535d20.
138. Burch R. Preventive migraine treatment. Continuum (Minneap Minn). 2021;27(3):613–32. https://doi.org/10.1212/con.0000000000000957.
139. Bavle A. Venlafaxine induced QTc interval prolongation in a therapeutic dose. Asian J Psychiatr. 2015;16:63–4. https://doi.org/10.1016/j.ajp.2015.06.001.
140. Sun H, Dodick DW, Silberstein S, Goadsby PJ, Reuter U, Ashina M, et al. Safety and efficacy of AMG 334 for prevention of episodic migraine: a randomised, double-blind, placebo-controlled, phase 2 trial. Lancet Neurol. 2016;15(4):382–90. https://doi.org/10.1016/S1474-4422(16)00019-3.
141. Goadsby PJ, Reuter U, Hallstrom Y, Broessner G, Bonner JH, Zhang F, et al. A controlled trial of erenumab for episodic migraine. N Engl J Med. 2017;377(22):2123–32. https://doi.org/10.1056/NEJMoa1705848.
142. Tepper S, Ashina M, Reuter U, Brandes JL, Dolezil D, Silberstein S, et al. Safety and efficacy of erenumab for preventive treatment of chronic migraine: a randomised, double-blind, placebo-controlled phase 2 trial. Lancet Neurol. 2017;16(6):425–34. https://doi.org/10.1016/S1474-4422(17)30083-2.
143. Dodick DW, Ashina M, Brandes JL, Kudrow D, Lanteri-Minet M, Osipova V, et al. ARISE: a phase 3 randomized trial of erenumab for episodic migraine. Cephalalgia. 2018;38(6):1026–37. https://doi.org/10.1177/0333102418759786.
144. Ashina M, Goadsby PJ, Reuter U, Silberstein S, Dodick D, Rippon GA, et al. Long-term safety and tolerability of erenumab: three-plus year results from a five-year open-label extension study in episodic migraine. Cephalalgia. 2019;39(11):1455–64. https://doi.org/10.1177/0333102419854082.
145. Silberstein SD, McAllister P, Ning X, Faulhaber N, Lang N, Yeung P, et al. Safety and tolerability of fremanezumab for the prevention of migraine: a pooled analysis of phases 2b and 3 clinical trials. Headache. 2019;59(6):880–90. https://doi.org/10.1111/head.13534.
146. Oakes TM, Kovacs R, Rosen N, Doty E, Kemmer P, Aurora SK, et al. Evaluation of cardiovascular outcomes in adult patients with episodic or chronic migraine treated with galcanezumab: data from three phase 3, randomized, double-blind, placebo-controlled EVOLVE-1, EVOLVE-2, and REGAIN studies. Headache. 2020;60(1):110–23. https://doi.org/10.1111/head.13684.
147. Smith TR, Spierings ELH, Cady R, Hirman J, Schaeffler B, Shen V, et al. Safety and tolerability of eptinezumab in patients with migraine: a pooled analysis of 5 clinical trials. J Headache Pain. 2021;22(1):16. https://doi.org/10.1186/s10194-021-01227-5.
148. Blumenfeld A, Hutchinson S, Pavlovic J, Best PJM, Monteith T, Ma J, et al. Post-hoc analysis of safety in phase 3 atogepant ADVANCE trial participants with or without cardiovas-

cular disease risk factors (P2-2.005). Neurology. 2022;98(18 Supplement):1583.
149. Schim J, Hutchinson S, Lipton R, Croop R, Stock E, Thiry A, et al. Rimegepant is safe and tolerable for the acute treatment of migraine in patients using preventive migraine medications: results from a long-term open-label safety study (2370). Neurology. 2021;96(15 Supplement):2370.
150. Depre C, Antalik L, Starling A, Koren M, Eisele O, Lenz RA, et al. A randomized, double-blind, placebo-controlled study to evaluate the effect of erenumab on exercise time during a treadmill test in patients with stable angina. Headache. 2018;58(5):715–23. https://doi.org/10.1111/head.13316.
151. Tepper S, Pascual J, Reuter U, Picard H, Hong F, Trotman M-L, et al. Analysis of blood pressure following short-term and long-term treatment with erenumab (P4.103). Neurology. 2018;90(15 Supplement):P4.103.
152. Kudrow D, Pascual J, Winner PK, Dodick DW, Tepper SJ, Reuter U, et al. Vascular safety of erenumab for migraine prevention. Neurology. 2020;94(5):e497–510. https://doi.org/10.1212/WNL.0000000000008743.
153. Saely S, Croteau D, Jawidzik L, Brinker A, Kortepeter C. Hypertension: a new safety risk for patients treated with erenumab. Headache. 2021;61(1):202–8. https://doi.org/10.1111/head.14051.
154. Goadsby PJ, Silberstein SD, Yeung PP, Cohen JM, Ning X, Yang R, et al. Long-term safety, tolerability, and efficacy of fremanezumab in migraine: a randomized study. Neurology. 2020;95(18):e2487–e99. https://doi.org/10.1212/WNL.0000000000010600.
155. Administration USFaD. FDA Drug Safety Communication: FDA strengthens warning that non-aspirin nonsteroidal anti-inflammatory drugs (NSAIDs) can cause heart attacks or strokes. 2015.
156. Chalaupka FD. Acute myocardial infarction with sumatriptan: a case report and review of the literature. Headache. 2009;49(5):762–4. https://doi.org/10.1111/j.1526-4610.2009.01409.x.
157. O'Quinn S, Davis RL, Gutterman DL, Pait GD, Fox AW. Prospective large-scale study of the tolerability of subcutaneous sumatriptan injection for acute treatment of migraine. Cephalalgia. 1999;19(4):223–31; discussion 00. https://doi.org/10.1046/j.1468-2982.1999.019004223.x.
158. Hall GC, Brown MM, Mo J, MacRae KD. Triptans in migraine: the risks of stroke, cardiovascular disease, and death in practice. Neurology. 2004;62(4):563–8. https://doi.org/10.1212/01.wnl.0000110312.36809.7f.
159. Dodick D, Lipton RB, Martin V, Papademetriou V, Rosamond W, MaassenVanDenBrink A, et al. Consensus statement: cardiovascular safety profile of triptans (5-HT agonists) in the acute treatment of migraine. Headache. 2004;44(5):414–25. https://doi.org/10.1111/j.1526-4610.2004.04078.x.
160. Elkind AH, Satin LZ, Nila A, Keywood C. Frovatriptan use in migraineurs with or at high risk of coronary artery disease. Headache. 2004;44(5):403–10. https://doi.org/10.1111/j.1526-4610.2004.04071.x.
161. Goldstein JA, Massey KD, Kirby S, Gibson M, Hettiarachchi J, Rankin AJ, et al. Effect of high-dose intravenous eletriptan on coronary artery diameter. Cephalalgia. 2004;24(7):515–21. https://doi.org/10.1111/j.1468-2982.2003.00713.x.
162. Muir DF, McCann GP, Swan L, Clark AL, Hillis WS. Hemodynamic and coronary effects of intravenous eletriptan, a 5HT1B/1D-receptor agonist. Clin Pharmacol Ther. 1999;66(1):85–90. https://doi.org/10.1016/S0009-9236(99)70057-3.
163. Diener HC. The risks or lack thereof of migraine treatments in vascular disease. Headache. 2020;60(3):649–53. https://doi.org/10.1111/head.13749.
164. Khan S, Amin FM, Christensen CE, Ghanizada H, Younis S, Olinger ACR, et al. Meningeal contribution to migraine pain: a magnetic resonance angiography study. Brain. 2019;142(1):93–102. https://doi.org/10.1093/brain/awy300.
165. Silberstein SD, Dodick DW. Migraine genetics: part II. Headache. 2013;53(8):1218–29. https://doi.org/10.1111/head.12169.
166. Olesen J. International classification of headache disorders. Lancet Neurol. 2018;17(5):396–7. https://doi.org/10.1016/S1474-4422(18)30085-1.
167. Klapper J, Mathew N, Nett R. Triptans in the treatment of basilar migraine and migraine with prolonged aura. Headache. 2001;41(10):981–4. https://doi.org/10.1046/j.1526-4610.2001.01192.x.
168. Artto V, Nissila M, Wessman M, Palotie A, Farkkila M, Kallela M. Treatment of hemiplegic migraine with triptans. Eur J Neurol. 2007;14(9):1053–6. https://doi.org/10.1111/j.1468-1331.2007.01900.x.
169. Whyte CA, Stillman MJ, Tepper SJ. Dihydroergotamine and its use in migraine with posterior fossa symptoms. Headache. 2010;50(9):1419–23. https://doi.org/10.1111/j.1526-4610.2010.01698.x.
170. Mathew PG, Krel R, Buddhdev B, Ansari H, Joshi SG, Spinner WD, et al. A retrospective analysis of triptan and DHE use for basilar and hemiplegic migraine. Headache. 2016;56(5):841–8. https://doi.org/10.1111/head.12804.
171. Roberto G, Raschi E, Piccinni C, Conti V, Vignatelli L, D'Alessandro R, et al. Adverse cardiovascular events associated with triptans and ergotamines for treatment of migraine: systematic review of observational studies. Cephalalgia. 2015;35(2):118–31. https://doi.org/10.1177/0333102414550416.
172. Ghanshani S, Chen C, Lin B, Duan L, Shen YA, Lee MS. Risk of acute myocardial infarction, heart failure, and death in migraine patients treated with triptans. Headache. 2020;60(10):2166–75. https://doi.org/10.1111/head.13959.
173. Rubio-Beltrán E, Labastida-Ramírez A, Haanes KA, van den Bogaerdt A, Bogers A, Zanelli E, et al. Characterization of binding, functional activity, and contractile responses of the selective 5-HT(1F) receptor agonist lasmiditan. Br J Pharmacol. 2019;176(24):4681–95. https://doi.org/10.1111/bph.14832.
174. Rubio-Beltran E, Chan KY, Danser AHJ, MaassenVanDenBrink A, Edvinsson L. Characterisation of the calcitonin gene-related peptide receptor antagonists ubrogepant and atogepant in human isolated coronary, cerebral and middle meningeal arteries. Cephalalgia. 2019;40(4):357–66. https://doi.org/10.1177/0333102419884943.
175. Shapiro RE, Hochstetler HM, Dennehy EB, Khanna R, Doty EG, Berg PH, et al. Lasmiditan for acute treatment of migraine in patients with cardiovascular risk factors: post-hoc analysis of pooled results from 2 randomized, double-blind, placebo-controlled, phase 3 trials. J Headache Pain. 2019;20(1):90. https://doi.org/10.1186/s10194-019-1044-6.
176. Martin VT, Ahmed Z, Hochstetler HM, Baygani SK, Dong Y, Hauck PM, et al. Tolerability and safety of lasmiditan treatment in elderly patients with migraine: post hoc analyses from randomized studies. Clin Ther. 2021;43(6):1066–78. https://doi.org/10.1016/j.clinthera.2021.04.004.
177. Chaitman BR, Ho AP, Behm MO, Rowe JF, Palcza JS, Laethem T, et al. A randomized, placebo-controlled study of the effects of telcagepant on exercise time in patients with stable angina. Clin Pharmacol Ther. 2012;91(3):459–66. https://doi.org/10.1038/clpt.2011.246.
178. Ho TW, Ho AP, Chaitman BR, Johnson C, Mathew NT, Kost J, et al. Randomized, controlled study of telcagepant in patients with migraine and coronary artery disease. Headache. 2012;52(2):224–35. https://doi.org/10.1111/j.1526-4610.2011.02052.x.
179. Voss T, Lipton RB, Dodick DW, Dupre N, Ge JY, Bachman R, et al. A phase IIb randomized, double-blind, placebo-controlled trial

of ubrogepant for the acute treatment of migraine. Cephalalgia. 2016;36(9):887–98. https://doi.org/10.1177/0333102416653233.
180. Hutchinson S, Silberstein SD, Blumenfeld AM, Lipton RB, Lu K, Yu SY, et al. Safety and efficacy of ubrogepant in participants with major cardiovascular risk factors in two single-attack phase 3 randomized trials: ACHIEVE I and II. Cephalalgia. 2021;41(9):979–90. https://doi.org/10.1177/03331024211000311.
181. Croop R, Goadsby PJ, Stock DA, Conway CM, Forshaw M, Stock EG, et al. Efficacy, safety, and tolerability of rimegepant orally disintegrating tablet for the acute treatment of migraine: a randomised, phase 3, double-blind, placebo-controlled trial. Lancet. 2019;394(10200):737–45. https://doi.org/10.1016/s0140-6736(19)31606-x.
182. ACOG Practice Bulletin No. 206 summary: use of hormonal contraception in women with coexisting medical conditions. Obstet Gynecol. 2019;133(2):396–9. https://doi.org/10.1097/AOG.0000000000003073.
183. Bousser MG, Conard J, Kittner S, de Lignieres B, MacGregor EA, Massiou H, et al. Recommendations on the risk of ischaemic stroke associated with use of combined oral contraceptives and hormone replacement therapy in women with migraine. The International Headache Society Task Force on Combined Oral Contraceptives & Hormone Replacement Therapy. Cephalalgia. 2000;20(3):155–6. https://doi.org/10.1046/j.1468-2982.2000.00035.x.
184. Prevention CfDCa. CDC contraceptive guidance for health care providers – US medical eligibility criteria for contraceptive use – combined hormonal contraceptives. Accessed 14 Oct 2021.

Migraine, Gastrointestinal Disorders, and the Brain-Gut-Microbiota Axis

15

Gretchen E. Tietjen

Introduction

Migraine is robustly associated with gastrointestinal (GI) symptoms and various GI disorders [1]. This chapter describes the epidemiological evidence linking migraine to nausea, vomiting and gastroparesis occurring with acute attacks, as well as to migraine syndromes of childhood where GI symptoms predominate (infantile colic, cyclic vomiting syndrome, abdominal migraine), and to comorbid GI conditions (irritable bowel disorder, peptic ulcer disease, celiac disease, inflammatory bowel disease) (Table 15.1). The putative mechanisms of the link between migraine and GI symptoms, syndromes, and conditions are reviewed, including as they pertain to the brain-gut-microbiota axis and its neural, endocrine, immune, and humoral bidirectional connections (Tables 15.1 and 15.2; Fig. 15.1). Treatment of migraine with pharmacologic and nonpharmacologic nonoral therapies, as well as with dietary alteration and supplementation, is discussed. The effect on migraine of therapies targeting GI syndrome and comorbid GI conditions are summarized in Table 15.1.

Questions

1. Several gastrointestinal (GI) syndromes (i.e., cyclic vomiting syndrome ad abdominal migraine) and GI conditions (irritable bowel syndrome, peptic ulcer disease, and celiac disease) are associated with migraine. The following statement(s) are true:
   A. Treatment of celiac disease with gluten free diet does not impact migraine severity
   B. Migraine treatments are often effective for cyclic vomiting syndrome and abdominal migraine
   C. The GI syndromes and conditions mentioned above are more common in males
   D. Mendelian randomization genetic studies suggest that migraine causes irritable bowel syndrome
   E. All of the above
2. The brain-gut-microbiota axis refers to bidirectional connections between these entities which integrate the functions of the central nervous, gastrointestinal, and immune systems in health and disease. The following statements are true:
   A. The brain influences the gut and microbiome via activation of the autonomic nervous system and HPA axis
   B. Increased gut permeability and inflammation are associated with imbalance in the microbiota composition (dysbiosis)
   C. Systemic release of microbial neurotransmitters, metabolites, and inflammatory cytokines impact the central nervous system
   D. CGRP has an important role in the communications between the brain, the gut and microbiome
   E. All of the above

G. E. Tietjen (✉)
University of Toledo College of Medicine and Life Sciences, Toledo, OH, USA

T. S. Monteith et al. (eds.), *Comprehensive Migraine Management*, https://doi.org/10.1007/978-3-031-86923-5_15

Table 15.1 Migraine-associated gastrointestinal disorders: prevalence, putative mechanisms, and treatment effects on migraine

Condition and prevalence	Migraine-related prevalence	Putative mechanisms	Effects of treatment on migraine/variant
Infantile colic Prevalence: 5–19% [11]	Precursor of migraine in adulthood Colic: 29–33% with maternal migraine [12, 134]; OR 1.7 (95%CI 1.3, 2.4) [12] Prevalence ratio 2.6 (95%CI 1.2, 5.5) [134] Frequency ≥15 d/month: OR 2.5 (95%CI 1.2, 5.3) [12] Colic history (hx): 73% with migraine v 27% w/o migraine [13]; OR 6.6 (95% CI 4.4, 10.0) Prospective cohort: Migraine at 18 y: 23% w colic hx v 11% w/o [14]; RR 2.8 (95%CI 1.2, 6.5) for migraine w colic hx. Risk for MO, not MA [14] Meta-analysis of migraine-colic link: OR 5.6 (95% CI 3.3, 9.5) [135]	Migraine has strong genetic underpinnings and colic may be early manifestation; crying may be related to increased sensitivity to stimuli and pain, and it has circadian aspect [72] Associated with (1) lower intestinal microbiota diversity, (2) fewer beneficial Lactobacillus species, (3) more gram negative (e.g., *E. coli*) species, (4) increased gut and systemic inflammatory markers [73]	Massage and reduction of environmental stimuli (lights, sounds) re-duces crying/colic [71, 139] Eliminating cow's milk protein in breastfed infants decreases colic [71] Probiotic *Lactobacillus reuteri* DSM17938 decreases crying, especially in breastfed infants with colic [140, 141]
Cyclic vomiting syndrome (CVS) Prevalence: 1–2% in children <14 y; mean age of onset 5 y [18, 20, 21] Prevalence: 2% in adults; mean age of onset 25 y [18, 22] F:M ratio 1:1 or slight female predominance in children [20, 23]	Precursor of migraine in adulthood CVS: predicts migraine in 46–71% [17, 25]	Autonomic: POTS, aberrant heart rate variability, increased gastric motility [76–79] Neuroendocrine etiology via HPA axis activation [80–82] Genetic: (1) Variants in *RYR2* encoding stress-induced calcium channel [83] (2) SNPs in gene encoding CB1 [84] (3) Mitochondrial polymorphisms [86–88] SPECT: possible generator in hypothalamus [91] fMRI: (1) increased salience connectivity to the mid-posterior insula (viscerosensory processing) v controls (2) diminished sensorimotor intrinsic connectivity v controls [92]	Acute [142–144]: Sumatriptan [145] Antiemetics, including aprepitant [103] Rehydration Preventive [143, 144]: 1st line: Tricyclic antidepressants [146–148] 2nd line: AEDs: including topiramate [149] Cyproheptadine [147] mitochondrial suppl: CoQ10, riboflavin, L-carnitine [89, 90, 148] CCB: Flunarizine [150] ß blocker: propranolol Aprepitant [103] Other: meditation, CBT, lifestyle modification [151]
Abdominal migraine (AM) Prevalence: 1–4% <15 y Onset: 3–10 y; resolved by 18 y F:M ratio 1.6:1 [20, 26, 28, 29]	Precursor of migraine: 70% of children will go on to develop migraine [30, 31]	Uncertain etiology Hypothesis: trigger-induced CNS arrousal with release of neuropeptides and neurotransmitters leads to GI dysregulation There is lower gastric and antral motility, and increased mucosal permeability [93, 94]	Acute: Triptans [152] Intravenous DHE [153] Preventive: Pizotifen RCT [154] Other: Flunarizine [150], propranolol, cyproheptadine [155]

(continued)

Table 15.1 (continued)

Condition and prevalence	Migraine-related prevalence	Putative mechanisms	Effects of treatment on migraine/variant
Irritable bowel syndrome (IBS) U.S. prevalence [131]: 4.7% by Rome IV criteria 8.6% by Rome III criteria F:M ratio 2:1	IBS: 17% in migraine Migraine: 25–50% with IBS vs 4–19% w/o IBS; OR 2.6 (95% CI 2.3, 3.1) for migraine in IBS;OR 3.4-fold higher for migraine subgroup <30 years old [39] Migraine in IBS: aOR 2.2 (95%CI 2.1, 2.4) in UK Biobank study [136]	Genetic: IBS causally related to migraine by MR analysis [40] Epigenetic: Migraine and IBS associated with early life stress related changes, e.g. central sensitization and GI dysbiosis [37, 95]	Treatment with tricyclic antidepressants and behavioral therapy for stress management are effective [156] Elimination diet showed improvement in migraine and IBS [157]
Peptic Ulcer Disease (PUD) Prevalence: 5–10% [132] lifetime 0.1–1.5% [133] yearly Incidence: 0.1–0.3% [132] yearly PUD in HP [41]: Incidence: 1% per year Incidence in US: 0.06% per year	Migraine in PUD: aOR 1.6 (95%CI 1.4, 1.8) in UK Biobank Study [136] Meta-analysis of HP prevalence: 45% w migraine v 33% w/o migraine; OR 1.9 (95%CI: 1.1, 3.5) [43]	Uncertain mechanism linking migraine with PUD/HP Immune/inflammatory changes in GI mucosa may activate trigeminal ganglia & other pain sensitive structures. Evidence: increased levels of IL-10 cytokine and CGRP in migraine and in HP and HP-induced PUD [97, 98]	HP eradication with antibiotics improved migraine symptoms, with full resolution of migraine in 28% at 12 months [158]. HP eradication + migraine tx decreased migraine disability more than migraine tx alone in RCT [159]. Avoid NSAIDs [42]
Celiac disease (CD) Global prevalence: Seroprevalence 1.4% Biopsy-based 0.7% [46] F:M ratio 3:1	Prevalence of HA in CD: 26% in adult CD OR 2.7 (95% CI 1.7, 4.3) 18% in pediatric CD OR 2.3 (95%CI 2.1, 2.5) [48] Prevalence of CD in HA: Adults: 4.4% in HA v 0.4% in Control Pediatric: 2.4% in HA, OR 1.7–8.3 for CD in HA [48] No association of migraine with CD in UK Biobank study [136]	Gluten-induced increase in proinflammatory cytokines and CGRP. CD-related vitamin and nutrient deficiency related to malabsorption. Occipital and parieto-occipital calcifications and white matter abnormalities in persons with CD and migraine; may be related to perivascular inflammation, abnormal vascular tone, brain hypoperfusion [57]	Gluten free diet (GFD) lead to total resolution of headaches in up to 75% adults and children [119] GFD in CD benefits migraine > TTH [120]
Inflammatory bowel disease (IBD) 1.3% in USA [50] F:M ratio 1.6:1	Migraine: 21–41% w IBD v 8–21% w/o IBD in small studies [51, 137, 138] Migraine/severe HA: 28% w IBD v 15% w/o IBD in 2015–2016 NHIS [51]; Prevalence ratio 1.6 (95%CI 1.4, 1.9) No association of migraine with IBD in UK Biobank study [136]	Uncertain mechanism Possible relationship to defects in absorption, immunity, and intestinal barrier function causing increase in microbial inflammatory metabolites with systemic diffusion of proinflammatory cytokines and endotoxins [100, 101]	No reports of reduction in migraine frequency or severity with improvements of IBD symptoms [1] Avoid NSAIDs [160], CGRP antagonists (CGRP protects intestinal mucosa in colitis models) [161] No contraindication for triptans, ditans, and acetaminophen

Abbreviations: *AEDs* anti-epileptic drugs, *AM* abdominal migraine, *aOR* adjusted odds ratio, *CBT* cognitive behavioral therapy, *CCB* calcium channel blocker, *CD* celiac disease, *CI* confidence interval, *CGRP* calcitonin gene-related peptide, *CNS* central nervous system, *CVS* cyclic vomiting syndrome, d day(s), *ELS* early life stress, *F:M* female:male, *fMRI* functional magnetic resonance imaging, *GFD* gluten-free diet, *GI* gastrointestinal, *HA* headache, *HP Helicobacter pylori*, *HPA* hypothalamus-pituitary-adrenal, *hx* history, *incl* including, *IBD* inflammatory bowel disease, *IBS* irritable bowel syndrome, *IL* interleukin, *m* month(s), *MO* migraine without aura, *MA* migraine with aura, *MR* Mendelian randomization, *NHIS* National Health Interview Survey, *NSAIDs* non-steroidal anti-inflammatory drugs, *OR* odds ratio, *POTS* postural orthostatic tachycardia syndrome, *PUD* peptic ulcer disease, *RCT* randomized, controlled trial, *RR* relative risk, *SPECT* single photon emission computer tomography, *TTH* tension-type headache, *tx* treatment, *UK* United Kingdom, *US* United States, *v* versus, *w* with, *w/o* without, *y* year(s)

Table 15.2 Brain-Gut-Microbiota Axis [9, 52–60]

Axis	Functional connections	
Brain–Gut	Brain ➔ Gut Neural (vagal efferents) and hormonal (HPA axis) systems influence intestinal immune cells, epithelial barrier cells, enteric neurons, smooth muscle cells, interstitial cells of Cajal, and enterochromaffin cells	Gut ➔ Brain Afferent spinal and vagal afferent nerves carry sensory info from ENS to NTS, which projects to LC, rostral ventrolateral medulla, amygdala, thalamus to influence emotional behavior, pain modulation, brain neurotransmitters Neuroimmunological signaling pathways Neuroendocrine signaling pathways
Brain–Microbiota	Brain ➔ Microbiota ANS and HPA axis activation (➔ release of glucocorticoids) regulate microbiota	Microbiota ➔ Brain Indirect pathways (systemic circulation): Regulation or release of neurotransmitters (5-HT, NA, dopamine, glutamate, GABA) Release of neuroactive metabolites, neuroprotective SCFAs (e.g., butyrate) Release of inflammatory cytokines ➔ HPA axis activation and trigeminal nociception Direct pathway: Stimulation of vagal and/or spinal nerves
Gut–Microbiota	Gut ➔ Microbiota Release of neurotransmitters in gut, shifts in inflammatory status, increased permeability of intestinal epithelial barrier, and other changes in gut function and environment modulate gut microbial behavior	Microbiota ➔ Gut Microbiota communicate with gut neuronal, glial, endocrine, and immune cells via microbial metabolites, such as SCFA and secondary bile acids. Example: microbial metabolites stimulate ECC synthesis of serotonin

Abbreviations: *5-HT* serotonin, *ANS* autonomic nervous system (parasympathetic and sympathetic), *ECC* enterochromaffin cells, *ENS* enteric nervous system, *GABA* gamma-aminobutyric acid, *HPA* hypothalamus-pituitary-adrenal axis, *LC* locus coeruleus, *NA* noradrenaline, *NTS* nucleus tractus solitarii, *SCFA* short chain fatty acids

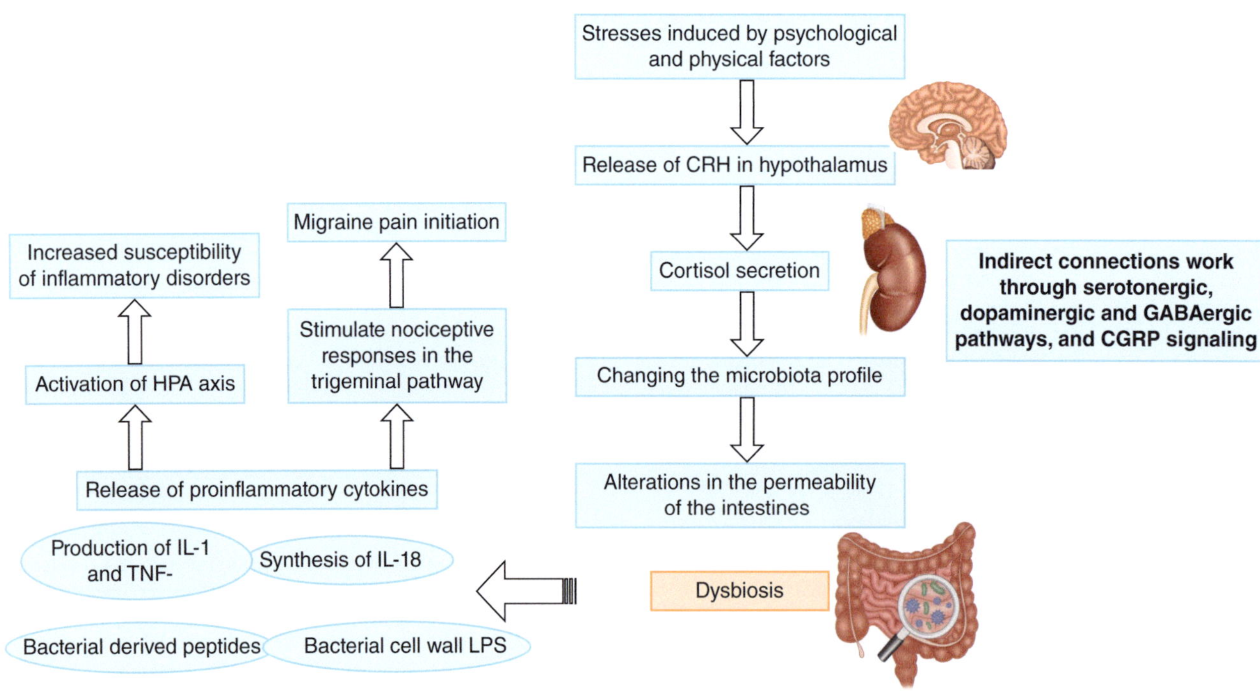

Fig. 15.1 The effects of the gut-microbiota on the brain via indirect signaling. (From Arzani et al. [57])

Epidemiology of Migraine and Gastrointestinal Symptoms and Disorders

Nausea, Vomiting, and Gastroparesis

The International Classification of Headache Disorders 3rd edition (ICHD-3) criteria for migraine without aura (1.1) [2] require either nausea and/or vomiting or photophobia and phonophobia "during headache", although nausea is also a well-recognized premonitory symptom. In a large US survey of persons with migraine, nausea occurred in 73% and vomiting in 29% [3]. In the Women's Health Study, nausea and/or vomiting were reported in about 65% of those with migraine [4]. In the Head-HUNT Study, odds ratio for nausea in headache was 3.2 (95% confidence interval [CI] 2.6–3.8), and it increased with headache frequency, reaching 6.7 (95% CI 5.2–8.5) for chronic migraine [5]. The age-adjusted prevalence of gastroparesis (delayed gastric emptying, characterized by abdominal pain, bloating, early satiety, and postprandial fullness) [6] per 100,000 persons was 9.6 (95% CI 1.8–17.4) for men and 37.8 (95% CI 23.3–52.4) for women [7]. It has, however, been reported to occur in 80% of persons with migraine [8], and in a study of 516 persons with gastroparesis, 37% reported migraine [9].

Infantile Colic

Migraine has been linked to infantile colic, defined as excessive crying and fussing (more than 3 hours per day, more than 3 days a week, and for more than 3 weeks) in a healthy, thriving infant [10]. Colic occurs in about one-fifth of infants [11] and typically abates by 3–4 months. It is included in the Appendix of the ICHD-3 as an episodic syndrome that may be related to migraine (1.6.4) [2]. Maternal migraine doubles the odds of colic [12] and colic predicts childhood migraine (in both retrospective and prospective studies) [13–15] as well as recurrent abdominal pain [16].

Cyclic Vomiting Syndrome

Cyclic vomiting syndrome (CVS) is classified in ICHD-3 as an episodic syndrome (and more specifically as a recurrent gastrointestinal disturbance) in children that may be related to migraine (1.6.1.1) [2]. It extends into adulthood in about 50% [17], or rarely, begins in adulthood [18]. CVS is characterized by recurrent attacks of intense nausea and vomiting, and often pallor and lethargy, which are usually stereotypical in the individual with regards to duration (usually lasting 2–48 hours), and timing of episodes (occurring every 6–8 weeks), and with complete resolution of symptoms between attacks [2, 19]. The prevalence is about 2% in children [20, 21] and adults [22]. In children <15 years old, studies have shown CVS to be either equally prevalent in males and females, or with a slight female predominance [20, 23]. It is hypothesized to be a part of the migrainous syndrome [24], or a precursor of migraine, predicting migraine in 46–71% of children with CVS [17, 25].

Abdominal Migraine

Abdominal migraine (AM) is also classified in ICHD-3 as an episodic recurrent gastrointestinal disturbance that may be related to migraine (1.6.1.2) [2]. It is described as an idiopathic disorder without headache, seen mainly in children (average onset age between 3 and 10 years old) [26] as recurrent attacks of moderate to severe midline abdominal pain, associated with vasomotor symptoms, nausea, vomiting, and pallor, lasting 2–72 hours and with no symptoms between attacks [27]. In children, the prevalence of AM is 1–4% with a female:male ratio of 1.6:1 [20, 28, 29]. Like CVS, it is a likely precursor of migraine given that 70% of children with AM will develop migraine or recurrent abdominal pain [30, 31].

Irritable Bowel Syndrome

Irritable bowel syndrome (IBS) is a chronic, recurrent functional gastrointestinal (GI) disorder characterized by abdominal pain, bloating, and altered bowel movements (diarrhea and/or constipation) [32]. Like migraine, IBS is heritable [33], prevalent [34], more common in women [34, 35], comorbid with anxiety and depression [36], and associated with stress, including early life stress (ELS) [37]. In adults, migraine is associated with IBS [38, 39]. A two-sample Mendelian randomization (MR) analysis suggested a causal relationship between IBS (exposure) and migraine (outcome) without evidence of reverse causation [40]. This does not, however, rule out modifiable risk factors linking the conditions.

Peptic Ulcer Disease and *Helicobacter pylori* Infection

Helicobacter pylori (HP) infection causes nearly all duodenal ulcers and at least 60% of gastric ulcers [41]. Use of NSAIDs, often used for migraine, is another independent peptic ulcer disease (PUD) risk factor, and it works in synergy with HP [42]. The one-year incidence of PUD is 1% in persons with HP, which is several-fold higher than in those without infection [41]. Migraine has been associated with HP, including in a meta-analysis of nearly 1000 patients [43], and with duodenal ulcers but not gastric ulcers [44].

Celiac Disease

Celiac disease (CD) is a female-predominant (3:1 female:male ratio), gluten-induced inflammatory autoimmune disorder of the small intestine, which untreated, leads to intestinal damage with malabsorption with symptoms of diarrhea, bloating, fatigue, and weight loss [45]. The global prevalence of biopsy-verified CD is 0.7%, about half of the prevalence for serological diagnosed cases [46]. Rare neurological manifestations include epilepsy, ataxia, encephalitis, neuropathy, and migraine-like headaches [47]. In adult and pediatric CD, odds of headache are elevated two- to threefold [48]. In children, idiopathic headache raises the odds of CD and may be the presenting symptom.

Inflammatory Bowel Disease

Inflammatory bowel disease (IBD) comprises Crohn's disease and ulcerative colitis, which are chronic autoimmune inflammatory conditions of the colon and small intestine characterized by diarrhea, rectal bleeding, abdominal pain, fatigue and weight loss [49]. The US prevalence of IBD is 1.3%, and 28% of persons with IBD have migraine [50, 51].

Mechanistic Role of the Brain-Gut-Microbiota Axis in Migraine and Associated GI Symptoms and Disorders

Brain-Gut-Microbiota Axis

The brain-gut-microbiota axis consists of neural, endocrine, immune and humoral connections between (1) the central nervous system (CNS), i.e., brain and spinal cord, (2) the gut, including the neuroendocrine regulatory system (NES) and immune cells in adjacent lymphoid tissue, and (3) the intestinal microbiota [52–56]. The NES regulates GI motility, secretion, absorption, visceral sensitivity, local immune defense, and appetite. It comprises the enteric nervous system (ENS) and endocrine cells of the mucosa, which produce neuropeptides/amines (including calcitonin gene-related peptide [CGRP], serotonin, vasoactive intestinal peptide, neuropeptide Y, substance P, somatostatin and ghrelin) [55]. The third component of the axis, the gut-microbiota on the intestinal surface, consists of 100 trillion one-cell microorganisms, predominantly bacteria. The brain-gut-microbiota axis, including the intestinal barrier, immune system, and neural connections develop in concert in the neonatal period, when colonization of the gut begins. Subsequent changes in the microbiota are predominantly influenced by diet, antibiotic use, stress hormones, and changes in gut function [34]. The bidirectional connections of the brain-gut-microbiota axis are outlined in Table 15.2 [9, 52–60]. Alterations in the microbiota composition, referred to as dysbiosis [61], may increase gut permeability, release of proinflammatory cytokines and stimulation of nociceptive responses in the trigeminovascular pathway [57, 61, 62]. CGRP has an important role in the bidirectional communications between the brain, the gut and microbiome, exerting influence on stress, immunity and inflammation (Fig. 15.1) [57]. Stress, a trigger for migraine, impacts the composition of the gut-microbiota, and in turn, communication between microbiota and the CNS influences stress reactivity and responses. CGRP, produced and secreted from enteric and central neurons, enhances acute inflammation via dilation of blood vessels, extravasation of inflammatory cells, and secretion of inflammatory cytokines, while suppressing inflammation in the later stages by inhibiting macrophages and lymphocytes [63]. CGRP-induced (1) mediation of neurogenic inflammation and (2) modulation of nociceptive input via receptor activation within pain-signaling pathways, intracranial arteries and mast cells, are recognized as being key in migraine pathogenesis. The discovery that antagonists to the CGRP ligand and receptor have proved effective in preventing and aborting migraine attacks support the central role of CGRP [64].

Migraine

Dysbiosis has been demonstrated in migraine, including in a metagenome-wide association study of elderly women [65]. Compared to healthy controls, the microbiota in migraine showed less biodiversity, fewer beneficial and more detrimental microorganisms. Studies in migraine suggest that dysbiosis is associated with (1) increased headache severity and duration [66], (2) chronic frequency (via upregulation of TNFα in trigeminal nociceptive system) [62], (3) markers of early atherosclerosis (e.g., higher body mass index, increased thickness of carotid intima-media, elevated glycosylated hemoglobin and tumor necrosis factor-alpha levels) [67] and (4) increased odds of food allergies, anxiety, fibromyalgia, and chronic pelvic pain [66].

Migraine-Related Nausea, Vomiting, and Gastroparesis

Nausea during headache in migraine is putatively secondary to pain, implicating trigeminal neurons and the nucleus tractus solitarius (NTS) [68]. Nausea preceding headache may be a primary event, with premonitory phase activation of the NTS, dorsal motor nucleus of vagus, nucleus ambiguus and periaqueductal gray [69]. Additionally, nausea and vomiting are common symptoms of gastroparesis (delayed gastric emptying), which occurs during and outside the migraine attack [70]. Gastric emptying and motility involve the CNS and ENS (with an alteration in serotonergic signaling), as well as the sympathetic autonomic nervous system, and the interstitial cells of Cajal interacting with smooth muscle cells [9].

The putative mechanisms relating migraine to gastrointestinal disorders in ICHD-3-defined episodic syndromes [2], i.e., infantile colic, cyclic vomiting syndrome, abdominal migraine are described below, and those that fall outside the ICHD-3 system, i.e., IBS, PUD and HP, CD, and IBD, are briefly summarized in Table 15.1.

Infant Colic

Visceral pain, intraluminal gas, and dysmotility, as well as psychological factors such as infant temperament and strained mother-infant interactions have been hypothesized to play a role in the pathogenesis of colic [71]. Colic's relationship to maternal migraine and its foreshadowing of childhood migraine suggests it may be an early sign of migraine with genetic underpinnings [72]. Colic has been associated with dysbiosis and increased gut and systemic inflammatory markers [73].

Cyclic Vomiting Syndrome

The pathogenesis of CVS is likely related to multiple factors acting alone or in concert with one another [74, 75]. Reports of increased gastric motility, postural orthostatic tachycardia, and aberrant heart rate variability in CVS supports autonomic underpinnings [76–79]. Neuroendocrinological origins of CVS have been suspected based on findings consistent with hypothalamic-pituitary-adrenal (HPA) stress axis activation [80–82]. In addition, variants in the ryanodine receptor 2 (*RYR2*) gene that encodes for stress-induced calcium channel function, was found in 24% of persons with CVS versus 5% of controls [83]. Variants have been associated with gut dysmotility and autonomic symptoms [83]. Further, CVS has been associated with single nucleotide polymorphisms in the CNR1 gene that encodes cannabinoid receptor type 1 (CB_1), which is primarily in the CNS [84]. Cannabis hyperemia syndrome, triggered by chronic high dose cannabis use, presents with symptoms reminiscent of CVS [85]. A study of mitochondrial polymorphisms demonstrated a possible [86, 87], but still uncertain [88], role in CVS pathogenesis, and treatment with mitochondrial supplements (riboflavin, L-carnitine, co-enzyme Q10) have shown efficacy [89, 90]. Similar to reports in migraine, a brain perfusion single photon emission photometry (SPECT) study done during the emetic phase of CVS demonstrated a possible generator in the hypothalamus [91]. Functional MRI studies in CVS (compared to controls) showed increased salience connectivity to the mid-posterior insula, an area involved in viscerosensory processing, as well as diminished sensorimotor intrinsic connectivity [92].

Abdominal Migraine

The etiology of abdominal migraine is uncertain. It has been hypothesized to be secondary to a triggered CNS release of neuropeptides and neurotransmitters causing GI dysregulation, such as lower gastric emptying rate and antral motility [93], and increased mucosal permeability [94]. A variant in the gene for RYR2, which is expressed throughout the alimentary tract, may have a role in the pathogenesis of abdominal migraine.

Irritable Bowel Syndrome

Mendelian randomization analysis demonstrates a genetic predisposition for migraine in persons with IBS [40]. Female predominance in both conditions suggests a role for reproductive hormones. The association of migraine and IBS with ELS and recurrent stress, alludes to epigenetic changes impacting the HPA axis and brain-gut-microbiota axis with inflammation-related increase in gut permeability and dysbiosis [37, 95]. Basic studies of ELS demonstrate its central effects on metabolism and actions of serotonin, noradrenaline, glutamate, and brain derived neurotrophic factor expression [95]. Early life stress also leads to central sensitization with hyperalgesia (including visceral hypersensitivity) and allodynia [96].

Peptic Ulcer Disease and *Helicobacter pylori*

The mechanism of the association of migraine with PUD and HP is uncertain but suggests possible immune and duodenal inflammatory changes activating the trigeminal ganglia and other pain-sensitive structures [97, 98].

Celiac Disease

Potential mechanisms of the association of celiac disease and migraine include gluten-induced increase in proinflammatory cytokines and CGRP and CD-related vitamin and nutrient deficiency [97]. Parietal and occipital calcifications and white matter abnormalities seen on imaging in persons with CD and migraine suggest possible perivascular inflammation, vascular tone abnormalities, brain hypoperfusion, or CNS folate deficiency [99].

Inflammatory Bowel Disease

The mechanism of the relationship between IBD and migraine is uncertain. Defects in absorption, immunity, and barrier function of the intestinal epithelium may lead to an increase in microbial inflammatory metabolites (cytokines, endotoxins) reaching the brain via systemic diffusion [100, 101].

Migraine Treatment in Persons with GI Symptoms and Conditions

Nausea, vomiting, gastroparesis, altered GI absorption, and difficulty swallowing in persons with migraine may necessitate the use of nonoral formulations. For acute migraine treatment, nonoral options include sumatriptan (subcutaneous [SC], intranasal [IN] liquid and powder), dihydroergatamine (DHE) (SC, IN, intramuscular [IM], and intravenous [IV]), and ketorolac (IN and IM) [102]. Antiemetics with probable efficacy in treating migraine as well as migraine-related nausea include prochlorperazine, promethazine, metoclopramide, chlorpromazine and droperidol [102], and all but droperidol are available in oral formulation. Aprepitant, an oral substance P/neurokinin A receptor antagonist, is effective in acute and preventive treatment of CVS (Table 15.1) [103], and has also been used to prevent DHE-induced nausea and emesis in persons being treated for medically refractory migrainous headache [104]. When nonoral routes are preferred, prochlorperazine and promethazine may be administered as rectal suppositories, and prochlorperazine, promethazine, metoclopramide, chlorpromazine, and droperidol can all be administered IM or IV. Antiemetics metoclopramide and prochlorperazine, each have multiple class 1 studies supporting acute efficacy for migraine when given intravenously [105], and, along with sumatriptan, are recommended by the American Headache Society as first-line migraine medications in the emergency department [106]. Metoclopramide lessens nausea via inhibition of dopamine D2 and serotonin 5-HT3 receptors in the area postrema, and its prokinetic properties are via agonism of dopaminergic, 5-HT4, and muscarinic acetylcholine receptors [107, 108]. The analgesic properties are putatively related to the suppression of the central response to trigeminal nociception [109]. Prochlorperazine, similar to promethazine and chlorpromazine, is a phenothiazine derivative, with antidopaminergic, antinoradrenergic, antihistaminergic, and anticholinergic properties [110].

Novel nonoral alternatives for prevention of episodic and chronic migraine include four monoclonal antibodies (mAbs) to CGRP that target the CGRP ligand (eptinezumab, fremanezumab, and galcanezumab) or receptor (erenumab) [102]. Erenumab, fremanezumab, and galcanezumab are administered as SC injections and eptinezumab as an IV infusion. They are administered monthly (fremanezumab, galcanezumab, erenumab) or quarterly (fremanezumab, eptinezumab). Several studies suggest that CGRP is important marker of upper gastrointestinal tract afferent fiber integrity and plays a role in gastric homeostasis, including protection from increased gastric secretion associated injury [111]. However, real-world studies across CGRP monoclonal antibodies do not show significant gastrointestinal adverse events, except for low rates of severe constipation for erenumab [112]. OnabotulinumtoxinA injections are FDA-approved for prevention of chronic migraine [102], and sometimes used in conjunction with CGRP mAbs.

Neuromodulatory devices are other nonoral options with FDA-clearance to be used for acute migraine therapy (electrical trigeminal nerve stimulation [eTNS], noninvasive vagal nerve stimulator [nVNS], remote electrical neuromodulation [REN], and single-pulse transcranial magnetic stimulation [sTMS]) and for migraine prevention (eTNS, nVNS, and sTMS) [102].

GI-Related Treatments for Migraine

A number of dietary alterations have shown promise in improving migraine. A recent trial in adults with chronic and episodic migraine showed robust reduction of migraine in those randomized to a 16-week long diet with increased n-3 eicosapentaenoic acid plus docosahexaenoic acid plus/minus reduced n-6 linoleic acid compared to a control diet of average intake of n-3 and n-6 fatty acids [113]. Data suggested that oxylipins in the active diets lowered the nociceptive state without changes in inflammatory mediators, such as prostaglandins and CGRP. In a 4-week randomized control trial (RCT) of a high fiber, low glycemic index diet compared to conventional prophylactic medication showed reduced frequency and severity of migraine in both groups at 90 days [114]. Both low-fat vegan diet [115] and low-lipid diet [116] (randomized cross-over trials) as well as ketogenic diet [117] (observation study) led to reduction in headache frequency and severity, whereas an RCT with ketone body supplementation did not [118]. Gluten free diets (GFD) improve migraine in celiac disease [119, 120], but benefit for migraine in persons with non-celiac gluten sensitivity is unproven. In addition, reduction of proinflammatory adipose tissue through weight loss may improve migraine, as supported by prospective observational studies of bariatric surgery in obese adults [121, 122] and a clinical trial of behavioral therapy and physical training in obese adolescents [123].

Vitamin D deficiency has been associated with migraine, and supplementation has beneficial effects on migraine frequency and severity, potentially through its effects on the gut-microbiota, or by reduction of HP counts [124, 125]. Dietary supplementation with probiotics, which decrease gastroparesis and repair "leaky gut", has been shown to reduce migraine in some [126–128], but not all [129], clinical studies. A recent RCT of the combined effects of probiotics (live microorganisms) and prebiotics (fermentable carbohydrates that selectively provide food for probiotics) taken twice daily for 12 weeks compared to placebo showed reduction in migraine frequency, use of painkillers, gastrointestinal problems, zonulin levels (marker of barrier permeability), and high sensitivity CRP levels [130].

Successful treatment of recurrent gastrointestinal disturbances, such as CVS and AM, with acute and preventive migraine therapies supports the hypothesis that they may be related to migraine (Table 15.1). Furthermore, treatment of GI conditions that are comorbid with migraine, such as IBS, PUD, and CD, often brings improvement of migraine (Table 15.1).

Conclusion

Epidemiological evidence links migraine to GI symptoms occurring with acute attacks (i.e., nausea, vomiting, and gastroparesis), to episodic syndromes of childhood with predominant GI symptoms (i.e., infantile colic, CVS, and AM), and to a number of GI conditions (i.e., IBS, PUD, CD, and IBD). Among the putative mechanisms linking migraine and GI symptoms/syndromes/conditions are those involved in the neural, endocrine, immune, and humoral bidirectional connections of the brain-gut-microbiota axis. The prominence of GI symptoms and comorbidities in persons with migraine necessitates that nonoral therapies, including medications and neuromodulation, be considered for acute attacks and prevention. Furthermore, data suggests that weight loss, certain diets (i.e., diets that are high in n-3/low in n-6 fatty acids, high in fiber/with low glycemic index, low in fat, or ketogenic), and dietary supplements (i.e.,vitamin D and prebiotics/probiotics) may improve migraine. Migraine may also improve with successful treatment of comorbid GI disorders such as IBS (tricyclic antidepressants, behavioral therapy, elimination diet), PUD (antibiotics), and CD (gluten-free diet). Further quality research is needed to clarify the mechanisms of the relationship of migraine to the GI system and to identify how to best use this information to improve migraine therapeutics.

Teaching Points

1. Nausea and gastroparesis occur in approximately three-quarters of persons with migraine, and treatment of GI symptoms and migraine pain with nonoral therapies may be needed.
2. Episodic syndromes of childhood, including infantile colic, cyclic vomiting syndrome (CVS), and abdominal migraine (AM), may represent variants of migraine, and, in the case of CVS and AM, may improve with migraine therapies.
3. A number of GI conditions, including irritable bowel syndrome, peptic ulcer disease, celiac disease, and inflammatory bowel disease are associated with migraine, which may improve with successful treatment of the GI condition.
4. The brain-gut-microbiota axis refers to neural, endocrine, immune, and humoral bidirectional connections between the central nervous system (CNS), the gut, and the intestinal microbiota. Dysbiosis has been identified in migraine and its associated GI conditions, but more quality research is needed to firmly establish the nature of the axis connections.
5. Dietary changes and use of supplements (vitamin D, prebiotics, and probiotics) have shown evidence of benefit for those with migraine, but more quality research is needed to identify the best strategies for targeting the gut and its microbiota in migraine therapeutics.

Case

Susan, a 24-year old woman, presents with worsening migraine without aura. Since losing her job 6 months ago, there has been a gradual increase in migraine headache frequency from 4 days/month to 15 days/month, as well as feelings of anxiety and depression. Migraine onset was at 15 years of age, during the time her parents were divorcing, and she recalls worsening of her father's alcohol abuse and her mother's migraine and depression. Susan has used triptans as needed since diagnosis, but now she is using more (18/month) and her response to them is inconsistent. Four months ago, she developed abdominal pain and diarrhea and was diagnosed with irritable bowel syndrome with diarrhea (IBS-D). On symptomatic treatment with antispasmodic hyoscine and obstipant lomodium, she experienced slight improvement. Her examination is remarkable for signs of cutaneous allodynia plus abdominal bloating and tenderness. Her clinical presentation was consistent with chronic migraine, medication overuse, and IBS-D. Screening suggests moderate anxiety and depression.

Case Discussion

Migraine and IBS are highly prevalent, female-predominant comorbid conditions, often linked to depression and anxiety. Both migraine and IBS are hereditary but also associated with environmental factors, such as stressful events, including adverse childhood experiences. Both disorders may be complicated by central sensitization, which is manifested by allodynia in migraine and visceral hypersensitivity in IBS. Since her IBS symptoms are not adequately treated with hyoscine and lomodium, cognitive behavioral therapy/stress management and initiation of daily tricyclic antidepressants are reasonable next steps for IBS, and may also improve migraine. Probiotic supplementation is also under study for both conditions. Susan was instructed to limit triptan use to 2 days per week.

Questions and Answers

1. Several gastrointestinal (GI) syndromes (i.e., cyclic vomiting syndrome and abdominal migraine) and GI conditions (irritable bowel syndrome, peptic ulcer disease, and celiac disease) are associated with migraine. The following statement(s) are true:
   A. Treatment of celiac disease with gluten-free diet does not impact migraine severity
   B. Migraine treatments are often effective for cyclic vomiting syndrome and abdominal migraine
   C. The GI syndromes and conditions mentioned above are more common in males
   D. Mendelian randomization genetic studies suggest that migraine causes irritable bowel syndrome
   E. All of the above

The correct answer is B. Both acute (e.g., triptans and DHE) and preventive (e.g., tricyclic antidepressants, propranolol, and cyproheptadine) migraine therapies may be used to treat cyclic vomiting syndrome and abdominal migraine (B).

A gluten-free diet has been shown to substantially improve migraine in up to 75% of adults and children with celiac disease (A). The cited GI syndromes and conditions are generally more common in women (C). Mendelian randomization studies suggest that irritable bowel syndrome may cause migraine (D).

2. The brain-gut-microbiota axis refers to bidirectional connections between these entities which integrate the functions of the central nervous, gastrointestinal, and immune systems in health and disease. The following statements are true:
   A. Autonomic nervous system and HPA axis
   B. Increased gut permeability and inflammation are associated with imbalance in the microbiota composition (dysbiosis)
   C. Systemic release of microbial neurotransmitters, metabolites and inflammatory cytokines impact the central nervous system
   D. CGRP has an important role in the communications between the brain, the gut and microbiome
   E. All of the above

The correct answer is E. The statements above describe key elements of the brain-gut-microbiota axis shown in Table 15.2. Dysbiosis has been associated with migraine and evidence suggests it may play a role via TNFα upregulation.

References

1. van Hemert S, Breedveld AC, Rovers JM, et al. Migraine associated with gastrointestinal disorders: review of the literature and clinical implications. Front Neurol. 2014;5:241.
2. Headache Classification Committee of the International Headache Society (IHS). The International Classification of Headache Disorders, 3rd edition. Cephalalgia. 2018;38:1–211.
3. Lipton RB, Stewart WF, Diamond S, Diamond ML, Reed M. Prevalence and burden of migraine in the United States: data from the American Migraine Study II. Headache. 2001;41:646–57.
4. Schürks M, Buring JE, Kurth T. Migraine, migraine features, and cardiovascular disease. Headache. 2010;50:1031–40.
5. Aamodt AH, Stovner LJ, Hagen K, Zwart JA. Comorbidity of headache and gastrointestinal complaints. The Head-HUNT Study. Cephalalgia. 2008;28(2):144–51.
6. Revicki DA, Camilleri M, Kuo B, et al. Development and content validity of a gastroparesis cardinal symptom index daily diary. Aliment Pharmacol Ther. 2009;30:670–80.
7. Jung HK, Choung RS, Locke GR 3rd, et al. The incidence, prevalence, and outcomes of patients with gastroparesis in Olmsted County, Minnesota, from 1996 to 2006. Gastroenterology. 2009;136(4):1225–33.
8. Aurora SK, Kori SH, Barrodale P, McDonald SA, Haseley D. Gastric stasis in migraine: more than just a paroxysmal abnormality during a migraine attack. Headache. 2006;46:57–63.
9. Aurora SK, Shrewsbury SB, Ray S, Hindiyeh N, Nguyen L. A link between gastrointestinal disorders and migraine: Insights into the gut-brain connection. Headache. 2021;61(4):576–89.
10. Wessel MA, Cobb JC, Jackson EB, et al. Paroxysmal fussing in infancy, sometimes called colic. Pediatrics. 1954;14:421–35.
11. Lucassen PL, Assendelft WJ, van Eijk JT, Gubbels JW, Douwes AC, van Geldrop WJ. Systematic review of the occurrence of infantile colic in the community. Arch Dis Child. 2001;84(5):398–403.
12. Gelfand AA, Buse DC, Cabana MD, Grimes B, Goadsby PJ, Allen IE. The Association between parental migraine and infant colic: a cross-sectional, web-based, U.S. survey study. Headache. 2019;59(7):988–1001.
13. Romanello S, Spiri D, Marcuzzi E, Zanin A, Boizeau P, Riviere S, et al. Association between childhood migraine and history of infantile colic. JAMA. 2013;309:1607–12.
14. Jan MM, Al-Buhairi AR. Is infantile colic a migraine-related phenomenon? Clin Pediatr (Phila). 2001;40(5):295–7.

15. Sillanpaa M, Saarinen M. Infantile colic associated with childhood migraine: a prospective cohort study. Cephalalgia. 2015;35:1246–51.
16. Savino F, Castagno E, Bretto R, Brondello C, Palumeri E, Oggero R. A prospective 10-year study on children who had severe infantile colic. Acta Paediatr Suppl. 2005;94(449):129–32.
17. Dignan F, Symon DN, Abu-Arafeh I, Russell G. The prognosis of cyclical vomiting syndrome. Arch Dis Child. 2001;84(1):55–7.
18. Gelfand AA. Episodic syndromes that may be associated with migraine: A.K.A. "the Childhood Periodic Syndromes". Headache. 2015;55(10):1358–64.
19. Drumm BR, Bourke B, Drummond J, et al. Cyclical vomiting syndrome in children: a prospective study. Neurogastroenterol Motil. 2012;24(10):922–7.
20. Abu-Arafeh I, Russell G. Cyclical vomiting syndrome in children: a population-based study. J Pediatr Gastroenterol Nutr. 1995;21(4):454–8.
21. Ertekin V, Selimoğlu MA, Altnkaynak S. Prevalence of cyclic vomiting syndrome in a sample of Turkish school children in an urban area. J Clin Gastroenterol. 2006;40(10):896–8.
22. Aziz I, Palsson OS, Whitehead WE, Sperber AD, Simrén M, Törnblom H. Epidemiology, clinical characteristics, and associations for Rome IV functional nausea and vomiting disorders in adults. Clin Gastroenterol Hepatol. 2019;17(5):878–86.
23. Sunku B, Li BUK. Cyclic vomiting syndrome: comorbidities and treatment. In: Faure C, Di Lorenzo C, Thapar N, editors. Pediatric neurogastroenterology. Wu GY, editor. Clinical Gastroenterology. New York: Springer; 2013. p. 391–400.
24. Tarantino S, Capuano A, Torriero R, et al. Migraine equivalents as part of migraine syndrome in childhood. Pediatr Neurol. 2014;51(5):645–9.
25. Moavero R, Papetti L, Bernucci MC, et al. Cyclic vomiting syndrome and benign paroxysmal torticollis are associated with a high risk of developing primary headache: a longitudinal study. Cephalalgia. 2019;39(10):1236–40.
26. Russell G, Abu-Arafeh I, Symon DN. Abdominal migraine: evidence for existence and treatment options. Paediatr Drugs. 2002;4(1):1–8.
27. Symon DN, Russell G. Abdominal migraine: a childhood syndrome defined. Cephalalgia. 1986;6(4):223–8.
28. Saps M, Nichols-Vinueza DX, Rosen JM, Velasco-Benítez CA. Prevalence of functional gastrointestinal disorders in Colombian school children. J Pediatr. 2014;164(3):542–5.e1.
29. Carson L, Lewis D, Tsou M, et al. Abdominal migraine: an under-diagnosed cause of recurrent abdominal pain in children. Headache. 2011;51:707–12.
30. Dignan F, Abu-Arafeh I, Russell G. The prognosis of childhood abdominal migraine. Arch Dis Child. 2001;84(5):415–8.
31. Spiri D, Rinaldi VE, Titomanlio L. Pediatric migraine and episodic syndromes that may be associated with migraine. Ital J Pediatr. 2014;40:92.
32. Goodoory VC, Houghton LA, Black CJ, Ford AC. Characteristics of, and natural history among, individuals with Rome IV functional bowel disorders. Neurogastroenterol Motil. 2021;34:e14268.
33. Henström M, D'Amato M. Genetics of irritable bowel syndrome. Mol Cell Pediatr. 2016;3(1):7.
34. Lovell RM, Ford AC. Global prevalence of and risk factors for irritable bowel syndrome: a meta-analysis. Clin Gastroenterol Hepatol. 2012;10(7):712–721.e4.
35. Kim YS, Kim N. Sex-gender differences in irritable bowel syndrome. J Neurogastroenterol Motil. 2018;24(4):544–58.
36. Lacy BE, Patel NK. Rome criteria and a diagnostic approach to irritable bowel syndrome. J Clin Med. 2017;6(11):99.
37. O'Mahony SM, Clarke G, Dinan TG, Cryan JF. Irritable bowel syndrome and stress-related psychiatric co-morbidities: focus on early life stress. Handb Exp Pharmacol. 2017;239:219–46.
38. Cole JA, Rothman KJ, Cabral HJ, Zhang Y, Farraye FA. Migraine, fibromyalgia, and depression among people with IBS: a prevalence study. BMC Gastroenterol. 2006;6:26.
39. Chang FY, Lu CL. Irritable bowel syndrome and migraine: bystanders or partners? J Neurogastroenterol Motil. 2013;19(3):301–11.
40. Chen J, Chen X, Xie Y, Sun Y, Wang X, Hesketh T. Irritable bowel syndrome and migraine: evidence from Mendelian randomization analysis in the UK Biobank. Expert Rev Gastroenterol Hepatol. 2021;15(10):1233–9.
41. Kuipers EJ, Thijs JC, Festen HP. The prevalence of Helicobacter pylori in peptic ulcer disease. Aliment Pharmacol Ther. 1995;9(Suppl 2):59–69.
42. Huang JQ, Sridhar S, Hunt RH. Role of Helicobacter pylori infection and non-steroidal anti-inflammatory drugs in peptic-ulcer disease: a meta-analysis. Lancet. 2002;359(9300):14–22.
43. Su J, Zhou XY, Zhang GX. Association between helicobacter pylori infection and migraine: a meta-analysis. World J Gastroenterol. 2014;20(40):14965–72.
44. Hormati A, Akbari N, Sharifipour E, et al. Migraine and gastric disorders: Are they associated? J Res Med Sci. 2019;24:60.
45. Shannahan S, Leffler DA. Diagnosis and updates in celiac disease. Gastrointest Endosc Clin N Am. 2017;27(1):79–92.
46. Singh P, Arora A, Strand TA, et al. Global prevalence of celiac disease: systematic review and meta-analysis. Clin Gastroenterol Hepatol. 2018;16(6):823–836.e2.
47. Rani U, Imdad A, Beg M. Rare neurological manifestation of celiac disease. Case Rep Gastroenterol. 2015;9(2):200–5.
48. Zis P, Julian T, Hadjivassiliou M. Headache associated with coeliac disease: a systematic review and meta-analysis. Nutrients. 2018;10(10):1445.
49. Ramos GP, Papadakis KA. Mechanisms of disease: inflammatory bowel diseases. Mayo Clin Proc. 2019;94(1):155–65.
50. Dahlhamer JM, Zammitti EP, Ward BW, Wheaton AG, Croft JB. Prevalence of inflammatory bowel disease among adults aged ≥18 years – United States, 2015. MMWR Morb Mortal Wkly Rep. 2016;65(42):1166–9.
51. Liu Y, Xu F, Wheaton AG, Greenlund KJ, Thomas CW. The association between inflammatory bowel disease and migraine or severe headache among US adults: findings from the National Health Interview Survey, 2015–2016. Headache. 2021;61(4):612–9.
52. Greenwood-Van Meerveld B, Johnson AC, Grundy D. Gastrointestinal physiology and function. Handb Exp Pharmacol. 2017;239:1–16.
53. Martin CR, Osadchiy V, Kalani A, Mayer EA. The brain-gut-microbiome axis. Cell Mol Gastroenterol Hepatol. 2018;6(2):133–48.
54. Dinan TG, Cryan JF. The microbiome-gut-brain axis in health and disease. Gastroenterol Clin N Am. 2017;46(1):77–89.
55. El-Salhy M, Solomon T, Hausken T, Gilja OH, Hatlebakk JG. Gastrointestinal neuroendocrine peptides/amines in inflammatory bowel disease. World J Gastroenterol. 2017;23(28):5068–85.
56. Zhu S, Jiang Y, Xu K, et al. The progress of gut microbiome research related to brain disorders. J Neuroinflammation. 2020;17(1):25.
57. Arzani M, Jahromi SR, Ghorbani Z, et al. Gut-brain axis and migraine headache: a comprehensive review. J Headache Pain. 2020;21(1):15.
58. Breit S, Kupferberg A, Rogler G, Hasler G. Vagus nerve as modulator of the Brain-Gut Axis in psychiatric and inflammatory disorders. Front Psych. 2018;9:44.
59. Mayer EA, Savidge T, Shulman RJ. Brain-gut microbiome interactions and functional bowel disorders. Gastroenterology. 2014;146(6):1500–12.

60. Socała K, Doboszewska U, Szopa A, et al. The role of microbiota-gut-brain axis in neuropsychiatric and neurological disorders. Pharmacol Res. 2021;172:105840.
61. DeGruttola AK, Low D, Mizoguchi A, Mizoguchi E. Current understanding of dysbiosis in disease in human and animal models. Inflamm Bowel Dis. 2016;22(5):1137–50.
62. Tang Y, Liu S, Shu H, Yanagisawa L, Tao F. Gut microbiota dysbiosis enhances migraine-like pain via TNFα upregulation. Mol Neurobiol. 2020;57(1):461–8.
63. Wei P, Keller C, Li L. Neuropeptides in gut-brain axis and their influence on host immunity and stress. Comput Struct Biotechnol J. 2020;18:843–51.
64. Tajti J, Szok D, Nyári A, Vécsei L. CGRP and CGRP-receptor as targets of migraine therapy: Brain Prize-2021. CNS Neurol Disord Drug Targets. 2021;21:460. https://doi.org/10.2174/1871527320666211011110307.
65. Chen J, Wang Q, Wang A, Lin Z. Structural and functional characterization of the gut microbiota in elderly women with migraine. Front Cell Infect Microbiol. 2020;9:470.
66. Georgescu D, Reisz D, Gurban CV, et al. Migraine in young females with irritable bowel syndrome: still a challenge. Neuropsychiatr Dis Treat. 2017;14:21–8.
67. Georgescu D, Iurciuc MS, Ionita I, et al. Migraine without aura and subclinical atherosclerosis in young females: is gut microbiota to blame? Medicina (Kaunas). 2019;55(12):786.
68. Kaube H, Keay KA, Hoskin KL, Bandler R, Goadsby PJ. Expression of c-*Fos*-like immunoreactivity in the caudal medulla and upper cervical cord following stimulation of the superior sagittal sinus in the cat. Brain Res. 1993;629:95–102.
69. Maniyar FH, Sprenger T, Schankin C, Goadsby PJ. The origin of nausea in migraine-a PET study. J Headache Pain. 2014;15(1):84.
70. Aurora SK, Papapetropoulos S, Kori SH, Kedar A, Abell TL. Gastric stasis in migraineurs: etiology, characteristics, and clinical and therapeutic implications. Cephalalgia. 2013;33(6):408–15.
71. Sung V. Infantile colic. Aust Prescr. 2018;41(4):105–10.
72. Qubty W, Gelfand AA. The link between infantile colic and migraine. Curr Pain Headache Rep. 2016;20(5):31.
73. de Weerth C, Fuentes S, Puylaert P, de Vos WM. Intestinal microbiota of infants with colic: development and specific signatures. Pediatrics. 2013;131(2):e550–8.
74. Li BUK, Balint J. Cyclic vomiting syndrome: evolution in our understanding of a brain-gut disorder. Adv Pediatr Infect Dis. 2000;47:117–60.
75. Redon S. Episodic syndromes that may be associated with migraine: what adult neurologists need to know. Rev Neurol (Paris). 2021;177(7):773–8.
76. Chelimsky TC, Chelimsky GG. Autonomic abnormalities in cyclic vomiting syndrome. J Pediatr Gastroenterol Nutr. 2007;44:326–30.
77. To J, Issenman R, Kamath M. Evaluation of neurocardiac signals in pediatric patients with cyclic vomiting syndrome through power spectral analysis of heart rate variability. J Pediatr. 1999;135:363–6.
78. Venkatesan T, Prieto T, Barboi A, et al. Autonomic nerve function in adults with cyclic vomiting syndrome: a prospective study. Neurogastroenterol Motil. 2010;22:1303–e339.
79. Hejazi R, Lavenbarg T, Pasnoor M, et al. Autonomic nerve function in adult patients with cyclic vomiting syndrome. Neurogastroenterol Motil. 2011;23:439–43.
80. Sato T, Uchigata Y, Uwadana N, et al. A syndrome of periodic adrenocorticotropin and vasopressin discharge. J Clin Endocrinol Metab. 1982;54:517–22.
81. Wolfe SM, Adler R. A syndrome of periodic hypothalamic discharge. Am J Med. 1964;36:956–67.
82. Taché Y, Martinez V, Million M, et al. Corticotropin-releasing factor and the brain-gut motor response to stress. Can J Gastroenterol. 1999;13(suppl. A):18A–25A.
83. Lee J, Wong SA, Li BU, Boles RG. NextGen nuclear DNA sequencing in cyclic vomiting syndrome reveals a significant association with the stress-induced calcium channel (RYR2). Neurogastroenterol Motil. 2015;27(7):990–6.
84. Wasilewski A, Lewandowska U, Mosinska P, et al. Cannabinoid receptor type 1 and mu-opioid receptor polymorphisms are associated with cyclic vomiting syndrome. Am J Gastroenterol. 2017;112(6):933–9.
85. Venkatesan T, Levinthal DJ, Li BUK, et al. Role of chronic cannabis use: cyclic vomiting syndrome vs cannabinoid hyperemesis syndrome. Neurogastroenterol Motil. 2019;31(suppl. 2):e13606.
86. Camilleri M, Carlson P, Zinsmeister AR, et al. Mitochondrial DNA and gastrointestinal motor and sensory functions in health and functional gastrointestinal disorders. Am J Physiol Gastrointest Liver Physiol. 2009;296:G510–6.
87. Wang Q, Ito M, Adams K, et al. Mitochondrial DNA control region sequence variation in migraine headache and cyclic vomiting syndrome. Am J Med Genet A. 2004;131(1):50–8.
88. Ye Z, Xue A, Huang Y, Wu Q. Children with cyclic vomiting syndrome: phenotypes, disease burden and mitochondrial DNA analysis. BMC Gastroenterol. 2018;181:104.
89. Boles RG. High degree of efficacy in the treatment of cyclic vomiting syndrome with combined co-enzyme Q10, L-carnitine and amitriptyline, a case series. BMC Neurol. 2011;11:102.
90. Boehnke C, Reuter U, Flach U, et al. High-dose riboflavin treatment is efficacious in migraine prophylaxis: an open study in a tertiary care centre. Eur J Neurol. 2004;11:475–7.
91. Redon S, Mareau C, Guedj E, Donnet A. Cyclic vomiting syndrome in adults and children: a hypothesis. Headache. 2017;57(6):943–51.
92. Ellingsen DM, Garcia RG, Lee J, et al. Cyclic vomiting syndrome is characterized by altered functional brain connectivity of the insular cortex: a cross-comparison with migraine and healthy adults. Neurogastroenterol Motil. 2017;29:1–5.
93. Devanarayana NM, Rajindrajith S, Benninga MA. Abdominal migraine in children: association between gastric motility parameters and clinical characteristics. BMC Gastroenterol. 2016;16:26.
94. Bentley D, Kehely A, al-Bayaty M, Michie CA. Abdominal migraine as a cause of vomiting in children: a clinican's view. J Pediatr Gastroenterol Nutr. 1995;21(suppl 1):S49–51.
95. O'Mahony SM, Marchesi JR, Scully P, et al. Early life stress alters behavior, immunity, and microbiota in rats: implications for irritable bowel syndrome and psychiatric illnesses. Biol Psychiatry. 2009;65(3):263–7.
96. Tietjen GE, Brandes JL, Peterlin BL, et al. Childhood maltreatment and migraine (part II). Emotional abuse as a risk factor for headache chronification. Headache. 2010;50(1):32–41.
97. Cámara-Lemarroy CR, Rodriguez-Gutierrez R, Monreal-Robles R, Marfil-Rivera A. Gastrointestinal disorders associated with migraine: a comprehensive review. World J Gastroenterol. 2016;22(36):8149–60.
98. Kang JW, Shin YI. The role of interleukin 10 in the associations between migraine and Helicobacter pylori infection. Pain Physician. 2013;16:E450.
99. D'Amico D, Rigamonti A, Spina L, Bianchi-Marzoli S, Vecchi M, Bussone G. Migraine, celiac disease, and cerebral calcifications: a new case. Headache. 2005;45(9):1263–7.
100. Fasano A, Shea-Donohue T. Mechanisms of disease: the role of intestinal barrier function in the pathogenesis of gastrointestinal autoimmune diseases. Nat Clin Pract Gastroenterol Hepatol. 2005;2:416–22.
101. Podolsky DK. Inflammatory bowel disease. N Engl J Med. 2002;347:417–29.

102. Ailani J, Burch RC, Robbins MS, Board of Directors of the American Headache Society. The American Headache Society Consensus Statement: update on integrating new migraine treatments into clinical practice. Headache. 2021;61(7):1021–39.
103. Cristofori F, Thapar N, Saliakellis E, et al. Efficacy of the neurokinin-1 receptor antagonist aprepitant in children with cyclical vomiting syndrome. Aliment Pharmacol Ther. 2014;40(3):309–17.
104. Chou DE, Tso AR, Goadsby PJ. Aprepitant for the management of nausea with inpatient IV dihydroergotamine. Neurology. 2016;87(15):1613–6.
105. Friedman BW, Irizarry E, Solorzano C, et al. Randomized study of IV prochlorperazine plus diphenhydramine vs IV hydromorphone for migraine. Neurology. 2017;89(20):2075–82.
106. Orr SL, Friedman BW, Christie S, et al. Management of adults with acute migraine in the Emergency Department: the American Headache Society evidence assessment of parenteral pharmacotherapies. Headache. 2016;56(6):911–40.
107. Lee A, Kuo B. Metoclopramide in the treatment of diabetic gastroparesis. Expert Rev Endocrinol Metab. 2010;5(5):653–62.
108. Bateman DN. Clinical pharmacokinetics of metoclopramide. Clin Pharmacokinet. 1983;8(6):523–9.
109. Dolgorukova A, Osipchuk AV, Murzina AA, Sokolov AY. The influence of metoclopramide on trigeminovascular nociception: possible anti-migraine mechanism of action. Neuroscience. 2020;425:123–33.
110. Din L, Preuss CV. Prochlorperazine. In: StatPearls. Treasure Island: StatPearls Publishing; 2021.
111. Evangelista S. Role of calcitonin gene-related Peptide in gastric mucosal defence and healing. Curr Pharm Des. 2009;15(30):3571–6. https://doi.org/10.2174/138161209789207024. PMID: 19860701.
112. Alex A, Vaughn C, Rayhill M. Safety and tolerability of 3 CGRP monoclonal antibodies in practice: a retrospective cohort study. Headache. 2020;60(10):2454–62.
113. Ramsden CE, Zamora D, Faurot KR, et al. Dietary alteration of n-3 and n-6 fatty acids for headache reduction in adults with migraine: randomized controlled trial. BMJ. 2021;374:n1448.
114. Evcili G, Utku U, Ogun MN, Ozdemir G. Early and long period follow-up results of low glycemic index diet for migraine prophylaxis. Agri. 2018;30(1):8–11.
115. Bunner AE, Agarwal U, Gonzales JF, Valente F, Barnard ND. Nutrition intervention for migraine: a randomized crossover trial. J Headache Pain. 2014;15(1):69.
116. Ferrara LA, Pacioni D, Di Fronzo V, et al. Low-lipid diet reduces frequency and severity of acute migraine attacks. Nutr Metab Cardiovasc Dis. 2015;25(4):370–5.
117. Di Lorenzo C, Coppola G, Sirianni G, et al. Migraine improvement during short lasting ketogenesis: a proof-of-concept study. Eur J Neurol. 2015;22(1):170–7.
118. Putananickal N, Gross EC, Orsini AL, et al. Efficacy and safety of exogenous beta-hydroxybutyrate for preventive treatment in episodic migraine: a single-centred, randomised, placebo-controlled, double-blind crossover trial. Cephalalgia. 2021:3331024211043792.
119. Hom GL, Hom BL, Kaplan B, Rothner AD. A single institution's experience of primary headache in children with celiac disease. J Child Neurol. 2020;35(1):37–41.
120. Ameghino L, Farez MF, Wilken M, Goicochea MT. Headache in patients with celiac disease and its response to the gluten-free diet. J Oral Facial Pain Headache. 2019;33:294–300.
121. Bond DS, Vithiananthan S, Nash JM, Thomas JG, Wing RR. Improvement of migraine headaches in severely obese patients after bariatric surgery. Neurology. 2011;76(13):1135–8.
122. Novack V, Fuchs L, Lantsberg L, Kama S, Lahoud U, Horev A, et al. Changes in headache frequency in premenopausal obese women with migraine after bariatric surgery: a case series. Cephalalgia. 2011;31(13):1336–42.
123. Verrotti A, Agostinelli S, D'Egidio C, Di Fonzo A, Carotenuto M, Parisi P, et al. Impact of a weight loss program on migraine in obese adolescents. Eur J Neurol. 2013;20(2):394–7.
124. Ghorbani Z, Togha M, Rafiee P, Ahmadi ZS, Rasekh Magham R, Haghighi S, et al. Vitamin D in migraine headache: a comprehensive review on literature. Neurol Sci. 2019;40(12):2459–77.
125. Bashir M, Prietl B, Tauschmann M, Mautner SI, Kump PK, Treiber G, et al. Effects of high doses of vitamin D3 on mucosa-associated gut microbiome vary between regions of the human gastrointestinal tract. Eur J Nutr. 2016;55(4):1479–89.
126. De Roos N, Giezenaar C, Rovers J, Witteman B, Smits M, Van Hemert S. The effects of the multispecies probiotic mixture Ecologic® Barrier on migraine: results of an open-label pilot study. Benefic Microbes. 2015;6(5):641–6.
127. Sensenig J, Johnson M, Staverosky T. Treatment of migraine with targeted nutrition focused on improved assimilation and elimination. Altern Med Rev. 2001;6(5):488–94.
128. Martami F, Togha M, Seifishahpar M, Ghorbani Z, Ansari H, Karimi T, et al. The effects of a multispecies probiotic supplement on inflammatory markers and episodic and chronic migraine characteristics: a randomized double-blind controlled trial. Cephalalgia. 2019;39(7):841–53.
129. de Roos NM, van Hemert S, Rovers JMP, Smits MG, Witteman BJM. The effects of a multispecies probiotic on migraine and markers of intestinal permeability-results of a randomized placebo-controlled study. Eur J Clin Nutr. 2017;71(12):1455–62.
130. Ghavami A, Khorvash F, Heidari Z, Khalesi S, Askari G. Effect of synbiotic supplementation on migraine characteristics and inflammatory biomarkers in women with migraine: results of a randomized controlled trial. Pharmacol Res. 2021;169:105668.
131. Palsson OS, Whitehead W, Törnblom H, Sperber AD, Simren M. Prevalence of Rome IV functional bowel disorders among adults in the United States, Canada, and the United Kingdom. Gastroenterology. 2020;158(5):1262–1273.e3.
132. Lanas A, Chan FKL. Peptic ulcer disease. Lancet. 2017;390(10094):613–24.
133. Sung JJ, Kuipers EJ, El-Serag HB. Systematic review: the global incidence and prevalence of peptic ulcer disease. Aliment Pharmacol Ther. 2009;29(9):938–46.
134. Gelfand AA, Thomas KC, Goadsby PJ. Before the headache: infant colic as an early life expression of migraine. Neurology. 2012;79(13):1392–6.
135. Gelfand AA, Goadsby PJ, Allen IE. The relationship between migraine and infant colic: a systematic review and meta-analysis. Cephalalgia. 2015;35:63–72.
136. Welander NZ, Olivo G, Pisanu C, Rukh G, Schiöth HB, Mwinyi J. Migraine and gastrointestinal disorders in middle and old age: a UK Biobank study. Brain Behav. 2021;11(8):e2291.
137. Chehel Cheraghi S, Ebrahimi Daryani N, Ghabaee M. A survey on migraine prevalence in patients with inflammatory bowel disease – a single centre experience. Middle East J Dig Dis. 2016;8(4):282–8.
138. Moisset X, Bommelaer G, Boube M, et al. Migraine prevalence in inflammatory bowel disease patients: a tertiary-care centre cross-sectional study. Eur J Pain. 2017;21(9):1550–60.
139. Field T. Pediatric massage therapy research: a narrative review. Children (Basel). 2019;6(6):78.

140. Sung V, D'Amico F, Cabana M, Chau K, Koren G, Savino F, et al. *Lactobacillus reuteri* to treat infant colic: a meta-analysis. Pediatrics. 2018;141:e20171811.
141. Ong TG, Gordon M, Banks SS, Thomas MR, Akobeng AK. Probiotics to prevent infantile colic. Cochrane Database Syst Rev. 2019;3(3):CD012473.
142. Gui S, Patel N, Issenman R, et al. Acute management of pediatric cyclic vomiting syndrome: a systematic review. J Pediatr. 2019;214:158–64.
143. Venkatesan T, Levinthal DJ, Tarbell SE, et al. Guidelines on management of cyclic vomiting syndrome in adults by the American Neurogastroenterology and Motility Society and the Cyclic Vomiting Syndrome Association. Neurogastroenterol Motil. 2019;31(Suppl 2):e13604.
144. Gelfand AA. Migraine and childhood periodic syndromes in children and adolescents. Curr Opin Neurol. 2013;26:262–8.
145. Hikita T, Kodama H, Kaneko S, et al. Sumatriptan as a treatment for cyclic vomiting syndrome: a clinical trial. Cephalalgia. 2011;31:504–7.
146. Prakash C, Clouse RE. Cyclic vomiting syndrome in adults: clinical features and response to tricyclic antidepressants. Am J Gastroenterol. 1999;94:2855–9.
147. Andersen JM, Sugerman KS, Lockhart JR, Weinberg WA. Effective prophylactic therapy for cyclic vomiting syndrome in children using amitriptyline or cyproheptadine. Pediatrics. 1997;100:977–81.
148. Boles RG, Lovett-Barr MR, Preston A, Li BU, Adams K. Treatment of cyclic vomiting syndrome with co-enzyme Q10 and amitriptyline, a retrospective study. BMC Neurol. 2010;10:10.
149. Sezer O, Sezer T. A new approach to the prophylaxis of cyclic vomiting: topiramate. J Neurogastroenterol Motil. 2016;22:656–60.
150. Kothare SV. Efficacy of flunarizine in the prophylaxis of cyclical vomiting syndrome and abdominal migraine. Eur J Paediatr Neurol. 2005;9:23–6.
151. Sagar RC, Sood R, Gracie DJ, et al. Cyclic vomiting syndrome is a prevalent and under-recognized condition in the gastroenterology outpatient clinic. Neurogastroenterol Motil. 2018;30:1–7.
152. Kakisaka Y, Wakusawa K, Haginoya K, et al. Efficacy of sumatriptan in two pediatric cases with abdominal pain-related functional gastrointestinal disorders: does the mechanism overlap that of migraine? J Child Neurol. 2010;25(2):234–7.
153. Raina M, Chelimsky G, Chelimsky T. Intravenous dihydroergotamine therapy for pediatric abdominal migraines. Clin Pediatr (Phila). 2013;52(10):918–21.
154. Symon DN, Russell G. Double blind placebo controlled trial of pizotifen syrup in the treatment of abdominal migraine. Arch Dis Child. 1995;72:48–50.
155. Napthali K, Koloski N, Talley NJ. Abdominal migraine. Cephalalgia. 2016;36:980–6.
156. Törnblom H, Drossman DA. Psychopharmacologic therapies for irritable bowel syndrome. Gastroenterol Clin N Am. 2021;50(3):655–69.
157. Aydinlar EI, Dikmen PY, Tiftikci A, Saruc M, Aksu M, Gunsoy HG, et al. IgG-based elimination diet in migraine plus irritable bowel syndrome. Headache. 2013;53:514–25.
158. Savi L, Ribaldone DG, Fagoonee S, Pellicano R. Is Helicobacter pylori the infectious trigger for headache?: a review. Infect Disord Drug Targets. 2013;13(5):313–7.
159. Faraji F, Zarinfar N, Zanjani AT, Morteza A. The effect of Helicobacter pylori eradication on migraine: a randomized, double blind, controlled trial. Pain Physician. 2012;15(6):495–8.
160. Hamdeh S, Micic D, Hanauer S. Review article: drug-induced small bowel injury. Aliment Pharmacol Ther. 2021;54(11–12):1370–88.
161. Reinshagen M, Flämig G, Ernst S, et al. Calcitonin gene-related peptide mediates the protective effect of sensory nerves in a model of colonic injury. J Pharmacol Exp Ther. 1998;286(2):657–61.

16 Migraine, Dysautonomia, Ehlers-Danlos Syndrome and Post-acute Sequalae of SARS-CoV-2 infection

Svetlana Blitshteyn

Introduction

Migraine is a complex neurologic disorder associated with systemic manifestations and multiple comorbidities. In this chapter dysautonomia, hypermobility spectrum disorders (HSD)/hypermobile Ehlers-Danlos syndrome (h-EDS), and post-acute sequelae of SARS-CoV-2 (PASC) are discussed as common migraine comorbidities. The autonomic nervous system (ANS) plays an important role in the pathophysiology of migraine, and therefore, dysfunction of the ANS, which is referred to as dysautonomia, can accompany headache either via various autonomic symptoms or a defined autonomic disorder, such as postural orthostatic tachycardia syndrome (POTS), neurocardiogenic syncope (NCS), orthostatic hypotension (OH) or orthostatic intolerance (OI).

Migraine and other primary and secondary headache disorders are highly prevalent in patients with HSD/h-EDS, which is associated with dysautonomia as one of its most common comorbidities [1]. Patients with HSD/h-EDS often present with severe, chronic and sometimes treatment-refractory, headaches, autonomic disorders, gastrointestinal dysfunction and allergic conditions that require a multidisciplinary diagnostic and treatment approaches to address the numerous symptoms and manifestations of the underlying connective tissue disorder [1]. Lastly, although many people recover from the acute SARS-CoV-2 infection, a number of patients experience persistent post-COVID symptoms and conditions lasting weeks to months as part of PASC, also known as Long COVID. Headache is a common symptom of PASC and may be more prevalent in the individuals with pre-existing migraine. These systemic migraine comorbidities require special consideration to reduce misdiagnosis, diagnostic delay, disability, and optimize management.

S. Blitshteyn (✉)
Department of Neurology, University at Buffalo Jacobs School of Medicine and Biomedical Sciences, Buffalo, NY, USA

Dysautonomia Clinic, Williamsville, NY, USA

Questions

1. A 35-year-old woman presents with intractable migraine, chronic dizziness, fatigue and nausea. Her MRI of the brain is unremarkable. Which diagnostic test is most likely to result in change of management that may improve headache and other symptoms?
   A. MRI of the cervical spine
   B. Upper endoscopy
   C. EEG
   D. Tilt table test
   E. Videonystagmography
2. A 25-year-old woman with chronic migraine reports difficulty maintaining employment due to headache, fatigue, difficulty concentrating described as "brain fog," and palpitations. Which of the following medications should be initiated in this patient?
   A. Topiramate
   B. Sertraline
   C. Propranolol
   D. Amitriptyline
   E. Valproate

Dysautonomia

Dysautonomia, a term that refers to dysfunction of the ANS, encompasses a wide variety of defined autonomic disorders, with the most common being POTS, NCS (also known as vasovagal syncope), and OH. OI is used when objective tests do not confirm a diagnosis of one of the common autonomic disorders in a clinical setting of symptoms that are precipitated by an upright position and relieved by recumbency. The diagnostic criteria of POTS, NCS and OH are outlined in Table 16.1 [2, 3]. Clinical features of common autonomic disorders are numerous and typically include orthostatic

T. S. Monteith et al. (eds.), *Comprehensive Migraine Management*, https://doi.org/10.1007/978-3-031-86923-5_16

Table 16.1 Diagnostic criteria for common autonomic disorders

Autonomic disorder	Diagnostic criteria
POTS [2]	1. HR increase ≥30 bpm within 10 min for adults (≥40 bpm for adolescents 12–19 years of age) of standing or TTT 2. Absence of OH 3. Symptoms of orthostatic intolerance for ≥3 months 4. Exclusion of other causes of postural tachycardia, such as dehydration, medication side effect and other medical conditions
NCS [1]	1. Transient loss of consciousness typically preceded by prodromal symptoms and signs, such as pallor, diaphoresis, nausea, abdominal discomfort, yawning, sighing, and hyperventilation that may occur up to 60 s prior to loss of consciousness. 2. A sudden fall in blood pressure, heart rate and cerebral hypoperfusion on standing or TTT
OH [3]	Sustained drop in blood pressure ≥20/10 mmHg within 3 min of standing or TTT

POTS Postural orthostatic tachycardia syndrome, *NCS* Neurocardiogenic syncope, *OH* Orthostatic hypotension, *HR* Heart rate, *bpm* Beats per minute, *TTT* Tilt table test

Table 16.2 Clinical features of common autonomic disorders

Review of systems	Clinical features
Cardiovascular	Orthostatic intolerance Postural tachycardia Orthostatic hypotension Postprandial hypotension Exercise intolerance Syncope Presyncope Palpitations Chest pain, pressure or discomfort
Neurologic	Headache, including migraine Dizziness or lightheadedness Cognitive dysfunction (a.k.a. "brain fog") Paresthesia Generalized weakness Neuropathic pain
Respiratory	Shortness of breath Hyperventilation
Gastrointestinal	Nausea Dysphagia Acid reflux Early satiety Abdominal fullness, distension or pain Gastric and intestinal dysmotility Diarrhea or constipation
Genitourinary	Urinary frequency, urgency or hesitancy Incomplete bladder emptying Urinary retention Overactive bladder Polyuria Nocturia Interstitial cystitis Erectile dysfunction Vaginal dryness Pelvic pain
Thermoregulatory	Hypohidrosis Hyperhidrosis Anhidrosis Gustatory sweating Heat intolerance Cold intolerance
Pupillomotor	Blurred vision Light sensitivity Dilated pupils
Secretomotor	Dry eyes Dry mouth
Constitutional	Fatigue Sleep disturbance Loss of appetite Weight loss or gain Pallor Flushing Diaphoresis Myalgia

intolerance, lightheadedness/dizziness, palpitations, headache, fatigue and cognitive dysfunction (Table 16.2).

Pre-COVID-19 pandemic, an estimated 500,000 to 3 million Americans, including 1 in 100 teenagers, may have had POTS [4, 5], but the prevalence is now significantly higher due to millions of people developing post-COVID POTS as part of PASC. At least 80% of patients with POTS are women between 15 and 50 years of age, but patients younger than 12 and older than 50 are also seen in specialty clinics. Although POTS is characterized by orthostatic tachycardia and orthostatic intolerance, neurologic symptoms, such as headache, fatigue, chronic dizziness, cognitive dysfunction (aka "brain fog") and sleep disturbance, are highly prevalent in this patient population.

The pathophysiology of POTS is thought to be largely heterogeneous and traditionally classified as neuropathic, hypovolemic and hyperadrenergic [6]. Recent exploration of the etiology of POTS implicated autoimmunity as one of its major mechanisms. Patients with POTS display a higher prevalence of various non-specific autoimmune markers, including anti-nuclear antibodies, and comorbid autoimmune disorders than the general population [7]. More specifically to the autonomic nervous system, ganglionic N-type and P/Q type acetylcholine receptor antibodies, alpha 1, beta 1 and beta 2 adrenergic antibodies, muscarinic M2 and M4 antibodies, angiotensin II type 1 receptor antibodies and opioid-like 1 receptor antibodies have been identified in patients with POTS [8–13]. Many of these antibodies have been also found in patients with chronic fatigue syndrome, small fiber neuropathy, complex regional pain syndromes and cardiovascular disorders—conditions that share some clinical features with POTS.

There is an intricate relationship between migraine and ANS, which plays a major role in the pathophysiology of migraine. Besides the cranial autonomic symptoms that may accompany migraine and other primary headache disorders, patients with migraine have significant abnormalities on the autonomic function tests with evidence of sympathetic hypofunction, sympathetic overactivity and decreased parasympathetic activity [14–16]. Patients with migraine also have a higher prevalence of the autonomic symptoms, such as dizziness, vertigo, syncope and orthostatic intolerance [17–19]. Thijs et al. found a higher lifetime prevalence of syncope (41%) in patients with migraine versus healthy controls (32%) and a higher prevalence of at least 5 or more syncope and orthostatic intolerance than people without migraine [18]. Conversely, headache—migraine in particular—is the most common comorbidity in patients with autonomic disorders, such as POTS and NCS, with the prevalence ranging between 27% and 96% [12, 20, 21]. In a large survey of 4835 patients with POTS, migraine headache was the most common comorbidity affecting 40% of patients [22].

Migraine and autonomic disorders may share a number of pathophysiologic mechanisms that involve the central nervous system, specifically the central autonomic networks, that are located in the dorsal medulla, hypothalamus, and the anterior cingulate cortex [23]. Brainstem dysregulation with possible neuroinflammation at the dorsal medulla is implicated as a possible mechanism in the pathophysiology of POTS [23] while migraine similarly involves dysfunction of the brainstem [24, 25]. In study of 291 patients with migraine, frequent syncope (OR 2.7) and OI (OR 2.0) were independent risk factors for high load of deep white matter lesions seen on MRI of the brain [26]. Additionally, it was determined that individuals with OI had a higher prevalence of high periventricular white matter lesion load (OR = 1.9), but there was no increased prevalence of orthostatic hypotension or POTS in that cohort of individuals with migraine [26]. A network sensitization has been suggested in both POTS and chronic migraine in a study that found photophobia and allodynia in both disorders, but only non-trigeminal sensory sensitization was observed in POTS patients compared to chronic migraine group that displayed both trigeminal and non-trigeminal sensory sensitization [27].

One of the main underlying mechanisms in autonomic disorders, such as POTS, NCS and OI, is hypovolemia, which may be due, in part, to the disturbance of the renin-angiotensin-aldosterone system and resultant abnormalities in sodium and water retention [28]. Hypovolemia may also be involved in generation or trigger of migraine headache [29]. Interestingly, Pogoda et al. found that patients who consumed a high sodium diet, whether by coincidence, preference or perhaps by noticing a beneficial effect on their symptoms, had lower migraine frequency [30]. The most plausible explanation is that decreased sodium consumption results in decreased plasma volume, which is then sensed by the cerebral vasculature, similarly to sensing changes in the barometric pressure or low blood glucose level. This decreased plasma volume—hypovolemia—may act as a possible precipitating factor in the genesis of migraine in susceptible patients [29].

Treatment of Postural Orthostatic Tachycardia Syndrome

Therapeutic approach to POTS consists of non-pharmacologic and pharmacologic treatment options. Pharmacotherapy includes first-line medications such as beta-blockers, which decrease resting and postural tachycardia by reducing sympathetic overactivity; fludrocortisone, a mineralocorticoid that augments retention of water and sodium and expands plasma volume; midodrine hydrochloride which is an apha-1 agonist that causes vasoconstriction and increased peripheral resistance, and other commonly used medications for the orthostatic intolerance, tachycardia and fatigue, such as pyridostigmine, ivabradine, clonidine, modafinil, methylphenidate or SSRI's [31].

Studies on pharmacotherapy in patients with POTS and migraine are lacking, but beta-blockers, such as a non-selective beta blocker propranolol 5–10 mg two to four times a day, or cardioselective beta blocker atenolol 12.5–25 mg daily to twice a day, are particularly useful in patients with POTS and migraine although a low dose needed to control POTS may be suboptimal for headache prevention while higher doses of beta-blockers may not be well-tolerated in patients with POTS, who are typically sensitive to medications. In the author's experience, fludrocortisone can sometimes trigger a headache exacerbation while tricyclics, such as amitriptyline and nortriptyline, at low doses are usually well-tolerated; high doses of tricyclics are to be avoided in patients with dysautonomia due to possible worsening of orthostatic intolerance, presyncope, postural tachycardia or orthostatic hypotension.

Non-pharmacologic treatment consists of increased fluid intake of at least 2.5 L per day and salt (sodium chloride) consumption via dietary and/or supplemental sodium chloride of at 7 to 10 g daily [31]. Compression garments, such as waist-high stockings and abdominal binders, can also be effective [32]. Avoiding dehydration, heat, prolonged sitting or standing, and medications that can exacerbate orthostatic symptoms is advised. A supine or sitting exercise program, utilizing swimming, recumbent bike or a rowing machine, is encouraged.

Therapeutic intervention for patients with autonomic disorders usually begin with non-pharmacologic approach consisting of plasma volume expansion via increased water and sodium consumption, utilization of compression garments, supine and recumbent exercise and avoidance of aggravating factors [31]. However, in many patients, non-pharmacologic therapy alone may be insufficient to improve symptoms, and therefore, a medication needs to be initiated. In some patients with medication-resistant POTS or in those with severe nausea, vomiting or other gastrointestinal symptoms, intravenous saline can be used effectively on as-needed basis [33]. In the author's experience, treatment of POTS can often improve headache frequency and severity. Conversely, when chronic migraine is effectively managed with prophylactic headache therapy, symptoms of POTS also tend to improve concurrently. This clinically observed correlation between migraine and POTS response to treatment reinforces the concept of shared pathophysiology of both disorders.

Hypermobility Spectrum Disorders and Ehlers-Danlos Syndrome

At least 25% of patients with POTS have comorbid h-EDS a hereditary connective tissue disorder that manifests with join hypermobility, joint pain, easily dislocated joints, skin fragility and other systemic and neurologic manifestations [1, 22]. HSD is a group of connective tissue disorders that similarly cause joint hypermobility, instability, injury, and pain as well as many other associated symptoms and manifestations, such as fatigue, headaches, GI problems, and autonomic dysfunction. The 2017 diagnostic criteria for h-EDS requires the presence of generalized joint hypermobility, as determined by the Beighton score, and other features, such as systemic manifestations of a connective tissue disorder (Fig. 16.1), positive family history and musculoskeletal complications such as chronic pain (multiple limbs or widespread pain), or joint dislocations or instability. Patients with typical clinical features who do not qualify for a diagnosis of h-EDS by the diagnostic criteria are usually diagnosed with HSD.

Migraine with and without aura is highly prevalent in patients with HSD and h-EDS who tend to have a more severe and disabling course of migraine than patients with migraine alone [34]. A significant number of patients with migraine have joint hypermobility, and 75% of patients with joint hypermobility syndrome have migraine compared to 43% in patients without joint hypermobility syndrome (adjusted odds ratio for the prevalence of migraine in joint hypermobility syndrome is 3.19) [35]. Additionally, migraine was noted to be the most prevalent headache disorder in patients with h-EDS occurring in greater than 80% of patients with headache [36]. It's important to note that patients with HSD and h-EDS may also have a higher prevalence of secondary headache due to increased intracranial hypertension (IIH), spontaneous intracranial hypotension (SIH), Chiari type I malformation, cranio-cervical instability (CCI), temporo-mandibular joint dysfunction (TMJ), cervical disk disease and obstructive sleep apnea [37]. Vascular EDS, which can be diagnosed via genetic testing, may be associated with a high prevalence of intracranial aneurysms, spontaneous cervical arterial dissection, carotid-cavernous fistula, carotid and vertebral artery dissections and other vascular complications.

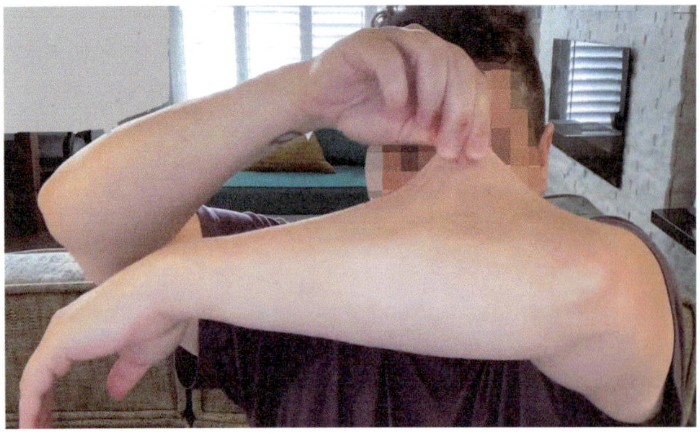

Fig. 16.1 Forty-four-year-old patient with migraine without aura, neurocardiogenic syncope, TMJ, narcolepsy, and hypermobile Ehlers-Danlos syndrome, demonstrating skin hyperextensibility

Mast cell activation syndrome (MCAS) is a complex multisystemic inflammatory disorder caused by inappropriate mast cell activation that can manifest with allergic symptoms, environmental and food intolerances, gastrointestinal symptoms and neurologic syndromes, such as migraine, dysautonomia and neuropathy [38, 39]. It was previously proposed that mast cells may be involved in the pathophysiology of migraine although confirmatory studies are lacking [40]. Clinically suspected MCAS can be sometimes difficult to confirm objectively, and diagnostic criteria continues to be debated regarding whether strict or loose diagnostic criteria should be used [39]. A triad of POTS, HSD/h-EDS and MCAS is commonly observed in clinical practice [41, 42]: treatment with antihistamines, such as loratadine, cetirizine, fexofenadine and famotidine, and mast cell stabilizing agents, such as cromolyn sodium, can improve a wide variety of mast-cell related symptoms, including headache, as observed in clinical practice. Although antihistamines are not recommended for acute and preventive migraine treatment specifically [43, 44], further studies are needed to delineate the role of mast cells and the efficacy of both inpatient and outpatient treatment with antihistamines in patients with migraine headache who are suspected to have MCAS.

Post-acute Sequalae of SARS-CoV-2

Coronavirus disease 2019 (COVID-19), caused by SARS-CoV-2 virus, is associated with various neurologic and autonomic manifestations in both hospitalized and non-hospitalized patients. While there are no uniform diagnostic criteria, the National Institutes of Health (NIH) and the Centers for Disease Control and Prevention (CDC) consider PASC to include persistent symptoms and post-COVID conditions experienced by people four or more weeks after initial coronavirus infection [45, 46]. The symptoms of PASC, which affects an estimated 10 to 35% of patients with COVID-19, a majority of whom are women, are numerous and multisystemic and can involve cardiovascular, neurologic and immunologic systems [47]. The most common symptoms of PASC include fatigue, cognitive dysfunction (aka "brain fog"), sensory disturbance and headache [48]. Although data on persistent headache characteristics attributed to COVID-19 continue to emerge, clinical observation by neurologists indicate the presence of many different headache types, some with migraine-like features [49]. Meinhardt et al. found SARS-CoV-2 proteins in trigeminal branches and the trigeminal ganglion pointing to an acquired activation of the trigeminovascular system by the SARS-CoV-2 infection [50, 51].

Multiple cases and large case series of patients presenting with new-onset ANS disorders after COVID-19 have been reported [52–57], and autonomic dysfunction appears to be one of the underlying mechanisms of PASC in general [58, 59]. In a case series of 20 patients with post-COVID POTS and other autonomic disorders, 30% had a history of intermittent autonomic symptoms, such as dizziness, syncope or palpitations, 20% had a remote history of concussion and 15% had a history of pre-existing migraine [56]. One study found that patients with a history of migraine who recovered from severe COVID-19 infection exhibited more long-term fatigue, but not headache, as post-COVID sequelae than those without migraine [60]. Another study showed that headache at the onset of acute COVID-19 infection was associated with a previous history of migraine and with the development of persistent post-COVID tension-type like headache and fatigue [61]. While studies on the pathophysiology and risk factors of PASC are ongoing, clinical experience suggests that a pre-existing history of migraine, minor autonomic symptoms, joint hypermobility and concussion, another known trigger of dysautonomia, might be possible risk factors for post-COVID autonomic disorders and PASC in general. As randomized controlled studies are not yet available to guide treatment decisions for PASC, the general approach may be to treat post-COVID headache as the primary headache it most closely resembles (e.g. migraine-like, tension-type like, etc). The choice to initiate preventive therapies can be based on overall headache frequency, severity, presence of other PASC-associated symptoms and principles of shared decision-making.

Conclusion

Common systemic migraine comorbidities include autonomic disorders, such as POTS, NCS, OH and OI, as well as HSD/h-EDS, MCAS and PASC. In clinical setting, these disorders may present a diagnostic and therapeutic challenge and require a high index of suspicion. Diagnosing and treating these comorbid disorders is necessary in order to effectively manage headache and reduce the symptom burden caused by these comorbidities. To this end, clinical trials are needed to determine the role of multidisciplinary care and various evidence-based acute and preventive migraine treatments in the setting of these systemic migraine comorbidities. Given the public health urgency associated with PASC, dedicated clinical investigations will also be needed to determine the best practices for management of headache and other clinical features of his highly prevalent and disabling condition.

Teaching Points

1. Common autonomic disorders, such as POTS, NCS, OH and OI, are comorbid with migraine and need to be diagnosed and treated.
2. In a patient with migraine and dizziness, palpitations, presyncope or syncope, a 10-minute stand test or a tilt table test should be obtained in order to assess for an autonomic disorder.
3. Treatment of dysautonomia with non-pharmacologic and pharmacologic therapies targeted to expand plasma volume, improve venous return and decrease sympathetic overactivity, should be implemented. Beta-blockers, such as a low dose of propranolol or atenolol, may be appropriate for treatment of migraine and autonomic symptoms.
4. Due to high prevalence of migraine and secondary headache disorders, HSD/h-EDS and should be considered in patients presenting with headache and generalized joint hypermobility, musculoskeletal complaints, systemic connective tissue manifestations or a positive family history of HSD/h-EDS.
5. Headache is one of the most common manifestations of PASC, and pre-existing migraine may be a possible risk factor for persistent headache and fatigue following an acute SARS-CoV-2 infection.

Case

A 30-year-old previously healthy woman with a history of episodic migraine without aura occurring approximately 4 times per year has been experiencing migraine twice a week in addition to severe fatigue, difficulty concentrating described as "brain fog," exercise intolerance and difficulty standing due to dizziness and palpitations for the past 6 months. She developed these symptoms after a mild COVID-19 infection. She does not take any medications and denies alcohol, tobacco and caffeine use. On exam, her supine heart rate is 92 beats per minute which increased to 125 beats per minute after standing quietly for 5 minutes without orthostatic hypotension. The patient complained of feeling dizzy while standing. The rest of the neurologic exam was unremarkable. Diagnostic investigations consisted of an unrevealing MRI of the brain without contrast, unremarkable 2D cardiac echocardiography, and a Holter monitor demonstrating an average heart rate of 82 bpm, with episodes of sinus tachycardia up to 160 beats per minute corresponding to the patient's recorded symptoms of dizziness and palpitations.

Case Discussion

In addition to exacerbation of pre-existing migraine headache, the patient has evidence of POTS as demonstrated by a greater than 30 beats per minute heart rate elevation from supine to standing position, stable blood pressure and symptoms of presyncope on a stand test. Both POTS and migraine can occur as part of PASC following COVID-19 infection. The treatment plan should include non-pharmacologic therapy for POTS, such as increased fluids intake of 2.5–3 L per day, sodium chloride intake of at least 7 g of salt (sodium chloride) per day with a combination of dietary salt and salt tablets, waist-high compression stockings and abdominal binders, and a supine or sitting exercise program using recumbent bike, rowing machine, floor exercise or swimming. If non-pharmacologic treatment is insufficient, which is often the case, first-line medication treatment options for POTS should be utilized, such as a low dose of a beta blocker (e.g. propranolol 5-10 mg twice a day as the starting dose). Alternatively, midodrine hydrochloride 2.5–5 mg three times a day can be tried. Additional pharmacotherapy may be used for migraine and POTS as necessary.

Questions and Answers

1. A 35-year-old woman presents with intractable migraine, chronic dizziness, fatigue and nausea. Her MRI of the brain is unremarkable. Which diagnostic test is most likely to result in change of management that may improve headache and other symptoms?
   A. MRI of the cervical spine
   B. Upper endoscopy
   C. EEG
   D. Tilt table test
   E. Videonystagmography

The correct answer is D. The tilt table test in a patient with migraine, dizziness, fatigue and chronic nausea may reveal a disorder of the autonomic nervous system, such as POTS, that has a different therapeutic approach from the one utilized for migraine headache alone. Diagnosing and treating POTS leads to improved symptoms, including headache, which is the most common comorbidity of POTS.

2. A 25-year-old woman with chronic migraine reports difficulty maintaining employment due to headache, fatigue, difficulty concentrating described as "brain fog," and palpitations. Which of the following medications should be initiated in this patient?
   A. Topiramate
   B. Sertraline
   C. Propranolol
   D. Amitriptyline
   E. Valproate

The correct answer is C. In this patient with chronic migraine and other symptoms, including palpitations, suspicion for an autonomic disorder is high. A beta blocker, such as propranolol, is a good choice of treatment for migraine and autonomic symptoms.

References

1. Brooks RS, Grady J, Lowder TW, Blitshteyn S. Prevalence of gastrointestinal, cardiovascular, autonomic and allergic manifestations in hospitalized patients with Ehlers-Danlos syndrome: a case-control study. Rheumatology (Oxford). 2021;60:4272–80.
2. Sheldon RS, Grubb BP II, Olshansky B, et al. Heart Rhythm Society expert consensus statement on the diagnosis and treatment of postural tachycardia syndrome, inappropriate sinus tachycardia, and vasovagal syncope. Heart Rhythm. 2015;2015(12):e41–63.
3. Freeman R, Weiling W, Axelrod F, et al. Consensus statement on the definition of orthostatic hypotension, neurally mediated syncope and the postural tachycardia syndrome. Clin Auton Res. 2011;21:69–72.
4. Robertson D. The epidemic of orthostatic tachycardia and orthostatic intolerance. Am J Med Sci. 1999;317:75–7.

5. Kizilbash SJ, Ahrens SP, Bruce BK, et al. Adolescent fatigue, POTS, and recovery: a guide for clinicians. Curr Probl Pediatr Adolesc Health Care. 2014;44:108–33.
6. Low PA, Sandroni P, Joyner M, et al. Postural tachycardia syndrome (POTS). J Cardiovasc Electrophysiol. 2009;20:352–8.
7. Blitshteyn S. Autoimmune markers and autoimmune disorders in patients with postural tachycardia syndrome (POTS). Lupus. 2015;24:1364–9.
8. Kharraziha I, Axelsson J, Ricci F, et al. Serum activity against G protein-coupled receptors and severity of orthostatic symptoms in postural orthostatic tachycardia syndrome. J Am Heart Assoc. 2020;9:e015989.
9. Gunning WT 3rd, Kvale H, Kramer PM, et al. Postural orthostatic tachycardia syndrome is associated with elevated G-protein coupled receptor autoantibodies. J Am Heart Assoc. 2019;8:e013602.
10. Watari M, Nakane S, Mukaino A, et al. Autoimmune postural orthostatic tachycardia syndrome. Ann Clin Transl Neurol. 2018;5:486–92.
11. Yu X, Li H, Murphy TA, Nuss Z, et al. Angiotensin II type 1 receptor autoantibodies in postural tachycardia syndrome. J Am Heart Assoc. 2018;7:e008351.
12. Thieben MJ, Sandroni P, Sletten DM, et al. Postural orthostatic tachycardia syndrome: the Mayo Clinic experience. Mayo Clin Proc. 2007;82:308–13.
13. Li H, Yu X, Liles C, et al. Autoimmune basis for postural tachycardia syndrome. J Am Heart Assoc. 2014;3:e000755.
14. Peroutka SJ. Migraine: a chronic sympathetic nervous system disorder. Headache. 2004;44:53–64.
15. Shechter A, Stewart WF, Silberstein SD, Lipton RB. Migraine and autonomic nervous system function: a population-based, case-control study. Neurology. 2002;58:422–7.
16. Gass JJ, Glaros AG. Autonomic dysregulation in headache patients. Appl Psychophysiol Biofeedback. 2013;38:257–63.
17. Vuković V, Plavec D, Galinović I, et al. Prevalence of vertigo, dizziness, and migrainous vertigo in patients with migraine. Headache. 2007;47:1427–35.
18. Thijs RD, Kruit MC, van Buchem MA, et al. Syncope in migraine: the population-based CAMERA study. Neurology. 2006;66:1034–7.
19. Blitshteyn S, Cheshire WP Jr. Syncope in migraine: the population-based CAMERA study. Neurology. 2007;68:878.
20. Ulas UH, Chelimsky TC, Chelimsky G, et al. Comorbid health conditions in women with syncope. Clin Auton Res. 2010;20:223–7.
21. Khurana RK, Eisenberg L. Orthostatic and non-orthostatic headache in postural tachycardia syndrome. Cephalalgia. 2011;31:409–15.
22. Shaw BH, Stiles LE, Bourne K, et al. The face of postural tachycardia syndrome – insights from a large cross-sectional online community-based survey. J Intern Med. 2019;286:438–48.
23. Blitshteyn S. Is postural orthostatic tachycardia syndrome (POTS) a central nervous system disorder? J Neurol. 2022;269:725–32. https://doi.org/10.1007/s00415-021-10502-z.
24. Goadsby PJ, Holland PR, Martins-Oliveira M, et al. Pathophysiology of migraine: a disorder of sensory processing. Physiol Rev. 2017;97:553–622.
25. Akerman S, Holland P, Goadsby P. Diencephalic and brainstem mechanisms in migraine. Nat Rev Neurosci. 2011;12:570–84.
26. Kruit MC, Thijs RD, Ferrari MD, et al. Syncope and orthostatic intolerance increase risk of brain lesions in migraineurs and controls. Neurology. 2013;80:1958–65.
27. Cortez MM, Millsap L, Brennan KC. Synergistic but separable sensory changes in postural tachycardia syndrome and chronic migraine. Clin Auton Res. 2021;31:263–71.
28. Raj SR. Postural tachycardia syndrome (POTS). Circulation. 2013;127:2336–42.
29. Blitshteyn S. Dietary sodium intake and migraine: is salt the answer? Headache. 2016;56:1210–1.
30. Pogoda JM, Gross NB, Arakaki X, et al. Severe headache or migraine history is inversely correlated with dietary sodium intake: NHANES 1999-2004. Headache. 2016;56:688–98.
31. Del Pozzi AT, Enechukwu M, Blitshteyn S. Postural orthostatic tachycardia syndrome in primary care: diagnosis, treatment and a case of African-American man presenting with POTS. BMJ Case Rep. 2019;12:e229824.
32. Bourne KM, Sheldon RS, Hall J, et al. Compression garment reduces orthostatic tachycardia and symptoms in patients with postural orthostatic tachycardia syndrome. J Am Coll Cardiol. 2021;77:285–96.
33. Ruzieh M, Baugh A, Dasa O, et al. Effects of intermittent intravenous saline infusions in patients with medication-refractory postural tachycardia syndrome. J Interv Card Electrophysiol. 2017;48:255–60.
34. Puledda F, Viganò A, Celletti C, et al. A study of migraine characteristics in joint hypermobility syndrome a.k.a. Ehlers-Danlos syndrome, hypermobility type. Neurol Sci. 2015;36:1417–24.
35. Bendik EM, Tinkle BT, Al-shuik E, et al. Joint hypermobility syndrome: a common clinical disorder associated with migraine in women. Cephalalgia. 2011;31:603–13.
36. Malhtra A, Pace A, Maya T, et al. Headache in hypermobility syndrome: a pain in the neck? Am J Med Genet. 2020;182:2902–8.
37. Henderson FC, Austin C, Benzel E, et al. Neurological and spinal manifestations of the Ehlers–Danlos syndromes. Am J Med Genet Part C Semin Med Genet. 2017;175C:195–211.
38. Afrin LB, Self S, Menk J, Lazarchick J. Characterization of mast cell activation syndrome. Am J Med Sci. 2017;353:207–15.
39. Afrin LB, Ackerley MB, Bluestein LS, et al. Diagnosis of mast cell activation syndrome: a global "consensus-2". Diagnosis (Berlin). 2020;8:137–52.
40. Baun M, Pedersen MH, Olesen J, et al. Dural mast cell degranulation is a putative mechanism for headache induced by PACAP-38. Cephalalgia. 2012;32:337–45.
41. Wang E, Ganti T, Vaou E, Hohler A. The relationship between mast cell activation syndrome, postural tachycardia syndrome, and Ehlers-Danlos syndrome. Allergy Asthma Proc. 2021;42:243–6.
42. Kohno R, Cannom DS, Olshansky B, et al. Mast cell activation disorder and postural orthostatic tachycardia syndrome: a clinical association. J Am Heart Assoc. 2021;10:e021002.
43. Loder E, Burch R, Rizzoli P. The 2012 AHS/AAN guidelines for prevention of episodic migraine: a summary and comparison with other recent clinical practice guidelines. Headache. 2012;52:930–45.
44. Marmura MJ, Silberstein SD, Schwedt TJ. The acute treatment of migraine in adults: the American Headache Society evidence assessment of migraine pharmacotherapies. Headache. 2015;55:3–20.
45. Collins FS. NIH launches new initiative to study "Long COVID". National Institutes of Health. 2021. https://www.nih.gov/about-nih/who-we-are/nih-director/statements/nih-launches-new-initiative-study-long-covid. Accessed 30 Mar 2021.
46. The Center for Disease Control. Evaluating and caring for patients with post-COVID conditions: interim guidance. 2021. https://www.cdc.gov/coronavirus/2019-ncov/hcp/clinical-care/post-covid-background.html
47. Rubin R. As their numbers grow, COVID-19 "long haulers" stump experts. JAMA. 2020;324:1381–3.
48. Salmon-Ceron D, Slama D, De Broucker T, et al. APHP COVID-19 research collaboration. Clinical, virological and imaging profile in patients with prolonged forms of COVID-19: a cross-sectional study. J Infect. 2021;82:e1–4.
49. Caronna E, Alpuente A, Torres-Ferrus M, Pozo-Rosich P. Toward a better understanding of persistent headache after mild COVID-19: three migraine-like yet distinct scenarios. Headache. 2021;61:1277–80.

50. Meinhardt J, Radke J, Dittmayer C, et al. Olfactory transmucosal SARS-CoV-2 invasion as a port of central nervous system entry in individuals with COVID-19. Nat Neurosci. 2021;24:168–75.
51. Caronna E, Ballvé A, Llauradó A, et al. Headache: a striking prodromal and persistent symptom, predictive of COVID-19 clinical evolution. Cephalalgia. 2020;40:1410–21.
52. Dani M, Dirksen A, Taraborrelli P, et al. Autonomic dysfunction in 'long covid': rationale, physiology and management strategies. Clin Med (Lond). 2021;21:e63–7. https://doi.org/10.7861/clinmed.2020-0896.
53. Novak P. Post COVID-19 syndrome associated with orthostatic cerebral hypoperfusion syndrome, small fiber neuropathy and benefit of immunotherapy: a case report. eNeurologicalSci. 2020;21:100276. https://doi.org/10.1016/j.ensci.2020.100276.
54. Miglis MG, Prieto T, Shaik R, Muppidi S, Sinn D, Jaradeh S. A case report of postural orthostatic tachycardia syndrome after COVID-19. Clin Auton Res. 2020;30:449–51. https://doi.org/10.1007/s10286-020-00727-9.
55. Kanjwal K, Jamal S, Kichloo A, Grubb BP. New-onset postural orthostatic tachycardia syndrome following coronavirus disease 2019 infection. J Innov Card Rhythm Manag. 2020;11:4302–4. https://doi.org/10.19102/icrm.2020.111102.
56. Blitshteyn S, Whitelaw S. Postural orthostatic tachycardia syndrome (POTS) and other autonomic disorders after COVID-19 infection: a case series of 20 patients. Immunol Res. 2021;69:205–11.
57. Shouman K, Vanichkachorn G, Cheshire WP, et al. Autonomic dysfunction following COVID-19 infection: an early experience. Clin Auton Res. 2021;31:385–94.
58. Radin JM, Quer G, Ramos E, et al. Assessment of prolonged physiological and behavioral changes associated with COVID-19 infection. JAMA Netw Open. 2021;4:e2115959.
59. Stute NL, Stickford JL, Province VM, et al. COVID-19 is getting on our nerves: sympathetic neural activity and haemodynamics in young adults recovering from SARS-CoV-2. J Physiol. 2021;599:4269–85.
60. Fernández-de-Las-Peñas C, Gómez-Mayordomo V, García-Azorín D, et al. Previous history of migraine is associated with fatigue, but not headache, as long-term post-COVID symptom after severe acute respiratory SARS-CoV-2 infection: a case-control study. Front Hum Neurosci. 2021;15:678472.
61. Fernández-de-Las-Peñas C, Gómez-Mayordomo V, Cuadrado ML, et al. The presence of headache at onset in SARS-CoV-2 infection is associated with long-term post-COVID headache and fatigue: a case-control study. Cephalalgia. 2021;41:1332–41.

Part IV

Lifestyle Modification, Trigger Management, and Integrative Medicine

Migraine and the Workplace

17

Olivia Begasse de Dhaem, Nim Lalvani, David Dodick, and Christine Lay

Introduction

Worldwide, migraine is the leading cause of disability in adults under age 50 years and the second leading cause of disability at all other ages [1, 2]. Migraine peaks during people's most productive years, which impacts their career and work decisions [3, 4]. In a qualitative survey of 81 participants with migraine on acute and/or preventive treatment, 90% of participants reported that migraine negatively impacted their lives [5]. Several domains of life were affected including work, cognitive function, and emotional health [5]. Around the globe, approximately one in four persons with migraine have moderate to severe disability ranging from 12% in Europe and 19% in Asia to up to 32.3% in North America and 22% in South America [6–9].

O. B. de Dhaem (✉)
Department of Neurology, University of Connecticut, Farmington, CT, USA

Institute for Headache and Brain Health, Greenwich, CT, USA

N. Lalvani
American Migraine Foundation, Mount Royal, NJ, USA

D. Dodick
Department of Neurology (Emeritus), Mayo Clinic, Phoenix, AZ, USA

C. Lay
Department of Neurology, University of Toronto, Toronto, ON, Canada

Questions

1. What is the proportion of migraine-related productivity loss at work related to presenteeism?
   A. 22%
   B. 57%
   C. 72%
   D. 89%
2. Migraine workplace education programs increase productivity via:
   A. Reducing absenteeism
   B. Decreasing stigma
   C. Increasing productivity at work
   D. All of the above

Factors Contributing to Migraine-Related Work Loss Productivity

Migraine-related disability is complex and multifactorial. It may present with difficulties in terms of problem-solving skills, speaking, driving, and ability to perform all expected work functions [10]. Factors that contribute to migraine-related disability include pain severity, migraine symptoms, unpredictability of attacks, emotional impact, maladaptive headache cognitions, comorbidities, lack of diagnosis and undermanagement, and stigma.

Not knowing when the next disabling attack will come is anxiety-provoking as it makes it virtually impossible to reliably plan work tasks. Because of fear of a potential next attack and the feeling of helplessness at preventing it, people may avoid work meetings and outings. It is a vicious cycle as social withdrawal may contribute to more severe symptoms [11]. In a qualitative survey of 81 participants with migraine, 52% reported a negative impact on their emotional health due to isolation, anxiety, frustration/anger, guilt, mood changes/irritability, and depression/hopelessness [5]. In addition to the physical inability to attend social events due

T. S. Monteith et al. (eds.), *Comprehensive Migraine Management*, https://doi.org/10.1007/978-3-031-86923-5_17

to migraine symptoms or fear of an attack, migraine is also isolating in the sense that it is difficult to feel understood by others [5]. Pain catastrophizing is also associated with migraine-related disability independently of migraine characteristics [12, 13].

Migraine comorbidities including depression, anxiety, and sleep disorders are independently associated with work absenteeism and presenteeism and increased disability [14–20]. In a survey study of 90 patients with migraine, every 5-point increase on the depressive symptom questionnaire (PHQ-9) and 4-point increase on the anxiety symptom questionnaire (GAD-7) was associated with over 3.5-fold increased odds of severe migraine-related disability [13]. Depressive and/or anxiety symptoms can be associated with increased migraine-related disability without meeting clinical threshold for major depressive disorder or generalized anxiety disorder [13].

Migraine remains largely underdiagnosed in the workplace. In a survey of 522 workers from 8 information technology companies in Korea, 74.7% of participants with migraine never consulted a physician for migraine [6]. In a survey of 2458 workers at an information technology firm in Japan, 72% of participants with migraine never consulted a doctor for migraine [11]. While 57% of participants with migraine never sought medical attention because they believed their migraine was not severe enough, 65% thought they could not manage their headaches by themselves [11]. Unfortunately, but not unexpectedly, underdiagnosis leads to undertreatment [21].

Stigma and Interactions Within the Workplace

People with migraine experience stigma at different levels in different settings. External stigma stems from interactions with colleagues, family, friends, healthcare providers; from institutions such as health insurance agencies and media; from our language—the word "headache" itself has a negative connotation [22, 23]. External stigma leads to discrimination, loss of status, loss of relationships and prejudice [24]. Stigma can be internalized and lead to anxiety, fear, guilt, or shame regarding one's disease and even to presenteeism and reduced pay [22, 25]. There is more stigma against chronic migraine than other neurological diseases such as epilepsy, stroke, multiple sclerosis and Parkinson's disease [26, 27]. Despite the significant disability of migraine, it is still viewed as an excuse. Based on a survey of almost 200,000 U.S. workers, only 22% of employers thought that migraine was a serious enough condition to warrant staying home from work [28]. In a web-based survey of a representative US sample of 2000 participants without migraine, 45.4% of participants who knew at least one person with migraine thought that migraine was easily treated, 32.4% answered that people with migraine exaggerated their symptoms, 35.5% thought that someone's migraine attacks were caused by their own unhealthy behavior(s), 39.1% thought that people with migraine hid their disease, 29% thought that people with migraine made things difficult for their coworkers and 31.1% thought that people use migraine as an excuse to get out of school or work commitments [29]. These answers were similar whether the participants knew coworkers, friends, family members or a combination of those with migraine [29].

Stigma correlates with the ability to work [24, 30]. In a study of 123 patients with episodic migraine, 123 patients with chronic migraine, and 62 patients with epilepsy, chronic migraine was associated with worse stigma scores on chronic illness compared to episodic migraine and epilepsy [24]. Internalized stigma was stronger for people with migraine compared to epilepsy and correlated with inability to work [24].

Personal Impact

The negative impact of migraine on people's productivity at work leads to significant personal consequences. Workers with migraine may be demoted or choose a job with lower pay and/or status due to the migraine-related limitations on their ability to work as productively as they would like [5]. For example, one of the study participants explained that she had to turn down a job that paid $15,000 more a year because it required her to travel to Europe and China. Long travels triggered very disabling migraine attacks that forced her to rest in the dark in the hotel room for a day afterwards [5]. In the Migraine in the Workplace Survey promoted on the social media of the Migraine Association of Ireland in July and August 2021, 22% of the 400 respondents had to change their profession due to migraine. In the US, only 37% of people with chronic migraine are employed full-time [31]. The disability of and stigma against migraine interfere with the ability of people with migraine to reach their full occupational potential and hence lead to a lower socioeconomic status. A lower socioeconomic status may be associated with more life stressors, less medical care, and worse migraine [32, 33].

Migraine is also associated with a lack of understanding by colleagues, impaired work relationships with colleagues, feelings of guilt for burdening colleagues and supervisor, low energy, and difficulty with concentration [34], [6]. In the Migraine in the Workplace Survey promoted on the social media of the Migraine Association of Ireland, when participants were asked what would be one change in their workplace that they felt would help them, the most common answer (30% of respondents) was awareness and understanding of their colleagues that migraine is not just a headache.

Economic Impact

Migraine-related productivity loss is costly to employers [35, 36]. Using data from 1999 and 2010 respectively, its annual cost to employers was estimated at $13 billion in the USA and €27 billion in Europe [37, 38]. Given inflation over time, these are now underestimations. Using more recent data from a case study at a Japanese information technology company, migraine is estimated to impair the work of 1 in 5 employees. Taking the company's 150,000 employees into account, this would be an estimated annual cost of $350 million [39].

The significant economic impact of migraine at work can sometimes be difficult to recognize and measure given that 89% of migraine-related productivity loss is due to presenteeism, i.e. coming to work during a migraine attack and pushing through without being able to be as productive as usual due to migraine symptoms [40]. Although workers with migraine have absences and have more short-term disability claims than those without migraine, presenteeism is estimated to cost employers three to ten times more than absences [40–42]. To date, there are still no standardized methods to measure presenteeism [36]. On average, people report being 46% effective when working during a migraine attack [43]. In a four-year-long study of 7959 employees at a large US health care system across six locations that assessed the prevalence and impact of 22 common health conditions, migraine was the second most costly condition in terms of presenteeism costing more than $2 million annually, after allergies [44]. From those results, it is estimated that migraine represents 16% of US workforce presenteeism with an estimated annual cost of $240 billion [44]. In a survey of 522 workers from 8 information technology companies in Korea, migraine prevalence was 18.2% and the estimated annual economic cost of migraine-related absenteeism and presenteeism per employee were $197.5 ± 686.1 and $837.7 ± 22.04 (mean ± standard deviation) respectively [6]. Those estimates were calculated from a modified Migraine Disability Assessment (MIDAS) questionnaire and the average daily wage in the information technology industry in Korea [6]. Based on the results of an online survey of 3624 active workers from different companies in Portugal, the estimated annual economic cost of migraine-related absenteeism and presenteeism per employee were $54.05 and $685.73 respectively [21]. Based on results of a survey of 2458 workers at an information technology company in Japan with a migraine prevalence of 17% and national statistics, it is estimated that the annual cost of presenteeism in Japan was estimated between $3.3 billion using MIDAS data for the estimation and $21.3 billion using Work Productivity and Activity Impairment data for the estimation [34].

The degree of disability and lost productive time correlates with increasing headache frequency, but there is no clear-cut separation in terms of disability and productivity loss between the current headache frequency criteria for episodic versus chronic migraine. Among the 5997 American Migraine Prevalence and Prevention study participants, the 29% with more than 10 headache days per month accounted for 49% of overall lost productive time [42]. In a study of 5916 employees at a car manufacturing factory in Turkey, workers with 10–14 headache days per month had on average 2 absences and 46 days with migraine-related impaired productivity per year compared to 3.5 days of absences and 87 days with decreased productivity for those with at least 15 days of headache per month [45]. Among the 836 American Registry for Migraine Research participants, there were no difference in terms of Work Productivity and Activity Impairment and Pain Interference scores between the group with 8–14 headache days per month compared to the group with 15–23 headache days per month [46]. However, the later had higher Migraine Disability Assessment Scale (MIDAS) scores [46].

Workplace Interventions

Migraine Education Programs at Work

As shown by six prospective cohort studies in the USA, migraine education programs in the workplace increase productivity by 29 to 36% in several ways. Such programs decrease absences by about 25%, decrease the number of days worked with a migraine attack by about 32%, increase productivity at work during a migraine attack by about 10%, and decrease stigma [35, 36, 47]. The type of education media varied from disease management program with phone access to a Nurse call-in line or virtual coaching, newsletters, computer-based modules, webinars, and lunch educational programs (led by a Neurologist, Psychologist, and Nurse). Migraine education programs have been shown to improve migraine diagnosis and treatment [48]. Without migraine education programs to raise awareness on migraine to all the employees including those without migraine, there is a significant burden on people with migraine to do the "migraine talk" and educate others on their disease [49].

Several programs exist currently to raise awareness, educate, and support people with migraine in the workplace including the Global Patient Advocacy Coalition (GPAC) Migraine Fitness at Work, Migraine at Work from the World Health Education Foundation, Migraine in the workplace from the Migraine Trust, and Migraine Friendly Workplace from the European Migraine & Headache Alliance. These programs can be a resource for employees, employers, and healthcare professionals.

Migraine Education and Management Programs at Work

As shown by six prospective cohort studies (two in the United States, one in Spain, one in Switzerland, one in France, and one in Japan), migraine education and management programs in the workplace improve productivity [36, 50]. Such programs decrease absences by 50 to 53%, increase productivity at work during a migraine attack by about 36 to 59%, and decrease the costs of migraine-related productivity loss [35, 50]. In general, the migraine education and management programs consist of three main steps: (1) company-wide education to raise migraine awareness, (2) voluntary and anonymous migraine evaluation for all interested employees, and (3) optional migraine management programs made available to employees diagnosed with migraine [35]. The investment required for migraine management programs in the workplace is widely variable as it depends on the local health care system, the way the medical evaluation and management is set up (e.g., using national healthcare services, virtual Nurse coaching, management through the company occupational health services, and referral to outside Physicians who work for the company) [35]. The Spanish Postal Service mailed a voluntary health survey to all its employees [51]. Those who screened positive for migraine were invited to the occupational health services for an evaluation and migraine management by a physician [51]. The migraine education and management program in the Spanish Postal Service reduced absences by 53%, increased productivity on days worked with migraine attack from 59% to 94.8%, which reduced the costs of migraine-related productivity loss from $38.96 down to $5.19 per migraine per employee (an almost 90% decrease) [51]. A Swiss pharmaceutical company launched a migraine awareness and management program in the workplace that started with company-wide emails, info booths, lectures, newsletters, brochures [50]. Employees were then invited to be anonymously and voluntarily evaluated for migraine via a teleneurology consult [50]. Those who were found to have migraine were offered treatment and virtual coaching sessions for 6 months [50]. The program cost about $1000 to the employer per participant for 6 months [50]. About half of the participants fully completed the program [50]. This program decreased absences by nearly 50% and increased productivity on migraine days at work (a reduction from 3.9 to 1.6 days per month with at least 50% reduced productivity at work due to migraine), which led to a total productivity benefit of 10.8 more workdays per year per employee, an almost 5 times positive return on investment [50]. The largest workplace headache education and management program to date was done in Japan. The Fujitsu Headache Project education modules were offered to all Fujitsu employees based in Japan and mandatory for supervisors [49]. The education modules created in partnership with the Global Patient Advocacy Coalition (GPAC) had a high participation rate: 73,432 (91%) employees completed the education program [49]. Participants were satisfied with the program: 61% found it to be useful and 30% found it to be very useful [49]. Most importantly, as a result of their participation in the education modules, 83% of employees without headache said they would change their attitude toward colleagues with headache disorders [49]. The Fujitsu Headache Project also offered consultations with a headache specialist for the employees who were interested [49]. 2971 (4%) employees sought headache consultation through program [49]. The program increased productivity for employees with moderate to severe headache by cutting down absences by 1.2 days per employee per year and cutting down days of presenteeism by 14 days per employee per year, which represented a 32-fold positive return on investment [49].

In addition, disclosing migraine to a supervisor can be difficult given the stigma associated with migraine [28]. Hence, migraine education and management programs in the workplace can help workers with migraine access treatment and resources without necessarily needing to disclose their migraine to their supervisor or coworkers [36].

Adaptations to the Work Environment and Demands

Adaptations to the culture and set-up of the workplace, quantitative, emotional, and social work demands may help [36]. Job satisfaction, social support (especially from supervisor), good work atmosphere, and sense of autonomy are positively associated with productivity and dedication and negatively associated with burnout [36]. Adaptations to the work environment such as natural lights, noise reduction, scent-free areas, access to water and restroom, regular breaks, air quality were also positively associated with productivity [36]. High quantitative work demands such as high workload, long work hours, inflexible schedule were negatively associated with productivity [36]. Night shift is also associated with lower migraine-related productivity and higher migraine frequency [52, 53]. Regarding social demands at work, a survey of 108 participants followed at a Headache Center in Serbia showed a positive association between MIDAS score and regular contact with at least 10 other people at work [54].

Table 17.1 Components of a migraine-friendly workplace

Education	Management	Work environment
• Education of the entire workforce regardless of headache status to raise awareness, increase understanding, break down stigma • Top-down approach with a lot of touch points over a continuous period of time	• Inclusion of migraine medications (that reduces disability) and efforts to reduce step therapy burden for self-insured employers and employers negotiating with commercial insurance • Migraine toolbox with acute treatment options with the least potential to disrupt function at work	• Supportive environment limiting unnecessary stress and work conflict, addressing stigma, increasing understanding • Scent-free, quiet areas, emphasis on natural light, proper ergonomics • Promotion of employees' autonomy and job satisfaction • Work accommodations (according to the ADA), such as flexible schedule, reduction in social demands on migraine days, avoidance of shift work/irregular schedule • Use of FMLA as needed

Clinical Practice Considerations

Asking patients open-ended questions about how migraine impacts their professional lives guides clinical management [5]. It leads to treatment optimization, more aggressive follow-up, better outcomes, and better satisfaction for both providers and patients [5]. For example, providers can start by asking:

- "If you didn't have migraine, how would your life be different?" [55]
- "How does migraine impact your life?" [5].

It is important for providers to understand patients' expectations of their current visit and their headache treatment, the professional/social/personal limitations and disability caused by migraine, the goals they want to achieve, the roadblocks, and what is important for them. As discussed above, migraine can come with internalized stigma and a feeling of guilt. During the visit, providers can acknowledge how difficult the situation can be for their patients, provide words of support, and emphasize how prevalent and disabling migraine is. They are not alone (Table 17.1).

Patients may need different acute treatment plans for different situations. While some therapies are effective and well tolerated, for some individuals, acute treatments may come with side effects that interfere with patients' ability to work. For example, lasmiditan and some triptans can be very helpful to treat an attack at home when patients can rest. Options with fewer side effects may be preferable in the workplace such as a different triptan, oral diclofenac, a combination of acetaminophen/aspirin/caffeine, a gepant, or a device such as remote electrical neuromodulation, non-invasive vagus nerve stimulation, single-pulse transcranial magnetic stimulation, or transcutaneous electrical nerve stimulation of the trigeminal and occipital nerves. In addition to acute treatment, preventive options should be considered when migraine attacks are frequent and/or disabling. Frequent use of acute treatment $\geq$15 days/month of acetaminophen and/or NSAIDs or $\geq$10 days/month of triptans, ergots, ditans, opioids, butalbital medications) can lead to medication overuse headache. Gepants are the only acute drug class that has been shown to reduce headache frequency when used daily and preclinical evidence supports its lack of propensity to lead to MOH.

It is important to ensure treatment optimization in terms of migraine and its comorbidities (depression, anxiety, sleep disorders, attention deficit hyperactivity disorder, vestibular disorders, etc.). Optimization of care can go a long way in improving migraine and significantly reducing the disability of migraine. Much can be done for our patients. Screening measures such as GAD-7, PHQ-9, and Insomnia Severity Index (ISI) forms can be easily completed prior to the visit. Providers must assess for new symptoms, red flags, medication side effects, and new or worsening medical comorbidities. It is always good to also screen for safety at home and work, trauma or history of abuse. There may also be social-environmental stressors for which social workers can provide support. It is helpful for providers to surround themselves with a multidisciplinary team of physical and occupational therapists, social workers, occupational specialists, and advocacy organizations. Psychologists can provide training on cognitive behavioral therapy and mindfulness to help patients develop healthy pain-coping mechanisms [56–58].

According to the Americans with Disabilities Act (ADA) and its 2008 amendment, it is important to know that migraine is a disability and people with migraine have the right to reasonable accommodations in the workplace, i.e. adaptations to help them perform their essential job functions despite the limitations due to their migraine attacks [59, 60]. Both employers and employees may need to work on job adaptations such as a flexible schedule, the ability to work from home when possible, a scent-free environment, optimization of desk ergonomics, or wearing light sensitivity glasses, for example [60–62]. There are publicly available online state regulations regarding the meal and rest breaks workers are entitled to have [63]. Providers can ensure patients know their rights and offer to provide medical information and letters to support their request for reasonable accommodations at work. If medical and comorbidities optimization and reasonable accommodations are not enough, a potential next step is the Family and Medical Leave Act (FMLA) which provides up to 12 weeks of job-protected, unpaid leave during any 12-month period for people with migraine currently employed by companies of at least 50 employees [60]. The unpaid time off does not have to be taken consecutively. Days off can be taken intermittently as needed [60].

Applying for disability is a last resort as it is financially and emotionally challenging, may make it very difficult to go back to the workplace later, and may interfere with patients' ability to get adequate medical care and coverage for treatment. Headache medicine providers can provide medical information and assist with completion of forms to support patients' requests for disability, but it is helpful to have a support network of occupational specialists, mental health specialists, and advocacy organizations that can support patients through all the complexities involved in applying for disability.

Conclusion

Migraine is prevalent, disabling, and costly in terms of personal impact and decreased work productivity. Headache medicine providers can help to counteract this by optimizing their patients' medical management and supporting them through challenging times. A goal of care includes educating people on their right to reasonable accommodations and providing them with letters if needed. It is important to raise awareness about migraine in the workplace. Further efforts are needed to develop works programs as a part of major advocacy efforts.

Teaching Points

1. Migraine is prevalent and disabling. Migraine-related disability is complex and multifactorial including its many symptoms, unpredictability, stigma, underdiagnosis and undertreatment, and its comorbidities.
2. The impact of migraine in the workplace is often missed because (1) of the stigma, (2) most migraine-related productivity loss is in terms of presenteeism (workers are present at work but not as productive as they normally would be due to the symptoms of their disease), and (3) since it is underdiagnosed and undertreated, it has a low claim-based prevalence and hence relatively low claim-based medical and pharmacy costs.
3. Healthcare professionals can help by providing support, raising awareness, empowering their patients through education and advocacy, and providing patients with different acute treatment options including some with limited side effect profile to use at work as needed to regain function.
4. Company-wide headache education and management programs in the workplace raise awareness, increase understanding, change attitudes, increase diagnosis, improve management, increase productivity, and hence benefit everyone.

Case

I was diagnosed with chronic migraine about 20 years ago when I was 15. I have had an attack nearly every day since. I have had to learn to live with migraine, not around it, to have any semblance of quality of life and a career.

As an editor and writer, I spend most of my days parked in front of a screen. I didn't feel comfortable disclosing my migraine diagnosis to previous employers until an attack or hospitalization forced my hand. The stigma attached to migraine and workplace policies, such as requiring a doctor's note for sick days or 8 am–5 pm work hours, forced me to come to work and push through despite my symptoms without disclosing my diagnosis. As a magazine editor, late-night press events were expected of me on top of a 40- to 50-hour work week. My migraine attacks became too severe and frequent to pursue in-person employment.

Hence, I transitioned to remote, contract work as a content producer in the health space. My current employment set-up allows for practical accommodations. I have a lot of flexibility in my work schedule without requiring doctor's notes. I have unlimited days off. I can turn my camera off during virtual meetings so that I can wear an ice hat or sit in a completely dark room. However, the emotional burden persists. I live in near-constant fear that migraine will steal more from my already limited quality of life, such as the inability to cook a meal, a relationship, or a holiday. Having to consistently "prove" my disease has cost me—and by extension, those companies—my best work.

Case Discussion

When asked to rate the intensity and disability of their migraine attack symptoms, patients with migraine ranked pain as the most disabling factor, followed by cognitive dysfunction second ("difficulty in thinking and worsening with mental effort"), followed by photo- and phono-phobia, and then nausea [10]. Migraine can negatively impact work productivity even on non-headache days. About 40% of people with migraine have interictal symptoms [11]. Even interictally, migraine is associated with cognitive dysfunction (such as deficits in attention, executive function, processing speed, and memory) in people during their peak productive years [12].

Acknowledgments We thank Kat Harrison for generously sharing and writing her story for the case presented in this chapter.

Questions and Answers

1. What is the proportion of migraine-related productivity loss at work related to presenteeism?
   A. 22%
   B. 57%
   C. 72%
   D. 89%.

The correct answer is D. One of the main reasons the impact of migraine in the workplace tends to be unnoticed is that people with migraine come to work despite all the symptoms of their disease. They want to work and prioritize work over the other aspects of their lives. Unfortunately, due to the many symptoms of the diseases, they aren't as productive as they normally would during a migraine attack, which leads to presenteeism. Presenteeism is seldom measured, doesn't have validated scale, and often goes unnoticed.

2. Migraine workplace education programs increase productivity via:
   A. Reducing absenteeism.
   B. Decreasing stigma.
   C. Increasing productivity at work.
   D. All of the above.

The correct answer is D. It is important for migraine education programs in the workplace to be promoted and offered to all employees to raise awareness, increase understanding, break down stigma, increase diagnosis and management, and as a result increase productivity via reduction in both absenteeism and presenteeism. Some workers may not know they have migraine and seek evaluation as a result of the education program. Some workers may receive suboptimal treatment and become empowered to self-advocate for better medical treatment as a result of participation in the education program. A company-wide education program help increase understanding and change people's attitudes toward colleagues with migraine. Stigma is independently associated with productivity loss and has to be addressed.

References

1. GBD 2016 Headache Collaborators. Global, regional, and national burden of migraine and tension-type headache, 1990–2016: a systematic analysis for the Global Burden of Disease Study 2016. Lancet Neurol. 2018;17(11):954–76.
2. Steiner TJ, Stovner LJ, Vos T, Jensen R, Katsarava Z. Migraine is first cause of disability in under 50s: will health politicians now take notice? J Headache Pain. 2018;19(1):17.
3. Burch RC, Buse DC, Lipton RB. Migraine: epidemiology, burden, and comorbidity. Neurol Clin. 2019;37(4):631–49.
4. Lipton RB, Stewart WF, von Korff M. Burden of migraine: societal costs and therapeutic opportunities. Neurology. 1997;48(3 Suppl 3):S4–9.
5. Estave PM, Beeghly S, Anderson R, Margol C, Shakir M, George G, et al. Learning the full impact of migraine through patient voices: a qualitative study. Headache. 2021;61(7):1004–20.
6. Kim BK, Cho SJ, Kim CS, Sakai F, Dodick DW, Chu MK. Disability and economic loss caused by headache among information technology workers in Korea. J Clin Neurol. 2021;17(4):546–57.
7. Henry P, Auray JP, Gaudin AF, Dartigues JF, Duru G, Lantéri-Minet M, et al. Prevalence and clinical characteristics of migraine in France. Neurology. 2002;59(2):232–7.
8. Lipton RB, Manack Adams A, Buse DC, Fanning KM, Reed ML. A Comparison of the Chronic Migraine Epidemiology and Outcomes (CaMEO) Study and American Migraine Prevalence and Prevention (AMPP) Study: demographics and headache-related disability. Headache. 2016;56(8):1280–9.
9. Peres MFP, Queiroz LP, Rocha-Filho PS, Sarmento EM, Katsarava Z, Steiner TJ. Migraine: a major debilitating chronic non-communicable disease in Brazil, evidence from two national surveys. J Headache Pain. 2019;20(1):85.
10. Raggi A, Covelli V, Leonardi M, Grazzi L, Curone M, D'Amico D. Difficulties in work-related activities among migraineurs are scarcely collected: results from a literature review. Neurol Sci. 2014;35(Suppl 1):23–6.
11. Kneipp SM, Beeber L. Social withdrawal as a self-management behavior for migraine: implications for depression comorbidity among disadvantaged women. ANS Adv Nurs Sci. 2015;38(1):34–44.
12. Holroyd K, Drew J, Cottrell C, Romanek K, Heh V. Impaired functioning and quality of life in severe migraine: the role of catastrophizing and associated symptoms. Cephalalgia. 2007;27(10):1156–65.
13. Seng EK, Buse DC, Klepper JE, Mayson SJ, Grinberg AS, Grosberg BM, et al. Psychological factors associated with chronic migraine and severe migraine-related disability: an observational study in a tertiary headache center. Headache. 2017;57(4):593–604.
14. Minen MT, Dhaem OBD, Diest AKV, Powers S, Schwedt TJ, Lipton R, et al. Migraine and its psychiatric comorbidities. J Neurol Neurosurg Psychiatry. 2016;87(7):741–9.
15. Beck A, Crain AL, Solberg LI, Unützer J, Glasgow RE, Maciosek MV, et al. Severity of depression and magnitude of productivity loss. Ann Fam Med. 2011;9(4):305–11.
16. Plaisier I, Beekman ATF, de Graaf R, Smit JH, van Dyck R, Penninx BWJH. Work functioning in persons with depressive and anxiety disorders: the role of specific psychopathological characteristics. J Affect Disord. 2010;125(1–3):198–206.
17. Lagerveld SE, Bültmann U, Franche RL, van Dijk FJH, Vlasveld MC, van der Feltz-Cornelis CM, et al. Factors associated with work participation and work functioning in depressed workers: a systematic review. J Occup Rehabil. 2010;20(3):275–92.
18. Hui S, Kuen A, Grandner MA. Trouble sleeping associated with lower work performance and greater healthcare costs: longitudinal data from Kansas State employee wellness program. J Occup Environ Med. 2015;57(10):1031–8.
19. Lantéri-Minet M, Radat F, Chautard MH, Lucas C. Anxiety and depression associated with migraine: influence on migraine sub-

jects' disability and quality of life, and acute migraine management. Pain. 2005;118(3):319–26.
20. Blumenfeld AM, Varon SF, Wilcox TK, Buse DC, Kawata AK, Manack A, et al. Disability, HRQoL and resource use among chronic and episodic migraineurs: results from the International Burden of Migraine Study (IBMS). Cephalalgia. 2011;31(3):301–15.
21. Lipton RB, Diamond S, Reed M, Diamond ML, Stewart WF. Migraine diagnosis and treatment: results from the American Migraine Study II. Headache. 2001;41(7):638–45.
22. Shapiro R. Migraine Stigma. Boston; 2019.
23. Gvantseladze K, Do TP, Hansen JM, Shapiro RE, Ashina M. The stereotypical image of a person with migraine according to mass media. Headache. 2020;60(7):1465–71.
24. Young WB, Park JE, Tian IX, Kempner J. The stigma of migraine. Preux PM, editor. PLoS One. 2013;8(1):e54074.
25. Cottrell CK, Drew JB, Waller SE, Holroyd KA, Brose JA, O'Donnell FJ. Perceptions and needs of patients with migraine. J Fam Pract. 2002;51(2):142–7.
26. Rao D, Choi SW, Victorson D, Bode R, Peterman A, Heinemann A, et al. Measuring stigma across neurological conditions: the development of the stigma scale for chronic illness (SSCI). Qual Life Res. 2009;18(5):585–95.
27. Cella D, Lai JS, Nowinski CJ, Victorson D, Peterman A, Miller D, et al. Neuro-QOL: brief measures of health-related quality of life for clinical research in neurology. Neurology. 2012;78(23):1860–7.
28. Stewart WF, Wood GC, Razzaghi H, Reed ML, Lipton RB. Work impact of migraine headaches. J Occup Environ Med. 2008;50(7):736–45.
29. 61st Annual Scientific Meeting American Headache Society® July 11–14 2019 Pennsylvania Convention Center Philadelphia, PA. Headache: J Head Face Pain. 2019;59(S1):1–208.
30. Shapiro R, Lipton R, Reiner P. EHMTI-0313. Factors influencing stigma toward persons with migraine. J Headache Pain. 2014;15(Suppl 1):E36.
31. Stewart WF, Wood GC, Manack A, Varon SF, Buse DC, Lipton RB. Employment and work impact of chronic migraine and episodic migraine. J Occup Environ Med. 2010;52(1):8–14.
32. Stewart WF, Roy J, Lipton RB. Migraine prevalence, socioeconomic status, and social causation. Neurology. 2013;81(11):948–55.
33. Peterlin BL, Scher AI. Migraine and the social selection vs causation hypotheses. Neurology. 2013;81(11):942–3.
34. Shimizu T, Sakai F, Miyake H, Sone T, Sato M, Tanabe S, et al. Disability, quality of life, productivity impairment and employer costs of migraine in the workplace. J Headache Pain. 2021;22(1):29.
35. Migraines Are a Serious Problem. Employers Can Help. [Internet]. [cited 2021 Nov 12]. Available from: https://hbr.org/2021/02/migraines-are-a-serious-problem-employers-can-help
36. Begasse de Dhaem O, Gharedaghi MH, Bain P, Hettie G, Loder E, Burch R. Identification of work accommodations and interventions associated with work productivity in adults with migraine: a scoping review. Cephalalgia. 2021;41(6):760–73.
37. Hu XH, Markson LE, Lipton RB, Stewart WF, Berger ML. Burden of migraine in the United States: disability and economic costs. Arch Intern Med. 1999;159(8):813–8.
38. Leonardi M, Raggi A, Ajovalasit D, Bussone G, D'Amico D. Functioning and disability in migraine. Disabil Rehabil. 2010;32(Suppl 1):S23–32.
39. New Hope for Migraine Sufferers – The New York Times [Internet]. [cited 2021 Nov 12]. Available from: https://www.nytimes.com/2020/01/06/well/live/new-hope-for-migraine-sufferers.html
40. Goetzel RZ, Long SR, Ozminkowski RJ, Hawkins K, Wang S, Lynch W. Health, absence, disability, and presenteeism cost estimates of certain physical and mental health conditions affecting U.S. employers. J Occup Environ Med. 2004;46(4):398–412.
41. Hemp P. Presenteeism: at work – but out of it. Harv Bus Rev. 2004;82(10):49–58, 155.
42. Stewart WF, Ricci JA, Chee E, Morganstein D, Lipton R. Lost productive time and cost due to common pain conditions in the US workforce. JAMA. 2003;290(18):2443–54.
43. Gerth WC, Carides GW, Dasbach EJ, Visser WH, Santanello NC. The multinational impact of migraine symptoms on healthcare utilisation and work loss. Pharmacoeconomics. 2001;19(2):197–206.
44. Allen D, Hines EW, Pazdernik V, Konecny LT, Breitenbach E. Four-year review of presenteeism data among employees of a large United States health care system: a retrospective prevalence study. Hum Resour Health. 2018;16(1):59.
45. Selekler HM, Gökmen G, Alvur TM, Steiner TJ. Productivity losses attributable to headache, and their attempted recovery, in a heavy-manufacturing workforce in Turkey: implications for employers and politicians. J Headache Pain. 2015;16:96.
46. Ishii R, Schwedt TJ, Dumkrieger G, Lalvani N, Craven A, Goadsby PJ, et al. Chronic versus episodic migraine: the 15-day threshold does not adequately reflect substantial differences in disability across the full spectrum of headache frequency. Headache J Head Face Pain. 2021;61(7):992–1003.
47. IHS-GPAC Fujitsu Case Study Impact Report. 2021.
48. Lipton RB, Bigal ME. Ten lessons on the epidemiology of migraine. Headache. 2007;47(Suppl 1):S2–9.
49. Ganesh K, Lazar A. The work of workplace disclosure: invisible chronic conditions and opportunities for design. Proc ACM Hum Comput Interact. 2021;5:10.1145/3449147.
50. Schaetz L, Rimner T, Pathak P, Fang J, Chandrasekhar D, Mueller J, et al. Employee and employer benefits from a migraine management program: disease outcomes and cost analysis. Headache. 2020;60(9):1947–60.
51. Vicente-Herrero M, Lainez M. Impacto de un programa de intervencion de la migrana en el medio laboral entre los trabajadores de correos. Medicina del Trabajo. 2006;15:12–22.
52. Sandoe CH, Sasikumar S, Lay C, Lawler V. The impact of shift work on migraine: a case series and narrative review. Headache. 2019;59(9):1631–40.
53. Kristoffersen ES, Waage S, Pallesen S, Bjorvatn B. Changes in work schedule affect headache frequency among Norwegian nurses: a 3-year-follow-up study. Occup Environ Med. 2024;81(4):191–200.
54. Mitrovic A, Sretenovic A, Stanic A. Contribution of twenty-one epidemiological factors to migraine disability. J Neurol Sci. 2013;333:e489–90.
55. Loder E. The approach to the headache patient. Stowe; 2021.
56. Thorn BE, Pence LB, Ward LC, Kilgo G, Clements KL, Cross TH, et al. A randomized clinical trial of targeted cognitive behavioral treatment to reduce catastrophizing in chronic headache sufferers. J Pain. 2007;8(12):938–49.
57. Seng EK, Holroyd KA. Behavioral migraine management modifies behavioral and cognitive coping in people with migraine. Headache. 2014;54(9):1470–83.
58. Wells RE, O'Connell N, Pierce CR, Estave P, Penzien DB, Loder E, et al. Effectiveness of mindfulness meditation vs headache education for adults with migraine: a randomized clinical trial. JAMA Intern Med. 2021;181(3):317–28.
59. The Americans with Disabilities Act Amendments Act of 2008 | U.S. Equal Employment Opportunity Commission [Internet]. [cited 2021 Nov 18]. Available from: https://www.eeoc.gov/statutes/americans-disabilities-act-amendments-act-2008

60. Shapiro RE. Migraine and disability rights. CONTINUUM Lifelong Learn Neurol. 2012;18(4):900.
61. Daly MC, Bound J. Worker adaptation and employer accommodation following the onset of a health impairment. J Gerontol B Psychol Sci Soc Sci. 1996;51(2):S53–60.
62. Work at Home/Telework as a Reasonable Accommodation | U.S. Equal Employment Opportunity Commission [Internet]. [cited 2021 Nov 18]. Available from: https://www.eeoc.gov/laws/guidance/work-hometelework-reasonable-accommodation
63. Minimum Length of Meal Period Required under State Law for Adult Employees in Private Sector 1 | U.S. Department of Labor [Internet]. [cited 2021 Nov 18]. Available from: https://www.dol.gov/agencies/whd/state/meal-breaks

Migraine Trigger Factors and Wellness in Clinical Practice

18

Ami Cuneo, Nina Riggins, Chace Shaw, and Teshamae S. Monteith

Introduction

Migraine is a brain disorder characterized by episodic attacks of disabling headaches with associated symptoms. Influenced by genetic and environmental factors, migraine is the leading cause of disability in individuals under 50 years of age and has a peak prevalence during highly productive years [1, 2].

A migraine trigger factor is defined as any event or exposure that, when present or withdrawn, increases the chance of an acute migraine attack, often within 48 hours [3, 4]. Trigger factors can be classified as modifiable versus unmodifiable, and external versus internal (Table 18.1) [5]. Trigger factors are experienced heterogeneously in individuals with migraine. No single trigger factor exists for all individuals, and for a person susceptible to a given trigger factor, not every exposure to that trigger factor results in an acute migraine attack [6, 7]. Even more, it appears some trigger factors must reach a cumulative effect to incite an acute migraine episode [8] (Fig. 18.1a, b).

For centuries, potential trigger factors for acute migraine attacks have been considered. Ancient texts speculated migraine attacks were related to harmful vapors from the body's humours affecting the brain [9, 10]. The strong genetic basis of migraine suggests a possible evolutionary advantage of sensitivity to migraine trigger factors, perhaps rooted in natural selection for traits promoting the ability to identify environmental dangers, thereby conferring a reproductive or survival benefit [11, 12]. Yet, individuals who are affected by migraine trigger factors have increased functional disability and headache intensity compared to those who are not susceptible [13, 14].

The twenty-first century marks a time of major advances in technology, as well as evolving lifestyles, modifications in work-life balance, consumption, and behaviors driven by cultural norms. For individuals with migraine, the social and professional consequences of trigger factors are important to explore [15, 16]. This chapter provides an update on common migraine trigger factors and clinical strategies for migraine management to improve patient well-being.

Questions

1. Which of the following is a complicating aspect of the study and management of migraine trigger factors?
   A. Overlap between migraine trigger symptoms and premonitory migraine symptoms
   B. Trigger heterogeneity
   C. Migraine trigger studies' overreliance on patient surveys
   D. All of the above
2. Which of the following common migraine trigger factors warrants work-up for secondary causes?
   A. Fasting
   B. Exertion
   C. Noise
   D. Fatigue

A. Cuneo (✉)
Department of Neurology, Headache Clinic, University of Washington, Seattle, WA, USA

N. Riggins
Headache Center of Excellence at the VA Palo Alto, Palo Alto, CA, USA

C. Shaw
Department of Psychiatry and Behavioral Sciences, Stanford University, Stanford, CA, USA

T. S. Monteith
Department of Neurology, Headache Division, Miller School of Medicine, University of Miami, Miami, FL, USA

T. S. Monteith et al. (eds.), *Comprehensive Migraine Management*, https://doi.org/10.1007/978-3-031-86923-5_18

Table 18.1 Common trigger factors and management

Trigger factor category	Trigger factor name	% Patients reporting trigger factor	Trigger factor management and recommendations
Lifestyle/behavioral	Stress	58%[153]–80% [5]	CBT, mindfulness-based stress reduction, relaxation, biofeedback [154, 155]
	Stress let-down	>3% [156]	Diaphragmatic breathing, guided imagery [155]
	Hunger/not eating	42%[157]–82% [158]	Frequent, small healthy meals [159, 160]
			Avoid skipping meals [154]
	Fatigue, lack of sleep, or overexertion[a]	22%[157]–79% [158] 36%[153]–74% [158]	Standard sleep hygiene recommendations [161]
			Evaluate for sleep disorders
			CBT for insomnia [89]
			Depression screening [161]
			Differentiate from prodrome with diary
	Change in sleep pattern	25%[162]–44% [163]	Standard sleep hygiene recommendations [164]
	Exercise[b]	20%[43]–42% [158]	Warm-up before exercise [165]
			Weight loss [165]
			Conditioning [165]
			Exercise 30–60 minutes 3–5 times per week(154)
	Head/neck pain/movements[a, b]	2%[43]–9% [162]	Use of ergonomic furniture [166]
			Rule out cervicogenic headache
	Sexual activity[b]	1%[157]–7% [162]	Pretreatment with indomethacin/NSAIDs/triptans
			Consider prophylactic therapies (e.g., beta-blockers)
			Reassurance after rule-out of secondary headache
			Sexual activity during migraine episode [167]
Hormonal	Hormonal fluctuations	78% [6]	Consider risks/benefits of HRT management
			Symptomatic therapy (e.g., in pregnancy, IVF, etc.)
	Menstruation	31%[157]–65% [5]	Consider mini-prophylaxis (NSAIDs, long-acting triptans), acute abortive therapy [168]
			Increase management of other trigger factors during menstrual period(98)
Sensory	Noise	39%[153]–75% [43]	Control exposure [138]
			Ear plugs
			Increase awareness of volume controls
	Visual stimulation[a]	27%[162]–75% [43]	Decrease the use of indoor fluorescent lights [166]
			Adjust flicker frequency on the computer screen [166]
			Intermittent use of tinted glasses to minimize exposure to adverse wavelength frequencies [169–172]
	Odors	26%[157]–75% [43]	Perfume-free work policies [166]
	Travel/driving	4%[43]–53% [153]	Consider use of antiemetics [173], NSAIDs [173], acute abortive therapy [173]
Environmental	Heat	30% [5]	Use fans to cool indoor environment [166]
	Weather/barometric pressure changes	17%[157]–53% [158]	Deliver barometric pressure information through media and smartphone apps to patients [174]
	Smoke	36%[5]–61% [158]	Restrict smoking indoors and near outdoor access doors [166]
Chemical	Specific foods/drinks	12%[153]–58% [158]	Migraine diary [154]
			Reduce consumption/make substitute
	Caffeine	14%[175]–30% [176]	Avoid overuse-withdrawal [177–179]
			Limit regular caffeine intake to <200 mg/day [92]
	Alcohol	4%[162]–42% [158]	Control exposure [98]
			Moderate consumption [180]
	Smoking	1%[43]–16% [157]	Smoking cessation [181]

[a]Potential premonitory symptom
[b]Red flag: Must rule out possible secondary headache etiologies in individuals experiencing these trigger factors

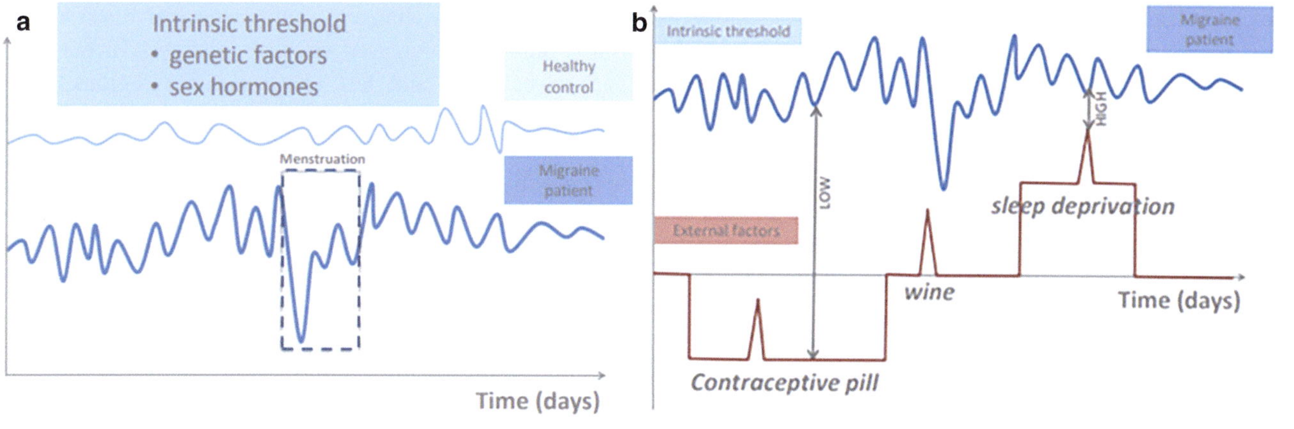

Fig. 18.1 (**a**) Intrinsic threshold for a migraine attack. The intrinsic threshold is affected by genetic factors and fluctuating hormone levels. (**b**). Influence of intrinsic threshold and external factors on risk of migraine attack. External trigger factors (e.g., exogenous hormone replacement, red wine, and alternations in sleep) in combination with an individual's intrinsic threshold may influence the chance of experiencing a migraine attack. (Courtesy of Dr. Gisela Terwindt, www.hoofdpijnonderzoek.nl)

Fig. 18.2 Phases of a migraine attack. The interictal phase is influenced by migraine attack trigger factors as well as environmental and genetic predisposition. The following premonitory, aura, headache, and postdrome phases involve a complex sequence of variable symptoms. (Credit: Andreou and Edvinsson. https://creativecommons.org/licenses/by/4.0/ No changes were made to the figure [26])

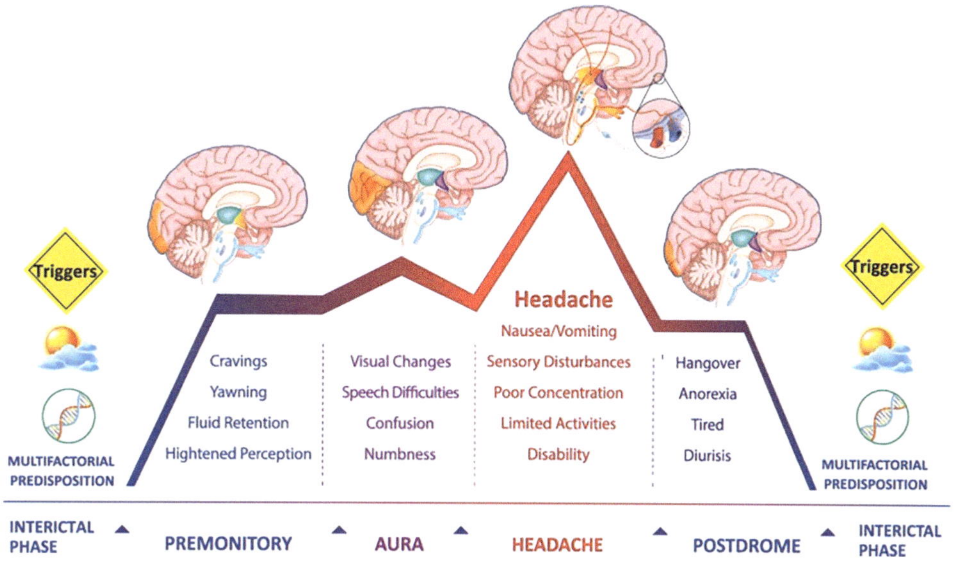

Pathophysiology of Migraine Trigger Factors

Migraine is a disorder of brain function. Individuals carrying a genetic predisposition for migraine are thought to have a hyperexcitable sensory processing system with increased signaling in several brain structures, including the hypothalamus, brainstem, and trigeminovascular system [17–23]. Recent brain connectome studies have hypothesized that migraine is a connectopathy, in which an imbalance between the demands of resources promoting network efficiency and the metabolic cost of wiring the migraine brain is present, leading to susceptibility to trigger factors [24, 25]. With this biological susceptibility to trigger factors, a multi-staged migraine attack ensues, including the proposed premonitory, aura, headache, and postdrome phases (Fig. 18.2) [26].

In classic pharmacological studies, glyceryl trinitrate infusion has been demonstrated to trigger functional activation of the brainstem, intra- and extra-cranial blood vessels, thalamus, and cortex, causing symptoms identical to those in spontaneous migraine attacks [27–29]. Trigger factors can be considered fluctuating migraine trigger threshold susceptibility-modulating factors (MTTSMF) [30], altering neuronal excitability and function, such that once a critical threshold is reached, a migraine headache and related symptoms follow [26, 31].

For example, in menstrual migraine, animal models and limited studies in humans suggest that cyclic fluctuations in sex hormone levels during the menstrual cycle may lower the threshold for migraine [32, 33]. Animal models have shown that fluctuations in estrogen result in increased susceptibility to cortical spreading depression, a pathophysiological mechanism underlying migraine aura as well as activation of the trigeminovascular system through the release of nociceptive compounds, such as calcitonin gene-related peptide and other inflammatory mediators [34–39]. This cortical hyperexcitability in the menstrual cycle may account for the increased migraine frequency seen after estrogen peaks and begins to decline in the perimenstrual days [40]. The role of progesterone is less clearly understood; though levels of estrogen and progesterone both decline around the time of menses, supplementation of estrogen (but not progesterone) has been shown to decrease the risk of migraine attack [41]. Additionally, menstrual migraine attacks occur more frequently in the setting of low magnesium levels, suggesting magnesium deficiency may be an additional exacerbating factor [42].

Interictal sensory stimulation (e.g., bright or fluorescent light, motion, loud sound, and odor) is another frequently reported trigger factor in individuals with migraine [43]. Neurophysiological studies have demonstrated a lack of habituation of evoked responses to repeated sensory stimuli in individuals with migraine [44, 45]. Several neuroimaging studies have been designed to elucidate the brain changes that occur as a consequence of migraine trigger factors. According to one study, olfactory stimulation causes functional neuroimaging changes in several odor-processing brain structures; during a migraine attack, these structures, in addition to the rostral pons, an area linked to migraine-related pain, show increased activity, suggesting a relationship between the trigemino-nociceptive and olfactory pathways in migraine pathophysiology (Fig. 18.3) [46]. Visually stressful stripe patterns can induce headaches in individuals with migraine, and prolonged stimulation may alter functional connectivity within the visual system and other networks [47]. In addition to functional changes, some structural brain alterations, including increased cortical thickness in the right parietal-occipital and left fronto-parietal regions, have been demonstrated in individuals with episodic migraine and interictal photosensitivity [48]. Taken together, it appears dysfunctional sensory networks and perhaps structural changes in individuals with migraine may either predispose to or are a consequence of sensory stimulation-triggered migraine attacks [49].

Stress is the most frequently perceived trigger factor, reported by up to 80% of individuals living with migraine and associated with migraine chronification [5, 50]. In animal studies, stress resilience is thought to play a role in the susceptibility to migraine attacks [51]. Stress perception may be a consequence of activation of the hypothalamic and amygdala circuits linked to the premonitory phase of migraine [52]. At the same time, stress let-down has been shown to be associated with headache onset, which may be related to the acute decrease in stress-related (anti-inflammatory and anti-nociceptive) glucocorticoid levels after a period of elevation from the activation of the hypothalamic-pituitary axis [53].

Sleep dysfunction has been associated with migraine, though the relationship is complex and incompletely understood [54, 55]. Migraine attacks may be related to changes in routine sleep schedule, including both over-sleeping and under-sleeping. Increasing evidence suggests an underlying physiologic relationship between sleep and migraine, with overlap in brainstem-cortical pathways involving anatomic structures (e.g., hypothalamus), critical neurotransmitters (e.g., serotonin, dopamine, and orexins), and the central nervous system's waste-removing glymphatic system [56].

Less is known about nutritional trigger factors; however, they are thought to induce migraine attacks through modulation of neuropeptides (e.g., glutamate, dopamine, and nor-

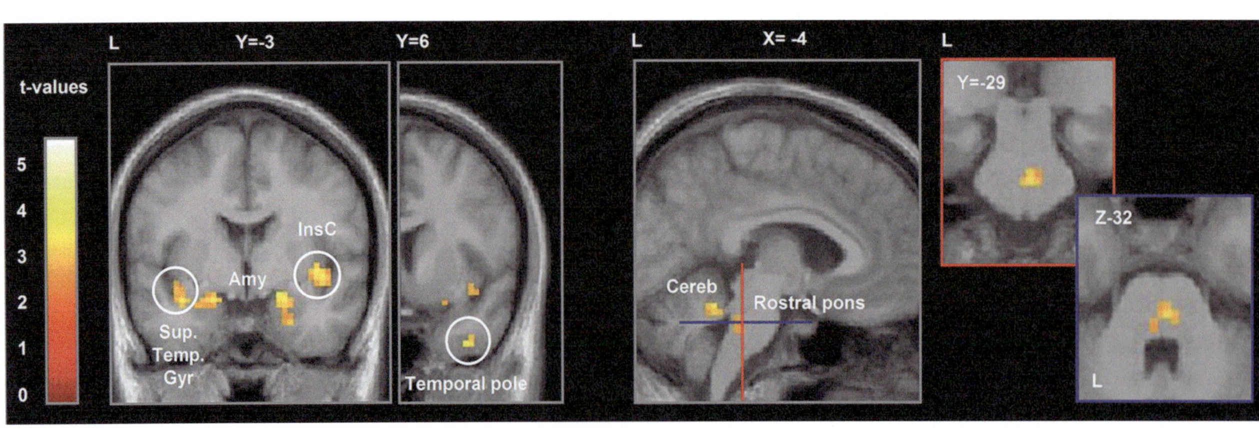

Fig. 18.3 Functional magnetic resonance (fMRI) imaging in individuals with migraine during an acute headache attack in response to olfactory stimulation. fMRI demonstrates significantly increased activation in the amygdala (Amy), insular (InsC), temporal pole, superior temporal gyrus (Sup Temp Gyr), rostral pons, and cerebellum (Cereb) compared with the participant's own data outside attacks, suggesting a relationship between the olfactory system and migraine-related pain. (Source: Stankewitz and May [46])

epinephrine), neuroreceptors (e.g., NMDA receptors), ion channels (e.g., sodium), vasodilation (e.g., from increased nitric oxide or histamine), glucose metabolism, and the activation of inflammatory cascades and the autonomic nervous system [57]. Additionally, specific trigger factors such as caffeine, an adenosine receptor antagonist, may act as both a migraine trigger factor and a treatment for a migraine attack [31, 58].

Migraine Trigger Factors Versus Premonitory Migraine Symptoms

A migraine trigger factor (i.e., any event or exposure that contributes to migraine attack onset) should be differentiated from a premonitory symptom, defined as a clinical manifestation of the early stage of an already-initiated migraine episode. Positron emission tomography (PET) imaging has identified nitroglycerin-triggered hypothalamic activation as part of the premonitory phase of migraine, [59] and alterations in hypothalamic-brainstem connectivity have been demonstrated [60]. However, in clinical practice, identifying a trigger factor versus a premonitory symptom may be challenging due to symptomatic overlap (Table 18.1) [61]. Fatigue, for instance, is a commonly perceived migraine trigger factor; however, yawning and somnolence are known brainstem-related dopaminergic premonitory symptoms [5, 59, 60, 62–64]. Other symptoms, such as light sensitivity and food cravings (e.g., chocolate), may also represent premonitory symptoms rather than true migraine trigger factors (Fig. 18.2) [65].

Integrating Advances for Clinical Practice

Clinically Relevant Trigger Factors

Trigger factors frequently are reported by individuals with migraine (Table 18.1) [5, 31]. Identification and management of trigger factors may be vital to patient care, as trigger factors' timing and cumulative effect may influence migraine outcomes (Fig. 18.1a, b) [57, 66]. Furthermore, certain trigger factors (e.g., exertion) may be associated with either a benign or dangerous secondary etiology of headache and require additional clinical workup.

Hormonal Fluctuations

Estrogen's triggering role in migraine attacks has been long suspected. In prepubertal children, the incidence of migraine is similar (<5%) for both males and females; however, following the puberty-related increase in estrogen in females, the cumulative incidence of migraine climbs to 43% and remains low in males [67, 68]. Migraine also is more prevalent during the reproductive years [69, 70]. Menses-related hormonal fluctuations are a frequently reported migraine trigger factor, affecting up to 78% of females living with migraine [6]. Some studies have suggested that migraine attacks related to the menstrual cycle have increased intensity, are more disabling and refractory to typical migraine treatments, and are longer in duration compared to non-menstrual migraine attacks [71, 72]. Other research has not demonstrated this correlation [73, 74]. Treatment strategies for menstrual migraine include short-term prevention with certain triptans, magnesium, estradiol, and naproxen [70].

Perceived Stress and Stress Let-Down

Studies have shown variable evidence for a causal relationship between perceived stress and the onset of an acute migraine episode [75–77]. Lipton et al. have demonstrated that the let-down from stress is predictive of an increased risk of a migraine attack, perhaps related to the consequences of a stressful period (e.g., possible missed medications, skipped meals, or disrupted sleep) [53]. An individual's comorbidities may also be considered. In a stress-sensitive individual, the ability to cope with stress appears contributory, [77] and the effect of stress may be increased in those with both migraine and depression [78]. Therefore, stress management is recommended for those experiencing stress-related migraine attacks [79, 80]. Behavioral approaches, such as cognitive behavioral therapy, biofeedback, and mindfulness techniques, may be helpful.

Sleep Dysfunction

Individuals with migraine often report sleep improves symptoms of an acute migraine attack. At the same time, disturbed sleep preceding, during, and following an acute migraine episode may occur [3, 56, 76, 81–83]. Decreased sleep efficiency in individuals suffering from migraine has been demonstrated, [84] and comorbid insomnia may be undiagnosed and undertreated [56, 85]. Furthermore, disordered breathing and snoring have been associated with morning-onset migraine attacks [86]. Additional studies have suggested that irregular sleeping patterns (e.g., related to shift work) may be associated with chronification of headache and increased migraine-related disability; however, meta-analyses remain inconclusive [87, 88]. Clinical recommendations include encouragement of healthy sleep practices, utilization of cognitive behavioral therapy for insomnia, and consideration of sleep medicine evaluation in those with suspicion of an underlying sleep disorder [89].

Nutrition

Foods and beverages are frequently reported migraine trigger factors. Dietary nitrites, found in cured and processed meats, can result in a migraine attack within hours [90–92].

Withdrawal of caffeine can trigger migraine attacks [93, 94]. Alcohol (particularly, red wine) is commonly cited [95, 96] though one European study reported alcohol alone had a low consistency of migraine provocation and may require the presence of other trigger factors for impact [8]. For many nutritional trigger factors, limited high-quality supportive data exist [9, 14, 97]. Furthermore, the relationship may be confounded by the premonitory phase of migraine, which independently may prompt a food craving (e.g., chocolate) prior to the onset of headache [98–100].

In the clinical setting, individuals with migraine should be encouraged to maintain a healthy, balanced diet, with an adequate supply of fresh fruits and vegetables, as well as nutritious sources of good fats and protein. Processed foods should be replaced with unprocessed foods with low glycemic indices [13, 94, 101–103]. Meal-skipping should be avoided. Though food trigger factors may be challenging to identify, elimination of specific foods may be associated with decreased frequency and severity of migraine headaches in some individuals [104–106].

Exercise

Exercise is an often-reported migraine trigger factor [5, 107]. Though individuals with migraine may be more prone to movement sensitivity at baseline, [108] studies have shown that regular exercise can decrease headache frequency, severity, and duration [109–112]. This apparent dichotomy may be influenced by confounding physical activity-related factors, such as physical stress, overheating, and fatigue, therefore complicating the clinical picture [9]. Additionally, physical activity avoidance may be related to premonitory phenomena, rather than representing a true migraine trigger factor [9, 113]. Therefore, patients with migraine may benefit from personalized exercise programs involving regular, sustainable, and enjoyable exercise to maximize the positive effects of exercise on neuroinflammatory, neurovascular, and psychological systems and improve headaches [114].

Barometric Pressure Changes

Up to 52% of individuals with migraine report weather and barometric pressure changes as migraine trigger factors [9]. A subset of those with migraine has been proposed to be more sensitive to meteorological variables (e.g., increased humidity and lower temperatures) [115]. However, the degree of influence of weather and barometric pressure changes on migraine remains inconclusive, as subjective weather perceptions and barometric weather changes have not correlated consistently with the occurrence of migraine attacks [116, 117].

Allergens

In a large population study comparing individuals with migraine to migraine-free cohorts, the migraine group had twice the likelihood of having allergies/hay fever [118]. Additionally, increased migraine pain intensity has been associated with allergic and inflammatory conditions [118, 119]. Mast cell activation is a hypothesized potential link [120] though the underlying pathophysiology is incompletely understood. Commercial IgG food sensitivity testing is increasingly available to test for allergies, sensitivities, and intolerances, but is not reliable. Furthermore, evidence for the elimination of diet-based IgG food sensitivity testing is limited, and large screening panels are not recommended [121, 122].

Environmental Pollutants, Tobacco, and Smoke Exposure

The influences of environmental exposures on populations with migraine are important social determinants of health. The potential role of long-term exposure to multiple ambient air pollutants on migraine prevalence and severity has been suggested but requires further study [123]. Though possible mechanisms of tobacco as a migraine trigger factor exist, current literature does not demonstrate a clear association [124–126]. Increased inhalation of tobacco smoke, however, has been associated with more severe headaches [127]. Decreasing first- and second-hand tobacco exposure is recommended for all patients due to the risk of systemic health effects.

Mapping and Predicting Migraine Trigger Factors in Clinical Practice

Historically, research regarding migraine trigger factors have been limited by studies affected by recall bias (e.g., surveys) [3, 4]. Recently, a validated questionnaire called the Headache Triggers Sensitivity and Avoidance Questionnaire (HTSAQ-SF) was developed to improve trigger factor identification in research and clinical practice [128]. In addition, digital diaries and smartphone applications (apps) can capture migraine trigger factors, pain characteristics, associated symptoms, treatment efficacy, and other factors [129–132]. Trigger-mapping apps may be used in prediction modeling to help individuals learn more about trigger factor identity, the degree of causality, and the additive effects of several trigger factors. An individual's accuracy in trigger factor prediction may also be determined [131, 133, 134]. Analyzed data can guide individuals with migraine, clinicians, and researchers in trigger management [133, 134]. Despite variable limitations (e.g., diary adherence and patient privacy in some headache apps), incorporating these approaches may lead to a new wave of individualized headache management options and perhaps provide insight into the underlying pathophysiology of migraine and trigger factors [133, 135, 136].

Managing Trigger Factors to Improve Wellness in Clinical Practice

Avoidance of migraine trigger factors is a standard clinical recommendation [137–140] though there is limited empirical support for this strategy. In recent years, some authors have proposed that trigger factor avoidance may lead to a fear-conditioning response, resulting in increased trigger factor potency [141–143]. In addition, concern has been raised that the unpredictable nature and prevalence of trigger factors, combined with a strategy of avoidance, may lead to restricted lifestyles for some individuals [5].

Though trigger factors may be challenging to manage, personalized recommendations (Table 18.1) should be offered to individuals with migraine, as tailored strategies may empower patients to gain an improved locus of control over migraine attacks [144]. Moreover, the clinician should aim to guide the patient toward general wellness. Protective factors should be identified. Aspects of individuals' social determinants of health should be addressed, as these may directly impact the risk of headaches [145]. Providing patient education on migraine and trigger pathophysiology should be considered [96]. An evidence-based, multi-modal approach to migraine should be implemented, including behavioral approaches, [80] strategies for nutrition, [14, 146, 147] exercise, [112, 148] improved sleep, [149] enhanced community/social support, and other means to promote brain health and healing [134, 150]. In general, the six pillars of lifestyle medicine (i.e., nutrition, physical activity, stress management, sleep, positive social connection, and risk reduction of substance use) should be emphasized to support migraine symptom management and patient wellness [151].

Conclusion

Migraine is a disabling, often lifelong condition influenced by genetic and environmental susceptibilities. Though trigger factors may be prevalent and unpredictable, the use of headache diaries and apps can help identify trigger factors and protective factors, as well as help evaluate treatment success. Emerging technologies, such as machine learning techniques, may also contribute to this field at individual and population-based levels [95].

Migraine has the potential to be treated successfully by prioritizing patient function and quality of life. A personalized approach that incorporates shared decision-making is imperative. Medical and psychological comorbidities, as well as social determinants of health, should be addressed. Comprehensive lifestyle strategies in combination with trigger factor management are integral to improving an individual's quality of life [152]. Above all, a sense of hope should be instilled in individuals suffering from migraine for optimal treatment success.

Teaching Points

1. Most individuals with migraine report experiencing migraine-trigger factors. A variable degree of evidence exists to support specific migraine trigger factors, and validation studies are needed.
2. Migraine pathophysiology involves several biochemical pathways resulting in increased susceptibility to exogenous and/or endogenous migraine trigger factors. Trigger factors may act cumulatively.
3. Migraine trigger factors and premonitory symptoms may overlap symptomatically; however, these are considered distinct.
4. Identification of migraine trigger factors and response to migraine-related interventions can be performed with the help of paper or electronic headache diaries and/or computer apps.
5. A comprehensive approach to management, including the identification and management of trigger factors, along with the adoption of appropriate pharmacologic and non-pharmacological interventions, is recommended.

Case

A 31-year-old woman with a history of episodic migraine presents with increased headache frequency, including six debilitating migraine days per month. Following a recent promotion at work and increased stress, she spends more time in video conferences, which she mentions is a migraine trigger factor for her. She asks for management suggestions.

Case Discussion

The treatment plan should be tailored to the patient. She reports trigger factors including screen time and stress. She should be advised to optimize ambient office lighting and sounds, consider the use of a blue-light screen filter and take breaks between meetings. To improve her stress, behavioral therapies to aid in relaxation (e.g., mindfulness) and to improve coping skills (e.g., cognitive behavioral therapy) should be offered. Other aspects to improve self-care include improvement in nutrition, sleep, and exercise. Acute and preventive medications may also be considered.

Questions and Answers

1. Which of the following is a complicating aspect of the study and management of migraine trigger factors?
   A. Overlap between migraine trigger symptoms and premonitory migraine symptoms.
   B. Trigger heterogeneity.
   C. Migraine trigger studies' overreliance on patient surveys.
   D. All of the above.

The correct answer is D. A wide range of migraine trigger factors is reported; however, variable degrees of evidence exist for particular trigger factors. Though migraine trigger factors and premonitory symptoms are considered distinct pathophysiological entities, they may appear clinically similar, and making a distinction can be challenging for the patient and provider. A challenge in attempting to elucidate the connections between migraine trigger factors and underlying migraine pathophysiology is based in part upon reliance on patient recall. Therefore, the use and further development of electronic, trigger-mapping apps may aid in obtaining a more accurate understanding of the relationships between particular trigger factors and migraine pathophysiology.

2. Which of the following common migraine trigger factors warrants work-up for secondary causes?
   A. Fasting.
   B. Exertion.
   C. Noise.
   D. Fatigue.

The correct answer is B. Migraine, by definition, may be worsened by or associated with avoidance of routine physical activity. Exertion is a commonly reported migraine trigger factor. In some cases, the distinction must be made between migraine, primary exertional headache, and a dangerous secondary etiology of headache (e.g., cerebral aneurysm). Therefore, additional workup may be required in individuals for whom exertion is a headache trigger factor.

References

1. Saylor D, Steiner TJ. The global burden of headache. Semin Neurol. 2018;38(2):182–90.
2. GBD 2016 Headache Collaborators. Global, regional, and national burden of migraine and tension-type headache, 1990–2016: a systematic analysis for the Global Burden of Disease Study 2016. Lancet Neurol. 2018;17(11):954–76.
3. Pellegrino ABW, Davis-Martin RE, Houle TT, Turner DP, Smitherman TA. Perceived triggers of primary headache disorders: a meta-analysis. Cephalalgia Int J Headache. 2018;38(6):1188–98.
4. Turner DP, Smitherman TA, Martin VT, Penzien DB, Houle TT. Causality and headache triggers. Headache. 2013;53(4):628–35.
5. Kelman L. The triggers or precipitants of the acute migraine attack. Cephalalgia Int J Headache. 2007;27(5):394–402.
6. van Casteren DS, Verhagen IE, Onderwater GL, MaassenVanDenBrink A, Terwindt GM. Sex differences in prevalence of migraine trigger factors: a cross-sectional study. Cephalalgia Int J Headache. 2021;41(6):643–8.
7. Aurora SK, Wilkinson F. The brain is hyperexcitable in migraine. Cephalalgia Int J Headache. 2007;27(12):1442–53.
8. Onderwater GLJ, van Oosterhout WPJ, Schoonman GG, Ferrari MD, Terwindt GM. Alcoholic beverages as trigger factor and the effect on alcohol consumption behavior in patients with migraine. Eur J Neurol. 2019;26(4):588–95.
9. Ferrari M, Haan J, Charles A, Dodick D, Sakai F. Oxford textbook of headache syndromes [Internet]. 2020 [cited 2022 Mar 16]. Available from: https://search.ebscohost.com/login.aspx?direct=true&scope=site&db=nlebk&db=nlabk&AN=2431728
10. Rose FC. The history of migraine from Mesopotamian to Medieval times. Cephalalgia Int J Headache. 1995;15(Suppl 15):1–3.
11. Loder E. What is the evolutionary advantage of migraine? Cephalalgia Int J Headache. 2002;22(8):624–32.
12. Gelfand AA, Loder E. Potential benefits of migraine-what is it good for? JAMA Neurol. 2019;76(3):250–1.
13. Yadav RK, Kalita J, Misra UK. A study of triggers of migraine in India. Pain Med Malden Mass. 2010;11(1):44–7.
14. Hindiyeh NA, Zhang N, Farrar M, Banerjee P, Lombard L, Aurora SK. The role of diet and nutrition in migraine triggers and treatment: a systematic literature review. Headache. 2020;60(7):1300–16.
15. Papakonstantinou D, Constantinos T. Workplace productivity loss as a result of absenteeism and presenteeism in chronic and episodic migraine: a scoping review. Int J Workplace Health Manag. 2021;15:38.
16. Steiner TJ, Stovner LJ, Vos T, Jensen R, Katsarava Z. Migraine is first cause of disability in under 50s: will health politicians now take notice? J Headache Pain. 2018;19(1):17.
17. Edvinsson L, Haanes KA. Views on migraine pathophysiology: where does it start? Neurol Clin Neurosci. 2020;8(3):120–7.
18. Goadsby PJ, Holland PR, Martins-Oliveira M, Hoffmann J, Schankin C, Akerman S. Pathophysiology of migraine: a disorder of sensory processing. Physiol Rev. 2017;97(2):553–622.
19. Akerman S, Holland PR, Goadsby PJ. Diencephalic and brainstem mechanisms in migraine. Nat Rev Neurosci. 2011;12(10):570–84.
20. Mulder EJ, Van Baal C, Gaist D, Kallela M, Kaprio J, Svensson DA, et al. Genetic and environmental influences on migraine: a twin study across six countries. Twin Res Off J Int Soc Twin Stud. 2003;6(5):422–31.
21. Karsan N, Goadsby PJ. Imaging the premonitory phase of migraine. Front Neurol. 2020;11:140.
22. de Tommaso M, Vecchio E, Quitadamo SG, Coppola G, Di Renzo A, Parisi V, et al. Pain-related brain connectivity changes in migraine: a narrative review and proof of concept about possible novel treatments interference. Brain Sci. 2021;11(2):234.
23. Holland PR, Barloese M, Fahrenkrug J. PACAP in hypothalamic regulation of sleep and circadian rhythm: importance for headache. J Headache Pain. 2018;19(1):20.
24. Silvestro M, Tessitore A, Caiazzo G, Scotto di Clemente F, Trojsi F, Cirillo M, et al. Disconnectome of the migraine brain: a "connectopathy" model. J Headache Pain. 2021;22(1):102
25. Tu Y, Zeng F, Lan L, Li Z, Maleki N, Liu B, et al. An fMRI-based neural marker for migraine without aura. Neurology. 2020;94(7):e741–51.
26. Andreou AP, Edvinsson L. Mechanisms of migraine as a chronic evolutive condition. J Headache Pain. 2019;20(1):117.
27. Afridi SK, Matharu MS, Lee L, Kaube H, Friston KJ, Frackowiak RSJ, et al. A PET study exploring the laterality of brainstem

activation in migraine using glyceryl trinitrate. Brain J Neurol. 2005;128(Pt 4):932–9.
28. Thomsen LL, Kruuse C, Iversen HK, Olesen J. A nitric oxide donor (nitroglycerin) triggers genuine migraine attacks. Eur J Neurol. 1994;1(1):73–80.
29. Bahra A, Matharu MS, Buchel C, Frackowiak RS, Goadsby PJ. Brainstem activation specific to migraine headache. Lancet Lond Engl. 2001;357(9261):1016–7.
30. Ferrari MD, Goadsby PJ, Burstein R, Kurth T, Ayata C, Charles A, et al. Migraine. Nat Rev Dis Primer. 2022;8(1):2.
31. Rothrock JF. The truth about triggers. Headache. 2008;48(3):499–500.
32. Ibrahimi K, van Oosterhout WPJ, van Dorp W, Danser AHJ, Garrelds IM, Kushner SA, et al. Reduced trigeminovascular cyclicity in patients with menstrually related migraine. Neurology. 2015;84(2):125–31.
33. Ferrari MD, Klever RR, Terwindt GM, Ayata C, van den Maagdenberg AMJM. Migraine pathophysiology: lessons from mouse models and human genetics. Lancet Neurol. 2015;14(1):65–80.
34. Sacco S, Ricci S, Degan D, Carolei A. Migraine in women: the role of hormones and their impact on vascular diseases. J Headache Pain. 2012;13(3):177–89.
35. Vetvik KG, MacGregor EA. Sex differences in the epidemiology, clinical features, and pathophysiology of migraine. Lancet Neurol. 2017;16(1):76–87.
36. Zhang X, Levy D, Kainz V, Noseda R, Jakubowski M, Burstein R. Activation of central trigeminovascular neurons by cortical spreading depression. Ann Neurol. 2011;69(5):855–65.
37. Zhang X, Levy D, Noseda R, Kainz V, Jakubowski M, Burstein R. Activation of meningeal nociceptors by cortical spreading depression: implications for migraine with aura. J Neurosci. 2010;30(26):8807–14.
38. Noseda R, Constandil L, Bourgeais L, Chalus M, Villanueva L. Changes of meningeal excitability mediated by corticotrigeminal networks: a link for the endogenous modulation of migraine pain. J Neurosci. 2010;30(43):14420–9.
39. Brennan KC, Romero Reyes M, López Valdés HE, Arnold AP, Charles AC. Reduced threshold for cortical spreading depression in female mice. Ann Neurol. 2007;61(6):603–6.
40. MacGregor EA. "Menstrual" migraine: towards a definition. Cephalalgia Int J Headache. 1996;16(1):11–21.
41. Krause DN, Warfvinge K, Haanes KA, Edvinsson L. Hormonal influences in migraine – interactions of oestrogen, oxytocin and CGRP. Nat Rev Neurol. 2021;17(10):621–33.
42. Mauskop A, Altura BT, Altura BM. Serum ionized magnesium levels and serum ionized calcium/ionized magnesium ratios in women with menstrual migraine. Headache. 2002;42(4):242–8.
43. Ierusalimschy R, Moreira Filho PF. Precipitating factors of migraine attacks in patients with migraine without aura. Arq Neuropsiquiatr. 2002;60(3-A):609–13.
44. Coppola G, Di Lorenzo C, Schoenen J, Pierelli F. Habituation and sensitization in primary headaches. J Headache Pain. 2013;14:65.
45. Brighina F, Palermo A, Fierro B. Cortical inhibition and habituation to evoked potentials: relevance for pathophysiology of migraine. J Headache Pain. 2009;10(2):77–84.
46. Stankewitz A, May A. Increased limbic and brainstem activity during migraine attacks following olfactory stimulation. Neurology. 2011;77(5):476–82.
47. Huang J, Zhu DC. Visually stressful striped patterns alter human visual cortical functional connectivity. Hum Brain Mapp. 2017;38(11):5474–84.
48. Chong CD, Starling AJ, Schwedt TJ. Interictal photosensitivity associates with altered brain structure in patients with episodic migraine. Cephalalgia. 2016;36(6):526–33.
49. Meylakh N, Henderson LA. Exploring alterations in sensory pathways in migraine. J Headache Pain. 2022;23(1):5.
50. Bigal ME, Lipton RB. Migraine chronification. Curr Neurol Neurosci Rep. 2011;11(2):139–48.
51. Kaufmann D, Brennan KC. The effects of chronic stress on migraine relevant phenotypes in male mice. Front Cell Neurosci. 2018;12:294.
52. Schulte LH, Menz MM, Haaker J, May A. The migraineur's brain networks: continuous resting state fMRI over 30 days. Cephalalgia Int J Headache. 2020;40(14):1614–21.
53. Lipton RB, Buse DC, Hall CB, Tennen H, Defreitas TA, Borkowski TM, et al. Reduction in perceived stress as a migraine trigger: testing the "let-down headache" hypothesis. Neurology. 2014;82(16):1395–401.
54. Dodick DW, Eross EJ, Parish JM, Silber M. Clinical, anatomical, and physiologic relationship between sleep and headache. Headache. 2003;43(3):282–92.
55. Freedom T, Evans RW. Headache and sleep. Headache. 2013;53(8):1358–66.
56. Vgontzas A, Pavlović JM. Sleep disorders and migraine: review of literature and potential pathophysiology mechanisms. Headache. 2018;58(7):1030–9.
57. Martin VT, Vij B. Diet and headache: part 2. Headache. 2016;56(9):1553–62.
58. Marmura MJ. Triggers, protectors, and predictors in episodic migraine. Curr Pain Headache Rep. 2018;22(12):81.
59. Maniyar FH, Sprenger T, Monteith T, Schankin C, Goadsby PJ. Brain activations in the premonitory phase of nitroglycerin-triggered migraine attacks. Brain J Neurol. 2014;137(Pt 1):232–41.
60. Schulte LH, May A. The migraine generator revisited: continuous scanning of the migraine cycle over 30 days and three spontaneous attacks. Brain J Neurol. 2016;139(Pt 7):1987–93.
61. Karsan N, Goadsby PJ. Biological insights from the premonitory symptoms of migraine. Nat Rev Neurol. 2018;14(12):699–710.
62. Barbanti P, Fofi L, Aurilia C, Egeo G. Dopaminergic symptoms in migraine. Neurol Sci Off J Ital Neurol Soc Ital Soc Clin Neurophysiol. 2013;34(Suppl 1):S67–70.
63. Giffin NJ, Ruggiero L, Lipton RB, Silberstein SD, Tvedskov JF, Olesen J, et al. Premonitory symptoms in migraine: an electronic diary study. Neurology. 2003;60(6):935–40.
64. Waelkens J. Domperidone in the prevention of complete classical migraine. Br Med J Clin Res Ed. 1982;284(6320):944.
65. Schulte LH, Jürgens TP, May A. Photo-, osmo- and phonophobia in the premonitory phase of migraine: mistaking symptoms for triggers? J Headache Pain. 2015;16:14.
66. Martin VT, Vij B. Diet and Headache: Part 1. Headache. 2016;56(9):1543–52.
67. Allais G, Chiarle G, Sinigaglia S, Airola G, Schiapparelli P, Benedetto C. Gender-related differences in migraine. Neurol Sci Off J Ital Neurol Soc Ital Soc Clin Neurophysiol. 2020;41(Suppl 2):429–36.
68. Stewart WF, Wood C, Reed ML, Roy J, Lipton RB, AMPP Advisory Group. Cumulative lifetime migraine incidence in women and men. Cephalalgia Int J Headache. 2008;28(11):1170–8.
69. Victor TW, Hu X, Campbell JC, Buse DC, Lipton RB. Migraine prevalence by age and sex in the United States: a life-span study. Cephalalgia Int J Headache. 2010;30(9):1065–72.
70. Maasumi K, Tepper SJ, Kriegler JS. Menstrual migraine and treatment options: review. Headache. 2017;57(2):194–208.
71. Andress-Rothrock D, King W, Rothrock J. An analysis of migraine triggers in a clinic-based population. Headache. 2010;50(8):1366–70.
72. MacGregor EA, Victor TW, Hu X, Xiang Q, Puenpatom RA, Chen W, et al. Characteristics of menstrual vs nonmenstrual migraine: a post hoc, within-woman analysis of the usual-care phase of a

nonrandomized menstrual migraine clinical trial. Headache. 2010;50(4):528–38.
73. Stewart WF, Lipton RB, Chee E, Sawyer J, Silberstein SD. Menstrual cycle and headache in a population sample of migraineurs. Neurology. 2000;55(10):1517–23.
74. Silberstein SD, Massiou H, McCarroll KA, Lines CR. Further evaluation of rizatriptan in menstrual migraine: retrospective analysis of long-term data. Headache. 2002;42(9):917–23.
75. Mäki K, Vahtera J, Virtanen M, Elovainio M, Keltikangas-Järvinen L, Kivimäki M. Work stress and new-onset migraine in a female employee population. Cephalalgia Int J Headache. 2008;28(1):18–25.
76. Chabriat H, Danchot J, Michel P, Joire JE, Henry P. Precipitating factors of headache. A prospective study in a national control-matched survey in migraineurs and nonmigraineurs. Headache. 1999;39(5):335–8.
77. Schoonman GG, Evers DJ, Ballieux BE, de Geus EJ, de Kloet ER, Terwindt GM, et al. Is stress a trigger factor for migraine? Psychoneuroendocrinology. 2007;32(5):532–8.
78. Hung CI, Liu CY, Wang SJ. Precipitating or aggravating factors for headache in patients with major depressive disorder. J Psychosom Res. 2008;64(2):231–5.
79. Sauro KM, Becker WJ. The stress and migraine interaction. Headache. 2009;49(9):1378–86.
80. Holroyd KA, Drew JB. Behavioral approaches to the treatment of migraine. Semin Neurol. 2006;26(2):199–207.
81. Kelman L, Rains JC. Headache and sleep: examination of sleep patterns and complaints in a large clinical sample of migraineurs. Headache. 2005;45(7):904–10.
82. Giffin NJ, Lipton RB, Silberstein SD, Olesen J, Goadsby PJ. The migraine postdrome: an electronic diary study. Neurology. 2016;87(3):309–13.
83. Alstadhaug K, Salvesen R, Bekkelund S. Insomnia and circadian variation of attacks in episodic migraine. Headache. 2007;47(8):1184–8.
84. Nayak C, Sinha S, Nagappa M, Nagaraj K, Kulkarni GB, Thennarasu K, et al. Study of sleep microstructure in patients of migraine without aura. Sleep Breath Schlaf Atm. 2016;20(1):263–9.
85. Zhu Z, Fan X, Li X, Tan G, Chen L, Zhou J. Prevalence and predictive factors for poor sleep quality among migraineurs in a tertiary hospital headache clinic. Acta Neurol Belg. 2013;113(3):229–35.
86. Bruni O, Russo PM, Violani C, Guidetti V. Sleep and migraine: an actigraphic study. Cephalalgia Int J Headache. 2004;24(2):134–9.
87. Leso V, Gervetti P, Mauro S, Macrini MC, Ercolano ML, Iavicoli I. Shift work and migraine: a systematic review. J Occup Health. 2020;62(1):e12116.
88. Sandoe CH, Sasikumar S, Lay C, Lawler V. The impact of shift work on migraine: a case series and narrative review. Headache. 2019;59(9):1631–40.
89. Smitherman TA, Walters AB, Davis RE, Ambrose CE, Roland M, Houle TT, et al. Randomized controlled pilot trial of behavioral insomnia treatment for chronic migraine with comorbid insomnia. Headache. 2016;56(2):276–91.
90. Henderson WR, Raskin NH. "Hot-dog" headache: individual susceptibility to nitrite. Lancet Lond Engl. 1972;2(7788):1162–3.
91. Cornwell N, Clarke L. Dietary modification in patients with migraine and tension-type heacache. Cephalalgia. 1991;11(11_suppl):143–4.
92. Sun-Edelstein C, Mauskop A. Foods and supplements in the management of migraine headaches. Clin J Pain. 2009;25(5):446–52.
93. Hoffmann J, Recober A. Migraine and triggers: post hoc ergo propter hoc? Curr Pain Headache Rep. 2013;17(10):370.
94. Finocchi C, Sivori G. Food as trigger and aggravating factor of migraine. Neurol Sci Off J Ital Neurol Soc Ital Soc Clin Neurophysiol. 2012;33(Suppl 1):S77–80.
95. Park JW, Chu MK, Kim JM, Park SG, Cho SJ. Analysis of trigger factors in episodic migraineurs using a smartphone headache diary applications. PLoS One. 2016;11(2):e0149577.
96. Mollaoğlu M. Trigger factors in migraine patients. J Health Psychol. 2013;18(7):984–94.
97. Wöber C, Brannath W, Schmidt K, Kapitan M, Rudel E, Wessely P, et al. Prospective analysis of factors related to migraine attacks: the PAMINA study. Cephalalgia Int J Headache. 2007;27(4):304–14.
98. Martin PR. Behavioral management of migraine headache triggers: learning to cope with triggers. Curr Pain Headache Rep. 2010;14(3):221–7.
99. Karsan N, Bose P, Newman J, Goadsby PJ. Are some patient-perceived migraine triggers simply early manifestations of the attack? J Neurol. 2021;268(5):1885–93.
100. Nowaczewska M, Wiciński M, Kaźmierczak W, Kaźmierczak H. To eat or not to eat: a review of the relationship between chocolate and migraines. Nutrients. 2020;12(3):608.
101. Abu-Salameh I, Plakht Y, Ifergane G. Migraine exacerbation during Ramadan fasting. J Headache Pain. 2010;11(6):513–7.
102. Al-Shimmery EK. Precipitating and relieving factors of migraine headache in 200 iraqi kurdish patients. Oman Med J. 2010;25(3):212–7.
103. Nazari F, Safavi M, Mahmudi M. Migraine and its relation with lifestyle in women. Pain Pract Off J World Inst Pain. 2010;10(3):228–34.
104. Özön AÖ, Karadaş Ö, Özge A. Efficacy of diet restriction on migraines. Noro Psikiyatr Ars. 2018;55(3):233–7.
105. Alpay K, Ertas M, Orhan EK, Ustay DK, Lieners C, Baykan B. Diet restriction in migraine, based on IgG against foods: a clinical double-blind, randomised, cross-over trial. Cephalalgia Int J Headache. 2010;30(7):829–37.
106. Bongiovanni D, Benedetto C, Corvisieri S, Del Favero C, Orlandi F, Allais G, et al. Effectiveness of ketogenic diet in treatment of patients with refractory chronic migraine. Neurol Sci Off J Ital Neurol Soc Ital Soc Clin Neurophysiol. 2021;42(9):3865–70.
107. Koppen H, van Veldhoven PLJ. Migraineurs with exercise-triggered attacks have a distinct migraine. J Headache Pain. 2013;14:99.
108. Martins IP, Gouveia RG, Parreira E. Kinesiophobia in migraine. J Pain. 2006;7(6):445–51.
109. Lemmens J, De Pauw J, Van Soom T, Michiels S, Versijpt J, van Breda E, et al. The effect of aerobic exercise on the number of migraine days, duration and pain intensity in migraine: a systematic literature review and meta-analysis. J Headache Pain. 2019;20(1):16.
110. Machado-Oliveira L, da Silva Gauto YO, de Santana Neto FJ, da Silva MG, Germano-Soares AH, Diniz PRB. Effects of different exercise intensities on headache: a systematic review. Am J Phys Med Rehabil. 2020;99(5):390–6.
111. Barber M, Pace A. Exercise and migraine prevention: a review of the literature. Curr Pain Headache Rep. 2020;24(8):39.
112. Varkey E, Cider A, Carlsson J, Linde M. Exercise as migraine prophylaxis: a randomized study using relaxation and topiramate as controls. Cephalalgia Int J Headache. 2011;31(14):1428–38.
113. Scharff L, Turk DC, Marcus DA. Triggers of headache episodes and coping responses of headache diagnostic groups. Headache. 1995;35(7):397–403.
114. Irby MB, Bond DS, Lipton RB, Nicklas B, Houle TT, Penzien DB. Aerobic exercise for reducing migraine burden: mechanisms, markers, and models of change processes. Headache. 2016;56(2):357–69.
115. Hoffmann J, Lo H, Neeb L, Martus P, Reuter U. Weather sensitivity in migraineurs. J Neurol. 2011;258(4):596–602.
116. Zebenholzer K, Rudel E, Frantal S, Brannath W, Schmidt K, Wöber-Bingöl C, et al. Migraine and weather: a prospective diary-based analysis. Cephalalgia Int J Headache. 2011;31(4):391–400.

117. Villeneuve PJ, Szyszkowicz M, Stieb D, Bourque DA. Weather and emergency room visits for migraine headaches in Ottawa. Canada Headache. 2006;46(1):64–72.
118. Buse DC, Reed ML, Fanning KM, Bostic R, Dodick DW, Schwedt TJ, et al. Comorbid and co-occurring conditions in migraine and associated risk of increasing headache pain intensity and headache frequency: results of the migraine in America symptoms and treatment (MAST) study. J Headache Pain. 2020;21(1):23.
119. Bektas H, Karabulut H, Doganay B, Acar B. Allergens might trigger migraine attacks. Acta Neurol Belg. 2017;117(1):91–5.
120. Levy D, Burstein R, Strassman AM. Mast cell involvement in the pathophysiology of migraine headache: a hypothesis. Headache. 2006;46(Suppl 1):S13–8.
121. Hunter JO. Food elimination in IBS: the case for IgG testing remains doubtful. Gut. 2005;54(8):1203. author reply 1203
122. Lavine E. Blood testing for sensitivity, allergy or intolerance to food. CMAJ Can Med Assoc J J Assoc Medicale Can. 2012;184(6):666–8.
123. Elser H, Morello-Frosch R, Jacobson A, Pressman A, Kioumourtzoglou MA, Reimer R, et al. Air pollution, methane super-emitters, and oil and gas wells in Northern California: the relationship with migraine headache prevalence and exacerbation. Environ Health Glob Access Sci Source. 2021;20(1):45.
124. Rausch JL, Fefferman M, Ladisich-Rogers DG, Menard M. Effect of nicotine on human blood platelet serotonin uptake and efflux. Prog Neuro-Psychopharmacol Biol Psychiatry. 1989;13(6):907–16.
125. Anderson KL, Pinkerton KE, Uyeminami D, Simons CT, Carstens MI, Carstens E. Antinociception induced by chronic exposure of rats to cigarette smoke. Neurosci Lett. 2004;366(1):86–91.
126. Taylor FR. Tobacco, Nicotine, and Headache. Headache. 2015;55(7):1028–44.
127. Iribarren C, Friedman GD, Klatsky AL, Eisner MD. Exposure to environmental tobacco smoke: association with personal characteristics and self reported health conditions. J Epidemiol Community Health. 2001;55(10):721–8.
128. Caroli A, Klan T, Gaul C, Kubik SU, Martin PR, Witthöft M. Types of triggers in migraine – factor structure of the Headache Triggers Sensitivity and Avoidance Questionnaire and Development of a New Short Form (HTSAQ-SF). Headache. 2020;60(9):1920–9.
129. Goadsby PJ, Constantin L, Ebel-Bitoun C, Igracki Turudic I, Hitier S, Amand-Bourdon C, et al. Multinational descriptive analysis of the real-world burden of headache using the Migraine Buddy application. Eur J Neurol. 2021;28(12):4184–93.
130. Vo P, Paris N, Bilitou A, Valena T, Fang J, Naujoks C, et al. Burden of migraine in Europe using self-reported digital diary data from the Migraine Buddy© application. Neurol Ther. 2018;7(2):321–32.
131. Vives-Mestres M, Casanova A. Modeling and visualizing two-way contingency tables using compositional data analysis: a case-study on individual self-prediction of migraine days. Stat Med. 2021;40(2):213–25.
132. Minen MT, Jaran J, Boyers T, Corner S. Understanding what people with migraine consider to be important features of migraine tracking: an analysis of the utilization of smartphone-based migraine tracking with a free-text feature. Headache. 2020;60(7):1402–14.
133. Spierings ELH, Donoghue S, Mian A, Wöber C. Sufficiency and necessity in migraine: how do we figure out if triggers are absolute or partial and, if partial, additive or potentiating? Curr Pain Headache Rep. 2014;18(10):455.
134. Peris F, Donoghue S, Torres F, Mian A, Wöber C. Towards improved migraine management: determining potential trigger factors in individual patients. Cephalalgia Int J Headache. 2017;37(5):452–63.
135. Seng EK, Prieto P, Boucher G, Vives-Mestres M. Anxiety, incentives, and adherence to self-monitoring on a mobile health platform: a naturalistic longitudinal cohort study in people with headache. Headache. 2018;58(10):1541–55.
136. Minen MT, Stieglitz EJ, Sciortino R, Torous J. Privacy issues in smartphone applications: an analysis of headache/migraine applications. Headache. 2018;58(7):1014–27.
137. Martin PR. Headache triggers: to avoid or not to avoid, that is the question. Psychol Health. 2000;15(6):801–9.
138. Martin PR, Reece J, Forsyth M. Noise as a trigger for headaches: relationship between exposure and sensitivity. Headache. 2006;46(6):962–72.
139. Schulman EA, Silberstein SD. Symptomatic and prophylactic treatment of migraine and tension-type headache. Neurology. 1992;42(3 Suppl 2):16–21.
140. Skaer TL. Clinical presentation and treatment of migraine. Clin Ther. 1996;18(2):229–45. discussion 228
141. Martin PR. Managing headache triggers: think "coping" not "avoidance". Cephalalgia Int J Headache. 2010;30(5):634–7.
142. Martin PR, Reece J, Callan M, MacLeod C, Kaur A, Gregg K, et al. Behavioral management of the triggers of recurrent headache: a randomized controlled trial. Behav Res Ther. 2014;61:1–11.
143. Turner DP, Lebowitz AD, Chtay I, Houle TT. Headache triggers as surprise. Headache. 2019;59(4):495–508.
144. Wöber C, Wöber-Bingöl C. Triggers of migraine and tension-type headache. Handb Clin Neurol. 2010;97:161–72.
145. Victorino CC, Gauthier AH. The social determinants of child health: variations across health outcomes – a population-based cross-sectional analysis. BMC Pediatr. 2009;9:53.
146. Woldeamanuel YW, Cowan RP. The impact of regular lifestyle behavior in migraine: a prevalence case-referent study. J Neurol. 2016;263(4):669–76.
147. Askarpour M, Yarizadeh H, Sheikhi A, Khorsha F, Mirzaei K. Associations between adherence to MIND diet and severity, duration and frequency of migraine headaches among migraine patients. BMC Res Notes. 2020;13(1):341.
148. Song TJ, Chu MK. Exercise in treatment of migraine including chronic migraine. Curr Pain Headache Rep. 2021;25(3):14.
149. Duman T, Dede ÖH, Uluduz D, Seydaoğlu G, Okuyucu E, Melek İ. Sleep changes during prophylactic treatment of migraine. Ann Indian Acad Neurol. 2015;18(3):298–302.
150. Ornish. Dean. Dr. dean ornish's program for reversing heart disease [Internet]. New York: Ivy Books; 2014 [cited 2022 Mar 16]. Available from: http://rbdigital.oneclickdigital.com
151. Merlo G, Vela A. Mental health in lifestyle medicine: a call to action. Am J Lifestyle Med. 2022;16(1):7–20.
152. Giannini G, Zanigni S, Grimaldi D, Melotti R, Pierangeli G, Cortelli P, et al. Cephalalgiaphobia as a feature of high-frequency migraine: a pilot study. J Headache Pain. 2013;14:49.
153. Zivadinov R, Willheim K, Sepic-Grahovac D, Jurjevic A, Bucuk M, Brnabic-Razmilic O, et al. Migraine and tension-type headache in Croatia: a population-based survey of precipitating factors. Cephalalgia Int J Headache. 2003;23(5):336–43.
154. Robblee J, Starling AJ. SEEDS for success: lifestyle management in migraine. Cleve Clin J Med. 2019;86(11):741–9.
155. Grazzi L, Andrasik F. Non-pharmacological approaches in migraine prophylaxis: behavioral medicine. Neurol Sci Off J Ital Neurol Soc Ital Soc Clin Neurophysiol. 2010;31(Suppl 1):S133–5.
156. Vives-Mestres M, Casanova A, Buse DC, Donoghue S, Houle TT, Lipton RB, et al. Patterns of perceived stress throughout the migraine cycle: a longitudinal cohort study using daily prospective diary data. Headache. 2021;61(1):90–102.
157. Deniz O, Aygül R, Koçak N, Orhan A, Kaya MD. Precipitating factors of migraine attacks in patients with migraine with and without aura. Pain Clin. 2004;16(4):451–6.
158. Spierings EL, Ranke AH, Honkoop PC. Precipitating and aggravating factors of migraine versus tension-type headache. Headache. 2001;41(6):554–8.

159. Dexter JD, Roberts J, Byer JA. The five hour glucose tolerance test and effect of low sucrose diet in migraine. Headache. 1978;18(2):91–4.
160. Turner DP, Smitherman TA, Penzien DB, Porter JAH, Martin VT, Houle TT. Nighttime snacking, stress, and migraine activity. J Clin Neurosci Off J Neurosurg Soc Australas. 2014;21(4):638–43.
161. Seo JG, Park SP. Significance of fatigue in patients with migraine. J Clin Neurosci Off J Neurosurg Soc Australas. 2018;50:69–73.
162. Karli N, Zarifoglu M, Calisir N, Akgoz S. Comparison of pre-headache phases and trigger factors of migraine and episodic tension-type headache: do they share similar clinical pathophysiology? Cephalalgia Int J Headache. 2005;25(6):444–51.
163. Fukui PT, Gonçalves TRT, Strabelli CG, Lucchino NMF, Matos FC, dos Santos JPM, et al. Trigger factors in migraine patients. Arq Neuropsiquiatr. 2008;66(3A):494–9.
164. Calhoun AH, Ford S. Behavioral sleep modification may revert transformed migraine to episodic migraine. Headache. 2007;47(8):1178–83.
165. Lane JC, Gulevich S. Exertional, cough, and sexual headaches. Curr Treat Options Neurol. 2002;4(5):375–81.
166. Friedman DI, De ver Dye T. Migraine and the environment. Headache. 2009;49(6):941–52.
167. Hambach A, Evers S, Summ O, Husstedt IW, Frese A. The impact of sexual activity on idiopathic headaches: an observational study. Cephalalgia Int J Headache. 2013;33(6):384–9.
168. Ansari T, Lagman-Bartolome AM, Monsour D, Lay C. Management of menstrual migraine. Curr Neurol Neurosci Rep. 2020;20(10):45.
169. Tatsumoto M, Eda T, Ishikawa T, Ayama M, Hirata K. Light of intrinsically photosensitive retinal ganglion cell (ipRGC) causing migraine headache exacerbation. Cephalalgia. 2013;1(2):33.
170. Noseda R, Kainz V, Jakubowski M, Gooley JJ, Saper CB, Digre K, et al. A neural mechanism for exacerbation of headache by light. Nat Neurosci. 2010;13(2):239–45.
171. Wilkins AJ, Nimmo-Smith I, Slater AI, Bedocs L. Fluorescent lighting, headaches and eyestrain. Light Res Technol. 1989;21(1):11–8.
172. Good PA, Taylor RH, Mortimer MJ. The use of tinted glasses in childhood migraine. Headache. 1991;31(8):533–6.
173. Tepper SJ, Silberstein SD, Rosen NL, Lipton RB, Dennehy EB, Dowsett SA, et al. The influence of migraine on driving: current understanding, future directions, and potential implications of findings. Headache. 2020;60(1):178–89.
174. Kimoto K, Aiba S, Takashima R, Suzuki K, Takekawa H, Watanabe Y, et al. Influence of barometric pressure in patients with migraine headache. Intern Med Tokyo Jpn. 2011;50(18):1923–8.
175. Mostofsky E, Mittleman MA, Buettner C, Li W, Bertisch SM. Prospective cohort study of caffeinated beverage intake as a potential trigger of headaches among migraineurs. Am J Med. 2019;132(8):984–91.
176. Nowaczewska M, Wiciński M, Kaźmierczak W. The ambiguous role of caffeine in migraine headache: from trigger to treatment. Nutrients. 2020;12(8):E2259.
177. Alstadhaug KB, Andreou AP. Caffeine and primary (migraine) headaches-friend or foe? Front Neurol. 2019;10:1275.
178. Alstadhaug KB, Ofte HK, Müller KI, Andreou AP. Sudden caffeine withdrawal triggers migraine – a randomized controlled trial. Front Neurol. 2020;11:1002.
179. Evans J, Richards J, Battisti A. Caffeine [Internet]. StatPearls; 2021. Available from: https://www.ncbi.nlm.nih.gov/books/NBK519490/
180. Panconesi A, Bartolozzi ML, Guidi L. Alcohol and migraine: what should we tell patients? Curr Pain Headache Rep. 2011;15(3):177–84.
181. Blau JN, Thavapalan M. Preventing migraine: a study of precipitating factors. Headache. 1988;28(7):481–3.

Sleep and Migraine

19

Angeliki Vgontzas

Introduction

Sleep disturbances are commonly reported by patients with migraine and present a clinical conundrum. Although some patients are diagnosed with a treatable sleep disorder, such as obstructive sleep apnea (OSA), others experience sleep disturbances likely interrelated with migraine (i.e., insomnia symptoms). The prevalence of sleep complaints and disorders is higher in those with greater headache burden, which suggests poor sleep may lead to chronification of migraine. Awareness of other conditions that cause nocturnal headaches such as cluster headaches, hypnic headaches, and secondary headaches associated with increased intracranial pressure is important but beyond the scope of this chapter.

Questions

1. Which of the following treatment strategies for insomnia are strongly supported by guidelines from the American Academy of Sleep Medicine and should be considered in patients with migraine and comorbid insomnia?
   A. Cognitive behavioral therapy for insomnia (CBT-I).
   B. Sleep hygiene.
   C. Melatonin 3–5 mg QHS.
   D. A and B.
   E. A, B, and C.
2. Which of the following statements regarding migraine and obstructive sleep apnea (OSA) is most accurate based on available evidence?
   A. Rates of OSA are higher in those with migraine and its treatment may improve headache frequency.
   B. Rates of OSA are higher in those with migraine but it is unknown whether treatment of OSA improves headache frequency.
   C. Rates of OSA are higher in those with chronic migraine and this is explained by comorbid obesity.
   D. Rates of snoring are higher in those with migraine but not diagnosed with OSA.
   E. There is no evidence to support that those with migraine are at higher risk of OSA than those without migraine.

What Is Sleep?

Sleep is a *reversible behavioral state or relative perceptual disengagement from and unresponsiveness to the environment* to which humans dedicate one-third of their lives [1]. Inadequate sleep duration is associated with worse cognitive performance, mood disorders, cardiovascular disease, and increased mortality [2, 3]. Other sleep parameters, such as sleep continuity, timing, and satisfaction/quality, also significantly impact health [4]. Good sleep is essential to well-being, and sleep complaints deserve clinical attention.

How Do We Assess Sleep?

This "complex amalgam of physiologic and behavioral processes" is assessed by clinical interviews, validated questionnaires, polysomnography (PSG), and actigraphy [1]. The clinical interview includes information on sleep/wake patterns, settings in which the symptoms occur, and bed partner's observations [5]. Because sleep complaints may be manifestations of other disorders (i.e., pulmonary, neurologic, and psychiatric), a general medical and psychiatric screen is often appropriate [6]. Validated questionnaires are widely used in clinical and research assessments of sleep dis-

A. Vgontzas (✉)
Department of Neurology, Brigham and Women's Hospital, Boston, MA, USA

T. S. Monteith et al. (eds.), *Comprehensive Migraine Management*, https://doi.org/10.1007/978-3-031-86923-5_19

Table 19.1 Sleep stages, EEG activity, and clinical correlates

Sleep stage	EEG activity/clinical correlate
Non-rapid eye movement (NREM)	
N1	EEG slows down from waking into this low-voltage, mixed-frequency wave stage
	Spend 1–7 min in the first cycle
	2–5% of total sleep
	Easily awoken from this stage of "light sleep"
N2	Typically follows N1, characterized by spindles and K complexes
	10–25 min in the first cycle
	45–55% of sleep
	Density of sleep spindles may be important for memory consolidation
N3	Characterized by delta waves, aka slow wave sleep or "restorative sleep"
	13–23% of sleep
	Lasts 20–45 min in the first cycle
REM sleep	Period of increased cortical activity and decreased tone of peripheral muscles (aside from the eyes)
	Last 1–5 min during the first cycle; longer in subsequent cycles
	20–25% of sleep
	Dreaming

orders (i.e., STOP-BANG screener for obstructive sleep apnea) or evaluate multi-dimensional sleep parameters (i.e., the Pittsburgh Sleep Quality Index) [7–10]. Sleep complaints may be prospectively tracked via validated daily diaries, where participants report on sleep parameters, daily activities, and sedating/stimulating substance intake. Polysomnography is the gold-standard objective measure of sleep and captures sleep stages (see Table 19.1). Actigraphy detects sleep parameters (i.e., duration and efficiency) by tracking arm movements in the naturalistic setting [11] but is less accurate in sleep continuity parameters than polysomnography [12].

Baseline Self-Reports

Adults and children with migraine report increased sleep complaints compared to those without migraine including difficulty falling and staying asleep, poor sleep quality, and lack of refreshment after sleep [13–23]. The MAST study of the US population reported that insomnia was the number one comorbidity associated with migraine [24]. Such findings are slightly attenuated but still significant when controlling for comorbid anxiety and depression [21, 25]. Sleep disturbances and poor sleep are more commonly reported in those with chronic rather than episodic migraine [15, 25–27] and for those with high-frequency rather than low-frequency episodic migraine [28], suggesting that sleep may be a marker of chronification.

Limited studies have investigated the time period over which sleep-migraine associations develop and the potential modifying effect of stress. Poor quality sleep (PSQI≥5) was associated with higher headache frequency over the following 6 weeks in a prospective cohort of adults with episodic migraine, and this was further worsened by moderate/high baseline scores of perceived stress [29]. Perceived stress is also a reported immediate precedent to headache days in those with episodic migraine [30] and, along with poor sleep, influences headache severity in those with chronic migraine [31, 32]. The exact timing of this relationship may be more nuanced; however, high stress may precede migraine by more than one day [31–33]. The relationship between sleep complaints and migraine over a longer time interval is not known, but the bidirectional risk between episodic migraine and incident clinical depression over a longer period (8–14 years) suggests that insomnia may also have a longer term influence [34, 35]. Longitudinal studies of migraine patients, incorporating measures of stress, sleep, and mood disorders, may provide insight into the now well-established cross-sectional reports on poor sleep quality [36].

Interindividual PSG Studies of Migraine (Interictal)

Polysomnography studies of patients with migraine [16, 18, 37–42] are of interest given that poor sleep may be a part of the migraine endophenotype but have been limited by design heterogeneity and small samples. A meta-analysis examining PSG studies in adults and children reported a modestly lower percentage of REM sleep in those with migraine versus controls in both adults and children [36]. The isolated finding of lower REM sleep in adults with migraine is difficult to interpret given the inclusion of patients across many life decades over which % of REM sleep is expected to change and the varying frequency of migraine. The more robust differences in the PSG of pediatric migraine patients (less total sleep time, more time awake at night, and shorter sleep latency) in addition to lower percentage of REM sleep is more convincing of a poor sleep endophenotype [36].

Studies Across the Migraine Attack

Retrospective studies report that along with stress, sleep changes are the most commonly identified migraine trigger [43]. Furthermore, two-thirds of patients report occasional headaches upon awakening [15, 22, 44, 45] with the frequency of early morning attacks increasing with age [46]. Early sleep changes may represent prodromal symptoms and, perhaps, early hypothalamic and brainstem activation [47, 48]. Inherently challenging PSG studies have reported increased awakenings and decreased amounts of slow-wave sleep in the nights before an attack in those with sleep-related attacks or morning attacks, without clear differences in sleep latency or total sleep time [16, 42]. A 6-week actigraphy study did not find differences in sleep duration, quality, and sleep latency the night before a migraine attack but did report lower sleep efficiency two nights prior to a migraine attack [49]. In those with chronic migraine, day-to-day variations in perceived stress may interact with poor sleep to confer migraine risk 2 days later [31]. Together, these studies suggest that decreased sleep efficiency may precede headache by several days, may differ by migraine subtype (episodic vs. chronic), and may be related to stress.

Sleep Disorders and Migraine

The comorbidity of sleep disorders and migraine has been previously reviewed [50] and is briefly summarized here for the most common sleep disorders (see Table 19.2).

Insomnia

Insomnia is defined as difficulty with sleep initiation or maintenance with daytime consequences despite adequate opportunity and circumstances to sleep [51]. It is the most prevalent sleep complaint, with approximately one-third of the population reporting an insomnia symptom [52] and 6% of the general population meeting a chronic insomnia diagnosis (insomnia 3x/week for 3 months or longer) [53]. Clinical samples of patients with chronic headaches (including chronic migraine, chronic tension-type headaches, and medication overuse headaches) reveal a high percentage of patients meeting ICSD criteria for co-occurring insomnia (67%) [54]. Rates for those not treated in specialized care clinics are unknown.

Obstructive Sleep Apnea (OSA)

Population-based studies have reported that adults with migraine report higher rates of snoring and are at higher risk for OSA (more so for chronic migraine) [25, 55] but have not reported increased rates of PSG-diagnosed OSA [41]. These apparent mixed results may be due to lower prevalence of OSA risk factors in general migraine populations (male sex, age >55). There is likely a subset of patients with migraine at higher risk for OSA (such as those with comorbid obesity) which should be considered to help differentiate the need for OSA evaluation.

Sleep-Related Bruxism

The correlation of bruxism with temporomandibular joint dysfunction (TMD), known to be comorbid with migraine, makes it a frequent anecdotal clinical observation [56]. Although most studies of sleep bruxism have not phenotyped headache, [57] one study in an orofacial pain clinic utilizing ICHD criteria found that sleep bruxism was associated with a diagnosis of chronic migraine, with a trend toward episodic

Table 19.2 International classification of sleep disorders-3 diagnostic criteria description and their association with migraine

Sleep disorder	ICSD-3 diagnostic criteria description	Association with migraine
Chronic insomnia	Difficulty with sleep initiation or maintenance with daytime consequences despite adequate opportunity and circumstances to sleep; occurs ≥3 times per week 3 months	Frequently report insomnia complaints 2/3 of patients with chronic headache disorders in clinical samples meet ICSD criteria for insomnia (67%) [54]
Obstructive sleep apnea	Signs/symptoms of sleep apnea (i.e., sleepiness, snoring, observed apnea) or an associated medical or psychiatric disorder (i.e., hypertension) coupled with five or more obstructive respiratory events per hour of sleep during PSG (i.e., AHI ≥ 5) or in absence of associated symptoms or disorders, AHI ≥ 15	Higher rates of snoring and higher risk for OSA on screeners (more so for chronic migraine) [25, 55] Rates of OSA, as diagnosed by polysomnography, not increased in a population-based study [41] Comorbid obesity may confer increased risk
Restless legs syndrome (RLS)	An urge to move the legs that primarily occurs in the evening with rest and is relieved by movement. Must be associated with distress, sleep disturbance, or impairment	The majority of 24 studies report an increased risk of RLS in those with migraine The effect size is much higher in case-control studies (approximately 4× higher in those with migraine than in controls) [62]
Sleep-related bruxism	Teeth grinding or clenching associated with an excessive sleep arousal activity	Frequent complaint Correlates with temporomandibular joint dysfunction (TMD) Prevalence rates are limited as headache type has not been well-characterized

migraine [58]. Small randomized controlled clinical trials of amitriptyline and propranolol in those with sleep-related bruxism (without migraine) have not yielded significant improvement in bruxism symptoms, and onabotulinum toxin-A trials have had modest results [59–61].

Restless Legs Syndrome (RLS)

A meta-analysis of 24 studies examining the association between migraine and restless legs syndrome reported that those with migraine have 4x the risk of RLS compared to controls (OR 4.2 (3.1–5.7)) [62]. Certain medications used for migraine management (i.e., antidopaminergic antinausea medications, antihistamines, and medications that increase serotonin) may exacerbate RLS.

Neurobiology of Sleep and Migraine

Neuroscientific evidence supports a shared pathophysiology between migraine and sleep disturbances although there have been limited direct studies linking the two. Key players include shared subcortical structures (such as the hypothalamus), common mediating signaling molecules (neurotransmitters, neuropeptides, and hormones), and the CNS waste removal system, the glymphatic system.

The hypothalamus plays an important role in initiating sleep and wakefulness via a "flip-flop switch," dysfunction of which has been noted in insomnia [63]. In migraine, PET imaging evidence supports early hypothalamic involvement in a migraine attack [48]. It is plausible that early hypothalamic involvement during the migraine prodrome mediates perceived sleep disturbances prior to an attack. Furthermore, neuropeptides under hypothalamic influence may be involved in sleep-migraine pathophysiology. Serotonin (5-HT) generally promotes wakefulness [63] and is released early in a migraine attack [64]—suggesting that serotonin release may contribute to or be a marker of the perception of sleep disturbance as a migraine trigger. Orexin is important for sleep-wakefulness and is elevated in the CSF of those with chronic migraine [65]; however, a randomized controlled trial of an orexin antagonist in humans had negative results [66]. Lastly, pituitary adenylate cyclase-activating peptide (PACAP) has been found to be elevated during migraine attacks [67] and is implicated in the activity of the retinohypothalamic tract in the suprachiasmatic nucleus of the hypothalamus, the "master clock" involved in circadian rhythm [68].

The glymphatic system is primarily active during sleep to remove interstitial waste [69], and cortical spreading depression in mice resulted in temporary impairment of glymphatic flow [70]. However, it is unknown whether chronic sleep disruption or CSD could result in the accumulation of more toxic substances and contribute to disease pathology.

Table 19.3 Suggested high-yield sleep history questions to be included in a migraine assessment

Questions on insomnia:
Do you have difficulty falling or staying asleep at night?
Do you wake up earlier in the morning than you would like?
This may be followed by questions on frequency, impact on daily functioning and screening for mood disorders
Questions screening for obstructive sleep apnea (modified from the STOP-BANG):
Do you snore loudly?
Has anyone observed you stop breathing while you sleep?
Do you feel fatigued or tired during the day?
Clinical suspicion should be higher in those who are obese (especially with BMI >35), older (>50), with hypertension, and male
Questions on sleep timing and regularity
What time do you usually go to sleep and wake?
Does this differ during weekdays and the weekend?

Clinical Evaluation of Sleep Complaints in Those with Migraine

A standardized approach to sleep complaints in those with migraine may help triage the need for referrals or further testing. Table 19.3 contains suggested high-yield questions for adults with migraine, modified from validated screeners [8, 10]. For children aged 2–18 years old, the 5-item BEARS screener, which includes questions on bedtime problems, excessive daytime sleepiness, awakenings during the night, regularity and duration of sleep, and sleep-disordered breathing, is recommended [71].

Considering Sleep in the Treatment of Migraine

The clinical impression is that migraine patients frequently report sleep disturbances and seek advice from their headache specialist or primary care provider. In addition to screening for sleep disorders, the next section provides clinical suggestions based on current available evidence. Please see Table 19.4.

Choosing a Preventive Migraine Medication

A preventive migraine medication is often selected based on attempts to address (or at least not exacerbate) comorbid symptomatology. For migraine patients with insomnia symptoms, consideration should be given in preventive medication selection.

Table 19.4 Considering insomnia in preventive medication choice

Category	Medication	Use in migraine	Influence on sleep
Tricyclic antidepressants	Amitriptyline	Low doses of 10–20 mg can be recommended; usually QHS [94]	Used off-label as an insomnia treatment
	Doxepin	Use documented in clinical practice [95]; not tested as a migraine preventive	Studied in 4 insomnia RCTs insomnia with moderate benefit on sleep outcomes
Neutraceuticals	Melatonin	Use as a preventive not graded by the AAN/AHS	Treatment for circadian rhythm disorders. AASM guidelines suggest that clinicians not use melatonin for the treatment of insomnia
		Efficacy reported in one abortive trial in children and adolescents (similar to taking a nap) [96] and as a preventive in one trial in adults	Timing may have unintended effects on the sleep phase
Beta-blockers		Propranolol and metoprolol are first-line preventive agents as graded by AAN/AHS	Limited evidence that lipophilic beta-blockers (i.e., propranolol, metoprolol, atenolol, and pindolol) carry insomnia as a side effect [97]
			Fatigue and bradycardia may compound the perception of daytime fatigue
Others	Valproic acid, topiramate, venlafaxine	First- and second-line preventive agents	May have sleep-inducing effects; recommend QHS use
	CGRP mAb and small molecule antagonists; onabotulinum toxinA	First-line preventive agents (onabotulinum toxin for chronic migraine only)	Unknown/not expected to affect sleep

Approach to Acute Migraine Management

Stimulating Medications

Caffeine is included in combination analgesic medications targeted for migraine. Consumption of a caffeinated beverage is also a patient-employed strategy perceived to be effective. In general, caffeine should be avoided after mid-afternoon given that its stimulating effects may linger for 6 hours [72]. However, individual responses to caffeine on headaches may differ, so sleep complaints should drive counseling [73]. Similarly, steroids, used to treat status migrainosus, should be dosed earlier in the day due to frequently reported sleep-disrupting side effects [74]. There is limited evidence suggesting that aspirin and ibuprofen may affect sleep continuity based on polysomnography [75]; however, sleep complaints are not commonly observed with modest use.

Sedating Medications

Several acute migraine medications may cause somnolence/sleepiness. Lasmiditan (5HT-1F agonist) causes sedation and dizziness in some and carries a driving restriction for 8 hours after dosing [76]. Sleepiness is a reported side effect of triptans; however, this may represent sleepiness associated with a migraine attack and not a direct pharmacologic effect [77]. The antihistamine diphenhydramine is sometimes used alongside antidopaminergic medications in acute care and outpatient settings to treat migraine despite limited supporting evidence [78]. Diphenhydramine is likely overused as a patient-initiated attempt to treat insomnia symptoms; however, its use does not improve PSG parameters and may worsen next-day psychomotor impairment [79]. Given the potential for diphenhydramine to contribute to fatigue in the postdrome, clinicians may want to inquire about its use and consider its avoidance.

Use of Sleep as an Abortive Treatment

Clinicians have historically observed that patients who slept during a migraine attack had faster resolution than those who did not [80]. Sedating medications or naps were intentionally used as an adjunctive analgesic strategy in acute settings [80, 81]. The use of napping is common in children under 8 years old (during 60% of attacks) and is less common in adolescence and adulthood [82]. The rates of daytime napping in adults with episodic migraine are similar to napping rates in the general US population (about one nap/week) and do not have an appreciable effect on subsequent actigraph-measured nightly sleep parameters or sleep quality [83]. Therefore, if feasible and preferred by the patient, a shorter daytime nap (<1 hour) may be a low-risk adjunct migraine treatment strategy. Of note, napping recommendations may differ in patients with chronic migraine who are likely at higher risk for the development of abnormal sleep patterns.

Initiating Behavioral Insomnia Treatments in Those with Migraine

Insomnia is underrecognized and undertreated in patients with migraine [17]. Multicomponent cognitive behavioral therapy for insomnia (CBT-I) is a strongly recommended treatment involving instruction on cognitive therapy strategies, education on sleep regulation, stimulus control, and sleep restriction therapy [84, 85]. In locations where face to face CBT-I is not feasible or there is a significant delay, clinicians can suggest starting with validated mobile apps, such as CBT-I Coach or Sleepio [86, 87]. In modest studies in adults and adolescents with comorbid chronic migraine and chronic insomnia, CBT-I showed significant reductions in headache frequency and improvement in sleep [88, 89]. The expectation is that insomnia complaints persist and fluctuate over many years and delays in treatment may result in a worse prognosis [90].

Sleep hygiene refers to recommendations on lifestyle and environmental factors that influence sleep and was designed as a treatment for insomnia but determined to be ineffective on its own [84, 91]. Although targeted advice (on caffeine intake, light, and noise) may be relevant to some migraine patients, there is limited evidence to support broad sleep hygiene recommendations. Sleep hygiene counseling reduced the duration and frequency of headaches in one study in children and adolescents with migraine, with the persistence of effect at 6 months follow-up [92]. One study of sleep hygiene counseling showed improvement in headache outcomes at a 6-week follow-up in women with chronic migraine [93]. It is important to note that sleep hygiene as a sole treatment is ineffective in adults with chronic insomnia and may delay access to more effective treatments [84]; therefore, it should not serve as a substitute for CBT-I referral.

Conclusion

Although there has been growing research on the relationship between sleep and migraine, clinically relevant questions remain unanswered. Most studies on sleep and migraine have utilized interviews or questionnaires, with few studies utilizing polysomnography or actigraphy [14, 36, 49]. Each methodology and population studied has provided a window into this complex bidirectional relationship. Screening of sleep disorders with appropriate referral and considering sleep when choosing migraine medications are initial steps. However, more research is needed to identify best practices for how to approach, set expectations, and counsel patients with migraine on sleep complaints.

Teaching Points

1. Patients with migraine report increased sleep complaints compared to those without migraine.
2. Limited studies of PSG suggest that pediatric migraine patients have consistent differences in objectively measured sleep. Larger baseline PSG studies in adults are needed.
3. One actigraphy study reported no differences in sleep parameters the night before a migraine attack and reduced efficiency two nights prior.
4. Migraine is comorbid with insomnia, restless legs syndrome, and sleep-related bruxism.
5. Although prevalence rates of OSA are not higher in those with migraine, some may be at higher risk, especially if they have comorbid obesity.
6. Low-dose amitriptyline may be a preferred preventive in those with migraine with insomnia symptoms.
7. Stimulating and sedating medications should be optimally timed.
8. A short daytime nap (<1 h) may be an adjunct to migraine abortive treatment.
9. Long duration naps should be avoided especially in those with chronic migraine.
10. Multicomponent CBT-I is supported by evidence for the treatment of insomnia; sleep hygiene as a sole treatment is not recommended.

Case

A 30-year-old patient presents with chronic migraine and is on amitriptyline, propranolol, and a CGRP-mAb. He continues to have milder daily headaches and 4–5 severe migraine headaches days per month. He has comorbid anxiety, treated with talk therapy. He notes significant difficulty in getting and staying asleep, without signs of sleep apnea. Sometimes, he feels so tired after work, that he will take a 4-hour nap at 5 PM or spend most of his weekend in bed. Melatonin and over-the-counter sleep aids work temporarily but inconsistently. On days he has a severe migraine, he takes Sumatriptan with diphenhydramine and metoclopramide in an attempt to put himself to sleep.

Case Discussion

The patient has comorbid chronic insomnia and chronic migraine and is at high risk for disability. Recommendations include psychiatric consult for anxiety (in addition to talk therapy) and multicomponent CBT-I. While referrals are pending, consider sleep hygiene counseling. This may include limiting daytime napping to <1 hour and not taking a nap after 3–4 PM, spending no more than 10 hours in bed at night, avoiding TV/phone use in bed at night, encouraging exercise in the middle of the day, and caffeine avoidance in the evening. You may consider increasing Amitriptyline, switching to Doxepin or a limited low-dose prescription of a longer acting benzodiazepine.

Acknowledgement I would like to thank my father, Alexandros N. Vgontzas, MD, Sc.D, Professor and Anthony Kales MD, University Chair in Sleep Disorders Medicine in the Department of Psychiatry and Biobehavioral Health at Penn State College of Medicine for his input on clinical management of sleep complaints.

Questions and Answers

1. Which of the following treatment strategies for insomnia are strongly supported by guidelines from the American Academy of Sleep Medicine and should be considered in patients with migraine and comorbid insomnia?
   A. Cognitive behavioral therapy for insomnia (CBT-I).
   B. Sleep hygiene.
   C. Melatonin 3–5 mg QHS.
   D. A and B.
   E. A, B, and C.

The correct answer is A. Multicomponent CBT-I is the preferred treatment for insomnia. Sleep hygiene, on its own, is not a proven strategy and may delay referral for CBT-I. Melatonin has evidence for phase disorders but not insomnia, and its timing may shift phase unintentionally.

2. Which of the following statements regarding migraine and obstructive sleep apnea (OSA) is most accurate based on available evidence?
   A. Rates of OSA are higher in those with migraine and its treatment may improve headache frequency.
   B. Rates of OSA are higher in those with migraine but it is unknown whether treatment of OSA improves headache frequency.
   C. Rates of OSA are higher in those with chronic migraine and this is explained by comorbid obesity.
   D. Rates of snoring are higher in those with migraine but not diagnosed with OSA.
   E. There is no evidence to support that those with migraine are at higher risk of OSA than those without migraine.

The correct answer is D. In population-based studies of those with migraine, rates of snoring are higher and those with migraine score higher on screens for OSA. However, one population-based study that evaluated migraine patients did not find an increased risk for OSA compared to the general population. Certain comorbidities of OSA with chronic migraine, such as obesity, put a subset of patients at higher risk.

References

1. Carskadon MA, Dement WC. Monitoring and staging human sleep. In: Kryger MH, Roth T, Dement WC, editors. Principles and practice of sleep medicine. 5th ed. St. Louis: Elsevier Saunders; 2011. p. 16–26.
2. Paruthi S, Brooks LJ, D'Ambrosio C, Hall WA, Kotagal S, Lloyd RM, et al. Recommended amount of sleep for pediatric populations: a consensus statement of the American Academy of Sleep Medicine. J Clin Sleep Med. 2016;12(6):785–6.
3. Watson NF, Badr MS, Belenky G, Bliwise DL, Buxton OM, Buysse D, et al. Recommended amount of sleep for a healthy adult: a joint consensus statement of the American Academy of Sleep Medicine and Sleep Research Society. Sleep. 2015;38(6):843–4.
4. Buysse DJ. Sleep health: can we define it? Does it matter? Sleep. 2014;37(1):9–17.
5. Kales A, Soldatos CR, Kales JD. Taking a sleep history. Am Fam Physician. 1980;22(2):101–7.
6. Basta M, Chrousos GP, Vela-Bueno A, Vgontzas AN. Chronic insomnia and stress system. Sleep Med Clin. 2007;2(2):279–91.
7. Ibanez V, Silva J, Cauli O. A survey on sleep questionnaires and diaries. Sleep Med. 2018;42:90–6.
8. Chung F, Subramanyam R, Liao P, Sasaki E, Shapiro C, Sun Y. High STOP-Bang score indicates a high probability of obstructive sleep apnoea. Br J Anaesth. 2012;108(5):768–75.
9. Buysse DJ, Reynolds CF 3rd, Monk TH, Berman SR, Kupfer DJ. The Pittsburgh Sleep Quality Index: a new instrument for psychiatric practice and research. Psychiatry Res. 1989;28(2):193–213.
10. Bastien CH, Vallieres A, Morin CM. Validation of the Insomnia Severity Index as an outcome measure for insomnia research. Sleep Med. 2001;2(4):297–307.
11. Martin JL, Hakim AD. Wrist actigraphy. Chest. 2011;139(6):1514–27.
12. Marino M, Li Y, Rueschman MN, Winkelman JW, Ellenbogen JM, Solet JM, et al. Measuring sleep: accuracy, sensitivity, and specificity of wrist actigraphy compared to polysomnography. Sleep. 2013;36(11):1747–55.
13. Bruni O, Fabrizi P, Ottaviano S, Cortesi F, Giannotti F, Guidetti V. Prevalence of sleep disorders in childhood and adolescence with headache: a case-control study. Cephalalgia. 1997;17(4):492–8.
14. Bruni O, Russo PM, Violani C, Guidetti V. Sleep and migraine: an actigraphic study. Cephalalgia. 2004;24(2):134–9.
15. Kelman L, Rains JC. Headache and sleep: examination of sleep patterns and complaints in a large clinical sample of migraineurs. Headache. 2005;45(7):904–10.
16. Goder R, Friege L, Fritzer G, Strenge H, Aldenhoff JB, Hinze-Selch D. Morning headaches in patients with sleep disorders: a systematic polysomnographic study. Sleep Med. 2003;4(5):385–91.
17. Zhu Z, Fan X, Li X, Tan G, Chen L, Zhou J. Prevalence and predictive factors for poor sleep quality among migraineurs in a tertiary hospital headache clinic. Acta Neurol Belg. 2013;113(3):229–35.
18. Budhiraja R, Roth T, Hudgel DW, Budhiraja P, Drake CL. Prevalence and polysomnographic correlates of insomnia comorbid with medical disorders. Sleep. 2011;34(7):859–67.
19. Odegard SS, Engstrom M, Sand T, Stovner LJ, Zwart JA, Hagen K. Associations between sleep disturbance and primary headaches: the third Nord-Trondelag Health Study. J Headache Pain. 2010;11(3):197–206.
20. Barbanti P, Fabbrini G, Aurilia C, Vanacore N, Cruccu G. A case-control study on excessive daytime sleepiness in episodic migraine. Cephalalgia. 2007;27(10):1115–9.
21. Kim J, Cho SJ, Kim WJ, Yang KI, Yun CH, Chu MK. Insufficient sleep is prevalent among migraineurs: a population-based study. J Headache Pain. 2017;18(1):50.
22. Rasmussen BK. Migraine and tension-type headache in a general population: precipitating factors, female hormones, sleep pattern and relation to lifestyle. Pain. 1993;53(1):65–72.
23. Gupta R, Bhatia MS, Dahiya D, Sharma S, Sapra R, Semalti K, et al. Impact of primary headaches on subjective sleep parameters among adolescents. Ann Indian Acad Neurol. 2008;11(3):164–9.
24. Buse DC, Reed ML, Fanning KM, Bostic R, Dodick DW, Schwedt TJ, et al. Comorbid and co-occurring conditions in migraine and associated risk of increasing headache pain intensity and headache frequency: results of the migraine in America symptoms and treatment (MAST) study. J Headache Pain. 2020;21(1):23.

25. Buse DC, Rains JC, Pavlovic JM, Fanning KM, Reed ML, Manack Adams A, et al. Sleep disorders among people with migraine: results from the chronic migraine epidemiology and outcomes (CaMEO) study. Headache. 2019;59(1):32–45.
26. Ferrari A, Leone S, Vergoni AV, Bertolini A, Sances G, Coccia CP, et al. Similarities and differences between chronic migraine and episodic migraine. Headache. 2007;47(1):65–72.
27. Peres MF, Stiles MA, Siow HC, Silberstein SD. Excessive daytime sleepiness in migraine patients. J Neurol Neurosurg Psychiatry. 2005;76(10):1467–8.
28. Lin YK, Lin GY, Lee JT, Lee MS, Tsai CK, Hsu YW, et al. Associations between sleep quality and migraine frequency: a cross-sectional case-control study. Medicine (Baltimore). 2016;95(17):e3554.
29. Vgontzas A, Li W, Mostofsky E, Mittleman MA, Bertisch SM. Baseline sleep quality, stress, and depressive symptoms, and subsequent headache occurrence in a six-week prospective cohort study of patients with episodic migraine. Headache. 2021;61(5):727–33.
30. Park JW, Chu MK, Kim JM, Park SG, Cho SJ. Analysis of trigger factors in episodic migraineurs using a smartphone headache diary applications. PLoS One. 2016;11(2):e0149577.
31. Houle TT, Butschek RA, Turner DP, Smitherman TA, Rains JC, Penzien DB. Stress and sleep duration predict headache severity in chronic headache sufferers. Pain. 2012;153(12):2432–40.
32. Lipton RB, Buse DC, Hall CB, Tennen H, Defreitas TA, Borkowski TM, et al. Reduction in perceived stress as a migraine trigger: testing the "let-down headache" hypothesis. Neurology. 2014;82(16):1395–401.
33. Wober C, Brannath W, Schmidt K, Kapitan M, Rudel E, Wessely P, et al. Prospective analysis of factors related to migraine attacks: the PAMINA study. Cephalalgia. 2007;27(4):304–14.
34. Swanson SA, Zeng Y, Weeks M, Colman I. The contribution of stress to the comorbidity of migraine and major depression: results from a prospective cohort study. BMJ Open. 2013;3(3):e002057.
35. Rist PM, Schurks M, Buring JE, Kurth T. Migraine, headache, and the risk of depression: prospective cohort study. Cephalalgia. 2013;33(12):1017–25.
36. Stanyer EC, Creeney H, Nesbitt AD, Robert Holland PR, Hoffmann J. Subjective sleep quality and sleep architecture in patients with migraine: a meta-analysis. Neurology. 2021;97:e1620.
37. Engstrom M, Hagen K, Bjork M, Stovner LJ, Stjern M, Sand T. Sleep quality, arousal and pain thresholds in tension-type headache: a blinded controlled polysomnographic study. Cephalalgia. 2014;34(6):455–63.
38. Nayak C, Sinha S, Nagappa M, Nagaraj K, Kulkarni GB, Thennarasu K, et al. Study of sleep microstructure in patients of migraine without aura. Sleep Breath. 2016;20(1):263–9.
39. Karthik N, Sinha S, Taly AB, Kulkarni GB, Ramachandraiah CT, Rao S. Alteration in polysomnographic profile in 'migraine without aura' compared to healthy controls. Sleep Med. 2013;14(2):211–4.
40. Vendrame M, Kaleyias J, Valencia I, Legido A, Kothare SV. Polysomnographic findings in children with headaches. Pediatr Neurol. 2008;39(1):6–11.
41. Kristiansen HA, Kvaerner KJ, Akre H, Overland B, Russell MB. Migraine and sleep apnea in the general population. J Headache Pain. 2011;12(1):55–61.
42. Engstrom M, Hagen K, Bjork M, Gravdahl GB, Sand T. Sleep-related and non-sleep-related migraine: interictal sleep quality, arousals and pain thresholds. J Headache Pain. 2013;14:68.
43. Pellegrino ABW, Davis-Martin RE, Houle TT, Turner DP, Smitherman TA. Perceived triggers of primary headache disorders: a meta-analysis. Cephalalgia. 2018;38(6):1188–98.
44. Alstadhaug K, Salvesen R, Bekkelund S. Insomnia and circadian variation of attacks in episodic migraine. Headache. 2007;47(8):1184–8.
45. Dexter JD. The relationship between stage III + IV + REM sleep and arousals with migraine. Headache. 1979;19(7):364–9.
46. Gori S, Lucchesi C, Morelli N, Maestri M, Bonanni E, Murri L. Sleep-related migraine occurrence increases with aging. Acta Neurol Belg. 2012;112(2):183–7.
47. Karsan N, Bose P, Newman J, Goadsby PJ. Are some patient-perceived migraine triggers simply early manifestations of the attack? J Neurol. 2021;268(5):1885–93.
48. Schulte LH, Allers A, May A. Hypothalamus as a mediator of chronic migraine: evidence from high-resolution fMRI. Neurology. 2017;88(21):2011–6.
49. Bertisch SM, Li W, Buettner C, Mostofsky E, Rueschman M, Kaplan ER, et al. Nightly sleep duration, fragmentation, and quality and daily risk of migraine. Neurology. 2020;94(5):e489–e96.
50. Vgontzas A, Pavlovic JM. Sleep disorders and migraine: review of literature and potential pathophysiology mechanisms. Headache. 2018;58(7):1030–9.
51. Sateia MJ. International classification of sleep disorders-third edition: highlights and modifications. Chest. 2014;146(5):1387–94.
52. Bixler EO, Kales A, Soldatos CR, Kales JD, Healey S. Prevalence of sleep disorders in the Los Angeles metropolitan area. Am J Psychiatry. 1979;136(10):1257–62.
53. Ohayon MM. Epidemiology of insomnia: what we know and what we still need to learn. Sleep Med Rev. 2002;6(2):97–111.
54. Sancisi E, Cevoli S, Vignatelli L, Nicodemo M, Pierangeli G, Zanigni S, et al. Increased prevalence of sleep disorders in chronic headache: a case-control study. Headache. 2010;50(9):1464–72.
55. Scher AI, Midgette LA, Lipton RB. Risk factors for headache chronification. Headache. 2008;48(1):16–25.
56. van der Meer HA, Speksnijder CM, Engelbert RHH, Lobbezoo F, Nijhuis-van der Sanden MWG, Visscher CM. The association between headaches and temporomandibular disorders is confounded by bruxism and somatic symptoms. Clin J Pain. 2017;33(9):835–43.
57. De Luca CG, Singh V, Conti P, Dick BD, Gozal D, Major PW, et al. Association between sleep bruxism and psychosocial factors in children and adolescents: a systematic review. Clin Pediatr (Phila). 2015;54(5):469–78.
58. Fernandes G, Franco AL, Goncalves DA, Speciali JG, Bigal ME, Camparis CM. Temporomandibular disorders, sleep bruxism, and primary headaches are mutually associated. J Orofac Pain. 2013;27(1):14–20.
59. Raigrodski AJ, Christensen LV, Mohamed SE, Gardiner DM. The effect of four-week administration of amitriptyline on sleep bruxism. A double-blind crossover clinical study. Cranio. 2001;19(1):21–5.
60. Huynh N, Lavigne GJ, Lanfranchi PA, Montplaisir JY, de Champlain J. The effect of 2 sympatholytic medications – propranolol and clonidine – on sleep bruxism: experimental randomized controlled studies. Sleep. 2006;29(3):307–16.
61. Ondo WG, Simmons JH, Shahid MH, Hashem V, Hunter C, Jankovic J. Onabotulinum toxin-A injections for sleep bruxism: a double-blind, placebo-controlled study. Neurology. 2018;90(7):e559–e64.
62. Schurks M, Winter A, Berger K, Kurth T. Migraine and restless legs syndrome: a systematic review. Cephalalgia. 2014;34(10):777–94.
63. Saper CB, Scammell TE, Lu J. Hypothalamic regulation of sleep and circadian rhythms. Nature. 2005;437(7063):1257–63.
64. Schuh-Hofer S, Richter M, Geworski L, Villringer A, Israel H, Wenzel R, et al. Increased serotonin transporter availability in the brainstem of migraineurs. J Neurol. 2007;254(6):789–96.
65. Sarchielli P, Rainero I, Coppola F, Rossi C, Mancini M, Pinessi L, et al. Involvement of corticotrophin-releasing factor and orexin-A in chronic migraine and medication-overuse headache: findings from cerebrospinal fluid. Cephalalgia. 2008;28(7):714–22.
66. Chabi A, Zhang Y, Jackson S, Cady R, Lines C, Herring WJ, et al. Randomized controlled trial of the orexin receptor antagonist filorexant for migraine prophylaxis. Cephalalgia. 2015;35(5):379–88.

67. Tuka B, Helyes Z, Markovics A, Bagoly T, Szolcsanyi J, Szabo N, et al. Alterations in PACAP-38-like immunoreactivity in the plasma during ictal and interictal periods of migraine patients. Cephalalgia. 2013;33(13):1085–95.
68. Holland PR, Barloese M, Fahrenkrug J. PACAP in hypothalamic regulation of sleep and circadian rhythm: importance for headache. J Headache Pain. 2018;19(1):20.
69. Iliff JJ, Wang M, Liao Y, Plogg BA, Peng W, Gundersen GA, et al. A paravascular pathway facilitates CSF flow through the brain parenchyma and the clearance of interstitial solutes, including amyloid beta. Sci Transl Med. 2012;4(147):147ra11.
70. Schain AJ, Melo-Carrillo A, Strassman AM, Burstein R. Cortical spreading depression closes paravascular space and impairs glymphatic flow: implications for migraine headache. J Neurosci. 2017;37(11):2904–15.
71. Owens JA, Dalzell V. Use of the 'BEARS' sleep screening tool in a pediatric residents' continuity clinic: a pilot study. Sleep Med. 2005;6(1):63–9.
72. Drake C, Roehrs T, Shambroom J, Roth T. Caffeine effects on sleep taken 0, 3, or 6 hours before going to bed. J Clin Sleep Med. 2013;9(11):1195–200.
73. Mostofsky E, Mittleman MA, Buettner C, Li W, Bertisch SM. Prospective cohort study of caffeinated beverage intake as a potential trigger of headaches among migraineurs. Am J Med. 2019;132(8):984–91.
74. Patel R, Belousov M, Jani M, Dasgupta N, Winokur C, Nenadic G, et al. Frequent discussion of insomnia and weight gain with glucocorticoid therapy: an analysis of Twitter posts. NPJ Digit Med. 2018:1.
75. Murphy PJ, Badia P, Myers BL, Boecker MR, Wright KP Jr. Nonsteroidal anti-inflammatory drugs affect normal sleep patterns in humans. Physiol Behav. 1994;55(6):1063–6.
76. Goadsby PJ, Wietecha LA, Dennehy EB, Kuca B, Case MG, Aurora SK, et al. Phase 3 randomized, placebo-controlled, double-blind study of lasmiditan for acute treatment of migraine. Brain. 2019;142(7):1894–904.
77. Goadsby PJ, Dodick DW, Almas M, Diener HC, Tfelt-Hansen P, Lipton RB, et al. Treatment-emergent CNS symptoms following triptan therapy are part of the attack. Cephalalgia. 2007;27(3):254–62.
78. Friedman BW, Cabral L, Adewunmi V, Solorzano C, Esses D, Bijur PE, et al. Diphenhydramine as adjuvant therapy for acute migraine: an emergency department-based randomized clinical trial. Ann Emerg Med. 2016;67(1):32–9 e3.
79. Katayose Y, Aritake S, Kitamura S, Enomoto M, Hida A, Takahashi K, et al. Carryover effect on next-day sleepiness and psychomotor performance of nighttime administered antihistaminic drugs: a randomized controlled trial. Hum Psychopharmacol. 2012;27(4):428–36.
80. Wilkinson M, Williams K, Leyton M. Observations on the treatment of an acute attack of migraine. Res Clin Stud Headache. 1978;6:141–6.
81. Wilkinson M. Treatment of the acute migraine attack – current status. Cephalalgia. 1983;3(1):61–7.
82. Aaltonen K, Hamalainen ML, Hoppu K. Migraine attacks and sleep in children. Cephalalgia. 2000;20(6):580–4.
83. Vgontzas A, Mostofsky E, Hagan K, Mittleman M, Bertisch S. Napping and headache outcomes in adults with episodic migraine: a six-week prospective cohort study. Boston: American Headache Society Annual Meeting Orlando, FL (Virtual); 2021.
84. Edinger JD, Arnedt JT, Bertisch SM, Carney CE, Harrington JJ, Lichstein KL, et al. Behavioral and psychological treatments for chronic insomnia disorder in adults: an American Academy of Sleep Medicine clinical practice guideline. J Clin Sleep Med. 2021;17(2):255–62.
85. van Straten A, van der Zweerde T, Kleiboer A, Cuijpers P, Morin CM, Lancee J. Cognitive and behavioral therapies in the treatment of insomnia: a meta-analysis. Sleep Med Rev. 2018;38:3–16.
86. Kuhn E, Weiss BJ, Taylor KL, Hoffman JE, Ramsey KM, Manber R, et al. CBT-I coach: a description and clinician perceptions of a mobile app for cognitive behavioral therapy for insomnia. J Clin Sleep Med. 2016;12(4):597–606.
87. Espie CA, Kyle SD, Williams C, Ong JC, Douglas NJ, Hames P, et al. A randomized, placebo-controlled trial of online cognitive behavioral therapy for chronic insomnia disorder delivered via an automated media-rich web application. Sleep. 2012;35(6):769–81.
88. Smitherman TA, Walters AB, Davis RE, Ambrose CE, Roland M, Houle TT, et al. Randomized controlled pilot trial of behavioral insomnia treatment for chronic migraine with comorbid insomnia. Headache. 2016;56(2):276–91.
89. Law EF, Wan Tham S, Aaron RV, Dudeney J, Palermo TM. Hybrid cognitive-behavioral therapy intervention for adolescents with co-occurring migraine and insomnia: a single-arm pilot trial. Headache. 2018;58(7):1060–73.
90. Morin CM, Jarrin DC, Ivers H, Merette C, LeBlanc M, Savard J. Incidence, persistence, and remission rates of insomnia over 5 years. JAMA Netw Open. 2020;3(11):e2018782.
91. Irish LA, Kline CE, Gunn HE, Buysse DJ, Hall MH. The role of sleep hygiene in promoting public health: a review of empirical evidence. Sleep Med Rev. 2015;22:23–36.
92. Bruni O, Galli F, Guidetti V. Sleep hygiene and migraine in children and adolescents. Cephalalgia. 1999;19(Suppl 25):57–9.
93. Calhoun AH, Ford S. Behavioral sleep modification may revert transformed migraine to episodic migraine. Headache. 2007;47(8):1178–83.
94. Burch R. Preventive migraine treatment. Continuum (Minneap Minn). 2021;27(3):613–32.
95. Parsekyan D. Migraine prophylaxis in adult patients. West J Med. 2000;173(5):341–5.
96. Gelfand AA, Ross AC, Irwin SL, Greene KA, Qubty WF, Allen IE. Melatonin for acute treatment of migraine in children and adolescents: a pilot randomized trial. Headache. 2020;60(8):1712–21.
97. Kostis JB, Rosen RC. Central nervous system effects of beta-adrenergic-blocking drugs: the role of ancillary properties. Circulation. 1987;75(1):204–12.

Further Reading

Leso V, Gervetti P, Mauro S, Macrini MC, Ercolano ML, Iavicoli I. Shift work and migraine: a systematic review. J Occup Health. 2020;62(1):e12116.

Sandoe CH, Sasikumar S, Lay C, Lawler V. The impact of shift work on migraine: a case series and narrative review. Headache. 2019;59(9):1631–40.

Role of Diet and Nutrition for Migraine

20

Nada Hindiyeh, David Walker, and Leon Moskatel

Introduction

Diet includes not only the specific foods and drinks regularly consumed but also the controlled restriction of nutrition for a particular purpose, such as weight management. Studies over the past decades have repeatedly indicated an association between diet and migraine, including showing that skipped meals, fasting, and the ingestion of particular fare can trigger migraine attacks.

Although a variety of common foods and beverages have been branded as triggers for migraine, conflicting evidence supports these claims. Moreover, several specialized diets have been proposed to reduce migraine burden, including not only elimination diets but also low-fat or ketogenic diets. However, inconsistent evidence supports their use. Furthermore, in the studies assessing these diets, it is unclear if the specialized diet directly or weight loss from the diet indirectly was responsible for migraine improvement. Indeed, weight loss, regardless of diet, has been shown to be beneficial in migraine prevention.

In this chapter, we review the evidence for dietary migraine attack triggers, specialized diets for migraine prevention, and weight loss as lifestyle treatment options for migraine.

Questions

1. Which phase of a migraine attack may be responsible for symptoms perceived to be migraine triggers such as food cravings?
   A. Premonitory phase.
   B. Aura phase.
   C. Headache phase.
   D. Prodrome phase.
2. To prevent migraine, which food or drinks should be completely eliminated?
   A. Chocolate.
   B. Alcohol.
   C. Gluten.
   D. None of the above.

What Not to Eat

Are Dietary Triggers Important?

Traditional migraine guidelines place a strong emphasis on avoidance of dietary triggers. Consequently, patients are commonly asked to track and eschew their migraine triggers. Foods may be triggers if a headache occurs in half or more instances within 1 day of exposure [1]. This, in part, stems from a seminal 1960 observational study that identified food as a migraine trigger in 25% of their migraine cohort [2]. Subsequent studies reported dietary triggers in 12–60% of people with migraine [1]. One of the largest retrospective observational studies to date evaluated 1207 patients with migraine diagnosed by the ICHD-2 criteria. About 76% identified food-triggered migraine attacks including 38% from alcohol and 27% noting specific foods as triggers [3]. The most commonly self-reported food triggers include chocolate, citrus fruits, nuts, ice cream, salami, tomatoes, onions, dairy products, meats, aged cheese, smoked fish, avocados, and bananas. Commonly reported beverage trig-

N. Hindiyeh (✉) · D. Walker · L. Moskatel
Department of Neurology, Stanford University, Palo Alto, CA, USA

T. S. Monteith et al. (eds.), *Comprehensive Migraine Management*, https://doi.org/10.1007/978-3-031-86923-5_20

gers include alcohol and coffee as well as constituent ingredients such as caffeine, monosodium glutamate (MSG), histamine, tyramine, nitrites, gluten, wheat, and aspartame [3–5]. However, dietary triggers of migraine remain a topic of debate as studies report conflicting outcomes, and the majority have questionable protocols including a high potential for recall bias.

Chocolate, frequently cited as a migraine trigger, has both studies to support and refute its causation of migraine. In a systematic review examining 25 articles, 23 reported chocolate as a trigger for headache only in a small percentage of participants ranging from 1.3 to 33% [6]. Moreover, the majority of these studies relied on potentially flawed retrospective recall. In the single study that did use an electronic diary to capture migraine triggers, chocolate was found to be a trigger factor in fewer than 1.5%. Two large double-blind provocation studies showed no significant difference in migraine attacks between the chocolate and placebo groups. A third, smaller study noted that 41.7% of people developed headaches after a chocolate injection and none after a placebo, but this was not statistically significant [6–9]. Consequently, given the delicious flavor profile and lack of quality evidence, avoidance of chocolate is not recommended.

Alcohol has also been examined as a causative agent of migraine with several cross-sectional studies reporting alcohol as a migraine trigger, while others have shown a decrease in attack frequency [5, 10]. Red wine, in particular, is most commonly cited as a migraine trigger with a rate as high as 77.8% in one large cross-sectional study [11]. In a provocation trial comparing wine to vodka, migraine attacks were significantly more likely after consumption of the former [12]. Furthermore, a prospective cohort study evaluating the association between headache on the day following alcohol consumption concluded that 1–2 drinks were not associated with an increased risk of headache, but 5 or more servings were [13].

Caffeine has also produced contradictory outcomes; it has been shown to trigger headache upon ingestion or withdrawal in some studies, while others have shown alleviation of headache. In a review of caffeine and headache, 21 of 25 studies reported caffeine as a migraine trigger in a small percentage of participants, ranging from 2.4 to 30%. In the two studies that evaluated caffeine withdrawal, a larger proportion of patients ranging from 10% to 30% reported this as a trigger. However, these studies are largely retrospective, and no provocative studies have been done on caffeine or its withdrawal in headaches [14]. Caffeine overuse has also been reported as a risk factor for the transformation of episodic to chronic migraine [15, 16].

Investigations have also evaluated caffeine as an acute migraine treatment. One prospective study compared 60 mg of intravenous caffeine to 2 g of intravenous magnesium, and although both were found to be effective in reducing migraine attack pain scores, caffeine was found to be significantly less effective than magnesium at 1 hour [17]. Several randomized controlled studies have shown the efficacy of combinations of caffeine with other analgesics [14]. When these studies are taken together, consistency with caffeine use appears key, and caffeine-containing analgesics can be effective for acute migraine although use should be limited to no more than 2 days a week to avoid medication overuse headache.

Other ingredients, such as MSG, have been evaluated in several randomized placebo-controlled trials [18]. MSG, the sodium salt of glutamate, is a flavor enhancer, and often blamed for post-prandial illness where headache can be prominent; glutamate, an important excitatory neurotransmitter, has been implicated in migraine pathophysiology [19, 20]. Studies where MSG was ingested with food, thought to decrease its absorption, found little evidence suggesting it as a migraine trigger. Conversely, 4 out of 5 provocation studies where MSG was dissolved in liquids in high concentrations were found to precipitate headaches. However, in those studies, blinding was possibly compromised as the distinctive flavor of MSG may have been recognizable [18]. Other ingredients have more conflicting studies, such as aspartame which has had two negative and two positive provocation studies [5].

Some people with migraine appear more susceptible to dietary triggers, likely due to genetic, biological, and environmental factors. Triggers may also be partial, additive, and synergistic in precipitating a migraine attack, and these factors are challenging to control.

The first stage of a migraine attack, the premonitory phase, has been well-established in up to 77% of people and is characterized by non-painful symptomatology, such as food cravings, thirst, fatigue, mood changes, yawning, changes in sleep and photophobia, that can precede the headache by up to 72 hours and is thought to be mediated by the hypothalamus [21, 22]. Consequently, it is postulated, for instance, that a craving for chocolate in the premonitory phase may be misconstrued as a migraine trigger [23]. Likewise, increased caffeine due to fatigue, sleepiness, and yawning during the premonitory phase may be misinterpreted as the actual trigger. Even a skipped meal may be the consequence of anorexia and gastroparesis in the premonitory phase as opposed to the trigger of a migraine attack [24].

Can Food Allergies Trigger Migraine?

Suspected food triggers are not synonymous with food allergies. Food allergies stem from the activation of antibodies in response to a specific allergen-containing food with reactions ranging from mild to severe. Identification of food allergies requires skin or serological testing.

There is no definitive way to test for food intolerances. Commercial tests that purport to identify intolerances through IgG levels to multiple foods are hampered by the absence of evidence to support this approach. Their claim that the removal of foods with high IgG levels can lead to symptomatic improvement is equally unfounded; the American Academy of Allergy, Asthma and Immunology does not support these tests [25].

In the headache treatment setting, elimination diets based on IgG testing of various foods have been done to evaluate these foods as migraine triggers. Three of these studies reported positive results after 4 weeks relative to controls, but that improvement disappeared at 12 weeks [26–29]. Migraine in these studies was self-reported and not diagnosed by ICHD criteria. As a result, there is insufficient evidence to suggest using IgG testing and elimination diets in migraine prevention. However, in a subset of migraine patients who report a clear, causative link between certain foods and migraine attacks, selective elimination is a reasonable consideration.

Specific elimination diets do have a place in the treatment of migraine for select cohorts, such as those with celiac disease, an immune-mediated reaction to gluten. In a meta-analysis estimating the prevalence of headache to be 26% in people with celiac disease, up to 75% of people reported headache improvement after initiation of a gluten-free diet [30].

What to Eat

Are Specific Diets Important?

Diet has been effectively utilized as an adjunct treatment for migraine. Patients may inquire about incorporating a specific diet into their daily routine but can hesitate as these can be time-consuming and significantly impact their lifestyle. Here, we review some of the most common and best-studied diets for migraine prevention.

Alterations in blood glucose have been implicated in migraine. The blood-glucose-raising potential of different carbohydrates is described through the glycemic index, a relative ranking system from 1 to 100. A glycemic index of 55 or less denotes a food with a low ability to raise blood glucose, while foods of 70 and above have a high ability to do so [31]. Patients with migraine may be more susceptible to irregularities in blood glucose; it is thought that by having a slower, steadier rise in glucose, a low-glycemic index diet prevents glucose fluctuations that contribute to migraine attacks. Weight loss can also result from this diet, and numerous studies suggest that this has a positive effect on migraine prevention [32].

An initial study has shown promise for this approach. About 350 patients in a randomized controlled study were assigned to follow either a low-glycemic index diet or regular preventive migraine medication. Both groups followed consistent frequency and timing of meals. Both cohorts had similar decreases in the Visual Analog Scale (VAS) and a reduction in headache days per month. However, this study suffered from the absence of a comparable placebo group [33].

The ketogenic diet is a low-carbohydrate, high-fat diet that purports to induce a state of ketosis, where the body's main energy source is ketone bodies rather than glucose. The ketogenic diet has shown efficacy in reducing the seizure burden in patients with refractory epilepsy and is now being investigated for migraine prevention [34]. The ketogenic diet may act by reducing cortical hyperexcitability which can then be applied to the migrainous hyperexcitable brain state [35, 36]. This mechanism of action in migraine has been lent credence by a small prospective study evaluating a 1-month ketogenic diet in patients with migraine. The authors reported normalization of evoked potentials and clinically, a reduction in attack frequency [37].

In a subsequent study, 96 overweight women with migraine were started on either a 6-month low-calorie diet (1200–1500 kcal) or a 1-month ketogenic very-low-calorie diet ($\leq$800 kcal) followed by a 5-month low-calorie diet. A significant reduction in migraine days and attack duration was observed in the keto diet group after 1 month, but this cohort regressed when they transitioned out of the keto diet. While both groups had a significant reduction in headache days as well as improvement in body mass index (BMI) at the 6-month mark, the more rapid improvement in the ketogenic diet group suggests this diet may have a separate mechanism in migraine reduction beyond weight loss [38].

A recent small study on patients with chronic migraine and medication-overuse headaches showed a striking reduction in migraine attack duration from 24 to 5.5 hours, frequency from 30 to 7.5 days a month, and rescue medication use from 30 to 6 days a month after 3 months; however, this study was an open-label and had no placebo control [39]. Conversely, a 12-week randomized controlled crossover trial of 16 participants comparing the ketogenic diet to an evidence-informed "anti-headache" diet (AHD) centered on the consumption of minimally processed foods, and reduced consumption of purported migraine triggers did not find a statistically significant difference between migraine frequency, severity, or duration. There was, however, a statistically significant improvement in quality of life (as assessed by the Migraine Specific Quality of Life Questionnaire) in the ketogenic diet while not in the AHD group. The majority of patients (69%) in this study had side effects from the ketogenic diet, with fatigue, stomach upset, and constipation as the most frequently reported. The side effect profile of the ketogenic diet can make adherence difficult, and patients must weigh the pros against the cons when deciding to follow this restrictive diet [40].

In contrast to diets that restrict carbohydrates and emphasize fats, a randomized, crossover dietary interventional trial of 83 participants compared the effects of a low-lipid diet against a normal-lipid diet on migraine frequency and severity. Both interventions had lower lipid intakes and calorie expenditures than participants' baseline consumption and both showed a reduction in migraine frequency although this was greater in the low-lipid group. Patients in the study lost an average of 1 kilogram suggesting that weight loss or energy expenditure reduction may also account for the migraine improvement [41].

In addition to low fat in the diet, a crossover study evaluated the combination of a 4-week vegan and low-fat diet followed by a 2- to 3-week food trigger elimination diet + vegan diet compared to a placebo group receiving supplements. Although no significant difference in headache frequency was noted, there was a significant reduction in acute migraine medication usage, reported pain, body weight, and lipid levels in the vegan cohort [42].

Omega-3 polyunsaturated fatty acids (PUFAs) are precursors to specialized lipid mediators known as resolvins which play a role in immunomodulation, resolution of inflammation, and have analgesic properties. Lipid mediators derived from omega-6 ($n-6$) fatty acids are generally regarded as pronociceptive, while those derived from omega-3 ($n-3$) are antinociceptive. A cross-sectional study of 12,317 people found that greater intake of PUFAs was associated with a lower prevalence of severe headaches or migraine [43].

A study of 182 participants with greater than 15 headache days a month evaluated three diets, a high $n-3$ diet (H3 diet), a high $n-3$ + low $n-6$ diet (H3-L6 diet), and an average $n-3$ and $n-6$ intake diet (control diet). Both the H3 and H3-L6 diet groups significantly reduced the number of total headache hours per day and headache days per month [44].

Both the Mediterranean and dietary approaches to stop hypertension (DASH) diets are promising for migraine prevention. The diets are similar, both promoting vegetables, fruits, lean meats, whole grains, nuts, and legumes and discouraging red meat and foods with added sugar. The Mediterranean diet focuses more on promoting healthy fats (e.g., olive oil and fish rich in omega-3 fatty acids), whereas the DASH diet focuses more on limiting sodium intake [45–47].

A study of 80 participants evaluating adherence to the Mediterranean diet or the DASH diet found that lower adherence to either diet was associated with more severe and frequent attacks [45]. Another study found that individuals with the highest adherence to the DASH diet had a 30% lower prevalence of severe headaches and decreased duration of headaches compared to those with the lowest adherence [46]. The DASH diet has also been evaluated against dietary advice in 102 women for 12 weeks, with a significant decrease in migraine frequency, duration, and depression scores in those in the DASH group [47].

A hybrid of the Mediterranean and DASH diets, the Mediterranean-DASH intervention for neurodegenerative delay (MIND) diet, has been associated with slower rates of cognitive decline and may help prevent migraine through its inclusion of foods with antioxidant properties (berries and green leafy vegetables) as well as anti-nociceptive $n-3$ fatty acids [48]. In a cross-sectional study of 266 participants, higher MIND diet scores were associated with a decreased likelihood to have severe headaches and decreased duration and frequency of headaches [49].

The studies discussed thus far focus on single nutrients or products when evaluating the dietary impact on migraine. The dietary diversity score (DDS) is often used to assess nutrient adequacy and overall diet quality. A lower DDS has been associated with greater adverse health such as metabolic syndrome and other chronic disorders [50, 51]. A cross-sectional study of 256 women found that subjects with a lower DDS had a higher likelihood to have higher pain severity and headache duration compared to the reference group [52].

Dehydration and water deprivation have been linked to headaches [53]. Increasing water intake is a benign dietary recommendation for migraine prevention. One proposed mechanism posits that increased water intake reduces osmolarity and balances the concentration of electrolytes, decreasing migraine severity [54]. A cross-sectional study of 256 women evaluated the impact of water intake on migraine and migraine disability assessment (MIDAS) after 30 days. Drinking more glasses of water per day was associated with less MIDAS score and pain. An average of 9.0 daily glasses of water was associated with no disability on the MIDAS scale and mild pain, compared to an intake of 7.5 glasses in the severely disabled group and 6.4 glasses in the severe pain group [55]. A prior RCT evaluated recommendations to increase water intake (1.5 L per day) against usual treatment and found a significant improvement in the migraine-specific quality of life in the intervention group compared to control although no significant change in headache frequency and medication use was reported [56].

Can Weight Loss Improve Migraine?

The relationship between obesity and primary headaches was first proposed in a 2003 prospective population-based study showing obese individuals had a fivefold increase in the relative risk of developing chronic daily headaches compared to normal-weight participants [57]. Obesity has since been established as an independent risk factor for headache development [58] as well as a risk factor in the chronification from episodic to chronic headaches [59]. A 2021 meta-analysis further demonstrated obesity as an overall risk factor for migraine [60].

A separate, previous meta-analysis that included 10 studies with 473 participants found that regardless of weight loss modality, such as bariatric surgery, behavioral interventions or specific diets, weight loss improved migraine burden including decreased frequency, pain severity, disability, and attack duration [61]. This improvement was not correlated with the degree of baseline obesity or degree of weight reduction.

The pathophysiology of the relationship between weight loss and migraine is likely multifactorial and requires further investigation. It is speculated that the negative energy balance from weight loss plays a role [61]. Energy restriction has been associated with a reduction in pro-inflammatory cytokines such as IL-6 and TNF-alpha which have been found to be elevated in people with migraine. It has also been associated with an increase in anti-inflammatory cytokines such as adipokines, adiponectin, and leptin which were found to be increased between migraine attacks and decreased during attacks [62]. Furthermore, alterations in hypothalamic neuropeptides that control energy expenditure and appetite regulation such as orexin A and serotonin are linked to both obesity and migraine [62].

Convergent studies hint that weight loss, regardless of method, may improve migraine in overweight or obese patients; however, further randomized, controlled studies are needed (Table 20.1).

Table 20.1 Common migraine diets and their descriptions

Diet	Description
Low-glycemic index	Glycemic index is a value assigned to carbohydrates corresponding to how quickly they raise blood glucose in comparison to pure glucose, which is assigned a value of 100. Low glycemic index is 55 or less, medium glycemic index, 56–69, and high glycemic index, 70 and above. Only carbohydrates are assigned a glycemic index value. This diet limits foods such as white bread, rice, pasta, potatoes, sweets, and sugary drinks [31, 33]
Ketogenic	A high-fat, low-carbohydrate, and moderate-protein intake diet that induces a state of ketosis, in which the body uses ketones as the major energy source [34–40]
Low-lipid	Lipid content <20% of the total daily energy intake [41]
Vegan	A plant-based diet that avoids any food that comes from animals, including dairy and eggs [42]
Omega-3 polyunsaturated fatty acids (PUFAs)	While not an entire diet, examples of foods containing PUFAs include fish and other seafood, seeds (flax seeds and chia seeds), nuts (walnuts), leafy vegetables, and plant oils [43, 44]
Dietary approaches to stop hypertension (DASH)	A diet promoted by the National Heart, lung and blood institute designed to prevent and control hypertension. It emphasizes reducing intake of sodium and saturated fats and recommends eating fruits, vegetables, low-fat dairy, whole grains, lean meats, legumes, and nuts [45–47]
Mediterranean	A diet based on the eating patterns of Mediterranean countries. It is similar to the DASH diet but encourages more consumption of olive oil and other sources of healthy fats, such as omega-3 fatty acids from fish. Both diets discourage red meats and foods with added sugar [45]
Mediterranean-DASH intervention for neurodegenerative delay (MIND)	A combination of the Mediterranean and DASH diet aimed at preventing cognitive decline that specifically highlights eating leafy greens and berries [48, 49]

Conclusion

Diet and nutrition play a significant role in migraine management though the evidence supporting specific food triggers and specialized diets remains mixed. Some foods, such as chocolate and alcohol, have conflicting studies regarding their influence as migraine triggers, while the premonitory phase of a migraine attack may often be mistaken for food cravings or triggers. Specialized diets, such as low-glycemic, ketogenic, low-lipid, and Mediterranean-based plans, show promise in reducing migraine burden, particularly for those with comorbidities such as obesity. Weight loss has been consistently shown to improve migraine outcomes, emphasizing the importance of dietary consistency and hydration. While elimination diets may benefit select patients with clear food-related triggers or conditions such as celiac disease, larger, more rigorous studies are needed to further establish the efficacy of these approaches in migraine prevention and management.

Teaching Points

1. Diet and nutrition can affect migraine.
2. The premonitory phase driven by the hypothalamus may be responsible for symptoms of food cravings (i.e., chocolate) and anorexia (skipped meals) traditionally perceived as migraine triggers.
3. Alcohol may be a migraine trigger when more than five drinks are consumed.

   Regularity in caffeine dose and usage is recommended, with the limitation of caffeine-containing analgesics to avoid medication-overuse headaches.
4. Elimination diets may be useful for cohorts of patients with comorbidities such as celiac disease.
5. Larger and more rigorous studies are needed to confirm the efficacy of specialized diets in migraine; however, consider:
   - (i) Diets that address patients' comorbid medical conditions (such as metabolic syndrome or cardiovascular disease).
   - (ii) Diets that are easy to implement such as increased water intake.
   - (iii) Diets that neurologists are already comfortable recommending, such as the MIND diet for protection against cognitive decline.
6. Weight loss may improve migraine, especially in people who are overweight or obese.

Case

A 36-year-old woman presents to your clinic for a follow-up of chronic migraine. She now reports a decrease in her headache frequency to an average of 10 migraine days a month and is currently on two preventive migraine treatments. Her comorbidities include obesity and asthma. She does not want to change her migraine medications but instead asks about what modifications she can make in her diet to further help decrease her migraine burden. She asks if there are any food triggers she should avoid and if any specific diets could be helpful for her.

Case Discussion

Diet and nutrition can affect migraine. Consistency with diet and hydration, including increased water intake can be helpful. Considering she is obese, weight loss may improve her migraine frequency. It is important for patients to discuss with a specialist what type of weight loss plan is appropriate for them. Specifically, based on research, a low-calorie diet or a ketogenic diet may be beneficial for her. Because alcohol is a potent migraine trigger, reducing or eliminating alcohol from the diet may be helpful. Likewise, if she drinks caffeine, regularity in dose can be helpful although excessive intake should be avoided (recommended dose of caffeine, maximum 200 mg/day).

Questions and Answers

1. Which phase of a migraine attack may be responsible for symptoms perceived to be migraine triggers such as food cravings?
   - A. Premonitory phase.
   - B. Aura phase.
   - C. Headache phase.
   - D. Prodrome phase.

The correct answer is A. The premonitory phase is the first phase of a migraine attack and is thought to be mediated by the hypothalamus. Hypothalamic activity may account for many premonitory symptoms up to 48 hours before the headache phase, thought to be migraine attack triggers such as food cravings, sleep disturbances, changes in mood, and thirst.

2. To prevent migraine, which food or drinks should be completely eliminated?
   A. Chocolate.
   B. Alcohol.
   C. Gluten.
   D. None of the above.

The correct answer is D. There is no evidence to suggest any particular food or drink should be completely eliminated to prevent migraine. Elimination of gluten may be effective in reducing migraine frequency and severity in people with celiac disease; however, there is no evidence that in those without celiac that elimination will completely prevent migraine.

References

1. Martin VT, Behbehani MM. Toward a rational understanding of migraine trigger factors. Med Clin North Am. 2001;85(4):911–41.
2. Lance JW. Observations on 500 cases of migraine and allied vascular headache. J Neurol Neurosurg Psychiatry. 2012;83(7):673–4.
3. Kelman L. The triggers or precipitants of the acute migraine attack. Cephalalgia. 2007;27(5):394–402.
4. Finocchi C, Sivori G. Food as trigger and aggravating factor of migraine. Neurol Sci. 2012;33(1):77–80.
5. Martin VT, Vij B. Diet and headache: Part 1. Headache J Head Face Pain. 2016;56(9):1543–52.
6. Nowaczewska M, Wiciński M, Kaźmierczak W, Kaźmierczak H. To eat or not to eat: a review of the relationship between chocolate and migraines. Nutrients. 2020;12(3):608.
7. Marcus DA, Scharff L, Turk D, Gourley LM. A double-blind provocative study chocolate as a trigger of headache. Cephalalgia. 1997;17(8):855–62.
8. Moffett AM, Swash M, Scott DF. Effect of chocolate in migraine: a double-blind study. J Neurol Neurosurg Psychiatry. 1974;37(4):445–8.
9. Gibb CM, Davies PT, Glover V, Steiner TJ, Rose FC, Sandler M. Chocolate is a migraine-provoking agent. Cephalalgia. 1991;11(2):93–5.
10. Hindiyeh NA, Zhang N, Farrar M, Banerjee P, Lombard L, Aurora SK. The role of diet and nutrition in migraine triggers and treatment: a systematic literature review. Headache J Head Face Pain. 2020;60(7):1300–16.
11. Onderwater GL, van Oosterhout WP, Schoonman GG, Ferrari MD, Terwindt GM. Alcoholic beverages as trigger factor and the effect on alcohol consumption behavior in patients with migraine. Eur J Neurol. 2019;26(4):588–95.
12. Littlewood J, Glover V, Davies PT, Gibb C, Sandler M, Rose FC. Red wine as a cause of migraine. Lancet. 1988;331(8585):558–9.
13. Mostofsky E, Bertisch SM, Vgontzas A, Buettner C, Li W, Rueschman M, Mittleman MA. Prospective cohort study of daily alcoholic beverage intake as a potential trigger of headaches among adults with episodic migraine. Ann Med. 2020;52(7):386–92.
14. Nowaczewska M, Wiciński M, Kaźmierczak W. The ambiguous role of caffeine in migraine headache: from trigger to treatment. Nutrients. 2020;12(8):2259.
15. Bigal ME, Lipton RB. Modifiable risk factors for migraine progression. Headache J Head Face Pain. 2006;46(9):1334–43.
16. Aguggia M, Saracco MG. Pathophysiology of migraine chronification. Neurol Sci. 2010;31(1):15–7.
17. Baratloo A, Mirbaha S, Kasmaei HD, Payandemehr P, Elmaraezy A, Negida A. Intravenous caffeine citrate vs. magnesium sulfate for reducing pain in patients with acute migraine headache; a prospective quasi-experimental study. Korean J Pain. 2017;30(3):176.
18. Obayashi Y, Nagamura Y. Does monosodium glutamate really cause headache?: A systematic review of human studies. J Headache Pain. 2016;17(1):1–7.
19. Kwok RH. Chinese-restaurant syndrome. N Engl J Med. 1968;278(14):796.
20. Moreno-Ajona D, Villar-Martínez MD, Goadsby PJ. Targets for migraine treatment: beyond calcitonin gene-related peptide. Curr Opin Neurol. 2021;34(3):363–72.
21. Laurell K, Artto V, Bendtsen L, Hagen K, Häggström J, Linde M, Söderström L, Tronvik E, Wessman M, Zwart JA, Kallela M. Premonitory symptoms in migraine: a cross-sectional study in 2714 persons. Cephalalgia. 2016;36(10):951–9.
22. Hindiyeh N, Hovren H. Advances in migraine therapeutics: the role of calcitonin gene-related peptide. In: Neurotherapeutics in the era of translational medicine. Academic; 2021. p. 181–201.
23. Hoffmann J, Recober A. Migraine and triggers: post hoc ergo propter hoc? Curr Pain Headache Rep. 2013;17(10):1–7.
24. Martins-Oliveira M, Tavares I, Goadsby PJ. Was it something I ate? Understanding the bidirectional interaction of migraine and appetite neural circuits. Brain Res. 2021:147629.
25. Bock SA. AAAAI support of the EACCI position paper on IgG4. J Allergy Clin Immunol. 2010;125(6):1410.
26. Aydinlar EI, Dikmen PY, Tiftikci A, Saruc M, Aksu M, Gunsoy HG, Tozun N. IgG-based elimination diet in migraine plus irritable bowel syndrome. Headache J Head Face Pain. 2013;53(3):514–25.
27. Alpay K, Ertaş M, Orhan EK, Üstay DK, Lieners C, Baykan B. Diet restriction in migraine, based on IgG against foods: a clinical double-blind, randomised, cross-over trial. Cephalalgia. 2010;30(7):829–37.
28. Mitchell N, Hewitt CE, Jayakody S, Islam M, Adamson J, Watt I, Torgerson DJ. Randomised controlled trial of food elimination diet based on IgG antibodies for the prevention of migraine like headaches. Nutr J. 2011;10(1):1–9.
29. Arroyave Hernández CM, Pinto ME, Hernández Montiel HL. Food allergy mediated by IgG antibodies associated with migraine in adults. Revista Alergia de Mexico. 2007;54(5)
30. Zis P, Julian T, Hadjivassiliou M. Headache associated with coeliac disease: a systematic review and meta-analysis. Nutrients. 2018;10(10):1445.
31. Monro JA, Shaw M. Glycemic impact, glycemic glucose equivalents, glycemic index, and glycemic load: definitions, distinctions, and implications. Am J Clin Nutr. 2008;87(1):237S–43S.
32. Evans CE, Greenwood DC, Threapleton DE, Gale CP, Cleghorn CL, Burley VJ. Glycemic index, glycemic load, and blood pressure: a systematic review and metaanalysis of randomized controlled trials. Am J Clin Nutr. 2017;105(5):1176–90.
33. Evcili G, Utku U, Ogun MN, Ozdemir G. Early and long period follow-up results of low glycemic index diet for migraine prophylaxis. Agri. 2018;30:8–11.
34. Klein P, Tyrlikova I, Mathews GC. Dietary treatment in adults with refractory epilepsy: a review. Neurology. 2014;83:1978–85.
35. Cantello R, Varrasi C, Tarletti R, et al. Ketogenic diet: electrophysiological effects on the normal human cortex. Epilepsia. 2007;48:1756–63.
36. Coppola G, Pierelli F, Schoenen J. Is the cerebral cortex hyperexcitable or hyperresponsive in migraine? Cephalalgia. 2007;27:1427–39.
37. Di Lorenzo C, Coppola G, Bracaglia M, Di Lenola D, Evangelista M, Sirianni G, Rossi P, Di Lorenzo G, Serrao M, Parisi V, Pierelli F. Cortical functional correlates of responsiveness to short-lasting preventive intervention with ketogenic diet in migraine: a multimodal evoked potentials study. J Headache Pain 2016;17(1):1–0.
38. Di Lorenzo C, Coppola G, Sirianni G, Di Lorenzo G, Bracaglia M, Di Lenola D, Siracusano A, Rossi P, Pierelli F. Migraine improve-

ment during short lasting ketogenesis: a proof-of-concept study. Eur J Neurol. 2015;22(1):170–7.

39. Bongiovanni D, Benedetto C, Corvisieri S, Del Favero C, Orlandi F, Allais G, Sinigaglia S, Fadda M. Effectiveness of ketogenic diet in treatment of patients with refractory chronic migraine. Neurol Sci. 2021;42(9):3865–70.
40. Haslam RL, Bezzina A, Herbert J, Spratt N, Rollo ME, Collins CE. Can ketogenic diet therapy improve migraine frequency, severity and duration? Healthcare (Basel). 2021;9(9):1105.
41. Ferrara LA, Pacioni D, Di Fronzo V, et al. Low-lipid diet reduces frequency and severity of acute migraine attacks. Nutr Metab Cardiovasc Dis. 2015;25:370–5.
42. Bunner AE, Agarwal U, Gonzales JF, Valente F, Barnard ND. Nutrition intervention for migraine: a randomized crossover trial. J Headache Pain. 2014;15:69.
43. Sanders AE, Shaikh SR, Slade GD. Long-chain omega-3 fatty acids and headache in the U.S. population. Prostaglandins Leukot Essent Fatty Acids. 2018;135:47–53.
44. Ramsden CE, Zamora D, Faurot KR, MacIntosh B, Horowitz M, Keyes GS, Yuan ZX, Miller V, Lynch C, Honvoh G, Park J, Levy R, Domenichiello AF, Johnston A, Majchrzak-Hong S, Hibbeln JR, Barrow DA, Loewke J, Davis JM, Mannes A, Palsson OS, Suchindran CM, Gaylord SA, Mann JD. Dietary alteration of n-3 and n-6 fatty acids for headache reduction in adults with migraine: randomized controlled trial. BMJ. 2021;374:1448.
45. Bakırhan H, Yıldıran H, Uyar CT. Associations between diet quality, DASH and Mediterranean dietary patterns and migraine characteristics. Nutr Neurosci. 2021;1-1:2324.
46. Mirzababaei A, Khorsha F, Togha M, Yekaninejad MS, Okhovat AA, Mirzaei K. Associations between adherence to dietary approaches to stop hypertension (DASH) diet and migraine headache severity and duration among women. Nutr Neurosci. 2020;23(5):335–42.
47. Arab A, Khorvash F, Kazemi M, Heidari Z, Askari G. Effects of the dietary approaches to stop hypertension (DASH) diet on clinical, quality of life, and mental health outcomes in women with migraine: a randomised controlled trial. Br J Nutr. 2021;1–28:1535.
48. Morris MC, Tangney CC, Wang Y, et al. MIND diet slows cognitive decline with aging. Alzheimers Dement. 2015;11(9):1015–22.
49. Askarpour M, Yarizadeh H, Sheikhi A, Khorsha F, Mirzaei K. Associations between adherence to MIND diet and severity, duration and frequency of migraine headaches among migraine patients. BMC Res Notes. 2020;13(1):341.
50. Azadbakht L, Mirmiran P, Azizi F. Dietary diversity score is favorably associated with the metabolic syndrome in Tehranian adults. Int J Obes. 2005;29(11):1361–7.
51. Kant AK, Schatzkin A, Ziegler RG. Dietary diversity and subsequent cause-specific mortality in the NHANES I epidemiologic follow-up study. J Am Coll Nutr. 1995;14(3):233–8.
52. Khorsha F, Mirzababaei A, Togha M, Mirzaei K. Association of dietary diversity score (DDS) and migraine headache severity among women. Neurol Sci. 2021;42(8):3403–10.
53. Arca KN, Halker Singh RB. Dehydration and headache. Curr Pain Headache Rep. 2021;25(8):56.
54. Sawka M. Chapter 4: Water. In: Dietary reference intakes for water, potassium, sodium, chloride, and sulfate. Natick: Army Research Institute of Environmental Medicine; 2005.
55. Khorsha F, Mirzababaei A, Togha M, Mirzaei K. Association of drinking water and migraine headache severity. J Clin Neurosci. 2020;77:81–4.
56. Spigt M, et al. A randomized trial on the effects of regular water intake in patients with recurrent headaches. Fam Pract. 2011;29(4):370–5.
57. Scher AI, Stewart WF, Ricci JA, Lipton RB. Factors associated with the onset and remission of chronic daily headache in a population-based study. Pain. 2003;106(1–2):81–9.
58. Bigal ME, Rapoport AM. Obesity and chronic daily headache. Curr Pain Headache Rep. 2012;16(1):101–9.
59. Bigal ME, Lipton RB. Obesity is a risk factor for transformed migraine but not chronic tension-type headache. Neurology. 2006;67(2):252–7.
60. Hatami M, Soveid N, Lesani A, Djafarian K, Shab-Bidar S. Migraine and obesity: is there a relationship? A systematic review and meta-analysis of observational studies. CNS Neurol Disord Drug Targets. 2021;20:863.
61. Di Vincenzo A, Beghetto M, Vettor R, Tana C, Rossato M, Bond DS, Pagano C. Effects of surgical and non-surgical weight loss on migraine headache: a systematic review and meta-analysis. Obes Surg. 2020;30(6):2173–85.
62. Kristoffersen ES, Børte S, Hagen K, Zwart JA, Winsvold BS. Migraine, obesity and body fat distribution – a population-based study. J Headache Pain. 2020;21(1):1–8.

Physical Activity, Exercise, and Migraine

21

Hope L. O'Brien and Eduard Tiozzo

Introduction

Despite recent improvements in the option for pharmacological management to improve migraine symptoms, there is still an unmet need. Implementation of an exercise regimen is recommended for patients with migraine, especially those who do not respond to medications or may choose to opt for a non-pharmacological solution to managing recurrent headaches [1]. The benefit of aerobic exercise and increased physical activity has been documented in chronic pain conditions including migraine [2–5]. However, there is no standardized protocol as to which type, amount, and intensity of activity is sufficient to improve migraine symptoms. In this chapter, the role of increased physical activity and exercise in migraine will be reviewed with suggested recommendations for patient management based on the evidence that exists.

Questions

1. Based on controlled trials of women with migraine, aerobic exercise resulted in which of the following?
   - A. Significant reduction of migraine frequency and intensity after 6 weeks of those who exercised compared to those who did not
   - B. Significant reduction of migraine intensity in those who exercised compared to those who did not
   - C. Significant improvement in frequency, duration, and intensity of migraine after 1 h of weekly exercises in those who exercised compared to those who did not
   - D. No significant improvement in intensity and frequency but a significant improvement in duration, among those who did exercise
   - E. No significant improvement in intensity and duration but a significant improvement in frequency, among those who did exercise
2. The long-term effects of exercise have been shown to
   - A. Elevate mood
   - B. Improve sleep
   - C. Manage weight
   - D. All the above
   - E. None of the above

H. L. O'Brien (✉)
Departments of Neurology, at the University of Cincinnati College of Medicine, Cincinnati, OH, USA

Headache Center of Hope, LLC, Cincinnati, OH, USA

E. Tiozzo
Department of Physical Medicine and Rehabilitation, at the University of Miami Miller School of Medicine, Miami, FL, USA

Defining Physical Activity and Exercise

Physical activity and exercise are often used interchangeably as the same term even though they represent different concepts. While physical activity includes any bodily movement that requires energy expenditure above resting level, exercise, as a subcategory of physical activity, includes bodily movements that are structured and planned [6]. Physical activity encompasses both occupational physical activity during working hours and leisure-time physical activity outside of work. A variety of leisure-time physical activities can include household work, driving, walking, and climbing stairs, as well as (structured) exercises such as aerobic exercise (repeated cyclic movements for an extended period, jogging, cycling, and swimming) and resistance exercise (muscle contraction activities that utilize weight machines, free weights, body weight, or elastic devices). Aerobic and resistance exercise represent different modalities, both responsible for improved health

T. S. Monteith et al. (eds.), *Comprehensive Migraine Management*, https://doi.org/10.1007/978-3-031-86923-5_21

and reduced risk of chronic symptoms and illnesses but through contrasting physiological adaptations [7, 8] and subsequently distinct clinical and public health benefits. While the benefits of aerobic exercise are exhibited through improved transport and utilization of oxygen via cardiac, pulmonary, and skeletal systems, the benefits of resistance exercise are achieved through enhanced muscle strength and power [7].

Physical Activity Guidelines

In order to educate and help people achieve minimal requirements for physical activity, various ways of prescribing the same levels have been used; from a metabolic equivalent task (i.e., MET; 500–1000 MET/week) to daily steps (10,000 steps; often recommended by medical establishment) and weekly active minutes which are commonly used in the national guidelines [9, 10]. Various US health-promoting organizations are unanimous with their minimum-minute recommendations for physical activity, needed for substantial health benefits [9]. In their updated 2008 Physical Activity Guidelines, the United States Department of Health and Human Services recommends that adults accumulate at least 150 min of moderate-intensity (i.e., moderate increases in heart rate and respiration that burns 3–6 times as much energy as at rest) or 75 min of vigorous-intensity (i.e., vigorous increases in heart rate and respiration that burns more than 6 times as much energy as at rest). In addition to 150 min of moderate-intensity or 75 min of vigorous-intensity aerobic activity, the same guidelines recommend adding muscle strengthening activities on at least 2 days a week that work all major muscle groups [11]. While the national health-promoting recommendations agree that the above-mentioned amounts and types of physical activity are sufficient to promote health, the American College of Sports Medicine (ACSM), the largest sports medicine and exercise organization in the world, goes a step further. In addition to aerobic and resistance exercises, the ACSM recommends flexibility and neuromotor exercises (e.g., Tai chi and yoga) on minimum 2 days a week [12]. The role of these types of exercise is to reduce the risk of falling and improve postural stability, mobility, and overall quality of life.

The specific exercise guidelines for migraine management do not exist and only serve as a general guide. Aerobic exercise is preferred over resistance exercise. An exercise program should include a warm-up period (to minimize triggering migraine attacks) at a tolerable, comfortable level, and with a suggested frequency of 2–3 times a week [13].

Proposed Biological Mechanisms of Exercise in Migraine

Exercise, with its multifarious health benefits, can be used for the management of several migraine comorbidities such as obesity, depression, anxiety, and sleep disturbance. Exercise has also been shown to improve self-esteem which can reduce symptoms of migraine [14]. Overall, it can be concluded that people who adhere to (aerobic) exercise may be more capable and competent in managing their migraine, more specifically frequency and duration of their migraine attacks. While the underlying biological mechanisms of exercise-specific benefits for migraine attacks remain unclear, speculations related to similar endogenous analgesic and anti-inflammatory effects exist [13].

During and after exercise, endogenous beta-endorphins are released into peripheral and central nervous systems. The release of substance P neuropeptide and beta-endorphin inhibits the transmission of pain in the peripheral nervous system, while in the central nervous system, it inhibits the release of amino acid gamma-aminobutyric acid (GABA), which can be beneficial for pain and migraine symptoms [15]. Baseline levels of β-endorphin have been shown to be lower in patients with migraine compared to individuals without migraine [16]. Exercise results in increased beta-endorphin levels [17] although it is unclear whether this exercise-induced increase corresponds to improvement of migraine symptoms.

In a non-controlled study of 40 women with "migrainosus" headache, a 6-week aerobic exercise performed 3 times a week, 40–50 min per session, at 60–80% of maximal heart rate, resulting in an increase in beta-endorphin which may have contributed to a decrease in headache days; from two to one headache day per month [18]. A brief and sudden feeling of euphoria, analgesia, and anxiolysis, otherwise known as "runner's high" is triggered by high-intensity endurance training and a corresponding increase in the endocannabinoid ligand anandamide (AEA) [19]. In patients with migraine, concentrations of AEA are significantly lower than normal controls, and exercise can have an important role in the modulation of pain processing through this endocannabinoid system [20]. It is important to note, however, that both beta-endorphin and AEA significantly increase when the anaerobic threshold is exceeded, meaning at moderate-to-high exercise intensity [20, 21]. This can pose a problem for migraine individuals, knowing that the accumulation of lactate, also occurring at higher intensities, can be related to higher migraine frequency [13, 22]. Otherwise, human studies on variations of AEA in migraine patients with exercise have been limited.

Lastly, exercise has been shown to reduce pro-inflammatory markers (e.g., C-reactive protein, tumor necrosis factor-alpha, interleukin-β (IL-β), IL-6, and IL-8) and increase anti-inflammatory markers (e.g., IL-6) [23], which can result in improvement of pain as seen in fibromyalgia but not in migraine [24]. Nonetheless, our understanding of the role of inflammation and its aggravating effects on migraine has increased and affords an opportunity for further research on the biochemical markers released during exercise and their impact on migraine attacks.

Migraine in Obesity

Both migraine and obesity are prevalent in the US population and represent two major public health problems [25]. Migraine affects one in ten and obesity one in three American adults [26, 27]. Both conditions are independent risk factors for cardiovascular disorders, particularly stroke [25], but the link between migraine and obesity has not always been clear. Early work suggested that being obese or overweight—even underweight—than normal weight (all estimated by the body mass index; BMI), was associated with migraine prevalence and frequency [28, 29]. Further studies indicated that abdominal obesity (estimated by the waist-hip ratio) is the type of obesity more associated with chronic daily headaches and higher frequencies of migraine attacks [30].

Adipose tissue distribution is dependent on genetics and environmental factors and thus varies with age, but the link between obesity indices and migraine appears to be multifactorial and not easily explained by only abdominal obesity and its proinflammatory state [31]. Regardless of the mechanisms, the current knowledge suggests that migraine prevalence occurs more commonly in women of reproductive age (2–3 greater than in men of the same age) and decreases after menopause (and men of a similar age). The same prevalence trend has been observed regardless of abdominal or total obesity prevalence [31]. For example, a study of patients with episodic and chronic migraine with a BMI ranging from 25 to 49.9 did not show a difference in monthly migraine days after behavioral weight loss that incorporated a progressive, home-based exercise [32].

In addition to the physiological, various other mechanisms have been explored to examine the obesity-migraine relationship: psychological (stress, depression, and anxiety) and behavioral (low physical activity, unhealthy eating habits such as skipping breakfast, irregular meals and high-fat diet, and sleep disorders) [30]. One of the overlapping mechanisms of obesity and migraine is a lack of physical activity. The role of low physical activity in the prevalence of obesity has been well-documented, but the role of low physical activity in migraine and within the context of obesity has received far less attention. Future research examining central and peripheral feeding and obesity pathways that overlap with migraine pathophysiology may elucidate mechanisms and new therapeutic strategies in migraine disorder.

Therapeutic Benefits of Aerobic Exercise in Migraine

The role of increased physical activity and exercise on migraine has been investigated through a wide range of methods with mixed results. In a cross-sectional study of 975 individuals, there was no relationship between physical activity and migraine [33]. However, other population studies showed those who were inactive or did not perform physical exercise were more likely to have recurrent migraine attacks [34, 35]. Additionally, inactivity was associated with migraine appearing later in development and associated with non-migraine headaches [36]. In a clinical trial of 327 individuals with migraine, a low level of physical activity was linked to increased migraine attacks [37]. Although it is unclear whether increased physical activity is linked to improvement of migraine symptoms, there is evidence to suggest low levels of physical inactivity are associated with higher migraine prevalence [34–37].

In a prospective study involving patients with transformed migraine followed by 1 year, those who responded to 30 min of regular exercise 3 days per week were found to have an improvement in headache frequency from chronic to episodic migraine [38]. In a 12-week, randomized control trial of 35 patients with episodic migraine randomized to either high-intensity interval training (HIT) for ~30 min, moderate exercise involving 45 min, 2 times per week versus control, those in the HIT group showed a greater probability (71%) of a positive effect on migraine days compared to the control group [39]. Those in the moderate exercise group had an "unlikely" benefit compared to the control group [39]. A prospective trial of patients with episodic migraine, 40 min of indoor cycling, 3 times a week for 12 weeks showed a reduction in migraine attacks and intensity [40].

A most recent prospective study of 94 participants showed that moderate-vigorous (aerobic) exercise at least 3 times per week, combined with migraine prevention for 6 weeks, resulted in a significant reduction of headache days when compared to those who were less active and on prevention therapy [38]. This difference was not seen when neither group was on prevention medication for migraine.

In a randomized controlled trial, 40 min of indoor cycling 3 times per week for 12 weeks reduced the number of migraine attacks but was not statistically different in the comparison group who performed relaxation or those on migraine prevention with topiramate after 6 months [39]. Similarly, after 12 weeks, individuals who performed aerobic exercises (fast-paced walking for 40 min) while taking amitriptyline had a significant improvement in frequency, intensity, and duration of headaches compared to those who were on amitriptyline alone [40].

There have been other controlled trials of women with migraine that show that moderate exercise improved pain intensity compared to those who did not exercise [41, 42]. Forty-five minutes of twice-weekly aerobic exercise (i.e., indoor gymnastics with music) followed by relaxation and psychological intervention resulted in a significant reduction in migraine intensity after 6 weeks [41]. After 8 weeks of an hour-long schedule of moderate exercise (i.e., walking, rowing, cycling, neck, and postural stretching) performed 3 times per week, there was a significant improvement in intensity, without difference in frequency or duration of those who exercised compared to those who did not exercise [42]. Furthermore, long-term effects of exercise in patients with migraine have also been shown to elevate mood, improve sleep, and manage weight [2–5, 40].

Therapeutic Benefits of Resistance Exercise in Migraine

The benefits of resistance exercise, as a primary countermeasure to age-related chronic diseases (i.e., cardiovascular disease, cancer, and type 2 diabetes), have been emerging [43]. Less represented in research, resistance exercise alone or combined with aerobic exercise—two concepts on the opposite end of an exercise continuum—has and adds multifaceted physiological and functional benefits. A recent review on the efficacy of different exercise modalities and intensities, in a head-to-head comparison, revealed that resistance exercise could be superior in reducing migraine burden than aerobic exercise [44]. It is worth noting that out of 27 studies less than 10% of the studies included resistance training whose regimen typically initiated with 2–3 sets of 12–15 repetitions at 45–60% of the maximum weight (considered low-to-moderate intensity). Mechanistically and compared to aerobic training, strength training could be more beneficial in reducing migraine burden due to its greater capacity to preserve lean muscle mass [45], and increased lean muscle mass has been inversely associated with migraine frequency [46].

Therapeutic Benefits of Yoga and Tai Chi in Migraine

Yoga and tai chi are popular mind-body therapies and have increasingly been used for health and a variety of medical conditions. Both therapies combine repetitive movements with an emphasis on controlled breathing, relaxation, and meditation. Randomized clinical trials implementing Yoga and tai chi have shown a reduction in headache frequency, and severity, as well as co-morbid conditions of anxiety and depression [47–50].

Limitations and Barriers to Exercise Implementation

Despite the potential benefits of migraine, exercise is reported as a trigger with as much as 57% of patients having pain worsened by regular activity [51, 52]. The ICHD-3 diagnostic criteria distinguish migraine from other types of primary headaches based on pain that is aggravation by activity [53]. For patients, suggesting exercise during a migraine attack seems unrealistic, and there is insufficient evidence to support exercise as an acute treatment [54, 55]. Fear of inducing a headache could lead to avoidance of an active lifestyle causing detrimental effects on overall health. Compared to those in the general population without headaches, migraine is associated with decreased cardiorespiratory fitness [56]. Low cardiorespiratory fitness has been recognized as an independent risk factor for mortality in adults [57]. Therefore, when presenting recommendations, it is important to distinguish between migraine and primary exercise headache (PEH); pain induced by or occurring during strenuous physical activity and lasting less than 48 h [51, 58].

Conclusion

In summary, much has been published regarding physical activity and exercise in migraine. However, the lack of randomized controlled trials and variation in the mode or type (i.e., running, jogging, and cycling), duration, and frequency of exercise makes comparison of these studies on the impact of migraine symptoms challenging [59, 60]. It is also unknown whether the addition of medication for migraine prevention and relaxation techniques amplifies the positive effects of exercise. There is some evidence that supports the role of light-to-moderate aerobic exercise, with or without medication, in reducing migraine symptoms and comorbid conditions. Furthermore, low to moderate resistance training may reduce similar symptoms. Therefore, based on the evidence, 30–50 min of moderate aerobic (or combined) exercise between 2 and 5 days per week [13, 18, 60–63] is a reasonable recommendation (see Table 21.1). However, future research should continue to examine the effect of different exercise modalities and their intensities to establish more conclusive and specific guidelines for migraine management.

Table 21.1 Physical activity/exercise specifics for migraine

	Prevent migraine attacks	Reduce risk of exercise-induced migraine attacks
Recommend	Start with 5- to 10-min warm-up Maintain moderate-intensity exercise lasting 30–50 min, 2–3 times per week Finish with 5- to 10-min cool-down/relaxation	Maintain hydration Minimize triggers that may aggravate a migraine attack
Avoid	Bouts of high-intensity exercise during migraine or when physically deconditioned	Excessive exposure to heat Dehydration

Teaching Points

1. Encourage patients to share how they include exercise in their daily routines.
2. Despite substantial literature on physical activity and exercise in migraine, study comparisons are challenging due to variability in exercise types, duration, and frequencies.
3. Light to moderate aerobic exercise in combination with prevention treatment or relaxation techniques can be beneficial in alleviating migraine and comorbid symptoms.
4. Current evidence for migraine management suggests 30–50 min of moderate aerobic or combined aerobic and resistance exercise practiced between 2 and 5 days per week.

Case

LM is a 49-year-old right-handed woman who presents with recurrent headaches described as unilateral in the left frontal location spreading posterior to the bi-occipital region. The pain lasts 4–7 h and is characterized as throbbing/stabbing pain in 7 out of 10 associated photophobia and nausea. The activity makes her headaches worse, and sleep alleviates her pain. She has had headaches similar to these since her 20 s occurring 2–3 times per month. However, over the past 6 weeks, the frequency has increased to 8 days per month, and the pain is no longer responding to sumatriptan 100 mg despite placement on propranolol by her PCP for migraine prevention, started 4 weeks ago. She denies symptoms of aura. She does not skip meals and drinks 30 ounces of fluids daily, including caffeinated coffee. She does not exercise and spends most of her time sitting in an office chair on Zoom meetings. On review of systems, she has difficulty falling asleep. Her past medical history is significant for vitamin D deficiency, and her co-morbid condition is significant for anxiety that has been well-controlled on venlafaxine 75 mg. She also takes vitamin D and melatonin for sleep. Family history is positive for migraine. She is divorced with two grown children, and she is not sexually active. She has made a New Year's resolution to get healthy and has met with a dietician. She realizes the importance of exercise but is concerned that increasing her physical activity will trigger or worsen her migraine attacks.

Subjective and Objective Examination

- Vitals—Afebrile. Pulse 82 regular, BP 137/81, BMI—35

GEN—No acute distress. Skin mottled

Neuro—Oriented x 4. PERRLA, EOMI. CN II—XII grossly intact. There is tightness over the bilateral trapezius and cervicospinal muscles. No gross motor deficits. N/5 strength in all distributions. Sensation fully intact. Coordination and gait normal

Case Discussion

Exercise Program Recommendation: Start with increasing her movement throughout the day. Implement stretching exercises such as Yoga or Tai chi, 2–3 days per week. Regular moderate aerobic activity starting with 5–10 min of a warm-up, followed by 20–30 min of moderate exercises, finishing with a 5–10-min cool-down or relation regimen is also an option. Prior to exercise, ensure hydration and avoid areas of excessive heat.

Questions and Answers

1. Based on controlled trials of women with migraine, aerobic exercise resulted in which of the following?
   A. Significant reduction of migraine frequency and intensity after 6 weeks of those who exercised compared to those who did not
   B. Significant reduction of migraine intensity in those who exercised compared to those who did not
   C. Significant improvement in frequency, duration, and intensity of migraine after 1 h of weekly exercises in those who exercised compared to those who did not

D. No significant improvement in intensity and frequency but a significant improvement in duration, among those who did exercise
E. No significant improvement in intensity and duration but a significant improvement in frequency, among those who did exercise

The correct answer is B. In two controlled trials of women participants, aerobic exercise followed by relaxation and psychological intervention resulted in the reduction of migraine intensity after 6 weeks; 1 h of exercise resulted in a significant difference in intensity but not frequency or duration, among those who did exercise compared to those who did not [41, 42].

2. The long-term effects of exercise have been shown to
   A. Elevate mood
   B. Improve sleep
   C. Manage weight
   D. All the above
   E. None of the above

The correct answer is D. Long-term effects of exercise in patients with migraine have been shown to elevate mood, improve sleep, and manage weight [2–5, 40].

References

1. Lipton RB, Munjal S, Buse DC, Alam A, Fanning KM, Reed ML, et al. Unmet acute treatment needs from the 2017 migraine in America symptoms and treatment study. Headache. 2019;59(8):1310–23.
2. Sullivan AB, Scheman J, Venesy D, Davin S. The role of exercise and types of exercise in the rehabilitation of chronic pain: specific or nonspecific benefits. Curr Pain Headache Rep. 2012;16(2):153–61.
3. Bigal ME, Lipton RB. The epidemiology, burden, and comorbidities of migraine. Neurol Clin. 2009;27(2):321–34.
4. Buse DC, Manack A, Serrano D, Turkel C, Lipton RB. Sociodemographic and comorbidity profiles of chronic migraine and episodic migraine sufferers. J Neurol Neurosurg Psychiatry. 2010;81(4):428–32.
5. Scher AI, Bigal ME, Lipton RB. Comorbidity of migraine. Curr Opin Neurol. 2005;18(3):305–10.
6. Caspersen CJ, Powell KE, Christenson GM. Physical activity, exercise, and physical fitness: definitions and distinctions for health-related research. Public Health Rep. 1985;100(2):126–31.
7. Hughes DC, Ellefsen S, Baar K. Adaptations to endurance and strength training. Cold Spring Harb Perspect Med. 2018;8(6):a029769.
8. Tiozzo E, Youbi M, Dave K, Perez-Pinzon M, Rundek T, Sacco RL, et al. Aerobic, resistance, and cognitive exercise training post-stroke. Stroke. 2015;46(7):2012–6.
9. Oja P, Titze S. Physical activity recommendations for public health: development and policy context. EPMA J. 2011;2(3):253–9.
10. Piercy KL, Troiano RP, Ballard RM, Carlson SA, Fulton JE, Galuska DA, et al. The physical activity guidelines for Americans. JAMA. 2018;320(19):2020–8.
11. Physical activity guidelines for Americans. 2nd ed. https://health.gov/sites/default/files/2019-09/Physical_Activity_Guidelines_2nd_edition.pdf. Washington, DC: U.S Department of Health and Human Services; 2018.
12. Garber CE, Blissmer B, Deschenes MR, Franklin BA, Lamonte MJ, Lee IM, et al. American College of Sports Medicine position stand. Quantity and quality of exercise for developing and maintaining cardiorespiratory, musculoskeletal, and neuromotor fitness in apparently healthy adults: guidance for prescribing exercise. Med Sci Sports Exerc. 2011;43(7):1334–59.
13. Amin FM, Aristeidou S, Baraldi C, Czapinska-Ciepiela EK, Ariadni DD, Di Lenola D, et al. The association between migraine and physical exercise. J Headache Pain. 2018;19(1):83.
14. Irby MB, Bond DS, Lipton RB, Nicklas B, Houle TT, Penzien DB. Aerobic exercise for reducing migraine burden: mechanisms, markers, and models of change processes. Headache. 2016;56(2):357–69.
15. Pilozzi A, Carro C, Huang X. Roles of beta-endorphin in stress, behavior, neuroinflammation, and brain energy metabolism. Int J Mol Sci. 2020;22(1):338.
16. Sicuteri F. Endorphins, opiate receptors and migraine headache. Headache. 1978;17(6):253–7.
17. Schwarz L, Kindermann W. Beta-endorphin, adrenocorticotropic hormone, cortisol and catecholamines during aerobic and anaerobic exercise. Eur J Appl Physiol Occup Physiol. 1990;61(3–4):165–71.
18. Koseoglu E, Akboyraz A, Soyuer A, Ersoy AO. Aerobic exercise and plasma beta endorphin levels in patients with migrainous headache without aura. Cephalalgia. 2003;23(10):972–6.
19. Sparling PB, Giuffrida A, Piomelli D, Rosskopf L, Dietrich A. Exercise activates the endocannabinoid system. Neuroreport. 2003;14(17):2209–11.
20. Schwarz L, Kindermann W. Changes in beta-endorphin levels in response to aerobic and anaerobic exercise. Sports Med. 1992;13(1):25–36.
21. Raichlen DA, Foster AD, Gerdeman GL, Seillier A, Giuffrida A. Wired to run: exercise-induced endocannabinoid signaling in humans and cursorial mammals with implications for the 'runner's high. J Exp Biol. 2012;215(Pt 8):1331–6.
22. Watanabe H, Kuwabara T, Ohkubo M, Tsuji S, Yuasa T. Elevation of cerebral lactate detected by localized 1H-magnetic resonance spectroscopy in migraine during the interictal period. Neurology. 1996;47(4):1093–5.
23. Scheffer DDL, Latini A. Exercise-induced immune system response: anti-inflammatory status on peripheral and central organs. Biochim Biophys Acta Mol basis Dis. 2020;1866(10):165823.
24. Bjersing JL, Dehlin M, Erlandsson M, Bokarewa MI, Mannerkorpi K. Changes in pain and insulin-like growth factor 1 in fibromyalgia during exercise: the involvement of cerebrospinal inflammatory factors and neuropeptides. Arthritis Res Ther. 2012;14(4):R162.
25. Bigal ME, Liberman JN, Lipton RB. Obesity and migraine: a population study. Neurology. 2006;66(4):545–50.
26. Lipton RB, Stewart WF, Diamond S, Diamond ML, Reed M. Prevalence and burden of migraine in the United States: data from the American Migraine Study II. Headache. 2001;41(7):646–57.
27. Tiwari A, Balasundaram P. Public health considerations regarding obesity. Treasure Island (FL): StatPearls; 2022.
28. Scher AI, Stewart WF, Ricci JA, Lipton RB. Factors associated with the onset and remission of chronic daily headache in a population-based study. Pain. 2003;106(1–2):81–9.
29. Bigal ME, Lipton RB. Obesity is a risk factor for transformed migraine but not chronic tension-type headache. Neurology. 2006;67(2):252–7.
30. Bond DS, Roth J, Nash JM, Wing RR. Migraine and obesity: epidemiology, possible mechanisms and the potential role of weight loss treatment. Obes Rev. 2011;12(5):e362–71.
31. Peterlin BL, Rapoport AM, Kurth T. Migraine and obesity: epidemiology, mechanisms, and implications. Headache. 2010;50(4):631–48.

32. Bond DS, Thomas JG, Lipton RB, Roth J, Pavlovic JM, Rathier L, et al. Behavioral weight loss intervention for migraine: a randomized controlled trial. Obesity (Silver Spring). 2018;26(1):81–7.
33. Rasmussen BK. Migraine and tension-type headache in a general population: precipitating factors, female hormones, sleep pattern and relation to lifestyle. Pain. 1993;53(1):65–72.
34. Queiroz LP, Peres MF, Piovesan EJ, Kowacs F, Ciciarelli MC, Souza JA, et al. A nationwide population-based study of migraine in Brazil. Cephalalgia. 2009;29(6):642–9.
35. Molarius A, Tegelberg A, Ohrvik J. Socio-economic factors, lifestyle, and headache disorders – a population-based study in Sweden. Headache. 2008;48(10):1426–37.
36. Varkey E, Hagen K, Zwart JA, Linde M. Physical activity and headache: results from the Nord-Trondelag Health Study (HUNT). Cephalalgia. 2008;28(12):1292–7.
37. Wober C, Brannath W, Schmidt K, Kapitan M, Rudel E, Wessely P, et al. Prospective analysis of factors related to migraine attacks: the PAMINA study. Cephalalgia. 2007;27(4):304–14.
38. Hagan KK, Li W, Mostofsky E, Bertisch SM, Vgontzas A, Buettner C, et al. Prospective cohort study of routine exercise and headache outcomes among adults with episodic migraine. Headache. 2021;61(3):493–9.
39. Varkey E, Cider A, Carlsson J, Linde M. Exercise as migraine prophylaxis: a randomized study using relaxation and topiramate as controls. Cephalalgia. 2011;31(14):1428–38.
40. Santiago MD, Carvalho Dde S, Gabbai AA, Pinto MM, Moutran AR, Villa TR. Amitriptyline and aerobic exercise or amitriptyline alone in the treatment of chronic migraine: a randomized comparative study. Arq Neuropsiquiatr. 2014;72(11):851–5.
41. Dittrich SM, Gunther V, Franz G, Burtscher M, Holzner B, Kopp M. Aerobic exercise with relaxation: influence on pain and psychological well-being in female migraine patients. Clin J Sport Med. 2008;18(4):363–5.
42. Narin SO, Pinar L, Erbas D, Ozturk V, Idiman F. The effects of exercise and exercise-related changes in blood nitric oxide level on migraine headache. Clin Rehabil. 2003;17(6):624–30.
43. McLeod JC, Stokes T, Phillips SM. Resistance exercise training as a primary countermeasure to age-related chronic disease. Front Physiol. 2019;10:645.
44. Woldeamanuel YW, Oliveira ABD. What is the efficacy of aerobic exercise versus strength training in the treatment of migraine? A systematic review and network meta-analysis of clinical trials. J Headache Pain. 2022;23(1):134.
45. Beavers KM, Ambrosius WT, Rejeski WJ, Burdette JH, Walkup MP, Sheedy JL, et al. Effect of exercise type during intentional weight loss on body composition in older adults with obesity. Obesity (Silver Spring). 2017;25(11):1823–9.
46. Caverni CN, da Costa AT, Simioni CG, Fukue RR, Tengan CH, Villa TR. Evaluation of body composition in patients with migraine on prophylactic treatment with topiramate. Heliyon. 2021;7(4):e06865.
47. Boroujeni MZ, Marandi SM, Esfarjani F, Sattar M, Shaygannejad V, Javanmard SH. Yoga intervention on blood NO in female migraineurs. Adv Biomed Res. 2015;4:259.
48. John PJ, Sharma N, Sharma CM, Kankane A. Effectiveness of yoga therapy in the treatment of migraine without aura: a randomized controlled trial. Headache. 2007;47(5):654–61.
49. Kisan R, Sujan M, Adoor M, Rao R, Nalini A, Kutty BM, et al. Effect of Yoga on migraine: a comprehensive study using clinical profile and cardiac autonomic functions. Int J Yoga. 2014;7(2):126–32.
50. Xie YJ, Hui SSC, Ho SC, Suen LKP. The effectiveness of 12-week Tai Chi training in the prophylaxis of episodic migraine: a pilot randomized controlled trial in Chinese women. Cephalalgia. 2017;37:334.
51. Park JW, Chu MK, Kim JM, Park SG, Cho SJ. Analysis of trigger factors in episodic migraineurs using a smartphone headache diary applications. PLoS One. 2016;11(2):e0149577.
52. Varkey E, Gruner Svealv B, Edin F, Ravn-Fischer A, Cider A. Provocation of migraine after maximal exercise: a test-retest study. Eur Neurol. 2017;78(1–2):22–7.
53. Headache Classification Committee of the International Headache Society (IHS) The International Classification of Headache Disorders, 3rd edition. Cephalalgia. 2018;38(1):1–211.
54. Darling M. The use of exercise as a method of aborting migraine. Headache. 1991;31(9):616–8.
55. Strelniker YM. Intensive running completely removes a migraine attack. Med Hypotheses. 2009;72(5):608.
56. Hagen K, Wisloff U, Ellingsen O, Stovner LJ, Linde M. Headache and peak oxygen uptake: the HUNT3 study. Cephalalgia. 2016;36(5):437–44.
57. Blair SN, Kohl HW 3rd, Paffenbarger RS Jr, Clark DG, Cooper KH, Gibbons LW. Physical fitness and all-cause mortality. A prospective study of healthy men and women. JAMA. 1989;262(17):2395–401.
58. Upadhyaya P, Nandyala A, Ailani J. Primary exercise headache. Curr Neurol Neurosci Rep. 2020;20(5):9.
59. Lemmens J, De Pauw J, Van Soom T, Michiels S, Versijpt J, van Breda E, et al. The effect of aerobic exercise on the number of migraine days, duration and pain intensity in migraine: a systematic literature review and meta-analysis. J Headache Pain. 2019;20(1):16.
60. Song TJ, Chu MK. Exercise in treatment of migraine including chronic migraine. Curr Pain Headache Rep. 2021;25(3):14.
61. Seok JI, Cho HI, Chung CS. From transformed migraine to episodic migraine: reversion factors. Headache. 2006;46(7):1186–90.
62. Hanssen H, Minghetti A, Magon S, Rossmeissl A, Rasenack M, Papadopoulou A, et al. Effects of different endurance exercise modalities on migraine days and cerebrovascular health in episodic migraineurs: a randomized controlled trial. Scand J Med Sci Sports. 2018;28(3):1103–12.
63. Varkey E, Cider A, Carlsson J, Linde M. A study to evaluate the feasibility of an aerobic exercise program in patients with migraine. Headache. 2009;49(4):563–70.

Dr. O'Brien is on the Speaker Bureau for AbbVie, Lilly and Pfizer and has received research support for clinical trials from AbbVie and Lilly. All funding has been received by the Headache Center of Hope Institution. She also receives editorial royalty fees from UpToDate.

Neuromodulation for Migraine

22

J. Lloyd and A. P. Andreou

Introduction

Pharmaceutical treatments for migraine have been the preferred treatment option for hundreds of years, with ergots recommended in 1868 and ergotamine isolated in 1918. More recent advances have led to migraine-specific, targeted treatments such as triptans and the calcitonin gene-related peptide (CGRP) monoclonal antibodies. However, pharmaceuticals require systemic administration, often resulting in off-target adverse events. Often, patients prefer non-pharmaceutical treatment options, while a significant percentage of chronic migraine (CM) patients may become refractory to pharmaceutical treatments.

In this chapter, we will discuss the currently available neuromodulation treatments for migraine [1, 2] as well as neuromodulation techniques applied at an experimental level, covering the biological rationale and mechanisms of action and the available clinical data. This will be split into three sections: non-invasive treatments targeting the peripheral nervous system, non-invasive treatments targeting the central nervous system, and invasive neuromodulation treatments (Fig. 22.1).

Questions

1. Which of the following is a neuromodulation device that the FDA cleared for the management of migraine, cluster headache, and hemicrania continua?
   A. Transcutaneous *supraorbital* neurostimulation
   B. Non-invasive vagus nerve stimulator
   C. *Remote electrical* neuromodulation
   D. External concurrent occipital and trigeminal neurostimulation
2. What are the contraindications to the use of non-invasive neuromodulation devices for migraine?
   A. Pacemaker
   B. Medication overuse headache
   C. Neuropathic pain
   D. All of the above

J. Lloyd
Headache Research-Wolfson CARD, Institute of Psychiatry, Psychology and Neuroscience, King's College London, London, UK

A. P. Andreou (✉)
Headache Research-Wolfson CARD, Institute of Psychiatry, Psychology and Neuroscience, King's College London, London, UK

Headache Centre, Guy's and St Thomas' NHS Foundation Trust, London, UK

T. S. Monteith et al. (eds.), *Comprehensive Migraine Management*, https://doi.org/10.1007/978-3-031-86923-5_22

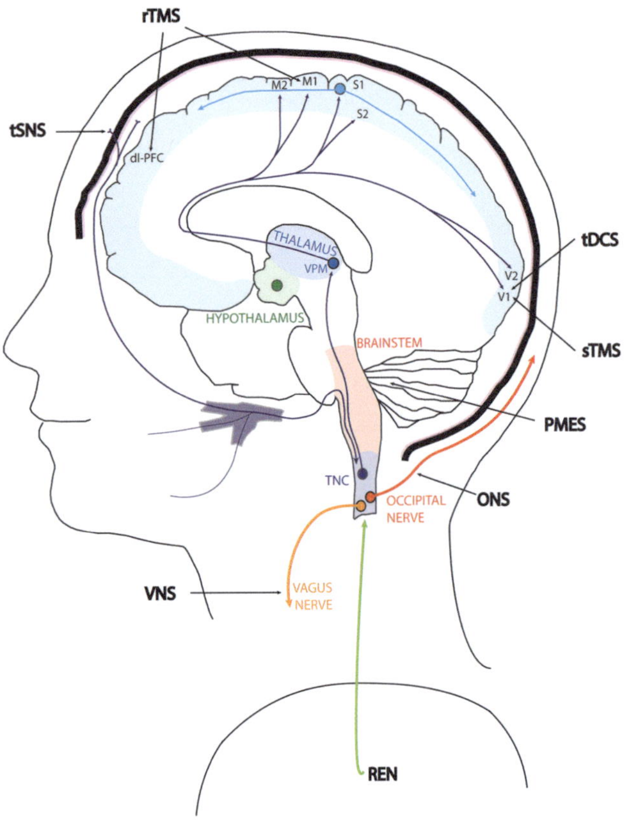

Fig. 22.1 Sites of action of neuromodulation treatments for migraine. **Brain nuclei**—dorsolateral prefrontal cortex (dl-PFC), primary motor cortex (M1), secondary motor cortex (M2), primary somatosensory cortex (S1), secondary somatosensory cortex (S2), trigeminal nucleus caudalis (TNC), Ventral posteromedial nucleus (VPM), primary visual cortex (V1), and secondary visual cortex (V2). **Invasive neuromodulation**—occipital nerve stimulation (ONS) and high frequency (>10 Khz) spinal cord stimulation (SCS). **Non-invasive neuromodulation**—percutaneous mastoid electrical stimulator (PMES), remote electrical neuromodulation (REN), single-pulse transcranial magnetic stimulation (sTMS), supraorbital nerve stimulator (tSNS), transcranial direct current stimulation (tDCS), repeated measures transcranial magnetic stimulation (rTMS), and vagus nerve stimulation (VNS)

Non-invasive Treatments Targeting the Peripheral Nervous System

Transcutaneous Supraorbital and Supratrochlear Nerve Stimulation

Transcutaneous supraorbital nerve stimulation (tSNS) refers to the application of electrical current over the skin covering the supraorbital and supratrochlear nerve at the region of the forehead. The first device is technically classified as external trigeminal neurostimulation (eTNS) and is a form of transcutaneous electrical nerve stimulation (TENS) known as Cefaly (CEFALY® Technology, Belgium; Fig. 22.2a) device. There is a second TENS device, Headterm-2 (EmeTerm, Canada; Fig. 22.2b). Both portable devices have been introduced as non-invasive tSNS methods that can be used by patients as home treatments for migraine management.

Biological Rationale and Mechanism of Action

The majority of investigations for tSNS have been with CEFALY.® The ophthalmic (V1) branch of the trigeminal nerve innervates the ethmoid and sphenoid sinuses, extra and intracranial vasculature (including the middle meningeal artery and the cerebral sinuses), the dura mater, and the skin of the upper portion of the face [3]. T is believed that the V1 branch is the primary somatosensory nerve activated during migraine attacks. In tSNS, electrodes are attached bilaterally to the forehead, and the transcutaneous electrical current directly stimulates the supraorbital (and supratrochlear) branches of the ophthalmic division of the trigeminal nerve. The tSNS device produces rectangular biphasic compensated impulses, a maximum intensity of 16 mA, a width of 250 μS, frequency of 60 Hz, with a progressive slope from 1 to 16 mA over 14 min.

This stimulation is thought to activate the non-nociceptive Aβ somatosensory afferents (producing paraesthesia) without activating Aδ- or C-nociceptive afferents (avoiding wind-up or central sensitisation) [4]. However, many patients report pain during stimulation with the tSNS device, suggesting that at least some C-fibres may be also activated. Stimulation of V1 trigeminal branches may improve migraine symptoms by inhibiting nociceptive trigeminal fibres through stimulation of large non-nociceptive fibres as per the gate control theory [5].

An 18-fluorodeoxyglucose positron emission tomography (FDG-PET) study evaluating the brain metabolic changes before and 3 months after treatment with tSNS in EM patients showed a reduction of the hypometabolism in frontotemporal areas, especially in the orbitofrontal (OFC) and rostral anterior cingulate cortices (rACC) [6]. Further functional neuroimaging brain research of migraine patients showed decreased activation of the ACC in response to trigeminal heat stimulation after tSNS. The use of somatosensory evoked potentials has shown that a 3-month supraorbital stimulation increases thalamocortical activity [7]. Taken together, this initial evidence may suggest an indirect neuromodulation effect of tSNS through the modulation of central pain-controlling areas.

Clinical Data

tSNS has been tested for the acute and preventive treatment of migraine. The use of tSNS as a migraine abortive treatment was initially studied in a prospective open-label trial. Thirty migraine attacks were treated with tSNS for 60 min in 30 patients. Mean pain intensity was significantly reduced in over 50% of the attacks at 1 and 2 h after treatment. No patients took rescue medication within the 2-h observation phase. The therapy seems well-tolerated by all patients [8].

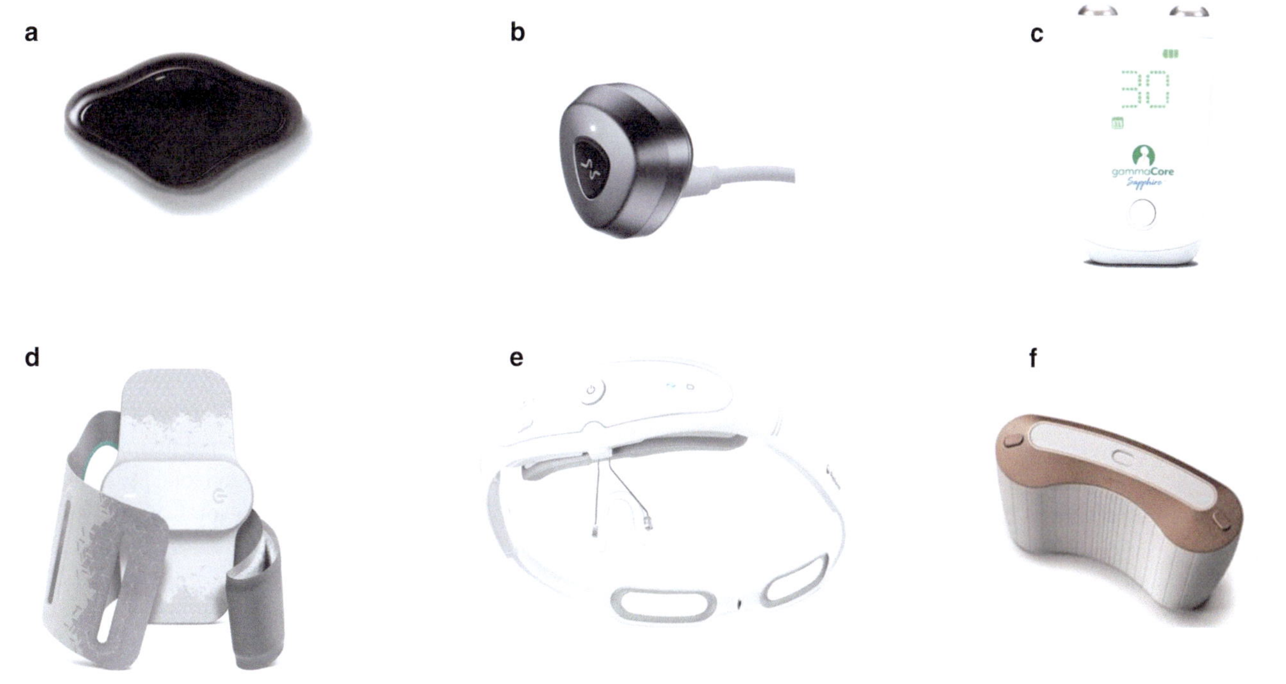

Fig. 22.2 Non-invasive neuromodulation devices cleared by the Food and Drug Administration for the treatment of migraine. Electrical trigeminal neurostimulator (**a**), transcutaneous electrical nerve stimulator (**b**), non-invasive vagal nerve stimulator (**c**), remote electrical neuromodulation (**d**), combined external occipital-trigeminal neurostimulator (**e**), and single-pulse transcranial magnetic stimulator (**f**) devices are depicted. (Images courtesy of Cefaly Technology (**a**); WAT Medical (**b**); electroCore (**c**); Theranica Bio-Electronics; image owned and released by Theranica-Bio-Electronics (**d**); Neurolief (**e**); eNeura (**f**). Image adapted with permission from [108])

In view of these promising initial findings, a double-blind, randomised, and sham-controlled study was subsequently conducted in a larger number of patients. One hundred and six patients with acute migraine attacks were treated in a randomised control trial (RCT) (ACME). Overall, the change in pain intensity at 1 hour compared to baseline was significant in the treated group compared to sham-treated (−59% vs −30%, respectively). Reduction in pain intensity was significant in migraine without aura but not in migraine with aura patients. Furthermore, it supported the safety and good tolerability of this therapy [9].

Following a 3-month pilot evaluation of the tSNS device as a preventive treatment for EM which showed positive initial results [10], one prospective, multi-centre, double-blinded, randomised, and sham-controlled trial (the PREMICE study) has been conducted. The trial included 67 patients with EM treated with 20 min per day of Cefaly® or sham stimulation over a period of 3 months. The patients in the Cefaly® treatment group reported a statistically higher reduction in monthly migraine days (from 6.9 to 4.8) than that of the sham group. Approximately, 40% of the patients experienced a 50% reduction in migraine days rate, which was significantly higher than the sham. In the tSNS group, there was a marked reduction in the number of migraine attacks, headache days, and acute abortive medication intake per month. No serious adverse events were noticed [11].

Additional open-label trials have taken place investigating the efficacy of the tSNS device, finding improvements in migraine days and acute medication consumption with no adverse events [12, 13]. Supraorbital nerve stimulation has also been shown to be more effective in combination with flunarizine than either treatment in isolation, showing a higher 50% responder rate with reductions in migraine intensity and acute medication consumption and no differences in adverse events reported [14].

Regarding the safety of the technique, a survey of 2313 migraine sufferers estimated adverse events (AE) and willingness to continue tSNS with the tSNS device over a 40-day trial period. The results confirmed that this mode of treatment is safe and well-tolerated for migraine patients and provided satisfaction to the majority of patients. The most common AEs were local painful paraesthesia, sleep disturbances, and headache worsening. Rarely reported adverse effects were nausea and vomiting, inability to keep the eyes open during the stimulation, increased tinnitus during the session, eye redness and tearing, skin irritation or allergic cutaneous reaction to the electrode gel, skin numbness, minor forehead pain, feeling of abrupt electrical variation, and tachycardia [15].

The second tSNS, the Headterm-2 device, has been tested in a small, randomised sham-controlled trial in an emergency department setting. Seventy-eight migraine patients (both with and without aura) were included in the study. Patients on the active arm received a 20-minute stimulation protocol (125 μs pulses at 50 Hz and 60 V). The primary clinical endpoint was a reduction at the VAS scale recorded 20 minutes and 2 hours post-treatment. The change in VAS scores from baseline was significantly different between the active and sham groups at both 20 minutes (51 vs 1, $P < 0.001$) and 2 hours (66 vs 10, $P < 0.001$) post-treatment, with the authors concluding to be an effective and economical treatment with few side effects [16]. Headterm-2 is now FDA-approved and available as a non-prescription treatment for migraine prevention. Larger studies are needed to confirm its efficacy in both the acute and preventive treatment of migraine.

Non-invasive Vagus Nerve Stimulation

Transcutaneous vagus nerve stimulation (nVNS) targets non-invasively the vagus nerve, which extends from the brainstem to the abdomen and communicates with a variety of muscles and organs along its entire length. In the field of headaches, nVNS aims to target non-invasively the cervical branch of the vagus nerve using a small handheld device to stimulate the nerve in the region of the neck (Gammacore, Fig. 22.2c), or a small device aiming to transcutaneously stimulate the auricular vagus nerve (NEMOS device).

Biological Rationale and Mechanism of Action

The vagus nerve, the Xth cranial nerve, arises from the medulla, containing both afferent sensory (80%) and efferent motor (20%) fibres. The vagus nerve provides parasympathetic innervation to the autonomic nervous system, involved in a variety of autonomic functions including the respiratory, cardiovascular, and nociceptive systems.

The exact mechanism by which nVNS yields pain relief is not well-understood. The stimulation is thought to activate low-threshold myelinated A-fibres, producing an antinociceptive effect on the second-order neurons of the spinothalamic and spino-reticular tracts within the trigeminocervical complex (TCC). VNS in animal models has been shown to modulate trigeminal activity, inhibiting the response of TCC neurons to trigeminal stimulation in 48% of neurons and facilitating activity in 29.5% of neurons and shown to be superior to sham at providing pain freedom up to 60 min post-stimulation and therapeutic benefit up to 120 min [17].

This inhibition of trigeminal neuronal activity may be mediated by opioidergic mechanisms, as it can be prevented through the application of a non-selective opioid receptor antagonist (Naloxone) and specific delta opioid receptor antagonist (SNC 162) [18]. This opioidergic recruitment may result in modulation of excitability in the TCC, as nVNS can suppress nitroglycerine (GTN)-driven glutamate release in the TCC [19], and subsequent expression of proteins associated with peripheral and central sensitisation in trigeminal neurons [20].

Stimulation of the vagus nerve has also been shown to have indirect central effects, inhibiting cortical spreading depression potentially shortening visual aura [21, 22]. In fMRI studies in humans, VNS increases the connectivity between the motor-related thalamus and anterior cingulate cortex/medial prefrontal cortex and decreases the connectivity between occipital cortex-related thalamus subregion and postcentral gyrus/precuneus [23].

Clinical Data on Migraine

nVNS has been tested for the acute and preventive treatment of migraine. Open-label studies suggested that nVNS could be a beneficial abortive migraine treatment. A study conducted in 48 patients who treated a total of 131 mild-to-moderate migraine attacks showed a pain-relief rate of 38.2% at 1 h and 51.1% at 2 h, whereas the pain-free rate was 17.6% at 1 h and 22.9% at 2 h [24]. When the effect of nVNS was assessed in moderate to severe migraine attacks, the pain-free rate at 2 h was 21% for the first treated attack, and the pain-free rate for all moderate or severe attacks was 22% [25]. When studied in a multicentre, randomised, double-blind, parallel-group, and sham-controlled study of 243 migraine patients (PRESTO trial), nVNS treatment did not meet the primary endpoint of pain-freedom at 2 h of the first treated attack (30.4% of patients from the verum group versus 19.7% of the sham group, $P = 0.067$). This is of little surprise given the low percentage of pain freedom in the two open-label studies. The verum group achieved positive but inconsistent results, in some of the secondary endpoints, including pain relief at 2 h but not at 30 or 60 min post-nVNS treatment [26].

Gammacore was also evaluated as a migraine preventative treatment in a multi-centre, double-blind, and sham-controlled pilot study in 59 patients with CM (the EVENT study). Again, the primary endpoint of the trial was not met at the end of the double-blind phase: the mean reduction in the number of headache days at month 2 was −1.4 (nVNS) vs. −0.2 (sham) ($\Delta = 1.2$; $P = 0.56$) [27]. Subsequently, a larger multi-centre, randomised, double-blind trial conducted in 322 EM patients confirmed the poor efficacy of the device in migraine prevention (the PREMIUM trial). At 12 weeks, the mean reductions in migraine days per month (primary outcome) were 2.26 for nVNS and 1.80 for sham ($P = 0.15$). The trial also highlighted issues with suboptimal adherence to treatment and poor sham, which may have biased the results of the study [28]. Real-world experience in a small group of patients has confirmed the lack of efficacy of nVNS as a preventative treatment in refractory patients with chronic migraine [29].

The NEMOS® device was evaluated in CM in a single-centre, prospective, double-blind, randomised, parallel-group, and controlled trial. The study consisted of a 4-week screening period ("baseline") followed by a 12-week randomised, double-blind, and parallel-group treatment period with either 1 Hz or 25 Hz nVNS with the NEMOS® device. The stimulation parameters were set as pulse width: 250 μs, frequency: 1 Hz or 25 Hz, and duty cycle: 30s on, 30s off. The primary outcome measure was the mean change in headache days per 28-day period. The study showed a significant decrease in headache days per 28 days from baseline to evaluation, which was significantly larger in the 1 Hz group than in the 25 Hz group. In the 1 Hz group, the reduction amounted to 7 headache days less than baseline per 28 days (36.4% reduction from baseline), whereas the 25 Hz group reached only −3.3 days (17.4% reduction from baseline). The number of responders (>50% improvement in headache days) was 29.4% in the 1 Hz group and 13.6% in the 25 Hz group. The number of days with the intake of acute headache medication as well as the migraine disability assessment (MIDAS) and HIT-6 scores was significantly reduced in both treatment groups, without any between-group differences. The most frequent treatment-related adverse events were local problems at the stimulation site, such as mild or moderate pain, paraesthesia, pruritus during or after stimulation, and erythema, ulcer, or scab. Treatment-related adverse events leading to the discontinuation of the study were stimulation site ulcers (accompanied by pain, paraesthesia, or pruritus) in two patients of the 1 Hz group and in on patient of the 25 Hz group [30]. The study findings suggest that auricular nVNS at 1 Hz for 4 h daily may be effective for CM prevention over a short period of time. The absolute reduction in headache days (7.0) and the difference between groups (2.7 headache days) is comparable to the effects of other licensed CM treatments, such as topiramate and onabotulinumtoxinA, although the 50% responders' rate is lower. The nVNS treatment also resulted in a meaningful improvement in the quality of life as assessed by MIDAS and HIT 6. The safety profile was favourable, and compliance with daily stimulation was high. In view of this promising initial data, this neuromodulation modality should be explored in future studies.

Remote Electrical Neuromodulation

Remote electrical neuromodulation (REN) applies transcutaneous electrical current to the peripheral primary afferent fibres, primarily the skin of the upper arm. The main REN device is the Nerivio (Nerivio, Theranica Bio-Electronics Ltd., Israel; Fig. 22.2d), a wearable, smartphone-controlled neurostimulation device. REN is a form of TENS technique that has been assessed in migraine and is the first non-cephalic form of neuromodulation for headache disorders.

Biological Rational and Mechanism of Action

The therapeutic effect of REN is based on the phenomenon of conditioned pain modulation (CPM), which is an intrinsic analgesic mechanism characterised by inhibition of pain in remote body regions after stimulation of C- and Aδ- sensory fibres above their depolarisation threshold but below the nociceptive threshold [31]. The postulated underlying mechanism of analgesia is the activation of descending inhibition pathways of the brainstem [31], particularly the opioidergic pathways of the ventrolateral periaqueductal grey [32] and rostral ventral medulla [33, 34], which reduce activity at the synapse of first- and second-order afferent fibres in the dorsal horn of the spinal cord. The company claims that REN's robust non-painful conditioning stimuli are sufficient to induce pain inhibition [35]. The stimulation protocol is a symmetrical, biphasic, and square pulse with a pulse width of 50–400 μs, modulated frequency of 80–120-Hz, and patient-controlled output current of up to 40 mA in a 45-min session.

Clinical Data

REN has been tested in the acute treatment of migraine. A prospective, double-blinded, randomised, crossover, and sham-controlled trial conducted on 71 migraine patients showed that treatment with Nerivio led to 50% pain reduction in 64% of participants compared to 26% of participants in the sham group. Approximately, one-third of participants became pain-free with Nerivio treatment compared to 6% of the placebo group. Better results were obtained if stimulation was started at the onset of a migraine attack (within 20 min of pain onset) [31].

Similar results emerged from another double-blind, randomised, and sham-controlled study conducted on 252 migraine patients. The primary endpoint was the change in the proportion of participants obtaining pain relief at 2 h post-treatment (30–45 min). Relief of the most bothersome symptoms (MBS) was also assessed as one of the key secondary endpoints. Active stimulation was significantly more effective than sham stimulation in achieving pain relief (66.7% vs. 38.8%), pain-freedom (37.4% vs. 18.4%), and MBS relief (46.3% vs. 22.2%) at 2 h post-treatment with sustained effect at 48 h post-treatment. Side effects were experienced by a small proportion of patients without any significant difference from the sham group. Device-related adverse events included warmth sensation, temporary arm/hand numbness, redness, itching, tingling, muscle spasms, and pain in the arm, shoulders, or neck. All device-related adverse events were mild and resolved within 24 h [35]. When compared to standard of care in a post-hoc analysis of 99 of the 252 patients, REN was shown to be more effective than "usual care," meaning specific acute migraine medications (e.g., triptans), non-specific acute medications (e.g., NSAIDS and acetaminophen), and no pharmacological treatments (84.4% of participants vs 68.9% had pain relief at 2 hours) [36].

A further recent open-label study of 126 chronic migraine patients found REN was an effective acute treatment for showing some pain relief at 2 and 24 hours post-treatment [37].

REN was recently FDA-cleared for preventive management of migraine.

External Occipital and Trigeminal Combined Neurostimulation

A peripherally acting neuromodulation treatment that combines both occipital and trigeminal external stimulation (COT-NS; Relivion device; Neurolief Ltd, Israel; Fig. 22.2e) has been recently approved by the FDA.

COT-NS is designed as another headband device that applies 6 points of stimulation; 4 to the ophthalmic branch of the trigeminal nerve over the forehead and 2 stimulation points to the occipital nerve over the crown of the head, with the intensity and stimulation pattern controlled via a smartphone app.

Biological Rational and Mechanism of Action

No preclinical studies have been performed aiming to highlight the mechanism of action of combined occipital and trigeminal neuromodulation. The principal is that neuromodulation of both the trigeminal and occipital peripheral fibres could influence the degree of activation of the ascending trigeminothalamic pathway, given their convergence on second-order neurons within the trigeminocervical complex [38]. However, preclinical studies are required to demonstrate the efficacy of the stimulating paradigms in actually suppressing the activation of second-order neurons.

Clinical Data

To date, only two randomised control trials have been carried out on the efficacy of eCOT-NS. The trial was a randomised, sham-controlled, double-blind, and multi-centre trial of 109 episodic migraine patients, with and without aura. Participants in the active arms of the study received up to a 60-minute stimulation (330–400 ms, 80-Hz stimulation pulse of up to 6 mA for the trigeminal nerve and up to 12 mA for the greater occipital nerve). Reduction of migraine headache at 2 hours after treatment was the primary endpoint. In the active arm, 23% more patients reported pain relief at 2 hours vs sham arm (60% vs 37%, $P = 0.018$), and the adverse events were not concluded to be serious or severe [39].

A further randomised, double-blind, and sham-controlled trial tested COT-NS on 55 chronic migraine patients (both with and without aura). The active group ($N = 27$) received 60-minute (± 20 mins) treatment (400 μs, 80 Hz stimulation pulses, of up to 6 mA to the trigeminal nerve and up to 12 mA for the occipital nerve). The relative change in VAS pain score was used as the primary endpoint and assessed at 1 hr., 2 hrs, and 24 hrs post-treatment. The percentage decreases in VAS at the 3 time points were all significantly different compared to the sham group (1 hr.: 42.8%, $P = 0.0002$, 2 hrs: 34.7%, $P = 0.0324$, 24 hrs: 37.0% $P = 0.0220$). They also reported no significant difference in AEs between the two testing groups [40].

The COT-NS device has been approved by the FDA for the acute treatment of migraine.

Non-invasive Neuromodulation Treatments Acting in the Central Nervous System

Transcranial Direct Current Stimulation

Transcranial direct current stimulation (tDCS) is a non-invasive, non-painful brain stimulation procedure, in which weak direct current (0.1–2 mA) is applied through the skull over cortical areas for 10–30 min. tDCS has been shown effective in neuropsychiatric and neurological conditions such as major depression, as well as, in enhancing learning and memory formation [41–45]. TDCS uses stimulation from a positive (anode) and negative (cathode) electrode placed over a target area to manipulate the membrane potential of neurons in the cortex. Anodal stimulation depolarises the neurons causing cortical excitation, whereas cathodal stimulation hyperpolarises the neurons decreasing excitation in the cortex [46]. TDCS has been used in experimental and small pilot studies in migraine. It should be noted that the treatment is not FDA-approved and requires patients to attend a neurophysiological setting to receive the treatment.

Biological Rationale and Mechanism of Action

TDCS has been used in migraine treatment due to increasing data supporting cortical altered functionality in patients during and between attacks [47–51]. Previous work showed that tDCS applied over the motor cortex of human subjects increases the excitability of the motor cortex in a glutamate-dependent manner [52, 53]. Application of direct current over mouse motor cortical slice has shown that DCS enhances synaptic response that depends on the N-methyl-D-aspartate receptor (NMDAR) and brain-derived neurotrophic factor [54]. A more recent important study looking at the molecular actions of tDCS suggested that tDCS-induced plasticity is mediated through astrocytic $Ca2+/IP3$ signalling [55].

In migraine patients in particular, an increase in grey matter volume of the lingual gyrus of the occipital lobe vs healthy controls has been shown, which was not related to the severity of the migraine [56]. Following tDCS treatment (28 days application to the verum, 1 mA for 20 mins) as well as a reduction of migraine days per month, there was also a parallel decrease in grey matter volume of the lingual gyrus vs sham-controls [57].

Clinical Data

Several small pilot studies have investigated tDCS as a prophylactic treatment for migraine. A pilot study treated ten patients with MO three times a week for 8 weeks, applying anodal tDCS to the visual cortex. A decrease in migraine attack frequency and duration (but not intensity) was seen following tDCS treatment compared to baseline as well as a decrease in analgesic intake [58]. An RCT by Antal et al. applied cathodal stimulation to the visual cortex of 26 patients three times a week for 6 weeks. They showed no change in the frequency of migraine attacks with tDCS treatment compared with the control group although the duration of attacks and the intensity and number of migraine days were reduced [59]. TDCS has been found to be effective when applied to the primary motor cortex (M1). Thirty-seven episodic migraine patients (17 sham) were given 20 sessions of consecutive days of 1 mA anodal stimulation for 20 minutes. Twelve weeks after treatment, there was a significant reduction in attack frequency and abortive use, with no serious adverse events [60]. Another RCT was carried out to compare stimulation sites using anodal stimulation 12× sessions of 2 mA for 20 minutes, applied to the M1 or dorsolateral prefrontal cortex in 13 refractory chronic migraine patients. Dorsolateral prefrontal cortex stimulation was more effective although both stimulations performed better than sham. Additionally, M1 stimulation caused more adverse events [61].

A further RCT treated ten migraine patients three times a week for 4 weeks. A significant reduction in the number and duration of attacks (but not the intensity) as well as the analgesic intake was seen when compared to the baseline. However, when compared with the control group, no differences were seen in the number, duration, or intensity of migraine attacks [62]. Similarly, a recent double-blind randomised study showed no efficacy of tDCS in patients with CM with medication overuse [63]. Another recent single-blind, randomised sham-controlled study in episodic migraine patients utilised self-administered anodal tDCS over the visual cortex and showed significant a decrease in the number of monthly migraine days but not in total headache days or anxiety and depression score [64].

Overall, it remains unclear how effective tDCS is in treating migraine due to the variety of stimulation sites and protocols, the small-scale studies conducted to date, and the lack of a sham control group.

Transcranial Magnetic Stimulation

TMS directly stimulates the underlying cortex using a copper electromagnetic coil to generate a magnetic pulse. The magnetic pulse passes unimpeded through the nonconductive scalp and skull but produces an electrical current in the electrically conductive neural tissue of the underlying cortex via electromagnetic induction. The current induced by the magnetic pulse is perpendicular to the coil surface due to magnetic flux, at a maximum on the cortical surface and directly proportional to the current passed through the coil. Direct stimulation of the TMS is highly localised to the cortex, as the magnetically induced electrical current rapidly dissipates from the electromagnetic coil, with the greatest current intensity within 1–2 cm of the coil [65]. There are different modes of TMS, single-pulse TMS (sTMS) and repeated TMS (rTMS), with theta burst stimulation being a type of rTMS as explained below. In this section, we will summarise data for both rTMS and sTMS although it should be noted that to date only sTMS has been approved for the treatment of migraine.

In general, the cortical response to TMS is dependent on the strength of the pulse applied. For example, single-pulse TMS (sTMS) applied below the motor endpoint potential (MEP) to the cortex caused facilitation of neuronal activity for ~500 ms followed by inhibition for several seconds. Stronger sTMS stimuli (>50%) caused an initial inhibition of neuronal activation for ~100–200 ms, followed by rebound facilitation [66]. sTMS-induced transient facilitation followed by inhibition was suggested to be caused by direct stimulation of excitatory axons which excite inhibitory neurons leading to a rebound inhibition via metabotropic gamma-aminobutyric acid (GABA) receptors [67].

Repeated Transcranial Magnetic Stimulation

Biological Rational and Mechanism of Action

rTMS refers to the application of trains of hundreds or thousands of magnetic pulses delivered to produce long-lasting modulation in the underlying neuronal tissue. The modulatory effect of the pulse trains can be variable depending on the frequency of pulses applied; low frequency (LF) firing (<1 Hz) has been shown to inhibit cortical activity, while high frequency (HF) firing (>1 Hz) produced facilitation of cortical activity.

Additionally, theta burst stimulation (TBS) uses high-frequency (50–100 Hz) bursts of pulses repeated at a lower frequency (5 Hz) to induce plasticity of the cortex [68]. The induced plasticity is believed to be similar to or greater than that induced by rTMS [69]. The stimulation protocol mirrors the 5 Hz theta stimulation pattern which is used to induce long-term potentiation in hippocampal brain slices [70]. Two protocols for TBS have been developed; continuous TBS (cTBS) applies bursts of pulses in an uninterrupted train, producing a long-term depression (LTD)-like depression in cortical excitability [71]. Intermittent TBS (iTBS) uses a period of bursts of pulses with a resting interval interspersed. This protocol produces a long-term potentiation (LTP)-like facilitation of cortical activity.

rTMS has been shown to affect pain thresholds in animal models and humans. High-frequency rTMS, applied over a large cortical area induced allodynia in rodent models [72]; however, when applied to the motor cortex of patients with chronic neuropathic pain, it resulted in a reduction of acute pain [73]. The site of the application appears to play an important role, as paired-pulse TMS applied to the secondary somatosensory cortex or the occipital cortex had no effect on human pain perception, but there was a facilitatory effect when applied to the somatosensory cortex and an inhibitory effect when applied to the medial frontal cortex [74].

However, in migraine with aura patients, paradoxical facilitation of cortical excitability was seen with 1 Hz (low-frequency) rTMS stimulation to the occipital [75], extra-striate [76], and motor cortices [77], which was not seen in healthy subjects. This facilitation supports the cortical hyperexcitability model of migraine. Brighina et al. (2005) suggested this may indicate a failure of GABAergic inhibition; however, it could additionally be due to lower stimulation thresholds for glutamatergic neurons [77]. The analgesic effect of rTMS applied to the motor cortex or dorsolateral prefrontal cortex can be blocked via the application of naloxone [78–80]. This suggests that top-down endogenous opioids may play a role in rTMS' analgesic effect.

As with LTD and LTP, the depression and facilitation of the motor cortex produced by TBS is dependent on NMDA receptor activity [81]. In the visual cortex, cTBS increased the threshold for producing visual phosphenes, consistent with a depression of cortical excitability; however, iTBS had no effect on the phosphene threshold [82].

Clinical Data rTMS

Several studies have been carried out to investigate rTMS as a prophylactic treatment for migraine. A case study of two patients in an RCT study for the treatment of major depressive disorder with rTMS reported an improvement in daily headaches. The patients had a prior diagnosis of daily headaches, unrelated to the major depression for which they were enrolled in the trial. When patients were given five treatments of rTMS (10 Hz, 3000 pulses per session, 120%) per week for 4–6 weeks to the left dorsolateral prefrontal cortex, they noted a reduction in migraine attack severity and frequency as well as improvement in depression scores, which persisted up to a month [83].

In a pilot study of 11 chronic migraine patients, rTMS (20 Hz, 10× 2 second trains, 90%) was applied to the prefrontal cortex in 12 sessions. rTMS reduced the number and severity of headache attacks as well as the amount of abortive medications, which was not seen in the placebo group. The authors speculated that outcomes may be due to the modulation of serotonergic systems or the cortico-limbic connections [84].

Armin et al. (2020) also investigated high-frequency rTMS applied to the left dorsolateral prefrontal cortex in an open-label study. Fourteen migraine patients (12 migraines without aura and 2 migraines with aura) were given five sessions of 900 rTMS pulses (5 Hz, 1× 3-minute train, 100%) over 1 week and compared against 19 control patients (17 migraines with aura and 2 migraines without aura) given a sham treatment (5 Hz, 1× 3-minute train, 50%). Improvements were seen in the attack frequency (3.1 reduction vs 1.5), the number of migraine days (3.8 days vs 2.8 days), and the impact of headache (15.3 reduction vs 6.1) [85]. The study concluded that rTMS is an attractive, well-tolerated option for migraine prophylaxis.

Misra et al. also found positive results using high-frequency rTMS to the left dorsolateral frontal cortex. About 51 patients (50 migraine without aura and 1 migraine with aura) who had at least seven attacks per month were given three sessions of 600 rTMS pulses (8 Hz, 10× 2 second trains, 70%). Significant improvements in attack frequency and severity were seen as well as a reduction in the number of acute medications. A visual analogue scale was used to asses patient headache; 50 patients (98%) reported a 50% improvement in the first and second weeks [86].

A further RCT study by the same group applied three sessions of 600 rTMS pulses (8 Hz, 10× 2 second trains, 70%) to the motor cortex (a hotspot for the right digiti minimi) in 100 patients (93 migraines without aura and 7 migraines with aura). Both rTMS and sham stimulation groups showed a reduction in headache frequency compared to baseline reaching the nadir in the first week, the rTMS group remained reduced until the fifth week, but the sham stopped being significant after the third week. Additionally, the severity and frequency of attacks as well as the functional disability and the analgesic consumption were improved in the rTMS group compared to the sham treatment group [87].

Prophylactic rTMS has been tested against botulinum toxin A injections in a small-scale pilot randomised study. Fourteen chronic migraine patients were given 12 sessions of high-frequency (10 Hz) stimulation over the M1 cortex. A comparable efficacy to botulinum toxin A injections was seen following the rTMS, for the first 8 weeks, however, dropped off by 12 weeks in the rTMS group [88].

However, several further RCTs have contradicted these studies, finding little effectiveness of rTMS as a treatment for migraine. A smaller RCT applied 1600 high-frequency rTMS pulses (10 Hz, 110%, 32× 5 second trains) to the dorsolateral prefrontal cortex of 14 chronic migraine patients in 23 sessions over 8 weeks. No significant improvement was seen in the rTMS-treated group; however, a significant improvement (58.1%) in headache days was seen in the sham-treated group [89].

Teepker et al. (2010) investigated low-frequency rTMS for the treatment of migraine, by applying 1000 pulses (1 Hz, 2× 500 pulse trains, 100%) over the vertex of 27 patients (14 migraines without aura and 13 migraines with aura) for 5 consecutive days. A reduction in headache days and migraine days was seen in the treatment group compared to baseline; however, this was not significant when compared to the sham treatment. No significant change was seen in either the intensity of the headache attacks or the amount of analgesics taken. They concluded that rTMS treatment is well-tolerated but not effective in the prevention of migraine [90].

Of the six RCTs discussed here, they each used very different stimulation protocols, making direct comparison difficult. The site, intensity, and parameters of the applied rTMS pulses differed significantly in each of the RCTs, any of which could be the deciding factor in the effectiveness of the treatment. The only consistent feature separating the successful and unsuccessful RCTs appears to be the intensity of the stimulus. The successful treatments all used stimulation intensity below the motor threshold, whereas the two unsuccessful RCTs both used stimulus intensity at, or above the motor threshold. rTMS may yet be proven to be an effective treatment for migraine; however, optimisation is still required to find the optimal stimulation protocol and placement [91].

Clinical Data TBS

At the time of writing, only two small studies have been published investigating the efficacy of TBS as a prophylactic treatment for migraine. The first was by Chen et al. (2016) who investigated continuous theta-burst stimulation in nine migraine patients. cTBS applied to the primary motor cortex was applied in 20 sessions over a 4-week period (3× 50 Hz pulses at 80% intensity, for 40 seconds with 200 ms intervals), and patients were monitored for a further 4 weeks following treatment. A reduction was seen in both headache (13.4 ± 10.1 days to 8.7 ± 10.1 days) and migraine days (8.6 ± 8.7 days to 1.0 ± 1.6 days) during and following treatment compared to baseline [92]. Sahu et al. (2019) applied intermittent TBS to the dorsolateral prefrontal cortex (dlPFC) of 20 migraine patients and compared outcomes in 21 patients receiving a sham treatment. iTBS sessions were given *bis in die* (20 trains of 600 pulses at 80% intensity with 3× 50 Hz pulse bursts and 8-second intervals) for a total of 10 sessions over 5 consecutive days, and patients were monitored for 12 weeks following treatment. A reduction in frequency, duration, and severity of migraine headaches was seen in the iTBS group compared to the sham group with the greatest reduction seen in the second week immediately following treatment. Both studies suggest that TBS may be a safe and effective prophylactic treatment for migraine; however, larger scale studies would be required to confirm these findings.

Single-Pulse Transcranial Magnetic Stimulation

Biological Rationale and Mechanism of Action

Early TMS devices could only produce single-pulse TMS (sTMS) or pairs of TMS pulses requiring time to recharge the capacitors. The first hand-held, self-treatment sTMS option was designed for the treatment of migraine. The spring TMS device (now branded as SAVI Dual™, *eNeura Inc;* Fig. 22.2f) is a small, portable device capable of outputting a 0.9 T magnetic pulse, inducing a current of approximately 4 mA/cm^2. The device can be used as an acute treatment ad libitum or as a prophylactic treatment starting at two sequential pulses bis in die titrated usually to a maximum of eight sequential pulses *ter in die*.

In rodents, sTMS activated inhibitory $GABA_B$ fibres in the upper cortical layers which in turn inhibit the activity of dendritic pyramidal neurons in layer V. Blocking $GABA_B$ receptors was shown to prevent the inhibitory effects of sTMS on the somatosensory cortex [93]. Specifically, in studies where the same stimulating sTMS parameters were used in migraine rodent models, sTMS was shown to block mechanically and chemically induced cortical spreading depression (CSD) and increase the threshold of activation of electrically induced CSD as well as inhibit glutamate-induced cortical neuronal activity [94, 95]. Both cortical actions were subsequently blocked via pre-application of GABA antagonists suggesting that sTMS enhances inhibitory GABAergic activity rather than directly suppressing excitatory glutamatergic neurons [96]. Several studies have also suggested that cortical TMS indirectly modulates the thalamus and hypothalamus [97]. In migraine models, sTMS has been shown to block both spontaneous and C-fibre activity of third-order neurons in the VPM thalamic nucleus, potentially by interacting with corticothalamic circuits [94, 95].

Clinical Data

In 2010, Lipton et al. carried out a randomised, double-blind, parallel-group, two-phase, sham-controlled, and multi-centre study investigating the efficacy of sTMS in the acute treatment of migraine. Eighty-two migraine with aura (MA) patients treated with at least one migraine attack with sTMS were compared against 82 MA patients treated with sham stimulation. Pain freedom at 2 h after treatment showed a 17% therapeutic gain in the sTMS versus the sham treatment. This appeared to be a sustained effect with a greater proportion of the sTMS group remaining pain-free 24-h and 48-h post-treatment. There were no reported serious adverse events, whereas minor side effects included headache, migraine, sinusitis, and paraesthesia and were not significantly different between the two treatment groups [98].

Several post-marketing studies have also looked at sTMS as a prophylactic treatment for migraine. Data from a 3-month UK post-market pilot program showed pain relief in 62% of 190 patients (both migraine with and without aura). Headache days per month were reduced in both episodic (EM) and patients with CM, and in addition to reduced attack duration, sTMS showed efficacy in relieving associated migraine symptoms and a reduction in disability scores [99]. Subsequently, the eNeura SpringTMS Post-Market Observational US Study of Migraine (ESPOUSE), a multi-centre, prospective, open-label, and observational study, involved 217 patients who used the sTMS device daily for 3 months. Overall, a significant reduction in headache days was seen (−2.75 ± 0.40 from a baseline of 9.06 days), and 46% of patients achieved at least a 50% response rate. There was also a reduction in acute medication use and HIT-6 disability scores [100].

sTMS' efficacy as a preventative treatment has also been studied specifically in adolescents (12–17 years old) in an open-label pilot. Twelve patients completed the trial, with a further nine failing to complete the study (the most common reason for not completing was not returning or completing the baseline headache diary). Patients were given 4× 0.9T pulses twice a day (two pairs of two pulses separated by 15-minute intervals) for 12 weeks, with further pulses available for acute treatment. Use of the device was reported as feasible and tolerable. There was also a significant reduction in headache days per month (−4.5 ± 1.7 days) and MIDAS score (−36 ± 14) [101].

A smaller study from Canada tested paired-pulse sTMS on 42 migraine patients (both MA and MO) as soon after the start of an attack as possible. After one round of two paired pulses of either high stimulation (50% of the maximum output) or low stimulation (30% maximum output) (using a Caldwell stimulator, max output; 2.3 T, 187 V), 69% of patients showed an improvement, 87% improvement after 2 rounds, and 82% after 3 rounds, suggesting a cumulative effect of sTMS. They also suggested a larger effect in MA patients as 100% (10/42) reported immediate pain relief. Finally, they suggested an autonomic effect, with heart rates dropping from 79.05 ± 10.27 to 72.89 ± 11.35 beats/min. However, this study was not well-controlled and lacked power. The common adverse events reported included light-headedness (3.7%), tingling (3.2%), and tinnitus (3.2%) [102].

Finally, a recent real-world evidence clinical audit in the UK investigated daily sTMS applications in difficult-to-treat migraine patients over the course of 12 months. One hundred and fifty-three high-frequency episodic and chronic migraine patients applied daily 0.9T sTMS pulses, initially 2 pulses twice a day titrated to a possible maximum of 6 pulses three times a day over the course of 11 weeks. At 3 months, 60% of patients responded to treatment with a reduction of 5.0 monthly headache days (from 18.0 to 13.0 days). At 12 months, 45% continued to have a sustained response to sTMS with reduced monthly headache days. Similarly, monthly migraine days and headache impact tests also showed a favourable sustained reduction [103].

Percutaneous Mastoid Electrical Stimulator

In percutaneous mastoid electrical stimulation (PMES), electrodes are attached bilaterally behind the ear. This is believed to stimulate the cerebellar fastigial nucleus. The stimulation consists of a 10 mA peak current, with a width of 90 μs at a frequency of 1.8 kHz; 45-minute sessions are applied daily for 3 months. The fastigial nucleus is a deep cerebellar nucleus with excitatory efferent projections to the vestibular nuclei of the brainstem.

Biological Rational and Mechanism of Action

Fastigial nucleus stimulation has been shown to inhibit the initiation of CSD and has been suggested to reduce cortical excitability [104], potentially by prolonging the opening of K-ATP channels [105]. Alternatively, it has also been suggested that PMES alters supraspinal brain stem structures, similarly to VNS and occipital nerve stimulation to induce descending pain modulation.

Clinical Data

To date, only two RCTs have been conducted in China. In the first prospective, multi-centre, randomised, double-blind, and sham-controlled trial of 80 episodic migraine patients, there was a significantly higher 50% response rate in those receiving 45 minutes daily percutaneous mastoid electrical stimulation compared to the sham group (71.3% vs 14.4%). Patients in the active arm also showed a 3.99 reduction in migraine days per month (vs −1.13 days in sham), with no reported adverse events, concluding that PMES was effective as a preventative treatment for migraine [106].

A further head-to-head study by the same group compared PMES with transcutaneous supraorbital nerve stimulation. In 90 patients, they found comparable effectiveness between the two stimulation protocols with no significant difference in migraine days per month (−2.85 and −3.5 for PMES and tSNS, respectively). The headache-related disability as tested through the headache impact test (HIT-6) showed supraorbital nerve stimulation as having significantly better outcomes than PMES. They concluded that both neuromodulation techniques were safe and efficacious, with comparable outcomes [107].

Invasive Neuromodulation Treatments

Occipital Nerve Stimulation

To stimulate the occipital nerve, usually two electrodes are implanted subcutaneously, at the back of the neck, across the branches of the greater and lesser occipital nerves. This technique has been applied by specialist centres in both migraine and cluster headaches in refractory patients.

Biological Rationale and Mechanism of Action

The greater occipital nerve (GON) arises from between the C1 and C2 vertebrae and provides innervation to the occipital scalp. The lesser occipital nerve rises from the C2 vertebrae and provides innervation to the skin of the lateral scalp posterior to the ear. About 60% of primary GON afferents have been shown to converge along with trigeminal afferents to the same second-order neurons in the TCC [109]. Supramaximal stimulation of the greater occipital nerve produces facilitation of second-order neurons in the TCC [109]. However, low-frequency stimulation (3 Hz) of the greater occipital nerve has been shown to not modulate the trigeminal system [110].

The rational for GON stimulation in the treatment of migraine is the convergence of both trigeminal and occipital nerves on the second-order neurons in the TCC. Stimulation of the occipital nerve modulates the TCC neurones' response to stimuli via inhibitory, GABA, and glycinergic transmission [111]. As well as altering trigeminal signalling at the TCC, stimulation of the occipital nerve has been shown to reduce the firing of the third-order ventral posteromedial thalamus, in a chronic migraine model [112]. Occipital nerve stimulation has been suggested to modulate the peripheral and central sensitisation present in migraine [113].

Clinical Data

Several large multicentre randomised control trials (RCTs) using implanted occipital nerve stimulation have been carried out. The ONSTIM RCT study compared occipital nerve stimulation (stimulation parameters: 0–10.5 V, 3–130 Hz, 60–450 μs) of three groups of patients: adjustable stimulation (0–10.5 V, 3–130 Hz, 60–450 μs, n = 33), a control group with a pre-set stimulation (1 minute per day stimulation, n = 17) and second control group that maintained medical management treatment (n = 17). After 3 months, 39% of the adjustable stimulation had a 50% improvement in headache days vs 6% of the pre-set group and 0% of the medical management group [114].

A further study of 105 patients given occipital nerve stimulation for 12 weeks found no difference on the primary endpoint (>50% reduction in daily visual analogue scale) vs the sham group (n = 52); however, in patients seeing a 30% reduction, there was a significant difference. Additionally, they showed significant improvements in headache days, migraine days, pain relief, and migraine-related disability compared to sham group [115].

Two further single-centre RCTs have also been carried out on occipital nerve stimulation for chronic migraine and both found the treatment to be safe and effective [116, 117]. To date, the treatment is offered to refractory migraine patients at specialised migraine or neuromodulation tertiary centres.

High-Frequency Spinal Cord Stimulation

High-frequency (>10 Khz) spinal cord stimulation (HF10 SCS) requires the invasive implant of an electrode over the spinal cord at the level of the second and third cervical vertebrae. Once the electrode is in place, it provides intermittent trains of five high-frequency tonic stimuli delivered at 500 Hz applied 40 times per second with a long pulse width of 1000 ms and 1000 ms interspike interval [4]. Unlike low-frequency stimulation, HF10 SCS does not induce paraesthesia.

Biological Rationale and Mechanism of Action

The mechanisms of action for high-frequency spinal cord stimulation are not well-understood. Paraesthesia is believed to be induced through the activation of Aβ-fibres within the dorsal horn of the spinal cord. HF10 SCS is believed to be able to selectively activate GABAergic inhibitory interneurons over the myelinated excitatory fibres of the dorsal column [118, 119]; this corroborates previous research suggesting that HF10 SCS inhibits wide dynamic range neurons [120, 121], which integrate nociceptive and innocuous somatosensory signalling, explaining the lack of paraesthesia and perhaps the anti-nociceptive effects.

Beyond the dorsal horn, there are brainstem structures associated with the descending brainstem modulation of spinal nociceptive circuits in the gate control theory of pain [5] that may be modulated by spinal cord stimulation. Beyond the brainstem, higher structures such as the thalamus and anterior cingulate cortex, may be potentially modulated by HF10 SCS [122]; however, at the current time, the evidence is too sparse to draw further conclusions. Currently, there are no headache-specific mechanistic studies into the actions of HF10 SCS, which is a massive limitation for the wider investigation of this treatment in refractory migraine patients.

Clinical Data

Four small studies have investigated FH10 SCS for chronic migraine. A retrospective study by Agostino et al. (2014) found that 82% of the 17 patients implanted with the HF10 SCS had a 30% decrease in mean headache intensity. Improvements were also seen in mean migraine days (decreased from 28 to 9 days), quality of life (increased from 3.3 to 7.2), and number of patients not requiring analgesics (increased from 0.0% to 37.5%). Three patients suffered from infection, requiring the removal of the stimulator, and three patients had lead migration requiring correction [123].

Arcioni et al. (2015) implanted 17 refractory chronic migraine patients with HF10 SCS. Fourteen patients continued the treatment for 6 months; 7 patients had a 30% improvement in headache days (average reduction of 12.9 ± 5.3 days). Improvements were also seen in medication intake (from 64% overusing triptans to 36%), HIT-6 score (decreased by 8.3), headache intensity, and frequency (decreased by 49% and 40%, respectively). Two patients had lead migration, one had a lead fracture, two patients had infections, and three reported discomfort from the implant [124].

Lambru et al. (2016) implanted HF10 SCS into four chronic migraine patients as well as two SUNA patients and one patient with cluster headaches. Followed up at a mean of 25 months, all four chronic migraine patients showed a 50% improvement in headache days, reverting to episodic migraine. One patient suffered a lead breakage resulting in worsening headaches, which was resolved following surgical replacement [125].

Finally, HF10 SCS was investigated in 20 further refractory chronic migraine patients. At 52 weeks post-implantation, 50% of patients achieved the primary outcome of a 50% reduction in monthly migraine days. Additionally, there was also improvement in headache-related disability [126].

Conclusion

The various neuromodulation devices and techniques discussed here provide a different treatment approach to the more commonly used pharmacological treatments of migraine.

Neuromodulation has been demonstrated to be safe and efficacious for the treatment of migraine both acutely and preventatively. Direct stimulation of the neuronal pathways associated with migraine, be that peripherally or centrally, allows for specific targeted treatment, resulting in fewer adverse events stemming from the treatment interacting with off-target areas, as is the case in systemically administered pharmaceuticals.

Despite advances being made in understanding the underlying mechanisms, much is still unknown regarding their precise mechanism of action in migraine, and much more research is required. As well as research being required for the mechanisms of action, the majority of the techniques discussed above only have a very small number of trials, and only a few devices have FDA clearance. Far more research is required to have a more conclusive idea of the effect of these techniques on the different types of migraines.

Teaching Points

1. There are six FDA-approved neuromodulation devices for migraine (Table 22.1). Neuromodulation techniques have been developed aiming to stop a migraine attack and/or to reduce the overall frequency of attacks.
2. Currently, available neuromodulation treatments for migraine can be split into three sections: non-invasive treatments targeting the peripheral nervous system, non-invasive treatments targeting the central nervous system, and invasive neuromodulation treatments.
3. Neuromodulation has been demonstrated to be safe and efficacious for the treatment of migraine both acutely and preventatively.

Case

A 34-year-old female is asking about non-medication migraine treatment as she is breastfeeding. She had previous treatment for depression with rTMS in the past with success. She would like to learn if a similar modality can be used.

Case Discussion

Single pulse TMS is an FDA-cleared option for acute and preventive management of migraine, for individuals 12 years of age and older. It can be successfully used during the period of breastfeeding as it provides a non-pharmacological alternative for the treatment of migraine with and without aura.

Table 22.1 FDA-approved non-invasive neuromodulation devices for primary headache disorders

	eTNS	TENS	sTMS	nVNS	REN	COT-NS
Target	Supraorbital and supratrochlear branches of the ophthalmic nerve		Cortical spreading depolarisation and thalamus	Vagus nerve (cervical), cortical spreading depolarisation, thalamus	Nociceptive receptors, conditioned pain modulation	Supraorbital and supratrochlear nerves, greater occipital nerves
Device commercial name	Cefaly	HeadaTerm 2	SAVI Dual	gammaCore	Nerivio	Relivion
Stimulation type	Electric	Electric	Magnetic	Electric	Electric	Electric
Indication	Migraine: acute and prevention	Prophylaxis of migraine in adults	Migraine: acute and prevention	Migraine: acute and prevention; acute episodic cluster headache and adjunctive episodic and chronic cluster prevention paroxysmal hemicrania and hemicrania continua prevention	Migraine: acute and prevention	Migraine: acute only
Paediatric/adolescent indication	None	None	Adolescent	Adolescent	Age 8 and older	None
Data on pregnancy	None	None	Survey study	–	Retrospective controlled survey	None

Source: Reproduced with permission from Practical Neurology, Tepper et al. [108]
Abbreviations: *eCOT-NS* combined supraorbital, supratrochlear, and greater occipital nerve stimulation, *eTNS* external trigeminal neurostimulation, *nVNS* non-invasive vagus nerve stimulation, *REN* remote electrical neuromodulation, *TMS* single-pulse transcranial magnetic stimulator, *TENS* transcutaneous electrical nerve stimulation

Questions and Answers

1. Which of the following is a neuromodulation device that the FDA cleared for the management of migraine, cluster headache, and hemicrania continua?
   A. Transcutaneous *supraorbital* neurostimulation.
   B. Non-invasive vagus nerve stimulator.
   C. *Remote electrical* neuromodulation.
   D. External concurrent occipital and trigeminal neurostimulation.

The correct answer is B. Non-invasive vagus nerve stimulator is FDA-cleared for the treatment of acute and preventive migraine, episodic cluster, and hemicrania. Transcutaneous supraorbital neurostimulation and remote electrical neuromodulation are FDA-cleared for acute and preventive management of migraine. External concurrent occipital and trigeminal neurostimulation is currently FDA-cleared for the management of acute migraine attacks.

2. What are the contraindications to the use of non-invasive neuromodulation devices for migraine?
   A. Pacemaker.
   B. Medication overuse headache.
   C. Neuropathic pain.
   D. All of the above.

The correct answer is A. Pacemaker is a contraindication to the use of non-invasive neuromodulation devices for migraine. Anxiety and previous use of different devices without side effects; effects are not contraindications for the use of devices for neuromodulation.

References

1. Andreou AP, Edvinsson L. Mechanisms of migraine as a chronic evolutive condition. J Headache Pain. 2019;20(1):117.
2. Lloyd J, Biloshytska M, Andreou AP, Lambru G. Noninvasive neuromodulation in headache: an update. Neurol India. 2021;69(12 Suppl 1):S183–S93.
3. Shankland WE. The trigeminal nerve. Part II: the ophthalmic division. Cranio. 2001;19(1):8–12.
4. Lambru G, Lanteri-Minet M. Neuromodulation in headache and facial pain management: principles, rationale and clinical data. Springer Nature; 2019.
5. Wall PD. The gate control theory of pain mechanisms: a re-examination and re-statement. Brain. 1978;101(1):1–18.
6. Magis D, D'Ostilio K, Thibaut A, De Pasqua V, Gerard P, Hustinx R, et al. Cerebral metabolism before and after external trigeminal nerve stimulation in episodic migraine. Cephalalgia. 2017;37(9):881–91.
7. Di Lenola D, Coppola G, Serrao M, Di Lorenzo C, Pierelli F. O024. Transcutaneous supraorbital nerve stimulation enhances somatosensory thalamic activity in migraine between attacks: a central mechanism of clinical efficacy? J Headache Pain. 2015;16(1):A160.

8. Chou DE, Gross GJ, Casadei CH, Yugrakh MS. External trigeminal nerve stimulation for the acute treatment of migraine: open-label trial on safety and efficacy. Neuromodulation. 2017;20(7):678–83.
9. Chou DE, Shnayderman Yugrakh M, Winegarner D, Rowe V, Kuruvilla D, Schoenen J. Acute migraine therapy with external trigeminal neurostimulation (ACME): a randomized controlled trial. Cephalalgia. 2019;39(1):3–14.
10. Gérardy P, Fabry D, Fumal A, Schoenen J. A pilot study on supra-orbital surface electrotherapy in migraine: PD. 22. Cephalalgia. 2009;29(1)
11. Schoenen J, Vandersmissen B, Jeangette S, Herroelen L, Vandenheede M, Gérard P, et al. Migraine prevention with a supraorbital transcutaneous stimulator: a randomized controlled trial. Neurology. 2013;80(8):697–704.
12. Russo A, Tessitore A, Conte F, Marcuccio L, Giordano A, Tedeschi G. Transcutaneous supraorbital neurostimulation in "de novo" patients with migraine without aura: the first Italian experience. J Headache Pain. 2015;16(1):69.
13. Di Fiore P, Bussone G, Galli A, Didier H, Peccarisi C, D'Amico D, et al. Transcutaneous supraorbital neurostimulation for the prevention of chronic migraine: a prospective, open-label preliminary trial. Neurol Sci. 2017;38(1):201–6.
14. Jiang L, Yuan DL, Li M, Liu C, Liu Q, Zhang Y, et al. Combination of flunarizine and transcutaneous supraorbital neurostimulation improves migraine prophylaxis. Acta Neural Scand. 2019;139(3):276–83.
15. Magis D, Sava S, d'Elia TS, Baschi R, Schoenen J. Safety and patients' satisfaction of transcutaneous supraorbital neurostimulation (tSNS) with the Cefaly® device in headache treatment: a survey of 2,313 headache sufferers in the general population. J Headache Pain. 2013;14(1):95.
16. Hokenek NM, Erdogan MO, Hokenek UD, Algin A, Tekyol D, Seyhan AUJTAJoEM. Treatment of migraine attacks by transcutaneous electrical nerve stimulation in emergency department: a randomize controlled trial. Am J Emerg Med. 2021;39:80–5.
17. Lyubashina O, Sokolov A, Panteleev S. Vagal afferent modulation of spinal trigeminal neuronal responses to dural electrical stimulation in rats. Neuroscience. 2012;222:29–37.
18. Hu B, Akerman S, Goadsby PJ. Characterization of opioidergic mechanisms related to the anti-migraine effect of vagus nerve stimulation. Neuropharmacology. 2021;195:108375.
19. Oshinsky ML, Murphy AL, Hekierski H, Cooper M, Simon BJ. Noninvasive vagus nerve stimulation as treatment for trigeminal allodynia. Pain. 2014;155(5):1037–42.
20. Hawkins JL, Cornelison LE, Blankenship BA, Durham PL. Vagus nerve stimulation inhibits trigeminal nociception in a rodent model of episodic migraine. Pain Rep. 2017;2(6):e628–e.
21. Chen S-P, Ay I, de Morais AL, Qin T, Zheng Y, Sadhegian H, et al. Vagus nerve stimulation inhibits cortical spreading depression. Pain. 2016;157(4):797.
22. De Icco R, Bitetto V, Martinelli D, Allena M, Guaschino E, Bottiroli S, et al. Noninvasive peripheral vagal nerve stimulation prevents migraine aura: a case report. Cephalalgia Rep. 2019;2:2515816319855607.
23. Zhang Y, Huang Y, Li H, Yan Z, Zhang Y, Liu X, et al. Transcutaneous auricular vagus nerve stimulation (taVNS) for migraine: an fMRI study. Reg Anesth Pain Med. 2021;46(2):145–50.
24. Barbanti P, Grazzi L, Egeo G, Padovan AM, Liebler E, Bussone G. Non-invasive vagus nerve stimulation for acute treatment of high-frequency and chronic migraine: an open-label study. J Headache Pain. 2015;16(1):61.
25. Goadsby P, Grosberg B, Mauskop A, Cady R, Simmons K. Effect of noninvasive vagus nerve stimulation on acute migraine: an open-label pilot study. Cephalalgia. 2014;34(12):986–93.
26. Tassorelli C, Grazzi L, de Tommaso M, Pierangeli G, Martelletti P, Rainero I, et al. Noninvasive vagus nerve stimulation as acute therapy for migraine: the randomized PRESTO study. Neurology. 2018;91(4):e364–e73.
27. Silberstein SD, Calhoun AH, Lipton RB, Grosberg BM, Cady RK, Dorlas S, et al. Chronic migraine headache prevention with non-invasive vagus nerve stimulation: the EVENT study. Neurology. 2016;87(5):529–38.
28. Diener H-C, Goadsby PJ, Ashina M, Al-Karagholi MA-M, Sinclair A, Mitsikostas D, et al. Non-invasive vagus nerve stimulation (nVNS) for the preventive treatment of episodic migraine: the multicentre, double-blind, randomised, sham-controlled PREMIUM trial. Cephalalgia. 2019;39(12):1475–87.
29. Trimboli M, Al-Kaisy A, Andreou AP, Murphy M, Lambru G. Non-invasive vagus nerve stimulation for the management of refractory primary chronic headaches: a real-world experience. Cephalalgia. 2018;38(7):1276–85.
30. Straube A, Ellrich J, Eren O, Blum B, Ruscheweyh R. Treatment of chronic migraine with transcutaneous stimulation of the auricular branch of the vagal nerve (auricular t-VNS): a randomized, monocentric clinical trial. J Headache Pain. 2015;16:543.
31. Yarnitsky D, Volokh L, Ironi A, Weller B, Shor M, Shifrin A, et al. Nonpainful remote electrical stimulation alleviates episodic migraine pain. Neurology. 2017;88(13):1250–5.
32. DeSantana J, Da Silva L, De Resende M, Sluka K. Transcutaneous electrical nerve stimulation at both high and low frequencies activates ventrolateral periaqueductal grey to decrease mechanical hyperalgesia in arthritic rats. Neuroscience. 2009;163(4):1233–41.
33. Kalra A, Urban M, Sluka K. Blockade of opioid receptors in rostral ventral medulla prevents antihyperalgesia produced by transcutaneous electrical nerve stimulation (TENS). J Pharmacol Exp Therap. 2001;298(1):257–63.
34. Bi Y, Wei Z, Kong Y, Hu L. Supraspinal neural mechanisms of the analgesic effect produced by transcutaneous electrical nerve stimulation. Brain Struct Funct. 2021;226(1):151–62.
35. Yarnitsky D, Dodick DW, Grosberg BM, Burstein R, Ironi A, Harris D, et al. Remote electrical neuromodulation (REN) relieves acute migraine: a randomized, double-blind, placebo-controlled, multicenter trial. Headache. 2019;59(8):1240–52.
36. Rapoport AM, Bonner JH, Lin T, Harris D, Gruper Y, Ironi A, et al. Remote electrical neuromodulation (REN) in the acute treatment of migraine: a comparison with usual care and acute migraine medications. J Headache Pain. 2019;20(1):83.
37. Grosberg B, Rabany L, Lin T, Harris D, Vizel M, Ironi A, et al. Safety and efficacy of remote electrical neuromodulation for the acute treatment of chronic migraine: an open-label study. Pain Rep. 2021;6(4):e966–e.
38. Bartsch T, Levy MJ, Knight YE, Goadsby PJ. Inhibition of nociceptive dural input in the trigeminal nucleus caudalis by somatostatin receptor blockade in the posterior hypothalamus. Pain. 2005;117(1–2):30–9.
39. Tepper SJ, Grosberg B, Daniel O, Kuruvilla DE, Vainstein G, Deutsch L, et al. Migraine treatment with external concurrent occipital and trigeminal neurostimulation—a randomized controlled trial. Headache. 2022;62(8):989–1001.
40. Daniel O, Tepper SJ, Deutsch L, Sharon RJP. External concurrent occipital and trigeminal neurostimulation relieves migraine headache: a prospective, randomized, double-blind, sham-controlled trial. Pain Ther. 2022;11(3):907–22.
41. Berlow YA, Zandvakili A, Carpenter LL, Philip NS. Transcranial direct current stimulation for unipolar depression and risk of treatment emergent mania: an updated meta-analysis. Brain Stimul. 2019;12(4):1066–8.
42. Alonzo A, Aaronson S, Bikson M, Husain M, Lisanby S, Martin D, et al. Study design and methodology for a multicentre, randomised controlled trial of transcranial direct current stimulation as a treatment for unipolar and bipolar depression. Contemp Clin Trials. 2016;51:65–71.

43. Fregni F, Boggio PS, Nitsche MA, Marcolin MA, Rigonatti SP, Pascual-Leone A. Treatment of major depression with transcranial direct current stimulation. Bipolar Disord. 2006;8(2):203.
44. Johnson JM, Durrant SJ. The effect of cathodal transcranial direct current stimulation during rapid eye-movement sleep on neutral and emotional memory. R Soc Open Sci. 2018;5(7):172353.
45. Saucedo Marquez CM, Zhang X, Swinnen SP, Meesen R, Wenderoth N. Task-specific effect of transcranial direct current stimulation on motor learning. Front Hum Neurosci. 2013;7:333.
46. Antal A, Kincses TZ, Nitsche MA, Bartfai O, Paulus W. Excitability changes induced in the human primary visual cortex by transcranial direct current stimulation: direct electrophysiological evidence. Investig Ophthalmol Visual Sci. 2004;45(2):702–7.
47. Brighina F, Cosentino G, Vigneri S, Talamanca S, Palermo A, Giglia G, et al. Abnormal facilitatory mechanisms in motor cortex of migraine with aura. Eur J Pain. 2011;15(9):928–35.
48. Gunaydin S, Soysal A, Atay T, Arpaci B. Motor and occipital cortex excitability in migraine patients. Can J Neurol Sci. 2006;33(1):63–7.
49. Werhahn K, Wiseman K, Herzog J, Foörderreuther S, Dichgans M, Straube A. Motor cortex excitability in patients with migraine with aura and hemiplegic migraine. Cephalalgia. 2000;20(1):45–50.
50. Aurora S, Al-Sayeed F, Welch K. The cortical silent period is shortened in migraine with aura. Cephalalgia. 1999;19(8):708–12.
51. Coppola G, Pierelli F, Schoenen J. Is the cerebral cortex hyperexcitable or hyperresponsive in migraine? Cephalalgia. 2007;27(12):1427–39.
52. Liebetanz D, Fregni F, Monte-Silva KK, Oliveira MB, Amâncio-dos-Santos Â, Nitsche MA, et al. After-effects of transcranial direct current stimulation (tDCS) on cortical spreading depression. Neurosci Lett. 2006;398(1–2):85–90.
53. Nitsche MA, Paulus W. Sustained excitability elevations induced by transcranial DC motor cortex stimulation in humans. Neurology. 2001;57(10):1899–901.
54. Fritsch B, Reis J, Martinowich K, Schambra HM, Ji Y, Cohen LG, et al. Direct current stimulation promotes BDNF-dependent synaptic plasticity: potential implications for motor learning. Neuron. 2010;66(2):198–204.
55. Monai H, Ohkura M, Tanaka M, Oe Y, Konno A, Hirai H, et al. Calcium imaging reveals glial involvement in transcranial direct current stimulation-induced plasticity in mouse brain. Nat Commun. 2016;7(1):1–10.
56. Gaist D, Hougaard A, Garde E, Reislev NL, Wiwie R, Iversen P, et al. Migraine with visual aura associated with thicker visual cortex. Brain. 2018;141(3):776–85.
57. Schading S, Pohl H, Gantenbein A, Luechinger R, Sandor P, Riederer F, et al. Tracking tDCS induced grey matter changes in episodic migraine: a randomized controlled trial. J Headache Pain. 2021;22(1):139.
58. Viganò A, D'Elia TS, Sava SL, Auvé M, De Pasqua V, Colosimo A, et al. Transcranial Direct Current Stimulation (tDCS) of the visual cortex: a proof-of-concept study based on interictal electrophysiological abnormalities in migraine. J Headache Pain. 2013;14(1):23.
59. Antal A, Kriener N, Lang N, Boros K, Paulus W. Cathodal transcranial direct current stimulation of the visual cortex in the prophylactic treatment of migraine. Cephalalgia. 2011;31(7):820–8.
60. Auvichayapat P, Janyacharoen T, Rotenberg A, Tiamkao S, Krisanaprakornkit T, Sinawat S, et al. Migraine prophylaxis by anodal transcranial direct current stimulation, a randomized, placebo-controlled trial. Med Assoc Thai. 2012;95(8):1003–12.
61. Andrade SM, de Brito Aranha REL, de Oliveira EA, de Mendonça CTPL, Martins WKN, Alves NT, et al. Transcranial direct current stimulation over the primary motor vs prefrontal cortex in refractory chronic migraine: a pilot randomized controlled trial. J Neurol Sci. 2017;378:225–32.
62. Rocha S, Melo L, Boudoux C, Foerster A, Araujo D, Monte-Silva K. Transcranial direct current stimulation in the prophylactic treatment of migraine based on interictal visual cortex excitability abnormalities: a pilot randomized controlled trial. J Neurol Sci. 2015;349(1–2):33–9.
63. Grazzi L, Usai S, Bolognini N, Grignani E, Sansone E, Tramacere I, et al. No efficacy of transcranial direct current stimulation on chronic migraine with medication overuse: a double blind, randomised clinical trial. Cephalalgia. 2020;40(11):1202–11.
64. Pohl H, Moisa M, Jung HH, Brenner K, Aschmann J, Riederer F, et al. Long-term effects of self-administered transcranial direct current stimulation in episodic migraine prevention: results of a randomized controlled trial. Neuromodulation Technol Neural Interface. 2021;24(5):890–8.
65. Epstein CM, Schwartzberg DG, Davey KR, Sudderth DB. Localizing the site of magnetic brain stimulation in humans. Neurology. 1990;40(4):666.
66. Moliadze V, Zhao Y, Eysel U, Funke K. Effect of transcranial magnetic stimulation on single-unit activity in the cat primary visual cortex. J Physiol. 2003;553(2):665–79.
67. Funke K, Benali A. Cortical cellular actions of transcranial magnetic stimulation. Restor Neurol Neurosci. 2010;28(4):399–417.
68. Huang Y-Z, Edwards MJ, Rounis E, Bhatia KP, Rothwell JC. Theta burst stimulation of the human motor cortex. Neuron. 2005;45(2):201–6.
69. Nyffeler T, Wurtz P, Lüscher H-R, Hess CW, Senn W, Pflugshaupt T, et al. Repetitive TMS over the human oculomotor cortex: comparison of 1-Hz and theta burst stimulation. Neurosci Lett. 2006;409(1):57–60.
70. Larson J, Wong D, Lynch G. Patterned stimulation at the theta frequency is optimal for the induction of hippocampal long-term potentiation. Brain Res. 1986;368(2):347–50.
71. Di Lazzaro V, Pilato F, Saturno E, Oliviero A, Dileone M, Mazzone P, et al. Theta-burst repetitive transcranial magnetic stimulation suppresses specific excitatory circuits in the human motor cortex. J Physiol. 2005;565(3):945–50.
72. Ambriz-Tututi M, Sánchez-González V, Drucker-Colín R. Transcranial magnetic stimulation reduces nociceptive threshold in rats. J Neurosci Res. 2012;90(5):1085–95.
73. Lefaucheur J-P, Jarry G, Drouot X, Ménard-Lefaucheur I, Keravel Y, Nguyen J-P. Motor cortex rTMS reduces acute pain provoked by laser stimulation in patients with chronic neuropathic pain. Clin Neurophysiol. 2010;121(6):895–901.
74. Kanda M, Mima T, Oga T, Matsuhashi M, Toma K, Hara H, et al. Transcranial magnetic stimulation (TMS) of the sensorimotor cortex and medial frontal cortex modifies human pain perception. Clin Neurophysiol. 2003;114(5):860–6.
75. Brighina F, Piazza A, Daniele O, Fierro B. Modulation of visual cortical excitability in migraine with aura: effects of 1 Hz repetitive transcranial magnetic stimulation. Exp Brain Res. 2002;145(2):177–81.
76. Fierro B, Ricci R, Piazza A, Scalia S, Giglia G, Vitello G, et al. 1 Hz rTMS enhances extrastriate cortex activity in migraine: evidence of a reduced inhibition? Neurology. 2003;61(10):1446–8.
77. Brighina F, Giglia G, Scalia S, Francolini M, Palermo A, Fierro B. Facilitatory effects of 1 Hz rTMS in motor cortex of patients affected by migraine with aura. Exp Brain Res. 2005;161(1):34–8.
78. Taylor JJ, Borckardt JJ, Canterberry M, Li X, Hanlon CA, Brown TR, et al. Naloxone-reversible modulation of pain circuitry by left prefrontal rTMS. Neuropsychopharmacology. 2013;38(7):1189–97.

79. Taylor JJ, Borckardt JJ, George MS. Endogenous opioids mediate left dorsolateral prefrontal cortex rTMS-induced analgesia. Pain. 2012;153(6):1219–25.
80. de Andrade DC, Mhalla A, Adam F, Texeira MJ, Bouhassira D. Neuropharmacological basis of rTMS-induced analgesia: the role of endogenous opioids. Pain. 2011;152(2):320–6.
81. Huang Y-Z, Chen R-S, Rothwell JC, Wen H-Y. The after-effect of human theta burst stimulation is NMDA receptor dependent. Clin Neurophysiol. 2007;118(5):1028–32.
82. Franca M, Koch G, Mochizuki H, Huang Y-Z, Rothwell JC. Effects of theta burst stimulation protocols on phosphene threshold. Clin Neurophysiol. 2006;117(8):1808–13.
83. O'Reardon JP, Fontecha JF, Cristancho MA, Newman S. Unexpected reduction in migraine and psychogenic headaches following rTMS treatment for major depression: a report of two cases. CNS Spectr. 2007;12(12):921–5.
84. Brighina F, Piazza A, Vitello G, Aloisio A, Palermo A, Daniele O, et al. rTMS of the prefrontal cortex in the treatment of chronic migraine: a pilot study. J Neurol Sci. 2004;227(1):67–71.
85. Amin R, Emara T, Ashour S, Hemeda M, Eldin NS, Hamed S, et al. The role of left prefrontal transcranial magnetic stimulation in episodic migraine prophylaxis. Egypt J Neurol Psychiatr Neurosurg. 2020;56(1):19.
86. Misra UK, Kalita J, Bhoi SK. High frequency repetitive transcranial magnetic stimulation (rTMS) is effective in migraine prophylaxis: an open labeled study. Neurol Res. 2012;34(6):547–51.
87. Misra UK, Kalita J, Bhoi SK. High-rate repetitive transcranial magnetic stimulation in migraine prophylaxis: a randomized, placebo-controlled study. J Neurol. 2013;260(11):2793–801.
88. Shehata HS, Esmail EH, Abdelalim A, El-Jaafary S, Elmazny A, Sabbah A, et al. Repetitive transcranial magnetic stimulation versus botulinum toxin injection in chronic migraine prophylaxis: a pilot randomized trial. J Pain Res. 2016;9:771–7.
89. Conforto AB, Amaro E Jr, Gonçalves AL, Mercante JP, Guendler VZ, Ferreira JR, et al. Randomized, proof-of-principle clinical trial of active transcranial magnetic stimulation in chronic migraine. Cephalalgia. 2014;34(6):464–72.
90. Teepker M, Hötzel J, Timmesfeld N, Reis J, Mylius V, Haag A, et al. Low-frequency rTMS of the vertex in the prophylactic treatment of migraine. Cephalalgia. 2010;30(2):137–44.
91. Mohamad Safiai NI, Mohamad NA, Basri H, Inche Mat LN, Hoo FK, Abdul Rashid AM, et al. High-frequency repetitive transcranial magnetic stimulation at dorsolateral prefrontal cortex for migraine prevention: a protocol for a systematic review of controlled trials. PLoS One. 2021;16(6):e0251528.
92. Chen P-R, Lai K-L, Fuh J-L, Chen S-P, Wang P-N, Liao K-K, et al. Efficacy of continuous theta burst stimulation of the primary motor cortex in reducing migraine frequency: a preliminary open-label study. J Chin Med Assoc. 2016;79(6):304–8.
93. Murphy SC, Palmer LM, Nyffeler T, Müri RM, Larkum ME. Transcranial magnetic stimulation (TMS) inhibits cortical dendrites. elife. 2016;5:e13598.
94. Andreou AP, Holland PR, Akerman S, Summ O, Fredrick J, Goadsby PJ. Transcranial magnetic stimulation and potential cortical and trigeminothalamic mechanisms in migraine. Brain. 2016;139(7):2002–14.
95. Lloyd JO, Chisholm KI, Oehle B, Jones MG, Okine BN, Al-Kaisy A, et al. Cortical mechanisms of single-pulse transcranial magnetic stimulation in migraine. Neurotherapeutics. 2020;17:1973.
96. Li X, Nahas Z, Kozel FA, Anderson B, Bohning DE, George MS. Acute left prefrontal transcranial magnetic stimulation in depressed patients is associated with immediately increased activity in prefrontal cortical as well as subcortical regions. Biol Psychiatry. 2004;55(9):882–90.
97. Amassian V, Mari Z, Sagliocco L, Hassan N, Maccabee P, Cracco JB, et al. Perception of phosphenes and flashed alphabetical characters is enhanced by single-pulse transcranial magnetic stimulation of anterior frontal lobe: the thalamic gate hypothesis. Perception. 2008;37(3):375–88.
98. Lipton RB, Dodick DW, Silberstein SD, Saper JR, Aurora SK, Pearlman SH, et al. Single-pulse transcranial magnetic stimulation for acute treatment of migraine with aura: a randomised, double-blind, parallel-group, sham-controlled trial. Lancet Neurol. 2010;9(4):373–80.
99. Bhola R, Kinsella E, Giffin N, Lipscombe S, Ahmed F, Weatherall M, et al. Single-pulse transcranial magnetic stimulation (sTMS) for the acute treatment of migraine: evaluation of outcome data for the UK post market pilot program. J Headache Pain. 2015;16(1):51.
100. Starling AJ, Tepper SJ, Marmura MJ, Shamim EA, Robbins MS, Hindiyeh N, et al. A multicenter, prospective, single arm, open label, observational study of sTMS for migraine prevention (ESPOUSE Study). Cephalalgia. 2018;38(6):1038–48.
101. Irwin SL, Qubty W, Allen IE, Patniyot I, Goadsby PJ, Gelfand AA. Transcranial magnetic stimulation for migraine prevention in adolescents: a pilot open-label study. Headache. 2018;58(5):724–31.
102. Clarke BM, Upton ARM, Kamath MV, Al-Harbi T, Castellanos CM. Transcranial magnetic stimulation for migraine: clinical effects. J Headache Pain. 2006;7(5):341–6.
103. Lloyd J, Hill B, Murphy M, Al-Kaisy A, Andreou A, Lambru G. Single-Pulse Transcranial Magnetic Stimulation for the preventive treatment of difficult-to-treat migraine: a 12-month prospective analysis. J Headache Pain. 2022;23(1):1–11.
104. Golanov EV, Reis DJ. Neuroprotective electrical stimulation of cerebellar fastigial nucleus attenuates expression of periinfarction depolarizing waves (PIDs) and inhibits cortical spreading depression. Brain Res. 1999;818(2):304–15.
105. Wang J, Dong W-W, Zhang W-H, Zheng J, Wang X. Electrical stimulation of Cerebellar Fastigial nucleus: mechanism of neuroprotection and prospects for clinical application against cerebral ischemia. CNS Neurosci Ther. 2014;20(8):710–6.
106. Juan Y, Shu O, Jinhe L, Na Y, Yushuang D, Weiwei D, et al. Migraine prevention with percutaneous mastoid electrical stimulator: a randomized double-blind controlled trial. Cephalalgia. 2016;37(13):1248–56.
107. Deng Y, Zheng M, He L, Yang J, Yu G, Wang J. A head-to-head comparison of Percutaneous Mastoid electrical stimulator and Supraorbital Transcutaneous stimulator in the prevention of migraine: a prospective, randomized controlled study. Neuromodulation Technol Neural Interface. 2020;23(6):770–7.
108. Tepper SJMP, Monteith T. Update on noninvasive neuromodulation for headache treatment. Pract Neurol (US). 2024;23(4):23–8.
109. Bartsch T, Goadsby PJ. Stimulation of the greater occipital nerve induces increased central excitability of dural afferent input. Brain. 2002;125(7):1496–509.
110. Jürgens T, Busch V, Opatz O, Schulte-Mattler W, May A. Low-frequency short-time nociceptive stimulation of the greater occipital nerve does not modulate the trigeminal system. Cephalalgia. 2008;28(8):842–6.
111. García-Magro N, Negredo P, Martin YB, Nuñez Á, Avendaño C. Modulation of mechanosensory vibrissal responses in the trigeminocervical complex by stimulation of the greater occipital nerve in a rat model of trigeminal neuropathic pain. J Headache Pain. 2020;21(1):96.
112. Walling I, Smith H, Gee LE, Kaszuba B, Chockalingam A, Barborica A, et al. Occipital nerve stimulation attenuates neuronal firing response to mechanical stimuli in the ventral posteromedial thalamus of a Rodent Model of chronic migraine. Neurosurgery. 2017;81(4):696–701.

113. Wodehouse T, Bahra A, Mehta V. Changes in peripheral and central sensitization in patients undergoing occipital nerve stimulation. Br J Pain. 2019;14(4):250–5.
114. Saper JR, Dodick DW, Silberstein SD, McCarville S, Sun M, Goadsby PJ. Occipital nerve stimulation for the treatment of intractable chronic migraine headache: ONSTIM feasibility study. Cephalalgia. 2011;31(3):271–85.
115. Silberstein SD, Dodick DW, Saper J, Huh B, Slavin KV, Sharan A, et al. Safety and efficacy of peripheral nerve stimulation of the occipital nerves for the management of chronic migraine: results from a randomized, multicenter, double-blinded, controlled study. Cephalalgia. 2012;32(16):1165–79.
116. Serra G, Marchioretto F. Occipital nerve stimulation for chronic migraine: a randomized trial. Pain Physician. 2012;15(3):245–53.
117. Slotty P, Bara G, Kowatz L, Gendolla A, Wille C, Schu S, et al. Occipital nerve stimulation for chronic migraine: a randomized trial on subthreshold stimulation. Cephalalgia. 2015;35(1):73–8.
118. Lee KY, Bae C, Lee D, Kagan Z, Bradley K, Chung JM, et al. Low-intensity, Kilohertz frequency spinal cord stimulation differently affects excitatory and inhibitory neurons in the Rodent Superficial Dorsal Horn. Neuroscience. 2020;428:132–9.
119. Arle JE, Mei L, Carlson KW, Shils JL. High-frequency stimulation of Dorsal Column Axons: potential underlying mechanism of paresthesia-free neuropathic pain relief. Neuromodulation Technol Neural Interface. 2016;19(4):385–97.
120. Cuellar JM, Alataris K, Walker A, Yeomans DC, Antognini JF. Effect of high-frequency alternating current on spinal afferent nociceptive transmission. Neuromodulation Technol Neural Interface. 2013;16(4):318–27.
121. Yakhnitsa V, Linderoth B, Meyerson BA. Spinal cord stimulation attenuates dorsal horn neuronal hyperexcitability in a rat model of mononeuropathy. Pain. 1999;79(2):223–33.
122. Bentley LD, Duarte RV, Furlong PL, Ashford RL, Raphael JH. Brain activity modifications following spinal cord stimulation for chronic neuropathic pain: a systematic review. Eur J Pain. 2016;20(4):499–511.
123. De Agostino R, Federspiel B, Cesnulis E, Sandor PS. High-cervical spinal cord stimulation for medically intractable chronic migraine. Neuromodulation Technol Neural Interface. 2015;18(4):289–96.
124. Arcioni R, Palmisani S, Mercieri M, Vano V, Tigano S, Smith T, et al. Cervical 10 kHz spinal cord stimulation in the management of chronic, medically refractory migraine: a prospective, open-label, exploratory study. Eur J Pain. 2016;20(1):70–8.
125. Lambru G, Trimboli M, Palmisani S, Smith T, Al-Kaisy A. Safety and efficacy of cervical 10 kHz spinal cord stimulation in chronic refractory primary headaches: a retrospective case series. J Headache Pain. 2016;17(1):66.
126. Al-Kaisy A, Palmisani S, Carganillo R, Wesley S, Pang D, Rotte A, et al. Safety and efficacy of 10 kHz spinal cord stimulation for the treatment of refractory chronic Migraine: a prospective long-term open-label study. Neuromodulation Technol Neural Interface. 2021;25:103.

Behavioral Interventions for Migraine

23

Rachel D. Best, Ivy Snyder, and Elizabeth K. Seng

Introduction

Behavioral interventions for migraine have been shown to be efficacious in reducing migraine frequency, severity, and disability [1–3]. There are a range of behavioral interventions available for migraine, including psychoeducation about changing one's behaviors, such as diet, sleep, exercise, and medication adherence; relaxation techniques; biofeedback, cognitive behavioral therapy; and third-wave therapies such as mindfulness-based cognitive therapy.

Migraine may be best conceptualized with a biopsychosocial approach (Fig. 23.1) [4]. The biopsychosocial approach posits that health and illness are influenced by one's mind, body, and environment. Accordingly, treatment for migraine should ideally target one's mind, body, and environment using a complementary and integrative approach. A complementary and integrative approach supplements medical and pharmacological treatment with behavioral treatments.

While the optimal treatment for migraine involves both pharmacotherapy and behavioral interventions, there are also instances in which behavioral interventions may serve as the primary treatment for migraine. Specifically, if patients prefer not to use pharmacological treatment if they do not respond to pharmacological treatment, or if they have medical contraindications that prevent them from taking pharmacological treatment [1]. The rest of this chapter reviews the most commonly used behavioral interventions for migraine.

The goal of this chapter is to review the empirically supported behavioral interventions for migraine, considerations for how to make a referral, and describe the different modalities in which behavioral interventions are implemented. By the end of this chapter, you should be familiar with the different types of behavioral interventions available for migraine and the modalities in which they are distributed, and you should be informed on considerations when making a referral.

Questions

1. Which of the following behavioral interventions have been shown to be efficacious in improving migraine outcomes?
   A. Cognitive behavioral therapy for migraine
   B. Relaxation training
   C. Mindfulness-based cognitive therapy
   D. All of the above
2. The stigma around mental health treatment may be a barrier to patients seeking behavioral interventions to manage their migraine
   A. True
   B. False

R. D. Best (✉)
Ferkauf Graduate School of Psychology, Yeshiva University, New York, NY, USA

I. Snyder
UCLA LGBTQ+ Healthcare Fellowship, UCLA Health, Los Angeles, CA, USA

E. K. Seng
Ferkauf Graduate School of Psychology, Yeshiva University, New York, NY, USA

Veterans Affairs Headache Centers of Excellence Research, Education, Evaluation, Engagement Center Activities Center for Headache (RE3ACH), West Haven, CT, USA

Saul R. Korey Department of Neurology, Albert Einstein College of Medicine, Bronx, NY, USA

Montefiore Headache Center, Montefiore Medical Center, Bronx, NY, USA

T. S. Monteith et al. (eds.), *Comprehensive Migraine Management*, https://doi.org/10.1007/978-3-031-86923-5_23

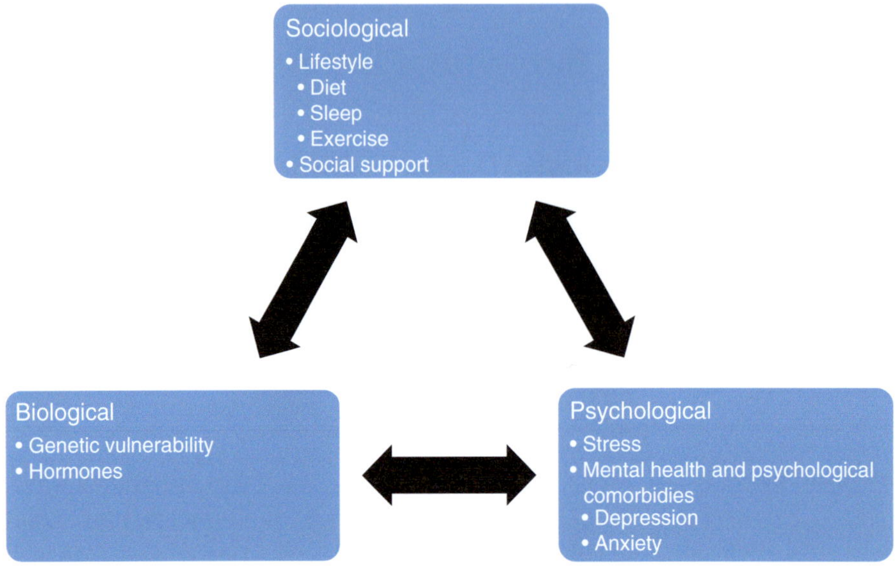

Fig. 23.1 Biopsychosocial model of migraine

Types of Behavioral Interventions

Lifestyle and Headache Education

Psychoeducation is a didactic-psychotherapeutic intervention that involves providing patients with information and skills that will help them better cope with their illness. Patients with migraine may benefit from psychoeducation about diet, exercise, sleep, medication adherence, and/or stress. Research indicates that low or stable alcohol and caffeine intake [5], hydration [6, 7], and consistent meals [8] lower the risk for migraine [9]. Aerobic exercise has been demonstrated to improve headache outcomes [10, 11]. Poor quality sleep, tiredness, excessive sleep, and restless sleep have all been associated with migraine attack onset [12–14]. Insomnia is comorbid with migraine and could worsen migraine symptoms [15]. Cognitive behavioral therapy for insomnia is the first-line recommended treatment for insomnia [16], and early trials suggest that cognitive behavioral therapy for insomnia in people with comorbid migraine and insomnia may improve both sleep and migraine symptoms [17]. Poor medication adherence, in the form of both overuse and underuse, may worsen headache outcomes [18, 19]. Psychoeducation, self-monitoring, and establishing a simple medication regimen may lead to improved medication adherence [19].

Stress

Stress has demonstrated a relationship with migraine attack onset [20]. Relationships between stress and migraine attack onset have varied in magnitude; for example, in one study, the presence of stress was associated with nearly double the odds of migraine attack onset, [21] whereas other studies have not found stress to be a significant predictor of headache [14]. Recent research has confirmed the presence of multiple stress-migraine attack profiles previously identified, including stress as a trigger/symptom (e.g., when high stress precedes migraine attacks), stress let-down (e.g., when a sudden decrease in stress precedes migraine attack, such as the first day of a vacation), and the lack of a relationship (e.g., for up to a third of people, there may be no relationship between stress and migraine attack onset) [20]. Recent research also indicates the extent to which stress is "surprising," or that the stressful events in one's day are unusual, maybe more important than mere stress level [5]. Stress management interventions, including relaxation, biofeedback, and cognitive behavioral therapy focused on stress reduction, have demonstrated efficacy in reducing migraine frequency [3]. Broadly speaking, reducing subjective stress experience seems to be associated with reduced migraine frequency in at least some patients. However, stress is likely not to be a relevant lifestyle factor for every person with migraine, and lifestyle interventions targeting stress management for migraine should be tailored to reflect that patient's patterns of stress and migraine attack onset.

Lifestyle factors may also contribute to the underlying neurological mechanisms of migraine. Stress is related to dysregulation in the hypothalamic-pituitary-adrenal (HPA) axis, and both stress and hypothalamic dysregulation have been associated with chronicity of migraine [22, 23]. Research has also suggested that oxidative stress may play a role, which can result from poor diet, stress, and poor sleep [24]. Furthermore, one study showed cognitive behavioral therapy (CBT) for migraine led to increased connectivity between the frontal lobe and the amygdala, and that increased frontal-amygdala connectivity was associated with fewer headache days per month [25].

Formal Behavioral Interventions

For some patients with migraine, provider education and self-guided lifestyle change is sufficient to produce meaningful changes in their behavior and migraine symptoms. However, for many patients with migraine, a behavioral specialist such as a psychologist can be useful in facilitating effective behavior change. Behavioral specialists should be considered in patients who require migraine prevention but are hesitant or unable to take medications, patients who are not receiving sufficient migraine frequency reduction with preventive medications, have higher levels of disability than expected based on migraine symptoms, or who have comorbid conditions such as insomnia or anxiety for which a behavioral provider could provide concomitant treatment [26].

Relaxation Training

Relaxation training is a systematic set of procedures intended to relax one's physical and mental state. The goal of relaxation training is to decrease activity in the sympathetic nervous system, minimizing the body's reaction to stress. Migraines are often related to stress [27]; thus, reducing stress may also reduce migraine and/ or its negative effects.

Relaxation training often includes deep breathing exercises and/or progressive muscle relaxation. Deep breathing exercises teach patients to breathe slowly and from their abdominals. Progressive muscle relaxation involves mindfully tightening and relaxing muscles throughout the body. This practice helps patients identify feelings of tension in the muscles and shows them how to relax them once they detect the tension.

Relaxation training is usually conducted in a clinic with a trained clinician over several sessions. These sessions are often supplemented by homework assignments. However, relaxation training can also be conducted via online instruction [28]. Studies have shown that engaging in relaxation techniques has led to reduced frequency of, and fewer severe, headaches [29]. Relaxation is often accompanied by other behavioral treatments, including biofeedback and CBT.

Biofeedback

Biofeedback is a technique that teaches patients to control their bodily functions by connecting them to electrical sensors while showing them how to regulate their physiological responses. Biofeedback is conducted by providing data on a variety of physiological functions, including brain waves, breathing, heart rate, muscle contraction, sweat gland activity, blood volume, and temperature. Muscles often tense in response to stress, anger, and anxiety. Muscle tension can be measured by electromyography (EMG). While receiving immediate feedback, participants are taught how to release muscle tension in their forehead, jaw, and/or shoulders. They can then apply these skills outside the clinic. Thermal biofeedback is one type of biofeedback that provides information on the temperature of one's hands. Hands often cool down in response to stress. During thermal biofeedback, a provider will guide the participant through feedback on the temperature of their fingers while showing them how to reduce their stress and regulate that temperature.

Biofeedback usually involves going to a clinic, often for multiple sessions, and working with a therapist. In these sessions, patients are attached to at least one machine that assesses their physiological functioning. The therapist will explain the data and instruct them on how to regulate their physiological functioning. Although biofeedback is primarily conducted in a clinic, there are a growing number of biofeedback devices meant to be used at home. These include apps attached to a mobile device or wearable devices. The FDA has approved Resperate, a portable device designed to promote slow breathing.

Biofeedback may directly reduce migraine symptoms. It may also increase self-efficacy and reduce secondary symptoms [30]. Biofeedback is often paired with relaxation training to show patients the physiological effects of the relaxation techniques. One study found that a combination of electromyography biofeedback, thermal biofeedback, and relaxation training significantly decreased the intensity and the frequency of migraine and reduced headache-related disability, psychological stress, depression, anxiety, and irritation [30]. A meta-analysis showed that biofeedback significantly reduced migraine frequency compared to waitlist controls; however, this reduction was not significant compared to patients who received relaxation training [31].

Cognitive Behavioral Therapies

Cognitive behavioral therapy (CBT) [32] refers to any talk therapy where the goal is to modify cognitions (thought patterns) and behaviors to reduce migraine attack frequency or improve quality of life while living with migraine. The underlying theory behind CBT is that thoughts, behaviors, and feelings constantly interact with one another. Thus, modifying one's thoughts or behaviors will have an impact on their thoughts, behaviors, and feelings. See Fig. 23.2 for a model of how thoughts, behaviors, and feelings may interact in the context of migraine. CBT is delivered by licensed mental health care providers at the doctoral (e.g., clinical psychology PhD, PsyD) or masters level (counselors and

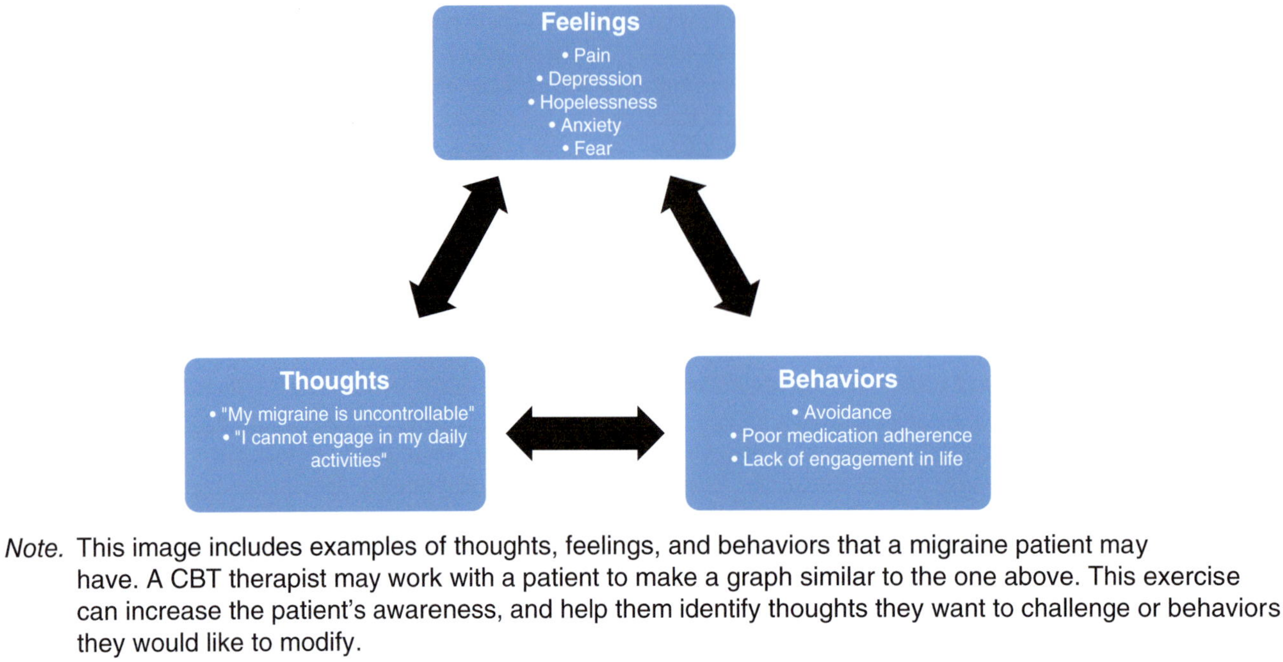

Fig. 23.2 Interaction of thoughts, feelings, and behaviors in migraine patients. *Note.* This image includes examples of thoughts, feelings, and behaviors that a migraine patient may have. A CBT therapist may work with a patient to make a graph similar to the one above. This exercise can increase the patient's awareness and help them identify thoughts they want to challenge or behaviors they would like to modify

social workers). Although originally developed to improve depressive symptoms, CBT has been applied to numerous diseases, including chronic pain, headache disorders, and migraine. CBT protocols [33] that have been developed for migraine and other headache disorders commonly focus on the following targets: (1) reducing stress; (2) reducing maladaptive pain cognitions; (3) modifying putative migraine triggers; (4) improving adherence to biomedical treatment strategies; and (5) reducing the burden of migraine. A case study utilizing CBT for migraine is included at the end of this chapter.

Cognitions Cognitive restructuring refers to the specific technique whereby a therapist guides a patient in identifying cognitive patterns, testing those cognitive patterns to determine if they are adaptive (e.g., leading to desired outcomes), identifying situations likely to produce maladaptive cognitions, and modifying maladaptive cognitions to improve responses to challenging situations. Cognitive restructuring in the context of migraine includes identifying the specific maladaptive cognitive patterns associated with migraine attack onset, higher intensity of migraine pain, hypervigilance for (and maladaptive avoidance of) possible migraine triggers, and lack of engagement in occupational, educational, social, or other role functioning. Promoting patients' resiliency can improve their functioning, regardless of the severity and frequency of pain [34].

The fear-avoidance model of pain is the theoretical basis for much of the cognitive restructuring that occurs in CBT for migraine [35–38]. In this model, a pain experience can be met by one of two cognitive responses: catastrophizing [39] considering the pain experience to be a "catastrophe" that will lead to one's life being ruined, or non-catastrophizing. When one does not catastrophize, one adaptively addresses any environmental factors contributing to the pain experience, makes informed judgments about activity engagement while in pain, and recognizes the time-limited nature of most pain courses. On the other hand, when the pain experience is met with catastrophizing, the patient begins a downward spiral of negative consequences: fear of pain, hypervigilance for pain experiences and potential triggers, lack of physical activity and social engagement, and depression. These negative consequences perversely increase the sensitivity to painful sensations, creating a cycle whereby catastrophizing fuels an expanding and worsening pain experience.

Behaviors The behavioral targets most commonly addressed in CBT for migraine [27–30] include relaxation strategies, sleep strategies, regular life behaviors (such as hydration, meals, and caffeine use), behavioral activation, and re-engagement with social, occupational, or educational roles. When setting goals for behavioral targets, basic motivational interviewing strategies are often used to select high-priority targets for change [40]. A high-priority change target should be one that is of high importance to the patient, and which the patient has high confidence they can modify in a relatively brief (often 2-week) period of time. For this reason, short-term realistic goals are often better first steps than long-term goals that may, on the surface, seem more important. For example, a patient may have dropped out of school because of their migraine disease, and they are no longer exercising. Although the goal of re-engaging with an educational role may be more important to reduce migraine disability in the long run, a short-term, more realistic behavioral activation goal of walking with a friend for 30 min, four mornings each week, can build self-efficacy through experiencing success. As the patient experiences success with smaller goals, their self-efficacy for migraine management increases, and they build the capacity and skills to tackle more challenging and long-term multi-component goals.

Third-Wave Therapies

Third-wave therapies include therapies that incorporate mindfulness and meditation techniques. There are some interventions that use mindfulness broadly, but there are also three specific third-wave therapies that have been adapted to use for migraine: mindfulness-based stress reduction, mindfulness-based cognitive therapy, and acceptance and commitment therapy.

Mindfulness-Based Stress Reduction (MBSR) Mindfulness-based stress reduction combines mindfulness practice and yoga to help patients gain better control of their mind and body, especially in reaction to stress. It was originally developed by Dr. Jon Kabat-Zinn and has been used to treat a variety of symptoms or conditions that are often related to stress, including chronic pain, anxiety, depression, high blood pressure, and sleep. MBSR treatment usually consists of eight weekly group sessions and sometimes a daylong mindfulness retreat. Randomized control trials found that compared to treatment as usual control group, MBSR decreased headache duration and headache-related disability and increased self-efficacy and mindfulness in migraine patients [41], increased quality of life and perceived pain perception in chronic headache patients [42], and reduced perceived stress and psychiatric symptoms for patients with tension headache [43]. A study that compared MBSR to stress management for headache (SFH) in episodic migraine patients found that patients who received MBSR treatment showed higher decreases in headache-related disability than controls [44]. Another RCT found that migraine patients who completed MBSR showed significantly more improvement in psychological symptoms, self-efficacy, and sensory pain perception compared to an active control [45]. MRI data demonstrate that MBSR improved cognitive efficiency (decreased parietal operculum and visual cortex activity and reduced resting connectivity of the dorsal anterior insula to posterior parietal cortex and visual cortex) in episodic migraine patients [46].

Mindfulness-Based Cognitive Therapy (MBCT) Mindfulness-based cognitive therapy combines mindfulness practices with cognitive behavioral therapy techniques to reduce maladaptive thought processes and perceived stress. MBCT usually consists of eight weekly group sessions with homework assignments. A randomized control trial showed that compared to a treatment-as-usual control group, headache patients who completed MBCT reported higher increases in self-efficacy and pain acceptance and decreases in pain catastrophizing and pain interference [47]. A study with migraine patients showed that those who received MBCT reported larger decreases in disability compared to those in a treatment-as-usual control condition [48].

Acceptance and Commitment Therapy (ACT) Acceptance and commitment therapy uses mindfulness techniques to increase acceptance and psychological flexibility. A randomized control trial showed that eight weekly group sessions of ACT decreased disability and affective distress in chronic pain patients when compared to a treatment-as-usual control group [49]. A study that included a single 5-h ACT workshop showed reduced symptoms of depression, general functioning, and disability in patients with comorbid migraine and depression [50]. Another randomized control trial showed that migraine patients who received eight sessions of group ACT reported a decrease in headache days and medication use [51]. While ACT does not reduce the pain experience, it does reduce disability and affective distress [52].

Considerations Involving Behavioral Interventions

How to Make an Effective Referral

There are many barriers to following through with a referral to behavioral treatment [53]. Barriers include lack of specific in-network referral (e.g., financial burden), lack of knowledge about behavioral treatments for migraine, and stigma associated with being referred to providers typically thought of as "mental health" providers. Headache providers should proactively attempt to cultivate a set of behavioral providers to whom they routinely refer. Behavioral providers could include psychologists, other licensed therapists such as social workers or counselors, physical and occupational therapists, nutritionists, and exercise physiologists. Although specific advanced training and expertise in treating migraine and headache disorders are ideal, many behavioral providers who have a solid base of training and expertise in their practice area are eager to cultivate new referral sources and are happy to seek out continuing education. For example, a psychologist, specially trained in working with health populations (a health psychologist), who has a background in relaxation and cognitive behavioral therapies would certainly be able to apply those skills to migraine and other headache disorders. By cultivating a set of behavioral specialists to whom you commonly refer, headache providers can begin to build networks of burgeoning headache experts in their geographic area.

Having a solid therapeutic alliance [54] is critical to making an effective referral and can mitigate barriers related to lack of knowledge and the perception that the referral is for mental health (instead of for migraine). The therapeutic alliance has three components: agreement on goals, agreement on tasks, and rapport. Although having a rapport with a patient is a good start, it is not sufficient to facilitate patient adherence to a treatment plan. If the patient and provider do not agree on the goal, the patient may not follow through with a referral. For example, a patient may have a goal of never experiencing another migraine attack, whereas the provider may have a goal of achieving pain freedom as quickly as possible when migraine attacks occur. In this case, the provider may have to use motivational interviewing techniques [40] to harness the patient's intrinsic motivation to set a functional goal, such as asking open-ended questions about how migraine impacts the patient's life and reflecting back how it is the intensity and duration of attacks that seem to be most problematic. Once patients and providers agree on goals, they may disagree on the tasks necessary to achieve those goals. If patients see only medication as an acceptable task for migraine management, this can be a major barrier to engaging in behavioral treatments. In these cases, using motivational interviewing to assess how important migraine management is for the patient, and asking permission to share both scientific and anecdotal evidence about the effectiveness of behavioral migraine treatments, can be useful. It is also useful to emphasize to patients that referrals for behavioral migraine treatments do not indicate that the provider does not believe the patient's migraine is real; in fact, the behavioral treatment referral indicates that the provider very much believes the patient is experiencing a significant neurological disease and that multidisciplinary care is the best way to address the patient's symptoms.

It is likely that most migraine patients would benefit from some form of behavioral intervention. Patients who have poor sleep, diet, exercise patterns, or excessive stress may be particularly good targets for referrals for behavioral interventions that target lifestyle changes. Patients who report noticeably high levels of migraine-related disability may be good targets for CBT or third-wave therapies. Behavioral interventions may be effective for patients with medication overuse headaches since pharmacological treatment leads to rebound headaches [55]. Furthermore, behavioral interventions can be used as primary care for patients who are not using migraine medication. This might be the case if medication proves inefficacious, patients do not want to take medication, they are unable to tolerate the medicine, or they are contraindicated, as may be the case for pregnant women [1].

Modality of Behavioral Interventions

Telehealth options may improve access to care for headaches. In one study of people with at least 4 headache days per month, participants indicated that they were most likely to pursue in-person or smartphone-based care for headaches rather than telephone-only options [56]. These responses were significantly associated with headache-related disability, suggesting that people with an increased impact of migraine are more likely to pursue care across in-person and smartphone options. During the COVID-19 pandemic, a study of migraine patients with high levels of migraine-related disability assessed perceptions of telemedicine for follow-up appointments: not only does telemedicine increase access to care for such patients, but patients also reported satisfaction with this visit modality overall, care outcomes were comparable to in-person care, and headache care providers were much more productive when compared to similar office visits [57]. A comparison of telehealth and in-person treatment can be found in Table 23.1.

Table 23.1 Behavioral modalities

Behavioral modality	Definition	Benefits	Barriers
Telehealth	Interventions conducted via video call, phone, Internet, or mobile device	Flexibility with location Less of a financial burden Evidence supports improved migraine outcomes	Requires a device Requires technological proficiency Technological difficulties
In-person	Interventions conducted in-person	Therapeutic alliance may be stronger Evidence supports improved migraine outcomes	Financial barrier Time-consuming Local availability

Conclusion

Migraine is not caused by lifestyle factors. However, for people with migraine, behavior changes can help reduce migraine symptoms and burden. Education about relevant lifestyle factors should be incorporated into routine migraine care. Providers should be cognizant that not all lifestyle factors are relevant for every patient; for example, although stress management has been useful for many patients with migraine, it may not be relevant for a substantial subset of migraine patients. For patients who require additional support with behavior change, have relevant comorbidities, or are continuing to experience migraine burden with effective prevention, referral to a formal behavioral treatment may be warranted. Providers should cultivate relationships with behavioral intervention providers and describe the rationale for the treatment to patients to facilitate follow-through with behavioral intervention referrals.

Teaching Points

1. Regulating the body's stress response through relaxation techniques or biofeedback training may improve migraine outcomes.
2. Formalized interventions such as cognitive behavioral therapy (CBT) and third-wave therapies are promising interventions for migraine patients who are open to psychological intervention.
3. Although psychological interventions may impact migraine outcomes, this does *NOT* mean that migraine is a psychological disease, or "in one's head."
4. When making a referral for a behavioral intervention, it is important to understand the patient's goals.

Case

Carla was referred to CBT therapy by her neurologist. Carla was experiencing approximately nine headache days per month, which she reported as extremely distressing and led to significant reductions in her quality of life. Carla's neurologist suggested that her migraines may be amplified by her current stressors, which include a recent split from a partner and a sudden decline in her father's health. Carla was the primary caregiver for her father and for her three teenage children, each of whom maintained multiple after-school activities. Carla's stress was high at baseline, with frequent exacerbations around her father's medical appointments and contact with her former partner. Carla's time was in high demand from all her family members, and she had minimal opportunity to relax. The only time she truly "turned off," she asserted, was when she was hit with a migraine attack. At such times, she engaged her rescue medication, relinquished responsibilities for her father to one of her children, retreated to her room, and remained in isolation until her pain receded to manageable levels, typically the next day. Carla remained fearful of these events, worrying her father or one of her children might have a health crisis while she was fully indisposed and was hypervigilant around pain onset and migraine prodrome even when her other stressors were relatively well managed.

Case Discussion

Carla's therapist began therapy with psychoeducation about the relationship between stress and migraine. Though many of Carla's stressors were fundamentally unchangeable, she was taught to identify times of stress exacerbation and to implement self-care strategies, including mindful observation of her thoughts. She was also taught to engage in some stress-reduction techniques, including diaphragmatic breathing, on a daily basis, to help lower her stress baseline. Carla's therapist also helped Carla challenge her maladaptive thought patterns, such as catastrophizing her migraine attacks, and her cognition that it was critical that she be the primary support for her entire family at all times. Carla and her therapist also worked on behavioral activation techniques such as engaging in physical activity within and outside the home, building social support, and creating a consistent schedule supporting her stress management.

By the end of treatment, Carla reported approximately four headache days per month. Additionally, she reported decreased psychological distress and increased quality of life.

Questions and Answers

1. Which of the following behavioral interventions have been shown to be efficacious in improving migraine outcomes?
   A. Cognitive behavioral therapy for migraine
   B. Relaxation training

C. Mindfulness-based cognitive therapy
D. All of the above

The correct answer is D. Cognitive behavioral therapy, relaxation training, and mindfulness-based cognitive therapy have all been shown to be efficacious in improving migraine outcomes, such as reduced pain, increased quality of life, decreased disability, increased pain flexibility, and improved medication adherence.

2. The stigma around mental health treatment may be a barrier to patients seeking behavioral interventions to manage their migraine
   A. True
   B. False

The correct answer is A. Stigma around mental health treatment may be a barrier to patients seeking behavioral interventions to manage their migraine. The stigma around mental health treatment may discourage patients from seeking help from a psychologist.

References

1. Buse CD, Andrasik F. Behavioral medicine for migraine. Neurol Clin. 2009;27(2):445–65.
2. Patel PS, Minen MT. Complementary and integrative health treatments for migraine. J Neuroophthalmol. 2019;39(3):360.
3. Penzien DB, Irby MB, Smitherman TS, Rains JC, Houle TT. Well-established and empirically supported behavioral treatments for migraine. Curr Pain Headache Rep. 2015;19(7):1–7.
4. Leonardi M, Raggi A, Grazzi L, D'Amico D. Disability, ICF biopsychosocial model and burden of migraine. J Headache Pain. 2015;16:1–2.
5. Turner DP, Lebowitz AD, Chtay I, Houle TT. Headache triggers as a surprise. J Head Face Pain. 2019;59(5):495–508.
6. Blau JN. Water deprivation: a new migraine precipitant. Headache. 2005;45(6):757–9.
7. Spigt M, Weerkamp N, Troost J, van Schayck CP, Knottnerus JA. A randomized trial on the effects of regular water intake in patients with recurrent headaches. Fam Pract. 2012;29(4):370–5.
8. Nas A, Mirza N, Hägele F, Kahlhöfer J, Keller J, Rising R, et al. Impact of breakfast skipping compared with dinner skipping on regulation of energy balance and metabolic risk. Am J Clin Nutr. 2017;105(6):1351–61.
9. Robblee J, Starling AJ. SEEDS for success: lifestyle management in migraine. Cleve Clin J Med. 2019;86(11):741–9.
10. La Touche R, Fernández Pérez JJ, Proy Acosta A, González Campodónico L, Martínez García S, Adraos Juárez D, et al. Is aerobic exercise helpful in patients with migraine? A systematic review and meta-analysis. Scand J Med Sci Sports. 2020;30(6):965–82.
11. Oliveira AB, Ribeiro RT, Mello MT, Tufik S, Peres MFP. Anandamide is related to clinical and cardiorespiratory benefits of aerobic exercise training in migraine patients: a randomized controlled clinical trial. Cannabis Cannabinoid Res. 2019;4(4):275–84.
12. Houle TT, Butschek RA, Turner DP, Smitherman TA, Rains JC, Penzien DB. Stress and sleep duration predict headache severity in chronic headache sufferers. Pain. 2012;153(12):2432–40.
13. Bertisch SM, Li W, Buettner C, Mostofsky E, Rueschman M, Kaplan ER, et al. Nightly sleep duration, fragmentation, and quality and daily risk of migraine. Neurology. 2020;94(5):e489–e96.
14. Peris F, Donoghue S, Torres F, Mian A, Wöber C. Towards improved migraine management: determining potential trigger factors in individual patients. Cephalalgia. 2017;37(5):452–63.
15. Rains JC. Sleep and migraine: assessment and treatment of comorbid sleep disorders. Headache. 2018;58(7):1074–91.
16. Schutte-Rodin S, Broch L, Buysse D, Dorsey C, Sateia M. Clinical guideline for the evaluation and management of chronic insomnia in adults. J Clin Sleep Med. 2008;4(5):487–504.
17. Smitherman TA, Kuka AJ, Calhoun AH, Walters ABP, Davis-Martin RE, Ambrose CE, et al. Cognitive-behavioral therapy for insomnia to reduce chronic migraine: a sequential Bayesian analysis. Headache. 2018;58(7):1052–9.
18. Lipton RB, Fanning KM, Serrano D, Reed ML, Cady R, Buse DC. Ineffective acute treatment of episodic migraine is associated with new-onset chronic migraine. Neurology. 2015;84(7):688–95.
19. Seng EK, Rains JA, Nicholson RA, Lipton RB. Improving medication adherence in migraine treatment. Curr Pain Headache Rep. 2015;19(6):1–7.
20. Vives-Mestres M, Casanova A, Buse DC, Donoghue S, Houle TT, Lipton RB, et al. Patterns of perceived stress throughout the migraine cycle: a longitudinal cohort study using daily prospective diary data. Headache. 2021;61(1):90–102.
21. Park J-W, Chu MK, Kim J-M, Park S-G, Cho S-J. Analysis of trigger factors in episodic migraineurs using a smartphone headache diary applications. PLoS One. 2016;11(2):e0149577.
22. Peres MFP, Del Rio MS, Seabra M, Tufik S, Abucham J, Cipolla-Neto J, et al. Hypothalamic involvement in chronic migraine. J Neurol Neurosurg Psychiatry. 2001;71(6):747–51.
23. Stubberud A, Buse DC, Kristoffersen ES, Linde M, Tronvik E. Is there a causal relationship between stress and migraine? Current evidence and implications for management. J Headache Pain. 2021;22(1):1–11.
24. Borkum JM. Brain energy deficit as a source of oxidative stress in migraine: a molecular basis for migraine susceptibility. Neurochem Res. 2021;46(8):1913–32.
25. Nahman-Averbuch H, Schneider VJ, Chamberlin LA, Kroon Van Diest AM, Peugh JL, Lee GR, et al. Alterations in brain function after cognitive behavioral therapy for migraine in children and adolescents. Headache. 2020;60(6):1165–82.
26. Singer AB, Buse DC, Seng EK. Behavioral treatments for migraine management: useful at each step of migraine care. Curr Neurol Neurosci Rep. 2015;15(4):14.
27. Sauro KM, Becker WJ. The stress and migraine interaction. Headache. 2009;49(9):1378–86.
28. Devineni T, Blanchard EB. A randomized controlled trial of an internet-based treatment for chronic headache. Behav Res Ther. 2005;43(3):277–92.
29. Mullally WJ, Hall K, Goldstein R. Efficacy of biofeedback in the treatment of migraine and tension type headaches. Pain Physician. 2009;12(6):1005–11.
30. Odawara M, Hashizume M, Yoshiuchi K, Tsuboi K. Real-time assessment of the effect of biofeedback therapy with migraine: a pilot study. Int J Behav Med. 2015;22(6):748–54.
31. Nestoriuc Y, Martin A, Rief W, Andrasik F. Biofeedback treatment for headache disorders: a comprehensive efficacy review. Appl Psychophysiol Biofeedback. 2008;33(3):125–40.
32. Beck AT. The past and future of cognitive therapy. J Psychother Pract Res. 1997;6(4):276.
33. Powers SW, Kashikar-Zuck SM, Allen JR, LeCates SL, Slater SK, Zafar M, et al. Cognitive behavioral therapy plus amitriptyline for chronic migraine in children and adolescents: a randomized clinical trial. JAMA. 2013;310(24):2622–30.
34. Stonnington CM, Kothari DJ, Davis MC. Understanding and promoting resiliency in patients with chronic headache. Curr Neurol Neurosci Rep. 2016;16(1):1–7.

35. Vlaeyen JW, Linton SJ. Fear-avoidance and its consequences in chronic musculoskeletal pain: a state of the art. Pain. 2000;85(3):317–32.
36. Holroyd KA, Cottrell CK, O'Donnell FJ, Cordingley GE, Drew JB, Carlson BW, et al. Effect of preventive (β blocker) treatment, behavioural migraine management, or their combination on outcomes of optimised acute treatment in frequent migraine: randomised controlled trial. BMJ. 2010:341.
37. Grinberg AS, Best RD, Min KM, Schindler EA, Koo BB, Sico JJ, et al. Cluster headache: clinical characteristics and opportunities to enhance quality of life. Curr Pain Headache Rep. 2021;25(10):1–6.
38. Klan T, Liesering-Latta E, Gaul C, Martin PR, Witthöft M. An integrative cognitive behavioral therapy program for adults with migraine: a feasibility study. Headache. 2019;59(5):741–55.
39. Sullivan MJ, Bishop SR, Pivik J. Pain catastrophizing scale (PCS) 1995. 2013.
40. Miller WR, Rollnick S. Motivational interviewing: helping people change. Guilford press; 2012.
41. Wells RE, Burch R, Paulsen RH, Wayne PM, Houle TT, Loder E. Meditation for migraines: a pilot randomized controlled trial. Headache. 2014;54(9):1484–95.
42. Bakhshani N-M, Amirani A, Amirifard H, Shahrakipoor M. The effectiveness of mindfulness-based stress reduction on perceived pain intensity and quality of life in patients with chronic headache. Global J Health Sci. 2016;8(4):142.
43. Omidi A, Zargar F. Effects of mindfulness-based stress reduction on perceived stress and psychological health in patients with tension headache. J Res Med Sci. 2015;20(11):1058.
44. Seminowicz DA, Burrowes SA, Kearson A, Zhang J, Krimmel SR, Samawi L, et al. Enhanced mindfulness-based stress reduction in episodic migraine: a randomized clinical trial with magnetic resonance imaging outcomes. Pain. 2020;161(8):1837–46.
45. Simshäuser K, Lüking M, Kaube H, Schultz C, Schmidt S. Is mindfulness-based stress reduction a promising and feasible intervention for patients suffering from migraine? A randomized controlled pilot trial. Complement Med Res. 2020;27(1):19–30.
46. Seminowicz DA, Burrowes SA, Kearson A, Zhang J, Krimmel SR, Samawi L, et al. Enhanced mindfulness based stress reduction (MBSR+) in episodic migraine: a randomized clinical trial with MRI outcomes. Pain. 2020;161(8):1837.
47. Day MA, Thorn BE, Ward LC, Rubin N, Hickman SD, Scogin F, et al. Mindfulness-based cognitive therapy for the treatment of headache pain: a pilot study. Clin J Pain. 2014;30(2):152–61.
48. Seng EK, Singer AB, Metts C, Grinberg AS, Patel ZS, Marzouk M, et al. Does mindfulness-based cognitive therapy for migraine reduce migraine-related disability in people with episodic and chronic migraine? A phase 2b pilot randomized clinical trial. Headache. 2019;59(9):1448–67.
49. Vowles KE, Wetherell JL, Sorrell JT. Targeting acceptance, mindfulness, and values-based action in chronic pain: findings of two preliminary trials of an outpatient group-based intervention. Cogn Behav Pract. 2009;16(1):49–58.
50. Dindo L, Recober A, Marchman JN, Turvey C, O'Hara MW. One-day behavioral treatment for patients with comorbid depression and migraine: a pilot study. Behav Res Ther. 2012;50(9):537–43.
51. Grazzi L, Bernstein C, Raggi A, Sansone E, Grignani E, Searl M, et al. ACT for migraine: effect of acceptance and commitment therapy (ACT) for high frequency episodic migraine without aura: a phase-II, multicentric, randomized, open-label study, vol. 22. AAN Enterprises; 2019. p. 10–004.
52. Mo'tamedi H, Rezaiemaram P, Tavallaie A. The effectiveness of a group-based acceptance and commitment additive therapy on rehabilitation of female outpatients with chronic headache: preliminary findings reducing 3 dimensions of headache impact. Headache. 2012;52(7):1106–19.
53. Langenbahn D, Matsuzawa Y, Lee YSC, Fraser F, Penzien DB, Simon NM, et al. Underuse of behavioral treatments for headache: a narrative review examining societal and cultural factors. J Gen Intern Med. 2021;36:3103–12.
54. Bordin ES. A working alliance based model of supervision. Couns Psychol. 1983;11(1):35–42.
55. Perlini C, Donisi V, Del Piccolo L. From research to clinical practice: a systematic review of the implementation of psychological interventions for chronic headache in adults. BMC Health Serv Res. 2020;20(1):1–17.
56. Minen MT, Szperka CL, Kaplan K, Ehrlich A, Riggins N, Rizzoli P, et al. Telehealth as a new care delivery model: the headache provider experience. Headache. 2021;61(7):1123–31.
57. Friedman DI, Rajan B, Seidmann A. A randomized trial of telemedicine for migraine management. Cephalalgia. 2019;39(12):1577–85.

Complementary and Integrative Medicine for the Treatment of Migraine

24

Brooklyn A. Bradley and Deena E. Kuruvilla

Introduction

Migraine is a disabling neurological condition characterized by headaches, photophobia, phonophobia, nausea, vomiting, and other neurological symptoms. The global incidence of migraine is approximately 10%; nonetheless, it is marginally higher in the United States at 12% [1]. The objectives of treatment for patients with migraine encompass a reduction in the frequency, duration, and severity of attacks [2]. Different management procedures such as mainstream pharmacological therapies, lifestyle counseling, neuromodulation, and complementary and integrative medicine should be used together to attain this outcome.

This chapter aims to review the complementary and integrative treatments which have evidence for migraine treatment. Physicians have witnessed the movement toward complementary and integrative medicine in the treatment of individuals with severe headaches and migraine. The National Institute of Health (NIH) describes complementary and integrative medicine (CIM) as a group of diverse medical and healthcare systems, practices, and products that are not generally considered conventional medicine [3]. According to the National Center for Complementary and Integrative Health, more than 30% of adults and 12% of children use healthcare approaches developed outside of conventional medicine to add to mainstream treatments [4]. Integrative medicine can be further categorized into natural products, mind-body medicine, and body-based practices.

Questions

1. A 24-year-old female with a history of depression, anxiety, and chronic migraine reports that she has had side effects to the following migraine preventive treatments—topiramate, valproic acid, botulinum toxin A, venlafaxine, nortriptyline, and propranolol. She reports she does not want to take any more prescription medications to treat migraine. Which of the following integrative medicine approaches would you avoid recommending?
   A. Acupuncture
   B. Daith piercing
   C. Magnesium
   D. Cognitive behavioral therapy
   E. Physical therapy consultation
2. A 35-year-old female with a long history of chronic migraine presents for follow-up. She has been receiving botulinum toxin for the prevention of migraine for 2 years now. She reports a 50% reduction in headache frequency and severity since starting the treatment. She would like to stop botulinum toxin and try something new in order to take a different approach. Acupuncture was the cure for her mother. Which of the following is your reply?
   A. I do not practice witchcraft
   B. Botulinum toxin is one of the only FDA-approved treatments for chronic migraine, and a sudden cessation could result in a sudden worsening of your headaches. Perhaps, we can discuss integrating acupuncture with botulinum toxin,
   C. Sure! Let's switch to acupuncture
   D. What worked for your mother may not work for you
   E. Why would you want to switch?!

B. A. Bradley · D. E. Kuruvilla (✉)
Department of Neurology, Westport Headache Institute, Westport, CT, USA

T. S. Monteith et al. (eds.), *Comprehensive Migraine Management*, https://doi.org/10.1007/978-3-031-86923-5_24

Nutraceutical Products

Riboflavin

Riboflavin is a cofactor that catalyzes the activity of flavoenzymes in the mitochondrial respiratory chain, and its insufficiency can produce mitochondrial dysfunction. The mechanism of riboflavin absorption in humans is through active transport, and it is chiefly absorbed in the upper ileum of the human intestine [2].

In an open-label Class III study, migraine patients received 400 mg/d of riboflavin over a 6-month period. A reduction from 4 to 2 monthly migraine days was found [5]. A Class I trial investigated the effects of combining riboflavin (400 mg/d), magnesium (600 mg/d), coenzyme Q10 (150 mg/d), plus a multivitamin-mineral component to placebo [6]. A Class II trial studied the effects of combining riboflavin 400 mg, magnesium 300 mg, and feverfew 100 mg in comparison to placebo which contained 25 mg riboflavin [7].

In a Class II study conducted in 2015 evaluating riboflavin compared to sodium valproate for the prevention of migraine, some adverse effects were weight gain, dizziness, and gastrointestinal problems. In addition, as riboflavin is mainly excreted in the urine, orange discoloration of urine can be common in patients taking high doses of riboflavin [2].

Magnesium

Magnesium participates as a cofactor in over 325 intracellular reactions, including enzyme activity, oxidative phosphorylation, and DNA synthesis [8]. Magnesium deficiency may develop from insufficient intake or increased excretion of magnesium in the gastrointestinal tract and urine [11]. Studies have suggested a relationship between magnesium deficiency and mild and moderate tension-type headaches and migraines [9].

Low amounts of magnesium in serum and cerebrospinal fluid may be the source [10, 11]. A systematic review of five RCTs in adult migraine patients illustrated potential evidence for the prevention of migraine with 600 mg magnesium dicitrate daily [9]. In a second study, a high oral dose of magnesium lowered the frequency of migraine attacks with 12 weeks of therapy [12]. The results confirmed the positive effect of 300 mg magnesium in a small sample of female patients with menstrual migraines [8].

The most common side effects of magnesium supplements include diarrhea and gastric effects though mild. Since magnesium has a relatively benign negative effect history, it may be appropriate in populations who are particularly vulnerable to the side effects of traditional drugs [9].

CoQ10

Coenzyme Q10 (CoQ10), also known as ubiquinone, is an antioxidant that acts against inflammatory markers of migraine. In addition, it has been found to lessen the expression of cytokines and matrix metalloproteinases (MMPs) [13]. CoQ10 participates in the electron transport chain of mitochondria, which ultimately accompanies its position in energy metabolism [14].

Six studies found no significant reduction in the severity of headaches during migraine attacks after taking CoQ10 for at least 6 weeks. In comparison to the control group, there was a statistically significant decrease in the duration of headache attacks with CoQ10 when compared to the control group [6, 15–19]. Past studies have shown that CoQ10 is effective as a method of prevention for migraine. The recommended dosage is 150 mg daily [14].

The side effects of CoQ10 may include insomnia, fatigue, nausea, diarrhea, and rare increases in liver function testing. There are limited reports on the adverse effects of CoQ10; however, there have been some cases of minor side effects such as diarrhea and chromaturia in studies that illustrated no significant difference compared to the group supplemented with CoQ10 [14].

Butterbur

Butterbur is scientifically designated as *Petasites hybridus*. It is a shrub that is cultivated in Europe and regions of Asia and North America. Butterbur has been found to be effective for migraine prevention but comes with risks [20].

Two Class I studies demonstrated that 50–75 mg twice a day led to a reduction in monthly migraine days. In the first study, monthly migraine days decreased by 60%, and this was statistically significant compared to placebo. The second Class I study found that monthly migraine days were reduced by 48% with a dose of 75 mg twice a day, by 36% for Petasites extract 50 mg twice a day and by 26% for the placebo group [20, 21].

Butterbur is effective for migraine prevention and can be offered to reduce monthly migraine days with caution [20]. Butterbur has been found to cause hepatic failure; therefore, its use is limited due to safety. This nutraceutical product needs to be free of pyrrolizidine alkaloids (PA) to ensure safety given possible hepatotoxicity. Concerns over hepatotoxicity have also caused The American Headache Society (AHS)/American Academy of Neurology (AAN) 2012 guidelines to be retired [22].

Feverfew

Feverfew (*Tanacetum parthenium)* is an herbaceous perennial native to Asia and is prevalent in the Balkans. It is a daisy-like plant used by the Greeks in the first century for inflammatory disorders [23]. The active ingredient parthenolide may impede migraine through its vascular smooth muscle relaxation and anti-inflammatory properties [24].

In a Class I study, the migraine frequency in patients administered with feverfew decreased from 4.76 by 1.9 attacks/month in the feverfew group and by 1.3 attacks in the placebo group [25]. In a Class II study, feverfew 6.25 mg TID was effective in reducing migraine frequency [20]. The recommended dosage is 100–300 mg up to four times a day with 0.2–0.4% parthenolide content [24].

Adverse effects include mouth ulceration and gastrointestinal symptoms. There is evidence of post-feverfew syndrome. Feverfew should not be discontinued abruptly, or withdrawal symptoms will occur such as insomnia, anxiety, and myalgia. Feverfew also has the potential to cause uterine contractions and is not recommended during pregnancy [24].

Omega-3

Omega-3 has anti-inflammatory properties that have made it a research concern for migraine prevention. Omega-3 fatty acids are constitutive of cell membrane phospholipids. Omega-3 fatty acids in vitro have been discovered to inhibit the production of proinflammatory cytokines from macrophages. This results in the reduction of inflammation and pain [26].

Omega-3 may be useful in treating chronic migraine although more studies are needed. Moreover, a recent systematic review of 11 studies investigating the effects of omega-3 on migraine frequency and severity showed no overall benefit [27]. A study showed that 2 months of supplementation with 1 gram of omega-3 fatty acids decreased migraine frequency. Patients also reported a 74% reduction in the duration of their individual headache [26].

Omega-3 adverse effects may include heartburn, loose stools, and nosebleeds. Some studies have shown that too much fish oil can cause an increase in metabolic weight as well. Over 3 grams per day may increase the risk of bleeding and weaken the immune system [22].

Vitamin D

Vitamin D deficiency is a global public health dilemma, as a total of 30–80% of children and adults have vitamin D deficiency around the world [28]. Vitamin D deficiency is associated with musculoskeletal disorders, cancer, autoimmune disorders, cardiovascular disorders, kidney disorders, mental disorders, and skin disorders [29].

In a study performed among postmenopausal patients with migraine and low levels of vitamin D, they discovered that with supplementation of vitamin D and calcium, the frequency and duration of migraine attacks decreased [30]. A 2018 randomized placebo-controlled double-blinded study found that vitamin D 100 μg daily for 24 weeks resulted in a reduction in migraine days overall [29, 31]. A study looking at simvastatin plus vitamin D for migraine prevention in adults with episodic migraine demonstrated that simvastatin plus vitamin D is an effective therapy for headache prevention in adults with episodic migraine [32].

Excessive levels of calcium in the blood because of Vitamin D supplementation may lead to adverse effects. These may include arrhythmias, hypercalcemia, metallic taste in the mouth, constipation, and dry mouth [33]. Vitamin D has a favorable safety profile and limited potential side effects, making it an effective and safe treatment for migraine [34].

Melatonin

Melatonin is a circadian pacemaker for sleep, in addition to operating as an antioxidant, antihypertensive, and sedative. It is generated from the pineal gland and is known as the "clock factor." [35] Levels of melatonin have been found to be low in migraine and cluster headache [36].

A randomized double-blind placebo-controlled study compared melatonin 3 mg, amitriptyline 25 mg, and placebo 1:1:1. After 3 months, migraine days per month were fewer in the melatonin and amitriptyline groups as compared to placebo [22]. In a small pilot study of 49 patients, there was a reduction in attack frequency after 6 months of therapy [36]. Oral melatonin 4 mg has shown efficacy in reducing headache frequency in patients with TTH and migraine [35, 36].

The adverse effects of melatonin include drowsiness, fatigue, dizziness, epigastralgia, anxiety, nightmares, pruritus, dry mouth, constipation, and alopecia. More severe effects, for instance, may be liver injuries and reproductive system dysfunction [35].

Mind-Body Medicine

Mindfulness and Meditation

Mindfulness and meditation focus on the ability to let go of judgment about the workings of the mind. Mindfulness training contrasts with classic meditation through the practice of both informal and formal self-reflection during the day rather than being confined to a specific time or place [37].

Several studies published in the last 3 years have evaluated the treatment of headaches with mindfulness-based stress reduction (MBSR), a standardized 8-week program. A 2015 study assessed MBSR plus medication treatment to medication treatment alone in 37 adults with 15+ days/month with chronic headache, where they were further classified as migraine or tension-type [38]. The MBSR group had less pain intensity and improved quality of life after the intervention compared with the control. Mindfulness may balance autonomic system dysregulation during a stressful episode [22].

Several studies have shed light on the use of mindfulness and meditation in patients with chronic headaches and migraine or tension-type headaches [39]. Adverse effects of mindfulness and meditation have not been reported.

Yoga

Yoga is a spiritual practice that is derived from the Hindu faith. Its foundation is formed upon breath control, simple meditation, and unique postures. This method is widely practiced in individuals with chronic migraine [40].

In 60 people with migraine history, an intensive ayurvedic treatment regimen followed by yoga daily for up to 90 days was compared to a control condition [41]. The control condition involved symptomatic use of NSAIDs [43]. The yoga/ayurvedic group improved from day 1 to day 90 on the Comprehensive Headache-related Quality of Life Questionnaire and a visual analogue scale [1–10] of headache intensity. A study of 32 women with migraine, assessed medication plus a 12-week yoga treatment program (3 sessions/week for 75 min each) to a medication-only control group [43]. This study showed a reduction in headache frequency, severity, and disability in the yoga group versus the control group [22].

No major side effects or risks were reported in the study. There have been rare case reports of mind/body treatments triggering psychosis; however, the only common occurrence is musculoskeletal side effects [22].

Manipulative and Body-Based Practices

Acupuncture

Acupuncture is the needling of specific points of the body, and it is one of the most widely used complementary therapies in the world. This method was originally developed as part of Chinese medicine with the intention of bringing the patient back to a phase of equilibrium [44].

In a 2016 Cochrane review with 22 trials, 41% of acupuncture patients had a 50% responder rate vs. 17% in placebo (acupuncture vs. no acupuncture). About 50% of acupuncture patients had a 50% responder rate vs. 41% in sham. Headache frequency, headache days, and headache scores 3–4 months after treatment were more favorable in patients receiving acupuncture [44].

Several large-scale observational studies have provided evidence that acupuncture is a relatively safe intervention. Some adverse effects such as pneumothorax are reported but rare. Between 8 and 11% of patients report minor side effects such as fatigue or temporary aggravation [44].

Chiropractic Maneuvers

Common chiropractic maneuvers include myofascial release, balanced ligamentous tension, and balanced membranous tension [45]. The goal of chiropractic therapy is realignment [22].

A recent RCT comparing chiropractic spinal manipulation vs. sham maneuver vs. medication treatment reported that all three groups had fewer monthly migraine days. The benefits could be attributed to a placebo effect [22]. Chiropractic maneuvers have been used for migraine prevention rather than acute treatment. Past studies have illustrated the use of eight chiropractic sessions over 6 months [22]. This improved migraine days per month; however, the effect of chiropractic manipulation may be most efficient when combined with mainstream medication [46].

Cervical artery dissection with high-velocity chiropractic manipulation is a reported adverse effect [22]. A 2017 retrospective chart review of cervical artery dissection over 4 years revealed that of 141 dissections, 12 patients had documented chiropractic manipulation immediately prior to onset of symptoms [47]. There was also a 2018 case report of a 32-year-old woman who died from a vertebral dissection and brainstem stroke following chiropractic manipulation [48].

Herbal Medicine

Menthol

Menthol is a component in peppermint oil that has been applicable in the treatment of pain-related conditions including headache [49]. Menthol is found in many topical medications, as it has peripheral and central analgesic effects [50].

An RCT investigating the efficacy of cutaneous application of menthol 10% solution for the abortive treatment of migraine reported a decrease in pain levels between the placebo and menthol groups in the first 2 h after administration. About 38.3% of migraine attacks treated with the study drug reported pain freedom 2 h after cutaneous application [49]. A pilot study determining whether topical menthol 6% gel (STOPAIN) will be efficacious in migraine attacks revealed a significant improvement in headache intensity by 2 h after gel application [51].

An RCT reported that following menthol application, subjects reported a burning sensation in the temporal region and aggravation because of menthol odor [49]. However, a previous patch test study of 4000 patients revealed that menthol and peppermint oil did not elicit an allergic or irritant response [52]. Menthol may be a safe and efficacious treatment in addition to mainstream medical therapy for the treatment of migraine attacks [49].

Lavender

Lavender essential oil has many applications, including its use as an anxiolytic drug, mood stabilizer, sedative, antihypertensive, antimicrobial, and analgesic agent [53]. The mechanism of action of lavender in the nervous system constitutes its anticholinergic, neuroprotective, and antioxidant activities [54].

A placebo-controlled clinical trial studying the efficacy of lavender essential oil inhalation for the treatment of migraine reported a statistically significant mean reduction of headache severity in the treatment group [53]. An RCT investigating the effect of lavender as prophylactic therapy for migraine revealed a statistically significant reduction in the Migraine Disability Assessment Scores (MIDAS) questionnaire compared to the baseline and control groups. The study also reported a reduction in the frequency and severity of migraine incidents by approximately 50% following lavender therapy [55].

The inhalation of lavender essential oil may be effective and safe in the acute management of migraine headaches [55].

Ginger

Ginger is a native plant of southeastern Asia that has been used in the management of motion sickness, dyspepsia, local pains, and vertigo. The product has also been found to be effective in normalizing blood pressure and strengthening the cardiovascular system [56]. Ginger acts as a nonsteroidal anti-inflammatory drug [57, 58].

An RCT evaluating the efficacy of ginger and sumatriptan in the abortive treatment of migraine attacks showed that after 2 h of using the combination, mean headache severity decreased. The efficacy of ginger powder and sumatriptan was comparable [56]. An RCT evaluating the potential of ginger to prevent migraine reported a decrease in the number of days with severe pain, and there was an analgesic use for acute migraine and duration of migraine attacks. However, there was no significant difference between ginger and placebo groups [59].

Ginger is often favorable for treatment as it does not have serious or frequent side effects reported with its use. An RCT comparing ginger and sumatriptan for migraine treatment revealed that the clinical adverse effects of ginger powder were less than sumatriptan [56].

Emerging Research

Green Light Therapy

Some patients are not able to control their pain or tolerate the side effects of many mainstream pharmacological strategies for treating migraines [60]. Emerging research has illustrated that migraine patients may benefit from green light therapy, a non-pharmacological approach [60].

In a study investigating the effects of a green light emitting diode (GLED) on the nociception in rodents, the researchers discovered that the light had a pain-modulating effect [61]. In this study, patients were divided into episodic (EM) and chronic (CM) migraine groups. There was approximately a 60% reduction in headache days each month with GLED [61].

The mechanism of GLED pain relief remains unknown; however, more research in this area would be beneficial as GLED could be used as a preventative strategy [60].

Cannabis

The use of marijuana in patients with migraine has been suggested based on the effects of cannabinoids on CBD1 receptors in the trigeminovascular system [62, 63]. Some of the factors that may contribute to individual responses to cannabis treatment include gender, type of cannabis, cannabidiol (CBD) content, tetrahydrocannabinol (THC) content, and dosage [64]. Preclinical studies have shown that the effects of cannabis and cannabinoids may be sex-dependent, where women exhibited increased antinociceptive sensitivity [65].

There is limited research on the efficacy of cannabis and cannabinoid derivatives for the treatment of migraine [64]. A study of cannabis treatment for migraine was conducted in 30 patients with medication overuse headache [66]. This study focused on nabilone, which is a synthetic cannabinoid. Nabilone was found to be more effective than ibuprofen in reducing migraine pain intensity and increased quality of life [66]. Another trial evaluated cannabinoids as a preventive and acute treatment for patients with chronic migraine and chronic cluster headaches. Patients were given either 19% THC or a combination of 0.4% THC + 9% CBD. An oral dose of 200 mg administered during a migraine attack decreased acute pain intensity by approximately 55% [67].

For providers recommending cannabis treatment to patients with migraine, it is vital to communicate the potential effects. In a review of the side effects of medical cannabinoid use, the most common included dizziness and gastrointestinal complaints such as nausea and vomiting [65]. Future research is warranted to measure the effects of medical marijuana not only on migraine headache intensity but also frequency in the adult population [63].

Conclusion

CIM may be most appropriate for patients who have experienced side effects, have difficulty tolerating mainstream medication, or have a preference for natural approaches. It is vital for providers to start a conversation about CIM treatments with their patients and discuss the available evidence-based data [37]. Overall, nutraceuticals, mind-body medicine, and body-based maneuvers have the most evidence for the prevention of migraine; however, providers should be well versed in the adverse consequences of each to counsel patients appropriately [3]. Treatments may have safety concerns if they are not being regulated. Complementary and integrative medicine should always be used in partnership with mainstream pharmacological therapy [36].

Teaching Points

1. Incorporate CIM treatments into discussions with patients by defining CIM, differentiating it from mainstream medical therapy, and emphasizing how these modalities can be used in conjunction with traditional therapies.
2. Stay informed on current research on CIM to better support your treatment decisions.
3. Highlight potential benefits of CIM for migraine during patient consults
4. Always emphasize the importance of consulting with a healthcare professional before starting any of the CIM modalities.
5. Work with patients to create personalized treatment plans.

Case

A 45-year-old female with a history of chronic migraine and anxiety presents for a routine follow-up for chronic migraine. She is on a migraine preventive regimen consisting of onabotulinumtoxin A, a calcitonin gene-related peptide antagonist, and nortriptyline.

She reports that she continues to have a significant disability related to migraine disease. She reports 20 migraine days per month on this regimen. The patient also mentions that medical marijuana was recently approved in her state.

Case Discussion

It is important for providers to have an open conversation about CIM treatments with the patient and support this dialogue with an evidence-based approach. The CARE mnemonic is a strategy that can be applied to this scenario, as it relates to exploring a patient's interest in CIM [37]. In this particular case, the use of the CARE mnemonic and having an open conversation about the limited evidence for the use of cannabis in headache disorders is relevant [37].

The CARE mnemonic highlights specific points to employ when discussing CIM with your patients [37] (Table 24.1). To satisfy C, the provider will want to consider that the patient has tried several preventative medications and still experiences disability and a high frequency of headaches. For A, the provider will create a safe space for this conversation to occur. To fulfill R, it would be significant to review medical cannabis and its potential adverse effects. For E, this patient has tried so many treatment combinations and preventative measures and is looking for a solution for chronic migraine [37].

The CARE mnemonic allows the patient and provider to have an open, non-judgmental dialogue about the risks and benefits of treatment options. This collaboration may help to strengthen trust between provider and patient and also improve the patient's overall quality of life [37].

Table 24.1 CARE mnemonic [37]

C	Conventional therapy experiences
A	Avoid judgment
R	Review integrative approaches and their limitations
E	Explore why the person is interested

Questions and Answers

1. A 24-year-old female with a history of depression, anxiety, and chronic migraine reports that she has had side effects to the following migraine preventive treatments—topiramate, valproic acid, botulinum toxin A, venlafaxine, nortriptyline, and propranolol. She reports she does not want to take any more prescription medications to treat migraine. Which of the following integrative medicine approaches would you avoid recommending?
   A. Acupuncture
   B. Daith piercing
   C. Magnesium
   D. Cognitive behavioral therapy
   E. Physical therapy consultation

The correct answer is B. There is no scientific evidence in the peer-reviewed literature to support the use of daith piercings for the treatment of any primary headache disorder. Positive results may be temporary and may be a result of a placebo response. In addition, patients are at a risk for infection and worsening of pain

2. A 35-year-old female with a long history of chronic migraine presents for follow-up. She has been receiving botulinum toxin for the prevention of migraine for 2 years now. She reports a 50% reduction in headache frequency and severity since starting the treatment. She would like to stop botulinum toxin and try something new in order to take a different approach. Acupuncture was the cure for her mother. Which of the following is your reply?
   A. I do not practice witchcraft.
   B. Botulinum toxin is one of the only FDA-approved treatments for chronic migraine, and a sudden cessation could result in a sudden worsening of your headaches. Perhaps, we can discuss integrating acupuncture with botulinum toxin,
   C. Sure! Let's switch to acupuncture!
   D. What worked for your mother may not work for you.
   E. Why would you want to switch?!

The correct answer is B. All of the approaches discussed throughout this chapter are complementary and integrative and should be used with conventional therapies.

References

1. Stewart WF, Shechter A, Rasmussen BK. Migraine prevalence. A review of population-based studies. Neurology. 1994;44:S17–23.
2. Thompson DF, Saluja HS. Prophylaxis of migraine headaches with riboflavin: a systematic review. J Clin Pharm Ther. 2017;42:394–403. https://doi.org/10.1111/jcpt.12548.
3. Wells RE, Bertisch SM, Buettner C, et al. Complementary and alternative medicine use among adults with migraines/severe headaches. Headache. 2011;51:1087–97. https://doi.org/10.1111/j.1526-4610.2011.01917.x.
4. Complementary, Alternative, or Integrative Health: What's In a Name? In: NCCIH. 2021. https://www.nccih.nih.gov/health/complementary-alternative-or-integrative-health-whats-in-a-name
5. Boehnke C, Reuter U, Flach U, et al. High-dose riboflavin treatment is efficacious in migraine prophylaxis: an open study in a tertiary care centre. Eur J Neurol. 2004;11:475–7. https://doi.org/10.1111/j.1468-1331.2004.00813.x.
6. Gaul C, Diener H-C, Danesch U. Improvement of migraine symptoms with a proprietary supplement containing riboflavin, magnesium and Q10: a randomized, placebo-controlled, double-blind, multicenter trial. J Headache Pain. 2015;16:32. https://doi.org/10.1186/s10194-015-0516-6.
7. Maizels M, Blumenfeld A, Burchette R. A combination of riboflavin, magnesium, and feverfew for migraine prophylaxis: a randomized trial. Headache. 2004;44:885–90. https://doi.org/10.1111/j.1526-4610.2004.04170.x.
8. Peikert A, Wilimzig C, Kohne-Volland R. Prophylaxis of migraine with oral magnesium: Results from a prospective, multi-center, placebo-controlled and double-blind randomized study. Cephalalgia. 1996;16:257–63. https://doi.org/10.1046/j.1468-2982.1996.1604257.x.
9. Maier JA, Pickering G, Giacomoni E, et al. Headaches and Magnesium: Mechanisms, Bioavailability, Therapeutic Efficacy and Potential Advantage of Magnesium Pidolate. Nutrients. 2020;12:2660. https://doi.org/10.3390/nu12092660.
10. Talebi M, Savadi-Oskouei D, Farhoudi M, et al. Relation between serum magnesium level and migraine attacks. Neurosciences (Riyadh). 2011;16:320–3.
11. Jain AC, Sethi NC, Balbar PK. A clinical electroencephalographic and trace element study with special reference to zinc, copper and magnesium in serum and cerebrospinal fluid (CSF) in cases of migraine. J Neurol. 1985;232(Suppl):161.
12. Facchinetti F, Sances G, Borella P, et al. Magnesium prophylaxis of menstrual migraine: effects on intracellular magnesium. Headache. 1991;31:298–301. https://doi.org/10.1111/j.1526-4610.1991.hed3105298.x.
13. Sanoobar M, Eghtesadi S, Azimi A, et al. Coenzyme Q10 supplementation ameliorates inflammatory markers in patients with multiple sclerosis: a double blind, placebo, controlled randomized clinical trial. Nutr Neurosci. 2015;18:169. https://doi.org/10.1179/1476830513Y.0000000106.
14. Sazali S, Badrin S, Norhayati MN, Idris NS. Coenzyme Q10 supplementation for prophylaxis in adult patients with migraine-a meta-analysis. BMJ Open. 2021a;11:e039358. https://doi.org/10.1136/bmjopen-2020-039358.
15. Dahri M, Hashemilar M, Asghari-Jafarabadi M, Tarighat-Esfanjani A. Efficacy of coenzyme Q10 for the prevention of migraine in women: a randomized, double-blind, placebo-controlled study. Eur J Integr Med. 2017;16:8–14. https://doi.org/10.1016/j.eujim.2017.10.003.
16. Dahri M, Tarighat-Esfanjani A, Asghari-Jafarabadi M, Hashemilar M. Oral coenzyme Q10 supplementation in patients with migraine: effects on clinical features and inflammatory markers. Nutr Neurosci. 2019;22:607–15. https://doi.org/10.1080/1028415X.2017.1421039.
17. Hajihashemi P, Askari G, Khorvash F, et al. The effects of concurrent Coenzyme Q10, L-carnitine supplementation in migraine prophylaxis: a randomized, placebo-controlled, double-blind trial. Cephalalgia. 2019;39:648–54. https://doi.org/10.1177/0333102418821661.
18. Nattagh-Eshtivani E, Dahri M, Hashemilar M, Tarighat-Esfanjani A. The effect of Coenzyme Q10 supplementation on serum levels of lactate, pyruvate, matrix metalloproteinase 9 and nitric oxide

in women with migraine. A double blind, placebo, controlled randomized clinical trial. Eur J Integr Med. 2018;21:70–6. https://doi.org/10.1016/j.eujim.2018.06.009.
19. Sándor PS, Di Clemente L, Coppola G, et al. Efficacy of coenzyme Q10 in migraine prophylaxis: a randomized controlled trial. Neurology. 2005;64:713–5. https://doi.org/10.1212/01.WNL.0000151975.03598.ED.
20. Holland S, Silberstein SD, Freitag F, et al. Evidence-based guideline update: NSAIDs and other complementary treatments for episodic migraine prevention in adults. Neurology. 2012;78:1346–53. https://doi.org/10.1212/WNL.0b013e3182535d0c.
21. Lipton RB, Göbel H, Einhäupl KM, et al. Petasites hybridus root (butterbur) is an effective preventive treatment for migraine. Neurology. 2004;63:2240–4. https://doi.org/10.1212/01.wnl.0000147290.68260.11.
22. Wells RE, Beuthin J, Granetzke L. Complementary and Integrative medicine for episodic migraine: an update of evidence from the last 3 years. Curr Pain Headache Rep. 2019;23:10. https://doi.org/10.1007/s11916-019-0750-8.
23. Pareek A, Suthar M, Rathore GS, Bansal V. Feverfew (Tanacetum parthenium L.): a systematic review. Pharmacogn Rev. 2011;5:103–10. https://doi.org/10.4103/0973-7847.79105.
24. Wider B, Pittler MH, Ernst E. Feverfew for preventing migraine. Cochrane Database Syst Rev. 2015;2015:CD002286. https://doi.org/10.1002/14651858.CD002286.pub3.
25. Pfaffenrath V, Diener HC, Fischer M, et al. The efficacy and safety of Tanacetum parthenium (feverfew) in migraine prophylaxis–a double-blind, multicentre, randomized placebo-controlled dose-response study. Cephalalgia. 2002;22:523–32. https://doi.org/10.1046/j.1468-2982.2002.00396.x.
26. Soveyd N, Abdolahi M, Bitarafan S, et al. Molecular mechanisms of omega-3 fatty acids in the migraine headache. Iran J Neurol. 2017;16:210–7.
27. Maghsoumi-Norouzabad L, Mansoori A, Abed R, Shishehbor F. Effects of omega-3 fatty acids on the frequency, severity, and duration of migraine attacks: A systematic review and meta-analysis of randomized controlled trials. Nutr Neurosci. 2018;21:614–23. https://doi.org/10.1080/1028415X.2017.1344371.
28. Andıran N, Çelik N, Akça H, Doğan G. Vitamin D deficiency in children and adolescents. J Clin Res Pediatr Endocrinol. 2012;4:25–9. https://doi.org/10.4274/jcrpe.574.
29. Mottaghi T, Khorvash F, Askari G, et al. The relationship between serum levels of vitamin D and migraine. J Res Med Sci. 2013;18:S66–70.
30. Thys-Jacobs S. Alleviation of migraines with therapeutic vitamin D and calcium. Headache. 1994;34:590–2. https://doi.org/10.1111/j.1526-4610.1994.hed3410590.x.
31. Gazerani P, Fuglsang R, Pedersen JG, et al. A randomized, double-blinded, placebo-controlled, parallel trial of vitamin D3 supplementation in adult patients with migraine. Curr Med Res Opin. 2019;35:715–23. https://doi.org/10.1080/03007995.2018.1519503.
32. Buettner C, Nir R-R, Bertisch SM, et al. Simvastatin and vitamin D for migraine prevention: a randomized controlled trial. Ann Neurol. 2015;78:970–81. https://doi.org/10.1002/ana.24534.
33. Razzaque MS. Can adverse effects of excessive vitamin D supplementation occur without developing hypervitaminosis D? J Steroid Biochem Mol Biol. 2018;180:81–6. https://doi.org/10.1016/j.jsbmb.2017.07.006.
34. Zhang Y-F, Xu Z-Q, Zhou H-J, et al. The Efficacy of vitamin D supplementation for migraine: a meta-analysis of randomized controlled studies. Clin Neuropharmacol. 2021;44:5–8. https://doi.org/10.1097/WNF.0000000000000419.
35. Long R, Zhu Y, Zhou S. Therapeutic role of melatonin in migraine prophylaxis. Medicine (Baltimore). 2019;98:e14099. https://doi.org/10.1097/MD.0000000000014099.
36. Bougea A, Spantideas N, Lyras V, et al. Melatonin 4 mg as prophylactic therapy for primary headaches: a pilot study. Funct Neurol. 2016;31:33–7. https://doi.org/10.11138/FNeur/2016.31.1.033.
37. Kuruvilla DE, Mehta A, Ravishankar N, Cowan RP. A patient perspective of complementary and integrative medicine (CIM) for migraine treatment: a social media survey. BMC Complement Med Ther. 2021;21:58. https://doi.org/10.1186/s12906-021-03226-0.
38. Bakhshani NM, Amirani A, Amirifard H, Shahrakipoor M. The effectiveness of mindfulness-based stress reduction on perceived pain intensity and quality of life in patients with chronic headache. Glob J Health Sci. 2015;8:142–51. https://doi.org/10.5539/gjhs.v8n4p142.
39. Motwani M, Kuruvilla D. Behavioral and integrative therapies for headache. In: Practical neurology. 2019. https://practicalneurology.com/articles/2019-may/behavioral-and-integrative-therapies-for-headache. Accessed 31 Oct 2021.
40. Anheyer D, Klose P, Lauche R, et al. Yoga for treating headaches: a systematic review and meta-analysis. J Gen Intern Med. 2020;35:846–54. https://doi.org/10.1007/s11606-019-05413-9.
41. Sharma VM, Manjunath NK, Nagendra HR, Ertsey C. Combination of Ayurveda and Yoga therapy reduces pain intensity and improves quality of life in patients with migraine headache. Complement Ther Clin Pract. 2018;32:85–91. https://doi.org/10.1016/j.ctcp.2018.05.010.
42. Ghlichloo I, Gerriets V. Nonsteroidal anti-inflammatory drugs (NSAIDs). In: StatPearls. StatPearls Publishing, Treasure Island. 2021.
43. Boroujeni MZ, Marandi SM, Esfarjani F, et al. Yoga intervention on blood NO in female migraineurs. Adv Biomed Res. 2015;4:259. https://doi.org/10.4103/2277-9175.172995.
44. Linde K, Allais G, Brinkhaus B, et al. Acupuncture for migraine prophylaxis. In: The Cochrane Collaboration, editor. Cochrane Database of systematic reviews. Chichester: Wiley; 2009. p. CD001218.pub2.
45. Ingold CJ, Ratay S. Osteopathic manipulative treatment: HVLA procedure – inhaled ribs. In: StatPearls. StatPearls Publishing, Treasure Island. 2021.
46. Cerritelli F, Ginevri L, Messi G, et al. Clinical effectiveness of osteopathic treatment in chronic migraine: 3-Armed randomized controlled trial. Complement Ther Med. 2015;23:149–56. https://doi.org/10.1016/j.ctim.2015.01.011.
47. Kennell KA, Daghfal MM, Patel SG, et al. Cervical artery dissection related to chiropractic manipulation: one institution's experience. J Fam Pract. 2017;66:556–62.
48. Turner RC, Lucke-Wold BP, Boo S, et al The potential dangers of neck manipulation & risk for dissection and devastating stroke: an illustrative case & review of the literature. Biomed Res Rev. 2018;2: 10.15761/BRR.1000110 https://doi.org/10.15761/BRR.1000110
49. Borhani Haghighi A, Motazedian S, Rezaii R, et al. Cutaneous application of menthol 10% solution as an abortive treatment of migraine without aura: a randomised, double-blind, placebo-controlled, crossed-over study. Int J Clin Pract. 2010;64:451–6. https://doi.org/10.1111/j.1742-1241.2009.02215.x.
50. Pan R, Tian Y, Gao R, et al. Central mechanisms of menthol-induced analgesia. J Pharmacol Exp Ther. 2012;343:661–72. https://doi.org/10.1124/jpet.112.196717.
51. St. Cyr A, Chen A, Bradley KC, et al. Efficacy and Tolerability of STOPAIN for a Migraine Attack. Front Neurol. 2015;6:11.
52. Kanerva L, Rantanen T, Aalto-Korte K, et al. A multicenter study of patch test reactions with dental screening series. Am J Contact Dermat. 2001;12:83–7.
53. Sasannejad P, Saeedi M, Shoeibi A, et al. Lavender essential oil in the treatment of migraine headache: a placebo-controlled clinical trial. Eur Neurol. 2012;67:288–91. https://doi.org/10.1159/000335249.

54. Koulivand PH, Khaleghi Ghadiri M, Gorji A. Lavender and the nervous system. Evid Based Complement Alternat Med. 2013;2013:e681304. https://doi.org/10.1155/2013/681304.
55. Rafie S, Namjoyan F, Golfakhrabadi F, et al. Effect of lavender essential oil as a prophylactic therapy for migraine: a randomized controlled clinical trial. J Herb Med. 2016;6:18–23. https://doi.org/10.1016/j.hermed.2016.01.003.
56. Maghbooli M, Golipour F, Moghimi Esfandabadi A, Yousefi M. Comparison between the efficacy of ginger and sumatriptan in the ablative treatment of the common migraine. Phytother Res. 2014;28:412–5. https://doi.org/10.1002/ptr.4996.
57. Chen L, Cai Z. The efficacy of ginger for the treatment of migraine: a meta-analysis of randomized controlled studies. Am J Emerg Med. 2021;46:567–71. https://doi.org/10.1016/j.ajem.2020.11.030.
58. Jolad SD, Lantz RC, Solyom AM, et al. Fresh organically grown ginger (Zingiber officinale): composition and effects on LPS-induced PGE2 production. Phytochemistry. 2004;65:1937–54. https://doi.org/10.1016/j.phytochem.2004.06.008.
59. Martins LB, Rodrigues AMDS, Monteze NM, et al. Double-blind placebo-controlled randomized clinical trial of ginger (Zingiber officinale Rosc.) in the prophylactic treatment of migraine. Cephalalgia. 2020;40:88–95. https://doi.org/10.1177/0333102419869319.
60. Martin LF, Patwardhan AM, Jain SV, et al. Evaluation of green light exposure on headache frequency and quality of life in migraine patients: a preliminary one-way cross-over clinical trial. Cephalalgia. 2021;41:135–47. https://doi.org/10.1177/0333102420956711.
61. Ibrahim MM, Patwardhan A, Gilbraith KB, et al. Long-lasting antinociceptive effects of green light in acute and chronic pain in rats. Pain. 2017;158:347–60. https://doi.org/10.1097/j.pain.0000000000000767.
62. Rhyne DN, Anderson SL, Gedde M, Borgelt LM. Effects of medical marijuana on migraine headache frequency in an adult population. Pharmacotherapy. 2016;36:505–10. https://doi.org/10.1002/phar.1673.
63. Akerman S, Holland PR, Goadsby PJ. Cannabinoid (CB1) receptor activation inhibits trigeminovascular neurons. J Pharmacol Exp Ther. 2007;320:64–71. https://doi.org/10.1124/jpet.106.106971.
64. Cuttler C, Spradlin A, Cleveland MJ, Craft RM. Short- and long-term effects of cannabis on headache and migraine. J Pain. 2020;21:722–30. https://doi.org/10.1016/j.jpain.2019.11.001.
65. Cooper ZD, Craft RM. Sex-dependent effects of cannabis and cannabinoids: a translational perspective. Neuropsychopharmacology. 2018;43:34–51. https://doi.org/10.1038/npp.2017.140.
66. Pini LA, Guerzoni S, Cainazzo MM, et al. Nabilone for the treatment of medication overuse headache: results of a preliminary double-blind, active-controlled, randomized trial. J Headache Pain. 2012;13:677–84. https://doi.org/10.1007/s10194-012-0490-1.
67. Baron EP, Lucas P, Eades J, Hogue O. Patterns of medicinal cannabis use, strain analysis, and substitution effect among patients with migraine, headache, arthritis, and chronic pain in a medicinal cannabis cohort. J Headache Pain. 2018;19:37. https://doi.org/10.1186/s10194-018-0862-2.

Part V

Migraine Management: Advances in Pharmacological and Interventional Therapies

Acute Migraine Treatment and Infusion Therapies

25

Michael J. Marmura

Introduction

Effective treatment of acute attacks is an essential part of overall migraine management. Acute treatment attempts to relieve or stop the progression of an attack. Acute treatment plans should consider not only the patient's diagnosis, symptoms, and any coexistent or comorbid conditions but also his or her expectations and goals. Integration with preventive and non-pharmacological treatment optimizes patient outcomes [1].

Migraine attacks are painful, with most reporting severe pain during many of their attacks [2]. Three-quarters of migraine patients have a reduced ability to function, and one-third require bed rest during migraine [3]. Associated symptoms of migraine complicate management, and the Food and Drug Administration (FDA) now requires that new acute therapies ameliorate patient-stated most bothersome symptoms (MBS). In addition to the associated symptoms of photophobia, phonophobia, and nausea/vomiting mentioned in migraine classification, MBS includes a wide range of potential problems such as vertigo or dizziness, cognitive symptoms, fatigue, osmophilia, or weakness [4]. Obtaining a complete history focusing on individual symptoms and their impact improves treatment adherence and effectiveness.

Questions

1. How do small molecule antagonists of calcitonin gene-related peptides (gepants) differ from triptans for the treatment of acute migraine?
   A. More rapid onset of effectiveness
   B. Higher rates of pain-freedom
   C. Better tolerability
   D. Higher risk of migraine recurrence
2. Which of the following treatments is most highly associated with medication overuse headaches?
   A. Barbiturate-containing combination therapies
   B. Gepants
   C. Nonsteroidal anti-inflammatory drugs
   D. Dihydroergotamine

Treatment of Migraine During the Premonitory Phase

Premonitory symptoms of migraine, or "prodrome," may precede acute attacks of headache by hours or even days. Common symptoms include changes in mood, food cravings or thirst, and yawning. Premonitory symptoms are common although most patients report hours, not days, of symptoms [5].

Two studies that found domperidone at the onset of premonitory symptoms was significantly more effective than a placebo in preventing the headache phase [6] and that a 40 mg dose was significantly more effective than a 20 mg dose [7]. Metoclopramide, an anti-dopaminergic and anti-emetic drug, may also treat migraine during prodrome [8] as evidenced by case reports [9].

M. J. Marmura (✉)
Department of Neurology, Thomas Jefferson University, Philadelphia, PA, USA

T. S. Monteith et al. (eds.), *Comprehensive Migraine Management*, https://doi.org/10.1007/978-3-031-86923-5_25

A few studies have investigated the role of acute migraine-specific treatments during the premonitory phase. A single small trial of DHE nasal spray (NS) during the migraine prodrome demonstrated statistically significant superiority over placebo in preventing the anticipated migraine attack [10]. Another study showed naratriptan, 2.5 mg at the time they knew migraine was inevitable, was effective [11]. A prospective, placebo-controlled study demonstrated that ubrogepant 100 mg was effective for preventing migraine in subjects with reliable premonitory symptoms [12].

Patients with clear triggers such as fasting or menstrual migraine may benefit from long-acting triptans [13, 14] prior to their attack. The fact that many patients are not reliably able to predict their migraine, and may not recognize their symptoms as warning signs, limits the usefulness of interventions during this phase [15].

Treatment of Migraine with Aura

The acute treatment of migraine with aura may differ from those without aura [16]. A pooled analysis of outcomes from clinical trials suggests sumatriptan 100 mg is less effective in patients with migraine with aura, unlike DHE and eletriptan which had similar effects in both groups [17, 18].

Clinical trials report mixed results from treating migraine with triptans during the aura phase. Early studies that evaluated the treatment of acute migraine during the aura phase using subcutaneous (SC) sumatriptan [19], zolmitriptan [20], and eletriptan [21] were negative. Other studies have shown the effectiveness of using oral sumatriptan 100 mg [22] and other triptans. A few case series have reported excellent safety and efficacy using triptans in patients with hemiplegic [23], basilar, or prolonged aura [24]. The effectiveness of acute medications such as triptans is unclear, but the evidence to date suggests it is safe to treat migraine during the aura phase.

Several treatments can treat prolonged aura based on case series and reports. These include sublingual nifedipine 10 mg [25], IV furosemide [26], the combination of IV prochlorperazine and magnesium sulfate [27], and IV divalproex sodium [28]. Ketamine nasal spray 25 mg reduced the severity and duration of hemiplegic deficits in one study [29], and the severity of prolonged migraine aura, but not duration, when compared to midazolam in a separate study [30].

Monitoring Frequency and Triggers

After starting acute treatment, patients can use their calendars to show the effectiveness of acute treatment and other factors such as recurrence [31].

Many factors prompt attacks in episodic migraine, and patients may be keen to learn about their triggers as a way to predict attacks. Patients may confuse premonitory symptoms such as food cravings or mood changes with triggers. Experimental triggers such as glyceryl trinitrate [32], prostaglandin E2 [33], histamine [34], and calcitonin gene-related peptide (CGRP) [35] provoke migraine in most susceptible individuals. However, “natural” triggers such as bright lights, weather changes, and stress are much less reliable [36]. Many common symptoms prior to migraine such as neck pain and tiredness are likely premonitory symptoms.

Clinical studies including systematic reviews confirm common triggers in migraine with stress, auditory stimuli, fatigue, fasting, and menses, the most commonly implicated [37, 38]. Patients with reliable triggers or premonitory symptoms may choose to treat early or make allowances for impending migraine. Yet attempts to avoid triggers are often not realistic [39] and may lead to reductions in physical activity or hinder adaptive strategies [40]. Keeping a headache journal may allow patients to discover unrecognized triggers amenable to treatment, such as caffeine withdrawal on weekends or menstrual migraine, or to help patients realize their perceived triggers are not as reliable as believed.

Treatment of Acute Migraine Headache

Treating headaches as early as possible can prevent their escalation and increase the drug’s effectiveness. Patients with migraine may respond to triptans and other migraine-specific medication both for mild and severe migraine episodes [41].

Medication for an acute attack can be specific or nonspecific. Nonspecific medications help control the pain and associated symptoms of migraine. Specific medications target migraine itself. Nonspecific acute headache medications include analgesics (NSAIDs and combination analgesics), antiemetics, opioids, corticosteroids, and dopamine antagonists. Specific acute headache medications include ergotamine, DHE, triptans, gepants, and ditans. Table 25.1 lists available migraine-specific medications.

Attack characteristics should influence the choice of acute treatments. Consider non-oral treatments in the presence of nausea, vomiting, or those with gastroparesis [42]. Develop a treatment strategy for headaches of different severity, utilizing one or more of these drug classes [43] that includes initial treatment, a backup treatment, and a rescue treatment.

Table 25.1 Currently available migraine-specific medications

Class	Drug	Formulations
Triptans	Almotriptan	6.25, 12.5 mg tablet
	Eletriptan	20, 40 mg tablet
	Frovatriptan	2.5 mg tablet
	Naratriptan	1, 2.5 mg tablet
	Rizatriptan	5, 10 mg tablet 5, 10 mg dissolving tablet
	Sumatriptan	25, 50, 100 mg tablet 5, 10, 20 mg nasal spray 10 mg + permeation enhancer nasal spray 22 mg nasal powder
	Zolmitriptan	2.5, 5 mg tablet 2.5, 5 mg dissolving tablet 2.5, 5 mg nasal spray
Ergotamine and derivatives	Ergotamine	1 mg tablet 2 mg sublingual 1 mg with 100 mg caffeine tablet 2 mg with 100 mg caffeine suppository
	Dihydroergotamine	1 mg ampule (IV, IM, or SC) 4 mg/mL nasal spray 1.45 mg nasal spray
Gepants	Rimegepant	75 mg dissolvable tablet
	Ubrogepant	50, 100 mg tablet
	Zavegepant	10 mg nasal spray
Ditans	Lasmiditan	50, 100 mg tablet. 200 mg also approved

Step Care and Stratified Care

The two basic strategies for the acute treatment of migraine are step care and stratified care [44]. In step care, patients with migraine progress through a sequence of medications, usually ordered by a combination of perceived safety, cost, and efficacy. The risk of this approach is delay in taking the necessary medication. Stratified care bases treatment selection on an initial assessment of illness severity. Highly effective medications proven for acute migraine treatment reduce disability due to attacks. In a randomized, double-blind, controlled trial that compared these approaches, stratified care was associated with better acute treatment efficacy [45]. For patients who are treated late (> 1 h), interventions encouraging patients to be treated earlier may improve efficacy and outcome [46]. The "traffic light" concept may be a useful way to explain these concepts to patients and guide acute medication selection. In this model, green means mild headache requiring no treatment or simple analgesics. Yellow denotes moderate pain suggesting the need to slow down and potentially use migraine-specific medication. A red light stands for a more disabling "have to stop" headache when sedating medication may be acceptable [47].

Migraine-Specific Medications

Ergotamine and Dihydroergotamine

Both ergotamine and dihydroergotamine (DHE) are agonists at the serotonin 5 HT1A, 5 HT1B, 5 HT1D, 5 HT1E, and 5 HT1F receptors [48]. Contraindications to the use of ergotamine tartrate or DHE include renal or hepatic failure, pregnancy, hypertension, sepsis, coronary, cerebral, and peripheral vascular disease. While both DHE and ergotamine inhibit the reuptake of noradrenaline at sympathetic nerve endings, DHE is a weaker arterial vasoconstrictor but almost as potent a venoconstrictor as ergotamine. DHE is less emetic and with less effect on the uterus than ergotamine.

Ergotamine

The majority of ergotamine studies show superiority to placebo although many did not comply with modern methodology [49]. In comparative studies, ergotamine is not superior to many nonspecific migraine treatments and inferior to triptans. Ergotamine plus caffeine was less effective than oral sumatriptan [50] or the combination of isometheptene, dichloralphenazone, and acetaminophen [51] and not significantly different from DHE NS [52] or naproxen sodium [53]. A crossover comparison of efficacy and preference for rizatriptan 10 mg versus ergotamine plus caffeine found rizatriptan superior to ergotamine plus caffeine in all endpoints [54].

Dihydroergotamine

Dihydroergotamine (DHE) is available in 1 mg/ml ampules, which can be administered intramuscularly (IM), subcutaneously (SC) or intravenously (IV), and as a nasal spray (NS). Placebo-controlled trials demonstrate superiority of DHE NS against placebo although the magnitude of the benefit was small to moderate [10, 55]. Two trials compared DHE NS to other treatments. One found no significant difference between DHE and ergotamine plus caffeine [52]. The other trial found that 6 mg of SC sumatriptan was significantly better than DHE 1 mg with the option for a second 1 mg dose of DHE NS 1 h later [56]. The bioavailability of NS is 40% of the same dose given IM. DHE NS often causes transient nasal stuffiness, dysgeusia, and nausea [57].

In outpatients with acute migraine, clinical opinion suggests that DHE SC and IM are relatively safe and effective. The risk of MOH due to DHE is unclear but in clinical experience, it is lower than with triptans or ergotamine. Several studies have evaluated newer delivery methods to improve the usefulness of DHE. A recently approved nasal formulation uses a new delivery system in addition to delivering DHE to the upper nasal cavity and improves absorption using hydroxyfluoroalkane gas. Pharmacokinetic studies show comparative bioavailability to IV or IM DHE, with a faster onset of action than existing DHE NS and good tolerability [58]. A second novel liquid, DHE nasal spray 2 mg STS101 achieves effective DHE plasma concentrations within 10 min and has superior consistency, plasma concentration, and time to C_{max} compared to generic DHE NS. Adverse events (AEs) were lower than IV DHE [59].

Another formulation using a dissolving microneedle patch appears to have a similar onset of action and bioavailability as DHE SC [60]. A sublingual film DHE is also under development [61].

Triptans

Triptans are selective 5-HT1B/1D agonists for the acute treatment of migraine. The first to be developed and tested was sumatriptan, followed by zolmitriptan, naratriptan, rizatriptan, almotriptan, eletriptan, and frovatriptan. The triptans have several advantages when compared with other migraine therapies. Triptans exhibit selective pharmacology, and simple and consistent pharmacokinetics, and have established efficacy based on large, well-designed, controlled trials [62]. There are multiple generic as well as non-oral formulations of triptans available. Treatment with triptan use improves outcomes compared to ergots, and most have equal or better results compared to nonspecific analgesics [63]. Guidelines recommend triptans as first-line acute therapies for those with moderate-severe migraine attacks who have not responded to simple analgesics or other non-opioid analgesics (including combination NSAIDs such as acetaminophen plus aspirin plus caffeine), assuming no contraindications [64, 65]. In spite of this, triptans remain underutilized in patients with episodic migraine, especially considering that opioid and barbiturate use is still common [66]. While the majority of patients respond well to treatment with triptans, a significant minority (30–40%) either cannot tolerate and/or do not find triptans effective [67].

Triptan contraindications include poorly controlled hypertension, vasospastic or ischemic coronary artery disease, and severe hepatic or renal disease. In patients at high risk for coronary artery disease, a cardiac evaluation is recommended, and consider giving the first dose in the office when the patient does not have migraine [68]. Drug labels list basilar or hemiplegic migraine as contraindications for triptan use although several studies have reported good outcomes and safety from using triptans in these patients [23, 69].

Common triptan AEs include transient tingling, flushing, neck pain, dizziness, or warm and hot sensations. Paresthesias or pain may occur in trigeminal or non-trigeminal areas [70]. Chest pain or tightness is a common side effect but does not typically represent cardiac disease [71]. A 2006 FDA alert warned about the potential risk of using triptans together with selective serotonin reuptake inhibitors or selective serotonin/norepinephrine reuptake inhibitors. However, subsequent review of the case reports failed to demonstrate causation [72], and large-scale data reviews show the issue is rare despite frequent co-prescribing [73].

In choosing between triptans, clinicians should consider factors such as efficacy, tolerability, patient preference, and the presence of significant nausea or vomiting. SC sumatriptan is the most rapid-acting and effective triptan. Sumatriptan and zolmitriptan have nasal spray formulations which are ideal for patients with severe nausea or vomiting, and both rizatriptan and zolmitriptan are available as orally disintegrating as well as conventional tablets. For oral triptans, rizatriptan 10 mg, eletriptan 80 mg, and almotriptan 12.5 mg may have greater efficacy [74]. Switching from one triptan to another is safe but not necessarily likely to improve outcomes or disability [75].

Multiple placebo-controlled trials have consistently shown that SC sumatriptan 4 and 6 mg is superior to placebo for headache relief and complete relief at 1 and 2 h [76–78]. AEs include injection-site reactions (43%), tingling (12%), and other known triptan side effects. A pooled analysis of placebo-controlled studies notes a number needed to treat 2.3 and 2.5, respectively, for the 6 and 4 mg doses of SC sumatriptan for patients with moderate-severe baseline pain. These results compare favorably to later studies using oral and nasal forms of the drug [79]. In trials comparing sumatriptan SC to DHE, 1- and 2-h data for headache relief and pain freedom favored sumatriptan, while 2—24-h recurrence rates favored DHE [56, 80].

Oral sumatriptan, in a dose of 100 mg, is significantly more effective than placebo for headache relief and complete relief at 2 and 4 h [81–83]. In a multidose study reporting 4-h outcomes, headache relief and pain freedom rates with the 50 mg dose were comparable to those reported with the 100 mg dose and superior to the 25 mg dose [84]. A formulation with a dispersible tablet was also significantly more effective than a placebo in achieving pain relief at 2 h [85].

Placebo-controlled trials support the efficacy of sumatriptan NS 10 and 20 mg for headache relief at 1 and 2 h [86, 87]. Significantly, more patients reported AEs with sumatriptan NS than with placebo, the most common being "taste disturbance."

A different formulation using a breath-powered device delivers dry powder sumatriptan more efficiently and the closing of the palate prevents users from swallowing the drug [88]. In a double-dummy, crossover, multi-attack study, this device which delivers 22 mg sumatriptan (11 mg in each nostril) demonstrated significant rates of pain relief and pain freedom compared to placebo and oral sumatriptan 100 mg as early as 15 min [89]. These differences were significant at time points from 15 to 90 min but not at 2 h (60.7% total migraine freedom for the nasal device vs. 56.7% oral sumatriptan). Abnormal taste and nasal discomfort were common AEs but rated as mild.

A version of sumatriptan 10 mg using a permeation enhancer demonstrates superior pharmacokinetic profiles with more rapid absorption than previous 20 mg nasal sprays [90]. At 2 h, this formulation provides significantly higher rates of free freedom, pain relief, and relief of MBS [91].

Combining sumatriptan with NSAIDs such as naproxen sodium [92, 93] improves efficacy. In two controlled trials, the single-tablet, fixed dose, combination of sumatriptan 85 mg with naproxen sodium 500 mg provided superior relief compared to placebo and either oral formulation alone. Early treatment within 1 h provided substantially more relief [94].

Almotriptan: Almotriptan was compared with placebo in three double-blind trials with doses ranging from 2 to 25 mg across the three trials. These trials supported the utility of 6.25 mg–25 mg. Sumatriptan 100 mg was used as an active comparator in one trial, and no differences were seen between drugs regarding efficacy although almotriptan was better tolerated [95, 96].

Eletriptan: Oral eletriptan is rapidly absorbed, with high bioavailability (50%) and a long half-life (5 h). Eletriptan is metabolized by the P450 3A4 system and is safe for use in patients taking MAO inhibitors. Eletriptan, 20, 40, and 80 mg, was effective in placebo-controlled trials [97–99]. Eletriptan 40 mg was more effective than 20 mg and had fewer side effects than the 80 mg dose. These studies show that eletriptan is more effective than placebo in achieving pain relief within 2 h following treatment. In comparative studies, eletriptan 40 mg appears statistically superior to 50 mg or 100 mg sumatriptan [100, 101].

Frovatriptan: Two randomized, placebo-controlled efficacy studies study the effectiveness of frovatriptan, with dose ranges between 0.5 mg and 5 mg. These studies found that frovatriptan 2.5 mg was significantly better than placebo in achieving headache relief at 2 h. All doses were significantly superior to placebo at 4 h, but only the 2.5 mg dose is available clinically [102, 103].

Naratriptan: Oral naratriptan differs from sumatriptan primarily in its longer half-life, longer T-max, higher oral bioavailability (70%), and lipophilicity. Two trials found a significant clinical benefit over placebo for the 1 mg and 2.5 mg doses at 4 h post-treatment [104, 105]. Relief rates with naratriptan were lower than the other oral triptans, but studies showed excellent tolerability for the 2.5 mg dose of naratriptan, with an AE rate close to that of placebo.

Rizatriptan: Rizatriptan has rapid oral absorption and high oral bioavailability at 45% for the 10 mg dose. Four double-blind trials found that rizatriptan was significantly better than placebo for headache relief and complete relief at 2 h; the doses ranged from 5 mg to 40 mg, with higher rates of relief reported with the higher doses [106–109]. Multiple studies have also established the efficacy of rizatriptan orally dissolving tablet [110, 111]. A new formulation awaiting approval containing rapid-release meloxicam 20 mg and rizatriptan 10 mg shows significant benefit compared to the individual ingredients and placebo [112, 113].

Zolmitriptan: In four randomized, controlled trials, zolmitriptan 2.5 mg or 5 mg tablets were significantly more effective than placebo for headache relief and complete relief at 2 and 4 h [114–116]. When compared to sumatriptan 25 and 50 mg w, both doses of zolmitriptan were either comparable or statistically superior to both doses of sumatriptan for headache relief, consistency of response, and 24-h headache relief rates [114]. Zolmitriptan orally disintegrating tablets 2.5 and 5 mg [117, 118] are also effective in achieving pain relief at 2 h (pain-free in 2 h and headache relief in 2 h).

Zolmitriptan nasal spray [119] response rates at 2 h for the 0.5, 1.0, 2.5, and 5-mg doses were 41, 55, 59, and 70%, respectively, compared with 30% for placebo (all $p < 0.001$) and 61% for zolmitriptan 2.5-mg tablet. In a second trial, zolmitriptan 5-mg nasal spray provided pain relief in some patients as early as 15 min onward [120]. The third study reported that zolmitriptan 5 mg was superior to placebo in achieving complete symptom relief (no pain and no migraine symptoms) at 30 min and thereafter [121].

Ditans (Lasmiditan)

Ditans are selective 5-HT1F agonists designed for acute migraine treatment. The characterization of the 5-HT1F receptor followed the introduction of sumatriptan and the discovery that triptans treat migraines by blocking the release of inflammatory neuropeptides such as CGRP rather than vasoconstriction [122]. Unlike triptans, ditans do not produce discernable vasoconstrictive effects and do not increase blood pressure [123]. Ditans are highly lipophilic and cross the blood-brain barrier after intravenous or oral administration, with a much greater CNS penetrance than any triptan [124].

Lasmiditan is a highly selective 1F agonist with a binding affinity over 400 times greater for 5-HT1F compared to 5-HT1B and 5-HT1D receptors [123]. Lasmiditan is the first and only ditan approved for acute migraine.

Multiple clinical trials have established the safety and effectiveness of lasmiditan for acute migraine treatment. Clinical trials examined three doses of lasmiditan (50, 100, and 200 mg) compared to placebo and specifically targeted subjects with cardiovascular risk factors [125]. Kuca et al. studied lasmiditan 100 and 200 mg against placebo, again with a majority of subjects (77.9%) having at least 1 cardiovascular risk factor [126]. For each study, all doses performed better than placebo for the primary endpoints of pain-freedom and relief of most bothersome symptoms at 2 h. While there were no significant differences between doses in each study, a subsequent meta-analysis showed superior efficacy with the 200 mg dose [127]. Lasmiditan effectiveness appears independent of previous triptan response [128], comorbidities [129], or concurrent preventive use [130].

Lasmiditan AEs appear related to its CNS penetration. Dizziness is the most commonly reported AE, and rates of severe dizziness are related to dose (0.3% at 50 mg, 0.7% at 100 mg, and 1.4% at 200 mg) [131]. Other common treatment-related AEs consisted of paresthesias, somnolence, fatigue, nausea, and weakness [132]. Lasmiditan causes significant driving impairment at 1.5 h in healthy volunteers, which resolves at 8 h [133]. Providers should counsel their patients to avoid operating a motor vehicle after taking lasmiditan. Adult recreational poly-drug users taking lasmiditan had higher rates of drug "liking" compared to placebo at all doses [134]. Drug liking with a 400 mg dose was similar to alprazolam but lower for the 100 and 200 mg doses. As a result, lasmiditan is a Schedule V controlled substance in the USA.

Small Molecule Antagonists of Calcitonin Gene-Related Peptide: Gepants

Multiple studies support the link between calcitonin gene-related peptide (CGRP) and migraine. Small molecule antagonists of CGRP, called gepants, effectively treat acute migraine pain and associated symptoms [135]. The development of gepants for migraine preceded monoclonal antibodies against CGRP. The first gepant, olegepant, was effective but not pursued due to its IV formulation [136]. Telcagepant showed promise to reduce migraine severity and associated symptoms and proved effective in a phase III trial [137]. Unfortunately, significant hepatoxicity occurred with frequent use, causing symptomatic disease in two subjects [138]. These complications spurred the development of monoclonal antibodies targeting CGRP. Second and third-generation gepants, including ubrogepant, rimegepant, atogepant, and zavegepant, do not cause hepatotoxicity. While the pivotal trials for gepant focused on the acute treatment of episodic migraine, they may be effective in chronic migraine. Gepants do not appear to cause MOH, suggesting a role in this population [139]. Despite the fact that CGRP is a potent vasodilator, there is no evidence that blocking CGRP increases the risk for those with stable cardiovascular disorders [140]. The FDA has issued updated post-marketing warnings of new or worsening hypertension and Raynaud's phenomenon with use of CGRP inhibitors.

Ubrogepant: Ubrogepant is effective for acute migraine as demonstrated by multiple phase III clinical trials. Dodick et al. compared oral 50 mg and 100 mg tablets of ubrogepant to placebo. Both doses of ubrogepant were more effective for pain freedom (21.2% with 100 mg and 19.2% with 50 mg) compared with placebo (11.8%) and relieving the most bothersome symptom (37.7% with 100 mg and 38.6% with 50 mg versus placebo 27.8%) [141]. Lipton et al. studied ubrogepant 25 and 50 mg versus placebo. More 50 mg ubrogepant-treated patients were pain-free at 2 h (21.8%) versus placebo (14.3%), with greater relief of the most bothersome symptom (38.9%) versus placebo (27.4%). Nausea was the most common AE with 50 mg ubrogepant and no serious AEs occurred [142]. The 25 mg dose was not significantly better than placebo.

Rimegepant: Multiple clinical trials demonstrate that rimegepant is effective for acute migraine. Lipton et al. studied oral rimegepant 75 mg tablets compared with placebo. At 2 h, the pain-free rates were 19.6% in the rimegepant group versus 12.0% for placebo, and patients treated with 75 mg rimegepant experienced greater relief of their most bothersome symptom (37.6%) versus placebo (25.2%) [143]. Croop et al. evaluated a 75-mg ODT of rimegepant versus placebo. Patients taking 75 mg rimegepant experienced greater pain relief (21.2%) versus placebo (10.9%) and greater relief of their most bothersome symptom (35.1% versus placebo 26.8%) [144].

Rimegepant was well tolerated with only 1.8% [143] and 2% [144] reporting nausea, the most common AE. No serious treatment-related AEs occurred in either study. Rimegepant is only available at 75 mg ODT. There is no safety data for doses higher than 75 mg per day. As with ubrogepant, do not use rimegepant in patients using strong CYP3A4 inhibitors or those with severe renal or hepatic impairment.

Zavegepant: Zavegepant is a third-generation intranasal gepant with rapid onset of action and good intranasal bioavailability [145]. In clinical trials, zavegepant 10 mg nasal spray was effective for acute migraine, with effectiveness starting as early as 15 min after administration [146].

Nonspecific Medications for Migraine

Using the stratified care approach, consider treating migraine attacks with no more than mild attack-related disability with nonspecific medications. In such cases, most people obtain headache relief with a simple analgesic, either alone or in combination with caffeine or other adjuvants.

Acetaminophen's efficacy, and the danger of Reye syndrome, make acetaminophen preferable to aspirin for children who have nonspecific headaches and are younger than 15 years of age [147]. Two placebo-controlled studies to assess acetaminophen's efficacy as monotherapy for the acute treatment of migraine have been performed: the earlier one failed to demonstrate a significant effect over placebo [148], and the second trial excluded patients who were severely disabled (requiring bed rest or vomiting >20% of the time) [149]. Acetaminophen was more effective than placebo at primary and secondary endpoints in the treatment of migraine pain but not in treating migraine-associated nausea. While acetaminophen 1000 mg alone is superior to placebo in the treatment of acute migraine, the NNT for pain-free response at 2 h is 12, which is inferior to most other commonly used analgesics [150].

Table 25.2 Common nonsteroidal anti-inflammatory drugs used in headache

Drug	Formulation and dose
Aspirin	Tablet and effervescent tablet: 500–1000 mg
Diclofenac	Tablet, soft gel: 50, 100 mg Oral solution: 50 mg Capsules: 18, 35 mg Liquid-filled capsules: 25 mg
Ibuprofen	Tablet, soft gel: 200–800 mg
Indomethacin	Tablet: 25, 50 mg Extended-release: 75 mg
Ketorolac	Tablet 10 mg Injection: 30, 60 mg Nasal spray: 31.5 mg
Naproxen	Tablet: 220, 250,500, 550 mg
Nabumetone	Tablet: 500, 750 mg
Piroxicam	Tablet: 10, 20 mg Sublingual: 40 mg
Celecoxib	Tablet: 100, 200 mg
AAC	Tablet: Acetaminophen 250 mg, aspirin 250 mg, caffeine 65 mg

Nonsteroidal Anti-inflammatory Drugs

At least, five different chemical classes of NSAIDs [151] have been used for headache treatment. These include salicylates, arylpropionic acids, aryl and heterocyclic acids, fenamic acids, and enolic acids. The major mechanism of action of NSAIDs is the differential inhibition of one of the two subtypes of the enzyme cyclooxygenase (COX1 and COX2), preventing prostaglandin synthesis [152].

NSAIDs are among the most commonly prescribed drugs in the world, but their use as anti-inflammatory, antipyretic, antithrombotic, and analgesic is often limited by their gastric toxicity secondary to the suppression of prostaglandin synthesis (mainly through inhibition of COX1 activity). The ratio of inhibition of COX1 to COX2 by NSAIDs determines the likelihood of specific AEs. NSAIDs such as aspirin and indomethacin with a high ratio have more AEs than naproxen, which has a low ratio [153].

Nonselective COX inhibitors inhibit both COX1 and COX2 and include aspirin, indomethacin, piroxicam, diclofenac, and ibuprofen. Selective COX2 inhibitors include meloxicam and celecoxib.

Several NSAIDs and analgesics are established, effective treatments for migraine based on controlled trials compared with placebo, and Table 25.2 lists the most commonly used NSAIDs for headaches.

Multiple trials support the superiority of aspirin (ASA) over placebo for migraine. Studies comparing 1000 mg effervescent ASA, 50 mg encapsulated sumatriptan, 400 mg ibuprofen, and placebo [154, 155] found that ASA was as effective as 50 mg sumatriptan and 400 mg ibuprofen in the treatment of migraine attacks although sumatriptan had the highest rate of pain freedom. In another study, dispersible ASA, at the dose of 900 mg, was superior to placebo in reducing migraine pain as early as 30 min [156]. ASA was superior to placebo and equal to the combination of acetaminophen-codeine in another study [157]. A multicenter trial that included 278 patients compared injectable lysine ASA (iLAS) to subcutaneous sumatriptan and placebo. Two hours following the administration of sumatriptan, iLAS, and placebo, 76.3%, 43.7%, and 14.3% of the patients, respectively, were pain-free. AEs were 7.6% for iLAS and 37.8% for sumatriptan [155]. ASA with or without antiemetics is effective for the acute treatment of migraine and in some patients may be as effective as triptans [158].

Ibuprofen is one of the most commonly used NSAIDs and more effective than placebo for acute migraine in multiple studies at doses of 200 and 400 mg. Only 400 mg was effective for relief of severe migraine attacks [159]. In comparative studies, ibuprofen was comparable to aspirin and celecoxib [154, 160, 161] but less effective than acetaminophen 250 mg, aspirin 250 mg, and caffeine 65 mg (AAC) [162].

Diclofenac is another effective NSAID for migraine which is available in multiple formulations. In one study, diclofenac potassium 50 and 100 mg both reduced pain intensity better than placebo, and the 100 mg dose significantly improved associated symptoms such as phonophobia, photophobia, and the need for rescue medication [163]. Diclofenac sodium soft-gel formulations are significantly more effective than placebo in achieving a 1-h headache reduction [164]. In a double-blind crossover trial, diclofenac potassium 50 and 100 mg was equally effective and better tolerated compared to sumatriptan 100 mg [165]. An oral solution with 50 mg diclofenac potassium achieved significant pain freedom at 2 h (25% vs. 10% placebo), with significant differences in pain relief starting at 30 min and superior 24-h sustained pain-free response compared to placebo [166].

Ketorolac is one of the most commonly used injectable medications for migraine (available as 15, 30, and 60 mg for IM injection). Small comparative trials suggest possible equivalence to some agents including diclofenac potassium oral solution [167–170]. A double-blind, placebo and active-comparator, crossover study compared ketorolac NS 31.5 mg, sumatriptan NS 20 mg, and placebo. Ketorolac NS was superior to placebo and non-inferior to sumatriptan for pain relief at 2 h [171].

Multiple placebo-controlled or comparative studies confirm the efficacy of various NSAIDs for acute migraine. NSAIDS with placebo-controlled studies demonstrating effectiveness include flurbiprofen 100 mg [172], naproxen 750 mg [173], naproxen sodium 825 mg followed by an additional 550 mg in 1 h [174], piroxicam sublingual 40 mg [175], and pirprofen 600 mg [176]. A new oral formulation of the COX-2 inhibitor celecoxib 120 mg is superior to placebo at 2 h for pain freedom and relief of most bothersome symptoms with excellent tolerability [177] and relatively low rates of gastric AEs similar to placebo [178]. Ketoprofen 75 or 150 mg was effective in one study showing comparable effectiveness to zolmitriptan 2.5 mg [179].

Combining NSAIDs with triptans can improve outcomes. Naproxen decreases the chances of migraine recurrence after using sumatriptan [92] and is an established combination for acute migraine [93]. A combination of rizatriptan and meloxicam designed to be rapidly absorbed has recently been for acute migraine [112, 113].

Multiple trials have affirmed the efficacy of AAC versus placebo for migraine attacks. All three studies excluded patients with severe disability (vomiting in a significant proportion of attacks or requiring bed rest in a significant proportion of attacks) and were positive versus placebo [180]. The effectiveness of AAC compares well to other antimigraine therapies, including triptans and other analgesics. In one trial, the combination of AAC was more effective than 50 mg sumatriptan for mild to moderate migraine [181]. In another randomized, controlled trial that included patients who usually used OTC medications to treat their headaches (migraine or tension-type headaches), the fixed combination of AAC was statistically significantly superior to the combination without caffeine, the individual components, or placebo [182]. Data suggests that the AAC combination is more effective than simple analgesics given as monotherapy.

Common NSAID AEs include GI upset, peptic ulcers and bleeding, abdominal pain, constipation, diarrhea, nausea, occasional paradoxical headache, lightheadedness, dizziness, somnolence, tinnitus, and fluid retention [49]. All NSAIDs are associated with an increased risk of peptic ulcer disease, the risk increasing with the dosage of the NSAID [183], and aggravation of existing gastrointestinal inflammatory disease. Contraindications to NSAIDs include active ulcer disease, gastritis, kidney disease, and bleeding disorders. The prolonged use of NSAIDs should be cautiously monitored due to cardiovascular concerns [184]. Assess those using NSAIDs other than acetaminophen for GI blood loss, renal dysfunction, worsening of hypertension, and aggravation of colitis. While it is unlikely that NSAIDs increase the risk of migraine chronification in those with low frequency, the potential for serious AEs with long-term frequent use requires clinicians to prescribe them judiciously [185].

Isometheptene and Isometheptene Combination Agents

The combination of acetaminophen, isometheptene (a sympathomimetic), and dichloralphenazone (a chloral hydrate derivative) is used in the treatment of migraine and tension-type headache [51, 186]. The initial dose is two capsules, with a maximum of five capsules per attack. In placebo-controlled trials, isometheptene attained borderline statistical significance in relieving migraine pain [186–188]. The combination was significantly more effective at reducing headache intensity and was associated with significantly less nausea and vomiting than ergotamine plus caffeine [51]. Isometheptene mucate plus acetaminophen plus dichloralphenazone was significantly more effective than placebo in two of three trials although the magnitude of the effect was relatively modest [189].

Contraindications include glaucoma, renal failure, significant hypertension, heart or liver disease, and use of MAO inhibitors. Common AEs include transient dizziness and skin rash. Multiple serious AEs presumably caused by vasoconstriction have been reported such as intracerebral hemorrhage [190], cerebral vasospasm, myocardial infarction, and autonomic dysreflexia [191].

Neuroleptics and Antiemetics

Dopamine antagonists in migraine provide relief as antiemetics or as adjunctive medication. Although it is unlikely that dopamine antagonism fully explains the effectiveness of neuroleptics, other antiemetics are not effective in treating acute migraine [192, 193]. While most studies have focused on their use as parenteral treatment, a few studies have specifically studied oral therapies. Exposure to dopamine antagonists has not been linked to MOH but may lead to movement disorders such as acute akathisia, Parkinsonism, tardive dyskinesia [194], and rarely neuroleptic malignant syndrome. Other notable AEs include sedation or dizziness, postural hypotension, cardiac QT prolongation, and increased prolactin release causing sexual dysfunction or galactorrhea [195].

Oral metoclopramide is an effective adjuvant medication for the treatment of migraine pain or nausea [196]. Metoclopramide decreases gastric atony and enhances the absorption of co-administered medications [197] and is available as tablets, syrup, and an injectable (dose 10–20 mg). Most studies of oral metoclopramide report its use in combination with other treatments such as aspirin [158] or triptans [198]. The usual dose in the outpatient setting is 10 mg oral or IM, as this dose appears as effective as higher doses up to 40 mg[199].

Prochlorperazine is an established treatment for refractory headaches but mostly in ED settings. In the outpatient setting, it is available at oral doses of 5 or 10 mg or 25 mg suppositories. In one study, buccal prochlorperazine at the dose of 3 mg was superior to 1 mg ergotamine plus caffeine 100 mg and placebo for relief of headache pain and migraine symptoms [200]. Treatment in combination with other acute medications such as triptans reduces nausea but is not proven to add to pain relief [201].

Promethazine is an alternative antiemetic with fewer extrapyramidal AEs but it does not enhance gastric emptying. Droperidol is effective parenterally for nausea and migraine. A study comparing 0.1 mg, 2.75 mg, 5.5 mg, and 8.25 mg IM versus placebo found that all doses 2.75 or greater provided significant relief at 2 h, with similar effectiveness among the three higher doses [202]. Other commonly used neuroleptics for acute headache or nausea include haloperidol [203], chlorpromazine, and perphenazine.

Barbiturate Hypnotics

Butalbital-containing agents were more commonly used for the treatment of headaches or migraine in the past. Available combinations with butalbital include formulations with acetaminophen alone, acetaminophen-caffeine, aspirin-caffeine, aspirin-caffeine-codeine, and acetaminophen-caffeine-codeine. Multiple studies have evaluated the use of butalbital-containing analgesics for tension-type headaches including ten separate controlled trials [204]. However, there is limited evidence for using butalbital for migraine. No randomized, placebo-controlled studies have established the efficacy of butalbital-containing agents in the treatment of acute migraine. Goldstein et al. compared butalbital plus aspirin plus caffeine plus codeine with butorphanol NS [205]. Butorphanol was superior in efficacy to the butalbital combination with codeine at 2 h, but differences between the two treatments were not significant at 4 h. Butalbital combined with codeine was associated with significantly fewer AEs than butorphanol NS[205].

While butalbital-containing analgesic use for headache remains common, serious AEs such as sedation, drowsiness, and dizziness may occur, in addition to the risks of excessive caffeine or acetaminophen leading to toxicity [206]. Butalbital combination analgesic use is strongly associated with conversion from episodic to chronic migraine [207]. Given the lack of evidence for use in migraine and the potential for serious AEs including dependence and worsening of migraine, limit or eliminate entirely butalbital-containing analgesic use in most patients.

Opioids

Clinicians should only consider opioids for rescue in migraine in those who have infrequent disabling migraines not responsive to standard medications or contraindications to other drugs. In trials of migraine, combinations containing codeine and acetaminophen are superior to placebo for pain relief but not pain freedom [157, 208]. In a comparative study, the combination was not superior to aspirin [157].

Butorphanol NS is a mixed mu agonist-antagonist opioid effective for treating acute migraine. Multiple placebo-controlled studies reported butorphanol NS pain relief within 30 and 60 min compared with placebo [209]. AEs were significant in the active group including dizziness (58%), nausea and/or vomiting (38%), and drowsiness (29%). After initial approval as an unscheduled drug, the manufacturer voluntarily reclassified butorphanol as a Schedule IV narcotic due to multiple reports of abuse and dependence. A failure to consider experiences of other formulations and the impact of using frequent opioids for migraine likely contributed to the initial enthusiasm for butorphanol [210], and newer acute guidelines do not recommend it [211].

Tramadol is an opioid with noradrenergic and serotoninergic activity among other sites. A combination of tramadol 75 mg and acetaminophen 650 mg was found to be more effective than placebo in one study. While the combination improved photophobia and phonophobia, it did not significantly relieve nausea [212].

Long-term opioid treatment for refractory migraine only helps a minority of patients and carries significant risk. Saper and colleagues [213] reported the results of a 5-year prospective study using sustained, long-acting opioids in the treatment of over 300 patients with intractable daily or almost-daily headaches. Of 160 patients treated for 3–5 years, only 23% demonstrated evidence of significant improvement. Up to 40% of patients showed some evidence of noncompliance (self-adjustment of doses, etc.) in the first year despite the highly structured program which required monthly or bimonthly visits during the entire study.

Patients with migraine often present with current or opioid use, even in tertiary settings [214]. Opioid users with migraine have higher morbidity, pain severity, and disability than non-users [215]. While the cause-effect relationship of these findings is not clear, opioid use is strongly associated with the development of chronic migraine. The critical threshold of opioid use predictive of transformation is 8 days, compared to 11 days for triptans [216]. A study of electronic health record (EHR) data found over half of patients with migraine received a prescription for opioids from their neurologist [217]. In one survey, over 36% of patients with migraine had opioids available to use as needed [218]. A history of opioid use significantly predicts triptan discontinuation [219]. Long-term, potentially permanent, and physiological problems due to opioid use include decreased gray matter, the release of pro-inflammatory peptides such as CGRP, activation of excitatory glutamate receptors, and endocrine abnormalities [220]. Multiple guidelines for acute migraine state that opioids should rarely, if ever, be used for migraine.

Other Acute Treatment (Octreotide, Corticosteroids, and Oxytocin)

Some preventive treatments may effectively treat acute migraine. Case reports suggested propranolol (40–80 mg) could treat acute migraine, but a placebo-controlled, double-blind study was negative [221]. Calcium channel blockers, such as IV verapamil, and sublingual nifedipine or flunarizine may treat aura [222] or headache [223]. Newer treatments such as eptinezumab may treat acute migraine with significant reductions on day one after infusion [224].

Multiple double-blind studies have assessed the efficacy of intranasal lidocaine for the acute treatment of migraine, with mixed results for its efficacy [225–227]. In one study, 4% lidocaine provided significant initial relief at 15 min, but recurrence in less than 1 h was very common [225]. Another study comparing 4% lidocaine to saline nasal spray placebo failed to show any relief [227].

Corticosteroids might have a role in migraine as adjuvant medication [228] or as a rescue for prolonged attacks [229]. Consider using oral corticosteroids as rescue therapy for patients with status migrainosus or to prevent migraine recurrence [230]. Hydrocortisone, dexamethasone, prednisone, and methylprednisolone are among the most commonly used oral treatments. The potential for serious AE such as avascular necrosis, hyperglycemia and weight gain, hypertension, and mood changes means that clinicians should use corticosteroids sparingly for patients with migraine.

Clinically, occasionally, we utilize muscle relaxants and anti-spasticity medications as acute migraine treatments, mainly for situations such as MOH or associated neck pain and spasms. These include anti-spasticity drugs such as baclofen or tizanidine and antispasmodics such as cyclobenzaprine. The evidence for any of these treatments in acute migraine is lacking although a small study reported successful treatment of MOH with the use of low-dose tizanidine before bedtime [231].

Octreotide, a long-acting somatostatin analogue, was effective in one double-blind, placebo-controlled trial against placebo. Octreotide 100 μg SC was superior to placebo at 2, 4, and 6 h in one study for pain relief [232] but in another, it showed no difference [233].

Guidelines and Treatment Principles for Acute Migraine Treatment

Several guidelines have proposed treatment algorithms with medication recommendations based on evidence-based therapies. These guidelines take into account the quality of the evidence as determined by blinded, placebo-controlled studies as well as clinical experience. Clinical trials for acute migraine now rely on placebo-controlled trials with primary outcomes of pain freedom and relief of most bothersome symptoms [234]. These studies recruit subjects with frequent but episodic migraine (2–8 per month) present for at least 1 year prior to inclusion and no known secondary cause of headache, typically using a parallel-group design.

Multiple guidelines stress the importance of individualizing treatment, based on potential benefits, risks, and cost [235]. For each acute therapy, treat at least two different attacks before deciding that a drug is ineffective. If there is no benefit from the drug, be sure that the dose is adequate and no other factors interfere with its effect. It may be necessary to change the formulation or route of administration or add an adjuvant. Consider changing the drug when the response is incomplete or too slow, the headache recurs, the results are inconsistent after an adequate trial at an adequate dose, or the AEs are bothersome.

For patients with infrequent attacks, mild-moderate pain and relatively low disability simple analgesics may be adequate. The AAC combination is likely more effective than simple analgesics alone. For patients with more severe or disabling attacks, triptans are the usual first-line therapy unless contraindicated. Clinicians can recommend lasmiditan or gepants in situations when multiple triptans are not effective or tolerated, or if patients cannot use triptans due to contraindications [236]. Lasmiditan may have greater efficacy than available gepants, but patients must agree to abide by the driving restriction after using. While these newer agents have different adverse event profiles, gepants and lasmiditan do not demonstrate superior efficacy to triptans [237]. Newer guidelines do not recommend using ergota-

Table 25.3 Principles of acute treatment

Use stratified care to select the most appropriate treatment for each attack
Treat early before the attack escalates
Avoid medication overuse, especially with triptans and combination analgesics
A headache calendar may help establish treatment effectiveness and recurrence
Use non-oral treatments for attacks with significant nausea or vomiting
Simple analgesics may treat milder, less disabling attacks
Triptans are first-line migraine-specific treatment for most unless contraindicated
Gepants are better tolerated compared to most migraine-specific medications
Consider rescue medication for severe or prolonged attacks

mine, opioids, and barbiturate-containing medications due to the availability of more effective and safer treatments [238]. Table 25.3 outlines several best practices for acute migraine treatment.

Clinical trials of acute medication for migraine investigate subjects with episodic migraine treating within a few hours of attack onset. Treating status migrainosus or prolonged migraine, such as in the emergency department (ED), requires a different approach. Highly effective treatments for acute migraine such as SC sumatriptan are equal to or less effective than parenteral treatments including prochlorperazine [239] or propofol [240] in this population. When treating patients with severe migraine or status migrainosus, consider previous acute treatments, comorbidities, overall migraine frequency and disability, and a discharge plan in case of migraine recurrence.

Several reviews have evaluated the evidence for various parenteral treatments for severe or prolonged migraine, often in the ED setting [241–244]. While the urgent setting complicates the process of doing high-quality clinical trials, there have been several placebo-controlled or comparative studies of various IV or IM treatments for migraine, either alone or in combination with other therapies.

Intravenous Therapies

Parenteral NSAIDs effectively treat migraine in infusion settings. Ketorolac is among the most effective treatments [245], especially in patients without previous opioid exposure [246]. In a pilot study of 74 subjects, IV ibuprofen 800 mg improved headache in 74% (17/23) compared to 48% (10/21) receiving placebo [247] for treatment of those with migraine lasting at least 2–72 h. Previous studies have demonstrated NSAIDs such as metamizole [248], lysine clonixinate [249], and diclofenac IM [250] are effective in this setting.

ED providers frequently use opioids for migraine in the ED despite recommendations, and until recently over half of patients presenting to the ED received them [251]. Meperidine with or without promethazine or hydroxyzine [167, 252, 253], tramadol [254], and hydromorphone [255] are among the most studied. Opioids are effective compared to placebo but with high rates of headache recurrence [244]. In comparative studies, the efficacy of opioids is usually equivalent to other agents such as ketorolac, and in one study, hydromorphone was inferior to prochlorperazine [256].

Corticosteroids in the ED both alleviate migraine pain and can reduce rates of migraine recurrence after discharge at 24–72 h. Most studies utilize 4–10 mg IV dexamethasone. In one study, a 10 mg dose significantly reduced recurrence at 48–72 h (58.3% vs. 12.9% placebo) [257], and in another, rates of recurrence were lower (38% vs. 13%) but did not meet statistical significance [258]. Other studies have been negative, and subjects receiving dexamethasone experience more AEs such as restlessness or drowsiness [259].

The role of dopamine antagonists is to eliminate nausea and improve migraine pain as monotherapy, or in combination as a pretreatment with DHE. Prochlorperazine IV is effective and has been proven superior to placebo [260], metoclopramide [261], IV magnesium [262], and ketorolac [263] in clinical studies. The evidence for metoclopramide IV is strong, with several studies showing superiority to placebo [264]. The usual dose is 10 mg, and higher doses are not necessary to work better [199]. Chlorpromazine [265], droperidol [266, 267], and haloperidol [268] are also effective. Drowsiness is the most common AE from neuroleptic treatment, but orthostatic hypotension may occur. Serious extrapyramidal reactions are uncommon but can cause significant distress. EKGs before and during treatment can recognize the development of cardiac QT prolongation.

The combination of neuroleptics and DHE provides superior pain relief to alternative infusion treatments in comparative studies. In one study, metoclopramide 5 mg and DHE 1 mg IV provided significant pain relief compared to ketorolac 60 mg IM [168]. In other studies, metoclopramide and DHE were equal to dexamethasone/metoclopramide [269], IV valproate [270] and superior to meperidine [271–273]. Pretreatment with prochlorperazine is also effective [274]. Magnesium IV may have a role as an infusion or ED treatment for migraine although not all studies report significant benefits. A few placebo-controlled studies report significant benefit [275, 276], but in other studies, the benefit was no greater than placebo [277]. Magnesium may benefit patients

Table 25.4 Parenteral medications for migraine

Drug	Dose	Clinical pearls
Dihydroergotamine	0.1–1 mg	Start at lower doses. Consider slow infusion over 1 h for sensitive patients. Pretreat with antiemetic. Monitor vital signs before and after treatment
Neuroleptics		May prolong the QT interval. Drowsiness, akathisia, and hypotension may occur
Prochlorperazine.	5–10 mg	CYP 3A4, 2D6 inhibitors may increase levels
Metoclopramide.	5–20 mg	May affect the oral absorption of other medications
Chlorpromazine.	6.25–25 mg	Hypotension, sedation very common
Droperidol.	0.625–2.5 mg	Do not use: QTc greater than 460
Haloperidol.	2–5 mg	Increased rate of movement disorders
Promethazine.	6.25–25 mg	Lower rates of akathisia
Other nonspecific		
Dexamethasone.	4–10 mg	May prevent migraine recurrence
Ketorolac.	15–30 mg	Use as adjunctive with neuroleptics, DHE
Magnesium.	1–2 g	May be more effective for migraine with aura
Sodium valproate.	400–1000 mg	Repeated infusions may be more effective
Lidocaine.	1–4 mg/min	Continuous infusion with telemetry monitoring
ketamine	0.1–1 mg/kg/hr	Diplopia, dizziness, and mood changes complicate management. Increase dose slowly

who have migraine with aura more than those without aura [278]. Flushing is the most common AE.

While clinicians frequently use anticonvulsants for migraine prevention, IV formulations may treat refractory acute migraine. A few open-label studies have described rapid improvement from the use of IV valproate sodium [279, 280]. One double-blind study of 90 adults with acute migraine evaluated a 400 mg dose of IV sodium valproate compared to 8 mg IV dexamethasone. Outcomes were similar in both groups with headache improvement at 0.5 h in 55% and 67.5% of patients in the sodium valproate and dexamethasone groups, respectively [281]. In other studies, treatments such as prochlorpromazine [282], metoclopramide, and ketorolac performed better in the ED setting for pain relief, and the combination of dihydroergotamine/metoclopramide was superior for preventing headache recurrence [270]. Case reports have noted the effectiveness of levetiracetam IV for acute migraine, but trials have yet to establish its effectiveness [283]

Most studies of lidocaine IV examine its effect in the inpatient setting [284, 285], but one study reported using a 1.5 mg/kg bolus and 1 mg/kg for 1 h showed effectiveness and long-term relief similar to ketorolac [286].

For severe, long-standing migraine, clinicians may choose to use ketamine IV in infusion and inpatient settings [287, 288], which may be effective even in those who fail to respond to other therapies. As an ED treatment, one study of low-dose ketamine (0.2 mg/kg IV) failed to relieve pain [289], and another showed inferiority to prochlorperazine [290]. Propofol has been utilized in ED settings for migraine, with studies showing effectiveness in open-label studies [291], and superiority to dexamethasone [292] and SC sumatriptan [293].

For patients presenting with severe, recurrent, and disabling migraine, the available evidence suggests parenteral neuroleptics, ketorolac, or other NSAIDs and DHE are probably effective. Consider using medications in combination, in particular antiemetics and DHE, for best results. Adjunctive medications such as corticosteroids, magnesium IV, and valproate IV may also improve pain or lower the chance of recurrence. While opioids are likely effective, the evidence suggests they are not superior to other treatments, and guidelines suggest only using them as a second-line therapy [241].

Table 25.4 summarizes the parenteral treatment of migraine in infusion or hospital settings with clinical pearls for each.

Inpatient Treatment of Migraine

Migraine is the most common cause of ED visits for headaches and the most common reason for admission [294]. Common indications for admission include status migranosus, intractable nausea and/or vomiting, failed outpatient treatment or frequent ED visits requiring inpatient pain or psychiatric management, and medical disease requiring careful observation [295]. Table 25.5 reviews major criteria for admission when hospitalization is most likely necessary and minor criteria which are not necessarily reasons for admission but could increase the likelihood of recommending it. The use of barbiturates or opioid-containing medications presents a major challenge as abrupt withdrawal can cause serious AEs. Expert consensus states overuse of either substance as a high priority for aggressive treatment and a clear imperative for inpatient treatment [296]. Although

Table 25.5 Admission criteria for migraine

Major	Minor
Intractable vomiting or dehydration	Intractable nausea or photophobia
Acute change in disability (missing school, may lose job)	Chronic disability (unable to work or attend school for >6 months)
Recurrent ED visits, no improvement with outpatient infusion	No improvement in outpatient care
Medication overuse including opioids or barbiturates	Medication overuse including triptans or analgesics
Status migrainosus	Daily headache
Unstable medical or psychiatric disorder	Chronic medical or psychiatric disorder

inpatient migraine treatment usually involves admission through an ED for 3 days or less, a longer treatment duration may benefit patients with long-standing RM. Studies reviewing hospitalization at specialized headache centers report longer lengths of stay for effective treatment, with a median of up to 13 days [297, 298]. While only a small minority of patients with migraine receive it, effective inpatient treatment improves pain, alleviates disability, and reduces analgesic use, with long-term benefits well beyond discharge [299].

Table 25.5 reviews commonly used parenteral treatments for migraine.

For inpatients with CM and RM, pharmacological treatment aims to treat migraine symptoms, withdraw overused medications, and improve responsiveness to treatment. DHE is one of the best-studied treatments with effects lasting weeks or months in several case series [300–302]. Most studies began DHE at lower doses and increased as tolerated up to 1 mg three times daily, usually in combination with metoclopramide or other antiemetics. DHE appears effective in treating MOH, and patients with triptan-related MO improve quickly [303].

Lidocaine IV can successfully treat CM with or without MOH [285, 304], with a length of treatment of about 7 days. Common AEs include nausea, blood pressure changes, visual hallucinations, and other psychiatric side effects [305]. Ketamine IV appears effective for RM in the inpatient setting [287, 306]. Complications such as nystagmus, confusion, or hallucinations usually respond to benzodiazepines or lowering the dose [287]. Other parenteral treatments consist of repetitive neuroleptics, corticosteroids, magnesium IV, levetiracetam, divalproex, or ketorolac [307]. A few studies have also described the use of propofol [308] and diphendydramine [309] for RM. Most centers recommend pharmacological treatment combined with a multi-disciplinary approach consisting of patent education, behavioral therapies such as biofeedback, preventive medication, and close follow-up after discharge [310, 311].

Conclusion

Effective acute treatments for migraine include triptans, ergotamine and DHE, NSAIDs, and combination analgesics. Gepants are effective for acute migraine and may have fewer AEs than triptans. Lasmiditan is an effective alternative to triptans, especially in non-responders or those with contraindications. For patients with severe, prolonged attacks such as status migrainosus, parenteral DHE, neuroleptics, dexamethasone, ketorolac, magnesium, and sodium valproate may be useful. Inpatient treatment of migraine is underutilized and may offer relief for those with severe migraine, disability, medication overuse, and those with significant medical or psychiatric comorbidities.

Teaching Points

1. Effective acute treatment is essential for migraine management and should be used early in the attack for most patients.
2. Customizing an acute treatment plan based on the attack with the availability of a back-up medication can improve patient outcomes.
3. Migraine-specific treatments such as triptans, gepants, dihydroergotamine, and lasmiditan are proven medications for migraine and can be used along with nonspecific therapies such as neuroleptics or anti-inflammatory drugs.
4. Parenteral therapies including dihydroergotamine, neuroleptics, anti-inflammatory drugs, and anticonvulsants can alleviate severe attacks such as status migrainosus.

Case

A 47-year-old woman presents for the evaluation and treatment of migraine. She began to have migraine as a teen with nausea, photophobia, phonophobia, and osmophobia. Her migraine worsened in her late 30 s and at one point had a daily headache, potentially exacerbated by rizatriptan overuse. Menstruation is her most notable trigger but she may have migraine before or during menses and cannot predict the day it will start. She currently has headaches 15 days per month, of which about ½ of them reach migraine intensity. She uses a combination of rizatriptan and ibuprofen for migraine. This combination is generally effective but she is rarely headache-free in the first few hours after taking it. She often needs to lie down after taking medication but generally feels better the next day.

Case Discussion

The treatment of acute migraine requires an assessment of treatment effectiveness and shared treatment decision-making with the patient. For patients with infrequent migraine, the best choice is the most effective therapy with relatively tolerable side effects. For patients with very frequent migraine, factors such as safety, potential for medication overuse, and migraine recurrence become more important. Other treatment considerations include the presence of reliable premonitory symptoms, consistent triggers such as menstruation, medical comorbidities, and patient preference such as choosing between oral and non-oral therapies. For the patient, in this case, one option would be to change the rizatriptan to another triptan which may be more effective such as SC sumatriptan or use a prescription nonsteroidal such as diclofenac potassium. Changing the treatment class from a triptan to dihydroergotamine, lasmiditan, or a gepant may also be effective. Calendaring may allow patients to better assess the reliability of perceived triggers to see if they may use acute treatment preemptively. Finally, some patients may benefit from a "rescue" acute treatment such as neuroleptic drugs for infrequent use to avoid suffering or the need for urgent visits to the emergency room.

Questions and Answers

1. How do small molecule antagonists of calcitonin gene-related peptide (gepants) differ from triptans for the treatment of acute migraine?
   A. More rapid onset of effectiveness
   B. Higher rates of pain-freedom
   C. Better tolerability
   D. Higher risk of migraine recurrence

The correct answer is C. In clinical trials, subjects using gepants had relatively lower rates of pain-freedom compared to most studies of triptans or lasmiditan. Triptans are available as an injection (sumatriptan) or nasal spray (zolmitriptan and sumatriptan). A potential benefit of gepants is their tolerability, with low rates of adverse events in clinical trials.

2. Which of the following treatments is most highly associated with medication overuse headaches?
   A. Barbiturate-containing combination therapies
   B. Gepants
   C. Nonsteroidal anti-inflammatory drugs
   D. Dihydroergotamine

The correct answer is A. In population-based studies, the risk of migraine progression among those using barbiturate-containing compound analgesics was higher than other acute migraine treatments including triptans and nonsteroidal anti-inflammatory drugs. The risk of medication overuse headache from using gepants is unknown, and dihydroergotamine is used for patients with status migranosus.

References

1. Ashina M, Buse DC, Ashina H, et al. Migraine: integrated approaches to clinical management and emerging treatments. Lancet. 2021;397(10283):1505–18.
2. Payne KA, Varon SF, Kawata AK, et al. The international burden of migraine study (IBMS): study design, methodology, and baseline cohort characteristics. Cephalalgia. 2011;31(10):1116–30.
3. Lipton RB, Silberstein SD. The role of headache-related disability in migraine management: implications for headache treatment guidelines. Neurology. 2001;56(6 Suppl 1):S35–42.
4. Hindiyeh NA, Kellerman DJ, Schmidt PC. Review of acute treatment of migraine trial results with the new FDA endpoints: design implications for future trials. Headache. 2019;59(5):819–24.
5. Pavlovic JM, Buse DC, Sollars CM, Haut S, Lipton RB. Trigger factors and premonitory features of migraine attacks: summary of studies. Headache. 2014;54(10):1670–9.
6. Waelkens J. Dopamine blockade with domperidone: bridge between prophylactic and abortive treatment of migraine? A dose-finding study. Cephalalgia. 1984;4(2):85–90.
7. Waelkens J, Caers I, Amery WK. Effects of therapeutic measures taken during the premonitory phase. In: Amery WK, Wauquier A, editors. The prelude to the migraine attack. London: Bailliere Tindall; 1986. p. 78–83.
8. Spierings EL. Practical aspects of the pharmacotherapy of headache. Compr Ther. 1992;18(1):36–41.
9. Rozen TD. Migraine prodrome: a nose on a face. Lancet. 2004;363(9408):517.
10. Massiou H. Dihydroergotamine nasal spray in prevention and treatment of migraine attacks: two controlled trials versus placebo. Cephalalgia. 1987;7(Suppl 6):440–1.
11. Luciani R, Carter D, Mannix L, Hemphill M, Diamond M, Cady R. Prevention of migraine during prodrome with naratriptan. Cephalalgia. 2000;20(2):122–6.
12. Dodick DW, Goadsby PJ, Schwedt TJ, et al. Ubrogepant for the treatment of migraine attacks during the prodrome: a phase 3, multicentre, randomised, double-blind, placebo-controlled, crossover trial in the USA. Lancet. 2023;402(10419):2307–16.
13. Latsko M, Silberstein S, Rosen N. Frovatriptan as preemptive treatment for fasting-induced migraine. Headache. 2011;51(3):369–74.
14. Silberstein SD, Elkind AH, Schreiber C, Keywood C. Randomized trial of frovatriptan for the intermittent prevention of menstrual migraine. Neurology. 2004;63:261–9.
15. Gago-Veiga AB, Pagán J, Henares K, et al. To what extent are patients with migraine able to predict attacks? J Pain Res. 2018;11:2083–94.
16. Hansen JM, Charles A. Differences in treatment response between migraine with aura and migraine without aura: lessons from clinical practice and RCTs. J Headache Pain. 2019;20(1):96.

17. Hansen JM, Goadsby PJ, Charles A. Reduced efficacy of sumatriptan in migraine with aura vs without aura. Neurology. 2015;84(18):1880–5.
18. Dodick DW, Lipton RB, Goadsby PJ, et al. Predictors of migraine headache recurrence: a pooled analysis from the eletriptan database. Headache. 2008;48(2):184–93.
19. Bates D, Ashford E, Dawson R, et al. Subcutaneous sumatriptan during the migraine aura. Neurology. 1994;44(9):1587–92.
20. Dowson A. Can oral 311C90, a novel 5HT1D agonist, prevent migraine headache when taken during an aura? Eur Neurol. 1996;36(Suppl 2):28–31.
21. Olesen J, Diener HC, Schoenen J, Hettiarachchi J. No effect of eletriptan administration during the aura phase of migraine. Eur J Neurol. 2004;11(10):671–7.
22. Aurora SK, Barrodale PM, McDonald SA, Jakubowski M, Burstein R. Revisiting the efficacy of sumatriptan therapy during the aura phase of migraine. Headache. 2009;49(7):1001–4.
23. Artto V, Nissilä M, Wessman M, Palotie A, Färkkilä M, Kallela M. Treatment of hemiplegic migraine with triptans. Eur J Neurol. 2007;14(9):1053–6.
24. Klapper J, Mathew N, Nett R. Triptans in the treatment of basilar migraine and migraine with prolonged aura. Headache. 2001;41(10):981–4.
25. Goldner JA, Levitt LP. Treatment of complicated migraine with sublingual nifedipine. Headache. 1987;27:484–6.
26. Rozen TD. Treatment of a prolonged migrainous aura with intravenous furosemide. Neurology. 2000;55(5):732–3.
27. Rozen TD. Aborting a prolonged migrainous aura with intravenous prochlorperazine and magnesium sulfate. Headache. 2003;43(8):901–3.
28. Rothrock JF. Successful treatment of persistent migraine aura with divalproex sodium. Neurology. 1997;27:484–6.
29. Kaube H, Herzog J, Käufer T, Dichgans M, Diener HC. Ketamine can stop aura in hemiplegic migraine. Cephalalgia. 2000;20(4):270.
30. Afridi SK, Giffin NJ, Kaube H, Goadsby PJ. A randomized controlled trial of intranasal ketamine in migraine with prolonged aura. Neurology. 2013;80(7):642–7.
31. Schulman E, McGeeney BE. Current concepts in refractory migraine. Curr Treat Options Neurol. 2013;15(1):40–55.
32. Afridi SK, Kaube H, Goadsby PJ. Glyceryl trinitrate triggers premonitory symptoms in migraineurs. Pain. 2004;110(3):675–80.
33. Antonova M, Wienecke T, Maubach K, Thomas E, Olesen J, Ashina M. The pharmacological effect of BGC20-1531, a novel prostanoid EP(4) receptor antagonist, in the prostaglandin E (2) human model of headache. J Headache Pain. 2011;12(5):551–9.
34. Yuan H, Silberstein SD. Histamine and migraine. Headache. 2018;58(1):184–93.
35. Cutrer FM, Mathew P. Calcitonin gene related peptide (CGRP)-provoked migraine-like attacks. Cephalalgia. 2010;30(10):1155–6.
36. Hougaard A, Amin FM, Hauge AW, Ashina M, Olesen J. Provocation of migraine with aura using natural trigger factors. Neurology. 2013;80(5):428–31.
37. Martin VT, Behbehani MM. Toward a rational understanding of migraine trigger factors. Med Clin North Am. 2001;85(4):911–41.
38. Kelman L. The triggers or precipitants of the acute migraine attack. Cephalalgia. 2007;27(5):394–402.
39. Marmura MJ. Triggers, protectors, and predictors in episodic migraine. Curr Pain Headache Rep. 2018;22(12):81.
40. Crombez G, Eccleston C, Van Damme S, Vlaeyen JW, Karoly P. Fear-avoidance model of chronic pain: the next generation. Clin J Pain. 2012;28(6):475–83.
41. Lipton RB, Cady RK, O'Quinn S, Hall CB, Stewart WF. Sumatriptan treats the full spectrum of headache in individuals with disabling IHS migraine. Headache. 1999;40:783–91.
42. Newman LC. Why triptan treatment can fail: focus on gastrointestinal manifestations of migraine. Headache. 2013;53(Suppl 1):11–6.
43. Silberstein SD. Appropriate use of abortive medication in headache treatment. Pain Mgt. 1991;4:22–8.
44. Lipton RB, Stewart WF, Stone AM, Lainez MJ, Sawyer JP. Stratified care vs step care strategies for migraine. The disability in strategies of care (DISC) study: a randomized trial. JAMA. 2000;284(20):2599–05.
45. Lipton RB, Stewart WF, Sawyer J. Stratified care is a more effective migraine treatment strategy than stepped care: results of a randomized clinical trial. Neurology. 2000;54:A14.
46. Lantéri-Minet M, Mick G, Allaf B. Early dosing and efficacy of triptans in acute migraine treatment: the TEMPO study. Cephalalgia. 2012;32(3):226–35.
47. Marissa Lagman-Bartolome A, Lay C. The traffic light of headache: simplifying acute migraine Management for Physicians and Patients Using the Canadian headache society guidelines. Headache. 2019;59(2):250–2.
48. Peroutka SJ. Developments in 5-hydroxytryptamine receptor pharmacology in migraine. Headache. 1990;30(Suppl 1):12.
49. Gray RN, McCrory DC, Eberlein K, Westman EC, Hasselblad V. Self-administered drug treatments for acute migraine headache. Prepared for the Agency for Health Care Policy and Research, Contract No. 290-94-2025. Available from the National Technical Information Service, Accession No. 127854. (Technical Review 2 4). 1999;February.
50. A randomized, double-blind comparison of sumatriptan and Cafergot in the acute treatment of migraine. The multinational Oral Sumatriptan and Cafergot comparative study group. Eur Neurol. 1991;31(5):314–22.
51. Yuill GM, Swinburn WR, Liversedge LA. A double-blind crossover trial of isometheptene mucate compound and ergotamine in migraine. Br J Clin Prac. 1972;26:76–9.
52. Hirt D, Lataste X, Taylor P. A comparison of DHE nasal spray and cafergot in acute migraine. Cephalalgia. 1989;9(Suppl 10):410–1.
53. Sargent JD, Baumel B, Peters K, et al. Aborting a migraine attack: naproxen sodium versus ergotamine plus caffeine. Headache. 1988;28(4):263–6.
54. Christie S, Gobel H, Mateos V, Allen C, Vrijens F, Shivaprakash M. Crossover comparison of efficacy and preference for rizatriptan 10 mg versus ergotamine/caffeine in migraine. Eur Neurol. 2003;49(1):20–9.
55. Bousser MG, Loria Y. Efficacy of dihydroergotamine nasal spray in the acute treatment of migraine attacks. Cephalalgia. 1985;5(Suppl 3):554–5.
56. Touchon J, Bertin L, Pilgrim AJ, Ashford E, Bes A. A comparison of subcutaneous sumatriptan and dihydroergotamine nasal spray in the acute treatment of migraine. Neurology. 1996;47(2):361–5.
57. Lataste X. Dihydroergotamine nasal spray. In: Ferrari MD, Lataste X, editors. Migraine and other headaches. Park Ridge: Parthenon; 1989. p. 249–60.
58. Shrewsbury SB, Jeleva M, Satterly KH, Lickliter J, Hoekman J. STOP 101: a phase 1, randomized, open-label, comparative bioavailability study of INP104, Dihydroergotamine Mesylate (DHE) administered Intranasally by a I123 precision olfactory delivery (POD(®)) device, in healthy adult subjects. Headache. 2019;59(3):394–409.
59. Albrecht D, Iwashima M, Dillon D, Harris S, Levy J. A phase 1, randomized, open-label, safety, tolerability, and comparative bioavailability study of intranasal Dihydroergotamine Powder (STS101), intramuscular Dihydroergotamine Mesylate, and intranasal DHE Mesylate spray in healthy adult subjects. Headache. 2020;60(4):701–12.

60. Tas C, Joyce JC, Nguyen HX, et al. Dihydroergotamine mesylate-loaded dissolving microneedle patch made of polyvinylpyrrolidone for management of acute migraine therapy. J Control Release. 2017;268:159–65.
61. Esim O, Ozkan CK, Kurbanoglu S, et al. Development and in vitro/in vivo evaluation of dihydroergotamine mesylate loaded maltodextrin-pullulan sublingual films. Drug Dev Ind Pharm. 2019;45(6):914–21.
62. Lipton RB, Bigal ME, Goadsby PJ. Double-blind clinical trials of oral triptans vs other classes of acute migraine medication – a review. Cephalalgia. 2004;24(5):321–32.
63. Cameron C, Kelly S, Hsieh SC, et al. Triptans in the acute treatment of migraine: a systematic review and network meta-analysis. Headache. 2015;55(Suppl 4):221–35.
64. Diener HC, Förderreuther S, Gaul C, et al. Prevention of migraine with monoclonal antibodies against CGRP or the CGRP receptor: addition to the S1 guideline: therapy of migraine attacks and prevention of migraine. Recommendations of the Germany Society of Neurology and the German Migraine and Headache Society. Neurol Res Pract. 2020;2:11.
65. VanderPluym JH, Halker Singh RB, Urtecho M, et al. Acute treatments for episodic migraine in adults: a systematic review and meta-analysis. JAMA. 2021;325(23):2357–69.
66. Lipton RB, Bigal M, Diamond M. Migraine prevalence, disease burden and the need for preventive therapy. Neurology. 2007;68:343–9.
67. Leroux E, Buchanan A, Lombard L, et al. Evaluation of patients with insufficient efficacy and/or tolerability to Triptans for the acute treatment of migraine: a systematic literature review. Adv Ther. 2020;37(12):4765–96.
68. Dodick D, Lipton RB, Martin V, et al. Consensus statement: cardiovascular safety profile of triptans (5-HT agonists) in the acute treatment of migraine. Headache. 2004;44(5):414–25.
69. Mathew PG, Krel R, Buddhdev B, et al. A retrospective analysis of triptan and dhe use for basilar and hemiplegic migraine. Headache. 2016;56(5):841–8.
70. Nahas SJ, Silberstein SD. Triptans: actions and reactions. Headache. 2008;48(4):611–3.
71. Dodick DW, Martin VT, Smith T, Silberstein S. Cardiovascular tolerability and safety of triptans: a review of clinical data. Headache. 2004;44(Suppl 1):S20–30.
72. Evans RW, Tepper SJ, Shapiro RE, Sun-Edelstein C, Tietjen GE. The FDA alert on serotonin syndrome with use of triptans combined with selective serotonin reuptake inhibitors or selective serotonin-norepinephrine reuptake inhibitors: American headache society position paper. Headache. 2010;50(6):1089–99.
73. Orlova Y, Rizzoli P, Loder E. Association of Coprescription of Triptan antimigraine drugs and selective serotonin reuptake inhibitor or selective norepinephrine reuptake inhibitor antidepressants with serotonin syndrome. JAMA Neurol. 2018;75(5):566–72.
74. Ferrari MD, Roon KI, Lipton RB, Goadsby PJ. Oral triptans (serotonin 5-$HT_{1B/1D}$ agonists) in acute migraine treatment: a metaanalysis of 53 trials. Lancet. 2001;358(9293):1668–75.
75. Serrano D, Buse DC, Kori SH, et al. Effects of switching acute treatment on disability in migraine patients using triptans. Headache. 2013;53(9):1415–29.
76. Cady RC, Ryan R, Jhingran P, O'Quinn S, Pait DG. Sumatriptan injection reduces productivity loss during a migraine attack: results of a double-blind, placebo-controlled trial. Arch Intern Med. 1998;158(9):1013–8.
77. Treatment of migraine attacks with sumatriptan. N Engl J Med. 1991;325(5):316–21.
78. Wendt J, Cady R, Singer R, et al. A randomized, double-blind, placebo-controlled trial of the efficacy and tolerability of a 4-mg dose of subcutaneous sumatriptan for the treatment of acute migraine attacks in adults. Clin Ther. 2006;28(4):517–26.
79. Derry CJ, Derry S, Moore RA. Sumatriptan (all routes of administration) for acute migraine attacks in adults – overview of Cochrane reviews. Cochrane Database Syst Rev. 2014;2014(5):Cd009108.
80. Winner P, Ricalde O, Leforce B, Saper J, Margul B. A double-blind study of subcutaneous dihydroergotamine vs subcutaneous sumatriptan in the treatment of acute migraine. Arch Neurol. 1996;53(2):180–4.
81. Pini LA, Sternieri E, Fabbri L, Zerbini O, Bamfi F. High efficacy and low frequency of headache recurrence after Oral sumatriptan. The Oral sumatriptan Italian study group. J Int Med Res. 1995;23(2):96–105.
82. Sargent J, Kirchner JR, Davis R, Kirkhart B. Oral sumatriptan is effective and well tolerated for the acute treatment of migraine: results of a multicenter study. Neurology. 1995;45(8):S10–4.
83. Tfelt-Hansen P, Henry P, Mulder LJ, Scheldewaert RG, Schoenen J, Chazot G. The effectiveness of combined oral lysine acetylsalicylate and metoclopramide compared with oral sumatriptan for migraine. Lancet. 1995;346(8980):923–6.
84. Pfaffenrath V, Cunin G, Sjonell G, Prendergast S. Efficacy and safety of sumatriptan tablets (25mg, 50mg, and 100mg) in the acute treatment of migraine: defining the optimum doses of oral sumatriptan. Headache. 1998;38(3):184–90.
85. Carpay HA, Dowson AJ. Sumatriptan fast-disintegrating/rapid-release tablets: viewpoints. Drugs. 2006;66(6):891–2.
86. Salonen R, Ashford E, Dahlof C, et al. Intranasal sumatriptan for the acute treatment of migraine. International intranasal Sumatriptan study group. J Neurol. 1994;241(8):463–9.
87. Ryan R, Elkind A, Baker CC, Mullican W, DeBussey S, Asgharnejad M. Sumatriptan nasal spray for the acute treatment of migraine: results of two clinical studies. Neurology. 1997;49:1225–30.
88. Tepper D. Breath-powered intranasal sumatriptan dry powder. Headache. 2016;56(4):817–8.
89. Silberstein S, Winner PK, McAllister PJ, et al. Early onset of efficacy and consistency of response across multiple migraine attacks from the randomized COMPASS study: AVP-825 Breath Powered(®) exhalation delivery system (Sumatriptan nasal powder) vs Oral sumatriptan. Headache. 2017;57(6):862–76.
90. Munjal S, Gautam A, Offman E, Brand-Schieber E, Allenby K, Fisher DM. A randomized trial comparing the pharmacokinetics, safety, and tolerability of DFN-02, an intranasal Sumatriptan spray containing a permeation enhancer, with intranasal and subcutaneous Sumatriptan in healthy adults. Headache. 2016;56(9):1455–65.
91. Lipton RB, Munjal S, Brand-Schieber E, Rapoport AM. DFN-02, Sumatriptan 10 mg nasal spray with permeation enhancer, for the acute treatment of migraine: a randomized, double-blind, placebo-controlled study assessing functional disability and subject satisfaction with treatment. CNS Drugs. 2019;33(4):375–82.
92. Krymchantowski AV. Naproxen sodium decreases migraine recurrence when administered with sumatriptan. Arq Neuropsiquiatr. 2000;58(2B):428–30.
93. Smith TR, Sunshine A, Stark SR, Littlefield DE, Spruill SE, Alexander WJ. Sumatriptan and naproxen sodium for the acute treatment of migraine. Headache. 2005;45(8):983–91.
94. Silberstein SD, Mannix LK, Goldstein J, et al. Multimechanistic (sumatriptan-naproxen) early intervention for the acute treatment of migraine. Neurology. 2008;71(2):114–21.
95. Pascual J, Falk RM, Piessens F, et al. Consistent efficacy and tolerability of almotriptan in the acute treatment of multiple migraine attacks.: results of a large, randomized, double-blind, placebo-controlled study. Cephalalgia. 2000;20(6):488–96.
96. Cabarrocas X, Zayas JM. Efficacy data on oral almotriptan, a novel 5HT1B/1D agonist. Headache. 1998;38(5):377.

97. Sheftell F, Ryan R, Pitman V. Efficacy, safety, and tolerability of oral eletriptan for treatment of acute migraine: a multicenter, double-blind, placebo-controlled study conducted in the United States. Headache. 2003;43(3):202–13.
98. Stark R, Dahlof C, Haughie S, Hettiarachchi J. Efficacy, safety and tolerability of oral eletriptan in the acute treatment of migraine: results of a phase III, multicentre, placebo-controlled study across three attacks. Cephalalgia. 2002;22(1):23–32.
99. Farkkila M. A dose-finding study of eletriptan (UK-116,044) (5-30 mg) for the acute treatment of migraine. Cephalalgia. 1996;16:387–8.
100. Goadsby PJ, Ferrari MD, Olesen J, et al. Eletriptan in acute migraine: a double-blind, placebo-controlled comparison to sumatriptan. Eletriptan Steering Committee. Neurology. 2000;54(1):156–63.
101. Diener HC, Ryan R, Sun W, Hettiarachchi J. The 40-mg dose of eletriptan: comparative efficacy and tolerability versus sumatriptan 100 mg. Eur J Neurol. 2004;11(2):125–34.
102. Rapoport A, Ryan R, Goldstein J, Keywood C. Dose range-finding studies with frovatriptan in the acute treatment of migraine. Headache. 2002;42(Suppl 2):S74–83.
103. Goldstein J, Keywood C. A study of the efficacy and safety of low doses of frovatriptan (VML251), a potent cerebroselective 5-hydroxytryptamine (5HT)1B/1D agonist in the acute treatment of migraine. Eur J Neurol. 1998;5(Suppl 3):S46–7.
104. Klassen A, Elkind A, Asgharnjad M, Webster C, Laurenza A. Naratriptan tablets are effective and well-tolerated in the acute treatment of migraine: results of a double-blind, placebo-controlled, parallel group trial. Headache. 1997;37(10):640–5.
105. Mathew NT, Peykamian M, Laurenza A, Austin R, Asgharnejad M. Efficacy and tolerability of naratriptan tablets in the treatment of migraine: results of a double-blind, placebo-controlled, crossover trial. Neurology. 1997;150:S35.
106. Cutler NR, Claghorn J, Sramek JJ, et al. Pilot study of MK462 in migraine. Cephalalgia. 1996;16(2):113–6.
107. Gijsman H, Kramer MS, Sargent J, et al. Double-blind, placebo-controlled, dose-finding study of rizatriptan (MK-462) in the acute treatment of migraine. Cephalalgia. 1997;17(6):647–51.
108. Teall J, Tuchman M, Cutler N, et al. Rizatriptan (MAXALT) for the acute treatment of migraine and migraine recurrence. A placebo-controlled, outpatient study (Rizatriptan 022 study group). Headache. 1998;38(4):281–7.
109. Visser WH, Lines CR, Reines SA, Group TRD-FS. Dose-finding studies of rizatriptan (MK-462) in the acute treatment of migraine. Cephalalgia. 1996;16:359–60.
110. Ahrens SP, Farmer MV, Williams DL, et al. Efficacy and safety of rizatriptan wafer for the acute treatment of migraine. Rizatriptan wafer protocol 049 study group. Cephalalgia. 1999;19(5):525–30.
111. Klapper JA, O'Connor S. Rizatriptan wafer–sublingual vs. placebo at the onset of acute migraine. Cephalalgia. 2000;20(6):585–7.
112. Jones A, O'Gorman C, Lipton R, Tepper S, Tabuteau H. Efficacy and safety of AXS-07 (MoSEIC Meloxicam-Rizatriptan) for the acute treatment of migraine: results from the INTERCEPT Phase 3, randomized, double-blind, placebo-controlled trial. Paper presented at: JOURNAL OF HEADACHE AND PAIN2021.
113. O'Gorman C, Jones A, TenHuisen K, et al. AXS-07 (MoSEIC™ Meloxicam/Rizatriptan): Novel oral therapeutic in clinical development for the acute treatment of migraine. Paper presented at: CEPHALALGIA2019.
114. Rapoport AM, Ramadan NM, Adelman JU, et al. Optimizing the dose of zolmitriptan (Zomig, 311C90) for the acute treatment of migraine: A multicenter, double-blind, placebo-controlled, dose range-finding study. 017 clinical trial study group. Neurology. 1997;49(5):1210–8.
115. Solomon GD, Cady RK, Klapper JA, Earl NL, Saper JR, Ramadan NM. Clinical efficacy and tolerability of 2.5mg zolmitriptan for the acute treatment of migraine. Neurology. 1997;49:1219–25.
116. Dahlof C, Diener HC, Goadsby PJ, et al. Zolmitriptan, a 5-HT1B/1D receptor agonist for the acute oral treatment of migraine: a multicentre, dose-range finding study. Eur J Neurol. 1998;5(6):535–43.
117. Charlesworth B, Dowson AJ, Purdy A, Becker W, Boes-Hansen S, Farkkila AM. Zolmitriptan nasal spray is fast-acting, effective and well tolerated in acute treatment of migraine. Neurology. 2002;
118. Loder E, Freitag FG, Adelman J, Pearlmand S, bu-Shakra S. Pain-free rates with zolmitriptan 2.5 mg ODT in the acute treatment of migraine: results of a large double-blind placebo- controlled trial. Curr Med Res Opin. 2005;21(3):381–9.
119. Charlesworth BR, Dowson AJ, Purdy A, Becker WJ, Boes-Hansen S, Farkkila M. Speed of onset and efficacy of zolmitriptan nasal spray in the acute treatment of migraine: a randomised, double-blind, placebo-controlled, dose-ranging study versus zolmitriptan tablet. CNS Drugs. 2003;17(9):653–67.
120. Dodick DW, Brandes J, Elkind A, Mathew N, Rodichok L. Speed of onset, efficacy and tolerability of zolmitriptan nasal spray in the acute treatment of migraine: a randomised, double-blind, placebo-controlled study. CNS Drugs. 2005;19:125–36.
121. Gawel M, Aschoff J, May A, Charlesworth BR. Zolmitriptan 5 mg nasal spray: efficacy and onset of action in the acute treatment of migraine – results from phase 1 of the REALIZE study. Headache. 2005;45:7–16.
122. Ahn AH, Basbaum AI. Where do triptans act in the treatment of migraine? Pain. 2005;115(1–2):1–4.
123. Rubio-Beltrán E, Labastida-Ramírez A, Haanes KA, et al. Characterization of binding, functional activity, and contractile responses of the selective 5-HT1F receptor agonist lasmiditan. Br J Pharmacol. 2019;176(24):4681–95.
124. Nelson DL, Phebus LA, Johnson KW, et al. Preclinical pharmacological profile of the selective 5-HT1F receptor agonist lasmiditan. Cephalalgia. 2010;30(10):1159–69.
125. Goadsby PJ, Wietecha LA, Dennehy EB, et al. Phase 3 randomized, placebo-controlled, double-blind study of lasmiditan for acute treatment of migraine. Brain. 2019;142(7):1894–904.
126. Kuca B, Silberstein SD, Wietecha L, Berg PH, Dozier G, Lipton RB. Lasmiditan is an effective acute treatment for migraine: a phase 3 randomized study. Neurology. 2018;91(24):e2222–32.
127. Yang Y, Sun Y, Gao B, Wang Z, Chen Z, Wang Z. Lasmiditan for acute treatment of migraine in adults: a systematic review and meta-analysis of Randomized Controlled Trials. CNS Drugs. 2020;34(10):1015–24.
128. Knievel K, Buchanan AS, Lombard L, et al. Lasmiditan for the acute treatment of migraine: subgroup analyses by prior response to triptans. Cephalalgia. 2020;40(1):19–27.
129. Clemow DB, Baygani SK, Hauck PM, Hultman CB. Lasmiditan in patients with common migraine comorbidities: a post hoc efficacy and safety analysis of two phase 3 randomized clinical trials. Curr Med Res Opin. 2020;36(11):1791–806.
130. Loo LS, Ailani J, Schim J, et al. Efficacy and safety of lasmiditan in patients using concomitant migraine preventive medications: findings from SAMURAI and SPARTAN, two randomized phase 3 trials. J Headache Pain. 2019;20(1):84.
131. Tepper SJ, Krege JH, Lombard L, et al. Characterization of dizziness after lasmiditan usage: findings from the SAMURAI and SPARTAN acute migraine treatment randomized trials. Headache. 2019;59(7):1052–62.
132. Krege JH, Rizzoli PB, Liffick E, et al. Safety findings from phase 3 lasmiditan studies for acute treatment of migraine: results from SAMURAI and SPARTAN. Cephalalgia. 2019;39(8):957–66.

133. Pearlman EM, Wilbraham D, Dennehy EB, et al. Effects of lasmiditan on simulated driving performance: results of two randomized, blinded, crossover studies with placebo and active controls. Hum Psychopharmacol. 2020;35(5):e2732.
134. Wilbraham D, Berg PH, Tsai M, et al. Abuse potential of Lasmiditan: a phase 1 randomized, placebo- and alprazolam-controlled crossover study. J Clin Pharmacol. 2020;60(4):495–504.
135. Negro A, Martelletti P. Gepants for the treatment of migraine. Expert Opin Investig Drugs. 2019;28(6):555–67.
136. Olesen J, Diener HC, Husstedt IW, et al. Calcitonin gene-related peptide receptor antagonist BIBN 4096 BS for the acute treatment of migraine. N Engl J Med. 2004;350(11):1104–10.
137. Ho AP, Dahlof CG, Silberstein SD, et al. Randomized, controlled trial of telcagepant over four migraine attacks. Cephalalgia. 2010;30(12):1443–57.
138. Ho TW, Connor KM, Zhang Y, et al. Randomized controlled trial of the CGRP receptor antagonist telcagepant for migraine prevention. Neurology. 2014;83(11):958–66.
139. Moreno-Ajona D, Perez-Rodriguez A, Goadsby PJ. Gepants, calcitonin-gene-related peptide receptor antagonists: what could be their role in migraine treatment? Curr Opin Neurol. 2020;33(3):309–15.
140. Favoni V, Giani L, Al-Hassany L, et al. CGRP and migraine from a cardiovascular point of view: what do we expect from blocking CGRP? J Headache Pain. 2019;20(1):1–7.
141. Dodick DW, Lipton RB, Ailani J, et al. Ubrogepant for the treatment of migraine. N Engl J Med. 2019;381(23):2230–41.
142. Lipton RB, Dodick DW, Ailani J, et al. Effect of ubrogepant vs placebo on pain and the most bothersome associated symptom in the acute treatment of migraine: the ACHIEVE II randomized clinical trial. JAMA. 2019;322(19):1887–98.
143. Lipton RB, Croop R, Stock EG, et al. Rimegepant, an Oral calcitonin gene-related peptide receptor antagonist, for migraine. N Engl J Med. 2019;381(2):142–9.
144. Croop R, Goadsby PJ, Stock DA, et al. Efficacy, safety, and tolerability of rimegepant orally disintegrating tablet for the acute treatment of migraine: a randomised, phase 3, double-blind, placebo-controlled trial. Lancet. 2019;394(10200):737–45.
145. Chaturvedula PV, Mercer SE, Pin SS, et al. Discovery of (R)-N-(3-(7-methyl-1H-indazol-5-yl)-1-(4-(1-methylpiperidin-4-yl)-1-oxopropan-2-yl)-4-(2-oxo-1, 2-dihydroquinolin-3-yl) piperidine-1-carboxamide (BMS-742413): a potent human CGRP antagonist with superior safety profile for the treatment of migraine through intranasal delivery. Bioorg Med Chem Lett. 2013;23(11):3157–3161.
146. Mercer SE, Chaturvedula PV, Conway CM, et al. Azepino-indazoles as calcitonin gene-related peptide (CGRP) receptor antagonists. Bioorg Med Chem Lett. 2021;31:127624.
147. Wenzel RG, Sarvis CA, Krause ML. Over-the-counter drugs for acute migraine attacks: literature review and recommendations. Pharmacotherapy. 2003;23(4):494–505.
148. Larsen BH, Christiansen LV, Andersen B, Olesen J. Randomized double-blind comparison of tolfenamic acid and paracetamol in migraine. Acta Neurol Scand. 1990;81(5):464–7.
149. Lipton RB, Baggish JS, Stewart WF, Codispoti M. Efficacy and safety of acetaminophen in the treatment of migraine: results of a randomized, double-blind, placebo-controlled, population-based study. Arch Intern Med. 2000;160:3486–92.
150. Derry S, Moore RA. Paracetamol (acetaminophen) with or without an antiemetic for acute migraine headaches in adults. Cochrane Database Syst Rev. 2013;2013(4):CD008040.
151. Pradalier A, Clapin A, Dry J. Treatment review: nonsteroid anti-inflammatory drugs in the treatment and long-term prevention of migraine attacks. Headache. 1988;28:550–7.
152. Lashbrook JM, Ossipov MH, Hunter JC, Raffa RB, Tallarida RJ, Porreca F. Synergistic antiallodynic effects of spinal morphine with ketorolac and selective COX1- and COX2-inhibitors in nerve-injured rats. Pain. 1999;82(1):65–72.
153. Wallace JL, Cirino G. The development of gastrointestinal-sparing nonsteroidal antiinflammatory drugs. Trends Pharmacol Sci. 1994;15:405–6.
154. Diener HC, Bussone G, de Liano H, et al. Placebo-controlled comparison of effervescent acetylsalicylic acid, sumatriptan and ibuprofen in the treatment of migraine attacks. Cephalalgia. 2004;24(11):947–54.
155. Diener HC. Efficacy and safety of intravenous acetylsalicylic acid lysinate compared to subcutaneous sumatriptan and parenteral placebo in the acute treatment of migraine. A double-blind, double-dummy, randomized, multicenter, parallel group study. The ASASUMAMIG study group. Cephalalgia. 1999;19(6):581–8.
156. MacGregor EA, Dowson A, Davies PT. Mouth-dispersible aspirin in the treatment of migraine: a placebo-controlled study. Headache. 2002;42(4):249–55.
157. Boureau F, Joubert JM, Lasserre V, Prum B, Delecoeuillerie G. Double-blind comparison of an acetaminophen 400mg-codeine 25mg combination versus aspirin 1000mg and placebo in acute migraine attack. Cephalalgia. 1994;14(2):156–61.
158. Kirthi V, Derry S, Moore RA, McQuay HJ. Aspirin with or without an antiemetic for acute migraine headaches in adults. Cochrane Database Syst Rev. 2010;14(4):CD008041.
159. Codispoti JR, Prior MJ, Fu M, Harte CM, Nelson EB. Efficacy of nonprescription doses of ibuprofen for treating migraine headache. A randomized controlled trial. Headache. 2001;41(7):665–79.
160. Misra UK, Jose M, Kalita J. Rofecoxib versus ibuprofen for acute treatment of migraine: a randomised placebo controlled trial. Postgrad Med J. 2004;80(950):720–3.
161. Saper J, Dahlof C, So Y, et al. Rofecoxib in the acute treatment of migraine: a randomized controlled clinical trial. Headache. 2006;46(2):264–75.
162. Goldstein J, Silberstein SD, Saper JR, Ryan RE Jr, Lipton RB. Acetaminophen, aspirin, and caffeine in combination versus ibuprofen for acute migraine: results from a multicenter, double-blind, randomized, parallel-group, single-dose, placebo-controlled study. Headache. 2006;46(3):444–53.
163. Dahlof C, Bjorkman R. Diclofenac-K (50 and 100mg) and placebo in the acute treatment of migraine. Cephalalgia. 1993;13(2):117–23.
164. Peroutka SJ, Lyon JA, Swarbrick J, Lipton RB, Kolodner K, Goldstein J. Efficacy of diclofenac sodium softgel 100 mg with or without caffeine 100 mg in migraine without aura: a randomized, double-blind, crossover study. Headache. 2004;44(2):136–41.
165. Group TD-K-SMS. Acute treatment of migraine attacks: efficacy and safety of a nonsteroidal anti-inflammatory drug, diclofenac/potassium, in comparison to oral sumatriptan and placebo. Cephalalgia. 1999;19:232–40.
166. Lipton RB, Grosberg B, Singer RP, et al. Efficacy and tolerability of a new powdered formulation of diclofenac potassium for oral solution for the acute treatment of migraine: results from the international migraine Pain assessment clinical trial (IMPACT). Cephalalgia. 2010;30(11):1336–45.
167. Davis CP, Torre PR, Williams C, et al. Ketorolac versus meperidine-plus-promethazine treatment of migraine headache: evaluations by patients. Am J Emerg Med. 1995;13(2):146–50.
168. Klapper J, Stanton JS. Ketorolac versus DHE and metoclopramide in the treatment of migraine headaches. Headache. 1991;31(8):523–4.
169. Shrestha M, Singh R, Moreden J, Hayes JE. Ketorolac vs chlorpromazine in the treatment of acute migraine without aura. A

prospective, randomized, double-blind trial. Arch Intern Med. 1996;156:1725–8.
170. Engel ER, Cheng J. IM ketorolac vs diclofenac potassium powder for oral solution for the acute treatment of severe migraine: a randomized controlled trial. Neurol Sci. 2020;41(3):537–42.
171. Rao AS, Gelaye B, Kurth T, Dash PD, Nitchie H, Peterlin BL. A randomized trial of ketorolac vs. Sumatripan vs. placebo nasal spray (KSPN) for acute migraine. Headache. 2016;56(2):331–40.
172. Awidi AS. Efficacy of flurbiprofen in the treatment of acute migraine attacks: a double-blind cross-over study. Curr Ther Res. 1982;32(3):492–7.
173. Andersson PG, Hinge HH, Johansen O, Andersen CU, Lademann A, Gotzsche PC. Double-blind study of naproxen vs placebo in the treatment of acute migraine attacks. Cephalalgia. 1989;9(1):29–32.
174. Johnson ES, Ratcliffe DM, Wilkinson M. Naproxen sodium in the treatment of migraine. Cephalalgia. 1985;5(1):5–10.
175. Nappi G, Micieli G, Tassorelli C, Viotti E, Altavilla T. Effectiveness of a piroxicam fast dissolving formulation sublingually administered in the symptomatic treatment of migraine without aura. Headache. 1993;33(6):296–300.
176. Guidotti M, Zanasi S, Garagiola U. Pirprofen in the treatment of migraine and episodic headache attacks: a placebo-controlled crossover clinical trial. J Int Med Res. 1989;17(1):48–54.
177. Lipton RB, Munjal S, Dodick DW, Tepper SJ, Serrano D, Iaconangelo C. Acute treatment of migraine with celecoxib Oral solution: results of a randomized, placebo-controlled clinical trial. J Pain Res. 2021;14:549–60.
178. Lipton RB, Munjal S, Tepper SJ, Iaconangelo C, Serrano D. A multicenter, randomized, double-blind, placebo-controlled study of the efficacy, tolerability, and safety of celecoxib Oral solution (ELYXYB) in acute treatment of episodic migraine with or without Aura. J Pain Res. 2021;14:2529–42.
179. Dib M, Massiou H, Weber M, Henry P, Garcia-Acosta S, Bousser MG. Efficacy of oral ketoprofen in acute migraine: a double-blind randomized clinical trial. Neurology. 2002;58(11):1660–5.
180. Lipton RB, Stewart WF, Ryan RE, Saper J, Silberstein S, Sheftell F. Efficacy and safety of the nonprescription combination of acetaminophen, aspirin, and caffeine in alleviating headache pain of an acute migraine attack: three double-blind, randomized, placebo-controlled trials. Arch Neurol. 1998;55:210–7.
181. Goldstein J, Silberstein SD, Saper JR, et al. Acetaminophen, aspirin, and caffeine versus sumatriptan succinate in the early treatment of migraine: results from the ASSET trial. Headache. 2005;45(8):973–82.
182. Diener HC, Pfaffenrath V, Pageler L, Peil H, Aicher B. The fixed combination of acetylsalicylic acid, paracetamol and caffeine is more effective than single substances and dual combination for the treatment of headache: a multicentre, randomized, double-blind, single-dose, placebo-controlled parallel group study. Cephalalgia. 2005;25(10):776–87.
183. Griffin MR, Piper JM, Daugherty JR, Snowden M, Ray WA. Nonsteroidal antiinflammatory drug use and increased risk for peptic ulcer disease in elderly persons. Ann Intern Med. 1991;114:257–63.
184. McGettigan P, Henry D. Cardiovascular risk and inhibition of cyclooxygenase: a systematic review of the observational studies of selective and nonselective inhibitors of cyclooxygenase 2. JAMA. 2006;296(13):1633–44.
185. Starling AJ, Hoffman-Snyder C, Halker RB, et al. Risk of development of medication overuse headache with nonsteroidal anti-inflammatory drug therapy for migraine: a critically appraised topic. Neurologist. 2011;17(5):297–9.
186. Ryan RE. A study of Midrin[R] in the symptomatic relief of migraine headache. Headache. 1974;14:33–42.
187. Diamond S, Medina JL. Isometheptene–a nonergot drug in the treatment of migraine. Headache. 1975;15(3):211–3.
188. Ogden HD. Controlled studies of a new agent in vascular headache. Headache. 1963;3(1):29–31.
189. Diamond S. Treatment of migraine with isometheptene, acetaminophen, and dichloralphenazone combination: a double-blind, crossover trial. Headache. 1976;15(4):282–7.
190. Campos CR, Yamamoto FI. Intracerebral hemorrhage in postpartum cerebral angiography associated with the use of isometheptene. Int J Gynaecol Obstet. 2006;95:151–2.
191. Wineinger M, Basford JR. Autonomic dysreflexia due to medication: misadventure in the use of an isometheptene combination to treat migraine. Arch Phys Med Rehabil. 1985;66(9):645–6.
192. Rowat BM, Merrill CF, Davis A, South V. A double-blind comparison of granisetron and placebo for the treatment of acute migraine in the emergency department. Cephalalgia. 1991;11(5):207–13.
193. Chappell AS, Bay JJ, Botzum GD, Cohen ML. Zatosetron, a 5HT3 receptor antagonist in a multicenter trial for acute migraine. Neuropharmacology. 1994;33(3–4):509–13.
194. Wijemanne S, Jankovic J, Evans RW. Movement disorders from the use of metoclopramide and other antiemetics in the treatment of migraine. Headache. 2016;56(1):153–61.
195. Marmura MJ. Use of dopamine antagonists in treatment of migraine. Curr Treat Options Neurol. 2012;14(1):27–35.
196. Matchar DB, Young WB, Rosenberg JA, et al. Evidence-based guidelines for migraine headache in the primary care setting: pharmacological management of acute attacks. Neurology. 2000; available from http://www.aan.com
197. Albibi R, McCallum RW. Metoclopramide: pharmacology and clinical application. Ann Intern Med. 1983;98:86–95.
198. Azzopardi TD, Brooks NA. Oral metoclopramide as an adjunct to analgesics for the outpatient treatment of acute migraine. Ann Pharmacother. 2008;42(3):397–402.
199. Friedman BW, Mulvey L, Esses D, et al. Metoclopramide for acute migraine: a dose-finding randomized clinical trial. Ann Emerg Med. 2011;57(5):475–82. e471
200. Sharma S, Prasad A, Nehru R, et al. Efficacy and tolerability of prochlorperazine buccal tablets in treatment of acute migraine. Headache. 2002;42(9):896–902.
201. Tietjen GE, Athanas K, Utley C, Herial NA, Khuder SA. The combination of naratriptan and prochlorperazine in migraine treatment. Headache. 2005;45(6):751–3.
202. Silberstein SD, Young WB, Mendizabal JE, Rothrock JF, Alam AS. Acute migraine treatment with the dopamine receptor antagonist, droperidol: results of a randomized, double-blind, placebo-controlled, multicenter trial. Neurology. 2003;60:315–21.
203. Honkaniemi J, Liimatainen S, Rainesalo S, Sulavuori S. Haloperidol in the acute treatment of migraine: a randomized, double blind, placebo controlled study. Neurology. 2004;62(7 Suppl5):A516.
204. Silberstein SD, McCrory DC. Butalbital-containing compounds for the treatment of tension-type and migraine headache. Headache. 2001;
205. Goldstein J, Gawel MJ, Winner P, et al. Comparison of butorphanol nasal spray and fiorinal with codeine in the treatment of migraine. Headache. 1988;38:516–22.
206. Wenzel RG, Sarvis CA. Do butalbital-containing products have a role in the management of migraine? Pharmacotherapy. 2002;22(8):1029–35.
207. Bigal ME, Lipton RB. Overuse of acute migraine medications and migraine chronification. Curr Pain Headache Rep. 2009;13(4):301–7.
208. Gawel MJ, Szalai JF, Stiglick A, Aimola N, Weiner M. Evaluation of analgesic agents in recurring headache compared with other clinical pain models. Clin Pharmacol Therapeut. 1990;47(4):504–8.
209. Diamond S, Freitag FG, Diamond ML, Urban G. Transnasal butorphanol in the treatment of migraine headache pain. Headache Qua. 1992;3(2):164–71.

210. Loder E. Post-marketing experience with an opioid nasal spray for migraine: lessons for the future. Cephalalgia. 2006;26(2):89–97.
211. Marmura MJ, Silberstein SD, Schwedt TJ. The acute treatment of migraine in adults: the american headache society evidence assessment of migraine pharmacotherapies. Headache. 2015;55(1):3–20.
212. Silberstein SD, Freitag FG, Rozen TD, et al. Tramadol/acetaminophen for the treatment of acute migraine pain: findings of a randomized, placebo-controlled trial. Headache. 2005;45(10):1317–27.
213. Saper JR, Lake AE, Hamel RH. Sustained, scheduled opioid therapy for patients with intractable headache: a 5-year prospective study. Presented to the American headache society, ACHE award lecture, Montreal, Quebec, June.
214. Minen MT, Lindberg K, Wells RE, et al. Survey of opioid and barbiturate prescriptions in patients attending a tertiary care headache center. Headache. 2015;55(9):1183–91.
215. Patel UK, Malik P, Shah D, et al. The opioid epidemic and primary headache disorders: a nationwide population-based study. Cureus. 2020;12:8.
216. Bigal ME, Lipton RB. Excessive opioid use and the development of chronic migraine. Pain. 2009;142(3):179–82.
217. Pressman AR, Buse DC, Jacobson AS, et al. The migraine signature study: methods and baseline results. Headache. 2021;61(3):462–84.
218. Lipton RB, Buse DC, Friedman BW, et al. Characterizing opioid use in a US population with migraine: results from the CaMEO study. Neurology. 2020;95(5):e457–68.
219. Wells RE, Markowitz SY, Baron EP, et al. Identifying the factors underlying discontinuation of triptans. Headache. 2014;54(2):278–89.
220. Tepper SJ. Opioids should not be used in migraine. Headache. 2012;52(Suppl 1):30–4.
221. Fuller GN, Guiloff RJ. Propranolol in acute migraine: a controlled study. Cephalalgia. 1990;10:229–33.
222. Hoffert MJ, Scholz MJ, Kanter RJC. A double-blind controlled study of nifedipine as an abortive treatment in acute attacks of migraine with aura. Cephalalgia. 1992;12(5):323–4.
223. Takeshima T, Nishikawa S, Takashashi K. Sublingual administration of flunarizine for acute migraine: will flunarizine take the place of ergotamine? Headache. 1988;28:602–6.
224. Lipton RB, Goadsby PJ, Smith J, et al. Efficacy and safety of eptinezumab in patients with chronic migraine: PROMISE-2. Neurology. 2020;94(13):e1365–77.
225. Maizels M, Scott B, Cohen W, Chen W. Intranasal lidocaine for treatment of migraine: a randomized, double-blind, controlled trial. JAMA. 1996;276(4):319–21.
226. Maizels M. Intranasal lidocaine for migraine in an outpatient population. Headache. 1998;38(5):391.
227. Blanda M, Rench T, Gerson LW, Weigand JV. Intranasal lidocaine for the treatment of migraine headache: a randomized, controlled trial. Acad Emerg Med. 2001;8(4):337–42.
228. Gallagher RM. Emergency treatment of intractable migraine. Headache. 1986;26:74–5.
229. Woldeamanuel YW, Rapoport AM, Cowan RPJC. The place of corticosteroids in migraine attack management: a 65-year systematic review with pooled analysis and critical appraisal. Cephalalgia. 2015;35(11):996–1024.
230. Saper JR. Chronic headache syndromes. Neurol Clin. 1989;7:387–412.
231. Smith TR. Low dose tizanidine combined with long-acting NSAIDs for detoxification from analgesic rebouns headache, a retrospective review. Cephalalgia. 2000;20(4):381.
232. Kapicioglu S, Gokce E, Kapicioglu Z, Ovali E. Treatment of migraine attacks with a long-acting somatostatin analogue (octreotide, SMS 201-995). Cephalalgia. 1997;17(1):27–30.
233. Levy MJ, Matharu MS, Bhola R, Meeran K, Goadsby PJ. Octreotide is not effective in the acute treatment of migraine. Cephalalgia. 2005;25(1):48–55.
234. Diener H-C, Tassorelli C, Dodick DW, et al. Guidelines of the international headache society for controlled trials of acute treatment of migraine attacks in adults. Cephalalgia. 2019;39(6):687–710.
235. Ailani J, Burch RC, Robbins MS, Board of Directors of the American Headache Society. The American Headache Society consensus statement: update on integrating new migraine treatments into clinical practice. Headache. 2021;61(7):1021–39.
236. American Headache Society. The American Headache Society position statement on integrating new migraine treatments into clinical practice. Headache. 2019;59(1):1–18.
237. Yang CP, Liang CS, Chang CM, et al. Comparison of new pharmacologic agents with Triptans for treatment of migraine: a systematic review and meta-analysis. JAMA Netw Open. 2021;4(10):e2128544.
238. Worthington I, Pringsheim T, Gawel MJ, et al. Canadian Headache Society Guideline: acute drug therapy for migraine headache. Can J Neurol Sci. 2013;40(S3):S1–3.
239. Kostic MA, Gutierrez FJ, Rieg TS, Moore TS, Gendron RT. A prospective, randomized trial of intravenous prochlorperazine versus subcutaneous sumatriptan in acute migraine therapy in the emergency department. Ann Emerg Med. 2010;56(1):1–6.
240. Moshtaghion H, Heiranizadeh N, Rahimdel A, Esmaeili A, Hashemian H, Hekmatimoghaddam S. The efficacy of propofol vs subcutaneous sumatriptan for treatment of acute migraine headaches in the emergency department: a double-blinded clinical trial. Pain Pract. 2015;15(8):701–5.
241. Orr SL, Friedman BW, Christie S, et al. Management of adults with acute migraine in the emergency department: the American headache society evidence assessment of parenteral pharmacotherapies. Headache. 2016;56(6):911–40.
242. Kelley NE, Tepper DE. Rescue therapy for acute migraine, part 1: triptans, dihydroergotamine, and magnesium. Headache. 2012;52(1):114–28.
243. Kelley NE, Tepper DE. Rescue therapy for acute migraine, part 2: neuroleptics, antihistamines, and others. Headache. 2012;52(2):292–306.
244. Kelley NE, Tepper DE. Rescue therapy for acute migraine, part 3: Opioids, NSAIDs, steroids, and post-discharge medications. Headache. 2012;52(3):467–82.
245. Taggart E, Doran S, Kokotillo A, et al. Ketorolac in the treatment of acute migraine: a systematic review. Headache. 2013;53(2):277–87.
246. Jakubowski M, Levy D, Goor-Aryeh I, Collins B, Bajwa Z, Burstein R. Terminating migraine with allodynia and ongoing central sensitization using parenteral administration of COX1/COX2 inhibitors. Headache. 2005;45(7):850–61.
247. Yuan H, Curran JG, Keith SW, Hopkins MM, Silberstein SD. Intravenous ibuprofen for acute treatment of migraine: a double-blind, randomized, placebo-controlled pilot study. Headache. 2021;
248. Bigal ME, Bordini CA, Speciali JG. Intravenous metamizol (Dipyrone) in acute migraine treatment and in episodic tension-type headache--a placebo-controlled study. Cephalalgia. 2001;21(2):90–5.
249. Krymchantowski AV, Carneiro H, Barbosa J, Jevoux C. Lysine clonixinate versus dipyrone (metamizole) for the acute treatment of severe migraine attacks: a single-blind, randomized study. Arq Neuropsiquiatr. 2008;66:216–20.
250. Engindeniz Z, Demircan C, Karli N, et al. Intramuscular tramadol vs diclofenac sodium for the treatment of acute migraine attacks in emergency department: a prospective, randomised, double–blind study. J Headache Pain. 2005;6(3):143–8.

251. Friedman BW, West J, Vinson DR, Minen MT, Restivo A, Gallagher EJJC. Current management of migraine in US emergency departments: an analysis of the National Hospital Ambulatory Medical Care Survey. Cephalalgia. 2015;35(4):301–9.
252. Larkin GL, Prescott JE. A randomized, double-blind, comparative study of the efficacy of ketorolac tromethamine versus meperidine in the treatment of severe migraine. Ann Emerg Med. 1992;21(8):919–24.
253. Belgrade M, Ling L, Schleevogt M, Ettinger M, Ruiz EJN. Comparison of single dose meperidine, butorphanol, and dihydroergotamine in the treatment of vascular headache. Neurology. 1989;39(4):590.
254. Alemdar M, Pekdemir M, Selekler HM. Single-dose intravenous tramadol for acute migraine pain in adults: a single-blind, prospective, randomized, placebo-controlled clinical trial. Clin Ther. 2007;29(7):1441–7.
255. Friedman BW, Irizarry E, Solorzano C, et al. Randomized study of IV prochlorperazine plus diphenhydramine vs IV hydromorphone for migraine. Headache. 2017;89(20):2075–82.
256. Cohen F, Friedman BW. A randomized study of IV prochlorperazine plus diphenhydramine versus IV hydromorphone for migraine-associated symptoms: a post hoc analysis. 2021;61(8):1227–33.
257. Baden EY, Hunter CJ. Intravenous dexamethasone to prevent the recurrence of benign headache after discharge from the emergency department: a randomized, double-blind, placebo-controlled clinical trial. CJEM. 2006;8(6):393–400.
258. Friedman B, Greenwald P, Bania T, et al. Randomized trial of IV dexamethasone for acute migraine in the emergency department. Neurology. 2007;69(22):2038–44.
259. Innes GD, Macphail I, Dillon EC, Metcalfe C, Gao M. Dexamethasone prevents relapse after emergency department treatment of acute migraine: a randomized clinical trial. CJEM. 1999;1(1):26–33.
260. Jones J, Sklar D, Dougherty J, White W. Randomized double-blind trial of intravenous prochlorperazine for the treatment of acute headache. JAMA. 1989;261(8):1174–6.
261. Jones J, Pack S, Chun E. Intramuscular prochlorperazine versus metoclopramide as single-agent therapy for the treatment of acute migraine headache. Am J Emerg Med. 1996;14(3):262–4.
262. Ginder S, Oatman B, Pollack M. A prospective study of i.v. magnesium and i.v. prochlorperazine in the treatment of headaches. J Emerg Med. 2000;18(3):311–5.
263. Seim MB, March JA, Dunn KA. Intravenous ketorolac vs intravenous prochlorperazine for the treatment of migraine headaches. Acad Emerg Med. 1998;5(6):573–6.
264. Colman I, Brown MD, Innes GD, Grafstein E, Roberts TE, Rowe BH. Parenteral metoclopramide for acute migraine: meta-analysis of randomised controlled trials. BMJ. 2004;329(7479):1369–73.
265. Bigal ME, Bordini CA, Speciali JG. Intravenous chlorpromazine in the emergency department treatment of migraines: a randomized controlled trial. J Emerg Med. 2002;23(2):141–8.
266. Silberstein SD, Young WB, Mendizabal J, Rothrock J, Alam A. Efficacy of intramuscular droperidol for migraine treatment: a dose response study. Headache Qua. 1999;10:55–7.
267. Wang SJ, Silberstein SD, Young WB. Droperidol treatment of status migrainosus and refractory migraine. Headache. 1997;37:377–82.
268. Honkaniemi J, Liimatainen S, Rainesalo S, Sulavuori S. Haloperidol in the acute treatment of migraine: a randomized, double-blind, placebo-controlled study. Headache. 2006;46(5):781–7.
269. Klapper JA, Stanton JS. The emergency treatment of acute migraine headache; a comparison of intravenous dihydroergotamine, dexamethasone, and placebo. Cephalalgia. 1991;11(Suppl 11):159–60.
270. Edwards KR, Norton J, Behnke M. Comparison of intravenous valproate versus intramuscular dihydroergotamine and metoclopramide for acute treatment of migraine headache. Headache. 2001;41(10):976–80.
271. Belgrade MJ, Ling LJ, Schleevogt MB, Ettinger MG, Ruiz E. Comparison of single-dose meperidine, butorphanol, and dihydroergotamine in the treatment of vascular headache. Neurology. 1989;39:590–2.
272. Scherl ER, Wilson JF. Comparison of dihydroergotamine with metoclopramide versus meperidine with promethazine in the treatment of acute migraine. Headache. 1995;35(5):256–9.
273. Carleton SC, Shesser RF, Pietrzak MP, et al. Double-blind, multicenter trial to compare the efficacy of intramuscular dihydroergotamine plus hydroxyzine versus intramuscular meperidine plus hydroxyzine for the emergency department treatment of acute migraine headache. Ann Emerg Med. 1998;32(2):129–38.
274. Callaham M, Raskin N. A controlled study of dihydroergotamine in the treatment of acute migraine headache. Headache. 1986;26:168–71.
275. Mauskop A, Altura BT, Cracco RQ, Altura BM. Intravenous magnesium sulfate rapidly alleviates headaches of various types. Headache. 1996;36(3):154–60.
276. Demirkaya S, Vural O, Dora B, Topcuoglu MA. Efficacy of intravenous magnesium sulfate in the treatment of acute migraine attacks. Headache. 2001;41(2):171–7.
277. Corbo J, Esses D, Bijur PE, Iannacconne R, Gallagher EJ. Randomized clinical trial of intravenous magnesium sulfate as an adjunctive medication for emergency department treatment of migraine headache. Ann Emerg Med. 2001;38(6):621–7.
278. Bigal ME, Bordini CA, Tepper SJ, Speciali JG. Intravenous magnesium sulphate in the acute treatment of migraine without aura and migraine with aura. A randomized, double-blind, placebo-controlled study. Cephalalgia. 2002;22(5):345–53.
279. Mathew NT, Kailasam J, Meadors L, Chernyschev O, Gentry P. Intravenous valproate sodium (depacon) aborts migraine rapidly: a preliminary report. Headache. 2000;40(9):720–3.
280. Shahien R, Saleh S, Bowirrat A. Intravenous sodium valproate aborts migraine headaches rapidly. Acta Neurol Scand. 2011;123(4):257–65.
281. Karimi N, Tavakoli M, Charati JY, Shamsizade M. Single-dose intravenous sodium valproate (Depakine) versus dexamethasone for the treatment of acute migraine headache: a double-blind randomized clinical trial. Clin Exp Emerg Med. 2017;4(3):138.
282. Tanen DA, Miller S, French T, Riffenburgh RH. Intravenous sodium valproate versus prochlorperazine for the emergency department treatment of acute migraine headaches: a prospective, randomized, double-blind trial. Ann Emerg Med. 2003;41(6):847–53.
283. Farooq MU, Majid A, Pysh JJ, Kassab MY. Role of intravenous levetiracetam in status migrainosus. J Headache Pain. 2007;8(2):143–4.
284. Rosen N, Silberstein S, Abbas MA. Effect of lidocaine infusion in the treatment of refractory chronic daily headache – a retrospective study. Neurology. 2006;66:A224.
285. Williams DR, Stark RJ. Intravenous lignocaine (lidocaine) infusion for the treatment of chronic daily headache with substantial medication overuse. Cephalalgia. 2003;23(10):963–71.
286. Gur STA, Ahiskalioglu EO, Aydin ME, Kocak AO, Aydin P, Ahiskalioglu A. Intravenous lidocaine vs. NSAIDs for migraine attack in the ED: a prospective, randomized, double-blind study. Eur J Clin Pharmacol. 2021;78(1):27–33.

287. Pomeroy JL, Marmura MJ, Nahas SJ, Viscusi ER. Ketamine infusions for treatment refractory headache. Headache. 2017;57(2):276–82.
288. Lauritsen C, Mazuera S, Lipton RB, Ashina S. Intravenous ketamine for subacute treatment of refractory chronic migraine: a case series. J Headache Pain. 2016;17(1):106.
289. Etchison AR, Bos L, Ray M, et al. Low-dose ketamine does not improve migraine in the emergency department: a randomized placebo-controlled trial. 2018;19(6):952.
290. Zitek T, Gates M, Pitotti C, et al. A comparison of headache treatment in the emergency department: prochlorperazine versus ketamine. Ann Emerg Med. 2018;71(3):369–77. e361
291. Krusz JC, Scott V. Topiramate in the treatment of chronic migraine and other headaches. Headache. 1999;39:363.
292. Soleimanpour H, Ghafouri RR, Taheraghdam A, et al. Effectiveness of intravenous dexamethasone versus propofol for pain relief in the migraine headache: a prospective double blind randomized clinical trial. BMC Neurol. 2012;12(1):1–7.
293. Krusz JC, Belanger J. Propofol--a highly effective treatment for acute headaches. Cephalalgia. 1999;19:358.
294. Lucado J, Paez K, Elixhauser A. Headaches in U.S. Hospitals and emergency departments, 2008: statistical brief #111. 2006.
295. Freitag FG, Lake A, Lipton RB, Cady R, Diamond S, Silberstein SD. Inpatient treatment of headache: an evidence-based assessment. United States Headache Guidelines Consortium. Headache. 2004;44:342–60.
296. Dougherty CO, Marmura MJ, Ergonul Z, Charleston LC, Szperka CL. Emergency and inpatient treatment of migraine: an American headache society survey. Br J Med Med Res. 2014;4(20):3800–13.
297. Lake AE III, Saper JR, Hamel RL. Comprehensive inpatient treatment of refractory chronic daily headache. Headache. 2009;49(4):555–62.
298. Diamond S, Freitag FG, Maliszewski M. Inpatient treatment of headache: long-term results. Headache. 1986;26:189–97.
299. Villarreal SS. A comparative study of selected patient variables as risk factors in hospitalization for chronic headache. Headache. 1995;35:349–54.
300. Raskin NH. Repetitive intravenous dihydroergotamine as therapy for intractable migraine. Neurology. 1986;36:995–7.
301. Nagy AJ, Gandhi S, Bhola R, Goadsby PJ. Intravenous dihydroergotamine for inpatient management of refractory primary headaches. Neurology. 2011;77(20):1827–32.
302. Silberstein SD, Silberstein JR. Chronic daily headache: prognosis following inpatient treatment with repetitive IV DHE. Headache. 1992;32:439–45.
303. Relja G, Granato A, Bratina A, Antonello RM, Zorzon M. Outcome of medication overuse headache after abrupt in-patient withdrawal. Cephalalgia. 2006;26(5):589–95.
304. Rosen N, Marmura M, Abbas M, Silberstein S. Intravenous lidocaine in the treatment of refractory headache: a retrospective case series. Headache. 2009;49(2):286–91.
305. Gil-Gouveia R, Goadsby PJ. Neuropsychiatric side effects of lidocaine: examples from the treatment of headache and a review. Cephalalgia. 2006;26:1399.
306. Lauritsen C, Mazuera S, Lipton RB, Ashina S. Intravenous ketamine for subacute treatment of refractory chronic migraine: a case series. J Headache Pain. 2016;17(1):1–5.
307. Robblee J, Grimsrud KW. Emergency department and inpatient management of headache in adults. Curr Neurol Neurosci Rep. 2020;20(4):1–9.
308. Mendes PM, Silberstein SD, Young WB, Rozen TD, Paolone MF. Intravenous Propofol in the treatment of refractory headache. Headache. 2002;42(7):638–41.
309. Swidan SZ, Lake AE III, Saper JR. Efficacy of intravenous diphenhydramine versus intravenous DHE-45 in the treatment of severe migraine headache. Curr Pain Headache Rep. 2005;9(1):65–70.
310. Lake AE, Saper JR, Madden SF, Kreeger C. Comprehensive inpatient treatment for intractable migraine: a prospective long-term outcome study. Headache. 1993;33:55–62.
311. Marmura MJ, Hou A. Inpatient management of migraine. Neurol Clin. 2019;37(4):771–88.

Calcitonin Gene-Related Peptide Antagonists in Acute Treatment of Migraine

26

Anjali Sundaramoorthy and Carrie Dougherty

Abbreviations

CRLR	Calcitonin receptor-like receptor,
IV	Intravenous
MOH	Medication overuse headache
NSAID	Nonsteroidal anti-inflammatory drug
RAMP-1	Receptor activity modifying protein 1

Introduction

Migraine is the most common neurological disorder, occurring in about 12% of the US population [1]. It is the second most common cause of disability worldwide [1]. Migraine is characterized by episodes of moderate to severe headaches with accompanying symptoms such as nausea, vomiting, photophobia, and phonophobia. Prior to the development of triptans, there were relatively few options, specifically development for acute treatment of migraine. The class of 5HT1B/D receptor agonists, termed triptans, revolutionized the treatment of migraine and has remained the standard of care since the approval of sumatriptan in the early 1990s. Prior to the 2019 approval of lasmiditan, the development of acute migraine medications was limited to novel routes of administration and reformulations of older medications, mostly triptans and NSAIDs. These medications did little to address the clinical limitations of triptans, which include poor tolerability, lack of consistent efficacy, and the potential for medication overuse headache (MOH).

Gepants are CGRP receptor antagonists. Identifying CGRP as a potential therapeutic target was a breakthrough for migraine treatment, but the trajectory of gepants development was rocky and required three decades to see fruition. The long-awaited debut of this class in late 2019 with ubrogepant, followed by rimegepant in quick succession, and zavegepant, the first non-oral gepant, represents a new era of migraine treatment. Atogepant will be discussed elsewhere as its indication is limited to migraine prevention.

A. Sundaramoorthy (✉)
Department of Neurology, Baylor Scott & White Health, Dallas, TX, USA

C. Dougherty
Department of Neurology, MedStar Georgetown University Hospital, Washington, DC, USA

Questions

1. Which patient would be the best candidate for acute treatment of migraine with a gepant?
   A. A 16-year-old girl with 3–5 migraines each month that respond to OTC NSAIDS
   B. A 37-year-old woman with 3–5 migraine days each month who responds well to rizatriptan and naproxen
   C. A 67-year-old man with migraine with aura 1–2 days each month and a history of ischemic stroke 3 months ago
   D. A 46-year-old woman with 7–9 migraine days each month, who had intolerable side effects in the past with sumatriptan and eletriptan
2. Which preventive migraine medication would require an adjusted dose of ubrogepant?
   A. Topiramate
   B. Amitriptyline
   C. Verapamil
   D. Valproate

Small Molecule CGRP-Targeted Therapies

CGRP is a vasodilatory neuropeptide that plays a key role in cerebrovascular regulation and in the trigeminovascular system [2]. Several clinically relevant observations support CGRP as a potential therapeutic target in migraine. Intravenous infusion of CGRP provokes a migraine-like

T. S. Monteith et al. (eds.), *Comprehensive Migraine Management*, https://doi.org/10.1007/978-3-031-86923-5_26

headache in patients with migraine [3]. CGRP levels are elevated during migraine exacerbation, and chronic migraine patients show persistently increased levels of CGRP even during pain-free intervals [3]. Conversely, the therapeutic benefit of triptans coincides with decreasing CGRP levels [4].

Receptor Pharmacology

Gepants target the CGRP receptor (CGRPR) (Fig. 26.1). The CGRPR consists of three subunits: calcitonin receptor-like receptor (CLR), receptor activity modifying protein 1(RAMP1), and receptor component protein (RCP) [5]. CLR is a G-protein-coupled receptor that must form a heterodimer with RAMP1 to bind CGRP. CGRP binds the cleft that is formed between CLR and RAMP1, activating the CGRPR. Once activated, RCP facilitates the coupling of the subunit of the G protein. This action initiates cAMP-dependent signaling in the cerebral vessel smooth muscle and ultimately vasorelaxation. Gepants are small nonpeptide molecules that compete for a binding pocket produced by the co-receptors RAMP-1 and CLR, components of the CGRP receptor. CGRP receptor antagonists block receptor activation and release of neuropeptides from sensory nerves in the periphery.

The first CGRP receptor antagonist that was shown to inhibit CGRP-mediated vasodilation was olcegepant [6]. Intravenous olcegepant was superior to placebo in 2-h pain relief for acute treatment of migraine, but given the limited clinical utility for IV administration, attention focused on the development of oral gepants [7]. Telcagepant, MK3207, and BI44370 were the first-generation oral gepants evaluated for acute treatment of migraine [8]. Telcagepant was well tolerated for acute migraine treatment, with efficacy superior to placebo and comparable to triptans [9]. Subsequent trials showed preventive benefits on par with

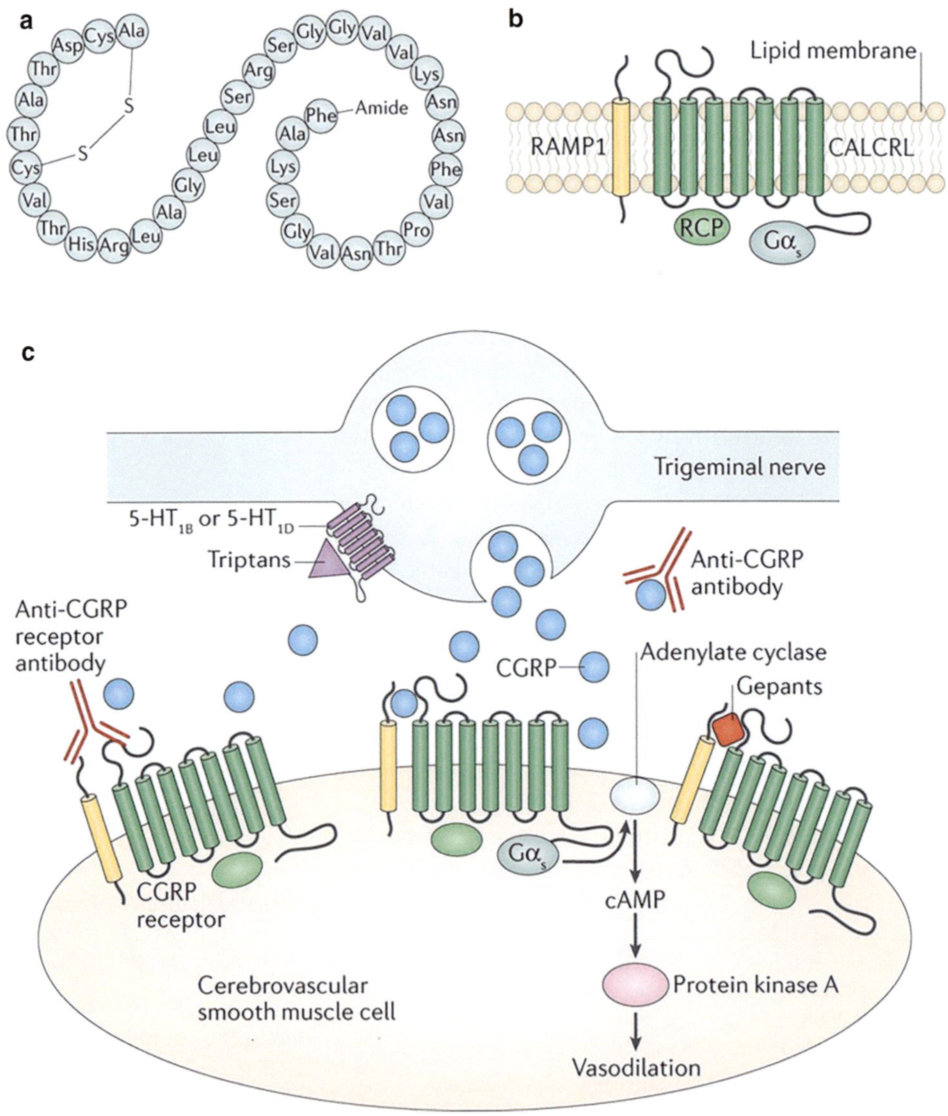

Fig. 26.1 (**a**) Amino acid structure of human α-type calcitonin gene-related peptide (CGRP). (**b**) The CGRP receptor complex, which consists of the two integral membrane proteins calcitonin receptor-like receptor (CALCRL) and receptor activity-modifying protein 1 (RAMP1) and two cytoplasmic proteins, receptor coupling protein (RCP) and the α-subunit of the G_S protein ($G\alpha_S$). (**c**) The targets for CGRP-related migraine therapies are illustrated in a CGRP-containing trigeminal nerve varicosity that innervates a cerebrovascular smooth muscle cell. 5-HT, 5-hydroxytryptamine receptor. (Source: Reprinted with permission from Edvinsson et al. [44])

topiramate [10, 11]. Unfortunately, trials of both telcagepant and MK3207 reported elevated alanine aminotransferase concerning hepatotoxicity [12, 13]. The toxic effect on the liver was attributed to the direct chemical structure of the first-generation molecules and not due to physiologic changes with CGRP antagonism. Further development of these molecules was shelved due to concerns of hepatotoxicity [4]. The proof of efficacy for CGRP-targeted therapies inspired the development of monoclonal antibodies to both CGRP and its receptor. Second-generation gepants, including rimegepant, ubrogepant, and atogepant, are structurally different from their predecessors and have not been associated with liver damage.

Ubrogepant

Ubrogepant is a small molecule CGRP receptor antagonist that was the first in its class to receive FDA approval for the acute treatment of migraine in adults on December 23, 2019. Two phase III trials established the safety and tolerability of ubrogepant in the acute treatment of migraine [14, 15].

These trials, ACHIEVE I and II, were randomized, double-blind, placebo-controlled, and parallel-group trials that assessed the safety and efficacy of ubrogepant at several doses in the acute treatment of migraine. ACHIEVE I evaluated ubrogepant 50 mg, 100 mg, or placebo, while ACHIEVE II also included a 25 mg dose [14, 15]. These studies demonstrated that both 50 mg and 100 mg of ubrogepant were superior to placebo in rates of 2 h pain freedom and freedom from the MBS when compared to placebo (Table 26.1). In ACHIEVE II, 25 mg failed to outperform placebo with respect to MBS freedom.

Ubrogepant is available in 50 mg or 100 mg tablets taken at the onset of headache with the option for a second dose taken 2 h later if needed. The maximum daily dose in a 24-h period is 200 mg. The safety of treating more than eight migraines per month has not been established. Ubrogepant has a peak plasma concentration at 1.5 h after ingestion. The elimination half-life is approximately 5–7 h [16]. Ubrogepant is metabolized through the liver and excreted through biliary, fecal, and renal routes. Dose adjustments for renal and/or hepatic impairment are required. It is not recommended for use in patients with end-stage renal disease, in pregnancy or while breastfeeding, and it is not approved for use in children.

Rimegepant

Rimegepant was approved for acute treatment of migraine on February 27, 2020, and then received an expanded indication as the first gepant for preventive treatment of episodic migraine in adults on May 27, 2021. A phase III double-blind, randomized, and placebo-controlled trial demonstrated that rimegepant was superior to placebo in achieving 2 h pain freedom and freedom from the most bothersome symptom (MBS) [16] (Table 26.1). An open-label safety trial with every other day and interim as-needed dosing demonstrated a reduction in migraine frequency over a 3-month period, indicating potential preventive benefit [18]. A subsequent placebo-controlled trial evaluating every other day dosing was superior at reducing monthly

Table 26.1 Results of primary endpoints of ubrogepant, rimegepant, and zavegepant pivotal trials [14, 15, 17, 22]

Ubrogepant (ACHIEVE I)	**Placebo**	**50 mg**	**100 mg**
% Patients with pain freedom at 2 h	11.8	19.2 ($p = 0.002$)	21.2 ($p < 0.001$)
% Patients with absence of MBS at 2 h	27.8	38.6 ($p = 0.002$)	37.7 ($p = 0.002$)
Ubrogepant (ACHIEVE II)	**Placebo**	**25 mg**	**50 mg**
% Patients with pain freedom at 2 h	14.3	20.7 ($p = 0.03$)	21.8 ($p = 0.01$)
% Patients with absence of MBS at 2 h	27.4	34.1 ($p = 0.07$)	38.9 ($p = 0.01$)
Rimegepant	**Placebo**	**75 mg**	
% Patients with pain freedom at 2 h	12.0%	19.6 ($p < 0.001$)	
% Patients with absence of MBS at 2 h	25.2%	37.6 ($p < 0.001$)	
Zavegepant	**Placebo**	**10 mg**	
% Patients with pain freedom at 2 h	15%	24% ($p < 0{\cdot}0001$)	
% Patients with absence of MBS at 2 h	31%	40% ($p = 0{\cdot}0012$)	

MBS most bothersome symptom, *h* hours

migraine days (−4.3 days vs. −3.5 days; $p < 0.010$) in patients with episodic migraine, with tolerability similar to placebo [19].

Rimegepant 75 mg oral disintegrating tablet dose is indicated for acute treatment at the onset of a migraine attack or every other day for prevention of episodic migraine. The maximum daily dose is 75 mg. The safety of using rimegepant more than 16 days per month has not been established. Rimegepant has a peak plasma concentration at 1.5 h after ingestion. The elimination half-life is approximately 11 h [20]. Rimegepant is metabolized through the liver and excreted through fecal and renal routes [20]. As with ubrogepant, it is not recommended for use in patients with severe hepatic impairment, end-stage renal disease, and in pregnancy or while breastfeeding, and it is not approved for use in children.

Zavegepant

Zavegepant is the first FDA-approved intranasal gepant for the acute treatment of migraine. Zavegepant is a third-generation, high affinity, selective and structurally unique, small molecule CGRP receptor antagonist. A nonoral, intranasal therapy is ideal in patients who experience severe nausea or vomiting or rapidly progressive head pain. A phase 2/3, double-blind, randomized, and placebo-controlled trial evaluated the safety and efficacy at three intranasal doses, 5 mg, 10 mg, and 20 mg vs. placebo in the acute treatment of migraine. Zavegepant 10 mg and 20 mg showed statistically superior results compared to placebo on the primary endpoints of 2 h pain freedom and 2 h MBS freedom. The most common adverse events were dysgeusia and nasal discomfort [21]. 10 mg was found to be the optimal dose.

A phase 3, double-blind, randomized, and placebo-controlled trial evaluated the safety and efficacy of zavegepant 10 mg in the treatment of moderate or severe migraine. In the study, 1405 patients were randomized to receive zavegepant 10 mg intranasal dose or placebo. Subjects were adults with a history of 2–8 moderate to severe migraine attacks per month. They self-administered 1 dose of zavegepant 10 mg nasal spray or placebo to treat one migraine attack. The coprimary efficacy endpoints were pain freedom at 2 h and pain relief from the MBS at 2 h. Zavegepant was found to be superior to placebo for the co-primary endpoints, pain freedom at 2 h (23.6% vs. 14.9%, $P < 0.001$) and freedom from the MBS at 2 h (39.6% vs. 31.3%, $P = 0.0012$). Secondary endpoints included pain relief at 15 min and 2 h, return to function at 30 min, and sustained pain relief through 48 h. The most commonly experienced adverse events were dysgeusia (20.5% vs. 4.7%), nasal discomfort (3.7% vs. 0.8%), and nausea (3.2% vs. 1.1%) [22].

Tolerability

The most common adverse events reported in clinical trials with ubrogepant were nausea, somnolence, dry mouth, and dizziness. All were reported in less than 5% of participants in each dosage group. No serious adverse events related to ubrogepant were reported in either pivotal trial [16]. In the rimegepant trials, nausea, abdominal pain, and dyspepsia occurred at a rate of <2% which is similar to placebo. Severe hypersensitivity reactions, including dyspnea and rash, have occurred with rimegepant in clinical studies, including delayed hypersensitivity [20].

Drug Interactions

Both rimegepant and ubrogepant are metabolized by CYP3A4 and P-gp and have potential drug-drug interactions. Neither medication should be administered in conjunction with strong CYP3A4 inhibitors [16, 20]. Adjusted dosing parameters are indicated for moderate CYP3A4 inhibitors, with a delay in repeat dosing to 48 h with rimegepant and a reduction to 50 mg in a 24-h period with ubrogepant. Concomitant administration with strong or moderate inducers of CYP3A can result in a significant reduction in drug exposure for both medications. It is recommended to avoid administration of rimegepant with CYP3A inducers [20]. Similarly, use of ubrogepant with strong CYP3A4 inducers is discouraged [16]. In the treatment of headache disorders, this is relevant for verapamil which is a moderate CYP3A4 inhibitor. When used in conjunction with potent P-gp inhibitors, rimegepant should not be redosed within 48 h, and ubrogepant should be limited to 50 mg with the option to redose with an additional 50 mg if needed [16, 20].

There are several potential drug-drug interactions with concomitant administration of zavegepant. Increased exposure to zavegepant may be seen with organic anion transporting polypeptide 1B3 (OATP1B3) or sodium taurocholate co-transporting polypeptide (NTCP inhibitors) concomitant administration. In contrast, OATP1B3 or NTCP inducers as well as decongestant concomitant administration may result in reduced exposure to zavegepant [22].

Cardiovascular Safety

CGRP is present throughout the cardiovascular system, and studies have shown that CGRP increases heart rate, cardiac contraction force, and coronary blood flow [20]. Given its vascular activity, studies gepants have included evaluations of unintended changes in vascular physiology. Preclinical animal models showed that inhibiting CGRP led to increased oxidative stress and neuronal cell loss in the setting of middle cerebral artery occlusion and carotid stenosis. This raised concerns that inhibiting CGRP would compromise compensatory vasodilation in the setting of ischemia. Several studies have investigated this concern [23–27]. One in vivo study on the effects of ubrogepant and atogepant on CGRP-induced relaxation in isolated middle meningeal, cerebral, and coronary arteries found that CGRP inhibited vasodilation but did not induce vasoconstriction. The effects were more potent in intracranial arteries than coronary arteries [23]. An investigation on the effect of gepants on cerebral ischemia showed increased infarct size and worse neurologic deficits in mice following the administration of olcegepant and rimegepant [24].

In a randomized placebo-controlled study of telcagepant in patients with stable coronary artery disease, there were no treatment-related changes in laboratory, vital signs, or electrocardiogram safety parameters, with the exception of a single telcagepant patient who experienced asymptomatic ST segment depression [25]. A double-blind, randomized, and placebo-controlled study of telcagepant in patients with stable or exercise-induced angina versus placebo [26]. Participants performed treadmill exercise at maximal serum concentration 2.5 h after treatment dose with no significant differences between treatment and placebo or ST-segment depression on EKG [26].

The pivotal clinical trials for rimegepant and ubrogepant excluded patients with clinically significant cerebrovascular or cardiovascular disease [14, 15, 17]. However, a post-hoc analysis from the ACHIEVE studies examined the safety and efficacy of ubrogepant in participants with cardiovascular risk factors. Participants were stratified as having no, low, or moderate-high cardiovascular risk and were assessed 48 h and 30 days after treatment [27]. The proportion of ubrogepant participants reporting a treatment-emergent adverse event was found to be comparable across risk categories and similar to placebo [27].

Ongoing studies are needed to assess the possible vascular effects of inhibiting CGRP activity. The FDA has issued updated post-marketing warnings of new or worsening hypertension and Raynaud's phenomenon with use of CGRP inhibitors. Providers should discuss the limitations of available safety information for the use of these medications in patients with elevated risk of ischemic events.

Comparing Gepants to Other Treatments

While rimegepant and ubrogepant have demonstrated efficacy compared to placebo in the acute treatment of migraine, they have not been evaluated in direct comparison to triptans. Meta-analyses have found that rimegepant and ubrogepant were less efficacious against placebo when compared to triptans [28, 29]. Triptans are associated with a higher rate of adverse events when compared to gepants.

In a real-world study, 29% of patients discontinued triptans due to intolerable side effects [30]. In clinical trials for rimegepant and ubrogepant, side effects were reported in less than 5% of participants and are generally considered mild [14, 15, 17]. This is reflected in the American Headache Society consensus statement on the role of new treatments in migraine management, which advises the use of gepants for patients with a lack of benefit or intolerable side effects to two oral triptans [31]. Comparisons of efficacy between lasmiditan, rimegepant, and ubrogepant were not statistically significant for 2 h pain freedom or pain relief; however, lasmiditan was associated with a higher risk of adverse events [28].

Combining Gepants with Triptans

Given the variability of migraine symptoms and the efficacy of various treatments, it is not uncommon in practice for patients to have multiple acute medications with varying routes of delivery or mechanisms of action. Combining antiemetics, nonsteroidal anti-inflammatory drugs, and triptans is common in clinical practice. Phase I trials evaluating the pharmacokinetics and hemodynamic effects of taking ubrogepant and sumatriptan or rimegepant and sumatriptan did not show any significant drug interactions or adverse events [32, 33]

In the ACHIEVE trials, subjects could be rescued with a triptan 2 h after the use of the study drug [14, 15]. The safety data from these trials showed that treatment-related adverse events were similar between those who took ubrogepant and a triptan versus those who took ubrogepant alone. This suggests that using a triptan ≥2 h after a gepant has no increased risk of side effects.

While the triptan-gepant combination appears to have no increased safety risk, it is unknown whether there is an additive benefit. The combination of sumatriptan and olcegepant was studied in a glyceryl trinitrate (GTN) mouse model of migraine [34]. Separately, both medications reduced GTN allodynia, but combining them did not result in any additional improvement as compared to either drug alone [34]. Acknowledging the limitations of this preclinical animal model suggests that combining these medications would provide additional benefits.

Combining Gepants with Monoclonal Antibodies Targeting CGRP or Its Receptor

Approval of gepants following the recent release of monoclonal antibodies targeting CGRP or its receptor has prompted consideration of combining acute and preventive treatments that have similar therapeutic targets. To date, the limited safety information on combining acute gepants with monoclonal antibodies to CGRP or its receptor has been reassuring [35–39]. An open-label long-term safety study of rimegepant included a subgroup of 13 patients on a stable dose of CGRP monoclonal antibodies (either erenumab, fremanezumab, or galcanezumab) who used rimegepant up to once daily as needed. Five patients reported on-treatment adverse events; all were considered mild-to-moderate, and none led to discontinuation [35]. Larger long-term studies are needed to confirm the safety of this combination. The next logical consideration in combination with CGRP therapies is whether an acute medication targeting the CGRP receptor is effective in the setting of a steady-state CGRP monoclonal antibody. A real-world study of the effectiveness of ubrogepant when combined with a CGRP monoclonal antibody showed that subjects still experienced high rates of pain reduction with ubrogepant (64.2% at 2 h and 84.5% at 4 h) [36]. Large-scale efficacy and safety studies are warranted, especially in high-risk groups.

Clinical Indications

Based on the AHS consensus statement, gepants are indicated as second-line options for acute treatment of migraine in adults [31]. Given that up to 30% of patients who use triptans do not obtain adequate pain relief, there is a clear unmet need for more effective therapy [40]. A post-hoc analysis of data from the ACHIEVE trials assessed the efficacy of ubrogepant in triptan-insufficient responders. Patients were stratified as triptan responders, triptan-insufficient responders, and triptan-naïve [40]. There was no difference in ubrogepant efficacy across the groups, suggesting that prior response to triptan was not predictive of response to gepant [41].

The pivotal clinical trials of ubrogepant and rimegepant required subjects to delay treatment until the pain was moderate to severe. In real-world clinical practice, patients are often instructed to take an abortive at the earliest onset of head pain for best efficacy. A phase III open-label extension trial demonstrated better efficacy of ubrogepant in the treatment of mild head pain as compared to moderate to severe [42].

Patients who use other acute migraine therapies such as NSAIDs and triptans frequently are at risk of developing medication overuse headache (MOH). Use of NSAIDs ≥15 days per month for greater than 3 months and use of triptans/ergots, combination analgesics, or opioids ≥10 days per month for greater than 3 months increases the risk of developing medication overuse headache [31]. Repeated treatment with gepants does not appear to confer this same risk. A preclinical study showed that ubrogepant 100 mg/kg in repeated effective doses did not produce cutaneous allodynia or latent sensitization when compared to sumatriptan [43]. This, in combination with daily and near-daily use of gepants for prevention, speaks against the risk of MOH with gepants use.

Conclusion

Gepants are a new class of acute treatment targeted to migraine pathophysiology [44]. Ubrogepant and rimegepant are currently FDA approved for the acute treatment of migraine. Several clinical trials have established their safety and efficacy in treating a migraine attack when compared to placebo. There are no direct comparisons, but meta-analyses suggest that gepants are less effective than triptans with regard to 2 h pain freedom and pain relief. Current evidence suggests that gepants are well tolerated, are not associated with an increased risk of adverse cardiovascular events, and appear unlikely to cause medication overuse headaches. An intranasal formulation, zavegepant, may be effective for acute migraine attacks of severe onset or associated with nausea and vomiting. Rimegepant and atogepant are approved for the prevention of episodic migraine, and atogepant has proven efficacy for the prevention of chronic migraine.

Teaching Points

1. CGRP is a vasoactive neuropeptide that has been shown to be important in migraine pathophysiology.
2. Small molecule CGRP receptor antagonists are termed "gepants."
3. Olcegepant and telcagepant are first-generation gepants that established their efficacy in migraine treatment; however, they were abandoned due to concerns over the route of administration and hepatotoxicity, respectively.
4. Second-generation gepants include rimegepant, ubrogepant, and atogepant and have not demonstrated any evidence of hepatoxicity in clinical trials to date.
5. Ubrogepant and rimegepant are approved for the acute treatment of migraine in adults.
6. Rimegepant is additionally approved for the prevention of episodic migraine in adults when dosed every other day.
7. Rimegepant and ubrogepant are metabolized by CYP3A4 and P-gp and have potential drug-drug interactions.
8. Atogepant is approved for preventive treatment of episodic migraine in adults; long-term safety studies and evaluation in chronic migraine are ongoing.
9. Gepants are well tolerated in clinical evaluations; nausea and somnolence are the most commonly reported adverse events in clinical trials.

10. Gepants are appropriate acute options for patients with contraindications or intolerance to triptans.
11. Zavegepant is a third-generation, first intranasally administered gepant, which may be helpful for attacks with sudden onset, nausea, or vomiting.

Case

A 44-year-old woman presents for evaluation of migraine. She describes her attacks as left-sided throbbing head pain associated with nausea, vomiting, and sensitivity to light. They typically last for 36–48 h and occur 2–4 times each month. Previously, she used sumatriptan 100 mg, which would alleviate her symptoms for 6–8 h, at which point the pain and associated symptoms would recur. She states sumatriptan was sedating, and she was uncomfortable taking a second dose of medication while at work because of the side effects. She tried naratriptan as an alternative but stated it was no better than over-the-counter NSAIDs.

Case Discussion

This patient has episodic migraine and needs an effective acute medication. She has tried two triptans but experienced either intolerable side effects or incomplete relief. In this case, in which a triptan did not pro vide enduring benefit and had side effects, a gepant would be a worthwhile next option. The long half-life of rimegepant ODT 75 mg might be preferred for attacks in which shorter acting medication did not provide sustained benefit. Additionally, the orally disintegrating tablet may be better tolerated than traditional PO formulations if there is associated vomiting.

Questions and Answers

1. Which patient would be the best candidate for acute treatment of migraine with a gepant?
   A. A 16-year-old girl with 3–5 migraines each month that respond to OTC NSAIDS
   B. A 37-year-old woman with 3–5 migraine days each month who responds well to rizatriptan and naproxen
   C. A 67-year-old man with migraine with aura 1–2 days each month and a history of ischemic stroke 3 months ago
   D. A 46-year-old woman with 7–9 migraine days each month, who had intolerable side effects in the past with sumatriptan and eletriptan

The correct answer is D. Acute gepants (rimegepant and ubrogepant) are best suited for patients with episodic migraine who have found triptans ineffective or intolerable. They are not indicated in children and have not been studied in patients with recent cerebrovascular accident.

2. Which preventive migraine medication would require an adjusted dose of ubrogepant?
   A. Topiramate
   B. Amitriptyline
   C. Verapamil
   D. Valproate

The correct answer is C. Verapamil is a CYP450 moderate CYP3A4 inhibitor and would increase exposure to ubrogepant. It is recommended to limit ubrogepant to 50 mg in 24 h if administered in conjunction with verapamil.

References

1. Burch RC, Buse DC, Lipton RB. Migraine: epidemiology, burden, and comorbidity. Neurol Clin. 2019;37(4):631–49.
2. McCulloch J, Uddman R, Kingman TA, Edvinsson L. Calcitonin gene-related peptide: functional role in cerebrovascular regulation. Proc Natl Acad Sci. 1986;83(15):5731–5.
3. Hansen JM, Hauge AW, Olesen J, Ashina M. Calcitonin gene-related peptide triggers migraine-like attacks in patients with migraine with aura. Cephalalgia. 2010;30(10):1179–86.
4. Juhász G, Zsombok T, Jakab B, Nemeth J, Szolcsányi J, Bagdy G. Sumatriptan causes parallel decrease in plasma calcitonin gene-related peptide (CGRP) concentration and migraine headache during nitroglycerin induced migraine attack. Cephalalgia. 2005;25(3):179–83.
5. Poyner DR, Sexton PM, Marshall I, et al. International Union of Pharmacology. XXXII. The mammalian calcitonin gene-related peptides, adrenomedullin, amylin, and calcitonin receptors. Pharmacol Rev. 2002;54:233–46. https://doi.org/10.1124/pr.54.2.233.
6. Petersen KA, Birk S, Doods H, Edvinsson L, Olesen J. Inhibitory effect of BIBN4096BS on cephalic vasodilatation induced by CGRP or transcranial electrical stimulation in the rat. Br J Pharmacol. 2004;143(6):697–704.
7. Olesen J, Diener HC, Husstedt IW, Goadsby PJ, Hall D, Meier U, Pollentier S, Lesko LM. Calcitonin gene–related peptide receptor antagonist BIBN 4096 BS for the acute treatment of migraine. N Engl J Med. 2004;350(11):1104–10.
8. de Vries T, Villalon CM, MaassenVanDenBrink A. Pharmacological treatment of migraine: CGRP and 5-HT beyond the triptans. Pharmacol Ther. 2020;211:107528.
9. Ho TW, Ferrari MD, Dodick DW, Galet V, Kost J, Fan X, Leibensperger H, Froman S, Assaid C, Lines C, Koppen H. Efficacy and tolerability of MK-0974 (telcagepant), a new oral antagonist of calcitonin gene-related peptide receptor, compared with zolmitriptan for acute migraine: a randomised, placebo-controlled, parallel-treatment trial. Lancet. 2008;372(9656):2115–23.
10. Ho TW, Connor KM, Zhang Y, Pearlman E, Koppenhaver J, Fan X, Lines C, Edvinsson L, Goadsby PJ, Michelson D. Randomized controlled trial of the CGRP receptor antagonist telcagepant for migraine prevention. Neurology. 2014;83(11):958–66.
11. Silberstein SD, Lipton RB, Dodick DW, Freitag FG, Ramadan N, Mathew N, Brandes JL, Bigal M, Saper J, Ascher S, Jordan DM. Efficacy and safety of topiramate for the treatment of chronic

migraine: a randomized, double-blind, placebo-controlled trial. Headache. 2007;47(2):170–80.
12. Ho TW, Ho AP, Ge Y, Assaid C, Gottwald R, MacGregor EA, Mannix LK, Van Oosterhout WP, Koppenhaver J, Lines C, Ferrari MD. Randomized controlled trial of the CGRP receptor antagonist telcagepant for prevention of headache in women with perimenstrual migraine. Cephalalgia. 2016;36(2):148–61.
13. Hewitt DJ, Aurora SK, Dodick DW, Goadsby PJ, Ge Y, Bachman R, Taraborelli D, Fan X, Assaid C, Lines C, Ho TW. Randomized controlled trial of the CGRP receptor antagonist MK-3207 in the acute treatment of migraine. Cephalalgia. 2011;31(6):712–22.
14. Lipton RB, Dodick DW, Ailani J, Lu K, Finnegan M, Szegedi A, Trugman JM. Effect of ubrogepant vs placebo on pain and the most bothersome associated symptom in the acute treatment of migraine: the ACHIEVE II randomized clinical trial. JAMA. 2019;322(19):1887–98.
15. Dodick DW, Lipton RB, Ailani J, Lu K, Finnegan M, Trugman JM, Szegedi A. Ubrogepant for the treatment of migraine. N Engl J Med. 2019;381(23):2230–41.
16. Allergan USA, Inc, Ubrelvy [package insert]; 2019.
17. Lipton RB, Croop R, Stock EG, Stock DA, Morris BA, Frost M, Dubowchik GM, Conway CM, Coric V, Goadsby PJ. Rimegepant, an oral calcitonin gene–related peptide receptor antagonist, for migraine. N Engl J Med. 2019;381(2):142–9.
18. McGinley JS, Gilbert JL, Thiry A, Croop R, Coric V, Lipton RB. Rimegepant 75 mg results in reductions in monthly migraine days: secondary analysis of a multicenter, open label long-term safety study of rimegepant for the acute treatment of migraine (1793). Neurology [Internet]. 2020 Apr [cited 2021 Dec 19];94 (15 Supplement) 1793. Available from: https://n.neurology.org/content/94/15_Supplement/1793.abstract.
19. Croop R, Lipton RB, Kudrow D, Stock DA, Kamen L, Conway CM, Stock EG, Coric V, Goadsby PJ. Oral rimegepant for preventive treatment of migraine: a phase 2/3, randomised, double-blind, placebo-controlled trial. Lancet. 2021;397(10268):51–60.
20. Biohaven, Inc, Nurtec [package insert]; 2020.
21. Croop R, Madonia J, Stock DA, Thiry A, Forshaw M, Murphy A, Coric V, Lipton RB. Zavegepant nasal spray for the acute treatment of migraine: a phase 2/3 double-blind, randomized, placebo-controlled, dose-ranging trial. Headache. 2022;62(9):1153–63.
22. Lipton RB, Croop R, Stock DA, Madonia J, Forshaw M, Lovegren M, Mosher L, Coric V, Goadsby PJ. Safety, tolerability, and efficacy of zavegepant 10 mg nasal spray for the acute treatment of migraine in the USA: a phase 3, double-blind, randomised, placebo-controlled multicentre trial. Lancet Neurol. 2023;22(3):209–17. https://doi.org/10.1016/S1474-4422(22)00517-8. Erratum in: Lancet Neurol. 2023 May;22(5):e7. https://doi.org/10.1016/S1474-4422(23)00107-2. Erratum in: Lancet Neurol. 2023 Aug;22(8):e9. https://doi.org/10.1016/S1474-4422(23)00245-4.
23. Rubio-Beltran E, Chan KY, Danser AJ, MaassenVanDenBrink A, Edvinsson L. Characterisation of the calcitonin gene-related peptide receptor antagonists ubrogepant and atogepant in human isolated coronary, cerebral and middle meningeal arteries. Cephalalgia. 2020;40(4):357–66.
24. Mulder IA, Li M, de Vries T, Qin T, Yanagisawa T, Sugimoto K, van den Bogaerdt A, Danser AJ, Wermer MJ, van den Maagdenberg AM, MaassenVanDenBrink A. Anti-migraine calcitonin gene–related peptide receptor antagonists worsen cerebral ischemic outcome in mice. Ann Neurol. 2020;88(4):771–84.
25. Behm MO, Blanchard RL, Murphy MG, Palcza JS, Harris DE, Butterfield KL, Smith WB, Preston RA, Chodakewitz JA, Krucoff MW. Effect of telcagepant on spontaneous ischemia in cardiovascular patients in a randomized study. Headache. 2011;51(6):954–60.
26. Chaitman BR, Ho AP, Behm MO, Rowe JF, Palcza JS, Laethem T, Heirman I, Panebianco DL, Kobalava Z, Martsevich SY, Free AL. A randomized, placebo-controlled study of the effects of telcagepant on exercise time in patients with stable angina. Clin Pharmacol Ther. 2012;91(3):459–66.
27. Hutchinson S, Silberstein SD, Blumenfeld AM, Lipton RB, Lu K, Yu SY, Severt L. Safety and efficacy of ubrogepant in participants with major cardiovascular risk factors in two single-attack phase 3 randomized trials: ACHIEVE I and II. Cephalalgia. 2021;19:03331024211000311.
28. Yang CP, Liang CS, Chang CM, Yang CC, Shih PH, Yau YC, Tang KT, Wang SJ. Comparison of new pharmacologic agents with triptans for treatment of migraine: a systematic review and meta-analysis. JAMA Netw Open. 2021;4(10):e2128544.
29. Ha DK, Kim MJ, Han N, Kwak JH, Baek IH. Comparative efficacy of oral calcitonin-gene–related peptide antagonists for the treatment of acute migraine: updated meta-analysis. Clin Drug Investig. 2021;11:1–4.
30. Wells RE, Markowitz SY, Baron EP, Hentz JG, Kalidas K, Mathew PG, Halker R, Dodick DW, Schwedt TJ. Identifying the factors underlying discontinuation of triptans. Headache. 2014;54(2):278–89.
31. Ailani J, Burch RC, Robbins MS, Board of Directors of the American Headache Society. The American Headache Society Consensus Statement: update on integrating new migraine treatments into clinical practice. Headache. 2021;61(7):1021–39.
32. Croop R, Ivans A, Anderson MS, Stringfellow J, Bertz R, Hanna M, Healy F, Stock DA, Coric V, Lipton RB. A phase 1 randomized study of hemodynamic effects and pharmacokinetic interactions during concomitant use of rimegepant and sumatriptan in healthy adults. Cephalalgia Rep. 2021;4:25158163211007922.
33. Jakate A, Boinpally R, Butler M, Lu K, McGeeney D, Periclou A. Evaluation of the pharmacokinetic interaction of ubrogepant coadministered with sumatriptan and of the safety of ubrogepant with triptans. Headache. 2020;60(7):1340–50.
34. Ernstsen C, Christensen SL, Olesen J, Kristensen DM. No additive effect of combining sumatriptan and olcegepant in the GTN mouse model of migraine. Cephalalgia. 2021;41(3):329–39.
35. Berman G, Croop R, Kudrow D, Halverson P, Lovegren M, Thiry AC, Conway CM, Coric V, Lipton RB. Safety of rimegepant, an oral CGRP receptor antagonist, plus CGRP monoclonal antibodies for migraine. Headache. 2020;60(8):1734–42.
36. Lipton RB, Contreras-De Lama J, Serrano D, Engstrom E, Poh W, Cadiou F, Adams A. COmbining UbRogepAnt and preventives for miGrainE (COURAGE) study using the migraine buddy application: a novel, entirely remote design for collecting real-world evidence. Headache. 2021;61(S1):100.
37. Mullin K, Kudrow D, Croop R, et al. Potential for treatment benefit of small molecule CGRP receptor antagonist plus monoclonal antibody in migraine therapy. Neurology. 2020;94:e2121–5.
38. Chiang CC, Arca KN, Dunn RB, et al. Real-world efficacy, tolerability, and safety of ubrogepant. Headache. 2021;61:620–7.
39. Jakate A, Blumenfeld AM, Boinpally R, et al. Pharmacokinetics and safety of ubrogepant when coadministered with calcitonin gene-related peptide-targeted monoclonal antibody migraine preventives in participants with migraine: a randomized phase 1b drug-drug interaction study. Headache. 2021;61:642–52.
40. Marcus SC, Shewale AR, Silberstein SD, Lipton RB, Young WB, Viswanathan HN, Doshi JA. Comparison of healthcare resource utilization and costs among patients with migraine with potentially adequate and insufficient triptan response. Cephalalgia. 2020;40(7):639–49.
41. Blumenfeld AM, Goadsby PJ, Dodick DW, Hutchinson S, Liu C, Finnegan M, Trugman JM, Szegedi A. Efficacy of ubrogepant

based on prior exposure and response to triptans: a post hoc analysis. Headache. 2021;61(3):422–9.
42. Lipton R, Dodick D, Goadsby P, et al. Ubrogepant is effective in the acute treatment of migraine with mild head pain. Neurology. 2020 April [cited 2021 Dec 19];94(15 Suppl):4726. Available at: https://n.neurology.org/content/94/15_Supplement/4726.abstract.
43. Navratilova E, Behravesh S, Oyarzo J, Dodick DW, Banerjee P, Porreca F. Ubrogepant does not induce latent sensitization in a preclinical model of medication overuse headache. Cephalalgia. 2020;40(9):892–902.
44. Edvinsson L, Haanes KA, Warfvinge K, et al. CGRP as the target of new migraine therapies — successful translation from bench to clinic. Nat Rev Neurol. 2018;14:338–50.

Established Oral and Newer Preventive Treatments

27

Shivang Joshi and Jessica R. Gautreaux

Introduction

Preventive therapy for migraine disease is an important step in the comprehensive approach to treating migraine disease. The main goal of using preventive therapy is, of course, to decrease migraine attacks. In addition, studies have shown that the use of preventive therapies can also improve quality of life and decrease disability for those living with migraine disease. Preventive therapies may have impacts on individual migraine attacks that do occur such as improved response to acute therapies or decreasing the severity of attacks [1–3].

As headache frequency has been recognized as a risk factor for transformation from episodic to chronic migraine [4], it is reasonable to consider that decreasing migraine attacks may prevent disease progression. There is some evidence that migraine disease may be impacted by making lifestyle modifications and avoiding triggers or entities that are recognized to potentially worsen migraine disease [5], but many patients will require an additional preventive modality.

Migraine preventive therapies have readily expanded over recent years from products taken orally on a daily basis to injectable medications administered monthly, to even non-invasive neuromodulation devices, giving patients more options than ever before to impact their migraine disease. This chapter will focus on oral preventive therapies for migraine management, as other preventive strategies have been discussed elsewhere.

Questions

1. Patient is a 43-year-old female with a history of migraine without aura. She is currently experiencing 9 days of migraine attacks per month. 7 out of her 9 headaches per month respond well to treatment with sumatriptan, but two persist despite triptan use with significant photophobia and nausea which interfere with her ability to function well at work. She has a history of asthma and has no other medical problems. She has been having difficulty sleeping which she thinks may be contributing to making her migraines worse. Which of the following is the best choice for an initial preventive for this patient?
   A. Erenumab
   B. Propranolol
   C. Ubrogepant
   D. Amitriptyline
   E. Eptinezumab
2. Which migraine therapy should be avoided in glaucoma?
   A. Topiramate
   B. Propranolol
   C. Amitriptyline
   D. Candesartan
   E. Rimegepant

When to Start a Preventive Therapy

The decision of when to add a preventive therapy to a patient's migraine treatment plan is, like many aspects of migraine care, one that must be individualized to each patient. Patients may benefit from non-pharmacological and pharmacological interventions or both in combination. For patients with severe attacks, which respond poorly to acute therapies, and cause significant disability, a preventive may be considered and offer great benefit even if these attacks are

S. Joshi (✉)
Headache Medicine, Community Neuroscience Services, University of Massachusetts, Westborough, MA, USA

J. R. Gautreaux
Children's Hospital New Orleans, Louisiana State University Health Sciences Center, New Orleans, LA, USA

T. S. Monteith et al. (eds.), *Comprehensive Migraine Management*, https://doi.org/10.1007/978-3-031-86923-5_27

rare. For patients with entities such as hemiplegic migraine or migraine with brainstem aura that can have significant neurological symptoms during attacks, prevention is usually offered even when attacks are not frequent. Patients who have less severe attacks with an effective acute treatment option may be able to tolerate a higher frequency of attacks before wanting to consider preventive therapy [1–3]. There are treatment guidelines that have made recommendations from the American Academy of Neurology, the American Headache Society, the Canadian Headache Society, and others, but these are not all consistent. The most recent consensus statement from the American Headache Society published in 2021 recommended that preventive treatment be considered in patients with any of the following:

- Migraine attacks >4 days per month
- >2 attacks that interfere with daily routines even with acute treatment
- There is a contraindication, failure, or overuse of acute treatment
- Acute treatments lead to adverse events
- Patient preference [6]

Daily Oral Preventive Agents

Though very recently, headache-specific therapies for migraine prevention have become available in the form of calcitonin gene-related peptide (CGRP) monoclonal antibodies and CGRP receptor antagonists, the standard of care for migraine prevention before their advent was the use of daily oral medications from several different medication classes including antiseizure medications, antihypertensives, and antidepressants. These therapies were not migraine-specific and were used for other disease states but over time were found to offer benefits for migraine disease. There are also a variety of neutraceuticals with some evidence for use in migraine prevention [7]. Despite the availability of newer therapies, it is typically recommended to begin preventive therapy with one of these oral agents with a long history of use and efficacy in migraine disease.

In 2012, the American Academy of Neurology and the American Headache Society developed guidelines for the common preventive therapies used at the time and rated these therapies based on the evidence available. Medications with two good quality studies supporting efficacy received a level A (effective) rating, one good quality study and two lower quality studies a level B (probably effective), one lower quality study and two lowest quality studies a level C (possibly effective), and a level U if data was insufficient or conflicting (Table 27.1) [8]. Of note, since the publications of these guidelines, higher quality evidence has become available for some agents as noted in the table; it is probable that the next revision of the guidelines will include a change in the level rating. Other headache societies such as the Canadian Headache Society have published guidelines that look beyond just the efficacy data available and also consider real-life use of the medications including side effect profiles, route of administration, and other factors to make their recommendations. The Canadian Headache Society has given a "strong" rating to metoprolol, propranolol, nadolol, candesartan, topiramate, amitriptyline, and gabapentin [9]. Table 27.1 lists each therapy by drug class and includes common dosing ranges and some common side effects though prescribers should refer to an appropriate comprehensive source for full prescribing considerations.

Adherence to a daily oral regimen for migraine prevention in general is low. A study looking at adherence to oral preventive therapy in chronic migraine showed rates of 26–29% at 6 months and 17–20% at 1 year [10]. When beginning an oral preventive agent, it is often important to start at a low dose and titrate up slowly [1, 3]. This approach can help to minimize side effects and improve tolerability which is often a cited reason for discontinuation or daily oral preventive [11]. Some patients may respond to a lower dose, but certainly, if there is a lack of efficacy, oral preventives should be maximized and continued for at least 6 weeks to see if there is benefit [1, 3]. This approach may mean it takes longer to see the full benefit of treatment, thus patients should be counseled regarding this factor as a perceived lack of efficacy is also a common reason for discontinuation of preventives.

Table 27.1 Oral preventive agents for migraine prevention

Medication	Dosing range	AAN/AHS guideline level of evidence [2, 8]	Common side effects
Antiseizure			
Divalproex sodium	500–1000 mg daily (can be given in divided dosing or single daily dosing if delayed release)	A	Weight gain, hair loss, nausea, fatigue, thrombocytopenia, hepatotoxicity—Does require monitoring
Topiramate	100 mg daily (or divided in twice daily dosing)	A	Weight loss, paresthesia, cognitive complaints/word-finding difficulty, nephrolithiasis
Gabapentin	900–3600 mg daily divided in three doses	U	Fatigue, dizziness

(continued)

Table 27.1 (continued)

Medication	Dosing range	AAN/AHS guideline level of evidence [2, 8]	Common side effects
Pregabalin	25–75 mg three times daily	U	Dizziness, somnolence nausea
Levetiracetam	500–1000 mg twice daily	None	Behavior change, irritability, aggression, fatigue
Antihypertensives			
Metoprolol	50 mg twice daily	A	Fatigue, dizziness, orthostasis, exercise intolerance
Propranolol	60 mg once or twice daily	A	Fatigue, dizziness, orthostasis, exercise intolerance
Candesartan	8–16 mg daily	B	Hypotension, dizziness
Lisinopril	10–40 mg daily	C	Hypotension, dizziness, cough
Verapamil	120–240 mg daily	U	Constipation, dizziness, hypotension
Antidepressants			
Amitriptyline	50 mg at bedtime	B	Fatigue, weight gain, dry mouth
Venlafaxine	75–225 mg XR daily	B	Insomnia, nausea, dizziness, sexual dysfunction
Duloxetine	60 mg daily	None	Nausea, weight loss, somnolence, fatigue, sexual dysfunction
Nortriptyline	50 mg daily	None	Drowsiness, dry mouth, dizziness, constipation
Gepant			
Atogepant	10–60 mg daily	A	Fatigue, nausea, constipation
Rimegepant	75 mg every other day	A	Nausea, indigestion
Other			
Cyproheptadine	4–8 mg once daily or divided twice daily	C	Drowsiness, weight gain
Memantine	10 mg twice daily	None	Dizziness, confusion, constipation
Neutraceuticals			
Magnesium	600–600 mg daily divided twice daily	B	GI disturbance
Riboflavin (vitamin B2)	400 mg daily	B	Discolors the urine to bright yellow
Feverfew	50–300 mg daily	B	Nausea, GI discomfort
CoQ10	300 mg daily	C	
Melatonin	3 mg at bedtime	None	

How to Choose Preventive Therapy

The decision regarding which preventive therapy is one that is best shared between both doctor and patient and should be individualized for each patient. Many patients with migraine disease have comorbidities that may be affected, both positively and negatively, by beginning a new therapy for migraine prevention. The potential effect of a migraine preventive on these comorbidities should be considered when choosing an agent, for example, a patient with migraine and low blood pressure may not be able to tolerate a beta-blocker. Conversely, a patient with anxiety may find a beta-blocker conveys benefit to both their anxiety and their migraine disease, making the beta-blocker a better choice than other preventive options. As with all decisions regarding medications, contraindications to individual agents must be considered (Table 27.2), for example, those with asthma are not good candidates for propranolol use. In patients with comorbidities who are taking other medications, drug interactions must be considered when choosing a migraine therapy as well as avoiding agents that can worsen a comorbid condition.

There is frequently some trial and error in finding a preventive agent that provides both efficacy and tolerability for each individual patient. For patients who prefer non-medicinal options entirely, devices and behavioral interventions may be most desirable. In clinical practice, it is not uncommon for many headache specialists to layer tools for migraine prevention in their treatment plans. It is important to use caution in regard to drug interactions, the risk for worsening side effects, and exacerbating comorbid conditions when using polypharmacy for migraine prevention. Combining a pharmaceutical agent with a behavioral therapy or device may limit these concerns.

With the CGRP monoclonal antibodies beginning a new era in migraine prevention, the American Headache Society published a consensus statement to guide the use of newer therapies in migraine treatment in 2021. According to the 2021 consensus statement, it was recommended that a monoclonal antibody should be considered in the following:

- Patients with 4–7 migraine days per month causing at least moderate disability *and* two unsuccessful 8-week

Table 27.2 Comorbidities and contraindications to consider in migraine prevention

Comorbidity	Therapy to avoid
Obesity	Divalproex sodium, amitriptyline, cyproheptadine
Postural orthostatic tachycardia syndrome	Beta-blockers, lisinopril, verapamil, candesartan
Depression	Beta-blockers
Constipation	Erenumab
Hypertension	Erenumab, venlafaxine, duloxetine
Renal impairment	Topiramate, venlafaxine, gabapentin, lisinopril, verapamil
Liver impairment	Divalproex sodium
Cardiac arrhythmia	Amitriptyline, nortriptyline, verapamil
Contraindication	
Asthma	Propranolol
Nephrolithiasis	Topiramate
Glaucoma	Topiramate
Pregnancy	Divalproex sodium, topiramate, lisinopril, candesartan, feverfew

trials of a traditional oral agent due to inability to tolerate or lack of efficacy

- Patients with 8–14 migraine days per month who have had two unsuccessful 8-week trials of a traditional oral agent due to inability to tolerate or lack of efficacy
- Patients with >15 migraine days per month (chronic migraine) who have *either* had two unsuccessful 8-week trials of a traditional oral agent due to inability to tolerate or lack of efficacy *or* inability to tolerate or lack of efficacy from two quarterly injections of onabotulinumtoxin A [6]

The American Headache Society published an updated position statement in 2024 advancing CGRP-targeting therapies as a first-line consideration for migraine prevention without a requirement for prior failure of other traditional classes of migraine preventive treatment. In general, traditional migraine therapies have been developed for other indications than migraine. Although there is similar efficacy, the tolerability of traditional preventives is of concern. In contrast to established oral preventive therapies, the evidence for CGRP-targeted therapies is supported by efficacy in the setting of multiple preventive failures, medication overuse, early separation from placebo, and responder rates of 50–75%. This position statement also helps further recognize migraine as a neurological disease, hopefully, helps reduce stigma, and allows patients to obtain targeted therapy [12].

Another significant factor in choosing a preventive option for patients is the coverage options offered by their insurance provider. It cannot be denied that newer therapies such as the CGRP monoclonal antibodies are typically very costly and may not be well-covered by insurance. Payors frequently require failed trials of preferred medications for the prevention of migraine before agreeing to coverage of the newer, more expensive therapies such as the CGRP-targeted therapies. Payers may also have preferred brands on their formulary that must be tried before another less preferred alternative can be used.

Goals and When to Wean Migraine Preventives

Common endpoints in studies of the efficacy of migraine preventives include a reduction in the number of migraine attacks, a decrease in the overall number of headache days, and the number of patients experiencing a 50% reduction in headache frequency. These are reasonable goals for use in the day-to-day clinical setting as well; however, other factors may also need to be considered. Patients using preventive therapies may have significant improvement in quality of life without a measurable decrease in headache days or attack frequency [13]. For example, a patient who was having eight severe migraine days per month that required him/her to miss work and activities of daily living may feel that preventive therapy has been very beneficial even if there are still eight attacks per month, but they are less severe, respond well to acute therapy, and do not interrupt activities of daily living any longer.

It is important when initiating preventive therapy of any type to counsel patients regarding appropriate expectations for treatment. Patients' goals and expectations for prevention as well as the provider's goals for treatment should be discussed. As mentioned previously in this chapter for many of the preventive therapies, it may take several weeks to months to see the desired benefit of treatment and improvements may increase over time. Though the CGRP monoclonal antibodies are thought to have a faster time to effect than an oral preventive, a 3-month course is typically recommended to determine the full benefit. It is also important to discuss that there may be benefits to preventive therapy even if the absolute number of headaches is only slightly decreased by prevention, for example, headache severity and related disability may decrease, or perhaps acute attacks begin to respond better to acute therapy again decreasing disability from the headache burden. Patients may discontinue treatments early in the course of therapy feeling they are ineffective if they are not aware of these factors, thus counseling patients regarding the time needed to see the benefit of preventives and of the many ways preventive therapy can affect their disease may improve adherence.

It is also important to inform patients that preventive therapy frequently can be weaned when patients are clinically doing better and is not always a permanent fixture in their migraine treatment regimen. It is this author's clinical experience that patients may be more willing to consider adding a preventive treatment to their migraine treatment plan when they understand that they are not committing to lifetime medication. There is little evidence to guide the decision of when to wean a preventive that has been beneficial to a patient, thus an individualized approach is suggested. For patients with less frequent migraines who respond well to an initial preventive, a 3–6-month course is typical before attempting a wean. On the other hand, patients with long-standing, high-frequency migraine that have been refractory to treatment, may be less willing to consider weaning from a preventive regimen that has offered them significant benefits after years of living with difficult-to-treat migraine disease. For these patients, a preventive regimen may remain in place long-term.

Drug-Drug Interactions

Understanding pharmacokinetic properties can help optimize migraine treatment. Treatment challenges may occur when patients present with multiple comorbid conditions such as diabetes, hypertension, depression, anxiety, chronic pain, and others. Polypharmacy can result in drug-drug interactions (DDI) that may result in adverse effects or decreased efficacy of a medication [14]. It is therefore important to have a basic understanding of the metabolism of drugs. We will review in brief common medications prescribed as well as newer pharmacological therapy for the treatment of migraines.

General Metabolism Considerations

Furanocoumarins found in grapefruit juice inhibit CYP3A4 and p-glycoprotein [15]. Polycyclic hydrocarbons in tobacco smoke can result in increased drug metabolism through enzyme induction of CYP1A1/CYP1A2 and CYP2E1 to a certain extent. Nicotine is metabolized in the liver by CYP2A4, and carbon monoxide can inhibit CYP enzymes in a dose-dependent manner [16]. There is also genetic polymorphism in certain ethnicities that leads to variable rates of drug metabolism. For example, p-glycoprotein expression is reduced in specific Asian and Caucasian populations [17].

Common Preventive Medications

Beta-Blockers

Beta-blockers such as propranolol, timolol, and nadolol nonselectively bind Beta 1 and Beta 2 receptors, while metoprolol selectively binds Beta 1. There are variable pharmacokinetic properties between them, for example, propranolol is highly protein-bound and likely to displace other protein-bound drugs. Propranolol has been associated with numerous DDIs including anti-diabetic medications, calcium channel blockers, cimetidine, digoxin, ergot alkaloids, NSAIDs, phenobarbital, HCTZ, rifampin, rizatriptan, and theophylline [18]. Metoprolol has a noteworthy DDI with paroxetine. Both modulate the CYP2D6 activity, and co-administration may result in bradycardia [19, 20]. In diabetic patients, there may be an increase in the risk of cardiovascular events and a higher incidence of severe hypoglycemia. Beta-blockers may mask the hypoglycemic effect [21]. In addition, exacerbation of COPD may occur with non-selective agents [22].

Antiepileptic Drugs

Divalproex Sodium

There is a teratogenic potential for the use of divalproex. It is also found in breast milk in low concentrations. It is primarily eliminated through hepatic metabolism. It is a CYP2C9 inhibitor and may decrease clearance of medications such as penem antibiotics, carbamazepine, and lamotrigine. Certain inhibitors of 2C9, 2A6, and 2B6 may decrease clearance resulting in increased toxicity. These medications include aspirin, fluoxetine, felbamate, isoniazid, and chlorpromazine [23, 24].

Topiramate

Topiramate may be found in breast milk in significant concentrations. It can also be found in CSF as it is assumed to cross the blood-brain barrier. It is not metabolized by the CYP pathways but is a weak inhibitor of CYP2C19 and a weak inducer of CYP3A4; substrates affected may include amitriptyline, cilostazol, and verapamil [25]. Dose modifications of ubrogepant are recommended when used with topiramate. Use of topiramate during pregnancy can lead to birth defects, including cleft lip and cleft palate. It is excreted predominantly unmetabolized by the kidneys. Topiramate in doses of 200 mg and higher may affect the efficacy of birth control pills as ethinyl estradiol levels may be decreased

[26]. There may be decreased clearance of metformin, resulting in lactic acidosis [27].

Antidepressant Medications

Amitriptyline and nortriptyline undergo hepatic metabolism. Concomitant use of SSRIs may result in anticholinergic toxicity. For example, they are polymorphic genetic mutations in individuals making them slow metabolizers of CYP2D6. The combination of tricylic anti-depressants and monoamine oxidase inhibitors should be avoided as this may result in serotonin syndrome. There may be an increased risk of bleeding with oral anticoagulants and warfarin due to decreased metabolism [28, 29]. Clinically, there is also a risk of unmasking hypomania. Similarly, venlafaxine should not be administered with MAOIs. It may also interact with drugs using the CYP2D6 pathway [30].

Calcium Channel Blockers

Verapamil undergoes extensive first-pass metabolism resulting in low oral bioavailability. Low levels have been reported in breast milk. Both verapamil and amlodipine undergo CYP3A4 metabolism. Both also modulate the P-glycoprotein transporter activity. Caution use with propranolol as there may be an increased risk of cardiovascular depression [31]. Clinically, verapamil has been associated with delay in colon transit resulting in constipation issues [32]. Myasthenia exacerbations and cardiac irregularities such as prolonged PR interval and AV block may occur [33].

Gepants

Rimegepant (acute and prevention) and atogepant (prevention for patients with episodic and chronic migraine) generally do not cross the blood-brain barrier. Rimegepant is metabolized by the CYP3A4. Rimegepant is a substrate of P-glycoprotein and BCRP, and there may be increased exposure to gepant with the use of verapamil, itraconazole, and novobiocin. Rimegepant DDIs include itraconazole and rifampin. Rimegepant has been studied in breastfeeding with no significant adverse effects noted [34, 35]. Atogepant interacts with strong CYP3A4 inhibitors and strong and moderate inducers as well as OATP inhibitors such as rifampin and cyclosporin [36]. Dose adjustment is recommended. Atogepant side effects include constipation and nausea.

Monoclonal Antibodies Targeting CGRP

These include erenumab, galcanezumab, fremanezumab, and eptinezumab. The molecular size is large. They are primarily metabolized through the reticuloendothelial system (RES) also known as the mononuclear phagocyte system. Binding to the neonatal Fc receptors in the RES pathway prevents clearance resulting in a long half-life allowing for less frequent dosing [37, 38].

Conclusion

Migraine prevention is just one component of the multifaceted approach to managing migraine disease but can provide significant improvement in the quality of life for patients living with migraine disease. Physicians and other healthcare providers have many tools at their disposal from which to choose to find an appropriate fit for each patient, and preventive treatment should be individualized taking into consideration patient preferences, side effect profiles, patient comorbidities, and insurance coverage of different agents. Migraine prevention is an area that has seen expansion in research and development over recent years, thus there is hope that the opportunity to improve migraine disease with both current and new preventive therapies will continue to grow. Important drug-drug interactions should be considered when considering migraine therapy. This may potentially lead to decreased adverse events and improved health outcomes.

Teaching Points

1. Managing migraine involves a comprehensive approach that includes acute and preventive pharmacological treatment, non-pharmacological, and neutraceutical treatments, as well as lifestyle considerations.
2. Choosing the appropriate preventive agent is a decision that should individualized to each patient taking all of the following into consideration: patient disability, patient preference, side effect profile, patient comorbidities, medication interactions, route of administration, and cost/insurance coverage.
3. Patients should receive anticipatory guidance regarding the goals of preventive therapy and expectations for the timing of the onset of benefit.
4. Both drug-drug interactions involving the CYP450 and drug-disease interactions should be considered when choosing a preventive medication.

Case

A 42-year-old woman with a history of migraine without aura, bipolar disorder, anxiety, depression, and a history of renal stones presents to the clinic concerned about an increased frequency of migraine attacks and adverse reactions to acute and preventive medications. She is also sometimes using marijuana for sleep and anxiety benefits. She is currently on 10 mg of rizatriptan for acute treatment and propranolol extended release 60 mg for prevention. Other medications include citalopram, and as needed alprazolam. Previous trials have included sumatriptan for acute, but this caused severe nausea and flushing sensation. Topiramate exacerbated renal stones and amitriptyline made the mood worse.

Case Discussion

The treatment plan should be tailored to this patient. There is a drug-drug interaction here where propranolol may increase the dose of rizatriptan by as much as 50%, per the product labeling. One may consider alternative preventive medication or lowering the dose of rizatriptan. Regardless of coming off propranolol, it should be tapered off. Alternative options may include adding a monoclonal antibody or a gepant for prevention. Limited data exists for using a gepant with a monoclonal antibody, but there appears to be no potential drug-drug interaction noted thus far. Patients should also be counseled on the rare potential of reversible cerebral vasoconstriction syndrome, in patients with migraine and the use of marijuana.

Questions and Answers

1. Patient is a 43-year-old female with a history of migraine without aura. She is currently experiencing 9 days of migraine attacks per month. 7 out of her 9 headaches per month respond well to treatment with sumatriptan, but two persist despite triptan use with significant photophobia and nausea which interfere with her ability to function well at work. She has a history of asthma and has no other medical problems. She has been having difficulty sleeping which she thinks may be contributing to making her migraine attacks worse. Which of the following is the best choice for an initial preventive for this patient?
   A. Erenumab
   B. Propranolol
   C. Ubrogepant
   D. Amitriptyline
   E. Eptinezumab

   The correct answer is D. Although CGRP-targeted therapies may be considered, this will not address her sleep concern. Propranolol is contraindicated in this patient due to asthma. Ubrogepant is not recommended as an agent for migraine prevention. Amitriptyline is a traditional oral agent that is a correct choice.
2. Which migraine therapy should be avoided in glaucoma?
   A. Topiramate
   B. Propranolol
   C. Amitriptyline
   D. Candesartan
   E. Rimegepant

   The correct answer is A. Topiramate should be generally avoided in glaucoma, as there is a reported increased risk of angle-closure glaucoma with topiramate use.

References

1. Silberstein SD. Preventive migraine treatment. Continuum. 2015;21(4):973–89.
2. Silberstein SD. Practice parameter: evidence-based guidelines for migraine headache (an evidence-based review): report of the quality standards Subcommittee of the American Academy of Neurology. Neurology. 2000;55(6):754–62.
3. Dodick DW, Silberstein SD. Migraine prevention. Pract Neurol. 2007;7(6):383–93.
4. Buse DC, Gresiman JD, Baigi K, Lipton RB. Migraine progression: a systematic review. Headache. 2019;59(3):306–38.
5. Agbetou M, Adoukonou T. Lifestyle modifications for migraine management. Front Neurol. 2022;18(13):719467.
6. Ailani J, Burch RC, Robbins MC, et al. The American Headache Society consensus statement: update on integrating new migraine treatments into clinical practice. Headache. 2021;61(7):1021–39.
7. Kuruvilla D, Wells RE. Evidence-based integrative treatments for headache. Headache. 2019;59(6):971–2.
8. Silberstein SD, Holland S, Freitag F, et al. Evidence-based guideline update: pharmacologic treatment for episodic migraine prevention in adults: report of the Quality Standards Committee of the American Academy of Neurology and the American Headache Society. Neurology. 2012;78(17):1337–45.
9. Pringsheim T, Davenport W, Mackie G, et al. Candian Headache Society guideline for migraine prophylaxis. Can J Neurol Sci. 2012;39(2 suppl 2):S1–S59.
10. Hepp Z, Dodick DW, Varon SF, et al. Adherence to oral migraine preventive medications among patients with chronic migraine. Cepalalgia. 2015;35(6):478–88.
11. Blumenfeld AM, Bloudek LM, Becker WJ, et al. Patterns of use and reasons for discontinuation of prophylactic medications for episodic migraine and chronic migraine: results from the second international burden of migraine study (IBMS-II). Headache. 2013;53(4):644–55. 2018;38(6):1038–1048
12. Charles AC, Digre KB, Goadsby PJ, Robbins MS, Hershey A, American Headache Society. Calcitonin gene-related peptide-targeting therapies are a first-line option for the prevention of migraine: an American Headache Society position statement update. Headache. 2024;64(4):333–41.
13. Tassorelli C, Diener H-C, Dodick DW, et al. Guidelines of the International Headache Society for controlled trials of pre-

ventive treatment of chronic migraine in adults. Cephalalgia. 2018;38(5):815–32.
14. Roberts AG, Gibbs ME. Mechanisms and the clinical relevance of complex drug-drug interactions. Clin Pharmacol. 2018;10:123–34.
15. Seden K, Dickinson L, Khoo S, Back D. Grapefruit-drug interactions. Drugs. 2010;70:2373–240716.
16. Zevin S, Benowitz NL. Drug interactions with tobacco smoking: an update. Clin Pharmacokinet. 1999;36:425–38.
17. Brambila-Tapia AJ. MDR1 (ABCB1) polymorphisms: functional effects and clinical implications. Rev Investig Clin. 2013;65:445–54.
18. Ferrari A, Sternieri E, Ferraris E, Bertolini A. Emerging problems in the pharmacology of migraine: interactions between triptans and drugs for prophylaxis. Pharmacol Res. 2003;48:1–9.
19. Goldberg MR, Sciberras D, De Smet M, et al. Influence of beta-adrenoceptor antagonists on the pharmacokinetics of rizatriptan,a 5-HT1B/1D agonist: differential effects of propranolol, nadolol and metoprolol. Br J Clin Pharmacol. 2001;52:69–76.
20. Stout SM, Nielsen J, Welage LS, et al. Influence of metoprolol dosage release formulation on the pharmacokinetic drug interaction with paroxetine. J Clin Pharmacol. 2011;51:389–96.
21. Tsujimoto T, Sugiyama T, Shapiro MF, Noda M, Kajio H. Risk of cardiovascular events in patients with diabetes mellitus on β-blockers. Hypertension. 2017;70:103–10.
22. Huang YL, Lai CC, Wang YH, et al. Impact of selective and nonselective beta-blockers on the risk of severe exacerbations in patients with COPD. Int J Chron Obstruct Pulmon Dis. 2017;12:2987–96.
23. Wen X, Wang JS, Kivisto KT, Neuvonen PJ, Backman JT. In vitro evaluation of valproic acid as an inhibitor of human cytochrome P450 isoforms: preferential inhibition of cytochrome P450 2C9 (CYP2C9). Br J Clin Pharmacol. 2001;52:547–53.
24. Bagnato F, Good J. The use of antiepileptics in migraine prophylaxis. Headache. 2016;56:603–15.
25. Patsalos PN. The pharmacokinetic profile of topiramate. Rev Contemp Pharmaco. 1999;10:155–62.
26. Rosenfeld WE, Doose DR, Walker SA, Nayak RK. Effect of topiramate on the pharmacokinetics of an oral contraceptive containing norethindrone and ethinyl estradiol in patients with epilepsy. Epilepsia. 1997;38:317–23.
27. Stage TB, Brøsen K, Christensen MM. A comprehensive review of drug-drug interactions with metformin. Clin Pharmacokinet. 2015;54:811–24.
28. Palaniyappan L, Insole L, Ferrier N. Combining antidepressants: a review of evidence. Adv Psychiatr Treat. 2009;15:90–9.
29. Carradori S, Secci D, Petzer JP. MAO inhibitors and their wider applications: a patent review. Expert Opin Ther Pat. 2018;28:211–26.
30. Holliday SM, Venlafaxine BP. A review of its pharmacology and therapeutic potential in depression. Drugs. 1995;49:280–94.
31. Hamann SR, Blouin RA, McAllister RG Jr. Clinical pharmacokinetics of verapamil. Clin Pharmacokinet. 1984;9:26–41.
32. Krevsky B, Maurer AH, Niewiarowski T, Cohen S. Effect of verapamil on human intestinal transit. Dig Dis Sci. 1992;37:919–24.
33. Swash M, Ingram DA. Adverse effect of verapamil in myasthenia gravis. Muscle Nerve. 1992;15:396–8.
34. Ubrelvy (ubrogepant). Full prescribing information. Madison: Allergan USA, Inc; 2020.
35. Nurtec ODT (rimegepant). Full prescribing information. New Haven: Biohaven Pharmaceuticals; 2020.
36. Goadsby PJ, Dodick DW, Ailani J, et al. Safety, tolerability, and efficacy of orally administered atogepant for the prevention of episodic migraine in adults: a double-blind, randomised phase 2b/3 trial. Lancet Neurol. 2020;19:727–37.
37. Zhou H, Mascelli MA. Mechanisms of monoclonal antibody-drug interactions. Annu Rev Pharmacol Toxicol. 2011;51:359–72.
38. Xu Y, Gabriel K, Wang Y, et al. A multi-center, open-label, pharmacokinetic drug interaction study of erenumab and a combined oral contraceptive in healthy females. CNS Drugs. 2019;33:513–22.

Monoclonal Antibodies to Calcitonin Gene-Related-Peptide and Its Receptor for Migraine Prevention

28

Olivia Kingsford, Shane Root, and Jennifer Robblee

Introduction

Despite its wide-reaching effect, migraine has historically been treated with nonspecific medications like anti-hypertensives, anti-epileptics, and antidepressants [1–3]. More recently, however, a protein called calcitonin gene-related peptide (CGRP) involved in the pathophysiology has led to medications targeting both the CGRP molecule itself and its receptor. In randomized controlled trials, they were found to be effective in the prevention of both episodic and chronic migraine. In addition, open-label extension and real-world data studies have confirmed favorable safety, tolerability profiles, and a positive impact on quality of life.

Questions

1. A 29-year-old female presents to clinic for follow-up for her chronic migraine. She has been on topiramate and amitriptyline in the past for migraine prevention, but she continues to have 15 headache days per month. She plans to get pregnant in the next year. Which of the following is the best option for her for migraine prevention?
   A. Erenumab
   B. Fremanezumab
   C. Eptinezumab
   D. Atogepant
   E. None of the above
2. A 55-year-old female presents to clinic for follow-up for her episodic migraine. She feels her current preventative medication is no longer effective. Her home medications include lisinopril, hydrochlorothiazide, metformin, and escitalopram. Which of the following would *not* be a good option for her?
   A. Rimegepant
   B. Erenumab
   C. Fremanezumab
   D. Atogepant
   E. Galcanezumab

Calcitonin Gene-Related Peptide and Migraine

CGRP is a 37 amino acid neuropeptide with two major forms, alpha and beta, first identified in rats in 1983 [4]. Alpha-CGRP is distributed in the nervous system, both centrally and peripherally, whereas beta-CGRP is found in enteric nerves and the pituitary gland [4, 5]. The alpha isoform is considered to be more relevant in the pathophysiology of migraine, given its predominant expression in trigeminal ganglia [6]. Additionally, alpha-CGRP was demonstrated to be the main mediator in cerebral artery dilation [7].

The efficacy of CGRP-targeted pharmaceutical therapies for migraine is largely attributable to the protein's localization to thin C-fibers and the CGRP receptor positive myelinated Aδ fibers [8]. The activation of dural C-fiber nociceptors leads to the release of CGRP, further sensitizing the nociceptors and activating adjacent Aδ pain fibers [9–11]. It is a potent vasodilator and affects multiple organ systems [12]. In the 1980s, it was found to be released along with Substance P in the setting of trigeminal ganglion stimulation, and an elevation of CGRP levels was seen in external jugular vein blood during migraine [13, 14].

CGRP is released in acute migraine attacks [15]. In 1993, sumatriptan was found to normalize CGRP levels

O. Kingsford · S. Root · J. Robblee (✉)
Lewis Headache Center, Department of Neurology, Barrow Neurological Institute, St. Joseph's Hospital and Medical Center, Phoenix, AZ, USA

T. S. Monteith et al. (eds.), *Comprehensive Migraine Management*, https://doi.org/10.1007/978-3-031-86923-5_28

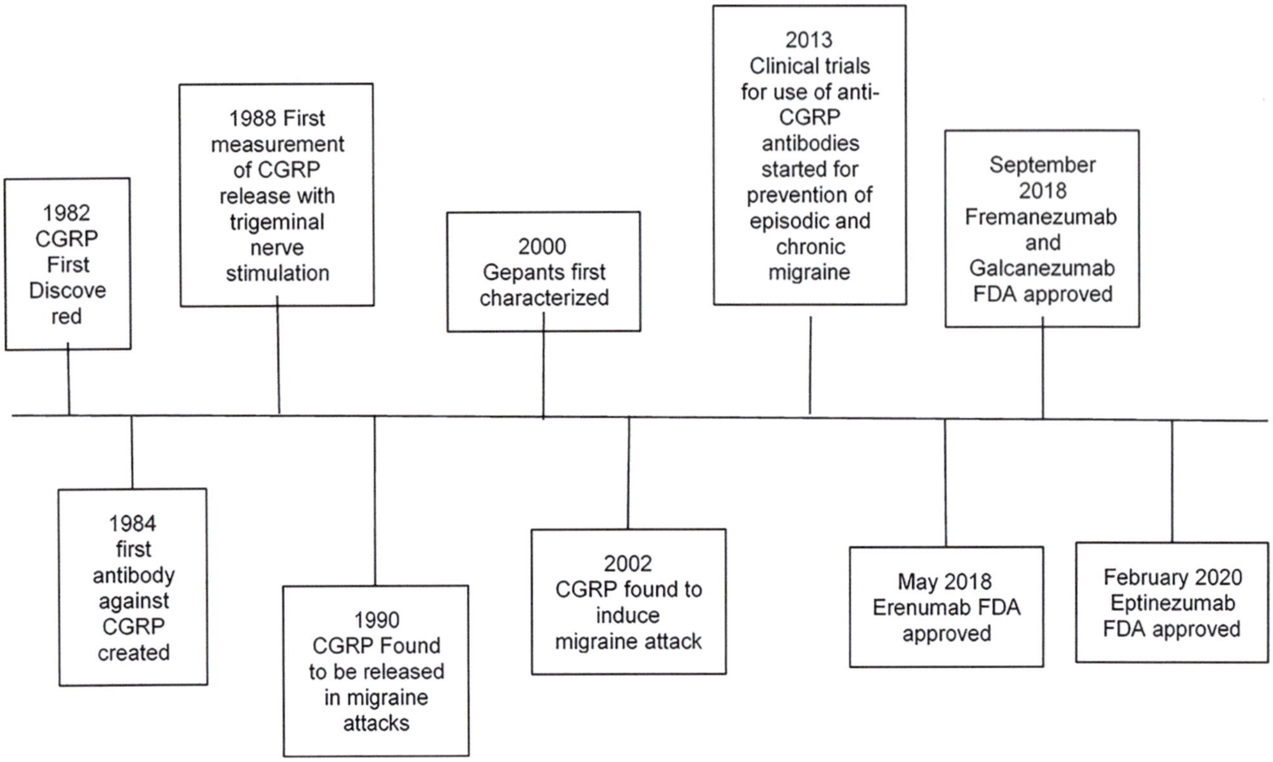

Fig. 28.1 Timeline of CGRP discovery and monoclonal antibody development

during acute migraine attacks along with resolving symptoms [16]. In 2002, one study found that infusion of CGRP could induce a migraine attack [17]. Small molecule CGRP receptor antagonists, known as "gepants," were the first medications targeting CGRP studied, but poor bioavailability and hepatotoxicity limited development of the first generation. Subsequently, monoclonal antibodies (mAbs) and the second generation of gepants have proven to be effective and well tolerated in the treatment of migraine. See Fig. 28.1 for a timeline of CGRP discovery and medication development [18–22].

CGRP Monoclonal Antibodies Versus Gepants

Important class differences exist between the CGRP mAbs and the small molecule CGRP antagonists (gepants). The monoclonal antibodies are significantly larger at approximately 150 kilodaltons than the small molecules (<1 kilodalton) [23]. The mAbs do not cross the blood–C-fibers–brain barrier in measurable quantities, so minimal central nervous system side effects are expected. The mAbs also have higher target specificity, which minimizes risk of off-target toxicity. The gepants carry a significantly shorter half-life (several minutes to hours), compared to the mAbs 3–6 week half-life. Neutralizing antibodies have been observed with the CGRP mAbs but not with use of the gepants, but this does not appear to be clinically relevant [24–27].

The first medications specifically targeted to the CGRP ligand or its receptor to receive FDA approval for migraine were the CGRP mAbs in 2018. The CGRP mAbs are indicated for the prevention of migraine only, unlike some of the gepants, which can be used for the acute treatment of migraine. Three of these medications, erenumab, fremanezumab, and galcanezumab, are self-administered subcutaneous injections. Eptinezumab is administered every 90 days as an intravenous infusion. Eptinezumab, fremanezumab, and galcanezumab inhibit the CGRP ligand, whereas erenumab is a monoclonal antibody against the CGRP receptor. See Table 28.1 for an overview of these medications. Dose, dosing frequency, side effect profile, and efficacy are reviewed in this chapter. Table 28.2 reviews key clinical trial, and Tables 28.3 and 28.4 will review data from post-market open-label trials.

Table 28.1 CGRP monoclonal antibodies with description of type of monoclonal antibody, its target, route of administration, dosing schedule, half-life, and reported side effects

	Erenumab	Fremanezumab	Galcanezumab	Eptinezumab
mAb type	Fully human IgG2	Humanized IgG2a	Humanized IgG4	Humanized IgG1
Target	CGRP Receptor	CGRP Ligand	CGRP Ligand	CGRP Ligand
Route	SC	SC	SC	IV
Dosing	70 mg, 140 mg monthly	225 mg monthly; 675 mg quarterly	240-mg loading dose, 120 mg monthly	100 mg, 300 mg quarterly
Half-life	28 days	31 days	27 days	27 days
Side Effects	Injection site irritation, allergic reaction, hypertension, constipation, alopecia	Injection site irritation, allergic reaction	Injection site irritation, allergic reaction	Allergic reaction, stuffy nose, sore throat
Other Indications	Post-Traumatic Headache Pending studies: pediatric migraine	Pending studies: pediatric migraine, post-traumatic headache, migraine interictal symptoms, and fibromyalgia	Cluster headache Pending studies: vestibular migraine	Pending studies: episodic cluster, medication overuse, pediatric migraine

mAb monoclonal antibody, *SC* subcutaneous, *IV* intravenous

Table 28.2 Summary of completed Phase 3 trials in episodic and chronic migraine

Medication	Trial name	*n*	Population	Dose	Monthly migraine days	50% Responder rate (%)
Erenumab	ARISE	577	EM	70 mg	−2.9	39.7
				Placebo	−1.8	29.5
	STRIVE	955	EM	70 mg	−3.2	50.0
				140 mg	−3.7	43.3
				Placebo	−1.8	26.6
	LIBERTY	246	EM (2–4 Rx)	140 mg	−1.8[a]	30
				Placebo	−0.2[a]	14
Fremanezumab	HALO-EM	875	EM	Monthly[c]	−4.2	47.7
				Quarterly[d]	−4.0	44.4
				Placebo	−2.7	27.9
	HALO-CM	1130	CM	Monthly[e]	−4.6[a]	40.8
				Quarterly[d]	−4.3[a]	37.6
				Placebo	−2.5[a]	18.1
	FOCUS	838	EM & CM	Monthly[c]	−4.1[b]	34
				Quarterly[d]	−3.7[b]	34
				Placebo	−0.6[b]	9
Galcanezumab	EVOLVE-1	862	EM	120 mg[f]	−4.73	62.3
				240 mg[g]	−4.57	60.9
				Placebo	−2.81	38.6
	EVOLVE-2	986	EM	120 mg[f]	−4.29	59.3
				240 mg[g]	−4.18	56.5
				Placebo	−2.28	36.0
	REGAIN	1118	CM	120 mg[f]	−4.83	35.1
				240 mg[g]	−4.62	37.0
				Placebo	−2.64	24.7
	CONQUER	463	EM or CM (2–4 Rx)	120 mg[f]	−4.14	37.7
				Placebo	−1.02	13.3
Eptinezumab[h]	PROMISE-1	898	EM	30 mg	−4.1	50.2
				100 mg	−3.9	49.8
				300 mg	−4.3	56.3
				Placebo	−3.1	37.4
	PROMISE-2	1121	CM	100 mg	−7.7	57.6
				300 mg	−8.2	61.3
				Placebo	−5.6	39.3
Atogepant	ADVANCE	834	EM	10 mg	−3.7	55.6
				30 mg	−3.9	58.7
				60 mg	−4.2	60.8
				Placebo	−2.5	29.0
Rimegepant	NCT03732638[i]	1591	EM	75 mg q2d	−4.3	49.1
				Placebo	−3.5	41.5

[a]Used adjusted mean change, [b]Least-square mean, [c]Monthly dosing is 225 mg each month, [d]Quarterly dosing was 675 mg every 3 months, [e]Monthly dosing was 675 mg month 1, 225 mg month 2, and 225 mg month 3, [f]240-mg loading dose followed by 120 mg monthly thereafter, [g]240-mg dose provided monthly, [h]Intravenous medication, [i]Phase 2/3 study

Rx Prior medications tried, *PND* Results pending, *BID* Twice daily, *QD* Once daily, *q2d* Once every other day

Table 28.3 Relative risk per 1000 exposed patients of adverse events for erenumab, fremanezumab, and galcanezumab reported to the FDA during the first 6 months of their availability

	Erenumab	Fremanezumab	Galcanezumab
Migraine	4.89	1.01	2.99
Headache	3.32	1.27	3.07
Drug ineffective	3.68	1.14	1.69
Nausea	2.94	0.91	1.09
Injection site pain	2.94	0.8	4.9
Injection site swelling	0.56	0.53	1.25
Injection site pruritus	0.26	0.63	1.14
Injection site erythema	0.58	0.71	1.58
Constipation	4.90	0.46	0.76
Fatigue	2.33	0.58	1.09
Cardiovascular disorder	0.02	–	–

Table 28.4 Review of post-market open-label trials

Drug(s) included	Study type	Year	*n*	Diagnosis	Primary outcome	Study duration	12-week MMD	12-week 50%RR	Adverse effects
G [28]	P	2023	191	EM, CM	MMD, 50%RR	12 months	5.5 ± 5.5 (EM) 7.4 ± 5.9 (CM)	69.8% (EM) 64.9% (CM)	constipation, ISR, dizziness, arthralgia, Raynaud
Er, F, G [29]	R	2022	104	CM	50%RR	24 weeks	13.9 (Er), 12.1 (G), 9.9 (F)	41% (Er), 46.2% (G), 53.8% (F)	GI, asthenia, edema
Er, F, G [30]	P	2022	864	EM, CM	reduction in headache days	6 months	N/A	64.9% (EM) 61.4% (CM)	N/A
Er, F, G [31]	P	2022	203	CM[b]	MMD	12 months	−8.2–12.1	36.4–56.8%	fatigue, ISR, constipation, muscle pain
Er, F, G [32]	R	2022	192	CM[a]	safety, MHD	12 months	−2.6	not listed	constipation, ISR
Er, F [33]	P	2022	19	CM[a]	MHD	9 months	−1.3 ± 4.9	not listed	none
Ep [34]	R	2022	128	CM	MIDAS	96 weeks	5.7	44.4%	constipation, asthenia, ISR
Er [35]	P	2022	164	CM	MMD	2 years	−7.5 at 6 months	31% at 6 months	constipation, flu-like symptoms, mood change
Er [36]	R	2022	166	EM, CM, MOH	MHD, acute Rx	6 months	−11.0	46.5%	constipation
Er [37]	P	2022	30	CM	MHD	6 months	15 (>65y) 12 (<65 yr)	N/A	constipation, ISR
Er [38]	R	2022	82	EM, CM[b]	reduction in headache days	6 months	−4.97	36.5%	N/A
Er [39]	P	2022	300	CM	MHD	52 weeks	−8.9	56.3%	constipation, nausea, fatigue. PE in one
Er [40]	R	2022	128	EM, CM	adverse effects	12 months	N/A	N/A	constipation, skin reactions, fatigue, sleep disturbances, nausea
Er [41]	P	2022	103	EM, CM[a]	MHD	3 months	−8	61.8%	constipation, tremors and tachycardia
F [42]	R	2022	1003	EM, CM[b]	N/A	6 months	−4.7 (EM) −7.9 (CM) −7.0 (MOH)	52.1% (EM) 58.3% (CM) 48.5% (MOH)	N/A
F [43]	P	2022	67	EM, CM	MHD	12 weeks	−9.4	76.5% (EM) 58.3% (CM)	N/A
G [44]	P	2022	43	EM, CM	MHD	6 months	7.44	72.09%	constipation, fatigue, acrocyanosis
G [45]	P	2022	156	CM[b]	MMD	3 months	N/A	41.7%	N/A

(continued)

Table 28.4 (continued)

Drug(s) included	Study type	Year	*n*	Diagnosis	Primary outcome	Study duration	12-week MMD	12-week 50%RR	Adverse effects
Er, F, G [46]	P	2021	52	EM, CM	MMD[d]	3 months	−10	N/A	constipation, muscle cramps, itching
G, Fr, Er [47]	P	2021	40	menstrual migraine	MMD	6 months	−3 in 6 months	N/A	N/A
G, Fr, Er [48]	P	2021	17	CM[a]	reduction in headache days	6 months	at 6 months −9 ± 9.4	N/A	N/A
Er, G [49]	P	2021	139	CM[b]	MHD, MOH	6 months	MOH 13.4 ± 7.6 non-MO −7.8 ± 7.2	63.6% MOH, 57.5% non-MO	N/A
Er, F, G [50]	R	2021	112	CM, NDPH, PPTH[c]	MHD	12 months	−2–3.2	not listed	ISR, constipation, fatigue, dizziness
Er [51]	R	2021	91	EM, CM[b]	MMD	12 months	5.0 ± 2.8	80.2%	N/A
Er [52]	OLE	2021	383	EM	MMD, Acute Rx, QOL	5 years	−5.3 (at year 5)	N/A	nasopharyngitis, URI, influenza, ligament rupture, osteoarthritis, uterine leiomyoma, adjustment disorder, DVT, breast cancer. 2 unrelated fatalities
Er [53]	R	2021	26	EM, CM[b]	MMD	12 months	−11.88	not listed	N/A
Er [54]	P	2021	75	CM	psychiatric predictors of negative outcomes	12 months	N/A	70.6%	N/A
Er [55]	P	2021	100	EM, CM	MMD	6 months	−3.8 ± 7.5	36%	constipation, fatigue, ISR
Er [56]	R	2021	18	EM, CM	MHD	1 year	−5.2 at 1 year	50% at 1 year	constipation
Er [57]	P	2021	98	CM[b]	Disability	12 months	−6.4	not listed	constipation
Er, F, G [58]	R	2020	77	CM	Adverse events, 50%RR	6 months	N/A	48.5%	constipation, ISR
Er [59]	P	2020	89	EM, CM[b]	MMD	6 months	−7	69.7%	constipation, ISR, pruritus, flu-like symptoms
Er [60]	P	2020	164	CM	MMD	6 months	−6.0	35%	constipation, flu-like symptoms, generalized aches, itchiness, ISR, spasms
Er [61]	R	2020	101	EM, CM	MHD	6 months	−6.5	34.9%	constipation
Er [62]	OLE	2019	235	EM	Safety	5 years	N/A	N/A	URI, sinusitis, influenza, back pain
G [63]	P	2018	135	EM, CM	MMD	12 months	−5.6 (120 mg) −6.5 (240 mg)	N/A	ISR, nasopharyngitis, URI, back pain, sinusitis

Acute Rx Change in acute medication use, *CM* chronic migraine, *EM* Episodic migraine, *Er* Erenumab, *Ep* Eptinezumab, *F* Fremanezumab, *G* Galcanezumab, *GI* GI symptoms, *MHD* Change in monthly headache days, *MMD* Change in monthly migraine days, *50%RR* 50% responder rate, *MOH* Medication overuse headache, *N/A* Not available, *NDPH* new daily persistent headache, *PE* Pulmonary Embolism, *PPTH* persistent post-traumatic headache, *QOL* Quality of life

[a]These studies included patients on OnabotulinumtoxinA

[b]These studies included patients with MOH demonstrating that CGRP monoclonal antibodies are effective in this population

[c]These studies include a pediatric population demonstrating efficacy in this population

[d]MMD looked at before, 3 and 12 months after starting CGRP mAb, and 1–3 months after stopping CGRP mAb

The CGRP Monoclonal Antibodies

Erenumab

Erenumab [AMG 334] was the first CGRP monoclonal antibody to be approved for migraine prevention by the FDA in May 2018. It is a fully human IgG2 monoclonal antibody targeting the CGRP receptor. It is a self-administered subcutaneous injection that comes as an autoinjector or prefilled syringe. Dosing is 70 mg or 140 mg per month. Adverse effects are injection site reaction, nasopharyngitis and upper respiratory infections, and constipation [24, 64]. Hypertension was seen in a post-market analysis, but not the double-blind randomized controlled trials [65]. Raynaud's phenomenon was also seen in post-market analysis. Dry natural rubber, a latex derivative, constitutes the needle shield within the white cap of the autoinjector as well as the gray needle cap of the prefilled syringe, so severe latex allergy should be considered.

There were three phase 3 trials that assessed the efficacy of erenumab in episodic migraine: ARISE, STRIVE, and LIBERTY with a later phase 3 EM and CM trial in a Japanese population. See Table 28.2 for a summary of these 3 trials leading to FDA approval.

The ARISE trial was a randomized, double-blind, placebo-controlled, phase 3 study that compared 70 mg to placebo[64]. The primary endpoint was a change in monthly migraine days (MMD), which showed a −2.9 change for the 70-mng dose as compared to 1.98 for placebo. The 50% responder rate for the 70-mg dose was 39.7% compared to 29.5% for placebo. Adverse events were upper respiratory tract infection, injection site pain, and nasopharyngitis.

The STRIVE trial was a multicenter, randomized, double-blind, placebo-controlled, parallel-group, phase 3 trial conducted at 121 sites across North America, Europe, and Turkey that compared 70-mg and 140-mg subcutaneous dosing to placebo for episodic migraine [24]. Primary endpoint was a change from baseline to months 4–6 in the mean number of headache days per month. MMD were reduced by 3.2 in the 70-mg group and 3.7 in the 140-mg group, as compared to 1.8 with placebo. A 50% or greater reduction of migraine days in 43% with 70-mg and in 50% with 140-mg dosing at the 4–6 month mark compared to 27% for placebo.

The LIBERTY trial was a double-blinded, placebo-controlled randomized trial involving 59 sites in 16 countries that compared the efficacy of 140-mg dosing to placebo in patients with episodic migraine for whom at least 2–4 other medications had been tried and found to be ineffective in reducing migraine days [66]. Primary endpoint was a 50% or greater reduction in the number of MMD during weeks 9–12. The 50% responder rate was 30% for 140 mg and 14% for placebo. The adjusted mean change for MMD days was −1.8 for 140 mg compared to −0.2 for placebo.

Erenumab has also been studied in chronic migraine. A double-blinded, placebo-controlled, randomized, phase 3 trial was completed in Japan comparing erenumab 70 mg to placebo in both episodic and chronic migraine. The subgroup analysis is now published for the chronic migraine subgroup [67]. In the chronic migraine subgroup, there was a comparison between patients with prior preventative trials and those with no prior preventative trials and those with the presence of a concomitant preventative medications. All of these sub-subgroups have a significant p-value for comparison of 70 mg to placebo. NCT02066415 is a phase 2 study that evaluated 70-mg and 140-mg dosing vs placebo over 12 weeks for patients aged 18–65 with chronic migraine [68]. The primary outcome was change in MMD, which demonstrated a 6.64 and 6.63 reduction for 70 mg and 140 mg, respectively, as compared to a 4.18 reduction for placebo. The 50% responder rates were 49.9% for 70 mg, 41.2% for 140 mg, and 23.5% for placebo. DRAGON is a phase 3 trial of 70 mg versus placebo in patients with migraine in Asia that is pending publication.

Erenumab is being evaluated for the treatment of other headache disorders and medical conditions as well. Monthly administration of erenumab 140 mg was found to result in a reduction of monthly migraine days for patients experiencing post-traumatic headache during an open-label, 12-week trial [69]. At the time of this writing, studies and trials are currently in progress evaluating the efficacy and tolerability of erenumab in chronic migraine and pediatric migraine.

Fremanezumab

Fremanezumab [TEV 48125] is a fully humanized IgG2a monoclonal antibody that potently and selectively binds to the CGRP ligand. It was approved by the FDA for migraine prevention in September 2018. It is a self-administered subcutaneous injection, with the option to take 225 mg once a month or 675 mg quarterly. It comes as an autoinjector or a prefilled syringe. The most common adverse effect seen in the trials was injection site reaction (pain, induration, erythema). Other adverse effects included nasopharyngitis and upper respiratory tract infections, dizziness, and nausea [27, 70]. Post-market analysis has also demonstrated hypertension and Raynaud's phenomenon.

The HALO studies evaluated fremanezumab: HALO-EM, evaluating its efficacy in episodic migraine, HALO-CM, evaluating its efficacy in chronic migraine, and HALO LTS, evaluating its effect long term [27, 70, 71]. A phase 3b study, FOCUS, evaluated patients with episodic and chronic migraine with 2–4 prior medication trials [72]. See Table 28.2 for a summary of these trials. After FDA approval, 2 phase 3 trials, one for EM and one for CM, were conducted in Japanese and Korean patients [73, 74].

The HALO-EM trial was a randomized, double-blind, placebo-controlled, parallel-group study involving 123 investigative sites in 9 countries [70]. Monthly doses of 225 mg vs quarterly doses of 675 mg (followed by two placebo doses) were compared to placebo over 12 weeks for patients with episodic migraine. There was a 4.2 and 4.0 reduction in MMD for monthly and quarterly dosing, respectively as compared to a 2.7 reduction for placebo. The 50% responder rates were 48% for monthly, 44% for quarterly, and 28% for placebo.

The HALO-CM trial was a randomized, double-blind, placebo-controlled, parallel-group trial involving 132 sites in 9 countries [27]. Monthly and quarterly dosing were compared to placebo. The monthly 225 mg had a loading dose of 657 mg for the first month. The quarterly dosing was 675 mg followed by 2 placebo months. The change from baseline in MMD was −4.6 for monthly, −4.3 for quarterly, and −2.5 for placebo. The 50% responder rates were 41% in monthly, 38% in quarterly, and 18% in placebo.

FOCUS was a randomized, double-blind, placebo-controlled phase 3b trial that enrolled 329 episodic migraine patients and 509 chronic migraine patients [72]. Monthly and quarterly dosing was compared to placebo with the primary outcome of reduction in MMD from baseline over 12 weeks. The primary outcome was significant with least-squares mean (LSM) of −4.2 for monthly, −3.7 for quarterly, and −0.6 for placebo. The 50% responder rates were 34% for both dosing schedules compared to 9% for placebo.

Investigation is currently underway to evaluate the efficacy and safety of fremanezumab in the treatment of pediatric migraine, post-traumatic headache, migraine interictal symptoms, and fibromyalgia.

Galcanezumab

Galcanezumab [LY2951742] is a fully humanized anti-CGRP IgG4 mAb that targets the CGRP ligand and binds with high affinity and high specificity. It was approved by the FDA for migraine prevention in September 2018. It is a self-administered subcutaneous injection with a loading dose of 240 mg followed by 120-mg dosing once a month. It comes as a prefilled syringe or pen. Adverse effects were injection site reactions, upper respiratory tract infections, sinusitis, and influenza [25, 75]. Post-market analysis has also demonstrated hypertension and Raynaud's phenomenon.

There were three studies that evaluated galcanezumab: "Evaluation of LY2951742 in the Prevention of Episodic Migraine" (EVOLVE) 1 and 2, and REGAIN. See Table 28.2 for a summary of these trials.

EVOLVE 1 was a double-blind, randomized, placebo-controlled that compared 120-mg and 240-mg dosing to placebo over 6 months for episodic migraine [25]. The 120-mg arm had a 240-mg loading dose followed by 120 mg monthly; the 240-mg arm was 240 mg monthly for 6 months. MMD were reduced by 4.73 for 120 mg and by 4.57 for 240 mg compared to a 2.81 reduction for placebo. The 50% responder rates were 62% for 120 mg, 60.9% for 240 mg, and 38.6% for placebo.

EVOLVE 2 was a phase 3, multicenter randomized, double-blinded, placebo-controlled trial for chronic migraine that also compared 120-mg and 240-mg dosing to placebo over 6 months, similar to EVOLVE-1 [75]. MMD were reduced by 4.29 for 120 mg and 4.18 for 240 mg as compared to a 2.28 reduction for placebo. 50% responder rates were 59.3% for 120 mg, 56.5% for 240 mg, and 36.0% for placebo.

REGAIN was a phase 3, double-blinded, randomized, placebo-controlled trial that compared 120-mg and 240-mg dosing to placebo over 3 months for chronic migraine [76]. The dosing was the same as for EVOLVE-1 and -2. MMD were reduced by 4.83 for 120 mg and 4.62 for 240 mg as compared to a 2.64 reduction for placebo. 50% responder rates were 35.1% for 120 mg, 37.0% for 240 mg, and 24.7% for placebo.

CONQUER is a newer phase 3b trial that looked at both episodic and chronic migraine in patients with 2–4 prior medication trials [77]. The 120-mg dose with 240-mg loading was compared to placebo. The primary outcome was change in MMD with 120 mg showing a −4.1.4 reduction in MMD compared to placebo of −1.0.

Galcanezumab 300 mg has an indication for prevention of cluster headache; the drug is currently being evaluated for its efficacy in treating vestibular migraine.

Eptinezumab

Eptinezumab [ALD 403] is a genetically engineered, desialylated, humanized a-CGRP IgG1 antibody that selectively and potently binds to alpha and beta forms of human CGRP. It is administered as 100 mg or 300 mg intravenously every 3 months. Adverse effects are hypersensitivity reaction and nasopharyngitis at similar rates to placebo [26, 78]. The formation of neutralizing antibodies was noted but was not clinically significant [26, 78].

Eptinezumab was studied in two phase 3 randomized controlled trials: "PRevention Of Migraine via Intravenous ALD403 Safety and Efficacy" (PROMISE) 1 and 2 trials [26, 78]. See Table 28.2 for a summary. PROMISE 1 was a phase 3, multicenter, randomized, double-blind, placebo-controlled, parallel-group study in episodic migraine [26]. Doses of 30 mg, 100 mg, and 300 mg every 3 months were compared to placebo over 12 weeks. It found that the 100-mg and 300-mg doses met the primary end point of reducing migraine days as compared to placebo[34]. The change in MMD was −4.1 for 40 mg, −3.9 for 100 mg, −4.3 for 300 mg, and −3.1 for placebo. The 50% responder rates were 50%, 50%, 56%, and 37% for 30 mg, 100 mg, 300 mg, and placebo, respectively.

PROMISE 2 was phase 3, multicenter, randomized, double-blind, placebo-controlled, parallel-group study in chronic migraine [78]. It compared 100-mg and 300-mg doses to placebo over 12 weeks. The change in MMD was −7.7 for 100 mg, −8.2 for 300 mg, and −5.6 for placebo. The 50% responder rates were 58%, 61%, and 39%, respectively, for 100 mg, 300 mg, and placebo.

There are three other recent phase III/IIIb trials in progress. DELIVER demonstrated efficacy in migraine patients with 2–4 prior ineffective treatments [79]. SUNLIGHT and SUNRISE focus on populations in Asia (China and Japan), but are pending completion. At the time of this writing, studies are underway to evaluate the efficacy of eptinezumab for its treatment of episodic cluster headache, medication overuse headache, and pediatric migraine.

Clinical Considerations

Safety

The overall safety of CGRP mAbs and gepants appears very favorable, especially when compared to antidepressants, antihypertensives, and anti-epileptic medications, which have been the mainstay of migraine prevention for decades. Across clinical trials, adverse events are generally comparable to placebo; injection site reactions were the most common adverse events, although discontinuation rates were overall uncommon. Although CGRP is a potent vasodilator and has demonstrated protective characteristics against hypertension in mouse models, there has been no evidence demonstrating clinically significant vasoconstriction by CGRP mAbs or gepants [80, 81]. Patients with a history of stable angina due to coronary artery disease were evaluated by way of treadmill exercise test immediately following administration of erenumab 140 mg with no difference in total exercise time or adverse events, compared with placebo [82].

Post-market studies have identified further adverse event patterns. As mentioned previously, post-market analysis of erenumab suggested concern of hypertension as an adverse effect, though no difference in hypertension adverse effects was observed during the double-blind treatment phase of erenumab 70 mg or 140 mg compared to placebo [64]. From the FDA Adverse Events Reporting System (FAESR), a retrospective study from the first 6 months of CGRP mAb use was reported as outlined in Table 28.3 [83]. They also noted that cardiovascular events were not in the top 10 adverse events for any of the CGRP mAbs and that serious outcomes were seen in <2% [83]. A more recent study found a 3.7% increase in the number of antihypertensive medications prescribed annually for all CGRP monoclonal antibodies [84]. Hypertension is now included on the FDA label for all 4 monoclonal antibodies [85–88].

Another study from FAERS looking at the fourth quarter of 2021 found that alopecia had a proportional reporting ratio of 4.29 for CGRP mAbs compared to all other drugs in FAERS, but similar to that for triptans and celecoxib [89]. A 2022 study looking at the Vigibase real-world data from the World Health Organization found 99 reports of Raynaud's phenomenon with CGRP mAbs with an information component (IC) of 3.3 (3.0–3.5), which they compared to triptans (IC 0.4 (0.1–0.6) and beta blockers (IC 0.5 (0.2–0.7) [90]. A retrospective study of 169 patients on CGRP antagonists found that 9 (5.3%) had microvascular complications including, 4 with worsening of prior Raynaud's, 4 with new onset Raynaud's including one with gangrene and autonecrosis, and one patients with known scleroderma experiencing worsening facial telangiectasia as well as digit acroosteolysis and subcutaneous calcinosis [91]. Raynaud's phenomenon has now been added to the label for all 4 CGRP mAbs [85–88].

Restricted Use During Pregnancy

Little data exists regarding the use of CGRP antagonists in the setting of pregnancy, though a dose-dependent relationship was observed between CGRP administration and the increase in systolic blood pressure, fetal growth retardation, and increased fetal mortality in pregnant rat models [92]. A total of 94 safety reports of human patients exposed to either erenumab, fremanezumab, or galcanezumab show no signal of disproportionate reporting for maternal toxicities, spontaneous abortions, or major birth defects when compared to the full database [93]. Regardless, the use of CGRP-related medications in both pregnancy and lactation is recommended against at the time of this writing while more data is gathered and evaluated. Specifically, the current recommendation is to stop CGRP mAbs at least 6 months prior to conception.

Adolescent and Pediatric Indications

At the time of this writing, migraine trials in pediatric and adolescent populations have not been performed and outcome data is limited. One retrospective multicenter study found that the CGRP mAbs were similarly effective and had similar side effects in adolescents as in adults [50]. In the interim, the Pediatric and Adolescent Headache special interest group of the American Headache Society published a manuscript to serve as Class IV evidence for guidelines for use in these populations [94] It is reasonable to consider the use of CGRP mAbs for pediatric and adolescent patients with frequent migraine or significant disability with cautious monitoring, but guidelines recommend appropriate prior pharmacologic and non-pharmacologic treatment trials [94]. Of note, clinical trials are currently underway to determine safety and efficacy.

Other Potential Considerations

According to the American Headache Society, there are additional conditions in which use of CGRP monoclonal antibodies is cautioned [94]. They caution use in those with a compromised blood–brain barrier, peripheral nerve injury, pregnancy, breastfeeding, cardiovascular disease, cerebrovascular disease, bone disease including osteopenia (especially pre-pubertal), and immunodeficiency. The reason for these cautions is that CGRP has many physiologic roles outside of migraine that include nervous system maturation or repair, utero-placental functions and vascular adaptations, neuro-immune axis, and vasodilation. Finally, there does appear to be benefit in medication overuse headache patients as well in refractory migraine based on many of the CGRP mAb clinical trials [25, 66, 72, 77, 78]. Despite the noted cautions, the strong evidence for these medication led to AHS releasing a position statement in 2024 stating that CGRP targeting medications should be considered first-line for the prevention of migraine [95].

OnabotulinumtoxinA and CGRP Inhibition

Concomitant use of onabotulinumtoxinA and CGRP mAb has also been evaluated, and, in fact, the American Headache Society consensus statement from 2021 considers this combination to be "probably effective" [96]. OnabotulinumtoxinA is a neurotoxin that acts as a presynaptic neuromuscular blocking agent but does affect CGRP [97]. It causes reversible muscle weakness when injected intramuscularly. The heavy chain binds to receptors on the C-fiber nerve terminal, is endocytosed into the cell as a vesicle, the light chain dissociates and enters the cytoplasm where it cleaves SNAP-25, which prevents vesicles containing peptides from fusing with the cell membrane and preventing the release of neuropeptides, including CGRP. As previously discussed, the activation of nociceptors on C-fibers is thought to be a mechanism of the pathophysiology of migraine, and by blocking neuropeptide release, onabotulinumtoxinA was theorized to prevent migraine attacks from occurring. Considering the CGRP monoclonal antibodies block activity of A-delta pain fibers, concomitant usage of onabotulinumtoxinA with a CGRP monoclonal antibody may act synergistically to prevent migraine pain by modulating both c-fibers and A-delta fibers (Fig. 28.2).

In a post-market study of erenumab, 83.2% of the 101 patients had been on onabotulinumtoxinA with 23% (10/43) of those with complete 6-month data reporting concurrent onabotulinumtoxinA use [61]. While no difference was found between the subgroup with concurrent onabotulinumtoxinA use versus those not on onabotulinumtoxinA, no adverse effect related to the combination was reported. A retrospective chart review of 257 patients on combo therapy of CGRP mAb and onabotulinumtoxinA showed that CGRP mAbs were discontinued in 23% compared to only 3% of onabotulinumtoxinA [100]. When compared to baseline with onabotulinumtoxinA only, monthly headache days were decreased at all visits over 6–12 months of combined treatment with good tolerance. Another retrospective review of 78 patients on both erenumab and onabotulinumtoxinA showed that compared to baseline on just onabotulinumtoxinA, patients had an 8.1 migraine headache day reduction with the addition of erenumab. A third retrospective study of 253 patients found that 72.5% reported a decrease in headache severity with the addition of a CGRP mAb to onabotulinumtoxinA [101]. In 66 patients with headache frequency data, MMD decreased by 10.9 with initial onabotulinumtoxinA addition, and by another 5.7 MMD reduction with CGRP mAb addition. None of these studies reported major adverse events.

Use of gepants with onabotulinumtoxinA is commonly done and felt to be safe, though studies are limited. Concomitant usage of ubrogepant and onabotulinumtoxinA was evaluated in a 46 patient subgroup of a post-market study on ubrogepant [102]. Between patients receiving onabotulinumtoxinA and those who were not, no differences were found in the responder rate or adverse event rate.

The pharmacokinetics of sumatriptan and patients' resting blood pressures were found to be unaffected with co-administration of sumatriptan 12-mg injection and erenumab 140 mg [103]. There is no current evidence to suggest that any of the CGRP mAbs have pharmacokinetic interactions with other drugs [104]. In fact, a phase 1 study showed no pharmacokinetic concerns when combining ubrogepant with erenumab or galcanezumab [105].

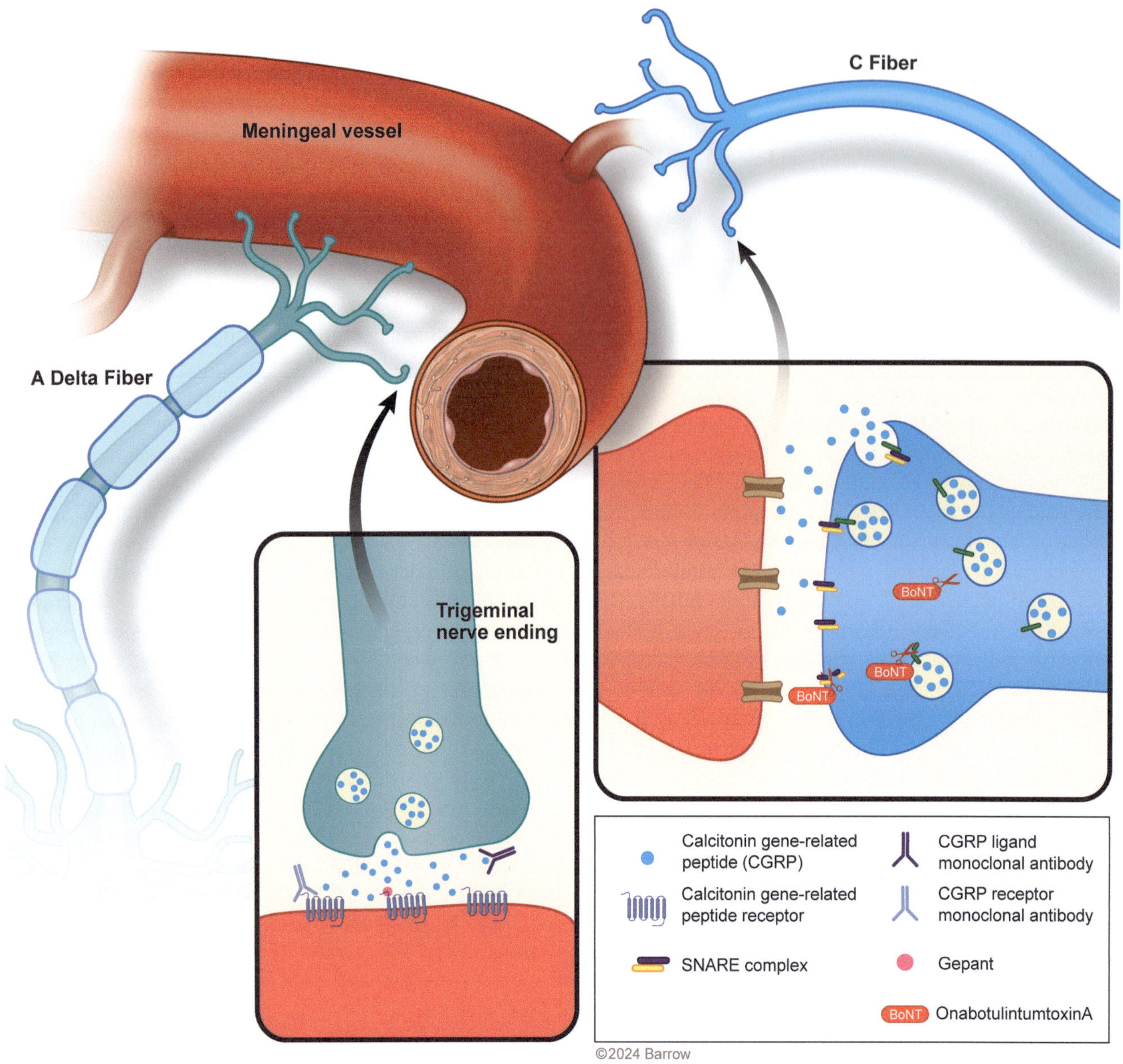

Fig. 28.2 Anatomical Sites of Action of CGRP inhibitors and onabotulinumtoxinA in migraine prevention. (Inspired by [9, 98, 99]). (Used with permission from Barrow Neurological Institute, Phoenix, Arizona)

Integration into Clinical Practice and Future Therapeutic

Numerous studies have shown that CGRP mAbs reduce healthcare utilization and emergency room visits. For migraine prevention, CGRP mAbs are considered first line according to the European Headache Federation guidelines, and likewise with physician attestation according to the American Headache Society consensus statement [95, 96, 106]. Numerous studies have shown that CGRP mAbs reduce healthcare utilization and emergency room visits. For migraine prevention, CGRP mAbs are considered first line according to the European Headache Federation guidelines, and likewise with physician attestation according to the American Headache Society consensus statement [96, 106]. At the time of this writing, there have been limited studies comparing the efficacy of CGRP inhibitors to previous migraine treatments. Reuter et al. performed a randomized, double-blind, active-controlled phase 4 trial of erenumab 70 mg or 140 mg versus Topiramate titrated to 50–100 mg per day [107]. They enrolled 777 patients with a 10.6% discontinuation rate in the erenumab group versus a 38.9% discontinuation rate in the topiramate group. The 50% response rate was 55.4% for erenumab compared to 31.2% for topiramate. The authors concluded that erenumab was effective and tolerable as compared to topiramate.

A meta-analysis by Frank et al. sought to compare the efficacy of the CGRP mAbs to topiramate or onabotulinumtoxinA [108]. They found all three classes demonstrated at least a 50% response rate as compared to placebo, with topiramate showing the greatest efficacy in terms of 50% responder rate, but also had the highest drop-out rate. A network meta-analysis compared the four CGRP mAbs with onabotulinumtoxinA or topiramate for chronic migraine [109]. They found that a single dose of eptinezumab, compared to placebo, was the most effective treatment with a mean difference of −2.60 days while fremanezumab 675/225/225 had the best responder rate compared to placebo, with an odd ratio of 2.96. Another meta-analysis for episodic migraine compared the four CGRP mAbs and topiramate, finding no difference in the reduction of MMD but that the CGRP mAbs had the better safety profile [110]. The number needed to treat (NNT) for CGRP mAbs was 6 compared to 7 for topiramate while the number needed to harm (NNH) was 130 for CGRP mAbs versus 9 for topiramate.

As the use of CGRP mAbs and gepants becomes more prevalent, head-to-head comparison of efficacy trials between them as well as compared to nonspecific oral medications and onabotulinumtoxinA are an avenue for future research to help decide when each should be used.

Pituitary adenylate cyclase activating polypeptide-38 (PACAP38) is a neuropeptide involved in neuroprotection, development, nociception, and inflammation. It has been found to induce severe migraine attacks and may be a promising target of future treatments for patients who do not respond to CGRP inhibition [111].

Conclusion

CGRP is a molecule thought to underlie the pathophysiology of migraine through its activation of the trigeminovascular system. CGRP inhibitors (monoclonal antibodies and small molecule inhibitors called gepants) are the first medications specifically designed for the prevention of migraine, advancing personalized medicine. Multiple randomized controlled trials have found that the monoclonal antibodies (erenumab, galcanezumab, fremanezumab, and eptinezumab) were safe and effective in reducing MMD for both episodic and chronic migraine. Further studies are needed to determine clinical predictors of drug response, concurrent use of various medication classes, as well as for head-to-head comparison for efficacy, tolerability, and cost effectiveness.

Teaching Points

1. The trigeminal vascular system, which has access to circulating antibodies, is likely the site of action of CGRP mAbs. Activation of C-fiber nociceptors in the dura is thought to lead to release of CGRP, further sensitizing nociceptors and potentially activating adjacent Aδ pain fibers.
2. Drugs targeting calcitonin gene-related peptide and its receptor have become an effective target for migraine prevention because of their role in migraine pathophysiology.
3. Four monoclonal antibodies targeting CGRP have been approved for migraine prevention. Erenumab, galcanezumab, and fremanezumab are monthly self-administered subcutaneously. Eptinezumab is administered as an intravenous infusion every 3 months.
4. The CGRP mAbs are overall safe medications, as compared to previously used preventative medications. Caution should be used in patients who become or are pregnant or are breastfeeding. Further studies are needed, but they may be an effective treatment in pediatric and adolescent patients as well.

Case

A 45-year-old male presents to the clinic for follow-up for his headache disorder. He has episodes of sudden onset intense pain with unilateral tearing and rhinorrhea on the left side of his face. Symptoms have improved with oxygen in the past. He is wondering if any of the monoclonal antibodies could be started to prevent these episodes from occurring?

Case Discussion

Galcanezumab can be started. It is important to be able to distinguish between migraine and other types of headache such as cluster headache. This patient's headaches are consistent with cluster headache. While the other monoclonal antibodies are being studied in cluster headache, at the time of writing, galcanezumab is the only monoclonal antibody approved for cluster headache prevention. The dose for cluster headache is higher than it is for migraine (300 mg per month).

Questions and Answers

1. A 29-year-old female presents to clinic for follow-up for her chronic migraine. She has been on topiramate and amitriptyline in the past for migraine prevention, but she continues to have 15 headache days per month. She plans to get pregnant in the next year. Which of the following is the best option for her for migraine prevention?
   A. Erenumab
   B. Fremanezumab
   C. Eptinezumab
   D. Atogepant
   E. None of the above

The correct answer is E. The use of CGRP-related medications in both pregnancy and lactation is recommended against at the time of this writing while more data is gathered and evaluated. In models with pregnant rats, a dose-dependent relationship was observed between CGRP administration and the increase in systolic blood pressure, fetal growth retardation, and increased fetal mortality. The current recommendation is to stop CGRP mAbs at least 6 months prior to conception.

2. A 55-year-old female presents to clinic for follow-up for her episodic migraine. She feels her current preventative medication is no longer effective. Her home medications include lisinopril, hydrochlorothiazide, metformin, and escitalopram. Which of the following would *not* be a good option for her?
   A. Rimegepant
   B. Erenumab
   C. Fremanezumab
   D. Atogepant
   E. Galcanezumab

The correct answer is B. Post-market analysis of erenumab revealed increased rates of hypertension that were not seen in the initial trials when compared to placebo. This patient is on multiple antihypertensive medications, so erenumab should be avoided to reduce the risk of worsening her hypertension.

References

1. Cutrer FM. Antiepileptic drugs: how they work in headache. Headache. 2001;41(Suppl 1):S3–10.
2. Fenstermacher N, Levin M, Ward T. Pharmacological prevention of migraine. BMJ. 2011;342:d583.
3. Silberstein SD. Preventive treatment of migraine. Trends Pharmacol Sci. 2006;27(8):410–5.
4. Rosenfeld MG, Mermod JJ, Amara SG, et al. Production of a novel neuropeptide encoded by the calcitonin gene via tissue-specific RNA processing. Nature. 1983;304(5922):129–35.
5. Sternini C. Enteric and visceral afferent CGRP neurons. Targets of innervation and differential expression patterns. Ann N Y Acad Sci. 1992;657:170–86.
6. Amara SG, Arriza JL, Leff SE, et al. Expression in brain of a messenger RNA encoding a novel neuropeptide homologous to calcitonin gene-related peptide. Science. 1985;229(4718):1094–7.
7. Jansen-Olesen I, Mortensen A, Edvinsson L. Calcitonin gene-related peptide is released from capsaicin-sensitive nerve fibres and induces vasodilatation of human cerebral arteries concomitant with activation of adenylyl cyclase. Cephalalgia. 1996;16(5):310–6.
8. Russell FA, King R, Smillie SJ, et al. Calcitonin gene-related peptide: physiology and pathophysiology. Physiol Rev. 2014;94(4):1099–142.
9. Pellesi L, Do TP, Ashina H, et al. Dual therapy with anti-CGRP monoclonal antibodies and botulinum toxin for migraine prevention: is there a rationale? Headache. 2020;60(6):1056–65.
10. Melo-Carrillo A, Strassman AM, Nir RR, et al. Fremanezumab-A humanized monoclonal anti-CGRP antibody-inhibits thinly myelinated (Adelta) but not unmyelinated (C) meningeal nociceptors. J Neurosci. 2017;37(44):10587–96.
11. Edvinsson JCA, Warfvinge K, Krause DN, et al. C-fibers may modulate adjacent Aδ-fibers through axon-axon CGRP signaling at nodes of Ranvier in the trigeminal system. J Headache Pain. 2019;20(1):105.
12. Poyner DR, Sexton PM, Marshall I, et al. International Union of Pharmacology. XXXII. The mammalian calcitonin gene-related peptides, adrenomedullin, amylin, and calcitonin receptors. Pharmacol Rev. 2002;54(2):233–46.
13. Goadsby PJ, Edvinsson L, Ekman R. Release of vasoactive peptides in the extracerebral circulation of humans and the cat during activation of the trigeminovascular system. Ann Neurol. 1988;23(2):193–6.
14. Goadsby PJ, Edvinsson L, Ekman R. Vasoactive peptide release in the extracerebral circulation of humans during migraine headache. Ann Neurol. 1990;28(2):183–7.
15. Goadsby PJ. Recent advances in understanding migraine mechanisms, molecules and therapeutics. Trends Mol Med. 2007;13(1):39–44.
16. Goadsby PJ, Edvinsson L. Joint 1994 Wolff Award Presentation. Peripheral and central trigeminovascular activation in cat is blocked by the serotonin (5HT)-1D receptor agonist 311C90. Headache. 1994;34(7):394–9.
17. Lassen LH, Haderslev PA, Jacobsen VB, et al. CGRP may play a causative role in migraine. Cephalalgia. 2002;22(1):54–61.
18. Edvinsson L, Haanes KA, Warfvinge K, et al. CGRP as the target of new migraine therapies—successful translation from bench to clinic. Nat Rev Neurol. 2018;14(6):338–50.
19. Teva Pharmaceuticals USA I. Ajovy (fremanezumab-vfrm). https://www.accessdata.fda.gov/drugsatfda_docs/label/2018/761089s000lbl.pdf. Accessed 16 July 2019.
20. AIMOVIG (erenumab-aooe) [prescribing information]. Amgen, Inc. 2018 (revised).
21. EMGALITY (galcanezumab-gnim) [prescribing information]. Eli Lilly and Company. 2018 (revised).
22. VYEPTI (epitinezumab-jjmr) [prescribing information]. Lundbeck. 2022 (revised).
23. Dodick DW. CGRP ligand and receptor monoclonal antibodies for migraine prevention: evidence review and clinical implications. Cephalalgia. 2019;39(3):445–58.
24. Goadsby PJ, Reuter U, Hallstrom Y, et al. A controlled trial of erenumab for episodic migraine. N Engl J Med. 2017;377(22):2123–32.
25. Stauffer VL, Dodick DW, Zhang Q, et al. Evaluation of galcanezumab for the prevention of episodic migraine: the EVOLVE-1 randomized clinical trial. JAMA Neurol. 2018;75(9):1080–8.
26. Ashina M, Saper J, Cady R, et al. Eptinezumab in episodic migraine: a randomized, double-blind, placebo-controlled study (PROMISE-1). Cephalalgia. 2020;40(3):241–54.

27. Silberstein SD, Dodick DW, Bigal ME, et al. Fremanezumab for the preventive treatment of chronic migraine. N Engl J Med. 2017;377(22):2113–22.
28. Vernieri F, Brunelli N, Marcosano M, et al. Maintenance of response and predictive factors of 1-year GalcanezumAb treatment in real-life migraine patients in Italy: the multicenter prospective cohort GARLIT study. Eur J Neurol. 2023;30(1):224–34.
29. Cantarelli L, Pestana Grafiña D, Gonzalez Perez A, et al. Efficacy and safety of erenumab, galcanezumab, and fremanezumab in the treatment of drug-resistant chronic migraine: experience in real clinical practice. Ann Pharmacother. 2023;57:416–24.
30. Barbanti P, Egeo G, Aurilia C, et al. Predictors of response to anti-CGRP monoclonal antibodies: a 24-week, multicenter, prospective study on 864 migraine patients. J Headache Pain. 2022;23(1):138.
31. Iannone LF, Fattori D, Benemei S, et al. Long-term effectiveness of three anti-CGRP monoclonal antibodies in resistant chronic migraine patients based on the MIDAS score. CNS Drugs. 2022;36(2):191–202.
32. Mechtler L, Saikali N, McVige J, et al. Real-world evidence for the safety and efficacy of CGRP monoclonal antibody therapy added to onabotulinumtoxinA treatment for migraine prevention in adult patients with chronic migraine. Front Neurol. 2021;12:788159.
33. Argyriou AA, Dermitzakis EV, Xiromerisiou G, et al. OnabotulinumtoxinA add-on to monoclonal anti-CGRP antibodies in treatment-refractory chronic migraine. Toxins. 2022;14:847.
34. Blumenfeld A, Ettrup A, Hirman J, et al. Long-term reductions in disease impact in patients with chronic migraine following preventive treatment with eptinezumab. BMC Neurol. 2022;22(1):251.
35. Andreou AP, Fuccaro M, Hill B, et al. Two-year effectiveness of erenumab in resistant chronic migraine: a prospective real-world analysis. J Headache Pain. 2022;23(1):139.
36. Alsaadi T, Noori S, Varakian R, et al. Real-world experience of erenumab in patients with chronic or episodic migraine in the UAE. BMC Neurol. 2022;22(1):221.
37. Cetta I, Messina R, Zanandrea L, et al. Comparison of efficacy and safety of erenumab between over and under 65-year-old refractory migraine patients: a pivotal study. Neurol Sci. 2022;43(9):5769–71.
38. Storch P, Burow P, Möller B, et al. Pooled retrospective analysis of 70 mg erenumab in episodic and chronic migraine: a two tertiary headache centers experience during clinical practice. Acta Neurol Belg. 2022;122(4):931–7.
39. Cullum CK, Do TP, Ashina M, et al. Real-world long-term efficacy and safety of erenumab in adults with chronic migraine: a 52-week, single-center, prospective, observational study. J Headache Pain. 2022;23(1):61.
40. Schenk H, Holle D, Nsaka M, et al. Twelve-month safety, tolerability and susceptibility to adverse events of prophylactic migraine therapy with erenumab: a retrospective real-world study. J Headache Pain. 2022;23(1):55.
41. Lowe M, Murray L, Tyagi A, et al. Efficacy of erenumab and factors predicting response after 3 months in treatment resistant chronic migraine: a clinical service evaluation. J Headache Pain. 2022;23(1):86.
42. Driessen MT, Cohen JM, Thompson SF, et al. Real-world effectiveness after initiating fremanezumab treatment in US patients with episodic and chronic migraine or difficult-to-treat migraine. J Headache Pain. 2022;23(1):56.
43. Barbanti P, Egeo G, Aurilia C, et al. Fremanezumab in the prevention of high-frequency episodic and chronic migraine: a 12-week, multicenter, real-life, cohort study (the FRIEND study). J Headache Pain. 2022;23(1):46.
44. Silvestro M, Tessitore A, Orologio I, et al. Galcanezumab effect on "whole pain burden" and multidimensional outcomes in migraine patients with previous unsuccessful treatments: a real-world experience. J Headache Pain. 2022;23(1):69.
45. Vernieri F, Altamura C, Brunelli N, et al. Rapid response to galcanezumab and predictive factors in chronic migraine patients: a 3-month observational, longitudinal, cohort, multicenter, Italian real-life study. Eur J Neurol. 2022;29(4):1198–208.
46. Gantenbein AR, Agosti R, Kamm CP, et al. Swiss QUality of life and healthcare impact assessment in a real-world erenumab treated migraine population (SQUARE study): interim results. J Headache Pain. 2022;23(1):142.
47. Silvestro M, Orologio I, Bonavita S, et al. Effectiveness and safety of CGRP-mAbs in menstrual-related migraine: a real-world experience. Pain Ther. 2021;10(2):1203–14.
48. Toni T, Tamanaha R, Newman B, et al. Effectiveness of dual migraine therapy with CGRP inhibitors and onabotulinumtoxinA injections: case series. Neurol Sci. 2021;42(12):5373–6.
49. Caronna E, Gallardo VJ, Alpuente A, et al. Anti-CGRP monoclonal antibodies in chronic migraine with medication overuse: real-life effectiveness and predictors of response at 6 months. J Headache Pain. 2021;22(1):120.
50. Greene KA, Gentile CP, Szperka CL, et al. Calcitonin gene-related peptide monoclonal antibody use for the preventive treatment of refractory headache disorders in adolescents. Pediatr Neurol. 2021;114:62–7.
51. Dinh BBK, Aziz WH, Terruzzi A, et al. Initial experience with novel CGRP-receptor inhibitor therapy in migraine in The United Arab Emirates: a retrospective observational study. BMC Neurol. 2021;21(1):486.
52. Ashina M, Goadsby PJ, Reuter U, et al. Long-term efficacy and safety of erenumab in migraine prevention: results from a 5-year, open-label treatment phase of a randomized clinical trial. Eur J Neurol. 2021;28(5):1716–25.
53. Maraia Z, Ricci D, Rocchi MBL, et al. Real-life analysis with erenumab: first target therapy in the episodic and chronic migraine's prophylaxis. J Clin Med. 2021;10(19):4425.
54. Bottiroli S, De Icco R, Vaghi G, et al. Psychological predictors of negative treatment outcome with Erenumab in chronic migraine: data from an open label long-term prospective study. J Headache Pain. 2021;22(1):114.
55. de Vries LS, Verhagen IE, van den Hoek TC, et al. Treatment with the monoclonal calcitonin gene-related peptide receptor antibody erenumab: a real-life study. Eur J Neurol. 2021;28(12):4194–203.
56. Eghtesadi M, Leroux E, Pagé G. Real-life response to erenumab in a therapy-resistant case series of migraine patients from the province of Québec, Eastern Canada. Clin Drug Investig. 2021;41(8):733–9.
57. Talbot J, Stuckey R, Crawford L, et al. Improvements in pain, medication use and quality of life in onabotulinumtoxinA-resistant chronic migraine patients following erenumab treatment – real world outcomes. J Headache Pain. 2021;22(1):5.
58. Alex A, Vaughn C, Rayhill M. Safety and tolerability of 3 CGRP monoclonal antibodies in practice: a retrospective cohort study. Headache. 2020;60(10):2454–62.
59. Ornello R, Casalena A, Frattale I, et al. Real-life data on the efficacy and safety of erenumab in the Abruzzo region, central Italy. J Headache Pain. 2020;21(1):32.
60. Lambru G, Hill B, Murphy M, et al. A prospective real-world analysis of erenumab in refractory chronic migraine. J Headache Pain. 2020;21(1):61.
61. Robblee J, Devick KL, Mendez N, et al. Real-world patient experience with erenumab for the preventive treatment of migraine. Headache. 2020;60(9):2014–25.
62. Ashina M, Goadsby PJ, Reuter U, et al. Long-term safety and tolerability of erenumab: three-plus year results from a five-year open-label extension study in episodic migraine. Cephalalgia. 2019;39(11):1455–64.

63. Camporeale A, Kudrow D, Sides R, et al. A phase 3, long-term, open-label safety study of Galcanezumab in patients with migraine. BMC Neurol. 2018;18(1):188.
64. Dodick DW, Ashina M, Brandes JL, et al. ARISE: a phase 3 randomized trial of erenumab for episodic migraine. Cephalalgia. 2018;38(6):1026–37.
65. Saely S, Croteau D, Jawidzik L, et al. Hypertension: a new safety risk for patients treated with erenumab. Headache. 2021;61(1):202–8.
66. Reuter U, Goadsby PJ, Lanteri-Minet M, et al. Efficacy and tolerability of erenumab in patients with episodic migraine in whom two-to-four previous preventive treatments were unsuccessful: a randomised, double-blind, placebo-controlled, phase 3b study. Lancet. 2018;392(10161):2280–7.
67. Hirata K, Sakai F, Takeshima T, et al. Efficacy and safety of erenumab in Japanese migraine patients with prior preventive treatment failure or concomitant preventive treatment: subgroup analyses of a phase 3, randomized trial. J Headache Pain. 2021;22(1):110.
68. Tepper S, Ashina M, Reuter U, et al. Safety and efficacy of erenumab for preventive treatment of chronic migraine: a randomised, double-blind, placebo-controlled phase 2 trial. Lancet Neurol. 2017;16(6):425–34.
69. Ashina H, Iljazi A, Al-Khazali HM, et al. Efficacy, tolerability, and safety of erenumab for the preventive treatment of persistent post-traumatic headache attributed to mild traumatic brain injury: an open-label study. J Headache Pain. 2020;21(1):62.
70. Dodick DW, Silberstein SD, Bigal ME, et al. Effect of fremanezumab compared with placebo for prevention of episodic migraine: a randomized clinical trial. JAMA. 2018;319(19):1999–2008.
71. Goadsby PJ, Silberstein SD, Yeung PP, et al. Long-term safety, tolerability, and efficacy of fremanezumab in migraine: a randomized study. Neurology. 2020;95(18):e2487–99.
72. Ferrari MD, Diener HC, Ning X, et al. Fremanezumab versus placebo for migraine prevention in patients with documented failure to up to four migraine preventive medication classes (FOCUS): a randomised, double-blind, placebo-controlled, phase 3b trial. Lancet. 2019;394(10203):1030–40.
73. Sakai F, Suzuki N, Kim BK, et al. Efficacy and safety of fremanezumab for episodic migraine prevention: multicenter, randomized, double-blind, placebo-controlled, parallel-group trial in Japanese and Korean patients. Headache. 2021;61(7):1102–11.
74. Sakai F, Suzuki N, Kim BK, et al. Efficacy and safety of fremanezumab for chronic migraine prevention: multicenter, randomized, double-blind, placebo-controlled, parallel-group trial in Japanese and Korean patients. Headache. 2021;61(7):1092–101.
75. Skljarevski V, Matharu M, Millen BA, et al. Efficacy and safety of galcanezumab for the prevention of episodic migraine: results of the EVOLVE-2 phase 3 randomized controlled clinical trial. Cephalalgia. 2018;38(8):1442–54.
76. Detke HC, Goadsby PJ, Wang S, et al. Galcanezumab in chronic migraine: the randomized, double-blind, placebo-controlled REGAIN study. Neurology. 2018;91(24):e2211–21.
77. Mulleners WM, Kim BK, Láinez MJA, et al. Safety and efficacy of galcanezumab in patients for whom previous migraine preventive medication from two to four categories had failed (CONQUER): a multicentre, randomised, double-blind, placebo-controlled, phase 3b trial. Lancet Neurol. 2020;19(10):814–25.
78. Lipton RB, Goadsby PJ, Smith J, et al. Efficacy and safety of eptinezumab in patients with chronic migraine: PROMISE-2. Neurology. 2020;94(13):e1365–77.
79. Ashina M, Lanteri-Minet M, Pozo-Rosich P, et al. Safety and efficacy of eptinezumab for migraine prevention in patients with two-to-four previous preventive treatment failures (DELIVER): a multi-arm, randomised, double-blind, placebo-controlled, phase 3b trial. Lancet Neurol. 2022;21(7):597–607.
80. Edvinsson L. CGRP receptor antagonists and antibodies against CGRP and its receptor in migraine treatment. Br J Clin Pharmacol. 2015;80(2):193–9.
81. Kimberly B, Butala N. Migraines and CGRP monoclonal antibodies: a review of cardiovascular side effects and safety profile. Int J Neurol Neurother. 2020;7:101.
82. Depre C, Antalik L, Starling A, et al. A randomized, double-blind, placebo-controlled study to evaluate the effect of erenumab on exercise time during a treadmill test in patients with stable angina. Headache. 2018;58(5):715–23.
83. Silberstein SD, Reshef S, Cohen JM, et al. Adverse events reported with therapies targeting the CGRP pathway during the first 6 months post-launch: a retrospective analysis using the FDA adverse events reporting system. Adv Ther. 2023;40(2):445–59.
84. Wang K, Fenton BT, Dao VX, et al. Trajectory of blood pressure after initiating anti-calcitonin gene-related peptide treatment of migraine: a target trial emulation from the veterans health administration. J Headache Pain. 2023;24:108. https://doi.org/10.1186/s10194-023-01640-y.
85. https://www.accessdata.fda.gov/drugsatfda_docs/label/2025/761063s010lbl.pdf
86. https://www.accessdata.fda.gov/drugsatfda_docs/label/2025/761089s030lbl.pdf
87. https://www.accessdata.fda.gov/drugsatfda_docs/label/2025/761077s026lbl.pdf
88. https://www.accessdata.fda.gov/drugsatfda_docs/label/2025/761119s009s012lbl.pdf
89. Woods RH. Alopecia signals associated with calcitonin gene-related peptide inhibitors in the treatment or prophylaxis of migraine: a pharmacovigilance study. Pharmacotherapy. 2022;42(10):758–67.
90. Gérard AO, Merino D, Van Obberghen EK, et al. Calcitonin gene-related peptide-targeting drugs and Raynaud's phenomenon: a real-world potential safety signal from the WHO pharmacovigilance database. J Headache Pain. 2022;23(1):53.
91. Breen ID, Brumfiel CM, Patel MH, et al. Evaluation of the safety of calcitonin gene-related peptide antagonists for migraine treatment among adults with Raynaud phenomenon. JAMA Netw Open. 2021;4(4):e217934.
92. Gangula PR, Dong YL, Wimalawansa SJ, et al. Infusion of pregnant rats with calcitonin gene-related peptide (CGRP)(8-37), a CGRP receptor antagonist, increases blood pressure and fetal mortality and decreases fetal growth. Biol Reprod. 2002;67(2):624–9.
93. Noseda R, Bedussi F, Gobbi C, et al. Safety profile of erenumab, galcanezumab and fremanezumab in pregnancy and lactation: analysis of the WHO pharmacovigilance database. Cephalalgia. 2021;41(7):789–98.
94. Szperka CL, VanderPluym J, Orr SL, et al. Recommendations on the use of anti-CGRP monoclonal antibodies in children and adolescents. Headache. 2018;58(10):1658–69.
95. Charles AC, Digre KB, Goadsby PJ, Robbins MS, Hershey A. Calcitonin gene-related peptide-targeting therapies are a first-line option for the prevention of migraine: An American Headache Society position statement update. Headache. 2024;64:333–41. https://doi.org/10.1111/head.14692.
96. Ailani J, Burch RC, Robbins MS, et al. The American Headache Society Consensus Statement: update on integrating new migraine treatments into clinical practice. Headache. 2021;61:1021.
97. Becker WJ. Botulinum toxin in the treatment of headache. Toxins. 2020;12(12):803.
98. Al-Hassany L, Goadsby PJ, Danser AHJ, et al. Calcitonin gene-related peptide-targeting drugs for migraine: how pharmacology might inform treatment decisions. Lancet Neurol. 2022;21(3):284–94.
99. Multani I, Manji J, Hastings-Ison T, et al. Botulinum toxin in the management of childrenwith cerebral palsy. Pediatr Drugs. 2019;21(4):261–81.

100. Blumenfeld AM, Frishberg BM, Schim JD, et al. Real-world evidence for control of chronic migraine patients receiving cgrp monoclonal antibody therapy added to onabotulinumtoxinA: a retrospective chart review. Pain Ther. 2021;10(2):809–26.
101. Cohen F, Armand C, Lipton RB, et al. Efficacy and tolerability of calcitonin gene-related peptide targeted monoclonal antibody medications as add-on therapy to onabotulinumtoxinA in patients with chronic migraine. Pain Med. 2021;22:1857.
102. Chiang CC, Arca KN, Dunn RB, et al. Real-world efficacy, tolerability, and safety of ubrogepant. Headache. 2021;61(4):620–7.
103. de Hoon J, Van Hecken A, Vandermeulen C, et al. Phase 1, randomized, parallel-group, double-blind, placebo-controlled trial to evaluate the effects of erenumab (AMG 334) and concomitant sumatriptan on blood pressure in healthy volunteers. Cephalalgia. 2019;39:100–10.
104. Szkutnik-Fiedler D. Pharmacokinetics, pharmacodynamics and drug-drug interactions of new anti-migraine drugs-Lasmiditan, gepants, and calcitonin-gene-related peptide (CGRP) receptor monoclonal antibodies. Pharmaceutics. 2020;12(12):1180.
105. Jakate A, Blumenfeld AM, Boinpally R, et al. Pharmacokinetics and safety of ubrogepant when coadministered with calcitonin gene-related peptide-targeted monoclonal antibody migraine preventives in participants with migraine: a randomized phase 1b drug-drug interaction study. Headache. 2021;61(4):642–52.
106. Sacco S, Bendtsen L, Ashina M, et al. European headache federation guideline on the use of monoclonal antibodies acting on the calcitonin gene related peptide or its receptor for migraine prevention. J Headache Pain. 2019;20(1):6.
107. Reuter U, Ehrlich M, Gendolla A, et al. Erenumab versus topiramate for the prevention of migraine–a randomised, double-blind, active-controlled phase 4 trial. Cephalalgia. 2022;42:108–18.
108. Frank F, Ulmer H, Sidoroff V, et al. CGRP-antibodies, topiramate and botulinum toxin type A in episodic and chronic migraine: a systematic review and meta-analysis. Cephalalgia. 2021;41(11–12):1222–39.
109. Yang CP, Zeng BY, Chang CM, et al. Comparative effectiveness and tolerability of the pharmacology of monoclonal antibodies targeting the calcitonin gene-related peptide and its receptor for the prevention of chronic migraine: a network meta-analysis of randomized controlled trials. Neurotherapeutics. 2021;18:2755.
110. Overeem LH, Raffaelli B, Mecklenburg J, et al. Indirect comparison of topiramate and monoclonal antibodies against CGRP or its receptor for the prophylaxis of episodic migraine: a systematic review with meta-analysis. CNS Drugs. 2021;35(8):805–20.
111. Rubio-Beltran E, Correnti E, Deen M, et al. PACAP38 and PAC1 receptor blockade: a new target for headache? J Headache Pain. 2018;19(1):64.

Chronic Migraine and Medication Overuse Headache

29

Mejgan G. Mukhtarzada and Teshamae S. Monteith

Introduction

Chronic migraine (CM) is a debilitating primary headache disorder, once considered a complication of migraine. CM has a global prevalence ranging from 1.4% to 2.2% [1]. It affects individuals in multiple domains, including on social, family, academic, and personal levels [2]. The exact mechanisms to explain progression to CM are unknown, and there is some debate regarding the classification of CM which is currently somewhat arbitrary. However, there are clinical distinctions between episodic migraine and CM, including comorbidity profiles, pharmacological response, disability, healthcare utilization, and quality of life [3]. Medication overuse (MOH) is often comorbid with CM and associated with significant disability and a risk of relapse. This chapter will mainly focus on the diagnosis and management of CM and MOH.

Questions

1. A 33-year-old woman presents for evaluation of daily headaches. She has a history of migraine with aura but has now developed increased frequency of headaches over the past year, with at least 4 days per week with headaches. She has been using combination butalbital, acetaminophen, caffeine tablets at least 12 days per month as well as naratriptan 10 days per month. Her headaches are usually (but not exclusively) left-sided and are typically moderate to severe intensity. The pain is described as a throbbing sensation and associated with light and sound sensitivity. She can have occasional nausea, but no vomiting with her headaches. What is the most appropriate next step in management?
   A. Change naratriptan to eletriptan
   B. Immediately stop all abortive medications
   C. Increase monthly sumatriptan quantity
   D. Start preventive therapy with topiramate
   E. Combine naproxen with sumatriptan
2. A 25-year-old female presents to your clinic with headache 20 days per month with an average intensity of 8–9/10 on the 0–10 pain scale (moderate to severe intensity). She has been experiencing this frequency of headaches for the past 1 year with progressive worsening. Her headaches are described as a throbbing sensation, in the temple region with a preference for the right side over the left. Her headaches are associated with light and sound sensitivity. She also has nausea with severe attacks. You diagnose her with chronic migraine without aura. She was previously on topiramate for about 3 weeks but developed significant paresthesias that were bothersome. Thus, this medication was stopped, and amitriptyline was initiated by another provider. This medication caused significant drowsiness within the first week, even at the lowest dose. What is the next best treatment option for chronic migraine prevention?
   A. Lamotrigine
   B. Valproic acid
   C. OnabotulinumtoxinA
   D. Propranolol
   E. Nortriptyline

Epidemiology

Typical prevalence estimates for CM range between 1.4% and 2.2% [1]. CM is 2.5–6.5 higher prevalence in women compared to men [1]. The one-year prevalence of migraine

M. G. Mukhtarzada
Department of Neurology, Geisinger Medical Center, Danville, PA, USA

T. S. Monteith (✉)
Department of Neurology, Headache Division, University of Miami, Miller School of Medicine, Miami, FL, USA

T. S. Monteith et al. (eds.), *Comprehensive Migraine Management*, https://doi.org/10.1007/978-3-031-86923-5_29

in the United States (USA) is 11.7–13.2% [4]. In the American Migraine Prevalence and Prevention (AMPP) Study, it was estimated that episodic migraine (EM) can transition to CM with a yearly chronification rate of 2.5% per year [5].

The Chronic Migraine Epidemiology and Outcomes (CaMEO) Study was a large web-based survey study of the US population. It recorded the course of individuals with EM and CM with assessments every 3 months over a one-year period. The study noted that there are numerous fluctuations between EM and CM at 3-month intervals. In the analysis of the CaMEO study, the majority of 5464 respondents with EM followed for 1 year remained as EM (94.6%) while 7.6% had CM [6]. Of the 526 respondents with CM, only 26.6% had CM during all periods assessed. Taken together, there are natural fluctuations, including periods of variation and stability, in self-reported headache frequency among individuals EM and CM [6].

Risk factors for progression may be both modifiable and nonmodifiable [2]. Several risk factors for increased transformation and reversion to CM include female sex, lower socioeconomic status, high baseline headache frequency, cutaneous allodynia, obesity, sleep disorders/snoring, psychiatric disease, chronic pain disorders, major life events, and excessive caffeine intake [7]. In addition, there are a number of factors associated with reversion to EM including lower baseline frequency, absence of cutaneous allodynia, adherence to migraine preventive drugs, discontinuation of overused acute medication, and physical experience [7].

It is imperative to recognize that the lack of adequate acute treatment can lead to a higher rate of conversion from episodic migraine (EM) to CM as well as analgesic overuse [8]. MOH affects about 60 million individuals worldwide [9]. In the USA, about 50% of individuals with CM meet the criteria of MOH [1, 10]. There is a higher prevalence of MOH in females compared to males (4:1) [11]. While the prevalence of MOH in children can range between 0.3% and 1% [12].

Barriers to Care and Public Health Considerations

CM has a significant burden on the individual and socioeconomic levels. Individuals with CM have almost two times higher disability scores than those with EM [13]. There are notable difficulties in attaining effective treatment of migraine. These barriers include inaccurate diagnosis, absence of correct medical consultation, and limited pharmacologic treatment provided, and the presence of medication overuse [14–16]. The AMPP also suggested that individuals with CM were more likely to receive an incorrect diagnosis and not be provided with specific medications for treatment [15]. Additionally, the CaMEO study evaluated barriers to care and indicated that individuals with CM were 41% more likely to be White, 52% to be female, and 34% more likely to be obese.

The International Burden of Migraine Study (IBMS) determined that CM has significantly greater direct and indirect medical costs compared to EM. Interestingly, the largest percentage for direct costs was pharmaceutical utilization [17]. MOH is also associated with significant socioeconomic concerns [18, 19]. MOH has higher overall costs compared to migraine headaches, which can be related to more medication use, lost productivity, more sick day leave, and overall increased healthcare use [20]. Thus, individuals with CM and MOH necessitate optimization of their migraine-specific treatments [21, 22].

Classification

Per the International Classification of Headache Disorders-3 (ICHD-3) criteria, CM is defined in an individual with headache occurring on 15 days or more per month for at least 3 months. At least 8 of these days must have characteristics of migraine with or without aura [23]. Although no longer considered a complication of migraine, some researchers hypothesize that CM develops into a separate entity clinically in individuals with predisposed EM [24].

In the Appendix of the ICHD-3, alternative criteria have been proposed pending further research validation, to distinguish between CM with pain free periods and continuous pain [23]. In addition, there is an argument that the threshold of migraine days for diagnosing CM should be reduced based on the disability that seems to occur at lower thresholds of approximately 8–14 headache days per month [25]. Others argue that CM can be readily distinguished from EM in pathophysiological studies and by treatment response; therefore, the 15-day threshold of headaches per month should remain as a part of the classification [26].

According to the ICHD-3 diagnostic criteria, MOH is classified as headache occurring 15 or more days per month for at least 3 months consecutively in a person with a preexisting primary headache disorder, who develops a new or worsening headache in association with frequent use of acute medication for pain relief [23]. Medications such as simple non-opioid analgesics including acetaminophen or nonsteroidal anti-inflammatory drugs (NSAIDS) can induce MOH when overuse occurs for at least 15 days per month for more than 3 months consecutively. If the acute medication is a triptan, ergotamine, opioid, or combination analgesic, MOH can be diagnosed if the overuse of acute medications occurs for 10 days or more per month for more than 3 months consecutively [27]. Although the diagnosis of MOH is based on these criteria, there is also a possibility that migraine progression may also be due to additional drivers (i.e., disease state) independent of analgesic overuse. Moreover, worsening of headache typically improves but not indefinitely after the cessation of the overused medication.

Pathophysiology

The pathophysiology of CM is not well understood but thought to involve numerous processes and multiple levels structurally and functionally. Interestingly, a study by Chalmer et al. did not find any genetic variants identified that give rise to migraine chronification [28]. The susceptibility to frequent attacks has been described as potentially a threshold problem [29]. Both protective factors as well as propagating factors may drive attack frequency.

A dysfunctional descending pain modulation network, as a consequence of repeat attacks, has also been proposed, in addition to peripheral and central sensitization. There may be altered states in the trigeminal and autonomic systems interictally that differ for EM and CM, evidenced by elevations of vasoactive neuropeptides. While studies may differ, those with CM have also been noted to have higher plasma levels of vasoactive neuropeptides, such as pituitary adenylate cyclase activating polypeptide-38 (PACAP-38), vasoactive intestinal peptide, and calcitonin gene-related peptide (CGRP) compared to patients with episodic migraine. Thus, these neuropeptides may be important intermediaries of neurovascular signaling [30, 31].

Trigeminal afferents described are sensitized in the proliferation of CM. CM may involve ascending trigeminal pathway sensitization within the brain known as central sensitization. The thalamus is implicated as a major contributor to central sensitization, evidenced by cutaneous allodynia [32, 33]. Also, it is thought that the sensitization of the trigeminal pathway, involving the trigeminovascular inputs, spinal trigeminal nucleus, thalamus, and sensory cortex in the brain becomes more continuous with the chronification of migraine [34]. This can contribute to both structural and functional changes in the brain, involving neuroplasticity, and can then lead to more frequent headache attacks [35, 36].

The changes studied using functional MRI support abnormal pain processing in CM. This is due to modifications in descending pain modulation [37, 38]. There have been many studies that show volume changes in the gray matter areas. These areas include the amygdala, dorsolateral prefrontal cortex, brainstem, and putamen [35, 39, 40]. Another study showed that individuals with CM had decreased volume in the hypothalamus [41]. This study showed that there was an association between the reduced size in CM individuals and frequency of headaches [41]. In addition, a functional imaging study using a brainstem-optimized protocol for high-resolution echo-planar imaging showed a stronger activation of the anterior right hypothalamus in CM compared to healthy controls [42].

The pathophysiology of medication overuse is highly complex. Imaging studies have shown that there are metabolic, functional, and structural changes in the brain of individuals with MOH [43]. It is hypothesized that there is a genetic predisposition to developing MOH. In humans, genetic risk factors include the brain-derived neurotrophic factor (BDNF) mutation Val66Met or polymorphisms in catechol-O-methyl-transferase (COMT) and serotonin transporter (SLC6A4) genes, but causality still needs to be determined [44, 45]. There may also be medication-specific pathways that are involved in MOH pathophysiology.

All acute treatments can theoretically cause MOH. However, there are certain medications that can lead to more frequent and quicker symptoms. Individuals who overuse triptans are more likely to develop MOH in comparison to individuals who use simple analgesics [46, 47]. Triptans, for example, have been shown to induce latent sensitization, which results in increased sensitivity to migraine triggers, cutaneous allodynia and increased plasma CGRP, and is speculated as a pathological basis for MOH [48].

In cortical and subcortical areas, triptans have also been shown to disrupt brain networks and increase susceptibility to cortical spreading depression (CSD) like response promoted by stress [49]. A functional MRI study of rats sensitized with sumatriptan indicated that there were many differences in networks of resting states including the default mode, autonomic, basal ganglia, salience, and sensorimotor networks [49]. Increased susceptibility to CSD has also been shown in animal models [50]. Also of note, after rats were sensitized with sumatriptan, blocking the signaling at the kappa opioid receptors in the amygdala appeared to prevent allodynia [51]. Thus, these may be possible pathways to consider when developing a preventive treatment that may result in MOH remission [52].

Electrophysiological studies have shown distinctions in those with MOH as compared to EM [53]. One study showed that in MOH sensory evoked potential amplitudes were the highest in those with the longest periods of chronification. The hyperexcitability may depend on the specific drug that is being overused. For example, those who overuse NSAIDs had higher amplitudes in somatosensory evoked potentials compared to those who overused triptans [53]. However, more research is needed to provide biological markers for optimal management and treatment of MOH.

Clinical Presentations of Chronic Migraine

In clinical practice, CM is often underdiagnosed. Individuals usually underreport their mild to moderate headache days, and only report days with severe headache [54]. Additionally, true headache-free or crystal-clear days may not be ade-

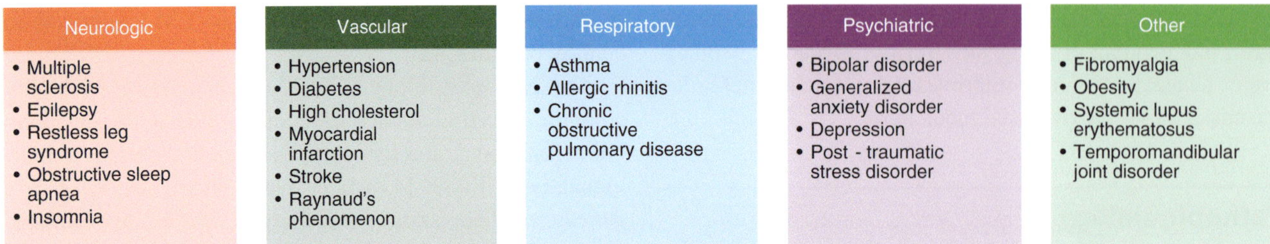

Fig. 29.1 Comorbidities of chronic migraine. (The figure was drafted from information provided: Burch et al. [2] and includes data from the American Migraine Prevalence and Prevention Study, Chronic Migraine Epidemiology and Outcomes (CaMEO) Study [4, 24])

quately quantified due to poor adherence to migraine diaries and as well as limited history-taking.

In CM, headache and associated features can be highly variable between attacks and within attacks. Headache may present with the typical unilateral and throbbing features or bilateral dull tension type-like headache with differing levels of associated migraine symptoms. For CM, both headache and other non-pain symptoms contribute to the symptom burden. In contrast to the acute attacks occurring in EM that are associated with well characterized multiphasic features (interictal and premonitory phase, aura, postdrome phases), phases occurring in CM are often less distinct. Taken together, non-headache symptoms such as fatigue, mood alternations, cognitive impairment, and vertigo can occur more frequently in the setting of CM [55].

The presence of certain comorbidities may add to the overall functional disability of individuals with CM. People with CM also have more medical comorbidities according to a large Scottish database [56]. In the study, 25 out of 31 conditions were more common in CM [56]. Figure 29.1 summarizes comorbidities of CM [2]. In addition to attaining medical history and features of the headache, physicians can also evaluate for "red flag" signs (such as abnormal neurologic exam or systemic symptoms which can point to a secondary headache disorder and lead to further diagnostic testing [7].

Medication Overuse Headache

An important modifiable risk factor for chronification is acute medication overuse. In the Migraine in American Symptoms and Treatment (MAST) study, a longitudinal, cross-sectional survey study of individuals with migraine in the USA, acute medication overuse was associated with greater rates of cutaneous allodynia, higher levels of pain intensity, and higher symptom severity scores [57]. Additionally, they are more likely to develop side effects from the medications overused. One study also showed acute medication overuse can negatively affect an individual's quality of life and their productivity [58].

Individuals with underlying risk factors such as stress, obesity, daily smoking, physical inactivity, and low socioeconomic status have greater risk of developing MOH [59]. Individuals who have a family history of MOH or substance overuse have an increased risk of developing MOH, as well [60]. A study by Lipton et al. found that inadequate acute treatment of EM was also associated with increased risk of chronification in the course of 1 year. Thus, improving acute treatment regimens is warranted for better CM outcomes [8].

Refractory Migraine

There have been several efforts to define refractory migraine, which is more common in people with CM. The European Headache Federation created an updated consensus definition to identify individuals with difficult-to-treat headaches [61]. The goal was to implement this definition in the clinical and research setting. The two major categories include resistant migraine and refractory migraine. Resistant migraine is defined as a migraine headache that remains debilitating regardless of some attempts of treatment (failure and/or contraindication to 3 drug classes of migraine preventive medication). These individuals should have a debilitating headache for at least 8 days per month for at least 3 months. However, refractory migraine is described as a migraine headache that remains debilitating even after maximal treatment attempts have been made (failure and/or contraindication to all classes of migraine prevention medications). Careful evaluation of refractory migraine is necessary to avoid missed diagnosis of other conditions known to cause persistent headache such as hemicrania continua, new daily persistent headache, intracranial hypertension, spontaneous intracranial hypotension, and cervicogenic headache.

Outpatient Treatment Options for Chronic Migraine

The goal of migraine care is to improve attack frequency, severity, and duration, as well as to improve functional disability. Individuals with migraine at risk for progression to CM should be identified and offered interventions to prevent

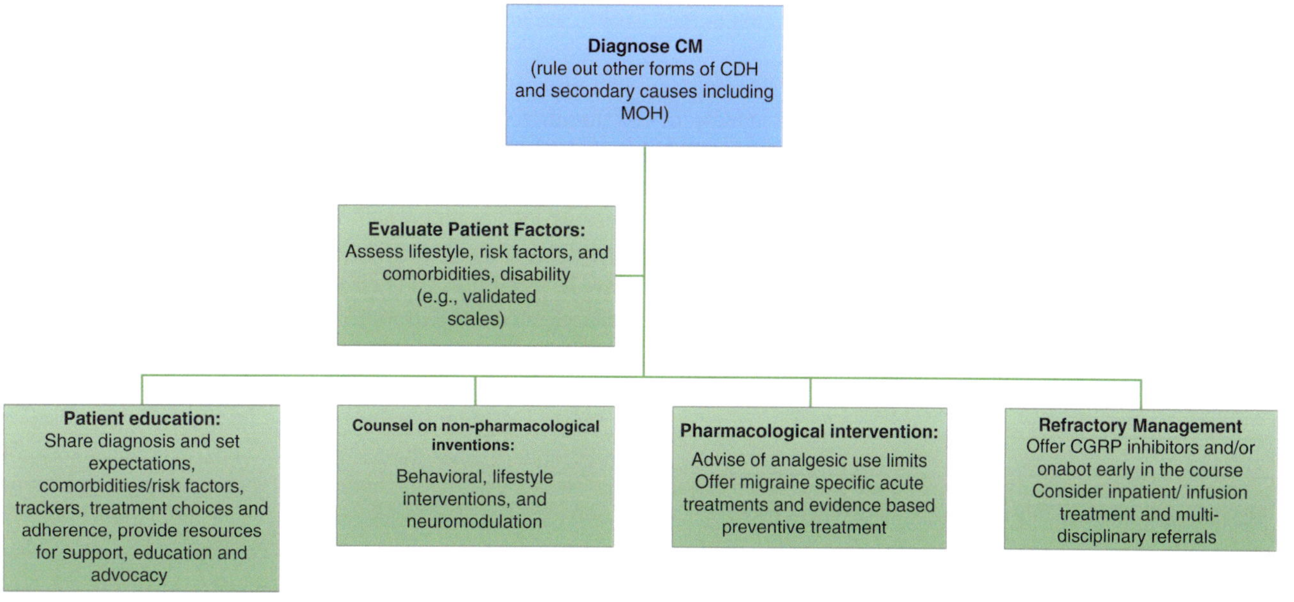

Fig. 29.2 Management of chronic migraine. After obtaining an accurate diagnosis of chronic migraine, it is important to identify potential lifestyle factors, risk factors, and comorbidities in addition to assessing disability and the impact of migraine. Patients should be educated on diagnosis, expectations, use of a diary/tracker, and appropriate use of acute analgesics. Patients should be offered both migraine-specific acute treatments and preventive therapies, including non-pharmacological and pharmacological interventions. Abbreviations: CDH Chronic daily headache, MOH Medication overuse headache, CM Chronic migraine, onabot OnabotulinumtoxinA

CM. When individuals are diagnosed with CM, multiple strategies are available for optimizing outcomes (Fig. 29.2).

Acute Treatment

Acute therapies for CM treatment are similar to those used for EM treatment and can include NSAIDS, other simple analgesics, and migraine-specific medications such as triptans, ergot derivatives, gepants, or a ditan [62]. Butalbital containing drugs and opiates should not be used as first line treatments in migraine and have a very limited role. In addition, they may strongly induce MOH and should not be used as first line [63]. Even 5 days of butalbital exposure per month is associated with migraine progression, which is more pronounced in women. The critical dose of exposure for opiates is 8 days per month and is more pronounced in men.

There have been reports that individuals with CM are less responsive to triptans [64]. Research has also suggested that individuals with CM have no improvement in disability based on their MIDAS score (Migraine Disability Assessment Test) with the addition of NSAIDs to their existing triptan regimen, but clinically it may be useful to do, especially when treatment is initiated early [65]. Overall, it is recommended that acute treatment should be limited to 2 days per week to avoid development of MOH, although MOH does not appear to be a concern for gepants use [66, 67]. Limiting the use can allow the preventive treatments to take effect, prevent progression of the headache frequency, and improve the individual's quality of life [62].

Preventive Treatment

Indication for migraine prevention occurs when there are at least 4 monthly headache days, to prevent CM. Continuation of oral migraine preventive medications in CM is low among the US population. A study by Hepp et al. found that persistence of oral migraine preventive agents from the time of initiation is low at six-month follow-up with an adherence of 25%, which decreases even further to 12% by 12 months. They also found that re-starting the treatment after it is discontinued or switching completely to another oral preventive occurs quite frequently. Additionally, the rates of discontinuation decline even further as patients alternate between additional oral migraine preventive agents [68]. The pharmacological interventions for prevention of CM are listed below [69]:

- Anti-convulsant (topiramate, divalproex sodium/valproate sodium)
- Anti-hypertensive medications such as beta blockers (metoprolol, propranolol, timolol, before atenolol or nadolol), as well as candesartan
- Anti-depressants including tricyclic anti-depressants (amitriptyline, nortriptyline) and serotonin-

norepinephrine reuptake inhibitors (venlafaxine, duloxetine)

- Other Level A or B treatments: (established efficacy or probably effective) according to American Academy of Neurology scheme for classification of evidence [70], fenoprofen, ibuprofen, ketoprofen, magnesium, riboflavin, feverfew, histamine
- Monoclonal antibodies targeting CGRP or its receptor including erenumab, fremenezumab, galcanezumab, or eptinezumab
- Small-molecules targeting the CGRP receptor (gepants) including atogepant
- OnabotulinumtoxinA

Of these, there are only a few that are considered highly effective prophylactic pharmacologic agents for CM.

Topiramate

Topiramate is an anticonvulsant that has a broad mechanism of action. It regulates neurotransmitter release of glutamate and gamma-Aminobutyric acid and modulates cell membrane ion channels. It also inhibits carbonic anhydrase isozymes [71]. There have been electrophysiological studies suggesting topiramate has actions on CSD and within the trigeminovascular system [72, 73].

There are multiple large clinical trials that have supported the safety and efficacy of topiramate for the preventive treatment of CM. In the TOP-CHROME study, doses of topiramate ranging from 50 to 200 mg per day were studied [74]. There was a significant reduction in the mean monthly migraine days compared to placebo [74]. In the Topiramate Chronic Migraine Study, those treated with topiramate at doses of around 100 mg daily had statistically significant reduction in migraine headache days relative to baseline (topiramate −5.6 vs placebo −4.1, $P = 0.032$) [75]. Topiramate was safe and well tolerated, with paresthesias being most common [75]. The INTREPID study was a multicenter, randomized, double-blind study that investigated topiramate in the prevention of migraine progression. In this study, topiramate did not prevent new-onset CM at 6 months, and however, it may have been due to a shorter observation period as well as low rates of transition in the placebo group [76]. However, there was a reduction in both headache and migraine headache days for those treated with topiramate.

In another study, topiramate was found to be effective treating individuals with CM with and without concurrent medication overuse. This may suggest that addressing the medication overuse and removal of acute therapies prior to initiation of prophylactic agents may not be fully warranted for effective treatment in CM [77]. A study by Silberstein et al. studied the benefit of adding propranolol to topiramate for treatment of CM individuals who were inadequately controlled on topiramate monotherapy. There was no reduction in migraine days with the addition of propranolol after a 6-month period [70]. The two CM clinical trials indicated that paresthesias were a common side effect of topiramate. In clinical practice, a discontinuation of topiramate is usually because of cognitive side effects. One study showed evidence that extended-release formulations of topiramate may have less cognitive side effects because of the stable, steady-state plasma concentrations [78]. The researchers performed verbal fluency studies which indicated less cognitive impairment with topiramate in the extended-release formulation compared to the immediate-release formulation. A subset of individuals treated with topiramate may experience weight loss. It is a carbonic anhydrase inhibitor, which may lead to the development of kidney stones. Acute angle glaucoma has been reported in case reports [79]. Topiramate may also increase the risk of osteoporotic fractures, and however, further studies are still needed [80].

OnabotulinumtoxinA

OnabotulinumtoxinA has been proven to be an effective preventive treatment for CM [81, 82]. Botulinum toxin is a proteolytic protein that is created by the bacteria, *Clostridium botulinum*. There are several antigenic distinct forms, A–G. This toxin is thought to work beyond inhibiting the neurotransmitter, acetylcholine, at the nerve endings located at the neuromuscular junction of skeletal muscle. Botulinum toxin binds to the afferent nerve terminals and is translocated from the synaptic vesicles to the cytosol. It then exits into the cytoplasm and cleaves the soluble N-ethylmaleimide-sensitive factor attachment protein receptor (SNARE) proteins which facilitate the release of neurotransmitters from the vesicle. By cleaving the SNARE proteins, the cell is prevented from releasing vesicles of CGRP, substance P, and glutamate [83]. OnabotulinumtoxinA may also have anti-nociceptive central effects through axonal transport where it can be absorbed peripherally and cleave SNARE proteins at the trigeminal ganglion and the trigeminal nucleus caudalis [84]. Research indicates that the anti-nociceptive effects of onabotulinumtoxinA may involve different sites of the trigeminal system and may also have interactions with the endogenous opioid system [85]. OnabotulinumtoxinA is the first FDA approved preventive treatment for CM when injected into extracranial dermatomes. This approval was granted based on promising results from two phase III clinical trials over a 24-week period as well as a 32-week open-label phase afterward.

In the Phase III REsearch Evaluating Migraine Prophylaxis Therapy 1 (PREEMPT I) study, the primary endpoint was the mean change from baseline in headache episodes at week

24. They found that there was no between-group difference. However, there was a significant decrease in total headache and migraine days, the total hours of headache and the frequency of moderate to severe headache days compared to baseline [81].

In the PREEMPT II trial, the primary endpoint was mean change in headache days per 28 days from baseline to weeks 21–24 after treatment. The study revealed that onabotulinumtoxinA was significantly superior to placebo for the primary endpoint (−9.0 onabotulinumtoxinA/−6.7 placebo, $P < 0.001$). It was also favored in all of the secondary endpoints including change from baseline in the frequency of migraine days, frequency of moderate/severe headache days, cumulative total headache hours on headache days, and frequency of use of acute headache medications such as triptans making it effective for the prophylaxis of headache in adults with CM [82]. Overall, adverse events were considered mild or moderate and discontinuation rates were low. The most common side effects were neck pain and muscular weakness, eyelid ptosis, myalgia, and musculoskeletal stiffness. In a cohort study of CM and MOH, the long-term benefits and safety of onabotulinumtoxinA treatment over a three-year period was evaluated with no serious adverse events reported [86]. Also, in an open-label prospective study, Generalized Anxiety Disorder questionnaires and Beck Depression Inventory II tests showed improvement in symptoms of anxiety and depression after treatment with onabotulinumtoxinA [87].

Additionally, there is much needed research in the utilization of healthcare resources in CM patients receiving preventive treatment for their headaches. A study by Hepp et al. showed that emergency department (ED) visits and hospitalizations for headaches were reduced greatly after onabotulinumtoxinA was started for prophylactic treatment. Interestingly, onabotulinumtoxinA was linked to lower ED visits compared to CM individuals who were started on oral migraine preventive medications [88].

CGRP-Targeted Therapies

There are several novel humanized monoclonal antibody treatments developed specifically for CM. These medications include fremanezumab [89], galcanezumab [90], and eptinezumab [91] which all target the CGRP ligand. Meanwhile, the drug erenumab is a fully humanized monoclonal antibody that targets the CGRP receptor [92].

These novel treatments are suggested to counteract the effects of excessive CGRP released during migraine attacks [93]. Erenumab, fremanezumab, and galcanezumab are administered subcutaneously whereas eptinezumab is the first intravenous anti-CGRP monoclonal antibody treatment. Each of the anti-CGRP pathway drugs has been proven effective and safe as CM prophylaxis in clinical trials. Additionally, a clinical trial supports the use of atogepant, an oral small molecule CGRP inhibitor, for preventive treatment of CM [94].

The combination of anti-CGRP inhibitors and onabotulinumtoxinA for CM is promising. Blumenfeld et al. conducted a retrospective, real-world study of 257 patients receiving onabotulinumtoxinA combined with either erenumab, galcanezumab, or fremanezumab. They determined that treatment was tolerated well with no new safety issues. In addition, individuals receiving this combination of therapies showed improvements in the headache frequency and migraine-related disability in comparison to individuals treated with onabotulinumtoxinA alone [95]. Given the limited options for preventive pharmacologic agents, further research is needed to find effective and safe preventive therapeutic targets for CM.

Management of Medication Overuse Headache

The management of MOH can vary from simple advice and education to medication discontinuation with physician monitoring, and/or early preventive treatment [96] (Fig. 29.3). Of note, the rate of relapse after successful withdrawal of the acute medication is high. Thus, individuals should have close follow-up [52]. In some cases, multimodal comprehensive interventions including infusion therapy and psychologists may be warranted. There have been several studies to determine the best strategies to treat MOH.

Preventive medications including topiramate, onabotulinumtoxinA, gepants, and anti-CGRP monoclonal antibodies can help reduce the frequency of migraine headaches and decrease acute medication use (Table 29.1). In addition to preventive treatment, patient education is beneficial. In one Italian study, individuals with MOH were provided standard preventive treatment in addition to a 15-minute educational session that discussed the importance of discontinuing overused medications. About 79% of those no longer had medication overuse and 69% had their headache frequency reduced by half at the two-month mark [97].

There have been several studies designed to determine the best strategy for treatment MOH. The Medication Overuse Treatment Strategy (MOTS) Trial was an open-label clinical trial that compared the efficacy of preventive treatment with or without switching acute overused medications [104]. All subjects were started on preventive medication and randomized to either switch the overused acute medication to an alternative acute medication (limited to 2 days or less per week) or they continued the overused medication without limiting the amount that was used. The results showed that starting an individual on a migraine preventive medication without switching or limiting the indi-

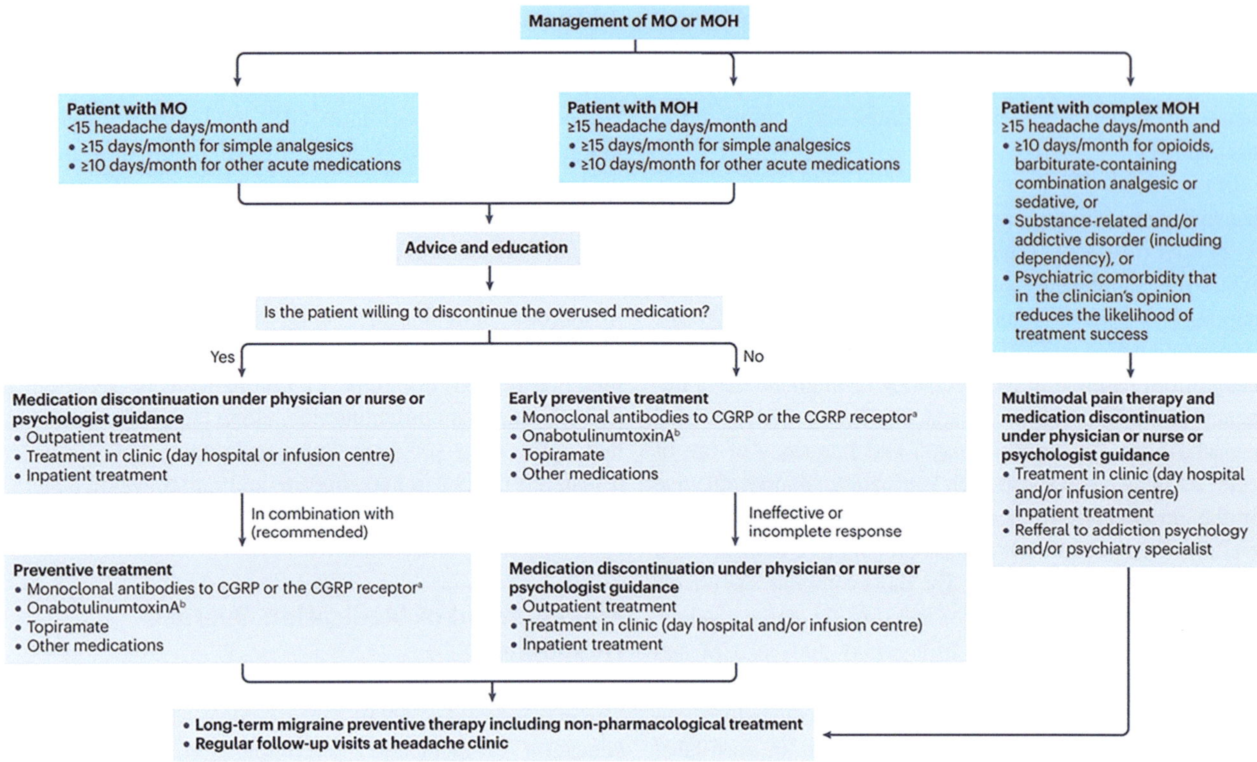

Fig. 29.3 Management of medication overuse headache. (This flowchart was reproduced with permission. Ashina et al. [96])

Table 29.1 Medications with preventive effect on chronic migraine and medication overuse or medication overuse headache assessed in post-hoc analyses of double-blind randomized placebo-controlled trials

Study	Treatment arms	Dose	Reduction in monthly migraine days	Elimination of medication overuse (%)[a]	Treatment duration	*n*
Diener et al. (2007) [74]	Topiramate	100 mg (daily)	−3.7[b]	–	16 weeks	23
	Placebo	NA	−0.5	–	16 weeks	23
Silberstein et al. (2013) [98]	OnabotulinumtoxinA	155–195 units (quarterly)	−8.2***	43.4**	6 months	445
	Placebo	NA	−6.2	31.8	6 months	459
Tepper et al. (2019) [99]	Erenumab	70 mg (monthly)	−6.6**	36.4**	3 months	77
	Erenumab	140 mg (monthly)	−6.6**	34.6**	3 months	78
	Placebo	NA	−3.5	17.7	3 months	113
Dodick et al. (2021) [100]	Galcanezumab	120 mg (monthly)	−4.8***	47.9[c]	3 months	177
	Galcanezumab	240 mg (monthly)	−4.5***	47.7[c]	3 months	175
	Placebo	NA	−2.3	29.6	3 months	344
Silberstein et al. (2020) [101]	Fremanezumab	225 mg (monthly)	−5.2***	60.6**	3 months	198
	Fremanezumab	675 mg (quarterly)	−4.8***	55.2*	3 months	201
	Placebo	NA	−2.8	46.3	3 months	188
Diener et al. (2021) [102]	Eptinezumab	100 mg (quarterly)	−8.4***	51.1[c]	6 months[d]	139
	Eptinezumab	300 mg (quarterly)	−8.6***	54.4[c]	6 months[d]	147
	Placebo	NA	−5.4	32.4	3 months[d]	145
Goadsby et al. (2022) [103]	Atogepant	60 mg (daily)	−7.5	41.8	3 months	170
	Atogepant	30 mg (daily)	−8.3	44.7	3 months	161
	Placebo	NA	−5.6	24.9	3 months	169

This table was reproduced with permission, originally produced in Ashina et al. [96]
NA Not applicable
***$P \leq 0.001$, **$P \leq 0.01$, *$P \leq 0.05$
[a]No longer fulfills criteria for medication overuse after 3 or 6 months
[b]Assessment over the last 4 weeks of the treatment; difference did not reach statistical significance ($P = 0.07$)
[c]P values not presented
[d]Assessment over last 3 months of the treatment period

vidual's acute medication was not inferior to switching or limiting the acute medication use. The study demonstrated that initiation of migraine preventive medication had decreased the moderate to severe headache days in CM individuals. However, there was no difference in the level of improvement between those individuals who continued to have acute medication overuse or not.

In another open-label, randomized clinical study, three outpatient interventions were evaluated for treatment of MOH: (1) withdrawal plus preventive treatment, (2) preventive treatment without withdrawal, or (3) withdrawal with optional preventive treatment 2 months after withdrawal [105]. While there were no differences in reduction of monthly migraine days, acute medication, or headache intensity, those randomized to the withdrawal plus preventive group were most likely to revert to episodic headache, as compared to the preventive group and the withdrawal group. All strategies were considered effective; however, the withdrawal plus preventive group had a remarkable rate of remission when followed at 6 months.

Inpatient Treatment Options for Chronic Migraine

When outpatient strategies are exhausted, some patients with CM with or without medication overuse may benefit from an inpatient admission. For patients without substantial comorbidities or disabilities, outpatient infusions for acute management may be efficacious [106]. Recommendations for an inpatient admission may be based on a history of refractoriness to outpatient preventive treatments or inadequate response to acute medications including migraine-specific therapies. In addition, other clinical scenarios that may warrant hospitalization include the presence of intractable nausea, vomiting or dehydration, barbiturate or opioid dependence needing detoxification, frequent emergency department (ED) visits, status migrainosus, or a medical condition or treatment that requires vigilant observation [107].

Although frequent ED visits result in most inpatient admissions for migraine, elective admissions are preferred as they allow for improved staffing and planning, instituting a therapeutic relationship, as well as creating expectations in terms of future treatments and objectives [108, 109]. The most frequently used intravenous acute medications include non-steroidal anti-inflammatories, neuroleptics, diphenhydramine, corticosteroids, magnesium, anticonvulsants, and migraine-specific treatments such as dihydroergotamine (DHE). The treatments can be introduced in a stepwise fashion or multiple medications from different classes may be started sequentially, depending on response to treatment [110]. In cases of refractory headache or the case of multiple psychiatric comorbidities, it is important to consider a multidisciplinary approach in the inpatient setting with the combination of behavioral therapies, including biofeedback, psychotherapy, or relaxation techniques in addition to medication treatments of migraine [111].

DHE is one of the most recognized treatments for the inpatient management of migraine [112]. In a study by Raskin et al., 55 patients with continuous headache for more than 2 months were treated with IV DHE at doses between 0.3 and 1 mg of IV DHE every 8 hours for 2 days. About 89% of those individuals were free of headache in 2 days [113]. DHE can be administered intermittently or less frequently. Continuous DHE infusion has been performed and has shown to be effective with fewer side effects [114].

It is important to discuss the side effects with patients ahead of time when administering DHE. Common side effects of DHE include nausea, which can be avoided with pretreatment with anti-emetics and slow titration of the drug as tolerated. Other sides effects are hypertension, diarrhea, chest tightness, and leg cramps [115]. Headache may worsen temporarily immediately after they receive the DHE which is not a predictor of poor response [116]. However, uncontrolled nausea is problematic [112]. Importantly, DHE is contraindicated in those with coronary or peripheral artery disease [117].

Continuous intravenous lidocaine infusion is also used for the inpatient treatment of CM [118, 119]. Side effects can include nausea, cerebellar findings, blood pressure fluctuations, sinus tachycardia, and cardiac arrhythmias, thus individuals should be monitored on continuous telemetry while receiving the infusion. Side effects are typically dose related and at higher doses, neuropsychiatric side effects such as hallucinations may occur. Toxicity can be prevented by checking serum lidocaine levels daily in order to ensure therapeutic levels are maintained [120].

Ketamine is a selective N-methyl-D-aspartate (NMDA) receptor antagonist, and it is controlled due to its abuse potential [121]. It is an anesthetic that has a role in the treatment of pain, depression, and CM [122]. One retrospective study assessed individuals with headache who received IV ketamine for up to 5 days in an inpatient setting. About 71.4% reported significant improvement in their headache by discharge and 27.3% had long-term benefit after discharge when seen in follow-up. Ketamine has neuropsychiatric side effects including confusion and hallucinations, thus must be administered with caution [123].

Non-pharmacologic Treatment Options

There are several promising non-pharmacologic treatment options available for individuals with intractable or pharmacologically non-responsive migraine headaches. These agents include non-invasive neurostimulation modalities and behavioral interventions [124]. Furthermore, given the varying comorbidities that can be seen in CM individuals, a multidisciplinary team treatment approach may be necessary. The team can include physical therapy, occupational therapy, and pain psychology. By facilitating a collaborative multidisciplinary team in practice, individuals can have a focus on all aspects including physical, environmental, and psychological triggers which can further facilitate treatment [108].

Conclusion

CM is a debilitating neurologic disorder that imposes substantial societal, economic, and individual burden characterized by higher disability and incidence of comorbidities compared to EM. Additionally, medication overuse is common among those with CM and can be associated with developing frequent headaches, medication side effects, and reduced quality of life.

Current treatment options for CM include risk factor and lifestyle modification, acute and preventive therapies, including as evidence-based treatments such as topiramate, onabotulinumtoxinA, CGRP receptor antagonists, and monoclonal antibodies to CGRP or its receptor. New emerging CM treatments such as neuromodulation also offer promising therapeutic approaches; however, further investigation is still needed. Given the high degree of burden, future research into this disabling disorder is highly warranted.

Teaching Points

1. Chronic migraine is a common and disabling disorder described in an individual with headache occurring on 15 days or more per month for 3 months or more (with at least 8 of these days having characteristics of migraine with or without aura).
2. The treatment of chronic migraine includes consideration of risk and lifestyle factors, avoidance of migraine attack triggers, use of prophylactic and abortive drugs, and non-drug treatment.
3. The recognition and management of comorbid disorders of chronic migraine may potentially optimize patient outcomes by improving overall quality of life.
4. Medication overuse is common among those with chronic migraine. It is associated with developing frequent headaches, medication side effects, reduced quality of life and should also properly be addressed to improve patient well-being and to reduce attack frequency.
5. The evidence to treat chronic migraine and medication overuse headache is the greatest with CGRP inhibitors, onabotulinumtoxinA, and topiramate.
6. Multiple therapeutic strategies are available for treatment of medication overuse headache, including acute withdrawal, withdrawal with preventive medication, and preventive medication with or without switching acute medications. Stratification to inpatient versus outpatient approaches should be guided by clinical factors, safety, and disability.

Case

A 27-year-old woman with a history of migraine presented for evaluation and management of frequent headaches. She reported having an onset of headaches at age 13. Initially, she had two to three episodes per month, described as moderate to severe, unilateral, throbbing headaches associated with sensitivity to light, sound, nausea and vomiting. Over the years, she had a slow increase in the frequency of her attacks, which has transformed to a daily pattern. Moreover, her acute medications have also increased to daily use. Over the past few years, she noted that between her severe migraine attacks, she had a constant mild to moderate headache that would partially respond to the NSAID/acetaminophen/caffeine combination pill. At the time of presentation, she reported taking the NSAID/acetaminophen/caffeine combination pill 3 times each day and a triptan for severe migraine attacks approximately 10 days per month.

Case Discussion

This patient has CM with MOH. CM was diagnosed since she experienced 15 or more days with headache each month, including at least 8 days on which she had severe migraine attacks. The patient also met criteria for overuse of triptans and for overuse of combination analgesics, each being used on 10 or more days per month. It is possible that the frequent use of acute medications led to MOH. The treatment of CM with medication overuse includes the use of migraine preventive therapy and reduction in the frequency of acute treatment used.

Questions and Answers

1. A 33-year-old woman presents for evaluation of daily headaches. She has a history of migraine with aura but has now developed increased frequency of headaches over the past year, with at least 4 days per week with headaches. She has been using combination butalbital, acetaminophen, caffeine tablets at least 12 days per month as well as naratriptan 10 days per month. Her headaches are usually (but not exclusively) left-sided and are typically moderate to severe intensity. The pain is described as a throbbing sensation and associated with light and sound sensitivity. She can have occasional nausea, but no vomiting with her headaches. What is the most appropriate next step in management?
   A. Change naratriptan to eletriptan
   B. Immediately stop all abortive medications
   C. Increase monthly sumatriptan quantity
   D. Start preventive therapy with topiramate
   E. Combine naproxen with sumatriptan

The correct answer is D. Start preventive therapy with topiramate. This patient has chronic migraine with medication overuse headache. It is important to restrict overused abortive agents, but it should not be done immediately, especially abrupt discontinuation of butalbital, which may cause seizures. Increasing the sumatriptan quantity is likely to make the problem worse and switching to a different triptan is unlikely to make a significant difference. The most reasonable option for this patient currently is to start a preventive therapy (such as topiramate) and counsel the patient to reduce use of abortive medications over time.

2. A 25-year-old female presents to your clinic with headache 20 days per month with an average intensity of 8–9/10 on the 0–10 pain scale (moderate to severe intensity). She has been experiencing this frequency of headaches for the past 1 year with progressive worsening. Her headaches are described as a throbbing sensation, in the temple region with a preference for the right side over the left. Her headaches are associated with light and sound sensitivity. She also has nausea with severe attacks. You diagnose her with chronic migraine without aura. She was previously on topiramate for about 3 weeks but developed significant paresthesias that were bothersome. Thus, this medication was stopped, and amitriptyline was initiated by another provider. This medication caused significant drowsiness within the first week, even at the lowest dose. What is the next best treatment option for chronic migraine prevention?
   A. Lamotrigine
   B. Valproic acid
   C. OnabotulinumtoxinA
   D. Propranolol
   E. Nortriptyline

The correct answer is C. The patient is diagnosed with chronic migraine without aura. Chronic migraine was diagnosed since she experienced 15 or more days with headache each month, including at least 8 days on which she had severe migraine attacks. There are 3 general preventive treatment options with Level A evidence for chronic migraine. These include topiramate, onabotulinumtoxinA, and CGRP inhibitors. The patient already tried topiramate for migraine prevention, however, the side effects were not tolerable for her. Out of all the options provided, onabotulinumtoxinA is the only treatment with the highest evidence for prevention of chronic migraine. There is no evidence to support the use of lamotrigine for migraine prevention, and valproic should be avoided in childbearing women. In addition, nortriptyline may also be associated with sedation although typically less so than amitriptyline.

References

1. Natoli JL, Manack A, Dean B, Butler Q, Turkel CC, Stovner L, et al. Global prevalence of chronic migraine: a systematic review. Cephalalgia. 2010;30(5):599–609.
2. Burch RC, Buse DC, Lipton RB. Migraine: epidemiology, burden, and comorbidity. Neurol Clin. 2019;37(4):631–49.
3. Lipton RB, Fanning KM, Buse DC, Martin VT, Reed ML, Manack Adams A, et al. Identifying natural subgroups of migraine based on comorbidity and concomitant condition profiles: results of the Chronic Migraine Epidemiology and Outcomes (CaMEO) Study. Headache. 2018;58(7):933–47.
4. Adams AM, Serrano D, Buse DC, Reed ML, Marske V, Fanning KM, et al. The impact of chronic migraine: the Chronic Migraine Epidemiology and Outcomes (CaMEO) Study methods and baseline results. Cephalalgia. 2015;35(7):563–78.
5. Scher AI, Stewart WF, Ricci JA, Lipton RB. Factors associated with the onset and remission of chronic daily headache in a population-based study. Pain. 2003;106(1–2):81–9.
6. Serrano D, Lipton RB, Scher AI, Reed ML, Stewart WBF, Adams AM, et al. Fluctuations in episodic and chronic migraine status over the course of 1 year: implications for diagnosis, treatment and clinical trial design. J Headache Pain. 2017;18(1):101.
7. Schwedt TJ. Chronic migraine. BMJ. 2014;348:g1416.
8. Lipton RB, Fanning KM, Serrano D, Reed ML, Cady R, Buse DC. Ineffective acute treatment of episodic migraine is associated with new-onset chronic migraine. Neurology. 2015;84(7):688–95.
9. Global Burden of Disease Study Collaborators. Global, regional, and national incidence, prevalence, and years lived with disability for 310 diseases and injuries, 1990–2015: a systematic analysis for the Global Burden of Disease Study 2015. Lancet. 2016;388:1545–602.
10. Westergaard ML, Glümer C, Hansen EH, Jensen RH. Prevalence of chronic headache with and without medication overuse: associations with socioeconomic position and physical and mental health status. Pain. 2014;155(10):2005–13.
11. Diener HC, Limmroth V. Medication-overuse headache: a worldwide problem. Lancet Neurol. 2004;3(8):475–83.
12. Lipton RB, Manack A, Ricci JA, Chee E, Turkel CC, Winner P. Prevalence and burden of chronic migraine in adolescents: results of the chronic daily headache in adolescents study (C-dAS). Headache. 2011;51(5):693–706.

13. Bigal ME, Rapoport AM, Lipton RB, Tepper SJ, Sheftell FD. Assessment of migraine disability using the migraine disability assessment (MIDAS) questionnaire: a comparison of chronic migraine with episodic migraine. Headache. 2003;43(4):336–42.
14. Post MW, Boosman H, van Zandvoort MM, Passier PE, Rinkel GJ, Visser-Meily JM. Development and validation of a short version of the Stroke Specific Quality of Life Scale. J Neurol Neurosurg Psychiatry. 2011;82(3):283–6.
15. Lipton RB, Serrano D, Holland S, Fanning KM, Reed ML, Buse DC. Barriers to the diagnosis and treatment of migraine: effects of sex, income, and headache features. Headache. 2013;53(1):81–92.
16. Lipton RB, Amatniek JC, Ferrari MD, Gross M. Migraine. Identifying and removing barriers to care. Neurology. 1994;44(6 Suppl 4):S63–8.
17. Messali A, Sanderson JC, Blumenfeld AM, Goadsby PJ, Buse DC, Varon SF, et al. Direct and indirect costs of chronic and episodic migraine in the United States: a web-based survey. Headache. 2016;56(2):306–22.
18. Bendtsen L, Munksgaard S, Tassorelli C, Nappi G, Katsarava Z, Lainez M, et al. Disability, anxiety and depression associated with medication-overuse headache can be considerably reduced by detoxification and prophylactic treatment. Results from a multicentre, multinational study (COMOESTAS project). Cephalalgia. 2014;34(6):426–33.
19. D'Amico D, Grazzi L, Curone M, Di Fiore P, Proietti Cecchini A, Leonardi M, et al. Difficulties in work activities and the pervasive effect over disability in patients with episodic and chronic migraine. Neurol Sci. 2015;36(Suppl 1):9–11.
20. Linde M, Gustavsson A, Stovner LJ, Steiner TJ, Barré J, Katsarava Z, et al. The cost of headache disorders in Europe: the Eurolight project. Eur J Neurol. 2012;19(5):703–11.
21. Bigal ME, Serrano D, Buse D, Scher A, Stewart WF, Lipton RB. Acute migraine medications and evolution from episodic to chronic migraine: a longitudinal population-based study. Headache. 2008;48(8):1157–68.
22. Lantéri-Minet M, Duru G, Mudge M, Cottrell S. Quality of life impairment, disability and economic burden associated with chronic daily headache, focusing on chronic migraine with or without medication overuse: a systematic review. Cephalalgia. 2011;31(7):837–50.
23. Headache Classification Committee of the International Headache Society. The international classification of headache disorders, 3rd edition. Cephalalgia. 2018;38:1–211.
24. Buse DC, Manack AN, Fanning KM, Serrano D, Reed ML, Turkel CC, et al. Chronic migraine prevalence, disability, and sociodemographic factors: results from the American Migraine Prevalence and Prevention Study. Headache. 2012;52(10):1456–70.
25. Ishii R, Schwedt TJ, Dumkrieger G, Lalvani N, Craven A, Goadsby PJ, et al. Chronic versus episodic migraine: the 15-day threshold does not adequately reflect substantial differences in disability across the full spectrum of headache frequency. Headache. 2021;61(7):992–1003.
26. Fischer-Schulte L, May A. The 15-day threshold in the definition of chronic migraine is reasonable and sufficient-five reasons for not changing the ICHD-3 definition. Headache. 2022;62(9):1231–3.
27. Headache Classification Committee of the International Headache Society (IHS). The international classification of headache disorders, 3rd edition (beta version). Cephalalgia. 2013;33(9):629–808.
28. Chalmer MA, Rasmussen AH, Kogelman LJA, Olesen J, Hansen TF, Consortium IHG, et al. Chronic migraine: genetics or environment? Eur J Neurol. 2021;28(5):1726–36.
29. May A, Schulte LH. Chronic migraine: risk factors, mechanisms and treatment. Nat Rev Neurol. 2016;12(8):455–64.
30. Cernuda-Morollón E, Larrosa D, Ramón C, Vega J, Martínez-Camblor P, Pascual J. Interictal increase of CGRP levels in peripheral blood as a biomarker for chronic migraine. Neurology. 2013;81(14):1191–6.
31. Pérez-Pereda S, Toriello-Suárez M, Ocejo-Vinyals G, Guiral-Foz S, Castillo-Obeso J, Montes-Gómez S, et al. Serum CGRP, VIP, and PACAP usefulness in migraine: a case-control study in chronic migraine patients in real clinical practice. Mol Biol Rep. 2020;47(9):7125–38.
32. Burstein R, Jakubowski M, Garcia-Nicas E, Kainz V, Bajwa Z, Hargreaves R, et al. Thalamic sensitization transforms localized pain into widespread allodynia. Ann Neurol. 2010;68(1):81–91.
33. Bigal ME, Ashina S, Burstein R, Reed ML, Buse D, Serrano D, et al. Prevalence and characteristics of allodynia in headache sufferers: a population study. Neurology. 2008;70(17):1525–33.
34. Su M, Yu S. Chronic migraine: a process of dysmodulation and sensitization. Mol Pain. 2018;14:1744806918767697.
35. Neeb L, Bastian K, Villringer K, Israel H, Reuter U, Fiebach JB. Structural gray matter alterations in chronic migraine: implications for a progressive disease? Headache. 2017;57(3):400–16.
36. Chou TM, Chen SP. Animal models of chronic migraine. Curr Pain Headache Rep. 2018;22(6):44.
37. Aurora SK, Barrodale PM, Tipton RL, Khodavirdi A. Brainstem dysfunction in chronic migraine as evidenced by neurophysiological and positron emission tomography studies. Headache. 2007;47(7):996–1003; discussion 4–7.
38. Mainero C, Boshyan J, Hadjikhani N. Altered functional magnetic resonance imaging resting-state connectivity in periaqueductal gray networks in migraine. Ann Neurol. 2011;70(5):838–45.
39. Bilgiç B, Kocaman G, Arslan AB, Noyan H, Sherifov R, Alkan A, et al. Volumetric differences suggest involvement of cerebellum and brainstem in chronic migraine. Cephalalgia. 2016;36(4):301–8.
40. Yu Y, Zhao H, Dai L, Su Y, Wang X, Chen C, et al. Headache frequency associates with brain microstructure changes in patients with migraine without aura. Brain Imaging Behav. 2021;15(1):60–7.
41. Chen Z, Chen X, Liu M, Ma L, Yu S. Volume of hypothalamus as a diagnostic biomarker of chronic migraine. Front Neurol. 2019;10:606.
42. Schulte LH, Allers A, May A. Hypothalamus as a mediator of chronic migraine: evidence from high-resolution fMRI. Neurology. 2017;88(21):2011–6.
43. Lai TH, Wang SJ. Neuroimaging findings in patients with medication overuse headache. Curr Pain Headache Rep. 2018;22(1):1.
44. Cargnin S, Viana M, Ghiotto N, Bianchi M, Sances G, Tassorelli C, et al. Functional polymorphisms in COMT and SLC6A4 genes influence the prognosis of patients with medication overuse headache after withdrawal therapy. Eur J Neurol. 2014;21(7):989–95.
45. Di Lorenzo C, Di Lorenzo G, Sances G, Ghiotto N, Guaschino E, Grieco GS, et al. Drug consumption in medication overuse headache is influenced by brain-derived neurotrophic factor Val66Met polymorphism. J Headache Pain. 2009;10(5):349–55.
46. Limmroth V, Katsarava Z, Fritsche G, Przywara S, Diener HC. Features of medication overuse headache following overuse of different acute headache drugs. Neurology. 2002;59(7):1011–4.
47. Thorlund K, Sun-Edelstein C, Druyts E, Kanters S, Ebrahim S, Bhambri R, et al. Risk of medication overuse headache across classes of treatments for acute migraine. J Headache Pain. 2016;17(1):107.
48. De Felice M, Ossipov MH, Wang R, Lai J, Chichorro J, Meng I, et al. Triptan-induced latent sensitization: a possible basis for medication overuse headache. Ann Neurol. 2010;67(3):325–37.
49. Becerra L, Bishop J, Barmettler G, Xie Y, Navratilova E, Porreca F, et al. Triptans disrupt brain networks and promote stress-induced CSD-like responses in cortical and subcortical areas. J Neurophysiol. 2016;115(1):208–17.

50. Green AL, Gu P, De Felice M, Dodick D, Ossipov MH, Porreca F. Increased susceptibility to cortical spreading depression in an animal model of medication-overuse headache. Cephalalgia. 2014;34(8):594–604.
51. Xie JY, De Felice M, Kopruszinski CM, Eyde N, LaVigne J, Remeniuk B, et al. Kappa opioid receptor antagonists: a possible new class of therapeutics for migraine prevention. Cephalalgia. 2017;37(8):780–94.
52. Diener HC, Dodick D, Evers S, Holle D, Jensen RH, Lipton RB, et al. Pathophysiology, prevention, and treatment of medication overuse headache. Lancet Neurol. 2019;18(9):891–902.
53. Coppola G, Curra A, Di Lorenzo C, Parisi V, Gorini M, Sava SL, et al. Abnormal cortical responses to somatosensory stimulation in medication-overuse headache. BMC Neurol. 2010;10:126.
54. Bigal ME, Sheftell FD, Tepper SJ, Rapoport AM, Lipton RB. Migraine days decline with duration of illness in adolescents with transformed migraine. Cephalalgia. 2005;25(7):482–7.
55. Vives-Mestres M, Casanova A, Silberstein SD, Hershey AD, Orr SL. Clinical factors associated with day-to-day peak pain severity in individuals with chronic migraine: a cohort study using daily prospective diary data. Headache. 2024;64(8):995–1004.
56. McLean G, Mercer SW. Chronic migraine, comorbidity, and socioeconomic deprivation: cross-sectional analysis of a large nationally representative primary care database. J Comorb. 2017;7(1):89–95.
57. Schwedt TJ, Alam A, Reed ML, Fanning KM, Munjal S, Buse DC, et al. Factors associated with acute medication overuse in people with migraine: results from the 2017 migraine in America symptoms and treatment (MAST) study. J Headache Pain. 2018;19(1):38.
58. Probyn K, Bowers H, Caldwell F, Mistry D, Underwood M, Matharu M, et al. Prognostic factors for chronic headache: a systematic review. Neurology. 2017;89(3):291–301.
59. Westergaard ML, Glümer C, Hansen EH, Jensen RH. Medication overuse, healthy lifestyle behaviour and stress in chronic headache: results from a population-based representative survey. Cephalalgia. 2016;36(1):15–28.
60. Mungoven TJ, Henderson LA, Meylakh N. Chronic migraine pathophysiology and treatment: a review of current perspectives. Front Pain Res (Lausanne). 2021;2:705276.
61. Sacco S, Braschinsky M, Ducros A, Lampl C, Little P, van den Brink AM, et al. European headache federation consensus on the definition of resistant and refractory migraine : developed with the endorsement of the European Migraine & Headache Alliance (EMHA). J Headache Pain. 2020;21(1):76.
62. Katsarava Z, Buse DC, Manack AN, Lipton RB. Defining the differences between episodic migraine and chronic migraine. Curr Pain Headache Rep. 2012;16(1):86–92.
63. Bigal ME, Lipton RB. Excessive acute migraine medication use and migraine progression. Neurology. 2008;71(22):1821–8.
64. Lipton RB, Chu MK. Conceptualizing the relationship between chronic migraine and episodic migraine. Expert Rev Neurother. 2009;9(10):1451–4.
65. Buse DC, Serrano D, Reed ML, Kori SH, Cunanan CM, Adams AM, et al. Adding additional acute medications to a triptan regimen for migraine and observed changes in headache-related disability: results from the American Migraine Prevalence and Prevention (AMPP) study. Headache. 2015;55(6):825–39.
66. Sun-Edelstein C, Rapoport AM. Update on the pharmacological treatment of chronic migraine. Curr Pain Headache Rep. 2016;20(1):6.
67. Kopruszinski CM, Navratilova E, Swiokla J, Dodick DW, Chessell IP, Porreca F. A novel, injury-free rodent model of vulnerability for assessment of acute and preventive therapies reveals temporal contributions of CGRP-receptor activation in migraine-like pain. Cephalalgia. 2021;41(3):305–17.
68. Hepp Z, Dodick DW, Varon SF, Chia J, Matthew N, Gillard P, et al. Persistence and switching patterns of oral migraine prophylactic medications among patients with chronic migraine: a retrospective claims analysis. Cephalalgia. 2017;37(5):470–85.
69. Charles AC, Digre KB, Goadsby PJ, Robbins MS, Hershey A; American Headache Society. Calcitonin gene-related peptide-targeting therapies are a first-line option for the prevention of migraine: An American Headache Society position statement update. Headache. 2024;64(4):333–41.
70. Silberstein SD, Dodick DW, Lindblad AS, Holroyd K, Harrington M, Mathew NT, et al. Randomized, placebo-controlled trial of propranolol added to topiramate in chronic migraine. Neurology. 2012;78(13):976–84.
71. Aurora SK, Brin MF. Chronic migraine: an update on physiology, imaging, and the mechanism of action of two available pharmacologic therapies. Headache. 2017;57(1):109–25.
72. Hoffman KM, Trawalter S, Axt JR, Oliver MN. Racial bias in pain assessment and treatment recommendations, and false beliefs about biological differences between blacks and whites. Proc Natl Acad Sci USA. 2016;113(16):4296–301.
73. Andreou AP, Goadsby PJ. Topiramate in the treatment of migraine: a kainate (glutamate) receptor antagonist within the trigeminothalamic pathway. Cephalalgia. 2011;31(13):1343–58.
74. Diener HC, Bussone G, Van Oene JC, Lahaye M, Schwalen S, Goadsby PJ, et al. Topiramate reduces headache days in chronic migraine: a randomized, double-blind, placebo-controlled study. Cephalalgia. 2007;27(7):814–23.
75. Silberstein SD, Lipton RB, Dodick DW, Freitag FG, Ramadan N, Mathew N, et al. Efficacy and safety of topiramate for the treatment of chronic migraine: a randomized, double-blind, placebo-controlled trial. Headache. 2007;47(2):170–80.
76. Lipton RB, Silberstein S, Dodick D, Cady R, Freitag F, Mathew N, et al. Topiramate intervention to prevent transformation of episodic migraine: the topiramate INTREPID study. Cephalalgia. 2011;31(1):18–30.
77. Diener HC, Dodick DW, Goadsby PJ, Bigal ME, Bussone G, Silberstein SD, et al. Utility of topiramate for the treatment of patients with chronic migraine in the presence or absence of acute medication overuse. Cephalalgia. 2009;29(10):1021–7.
78. Johnson J, Brittain S, Schwabe S. Cognitive effects of extended-release once-daily SPN-538 (Trokendi XR™) vs bid immediate-release topiramate (TPM-IR, Topamax®) in healthy volunteers. Neurology. 2014;82:S43-002.
79. Cole KL, Wang EE, Aronwald RM. Bilateral acute angle-closure glaucoma in a migraine patient receiving topiramate: a case report. J Emerg Med. 2012;43(2):e89–91.
80. Shen C, Chen F, Zhang Y, Guo Y, Ding M. Association between use of antiepileptic drugs and fracture risk: a systematic review and meta-analysis. Bone. 2014;64:246–53.
81. Aurora SK, Dodick DW, Turkel CC, DeGryse RE, Silberstein SD, Lipton RB, et al. OnabotulinumtoxinA for treatment of chronic migraine: results from the double-blind, randomized, placebo-controlled phase of the PREEMPT 1 trial. Cephalalgia. 2010;30(7):793–803.
82. Diener HC, Dodick DW, Aurora SK, Turkel CC, DeGryse RE, Lipton RB, et al. OnabotulinumtoxinA for treatment of chronic migraine: results from the double-blind, randomized, placebo-controlled phase of the PREEMPT 2 trial. Cephalalgia. 2010;30(7):804–14.
83. Schaefer SM, Gottschalk CH, Jabbari B. Treatment of chronic migraine with focus on botulinum neurotoxins. Toxins (Basel). 2015;7(7):2615–28.
84. Matak I, Bölcskei K, Bach-Rojecky L, Helyes Z. Mechanisms of botulinum toxin type A action on pain. Toxins (Basel). 2019;11(8):459.

85. Drinovac Vlah V, Filipović B, Bach-Rojecky L, Lacković Z. Role of central versus peripheral opioid system in antinociceptive and anti-inflammatory effect of botulinum toxin type A in trigeminal region. Eur J Pain. 2018;22(3):583–91.
86. Guerzoni S, Pellesi L, Baraldi C, Cainazzo MM, Negro A, Martelletti P, et al. Long-term treatment benefits and prolonged efficacy of onabotulinumtoxinA in patients affected by chronic migraine and medication overuse headache over 3 years of therapy. Front Neurol. 2017;8:586.
87. Boudreau GP, Grosberg BM, McAllister PJ, Lipton RB, Buse DC. Prophylactic onabotulinumtoxinA in patients with chronic migraine and comorbid depression: an open-label, multicenter, pilot study of efficacy, safety and effect on headache-related disability, depression, and anxiety. Int J Gen Med. 2015;8:79–86.
88. Hepp Z, Rosen NL, Gillard PG, Varon SF, Mathew N, Dodick DW. Comparative effectiveness of onabotulinumtoxinA versus oral migraine prophylactic medications on headache-related resource utilization in the management of chronic migraine: retrospective analysis of a US-based insurance claims database. Cephalalgia. 2016;36(9):862–74.
89. Silberstein SD, Dodick DW, Bigal ME, Yeung PP, Goadsby PJ, Blankenbiller T, et al. Fremanezumab for the preventive treatment of chronic migraine. N Engl J Med. 2017;377(22):2113–22.
90. Detke HC, Goadsby PJ, Wang S, Friedman DI, Selzler KJ, Aurora SK. Galcanezumab in chronic migraine: the randomized, double-blind, placebo-controlled REGAIN study. Neurology. 2018;91(24):e2211–e21.
91. Dodick DW, Lipton RB, Silberstein S, Goadsby PJ, Biondi D, Hirman J, et al. Eptinezumab for prevention of chronic migraine: a randomized phase 2b clinical trial. Cephalalgia. 2019;39(9):1075–85.
92. Tepper S, Ashina M, Reuter U, Brandes JL, Doležil D, Silberstein S, et al. Safety and efficacy of erenumab for preventive treatment of chronic migraine: a randomised, double-blind, placebo-controlled phase 2 trial. Lancet Neurol. 2017;16(6):425–34.
93. Bigal ME, Walter S, Rapoport AM. Therapeutic antibodies against CGRP or its receptor. Br J Clin Pharmacol. 2015;79(6):886–95.
94. Pozo-Rosich P, Ailani J, Ashina M, Goadsby PJ, Lipton RB, Reuter U, et al. Atogepant for the preventive treatment of chronic migraine (PROGRESS): a randomised, double-blind, placebo-controlled, phase 3 trial. Lancet. 2023;402(10404):775–85.
95. Blumenfeld AM, Frishberg BM, Schim JD, Iannone A, Schneider G, Yedigarova L, et al. Real-world evidence for control of chronic migraine patients receiving CGRP monoclonal antibody therapy added to onabotulinumtoxinA: a retrospective chart review. Pain Ther. 2021;10(2):809–26.
96. Ashina S, Terwindt GM, Steiner TJ, Lee MJ, Porreca F, Tassorelli C, et al. Medication overuse headache. Nat Rev Dis Primers. 2023;9(1):5. https://doi.org/10.1038/s41572-022-00415-0. PMID: 36732518.
97. Rossi P, Faroni JV, Nappi G. Short-term effectiveness of simple advice as a withdrawal strategy in simple and complicated medication overuse headache. Eur J Neurol. 2011;18(3):396–401.
98. Silberstein SD, Blumenfeld AM, Cady RK, Turner IM, Lipton RB, Diener HC, et al. OnabotulinumtoxinA for treatment of chronic migraine: PREEMPT 24-week pooled subgroup analysis of patients who had acute headache medication overuse at baseline. J Neurol Sci. 2013;331(1–2):48–56.
99. Tepper SJ, Diener HC, Ashina M, Brandes JL, Friedman DI, Reuter U, et al. Erenumab in chronic migraine with medication overuse: subgroup analysis of a randomized trial. Neurology. 2019;92(20):e2309–e20.
100. Dodick DW, Doty EG, Aurora SK, Ruff DD, Stauffer VL, Jedynak J, et al. Medication overuse in a subgroup analysis of phase 3 placebo-controlled studies of galcanezumab in the prevention of episodic and chronic migraine. Cephalalgia. 2021;41(3):340–52.
101. Silberstein SD, Cohen JM, Seminerio MJ, Yang R, Ashina S, Katsarava Z. The impact of fremanezumab on medication overuse in patients with chronic migraine: subgroup analysis of the HALO CM study. J Headache Pain. 2020;21(1):114.
102. Diener HC, Marmura MJ, Tepper SJ, Cowan R, Starling AJ, Diamond ML, et al. Efficacy, tolerability, and safety of eptinezumab in patients with a dual diagnosis of chronic migraine and medication-overuse headache: subgroup analysis of PROMISE-2. Headache. 2021;61(1):125–36.
103. Goadsby PJ, Friedman DI, Holle-Lee D, Demarquay G, Ashina S, Sakai F, et al. Efficacy of atogepant in chronic migraine with and without acute medication overuse in the randomized, double-blind, phase 3 PROGRESS trial. Neurology. 2024;103(2):e209584.
104. Schwedt TJ, Hentz JG, Sahai-Srivastava S, Murinova N, Spare NM, Treppendahl C, et al. Patient-centered treatment of chronic migraine with medication overuse: a prospective, randomized, pragmatic clinical trial. Neurology. 2022;98(14):e1409–e21.
105. Carlsen LN, Munksgaard SB, Nielsen M, Engelstoft IMS, Westergaard ML, Bendtsen L, et al. Comparison of 3 treatment strategies for medication overuse headache: a randomized clinical trial. JAMA Neurol. 2020;77(9):1069–78.
106. Zeeberg P, Olesen J, Jensen R. Efficacy of multidisciplinary treatment in a tertiary referral headache centre. Cephalalgia. 2005;25(12):1159–67.
107. Solomon GD, Cady RK, Klapper JA, Ryan RE. Standards of care for treating headache in primary care practice. National Headache Foundation. Cleve Clin J Med. 1997;64(7):373–83.
108. Sahai-Srivastava S, Sigman E, Uyeshiro Simon A, Cleary L, Ginoza L. Multidisciplinary team treatment approaches to chronic daily headaches. Headache. 2017;57(9):1482–91.
109. Lai TH, Wang SJ. Update of inpatient treatment for refractory chronic daily headache. Curr Pain Headache Rep. 2016;20(1):5.
110. Marmura MJ, Hou A. Inpatient management of migraine. Neurol Clin. 2019;37(4):771–88.
111. Lake AE, Saper JR, Hamel RL. Comprehensive inpatient treatment of refractory chronic daily headache. Headache. 2009;49(4):555–62.
112. Nagy AJ, Gandhi S, Bhola R, Goadsby PJ. Intravenous dihydroergotamine for inpatient management of refractory primary headaches. Neurology. 2011;77(20):1827–32.
113. Raskin NH. Repetitive intravenous dihydroergotamine as therapy for intractable migraine. Neurology. 1986;36(7):995–7.
114. Ford RG, Ford KT. Continuous intravenous dihydroergotamine in the treatment of intractable headache. Headache. 1997;37(3):129–36.
115. Silberstein SD, Schulman EA, Hopkins MM. Repetitive intravenous DHE in the treatment of refractory headache. Headache. 1990;30(6):334–9.
116. Eller M, Gelfand AA, Riggins NY, Shiboski S, Schankin C, Goadsby PJ. Exacerbation of headache during dihydroergotamine for chronic migraine does not alter outcome. Neurology. 2016;86(9):856–9.
117. Silberstein SD, Young WB. Safety and efficacy of ergotamine tartrate and dihydroergotamine in the treatment of migraine and status migrainosus. Working Panel of the Headache and Facial Pain Section of the American Academy of Neurology. Neurology. 1995;45(3 Pt 1):577–84.
118. Schwenk ES, Walter A, Torjman MC, Mukhtar S, Patel HT, Nardone B, et al. Lidocaine infusions for refractory chronic migraine: a retrospective analysis. Reg Anesth Pain Med. 2022;47(7):408–13.

119. Williams DR, Stark RJ. Intravenous lignocaine (lidocaine) infusion for the treatment of chronic daily headache with substantial medication overuse. Cephalalgia. 2003;23(10):963–71.
120. Gil-Gouveia R, Goadsby PJ. Neuropsychiatric side-effects of lidocaine: examples from the treatment of headache and a review. Cephalalgia. 2009;29(5):496–508.
121. Yuan H, Natekar A, Park J, Lauritsen CG, Viscusi ER, Marmura MJ. Real-world study of intranasal ketamine for use in patients with refractory chronic migraine: a retrospective analysis. Reg Anesth Pain Med. 2023;48(12):581–7.
122. Moshtaghion H, Heiranizadeh N, Rahimdel A, Esmaeili A, Hashemian H, Hekmatimoghaddam S. The efficacy of propofol vs. subcutaneous sumatriptan for treatment of acute migraine headaches in the emergency department: a double-blinded clinical trial. Pain Pract. 2015;15(8):701–5.
123. Pomeroy JL, Marmura MJ, Nahas SJ, Viscusi ER. Ketamine infusions for treatment refractory headache. Headache. 2017;57(2):276–82.
124. Ailani J, Burch RC, Robbins MS, Board of Directors of the American Headache Society. The American Headache Society Consensus Statement: update on integrating new migraine treatments into clinical practice. Headache. 2021;61(7):1021–39.

30 Procedures for the Treatment of Migraine

Regina Krel and Paul G. Mathew

Introduction

Migraine is a primary headache disorder, which is characterized by repeated attacks of severe, throbbing pain with a duration of 4–72 hours. Migraine typically involves photophobia, phonophobia, nausea, and vomiting. According to the International Classification of Headache Disorders 3 (ICHD-3), a diagnosis of chronic migraine requires the presence of 15 or more headache days per month for 3 months, of which 8 days are associated with migraine features [1].

Migraine remains the second largest cause of the world's disability and first among women of childbearing age based on the Global Disease Burden study in 2019 [2]. Although oral preventive medications can reduce the frequency of attacks, use can be limited by contraindications due to medical conditions and/or drug–drug interactions. In addition, oral preventive medications can have poor tolerability, limited effectiveness, and can lose efficacy over time.

In-office procedures have become integral in treatment regimens for migraine. OnabotulinumtoxinA (BTX) gained approval by the United States Food and Drug Administration (FDA) in 2010 for the preventive treatment of chronic migraine in adults. In addition to BTX, other in-office procedures such as sphenopalatine ganglion (SPG) blocks and peripheral nerve blocks (PNB) have demonstrated varying degrees of efficacy for the acute, rescue, and preventive treatment of migraine. The goal of this chapter is to review common procedures used to treat migraine.

R. Krel (✉)
Hackensack Meridian School of Medicine, Nutley, NJ, USA

Department of Neurology, Hackensack University Medical Center, Headache Center at the Neuroscience Institute, Hackensack, NJ, USA

P. G. Mathew
Harvard Medical School, Boston, MA, USA

Department of Neurology, Mass General Brigham Health, Foxborough, MA, USA

Department of Neurology, Atrius Health, Quincy, MA, USA

Questions

1. Which patient would benefit from starting treatment with BTX for the prevention of migraine?
   A. An 18-year-old woman who is suffering from 7 days of headache per month, usually around menses, and is currently using ibuprofen or acetaminophen without much relief.
   B. A 36-year-old man with 18 days of headache per month for the last 6 months who is using sumatriptan four times per week and is also on topiramate after having previously tried nortriptyline and magnesium supplementation.
   C. A 75-year-old man with a remote history of migraine-type headaches in his teenage years who developed headache recurrence last year. Headaches occur 3 times per month and are typically vice-like, bilateral, with no photophobia, phonophobia, nausea, or vomiting. Headache may last 1–2 hours and resolve with acetaminophen.
   D. All of the above
2. Which of the following best describes the PREEPMT BTX injection paradigm for the treatment of chronic migraine?
   A. 155 units into 31 injection sites every 16 weeks
   B. 155 units into 31 injection sites every 12 weeks
   C. 200 units into 21 injection sites every 16 weeks
   D. 155 units into 36 injection sites every 12 weeks
   E. 155 units into 31 injection sites at physician-selected intervals

Onabotulinumtoxin Type A

BTX received approval from the Food and Drug Administration (FDA) for the preventive treatment of chronic migraine in 2010. Through SNARE-dependent processes, BTX inhibits the exocytosis of motor and sensory neuropeptides, as well as

T. S. Monteith et al. (eds.), *Comprehensive Migraine Management*, https://doi.org/10.1007/978-3-031-86923-5_30

the insertion of peripheral membrane receptors that are integral in pain transmission from the periphery to the brain. BTX can decrease exocytosis of pro-inflammatory and excitatory molecules including substance P, calcitonin gene-related peptide, and glutamate from primary afferent C-fibers that transmit nociceptive pain, which can propagate peripheral and central sensitization. BTX also decreases the insertion of pain-sensitive ion channels such as transient receptor potential cation channel subfamily V member 1 (TRPV1) into the membranes of nociceptive neurons, which is likely enhanced in the sensitized neuron [3]. It is also thought that BTX alters inflammatory gene expression and immune cellular responses in patients with chronic migraine [3, 4].

PREEMPT 1 (Phase 3 REsearch Evaluation Migraine Prophylaxis Therapy) and PREEMPT 2 are two randomized double-blind placebo-controlled pivotal clinical trials that established the efficacy, safety, and tolerability of BTX for chronic migraine prevention. Patients received 155 units of BTX at fixed injection sites at 12-week intervals. Patients were assessed for a mean reduction in headache days at 24 weeks [5, 6]. The pooled data from the trial demonstrated a statistically significant reduction in headache days compared to the placebo group (−8.4 vs. −6.6, $p < 0.001$) [7].

The primary endpoint for these trials was headache reduction at 24 weeks. In addition, a 2014 study by Silberstein et al. found that 49% of patients had a 50% reduction in headache days per month after the first round of injections, but 11% and 10% of patients were first responders after their second and third rounds of injections, respectively [3]. As such, patients should receive at least 2–3 rounds of BTX injections at 12-week intervals in order to determine efficacy prior to discontinuation. In addition to proven efficacy, BTX has a favorable tolerability profile compared to oral therapies, and may be a good option for patients who are prone to side effects, have medication contraindications, or are averse to taking daily medication given the 12-week injection schedule. Common side effects following Botox injections include transient neck pain, headache, muscle weakness, and ptosis [5, 6, 8, 9].

The current FDA-approved BTX chronic migraine treatment paradigm is a standardized dose of 155 units administered in equally divided doses across 31 injection sites in 7 muscle groups (corrugators, procerus, frontalis, temporalis, occipitals, cervical paraspinals, and trapezius muscles) (Fig. 30.1). The 7 muscle groups included in the treatment paradigm involve peripheral sensory innervation by the trigeminal, occipital, and cervical sensory nerves. While doses

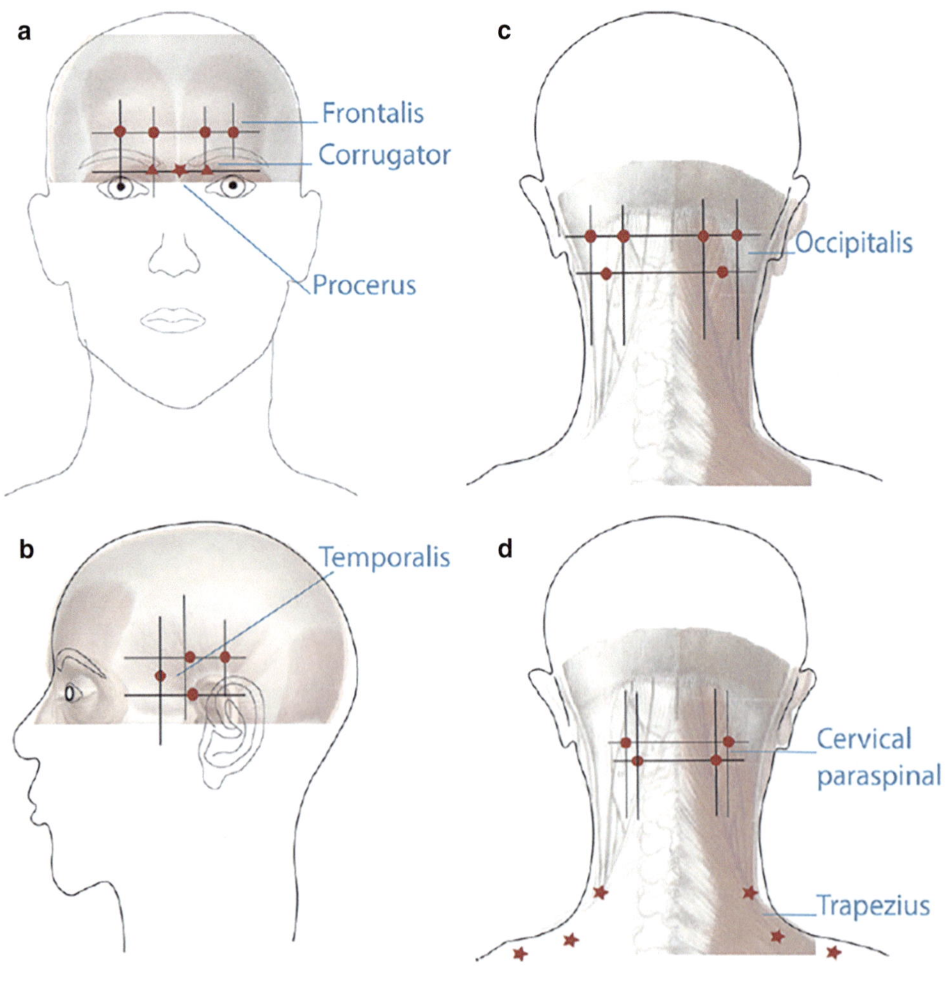

Fig. 30.1 Current FDA-approved BTX chronic migraine treatment paradigm is a standardized dose of 155 units administered in equally divided doses across 31 injection sites in 7 muscle groups (corrugators, procerus, frontalis, temporalis, occipitals, cervical paraspinals, and trapezius muscles)

below the established 155 unit protocol have not been found to result in significant reduction of headache days, there is evidence to support the use of higher doses, up to 195 units [8, 10]. One consideration for the use of higher BTX doses stems from "wear-off" phenomenon, which is loosely defined as when patients experience a positive response to BTX, but subsequently experience a decrease in efficacy days to weeks prior to their next treatment. Incrementally, increasing the dose from 155 units to up to 195 units at 12-week intervals may help reduce this phenomenon [11].

When evaluating a patient with migraine, it is important to note comorbid conditions, which can potentially exacerbate migraine. For example, temporomandibular disorders (TMD) tend to be more prevalent in patients with migraine than the general population, and may contribute to migraine chronification [12]. In patients with chronic migraine and TMD, performing BTX injections in the muscles of mastication, including the masseters, off-label in addition to the standard 155-unit chronic migraine paradigm, could be considered, which can be an effective dual therapy [13]. Cervical dystonia, hyperhidrosis, and hemifacial spasm are other conditions for which additional BTX injection sites could be considered.

Up until 2018, BTX has been the only FDA-approved treatment specifically for patients with chronic migraine. In 2018, the first calcitonin gene-related peptide (CGRP) monoclonal antibodies (MAbs) were FDA-approved for the treatment of migraine, and eventually received indications for the prevention of both episodic and chronic migraine in adults. CGRP MAbs are thought to act by preventing the activation of Aδ-fibers via reduction of CGRP. In comparison, BTX is thought to exert its effects on the C-fiber pathways [14]. It is therefore feasible that combined therapy with BTX and CGRP MAbs can be an effective treatment regimen for patients with refractory chronic migraine. A retrospective chart review of 257 patients who were receiving treatment with BTX and CGRP MAbs demonstrated efficacy and safety with concomitant use [15]. Similarly, combination therapy with BTX and gepants used for preventive therapy (atogepant, rimegepant) is likely more effective than monotherapy in reducing migraine days per month in patients with chronic migraine [16].

Sphenopalatine Ganglion Blocks

Intranasal sphenopalatine ganglion block. The sphenopalatine ganglion (SPG) block is a therapeutic target for migraine and cluster and involves the application of local anesthetics with a catheter or cotton tip. The SPG, a large extracranial parasympathetic ganglion with multiple neural connections (autonomic, motor, sensory), lies at a variable depth beneath the mucosal surface in the pterygopalatine fossa (exposed here for visualization) (Fig. 30.2) [17].

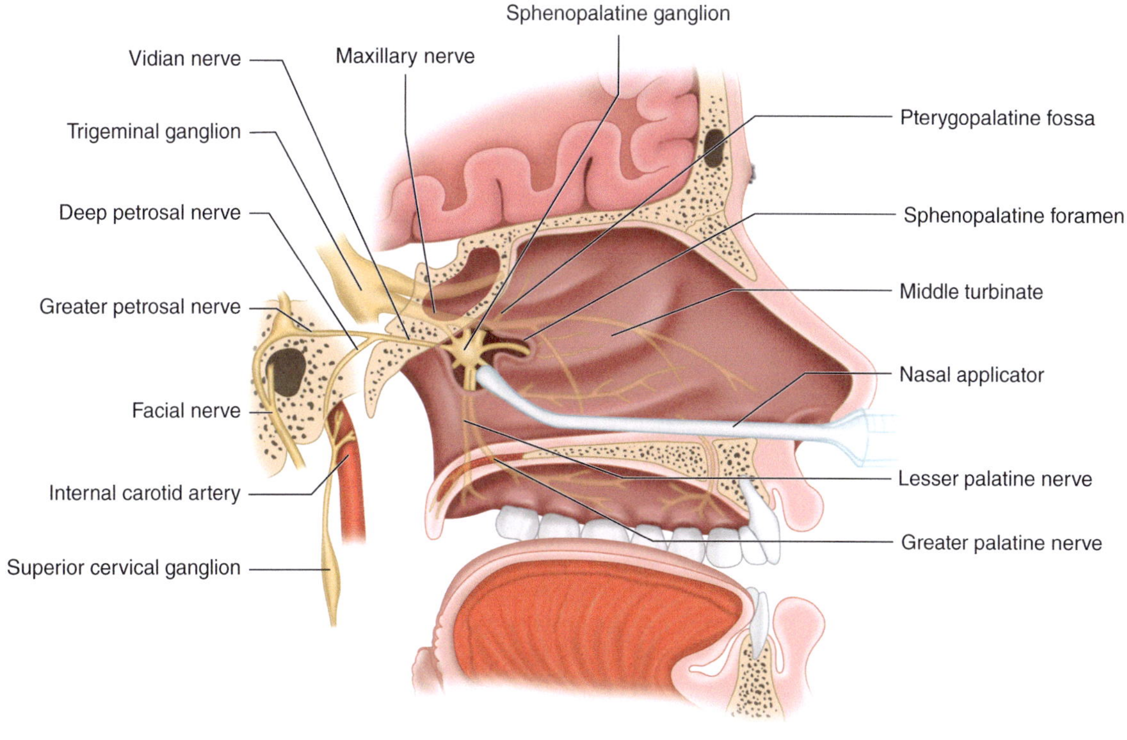

Fig. 30.2 Sphenopalatine ganglion anatomy. The SPG lies at a variable depth beneath the mucosal surface of the lateral wall of the nares

The autonomic features that are ipsilateral to the pain in cluster headache have long suggested the involvement of the SPG in headache and facial pain disorders [18]. There is data to suggest that SPG blocks can be useful for the treatment of cluster headache, migraine, and trigeminal neuralgia [19]. There are numerous techniques for performing SPG blocks. One of the oldest techniques was devised by Sluder around 1908, and involves the use of a needle to inject cocaine for the treatment of "Sluder's Neuralgia," which was a term used to describe a symptom complex consisting of neuralgic, motor, sensory, and gustatory manifestations that he attributed to the SPG [20]. An American Headache Society Survey revealed that in clinical practice, two of the most commonly utilized techniques involve the use of commercially available intranasal catheters that deliver local anesthetic transnasally to the SPG. The SphenoCath was used by 42.8% of responders, and the TX360 was used by 41.8% of responders (both devices are used off-label). Ease of use was the most common answer for why catheter-based devices were chosen. The Q-tip technique, which was used by 17.7% of responders, involves the insertion of a cotton swab soaked with local anesthetic into the nasal cavity. Variability also exists regarding which medications are utilized with 2% lidocaine being the most common, and 0.5% bupivacaine being the second most commonly used anesthetic [21].

There is limited data supporting the use of SPG blocks. A double-blind placebo-controlled trial assessed the repetitive use of SPG blocks using a catheter device for the treatment of chronic migraine. The protocol involved performing blocks twice weekly for a total of 6 weeks with 0.5% bupivacaine. Statistically significant pain relief was seen at 15- and 30-minute intervals and was sustained at 24 hours when compared to the placebo group. The procedure was well tolerated, and the most common side effect was bad taste if the anesthetic was swallowed, which can result in oral numbness and lacrimation [22]. In addition to performing the in-office procedure, SPG blockade can be performed via a self-administered method, which allows patients to perform the procedure in the comfort of their own home without the need for an appointment. This technique involves the use of an anesthetic nasal spray that is delivered while in the supine position. In one study, patients used self-administered SPG blocks once a month for prevention, and up to four additional administrations as needed for acute treatment. In this study, 66 patients utilized this treatment for prevention, and 79% of patients saw a reduction in headache frequency or severity at their 3-month follow-up. Out of 53 patients who used this method for rescue, 75% of the patients also noted a reduction in headache severity [23]. Further research is needed to establish optimal treatment protocols in terms of technique, medications, and dosing.

Peripheral Nerve Blocks

Cranial peripheral nerve blocks (PNB) are in-office procedures, which can provide rapid relief for acute treatment, disrupt a refractory headache cycle, and be used for prevention. In patients who have contraindications to multiple medications or in whom polypharmacy is limited due to drug–drug interactions, PNB can be a safe and effective treatment option [24]. PNB involves the injection of a local anesthetic, with or without steroids, in the distribution of the desired nerve. Commonly injected peripheral nerves for the treatment of headache disorders include the occipital (greater, lesser, and third), supraorbital, supratrochlear, infraorbital, and auriculotemporal nerves. The most common adverse reactions include bleeding, injection site pain, numbness, and lightheadedness [25].

Occipital Nerve Blocks

Upon review of the American Headache Society Interventional Procedure Survey (AHS-IPS), the most common indications for performing an occipital nerve block (ONB) were headache localized to the occiput, a positive occipital Tinel's sign on examination, and a prior positive response to PNB. Similarly to SPG blocks, the most commonly used medications were lidocaine and bupivacaine [25]. There is significant variability in terms of time intervals between injections, the volume of medication utilized, and the use of steroids. The indication with the most evidence to support the use of steroids with ONB is for the treatment of cluster headache [26].

The Procedural Headache Medicine Section of the American Headache Society (IPS-AHS) published expert consensus recommendations in an attempt to provide guidance in performing PNB and establish some uniformity. To perform occipital nerve blocks, the occiput is palpated, and the inion and mastoid process are identified. The skin is then prepped with alcohol and anesthetic volumes between 1.5 and 3 cc per nerve can be injected (Fig. 30.3). Care should be taken to confirm that the needle was not advanced intravascularly by obtaining a negative aspiration before injecting. This is particularly important when injecting particulate steroids, which have the potential to embolize [27].

In terms of data supporting the use of occipital nerve blocks for the treatment of chronic migraine, a meta-analysis demonstrated limited evidence that GONBs reduce headache frequency and intensity compared to placebo. There was even less evidence to support adding steroids. In the included randomized control trials (RCT), the change in migraine frequency was −4.45 days during the first month (95% CI: −6.56 to −2.34 days) and −5.49 during the second month (95% CI −8.94 to −2.03 days) [28]. The quality of

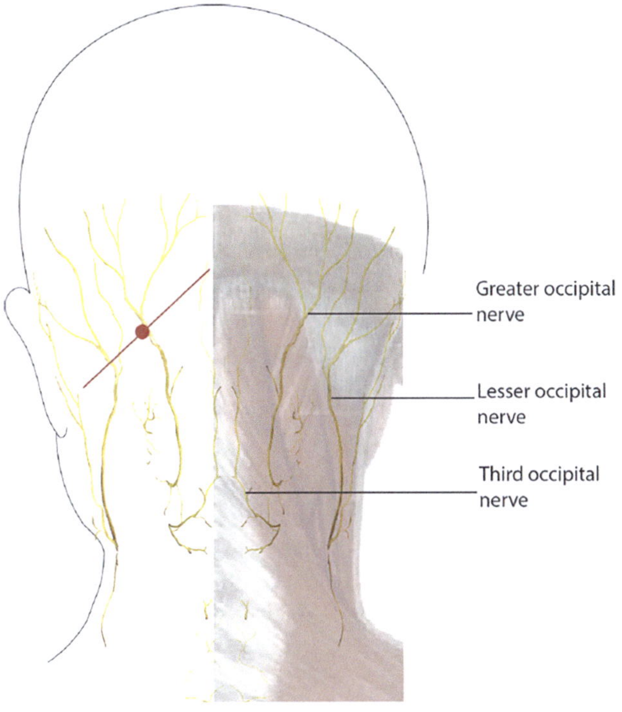

Fig. 30.3 Needle enters skin at red dot and is inserted along the red line toward the inion and then pulled back to ensure that there is no blood return. Medication (1.5–3 cc) is then delivered along the red line as the needle is withdrawn. The needle is removed, and the process repeated along the red line in the opposite direction toward the mastoid, delivering another 1.5–3 cc of medication

evidence was thought to be low due to small sample sizes, substantial risk of bias, and imprecision. Similar conclusions were drawn by Barad et al. in a systematic review that screened 1195 studies, assessed 352 full text articles, and included 16 randomized controlled trials that met the inclusion criteria [29].

Traditionally, ONBs are used to treat occipital neuralgia (ON), which is comorbid with migraine. ON is recurring paroxysmal shooting or stabbing pain that radiates from the skull base toward the apex in the case of greater occipital nerve involvement or toward the ipsilateral temple in the case of lesser occipital nerve involvement. It can present unilaterally or bilaterally. In addition to pain, ON can involve numbness, paresthesia, and cutaneous allodynia in the distribution of the involved nerves. On physical examination, percussion along the skull base may elicit an Occipital Tinel's sign, which can be positive in 75% of patients with ON [30]. Based on the ICHD 3 criteria for diagnosing occipital neuralgia, pain should be temporarily relieved by ONBs [1]. Regarding the prevalence of ON, a community-based headache clinic study involving 800 patients who presented with a chief complaint of headache demonstrated that approximately 25% of patients had a diagnosis of ON. Among these patients with ON, 85% also had a coexisting headache disorder, most commonly chronic migraine. These data would suggest that ON can exacerbate, and at times result in the chronification of concurrent headache disorders [30]. In addition, there is data to suggest that large volume ONBs (6 cc/side) can result in remission of ON pain for weeks, months, or even years. A hypothesis for this long duration of benefit is that the large volume injection has a hydrodissecting effect of the muscle, connective tissue, and other structures that are adjacent to the affected nerve, resulting in hydrodynamic nerve decompression [31].

Trigeminal Nerve Branch Blocks

Indications for blockade of distal trigeminal nerve branches (supraorbital, supratrochlear, infraorbital, and auriculotemporal nerve) include location of acute head pain, prior injection response, and presence of local tenderness. One study reported an 80% reduction in acute symptoms with supratrochlear and supraorbital blockade in 70 women with migraine. In cases of focal head trauma or at times spontaneously, these distal trigeminal branches can become compressed/irritated resulting in focal neuralgias, which, like occipital neuralgia, can at times be responsive to nerve blocks in which volume-dependent decompression may result in pain remission of long duration [32].

To perform supraorbital and supratrochlear nerve blocks, the supraorbital ridge is palpated, and the supraorbital (superior, mid-pupillary) and supratrochlear (superior, medial) notches are identified. The skin is then prepped with alcohol and volumes between 0.5 and 1 cc can be injected in the regions of notches, infiltrating the proximal areas of the desired nerve (Fig. 30.4). Care should be taken not to inject steroids in cosmetic areas like the forehead, as steroids can cause atrophy and disfigurement.

To perform auriculotemporal nerve blocks, the temporal artery is located at the level of the tragus and the nerve is typically 1–2 cm anterior to the artery. The skin is then prepped with alcohol, and volumes between 0.5 and 3 cc can be injected above the posterior part of the zygoma infiltrating in the area of the auriculotemporal nerve (Fig. 30.5). Care should be taken not to inject steroids in cosmetic areas like the temples, as steroids can cause atrophy and disfigurement [27].

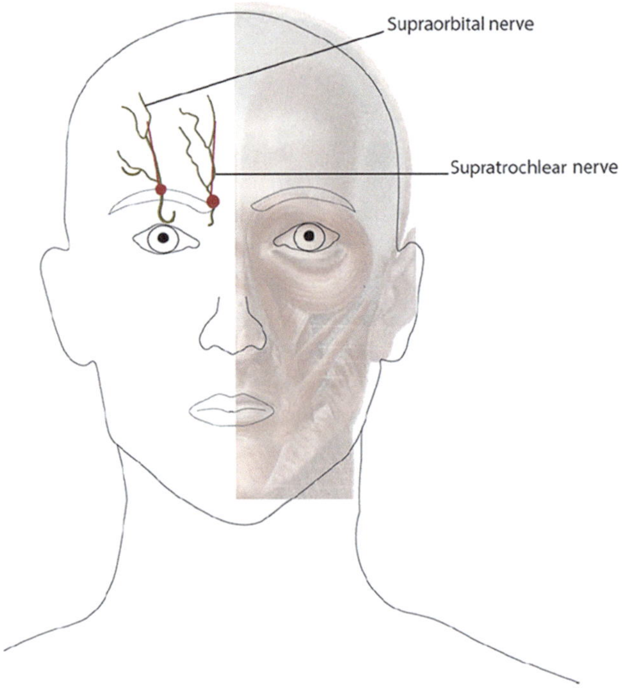

Fig. 30.4 Using direct palpation, the supraorbital foramen is identified and the needle is inserted into the red dots (superomedial corner of the orbit for supratrochlear nerve and the mid-pupillary line for the supraorbital nerve) infiltrating in the areas of supraorbital and supratrochlear nerves and being careful to remain superficial throughout the entire process

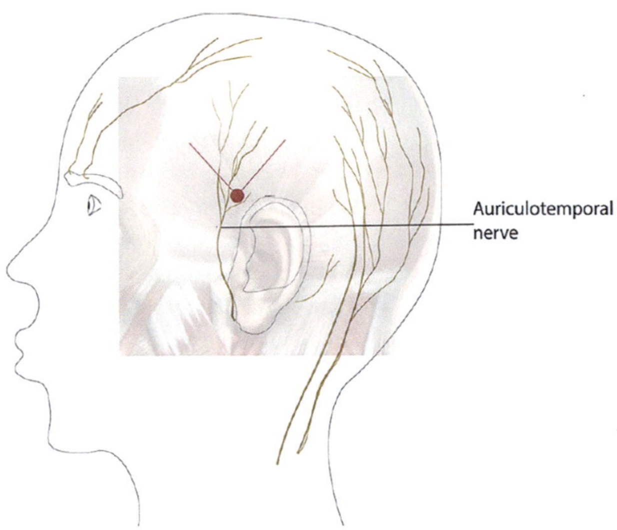

Fig. 30.5 Using direct palpation, the temporal artery pulse is located, and the skin prepared with alcohol. Next, the needle is inserted into the red dot (anterior to the temporal artery above the posterior part of the zygoma) infiltrating in the area of the auriculotemporal nerve and again being careful to remain superficial throughout the entire process

Acupuncture

Acupuncture is a non-pharmacologic treatment that has been used to treat a myriad of conditions, but is most commonly utilized for chronic pain management. Acupuncture is performed by applying small needles to specific points of the body to help improve the function of a specific system. The basis of acupuncture is to restore the balance of Qi or "vital energy." Qi is a culmination of 5 elements, which are wood, fire, water, earth, and metal. Acupuncture is aimed at opening blockage or decreasing excess of flow in this "vital energy" [33]. There has growing data to support its use in the treatment of migraine, although the exact mechanism of action is not fully understood. A systematic review of the use of acupuncture in migraine management demonstrated varying degrees of pain reduction and improvement of quality of life. Although additional clinical trials are needed to better assess the utility of acupuncture, it is a relatively safe non-pharmacological modality that can be in the adjunctive treatment of migraine [34].

Conclusion

Although there are many therapeutic options for the management of migraine, procedures can be an effective option to augment any treatment plan. Most procedures can be performed safely in an office setting, require little to no downtime for the patient, and involve minimal risk. Interventional techniques can be useful tools for patients who do not adequately respond, cannot tolerate, or have contraindications to conventional pharmacological treatments.

Teaching Points

1. In-office procedures can be safe and effective options for the treatment of patients with migraine, particularly in cases that involve poor tolerability, low efficacy, and/or contraindications to oral medications.
2. BTX has demonstrated favorable efficacy and tolerability since its FDA approval for the treatment of chronic migraine in 2010. In assessing efficacy, at least 2–3 injection series should be performed before discontinuing treatment as delayed responses to treatment can occur in a subset of patients.

(continued)

3. For the treatment of refractory chronic migraine, combination therapy with BTX and CGRP-based therapies including monoclonal antibodies and gepants should be considered.
4. There are a variety of peripheral nerve block techniques, most commonly targeting the greater occipital nerve block, for the treatment of migraine.
5. Patients with chronic migraine can also present with occipital neuralgia, and large volume occipital nerve blocks, which are both diagnostic and therapeutic, should be considered early in the course of treatment based on the index of clinical suspicion.

Case

A 41-year-old right-handed woman has a 15-year history of migraine without aura. Over the past 2 years, her headaches have gradually increased in frequency and have been occurring approximately 20 days per month over the past 6 months. She has tried amitriptyline, which she could not tolerate due to severe dry mouth and constipation. She has also tried topiramate with initial benefit, but this medication became less effective over time, and cognitive issues prevented further titration of her dose. Propranolol was avoided due to a past medical history of asthma and depression. She is frustrated that she continues to experience frequent headaches and is reluctant to try more oral preventive medications due to the risk of side effects.

Case Discussion

This patient has headache greater than 15 days per month for 3 consecutive months, and thus fulfills criteria for the diagnosis of chronic migraine without aura. Preventive medication use of amitriptyline, topiramate, and propranolol has been limited by intolerance, ineffectiveness, and contraindications. A next step in management for her would be the discussion for the use of BTX for chronic migraine prevention. BTX is approved for the preventive treatment of chronic migraine in adults.

Questions and Answers

1. Which patient would benefit from starting treatment with BTX for the prevention of migraine?
   A. An 18-year-old woman who is suffering from 7 days of headache per month, usually around menses, and is currently using ibuprofen or acetaminophen without much relief.
   B. A 36-year-old man with 18 days of headache per month for the last 6 months who is using sumatriptan four times per week and is also on topiramate after having previously tried nortriptyline and magnesium supplementation.
   C. A 75-year-old man with a remote history of migraine-type headaches in his teenage years who developed headache recurrence last year. Headaches occur 3 times per month and are typically vice-like, bilateral, with no photophobia, phonophobia, nausea, or vomiting. Headache may last 1–2 hours and resolve with acetaminophen.
   D. All of the above

The correct answer is B. This is a patient with chronic migraine, who previously tried a few preventive medications for migraine. Choice A is consistent with episodic migraine and menstrual migraine; prior trials to treat episodic migraine were negative although new trials are ongoing. Choice C is consistent with tension-type headache; there is no evidence that BTX is effective for this diagnosis.

2. Which of the following best describes the PREEPMT BTX injection paradigm for the treatment of chronic migraine?
   A. 155 units into 31 injection sites every 16 weeks
   B. 155 units into 31 injection sites every 12 weeks
   C. 200 units into 21 injection sites every 16 weeks
   D. 155 units into 36 injection sites every 12 weeks
   E. 155 units into 31 injection sites at physician-selected intervals

The correct answer is B. Choice B describes the PREEMPT protocol which was tested in the PREEMPT I and PREEMPT II clinical trials and demonstrated efficacy for chronic migraine prevention with the use of BTX. Larger quantities up to 195–200 units may be considered; however, injection site locations would be greater than 31 sites (up to 9 additional injection sites).

References

1. ICHD-3 The International Classification of Headache Disorders 3rd edition. (n.d.). Retrieved from https://www.ichd-3.org/
2. Steiner TJ, Stovner LJ, Jensen R, Uluduz D, Katsarava Z. Migraine remains second among the world's causes of disability, and first among young women: findings from GBD2019. J Headache Pain. 2020;21(1)
3. Burstein R, Blumenfeld AM, Silberstein SD, Manack Adams A, Brin MF. Mechanism of action of OnabotulinumtoxinA in chronic migraine: a narrative review. Headache. 2020;60(7):1259–72.
4. Gfrerer L, Xu W, Austen W, Ashina S, Melo-Carrillo A, Longhi MS, Adams AM, Houle T, Brin MF, Burstein R. OnabotulinumtoxinA alters inflammatory gene expression and immune cells in chronic headache patients. Brain. 2021;145(7):2436–49.
5. Aurora S, Dodick D, Aurora S, Turkel C, et al. OnabotulinumtoxinA for treatment of chronic migraine: results from the double-blind, randomized, placebo-controlled phase of the PREEMPT 1 trial. Cephalalgia. 2010;30(7):793–803.
6. Diener H, Dodick D, Aurora S, Turkel C, et al. OnabotulinumtoxinA for treatment of chronic migraine: results from the double-blind, randomized, placebo-controlled phase of the PREEMPT 2 trial. Cephalalgia. 2010;30(7):804–14.
7. Dodick D, Turkel C, DeGryse RE, et al. OnabotulinumtoxinA for treatment of chronic migraine: pooled results from the double blind, randomized, placebo-controlled phases of the PREEMPT clinical program. Headache J Head Face Pain. 2010;50(6):921–36.
8. Blumenfeld AM, Silberstein SD, Dodick DW, Aurora SK, Brin MF, Binder WJ. Insights into the functional anatomy behind the PREEMPT injection paradigm: guidance on achieving optimal outcomes. Headache J Head Face Pain. 2017;57(5):766–77.
9. Rothrock J, Adams A, Lipton R, et al. FORWARD study: evaluating the comparative effectiveness of OnabotulinumtoxinA and topiramate for headache prevention in adults with chronic migraine. Headache J Head Face Pain. 2019;59(10):1700–13.
10. Naprienko MV, Smekalkina LV, Surnova EA. Efficacy of different doses of botox in treatment of chronic migraine. Zhurnal Nevrologii I Psikhiatrii Im. S.S. Korsakova. 2017;117(8):44.
11. Masters-Israilov A, Robbins M. OnabotulinumtoxinA wear-off phenomenon in treatment of chronic migraine. Headache J Head Face Pain. 2019;59(10):1753–61.
12. Latysheva NV, Platonova AS, Filatova EG. Temporomandibular disorder and cervicalgia: pathophysiology underlying the comorbidity with chronic migraine. Zhurnal Nevrologii I Psikhiatrii Im. S.S. Korsakova. 2019;119(1):17.
13. Mor N, Tang C, Blitzer A. Temporomandibular myofacial pain treated with botulinum toxin injection. Toxins. 2015;7(8):2791–800.
14. Silvestro M, Tessitore A, Scotto di Clemente F, Battista G, Tedeschi G, Russo A. Additive interaction between onabotulinumtoxin-A and erenumab in patients with refractory migraine. Front Neurol. 2021;12
15. Blumenfeld AM, Frishberg BM, Schim JD, Iannone A, Schneider G, Yedigarova L, Manack Adams A. Real-world evidence for control of chronic migraine patients receiving CGRP monoclonal antibody therapy added to onabotulinumtoxinA: a retrospective chart review. Pain Ther. 2021;10(2):809–26.
16. Melo-Carrillo A, Strassman AM, Schain AJ, Adams AM, Brin MF, Burstein R. Combined onabotulinumtoxinA/atogepant treatment blocks activation/sensitization of high-threshold and wide-dynamic range neurons. Cephalalgia. 2021;41(1):17–32.
17. https://practicalneurology.com/articles/2021-may/sphenopalatine-blocks-without-catheter
18. Láinez MJA, Marti AS. Sphenopalatine ganglion stimulation in cluster headache and other types of headache. Cephalalgia. 2016;36(12):1149–55.
19. Binfalah M, Alghawi E, Shosha E, Alhilly A, Bakhiet M. Sphenopalatine ganglion block for the treatment of acute migraine headache. Pain Res Treat. 2018;2018:1–6.
20. Ahamed SH, Jones NS. What is Sluder's neuralgia? J Laryngol Otol. 2003;117(6):437–43.
21. Burkett JG, Robbins MS, Robertson CE, Mete M, Saikali NP, Halker Singh RB, Ailani J. Sphenopalatine ganglion block in primary headaches. Neurol Clin Pract. 2019;10(6):503–9. https://doi.org/10.1212/cpj.0000000000000773.
22. Cady R, Saper J, Dexter K, Manley HR. A double-blind, placebo-controlled study of repetitive Transnasal sphenopalatine ganglion blockade with TX360® as acute treatment for chronic migraine. Headache J Head Face Pain. 2014;55(1):101–16.
23. Bobker SM. Retrospective chart review: the feasibility of a self-administered nasal spray targeting the sphenopalatine ganglion (SPG) in treatment of chronic migraine. J Anesth Anesthet Drugs. 2022;2(1):1–5.
24. Hascalovici JR, Robbins MS. Peripheral nerve blocks for the treatment of headache in older adults: a retrospective study. Headache J Head Face Pain. 2016;57(1):80–6.
25. Blumenfeld A, Ashkenazi A, Grosberg B, Napchan U, Narouze S, Nett B, Lipton RB. Patterns of use of peripheral nerve blocks and trigger point injections among headache practitioners in the USA: results of the American Headache Society Interventional Procedure Survey (AHS-IPS). Headache J Head Face Pain. 2010;50(6):937–42.
26. Ashkenazi A, Blumenfeld A, Napchan U, Narouze S, Grosberg B, Nett R, Lipton RB. Peripheral nerve blocks and trigger point injections in headache management – a systematic review and suggestions for future research. Headache J Head Face Pain. 2010;50(6):943–52.
27. Blumenfeld A, Ashkenazi A, Napchan U, Bender SD, Klein BC, Berliner R, Robbins MS. Expert consensus recommendations for the performance of peripheral nerve blocks for headaches – a narrative review. Headache J Head Face Pain. 2013;53(3):437–46.
28. Velásquez-Rimachi V, Chachaima-Mar J, Cárdenas-Baltazar EC, Loayza-Vidalon A, Morán-Mariños C, Pacheco-Barrios K, Posso M, Alva-Díaz C. Greater occipital nerve block for chronic migraine patients: a meta-analysis. Acta Neurol Scand. 2022;146(2):101–14.
29. Barad M, Ailani J, Hakim SM, Kissoon NR, Schuster NM. Percutaneous interventional strategies for migraine prevention: a systematic review and practice guideline. Pain Med. 2022;23(1):164–88.
30. Mathew PG, Najib U, Khaled S, Krel R. Prevalence of occipital neuralgia at a community hospital-based headache clinic. Neurol Clin Pract. 2019;11(1):6–12.
31. Austen WG Jr, Remy K, Packowski K, Hazewinkel MH, Gfrerer L, Mathew PG. Refractory occipital neuralgia treatment with nerve decompression surgery: a case series. Front Neurol. 2023;14:1284101. https://doi.org/10.3389/fneur.2023.1284101.
32. Mathew PG, Cooper W. The diagnosis and management of post-traumatic headache with associated painful cranial neuralgias: a review and case series. Curr Pain Headache Rep. 2021;25(8):54.
33. Van Hal M, Dydyk AM, Green MS. Acupuncture. In: StatPearls [Internet]. Treasure Island: StatPearls Publishing; 2022. p. 2023.
34. Naguit N, Laeeq S, Jakkoju R, Reghefaoui T, Zahoor H, Yook JH, Rizwan M, Shahid NUA, Mohammed L. Is acupuncture safe and effective treatment for migraine? A systematic review of randomized controlled trials. Cureus. 2022;14(1):e20888. https://doi.org/10.7759/cureus.20888.

Part VI

Migraine Across the Lifespan and Special Populations

Pediatric Management of Migraine

31

Ankita Ghosh and Andrew D. Hershey

Introduction

Headaches are a frequent symptom found in children and adolescents. Globally, nearly 60% of children experience significant headaches with a prevalence of 1%–3% of migraine in 3–7 years old, 4%–11% in 7–11 years old, and 8%–23% by age 15 years [1]. The clinician's initial task is to rule out all the underlying secondary causes of headaches by taking a thorough headache history and by doing a neurological examination. In childhood, the most common, recurrent, primary headache disorder brought to medical attention is migraine. Primary headache disorders are diseases in themselves and are not caused by a secondary etiology, and are diagnosed based on criteria by the International Classification of Headache disorders, third edition [2]. This chapter aims to improve the approach to diagnosing primary headache disorders, to ruling out secondary headache causes, to increase the recognition of different subtypes of migraine and episodic syndromes, and to recommend evidence-based management for migraine.

Questions

1. An 18-year-old female with a 5-year history of migraine headaches presented to the emergency room with a severe headache which developed earlier in the day associated with left-sided weakness on her examination. She has several other family members with similar symptoms. Workup, including imaging studies, is normal. Which is the most common genetic cause for this patient's presentation?
   A. CACNA1A
   B. ATP1A2
   C. ATP1A3
   D. PRRT2
   E. SCN1A
2. Until what age does alternating hemiplegia of childhood generally occur?
   A. 24 months
   B. 12 months
   C. 15 months
   D. 18 months
   E. 3 years

Epidemiology and Impact of Pediatric Migraine

Onset of migraine with aura peaks around 5 years of age in males (6.6/1000 person-years); the migraine without aura peaks between ages 10 and 11 years (10/1000 person-years) [28]. In females, the onset of migraine with aura peaks

A. Ghosh (✉)
Division of Neurology, University of Tennessee Health Science Center, Memphis, TN, USA

A. D. Hershey
Division of Neurology, Cincinnati Children's Hospital, Cincinnati, OH, USA

Department of Pediatrics, University of Cincinnati College of Medicine, Cincinnati, OH, USA

T. S. Monteith et al. (eds.), *Comprehensive Migraine Management*, https://doi.org/10.1007/978-3-031-86923-5_31

between ages 12 and 13 years (14.1/1000 person-years); migraine without aura peaks between ages 14 and 17 years (18.9/1000 person-years) [3]. The prevalence of migraine in children is approximately 5% by age 10 [4], and it increases further over the course of adolescence. Prior to puberty, migraine affects both sexes equally. By late adolescence, migraine affects more girls than boys [4].

When a child presents with a headache, it is imperative to assess how the headache is impacting the individual's life. While most children experience infrequent headaches, there is a subset who can have chronic headaches, which increases the risk for academic difficulties, emotional problems, anxiety, and depression. Children with migraine miss more school days. Nausea with attacks is the strongest predictor of missing school [1]. Measuring migraine-associated disability by using the PedMIDAS questionnaire in children and adolescents is important for determining the appropriate level of treatment intervention and for following treatment response over time.

Approach to Headache History Taking

A properly obtained history can differentiate various headache types and underlying etiologies. It is the key to appropriate treatment. The interview process and evaluation need to be developmentally appropriate. Having a parent/guardian in the room with the patient helps in obtaining family history and other essential parts of medical history, but it could also be challenging as sometimes parents are inclined to give their child's headache history themselves. It is essential to give the message before starting the interview that the child is the focus of the visit and the parent(s)/guardians are there to support and help them.

A planned and systematic approach to taking the pediatric headache history is essential. A headache questionnaire increases the efficiency of history taking because it allows the patient and parent(s)/guardian(s) to think about the headache characterization and concerns before the conversation starts (Table 31.1). Answers should then be reviewed during the interview. Particular attention should be paid to the following characterization, associated symptoms, red flags, and disability.

Table 31.1 Questions for headache history taking

1. At what age did you start having any headaches?
2. What are triggers for your headache?
(a) Stress
(b) Less/more sleep
(c) Skipping meals
(d) Weather
(e) Menstruation
(f) Caffeine
(g) School work
3. Do you experience any of these symptoms before your headache starts?
(a) Tiredness
(b) Irritability
(c) Sunken eyes
(d) Flushed face
(e) Mood changes
(f) Food craving
4. Do you experience any "warning signs" that your headache is going to start?
5. Where does your head hurt?
6. What does the pain feel like?
(a) Throbbing
(b) Squeezing
(c) Stabbing
(d) Pinching
(e) Pressure
(f) Constant
7. Do you have any of these symptoms with your headache?
(a) Nausea
(b) Vomiting
(c) Light sensitivity
(d) Sound sensitivity
(e) Smell sensitivity
8. How many hours does your shortest and longest headache last for?
9. On a scale of 0–10, how do you rate your pain for mild headache and worse headache? (0 = no pain, 5 = moderate pain, 10 = worst pain)
10. How often does the headache occur?
(a) <1/month
(b) 1/week
(c) >3/week
(d) Daily
(e) Always
11. Does your headache:
(a) Gets worse when you stand up or lay down
(b) Gets worse when you cough or strain
(c) Wakes you up at night
(d) Gets better with sleep
12. Allodynia symptoms—Does it hurt to:
(a) Comb hair
(b) Take a shower
(c) Wash your face
(d) Wear ponytail
(e) Wear glasses, hats, headbands, headphones, tight clothing
13. Are you able to function at school with headaches?
14. Any pattern to your headache?

Headache Characterization

For location, ask the patient to point out the locations where their typical headache starts. There is an increased incidence of bilateral locations, especially frontal or bitemporal in children and adolescents with migraine. In the emergency department setting, occipital headache with abnormal neurology examination has been associated with pediatric brain tumors [5, 6]. In the clinical setting, the child who has recurrent occipital headaches but a normal neurologic examination and history consistent with migraine does not appear to be at increased risk of underlying pathology [7]. In addition, it is important to ask the frequency of all the types of headaches. Adolescents can be asked to rate their headaches on a numerical pain scale of 0–10. For younger children, a face pain scale can be used to assess the severity of the headaches. The headaches in children may be shorter in duration. It can last anywhere from 2 to 72 hours when untreated or undertreated.

Headaches occurring after specific triggers may also help families to characterize and recognize the pattern in younger patient population. Sleep disturbance is the most common trigger for migraine in children [8]. Other consistent triggers noted are skipping meals, stress, dehydration, menstrual cycle, and weather changes. Although recent studies suggest that migraine triggers are less common and less consistent than previously thought [9, 10], the consistency of triggers can clue toward the diagnosis itself [11].

Associated Symptoms

Oftentimes, a child may be unaware of the prodrome and the postdromal symptoms; however, parent(s)/guardians might notice changes in their behavior (Table 31.1). One-quarter of children with migraine experience aura [5]. The typical aura could be visual, sensory, or dysphasic. Visual aura is the most frequent in children and adolescents [12]. Children frequently describe it as brightly colored lights or moving lights. Less frequently they describe "negative" visual auras such as distorted images, scotomas, visual field defects [13]. Sensory aura is the second most common aura in children. They can describe paresthesia starting in the upper extremities and spreading to one part of the body and face. Dysphasic aura is one of the least common forms.

Nausea, vomiting, sensitivity to light, and sensitivity to sounds are part of the diagnostic criteria for migraine. Children and adolescents may also report lightheadedness, stomachache, confusion, and fatigue associated with headaches. Cranial autonomic symptoms such as conjunctival injection, lacrimation, nasal congestion, and rhinorrhea are common in younger children, and these symptoms are usually bilateral [14].

Red Flags

Secondary headaches can be seen in almost 2%–3% of children presenting to the emergency department and 1% of patients presenting to the primary care setting [15]. If the child is complaining of waking up at night because of headaches, change in severity and pattern of headaches, then potential secondary causes should be explored. The acronym SNOOP10Y (Table 31.2) may be a useful memory aid to ensure that secondary etiologies are not being overlooked. If there is any suspicion of secondary etiology, proper investigations such as Magnetic Resonance Imaging (MRI), electroencephalogram (EEG), and lumbar puncture (LP) should be considered. This acronym is adapted from the SNOOP10 mnemonic for secondary etiologies of adult headaches [16–18].

Table 31.2 Red flags—SNNOOP10Y

Signs or symptoms to consider secondary causes for headache
1. **S**ystemic symptoms—Fever, weight loss
2. **N**eoplasm history
3. **N**eurological signs on examination
Abnormal gait examination, macrocephaly, ataxia, papilledema, decreased consciousness, nystagmus, and other visual disturbances
4. **O**nset sudden—Thunderclap headaches raising concerns for subarachnoid hemorrhage and reversible cerebral vasoconstriction syndrome
5. **O**nset in sleep—Headaches occurring early in the morning or during sleep have been related to increased intracranial pressure
6. **P**attern change
7. **P**ositional exacerbation—Worse supine (raised intracranial pressure) or worse standing (CSF leak)
8. **P**recipitated by Valsalva—May indicate raised intracranial pressure
9. **P**apilledema—Raised intracranial pressure because of neoplasms, idiopathic intracranial hypertension
10. **P**rogressively worsening headaches—Raises concern for secondary headaches
11. **P**arents—Lack of family history—Children with migraine often have a family history of headaches. When no family history of headache is obtained, then secondary etiology for headaches should be ruled out
12. **P**ost-traumatic headache
13. **P**ainkiller medicine overuse—Medication overuse headache (MOH) is not an uncommon secondary cause of headaches found in adolescents with migraine. It is important to screen for MOH as it is a relatively straightforward treatable secondary headache [16]
14. **P**ainful eyes—Can be consistent with ophthalmoplegic migraine, or autoimmune conditions like Tolosa hunt syndrome or multiple sclerosis
15. **P**rolonged or persistent aura
16. **Y**oung age of headache onset—Prevalence of secondary headaches have been found more often in patients younger than 6 years of age [79]

Additional Components of Headache History

A thorough family history of headaches is common for primary headache disorders. In families of children with migraine, 50%–90% of relatives also have migraine [19]. The headache history also needs to include a detailed review of systems and past medical history to identify warnings. The medical history in the pediatric population should include details concerning pregnancy, labor and delivery, growth and development, previous injuries, operations, hospitalizations, serious illnesses, drug allergies, current medications, and use of illicit drugs or alcohol.

Comorbid Conditions

Particular attention should be paid to aggravating features such as anxiety, depression, nervousness, and psychological stressors. Children with migraine have a high prevalence of sleep disturbances such as insomnia, snoring, night terror, nightmare, and bruxism [20]. There is also a positive association between attention deficit hyperactivity disorder (ADHD) and migraine [21].

Physical Examination

The most sensitive indicator of a need for further assessment is the neurological examination [22]. A detailed physical, neurological, and comprehensive headache examination must be performed. Special attention should be paid to head circumference in younger children, and if significantly enlarged, then causes of macrocephaly should be explored. Gait should be assessed as patients with posterior fossa tumors can have ataxic gait. It is best to perform a fundoscopy examination with minimal lights turned on to minimize withdrawal. A comprehensive headache exam may further help identify contributors to the headache etiology [22]. This should include palpation of sinuses to assess for focal tenderness, examine the jaw for tenderness or clicking to assess for temporomandibular joint dysfunction, and auscultation of eyes and temples for cranial bruit, which indicates underlying vascular etiology. Beighton scale for hypermobility must also be performed as there is a positive association of migraine and increased migraine disability with joint hypermobility syndrome [23–25].

Types of Migraine in Children and Adolescents

Classification

In 1988, the International Headache Society (IHS) proposed a standardized criteria for classification of headache disorders called the International Classification of Headache Disorders I (ICHD-I), which was based on experts' opinion. However, several studies found that ICHD-I was unable to diagnose a large fraction of children with migraine as pediatric migraine is shorter in duration and mostly observed bitemporal or bifrontal [26–29]. The criticisms of the ICHD-I criteria led to the establishment of a new edition in 2004 (ICHD-2). Several updates were made, including changing the minimum headache duration to 2 to 72 hours (instead of 4–72); however, a duration of less than 2 hours still required diary corroboration and the inference of photophobia and phonophobia by parental observation. Assessment of the criteria still demonstrated deficits [30–32]. In 2013, the IHS published the ICHD-3. These criteria remain the current standard of diagnosis for primary and secondary headache disorders.

Migraine Phases in Pediatric Age Groups

The pathophysiology of migraine in children and adolescents is thought to be the same as in adults. Moreover, the clinical phenotype of prodromal symptoms in both adults and children is similar [33]. The most commonly noted symptoms are tiredness, mood changes, and yawning [33–35]. This progresses to typical features of migraine with or without aura as described in ICHD-3 (Table 31.3). A diagnosis of probable migraine should be considered when patients suffer from migraine-like attacks but missing one of the features required to fulfill the diagnostic criteria.

Phenotypic features of migraine in children and adolescents may vary from adults in terms of shorter headache duration and bilateral headache location (usually frontal and bitemporal). Most of the children and adolescents have a prodrome and postdrome phase of less than 12 hours [36–38]. Children with migraine with aura have a longer postdrome phase when compared to migraine without aura [37].

Table 31.3 ICHD-3 criteria for migraine without aura and migraine with aura

Migraine without aura:
At least five attacks lasting for 2–72 hours have ≥2 features:
(a) Moderate-severe pain intensity
(b) Aggravation by routine physical activity
(c) Pulsating quality
(d) Bilateral location (vs. unilateral location noted in adults)
Headaches associated with ≥1 symptom:
(a) Nausea and/or vomiting
(b) Photophobia and phonophobia
Migraine with aura:
Headache fulfilling the criteria for migraine with ≥1 reversible symptom:
Visual
Sensory
Speech/language
Plus ≥3 of these characteristics:
≥1 aura symptom lasting for ≥5 min
Each aura lasting from 5 to 60 min
Aura is followed by a headache within 60 min
≥2 aura occurs in succession
≥1 symptom is unilateral
≥1 symptom is positive (scintillations, pins/needles)

Hemiplegic Migraine

Hemiplegic migraine is classified as a type of migraine with aura with true motor weakness. The headache is often contralateral to weakness. Hemiplegia is often associated with reversible visual, sensory, or dysphasic auras. In rare cases, patients have been reported to have loss of consciousness, coma, confusion, fever, and Cerebrospinal fluid (CSF) pleocytosis. Hemiplegic migraine is further subclassified based on the familial (FHM) or sporadic nature of the diagnosis. Three genetic loci have been identified. In FHM type 1 (the most common type), there is a mutation in the CACNA1 gene (coding for calcium channel) on chromosome 19 [39]; in FHM2, there are mutations in the ATP1A2 gene (coding for K/Na ATPase) on chromosome 1 [40]; and in FHM3, there are mutations in the SCN1A gene (coding for sodium channel) on chromosome 2 [41].

Migraine with Brainstem Aura

It is characterized by recurrent attacks of aura originating from the brainstem which include dysarthria, vertigo, tinnitus, hyperacusis, diplopia, ataxia, and a decreased level of consciousness. The syndrome affects adolescents more frequently than adults. Formerly, this has been referred to as basilar migraine and basilar type migraine but was changed to migraine with brainstem aura to reflect the neurological nature of the symptoms and not to be due to vascular changes.

Episodic Syndromes that May Be Associated with Migraine

Previously episodic syndromes were referred to as "periodic syndromes." These are certain disorders which tend to affect children more often than adults who have a history of migraine with or without aura or who have a genetic predisposition for migraine. ICHD III includes cyclic vomiting, abdominal migraine, benign paroxysmal vertigo, and benign paroxysmal torticollis in the main criteria. Infantile colic, alternating hemiplegia of childhood, and vestibular migraine are included within the appendix. Additional periodic syndromes may include motion sickness, sleepwalking, sleep talking, and night terrors [19].

Cyclic Vomiting Syndrome

Cyclic vomiting syndrome (CVS) commonly occurs in toddlers and younger children but can also occur in adolescents (as seen in case 2) and occurs less commonly in adults. The pathophysiology of this syndrome remains unknown. CVS is characterized by stereotypical recurrent episodes of intense nausea and vomiting. In general, episodes tend to begin at night or in the early morning hours and can last an average of 24–48 hours and sometimes even up to 7–10 days [42]. Patients can have prodromal symptoms of pallor, anorexia, and abdominal discomfort followed by severe vomiting and dehydration. Mostly, patients and their families tend to identify the triggers for CVS. Patients feel normal between every episode. Evaluation for inborn errors of metabolism should be considered if toddlers present with this syndrome, and chronic cannabis use should be ruled out in adolescents as cannabinoid hyperemesis syndrome can mimic CVS [43]. Migraine prophylaxis can be effective in decreasing the frequency and severity of attacks [19].

Abdominal Migraine

The mean age of onset of abdominal migraine is reported to be 7 years, and the estimates of the prevalence in childhood range from 2.4% to 4.1% [44]. It is characterized by recurrent moderate-severe periumbilical, or midline abdominal pain accompanied by nausea, vomiting, pallor, or anorexia, lasting for 2–72 hours when untreated. Episodes of abdominal pain are separated by symptom-free intervals of weeks to months. These children have a history of migraine or a family history of migraine, but headache is minimal or absent during an episode of abdominal migraine [44]. Nasal sumatriptan may be effective in treating acute episodes of abdominal pain [45]. Propranolol and cyproheptadine have been shown to be effective prophylactics [45, 46]. Note that if the patient reports a headache during these attacks, then it is no longer abdominal migraine, but most likely migraine.

Benign Paroxysmal Vertigo and Paroxysmal Torticollis

Both these disorders occur in younger children. Children suffering from benign paroxysmal vertigo develop sudden unsteadiness lasting for only a few minutes. Children usually grab on to something for steadiness. It can be associated with nystagmus and vomiting. Benign paroxysmal torticollis is characterized by head tilt, vomiting, and ataxia that lasts hours to days. Small case study showed a mutation in the calcium channel gene CACNA1A, which can also cause familial hemiplegic migraine [47].

Infantile Colic

Children with migraine are more likely to have been colicky as babies, and women with migraine are more likely to have a baby with colic [48, 49]. Data suggest that colicky babies are more sensitive to sound and smell and cry most in the evenings and at night [50]. It is included in the appendix of ICHD-3 as one of the episodic syndromes that may be associated with migraine, and hence further studies are needed to confirm this association.

Alternating Hemiplegia of Childhood

Alternating hemiplegia of childhood (AHC) is a peculiar heterogeneous neurodevelopmental disorder characterized by a constellation of paroxysmal neurological manifestations, among which recurrent episodes of hemiplegia involving either side of the body and alternating in laterality are the hallmark of this disease [51]. Patients can also exhibit involuntary movements such as choreoathetoid movements, dystonic posturing, and nystagmus. These episodes occur before 18 months of age with a median age of onset of 3–5 months [52]. A relationship with migraine has been suggested on clinical grounds, and hence it is included in the appendix of ICHD 3 as one of the episodic syndromes that may be associated with migraine. Further research is needed to confirm the association. Up to 50% of these patients can develop seizures, and the possibility of AHC being one of the epilepsy syndromes cannot be ruled out. Mutations in the ATP1A3 gene (encoding the sodium-potassium (Na^+/K^+) ATPase α3 subunit) are likely to be responsible for at least 70% of cases [52].

Headache-Related Disability

Youths with headaches report frequent school absences, poorer school performance, and lower quality of life than youths with other conditions [53]. Headache-related disability can be assessed by the Pediatric Migraine Disability assessment questionnaire (PedMIDAS) from both parents/guardians and the patient [54]. PedMIDAS questionnaire is a six-question validated instrument for measuring headache-related disability in children and adolescents. This questionnaire can be downloaded online from Cincinnati Children's website. (https://www.cincinnatichildrens.org/service/h/headache-center/pedmidas).

Management of Migraine

Most of the patients who present to the clinic for evaluation of headaches are suffering from migraine. Updated guidelines for acute and preventative treatment of pediatric migraine were published in 2019 (Tables 31.4 and 31.5).

Table 31.4 AAN/AHS 2019 pediatric migraine acute treatment guideline

1. Evaluation
(a) Clinicians should diagnose a specific headache type (primary, secondary, or another headache syndrome)
(b) Ask about premonitory and aura symptoms, headache semiology, associated symptoms, and pain-related disability to improve diagnostic accuracy for migraine and appropriately counsel the patient
2. Acute migraine treatment recommendation
(a) Counsel that acute migraine treatments are more likely to be effective when used earlier in the migraine attack, when pain is still mild
(b) Counsel patients and families that a series of medications may need to be used to find treatments that most benefit the patient
(c) Instruct patients and families to use the medication that best treats the characteristics of each migraine to provide the best balance of efficacy, side effects, and patient preference
(d) for adolescents with migraine, clinicians should prescribe sumatriptan/naproxen OT (10/60, 30/180, 85/500 mg), zolmitriptan NS (5 mg), sumatriptan NS (20 mg), rizatriptan ODT (5 or 10 mg), or almotriptan OT (6.25 or 12.5 mg) to reduce headache pain
(e) Offer an alternate triptan, if 1 triptan fails to provide pain relief, to find the most effective agent to reduce migraine symptoms
(f) Clinicians may prescribe a nonoral route when a headache peaks in severity quickly, is accompanied by nausea or vomiting, or oral formulations fail to provide pain relief

(continued)

Table 31.4 (continued)

(g) Clinicians should counsel patients and families that if their headache is successfully treated by their acute migraine medication, but the headache recurs within 24 hours of their initial treatment, taking a second dose of acute migraine medication can treat the recurrent headache

(h) in adolescents whose migraine is incompletely responsive to a triptan, clinicians should offer ibuprofen or naproxen in addition to a triptan to improve migraine relief

3. Treatment of associated symptoms

(a) for children and adolescents with migraine who experience prominent nausea or vomiting, clinicians should offer additional antiemetic treatments

4. Lifestyle management:

(a) Counsel children and adolescents with migraine and their families about migraine-healthy habits, including lifestyle modification, identification of migraine triggers/aggravating factors, and avoidance of medication overuse

(b) Clinicians should make collaborative agreements with children and adolescents with migraine and their families on treatment goals that are individualized to the patient

(c) Counsel children and adolescents with migraine and their families to maintain a headache diary to monitor their response to treatments

5. Medication overuse headache counseling

(a) Counsel patients and families to use no more than 14 days of ibuprofen or acetaminophen per month, no more than 9 days of triptans per month, and no more than 9 days per month of any combination of triptans, analgesics, or opioids for more than 3 months to avoid medication overuse headache

6. Contraindications to triptan use

(a) Clinicians must not prescribe triptans to those with a history of ischemic vascular disease or accessory conduction pathway disorders to avoid the morbidity and mortality associated with aggravating these conditions

(b) Clinicians should counsel adolescent patients with migraine with aura that taking their triptan during a typical aura is safe, but that the triptan may be more effective if taken at the onset of head pain

(c) Clinicians may consider referral of children and adolescents with hemiplegic migraine or migraine with brainstem aura who do not respond to other treatments to a headache specialist to find effective treatment

Table 31.5 AAN/AHS guideline for pediatric migraine prevention

1. Patient and family education regarding preventive treatment

(a) Counsel patients and families that lifestyle and behavioral factors may influence headache frequency

(b) Educate patients and families to identify and modify migraine contributors that are potentially modifiable

(c) Discuss the potential role of preventive treatments in children and adolescents with medication overuse headaches, frequent headaches, or migraine-related disability or both

2. Initiating treatment

(a) Inform patients and caregivers that in clinical trials of preventive treatments for pediatric migraine, many children and adolescents who received placebo improved, and most preventive medications were not superior to placebo

(b) Acknowledging the limitations of currently available evidence, clinicians should engage in shared decision-making regarding the use of short-term treatment trials (a minimum of 2 months) for those who could benefit from preventive treatment

(c) Discuss the evidence for amitriptyline combined with CBT for migraine prevention, inform patients of the potential side effects of amitriptyline including the risk of suicide, and work with families to identify providers who can offer this type of treatment

(d) Discuss the evidence for topiramate for migraine prevention in children and adolescents and its side effects in this population

(e) Discuss the evidence for propranolol for migraine prevention and its side effects in children and adolescents

3. Counseling for patients with childbearing potential

(a) Consider the teratogenic effect of topiramate and valproate in their choice of migraine prevention therapy recommendations to patients of childbearing potential

(b) Clinicians who offer topiramate or valproate for migraine prevention to patients of childbearing potential must counsel these patients about potential effects on fetal/childhood development

(c) Clinicians who prescribe topiramate for migraine prevention to patients of childbearing potential must counsel these patients about the potential of this medication to decrease the efficacy of oral combined hormonal contraceptives, particularly at doses over 200 mg daily

(d) Clinicians who prescribe topiramate or valproate for migraine prevention to patients of childbearing potential should counsel patients to discuss optimal contraception methods with their health care provider during treatment

(e) Clinicians must recommend daily folic acid supplementation to patients of childbearing potential who take topiramate or valproate

4. Monitoring and stopping medications

(a) Clinicians must periodically monitor medication effectiveness and adverse events when prescribing migraine preventive treatment

(b) Clinicians should counsel patients and families about the risks and benefits of stopping preventive medication once good migraine control is established

5. Mental illness in children and adolescents with migraine

(a) Children and adolescents with migraine should be screened for mood and anxiety disorders because of the increased risk of headache persistence

(b) In children and adolescents with migraine who have comorbid mood and anxiety disorders, clinicians should discuss management options for these disorders

Lifestyle Modifications

Lifestyle modifications should be discussed with every child and family. It is the most important aspect of migraine management. In one review of 47 studies of pediatric patients, stress, sleep, obesity, and diet were all identified as important factors associated with increasing migraine attack frequency, severity, and duration [55].

Reduction in headache frequency has been seen with proper sleep hygiene [56]. Getting sufficient sleep and keeping consistent bedtime and wake-up times are most important. About 10–13 hours of sleep is recommended for youths aged 3–5 years, 9–12 hours of sleep is recommended for youths aged 6–12 years, and 8–10 hours of sleep is recommended for adolescents aged 13–18 years [57].

Dehydration could be a trigger for headaches in people with migraine. In a small, randomized control trial in adults, increased water intake was associated with reduced headache severity [58]. More than six cups of fluids per day for children 6 years and older and more than eight cups of fluids per day for children 9 years and older should be recommended [59]. Skipping meals could be a trigger for attacks and hence should be avoided [60]. Patients should be advised to eat a balanced meal containing green vegetables, protein, and dairy, which are rich sources of vitamin D and coenzyme Q10. Caffeine withdrawal is a known migraine trigger. Children and adolescents should be advised to either total caffeine avoidance or age-appropriate use. Weight loss and regular exercise have proven to be beneficial in reducing migraine frequency in adults and children [61, 62].

Acute Treatment

The goal of acute migraine treatment is to obtain consistent and effective relief of headache pain and the associated symptoms of migraine with minimal side effects so that patients can return to normal function. Educating the child and family about how to treat their headaches is an important aspect of care so that triggering factors can be identified and avoided. Acute treatment plans should be formulated in collaboration with the child and parents during the visit. Every child should be provided with a school letter stating the need for prompt medication administration at the onset of symptoms. The mainstay of treatment for acute attacks is oral analgesics if used in appropriate doses at the onset or early phase of headache symptoms.

When using these medications, caution must be provided to avoid overuse. Guideline (Table 31.4) recommends using Ibuprofen 7.5–10 mg/kg, for all children and adolescents with headaches. Acetaminophen 15 mg/kg was also found to be effective in a double-blind crossover study of 88 children, aged 4 to 15.8 years, however, ibuprofen provided faster relief [63]. Other nonsteroidal anti-inflammatory drugs (NSAID) like Naproxen, diclofenac, and ketorolac can also be effective [64].

For children who are at least 6 years of age and have severe attacks refractory to analgesics, triptan should be considered as a second tier of treatment plan. If one triptan does not provide sufficient relief, an alternative triptan choice can be provided as outlined in the guideline. The route of administration depends on various factors such as pill swallowing ability, severe nausea and vomiting associated with headaches, and how rapidly the headache reaches its maximum severity. Rizatriptan is the only triptan that has been approved by the US FDA for children aged 6 years and above; however, other triptans have been studied in this age group and were found effective and safe. Other triptans which gained US FDA approval for the treatment of migraine in adolescents 12 years or older are almotriptan, which is available in oral tablet form, sumatriptan-naproxen combination medication, and zolmitriptan nasal spray. In the author's experience and practice, the dosing of triptans can be guided by the child's weight. Most clinicians administer the lower strength triptan for children who weigh less than 30 kg and higher strength triptans for children who weigh more than 30 kg [11]. If triptans alone do not provide complete relief from migraine symptoms, then combining analgesics and triptans should be the next step in management. Sumatriptan and naproxen combination pills have been shown to be effective in treating acute attacks of migraine in adolescents, and it is FDA approved for youths aged 12 and above [65, 66].

Preventive Management of Migraine

The goal of preventive management for migraine is to decrease headache frequency. Migraine preventive therapy should be considered when patients suffer from frequent attacks or prolonged, debilitating frequent attacks refractory to acute therapies. However, pediatric pharmacological medication trials have been challenging due to high placebo rates in children.

To date, topiramate is the only FDA-approved treatment for migraine prevention in pediatric populations, 12 years and older. The Childhood and Adolescent Migraine Prevention Medication (CHAMP) trial has provided a new perspective into the migraine preventive management [67]. This NIH-funded large multisite, randomized, double-blind trial incorporated children and adolescents aged 8–17 years with migraine who had PedMIDAS score of at least 10. Children with continuous headache, medication overuse headache and psychiatric illness, severe disability with PedMIDAS score of 140 or above, or a previous adequate trial of either of the medications were excluded from the study. Participants were administered either amitriptyline (1 mg/kg/day), topiramate (2 mg/kg/day), or placebo [67, 68]. This study was discontinued early as more than half of the patients in each treatment arm met the primary endpoint

Table 31.6 Evidence-based preventive treatment for pediatric migraine

Medicine	Dosage	Side effects	Highest level of evidence (American Academy of Neurology) AAN classes
(a) Topiramate	2–3 mg/kg/d; maximum dose 200 mg/day	Common S/E: Paresthesia, somnolence, weight loss, fatigue, cognitive impairment, decreased perspiration, nervousness, nausea Serious S/E: Renal stones, depression, angle closure glaucoma	Class I[a]
(b) Propranolol	0.5 mg/kg/d to 4 mg/kg/d divided in three doses; maximum 120 mg/day	Common S/E: Sedation, hypotension, bradycardia, weight gain Serious S/E: May worsen depression and exercise-induced asthma	Class III[a]
(c) Amitriptyline	1 mg/kg/d (at bedtime)	Common S/E: Drowsiness, constipation, agitation Serious S/E: Ventricular arrythmia, QT prolongation	Class I[a]
(d) Divalproex sodium	15–30 mg/kg/day; maximum dose 1000 mg/day	Common S/E: Nausea, vomiting, weight and appetite changes, alopecia Serious S/E: Hepatotoxicity, pancreatitis, thrombocytopenia, teratogenicity	Class II[a]
(e) Levetiracetam	20–40 mg/kg/d divided in two doses: Maximum dose 3000 mg/day	Common S/E: Somnolence, nausea, vomiting, aggressive behavior Serious S/E: Depression, psychosis	Class I [80]
(f) Cyproheptadine	0.25–0.5 mg/kg/d, divided q8-q12h, maximum dose: 16 mg/day	Common S/E: Dizziness, fatigue, weight gain	Class IV [81]
(g) Riboflavin (vitamin B2)	200–400 mg/day, either once daily or divided twice daily	Bright yellow urine discoloration	Class I (negative trial) [70]
(h) Coenzyme Q10	100–200 mg/day	Gastrointestinal upset	Class II [71]
(i) Melatonin	0.3 mg/kg/d given at bedtime, maximum 10 mg/day	Sedation	Class II [82]

Recommendations with "a" are addressed in the 2019 American Academy of Neurology (AAN) guidelines

of at least 50% reduction in headache frequency at the 24-week time point and higher sets of side effects found in the group receiving amitriptyline and topiramate. The findings from the CHAMP trial prompt us to discuss the options more openly with families and patients so that they may make a more informed decision about their treatment plan, as recommended in the 2019 American Academy of Neurology guideline for preventive management (Table 31.5).

In clinical practice, there has been increasing emphasis on the optimization of preventive medications with the fewest side effects and stopping the medication when migraine frequency decreases. There is no evidence to indicate which therapy could be used as first line. It is important that once preventive treatment is started, clinician monitors response, adherence, and side effects to these medications (Table 31.6). In another pediatric study, the use of amitriptyline along with cognitive behavioral therapy was superior to using amitriptyline alone; however, amitriptyline has a warning for suicidal thoughts [69]. Nutraceuticals such as riboflavin, coenzyme q10, Vitamin D3, and magnesium have evidence for safety and mixed results for efficacy in children with migraine [70–72]. In addition, calcitonin gene-related peptide inhibitors are currently being investigated for migraine prevention, which if positive may provide substantial relief to children and adolescents living with migraine.

Neuromodulation Devices for Children and Adolescents

There are several neuromodulation devices that are cleared by the US Food and Drug Administration (FDA) and can be used in pediatric and adolescent populations. The transcranial magnetic stimulator (eNeura) generates a single magnetic pulse that generates a 0.9 T magnetic field for 0.01 of a second. It has been recently approved for both the acute treatment and prevention of migraine in children 12 years and older [73]. Remote electrical neuromodulation (REN) device (Nerivio) is another device which has been recently FDA cleared for acute and preventive migraine treatment for children ≥12 years [74]. This device can be placed on the upper arm for 45 minutes for acute relief or every other day for prevention. Transcutaneous vagal nerve stimulator (gammaCore) is another FDA-cleared device for children ≥12 years and older. The device provides electrical stimulation (maximum delivery of 40 millivolts and 60 milliamps output current) when applied to the neck. To date, the external trigeminal nerve stimulator (Cefaly) and the external combined occipital and trigeminal neuromodulator (Relivion) are not FDA cleared for children.

Transition of Care

Unsuccessful transitioning of young adults with migraine could lead to disruption of care and negative outcomes. A consensus statement from Neurology suggests three phases for successful transition: (a) transition planning, (b) patient education, and (c) transition readiness [75]. The goal during transition is to expand patients' personal knowledge of their condition and introduce the concept of self-management and self-advocacy [76]. The Transition Readiness Assessment Questionnaire (TRAQ) is considered the best validated transition readiness tool [77]. Patients should be encouraged to fill out this questionnaire independently to assess transition readiness. During the transition period, an adult headache provider should be identified and provided a transfer packet with the patient's headache history, treatment plans, comorbid conditions, including anxiety and depression, and any nonpharmacological treatment received in past [78].

Conclusion

Migraine is common in children; however, it is often underdiagnosed and undertreated. A systematic approach to the history, which includes an assessment of behavioral change and functional loss, may improve the diagnostic yield. To decrease the patient's disability associated with migraine, it would be best to strategize the treatment plan based on first-line, second-line, and third-line treatments. Existing data suggest that most children and adolescents with migraine will improve with multimodal care such as cognitive behavioral therapy, lifestyle modifications, nonpharmacological interventions along with pill-based treatment. Treatment decisions should be made using a shared decision-making approach.

Teaching Points

1. Parents can be inclined to give the patient's headache history. It is essential to give the message before starting the interview that the child is the focus of the visit and the parent(s)/guardians are there to support and help them during the interview process.
2. Phenotypic features of migraine in children and adolescents may vary from adults in terms of shorter headache duration and bilateral headache location.
3. Episodic syndromes (such as cyclic vomiting syndrome, abdominal migraine, benign paroxysmal torticollis and vertigo, alternating hemiplegia of childhood, and infantile colic) tend to affect children more often than adults. These children have a history of migraine with or without aura or have a genetic predisposition for migraine.

Case

An 8-year-old boy presents to the emergency department (ED) with eight attacks of intense vomiting, 3–4 times in an hour lasting for at least 2–3 hours, recurring after 2 weeks of normal functioning. ED physician consults for management.

Case Discussion

Patient has cyclic vomiting syndrome. During the acute phase, oral hydration should be encouraged, and intravenous fluid resuscitation should be provided if needed along with antiemetics such as ondansetron. Preventively, the first-line treatment for children greater than 5 years old is amitriptyline (0.5–1 mg/day). In children under 5 years old, cyproheptadine (0.25–0.5 mg/kg/day divided twice daily or once nightly) is considered first-line treatment.

Questions and Answers

1. An 18-year-old female with a 5-year history of migraine headaches presents to emergency room with a severe headache which developed earlier in the day associated with left-sided weakness on her examination. She has several other family members with similar symptoms. Workup, including imaging studies, is normal.

Which is the most common genetic cause for this patient's presentation?

A. CACNA1A
B. ATP1A2
C. ATP1A3
D. PRRT2
E. SCN1A

The correct answer is A. This patient's presentation is concerning familial hemiplegic migraine (FHM) given the findings on examination and positive family history. The most common types of FHM are transmitted in an autosomal dominant pattern, and the most common genetic mutation found in these patients is CACNA1A (calcium channelopathy).

2. Until what age alternating hemiplegia of childhood can occur?

A. 24 months
B. 12 months
C. 15 months
D. 18 months
E. 3 years

The correct answer is D. Alternating hemiplegia of childhood should occur by 18 months of age. ATP1A3 is the most common channelopathy noted in these patients.

References

1. Victor T, Hu X, Campbell J, Buse D, Lipton R. Migraine prevalence by age and sex in the United States: a life-span study. Cephalalgia. 2010;30(9):1065.
2. Headache Classification Committee of the International Headache Society (IHS). The international classification of headache disorders, 3rd edn. Cephalalgia. 2018;38(1):1.
3. Lima M, Padula N, Santos L, Oliveira L, Agapejev S, Padovani C. Critical Analysis of the International Classification of Headache Disorders Diagnostic Criteria (ICHD I-1988) and (ICHD II-2004), for migraine in children and adolescents. Cephalalgia. 2005;25(11)
4. Stewart WF, Linet MS, Celentano DD, van Natta M, Ziegler D. Age- and sex-specific incidence rates of migraine with and without visual aura. Am J Epidemiol. 1991;134(10):1111.
5. Conicella E, Raucci U, Vanacore N, Vigevano F, Reale A, Pirozzi N, et al. The child with headache in a pediatric emergency department. Headache J Head Face Pain. 2008;48(7):1005.
6. Lewis DW, Qureshi F. Acute headache in children and adolescents presenting to the emergency department. Headache J Head Face Pain Pain. 2000;40(3):200.
7. Bear JJ, Gelfand AA, Goadsby PJ, Bass N. Occipital headaches and neuroimaging in children. Neurology. 2017;89(5):469.
8. Hershey AD. Current approaches to the diagnosis and management of paediatric migraine. Lancet Neurol. 2010;9(2):190–204.
9. Casanova A, Vives-Mestres M, Donoghue S, Mian A, Martin PR. An observational study of self-reported migraine triggers and prospective evaluation of the relationships with occurrence of attacks enabled by a smartphone application (App). Headache. 2022;62(10):1406–15.
10. Hoffmann J, Recober A. Migraine and triggers: post hoc ergo propter hoc? Curr Pain Headache Rep. 2013;17(10):370.
11. Orr SL. Headache in children and adolescents. Continuum (Minneap Minn). 2024;30(2):438–72.
12. Balestri M, Papetti L, Maiorani D, Capuano A, Tarantino S, Battan B, et al. Features of aura in paediatric migraine diagnosed using the ICHD 3 beta criteria. Cephalalgia. 2018;38(11):1742.
13. Ulrich V, Olesen J, Gervil M, Russell M. Possible risk factors and precipitants for migraine with aura in discordant twin-pairs: a population-based study. Cephalalgia. 2000;20(9):821.
14. Gelfand AA, Reider AC, Goadsby PJ. Cranial autonomic symptoms in pediatric migraine are the rule, not the exception. Neurology. 2013;81(5):431.
15. Kernick D, Stapley S, Campbell J, Hamilton W. What happens to new-onset headache in children that present to primary care? A case-cohort study using electronic primary care records. Cephalalgia. 2009;29(12):1311.
16. Do TP, Remmers A, Schytz HW, Schankin C, Nelson SE, Obermann M, et al. Red and orange flags for secondary headaches in clinical practice. Neurology. 2019;92(3):134.
17. Pearls DD. Headache. Semin Neurol. 2010;30:01.
18. Szperka C. Headache in children and adolescents. CONTINUUM Lifelong Learn Neurol. 2021;27(3)
19. Wolff's Headache and Other Head Pain. Arch Neurol. 2009;66:4.
20. Miller VA, Palermo TM, Powers SW, Scher MS, Hershey AD. Migraine headaches and sleep disturbances in children. Headache J Head Face Pain. 2003;43(4):362.
21. Salem H, Vivas D, Cao F, Kazimi IF, Teixeira AL, Zeni CP. ADHD is associated with migraine: a systematic review and meta-analysis. Eur Child Adolesc Psychiatry. 2018;27:27(3).
22. Lewis DW, Ashwal S, Dahl G, Dorbad D, Hirtz D, Prensky A, et al. Practice parameter: evaluation of children and adolescents with recurrent headaches: report of the Quality Standards Subcommittee of the American Academy of Neurology and the Practice Committee of the Child Neurology Society. Neurology. 2002;59(4)
23. Puledda F, Viganò A, Celletti C, Petolicchio B, Toscano M, Vicenzini E, et al. A study of migraine characteristics in joint hypermobility syndrome a.k.a. Ehlers–Danlos syndrome, hypermobility type. Neurol Sci. 2015;36(8):1417.
24. Bendik EM, Tinkle BT, Al-shuik E, Levin L, Martin A, Thaler R, et al. Joint hypermobility syndrome: a common clinical disorder associated with migraine in women. Cephalalgia. 2011;31(5):603.
25. Ghosh A, Horn PS, Kabbouche Samaha M, Kacperski J, LeCates SL, White S, et al. Characterization of migraine in children and adolescents with generalized joint hypermobility: a case-control study. Neurol Clin Pract. 2023;13(5):e200188.
26. Linder SL. Understanding the comprehensive pediatric headache examination. Pediatr Ann. 2005;34(6):442.
27. Wöber-Bingöl C, Wöber C, Karwautz A, Vesely C, Wagner-Ennsgraber C, Amminger G, et al. Diagnosis of headache in childhood and adolescence: a study in 437 patients. Cephalalgia. 1995;15(1):13.
28. Cano A, Palomeras E, Alfonso S, Ortega D, Sanz P, Fossas P. Migraine without aura and migrainous disorder in children; International Headache Society (IHS) and revised IHS criteria. Cephalalgia. 2000;20(7)
29. Metsähonkala L, Sillanpää M. Migraine in children – an evaluation of the IHS criteria. Cephalalgia. 1994;14(4):285.
30. Winner P, Martinez W, Mate L, Bello L. Classification of pediatric migraine: proposed revisions to the IHS criteria. Headache J Head Face Pain Pain. 1995;35(7):407.
31. Bigal ME, Rapoport AM, Tepper SJ, Sheftell FD, Lipton RB. The classification of chronic daily headache in adolescents –a comparison between the second edition of the international classification of headache disorders and alternative diagnostic criteria. Headache J Head Face Pain. 2005;45(5)
32. Hershey AD, Winner P, Kabbouche MA, Gladstein J, Yonker M, Lewis D, et al. Use of the ICHD-II criteria in the diagnosis of pediatric migraine. Headache J Head Face Pain Pain. 2005;45(10):1288.
33. Arruda MA, Bigal ME. Migraine and migraine subtypes in preadolescent children: association with school performance. Neurology. 2012;79(18):1881.
34. Karsan N, Prabhakar P, Goadsby PJ. Characterising the premonitory stage of migraine in children: a clinic-based study of 100 patients in a specialist headache service. J Headache Pain. 2016;17(1):94.
35. Cuvellier JC, Mars A, Vallée L. The prevalence of premonitory symptoms in paediatric migraine: a questionnaire study in 103 children and adolescents. Cephalalgia. 2009;29(11):1197.
36. Giffin NJ, Ruggiero L, Lipton RB, Silberstein SD, Tvedskov JF, Olesen J, et al. Premonitory symptoms in migraine: an electronic diary study. Neurology. 2003;60(6):935.
37. Mamouri O, Cuvellier JC, Duhamel A, Vallée L, Nguyen The Tich S. Postdrome symptoms in pediatric migraine: a questionnaire retrospective study by phone in 100 patients. Cephalalgia. 2018;38(5):943.

38. Karsan N, Peréz-Rodríguez A, Nagaraj K, Bose PR, Goadsby PJ. The migraine postdrome: spontaneous and triggered phenotypes. Cephalalgia. 2021;41(6):721.
39. Joutel A, Bousser MG, Biousse V, Labauge P, Chabriat H, Nibbio A, et al. A gene for familial hemiplegic migraine maps to chromosome 19. Nat Genet. 1993;5(1):40.
40. de Vries B, Frants RR, Ferrari MD, van den Maagdenberg AMJM. Molecular genetics of migraine. Hum Genet. 2009;126:1.
41. Dichgans M, Freilinger T, Eckstein G, Babini E, Lorenz-Depiereux B, Biskup S, et al. Mutation in the neuronal voltage-gated sodium channel SCN1A in familial hemiplegic migraine. Lancet. 2005;366(9483):371.
42. Li BUBJ. Cyclic vomiting syndrome: evolution in our understanding of a brain-gut disorder. Adv Pediatr Infect Dis. 2000:117–60.
43. Allen JH. Cannabinoid hyperemesis: cyclical hyperemesis in association with chronic cannabis abuse. Gut. 2004;53(11):1566.
44. Catto-Smith AG, Ranuh R. Abdominal migraine and cyclical vomiting. Semin Pediatr Surg. 2003;12(4):254.
45. Abu-Arafeh I, Russell G. Prevalence and clinical features of abdominal migraine compared with those of migraine headache. Arch Dis Child. 1995;72(5):413.
46. Russell G, Abu-Arafeh I, Symon DNK. Abdominal migraine. Pediatr Drugs. 2002;4:1.
47. Giffin NJ, Benton S, Goadsby PJ. Benign paroxysmal torticollis of infancy: four new cases and linkage to CACNA1A mutation. Dev Med Child Neurol. 2002;44(07):490.
48. Jan MMS, Al-Buhairi AR. Is infantile colic a migraine-related phenomenon? Clin Pediatr (Phila). 2001;40(5):295.
49. Romanello S, Spiri D, Marcuzzi E, Zanin A, Boizeau P, Riviere S, et al. Association between childhood migraine and history of infantile colic. JAMA. 2013;309(15):1607.
50. Gelfand AA, Thomas KC, Goadsby PJ. Before the headache: infant colic as an early life expression of migraine. Neurology. 2012;79(13):1392.
51. Rosewich H, Weise D, Ohlenbusch A, Gartner J, Brockmann K. Phenotypic overlap of alternating hemiplegia of childhood and CAPOS syndrome. Neurology. 2014;83(9):861.
52. Sweney MT, Silver K, Gerard-Blanluet M, Pedespan JM, Renault F, Arzimanoglou A, et al. Alternating hemiplegia of childhood: early characteristics and evolution of a neurodevelopmental syndrome. Pediatrics. 2009;123(3):e534.
53. Powers SW, Patton SR, Hommel KA, Hershey AD. Quality of life in childhood migraines: clinical impact and comparison to other chronic illnesses. Pediatrics. 2003;112(1 Pt 1):e1–5.
54. Hershey A, Powers S, Vockell AL, LeCates S, Segers A, Kabbouche M. Development of a patient-based grading scale for PedMIDAS. Cephalalgia. 2004;24(10):844.
55. Dasari VR, Clark AJ, Boorigie ME, Gerson T, Connelly MA, Bickel JL. The influence of lifestyle factors on the burden of pediatric migraine. J Pediatr Nurs. 2021;57:79–83.
56. Bruni O, Galli F, Guidetti V. Sleep hygiene and migraine in children and adolescents. Cephalalgia. 1999;19(25_suppl):57.
57. Paruthi S, Brooks LJ, D'Ambrosio C, Hall WA, Kotagal S, Lloyd RM, et al. Recommended amount of sleep for pediatric populations: a consensus statement of the American Academy of Sleep Medicine. J Clin Sleep Med. 2016;12(6):785–6.
58. Spigt MG, Kuijper EC, Schayck CP, Troost J, Knipschild PG, Linssen VM, et al. Increasing the daily water intake for the prophylactic treatment of headache: a pilot trial*. Eur J Neurol. 2005;12(9):715.
59. Dietary reference intakes for water, potassium, sodium, chloride, and sulfate. Washington, DC: National Academies Press; 2005.
60. Marmura MJ. Triggers, protectors, and predictors in episodic migraine. Curr Pain Headache Rep. 2018;22(12)
61. Torres-Ferrus M, Vila-Sala C, Quintana M, Ajanovic S, Gallardo VJ, Gomez JB, et al. Headache, comorbidities and lifestyle in an adolescent population (the TEENs study). Cephalalgia. 2019;39(1):91.
62. Lemmens J, de Pauw J, van Soom T, Michiels S, Versijpt J, van Breda E, et al. The effect of aerobic exercise on the number of migraine days, duration and pain intensity in migraine: a systematic literature review and meta-analysis. J Headache Pain. 2019;20(1)
63. Hamalainen ML, Hoppu K, Valkeila E, Santavuori P. Ibuprofen or acetaminophen for the acute treatment of migraine in children: a double-blind, randomized, placebo-controlled, crossover study. Neurology. 1997;48(1):103.
64. Marmura MJ, Silberstein SD, Schwedt TJ. The acute treatment of migraine in adults: the American headache society evidence assessment of migraine pharmacotherapies. Headache J Head Face Pain Pain. 2015;55(1):3.
65. Derosier FJ, Lewis D, Hershey AD, Winner PK, Pearlman E, Rothner AD, et al. Randomized trial of sumatriptan and naproxen sodium combination in adolescent migraine. Pediatrics. 2012;129(6):e1411–20.
66. Winner P, Linder S, Hershey AD. Consistency of response to sumatriptan/naproxen sodium in a randomized placebo-controlled, cross-over study for the acute treatment of migraine in adolescence. Headache J Head Face Pain Pain. 2015;55(4):519–28.
67. Hershey ADPSCCEDCLKL, et al. The childhood and adolescent migraine prevention (CHAMP) study: a report on baseline characteristics of participants. Headache. 2016:859–70.
68. Hershey ADPSW, CCS. Childhood and Adolescent Migraine Prevention (CHAMP) study: a double-blinded, placebo-controlled, comparative effectiveness study of amitriptyline, topiramate, and placebo in the prevention of childhood and adolescent migraine. Headache. 2013;53:799–816.
69. Powers SW, Kashikar-Zuck SM, Allen JR, LeCates SL, Slater SK, Zafar M, et al. Cognitive behavioral therapy plus amitriptyline for chronic migraine in children and adolescents. JAMA. 2013;310(24):2622.
70. MacLennan SC, Wade FM, Forrest KML, Ratanayake PD, Fagan E, Antony J. High-dose ribof lavin for migraine prophylaxis in children: a double-blind, randomized, placebo-controlled trial. J Child Neurol. 2008;23(11):1300.
71. Slater SK, Nelson TD, Kabbouche MA, LeCates SL, Horn P, Segers A, et al. A randomized, double-blinded, placebo-controlled, crossover, add-on study of CoEnzyme Q10 in the prevention of pediatric and adolescent migraine. Cephalalgia. 2011;31(8):897.
72. Schoenen J, Jacquy J, Lenaerts M. Effectiveness of high-dose riboflavin in migraine prophylaxis A randomized controlled trial. Neurology. 1998;50(2):466.
73. Irwin SL, Qubty W, Allen IE, Patniyot I, Goadsby PJ, Gelfand AA. Transcranial magnetic stimulation for migraine prevention in adolescents: a pilot open-label study. Headache J Head Face Pain Pain. 2018;58(5):724–31.
74. Monteith TS, Stark-Inbar A, Shmuely S, Harris D, Garas S, Ironi A, et al. Remote electrical neuromodulation (REN) wearable device for adolescents with migraine: a real-world study of high-frequency abortive treatment suggests preventive effects. Front Pain Res (Lausanne, Switzerland). 2023;4:1247313.
75. Brown LW, Camfield P, Capers M, Cascino G, Ciccarelli M, de Gusmao CM, et al. The neurologist's role in supporting transition to adult health care. Neurology. 2016;87(8):835–40.
76. O'Brien HL, Cohen JM. Young adults with headaches: the transition from adolescents to adults. Headache J Head Face Pain Pain. 2015;55(10):1404–9.
77. Wood DL, Sawicki GS, Miller MD, Smotherman C, Lukens-Bull K, Livingood WC, et al. The transition readiness assessment ques-

tionnaire (TRAQ): its factor structure, reliability, and validity. Acad Pediatr. 2014;14(4):415–22.
78. Orr SL, Gelfand AA, Hranilovich J, Irwin SL, Kabbouche M, Lagman-Bartolome AM, et al. The development of the medical transfer packet for transition of care of the pediatric patient with headache. Headache J Head Face Pain Pain. 2020;60(10):2589–91.
79. Raieli V, Eliseo M, Pandolfi E, la Vecchia M, la Franca G, Puma D, et al. Recurrent and chronic headaches in children below 6 years of age. J Headache Pain. 2005;6(3):135.
80. Montazerlotfelahi H, Amanat M, Tavasoli AR, Agah E, Zamani GR, Sander JW, et al. Levetiracetam for prophylactic treatment of pediatric migraine: a randomized double-blind placebo-controlled trial. Cephalalgia. 2019;39(12):1509–17.
81. Lewis DW, Diamond S, Scott D, Jones V. Prophylactic treatment of pediatric migraine. Headache. 2004;44(3):230–7.
82. Gelfand AA, Qubty W, Patniyot I, Grimes B, Pletcher MJ, Goadsby PJ, et al. Home-based trials in adolescent migraine. JAMA Neurol. 2017;74(6):744.

32 Migraine Through a Woman's Life

Addie M. Peretz, Huma U. Sheikh, and Catherine S. Stika

Introduction

Migraine is a disorder predominantly impacting women, occurring around 2–3 times more often among women than men [1–3]. It is also the most disabling condition affecting young women [4], with a negative impact on multiple facets of life, from cognitive and emotional health to work, family, and social life [5]. Hormonal epochs throughout an individual's life can distinctly influence the frequency and burden of migraine attacks [6, 7]. The difference in prevalence between sexes begins around menarche, with the prevalence of migraine among women continuing to increase as women age, reaching a peak of around 25% during childbearing years, worsening during perimenopause [8], and potentially decreasing after menopause [9]. Despite the high prevalence of migraine among women, the mechanisms underlying sex disparities in migraine are understudied [10]. We will review the influence of sex on the epidemiology, pathophysiology, and treatment considerations over distinct hormonal epochs of an individual's life.

A. M. Peretz (✉)
Clinical Associate Professor of Neurology, Stanford University, Stanford, CA, USA

H. U. Sheikh
Mt Sinai Neurology Department, Icahn School of Medicine, New York, NY, USA

C. S. Stika
Department of Obstetrics and Gynecology, Northwestern University Feinberg School of Medicine, Chicago, IL, USA

Questions

1. Compared to men, women with migraine tend to experience which of the following?
   A. Greater disability from migraine attacks.
   B. Longer lasting migraine attacks.
   C. More frequent migraine attacks.
   D. Increased frequency of accompanying symptoms such as nausea.
   E. Decreased responsiveness to treatments.
   F. Increased risk of transformation from episodic to chronic migraine.
   G. All of the above.
2. A 28-year-old woman with a history of migraine without aura currently takes ubrogepant as her migraine rescue medication. She is planning to try to conceive and asks what is the next best step?
   A. Order an MRI of the brain.
   B. Reassure her that it is safe to continue taking ubrogepant as a migraine rescue medication during pregnancy.
   C. Advise her to stop ubrogepant and start fioricet prior to trying to conceive.
   D. Advise her to stop ubrogepant and instead try acetaminophen or metoclopramide for migraine.

Sex-Based Epidemiology of Migraine

Characteristics of migraine can be distinct among women compared with men. Women with migraine experience greater disability from migraine attacks. This increased burden from migraine manifests as longer and more frequent headaches, increased frequency of accompanying symptoms such as nausea and osmophobia, and increased side effects from medications, along with decreased responsiveness to treatments among women compared with men. Female sex is also a risk factor for the transformation of migraine from episodic to

T. S. Monteith et al. (eds.), *Comprehensive Migraine Management*, https://doi.org/10.1007/978-3-031-86923-5_32

chronic migraine, which occurs among an estimated 2.5–3% of patients with episodic migraine each year [1, 5, 11].

While most migraine comorbidities are not necessarily sex-specific, some comorbidities have a higher prevalence among women, and it is important to address these in conjunction with migraine management. Migraine is comorbid with multiple medical and psychiatric disorders including epilepsy, stroke, multiple sclerosis, asthma, allergic rhinitis, and mood disorders including depression and anxiety [11]. Additional potential comorbid disorders, with a high prevalence among women with migraine and unique to the female sex include endometriosis [12], premenstrual syndrome [13], and polycystic ovarian syndrome [14].

Influence of Sex Differences on the Migraine Brain

Many sex-specific factors influence the manifestation of migraine. These include and are not limited to reproductive hormones, genetic and epigenetic factors, environmental stressors, and psychosocial factors [10]. Imaging studies have demonstrated sex-influenced structural differences in the brain, including differences in gray matter thickness in the hippocampus, basal ganglia, and amygdala at various points in the menstrual cycle [15]. Ovarian hormonal influences have profound pathophysiologic implications for the migraine brain; this is clearly demonstrated by the manner in which hormonal epochs influence migraine frequency and severity.

Sex hormones modulate the production and metabolic pathways of several neurotransmitters and hormones including calcitonin gene-related peptide (CGRP), serotonin, glutamate, noradrenalin, nitric oxide (NO), and endogenous opioids. Multiple studies have demonstrated that CGRP, an important target of pharmacotherapy for migraine, is influenced by reproductive hormones, and CGRP signaling exhibits sex differences. Among postmenopausal women, CGRP is decreased, and during pregnancy, CGRP levels are increased [6, 16–18].

Estrogen is generally excitatory, facilitating serotonergic and glutamatergic tone and inhibiting GABAergic and noradrenergic tone; this, in turn, can play a role in pain processes and endothelial vasculature. Estrogens' role in migraine is further evidenced by receptor localization in key areas of migraine pathophysiology including over the whole brain and in the trigeminovascular system. In a rat model, estrogen receptor expression in the female trigeminal ganglion was found to be higher than in the male trigeminal ganglion, highlighting a region where estrogen may have a modulatory role in migraine [19].

Oxytocin, a neuropeptide with antinociceptive effects, is of particular interest as a potential target for migraine treatments and for its likely critical role in menstrually related migraine. Evidence for oxytocin's potential role in menstrual migraine include oxytocin level modulation by estrogen and the location of oxytocin receptors in the trigeminal ganglia and other migraine-related brain regions [20]. Oxytocin has also been shown to suppress migraine attacks.

A hypothesis proposed by Krause et al. seeks to explain the underpinnings of estrogen's influence on the migraine brain, "estrogen influences the balance of factors related to migraine susceptibility within the trigeminal ganglia. In the presence of estrogen, migraine symptoms that involve the trigeminal pathway are suppressed and a drop in estrogen levels as a result of different physiological or pharmacological states would shift the balance to migraine vulnerability and decrease the threshold for an attack without aura to occur. Although this view is somewhat simplistic, it predicts that effective treatment for menstrual migraine attacks could involve the suppression of CGRP (with antibodies or gepants) or administration of oxytocin agonists in the perimenstrual period" [21].

Hormonal Epochs (Both Endogenous and Exogenous) and Migraine

Menstruation, with ovarian hormone fluctuations and specifically a dramatic drop in estrogen in the late luteal phase, is a common trigger for migraine attacks [22]. During pregnancy, over 80% of women, particularly those with migraine without aura, experience an improvement in migraine, especially in the second and third trimesters [23–25]. The lack of dramatic hormonal fluctuations and the progressive increase in estradiol during pregnancy (roughly a 500-fold increase in estradiol from early follicular phase to term) may be responsible for the improvement many pregnant women experience in their migraine attack burden. With the abrupt fall in placental estrogens after delivery, migraine tends to recur within the first few weeks postpartum [23, 26]. Later in life, perimenopause can trigger increased migraine attacks due to erratic hormonal fluctuations [27]. The transition to menopause can last years in some individuals, and migraine attacks in perimenopause are characterized by their unpredictable frequency, increased severity, and decreased response to treatment [8]. Postmenopause, these fluctuations resolve, and with stable, low estradiol concentrations, some individuals experience improvement in their migraine attacks.

Gender-Affirming Hormone Therapy

Despite an increase in the transgender population, research into the unique headache diagnostic and treatment needs is lacking. Epidemiologically, clinical studies thus far have demonstrated an increased prevalence of migraine among male-to-female transexuals under estrogen therapy, mirroring that of cisgender women [28].

Menstruation

Menstrually associated migraine attacks have been characterized in the appendix of the International Classification of Headache Disorders under two diagnostic categories—pure menstrual migraine and menstrually related migraine with or without aura. Diagnosis relies upon careful tracking of menstruation and migraine symptoms to identify a pattern of migraine attacks that consistently correlate with menstruation. Pure menstrual migraine is defined by attacks of migraine occurring strictly between two days before and 3 days after the onset of menstruation on at least 2 out of 3 menstrual cycles. Menstrually related migraine is inclusive of both pure menstrual migraine attacks along with attacks that occur at other times of the menstrual cycle. Migraine attacks occurring peri-menstrually are characterized by greater disability and are often more refractory to treatment compared with migraine attacks not associated with menstruation. Figure 32.1 highlights the many hormonal fluctuations that occur over the course of the menstrual cycle.

Ovulation Induction and IVF

There is a paucity of studies examining the impact of fertility treatments on migraine prevalence and severity. To date, one small retrospective study analysis of women undergoing in vitro fertilization suggested that women with migraine suffered from increased headache attacks compared with women without a history of migraine [7, 13]. However, given the elevated estradiol levels achieved with ovulation induction, typically 1000 to 3000 pg/mL compared to 200–300 pg/mL with a spontaneous ovulation, it is physiologically plausible that migraineurs would experience increased headaches with these fluctuations. Additional research is needed to elucidate the impact of fertility treatments on migraine attack burden and ultimately to help patients navigate migraine and reproduction.

Diagnostic Considerations for Headache During Pregnancy

While migraine is certainly a reasonable diagnostic consideration for headaches occurring during pregnancy especially in light of the higher migraine prevalence among women of childbearing age, secondary etiologies should be considered. In a small retrospective study of 140 pregnant women presenting to the Emergency Department with an acute headache, for whom Neurology was consulted, nearly 60% of the headaches were diagnosed as migraine attacks, although the second most common diagnosis among nearly 18% of patients was hypertensive disorders such as pre-eclampsia and Posterior Reversible Encephalopathy Syndrome (PRES). Risk factors for a secondary headache include the absence of a prior headache history, the presence of hypertension, fever, and abnormal neurologic findings [30]. Many physiologic changes occur during pregnancy, such as decreased systemic vascular residence, which can lead to increased venous stasis and a hypercoagulable state, especially in the third trimester and postpartum, which can predispose to secondary headaches [31].

It should be noted that patients with a history of migraine are at higher risk for adverse maternal and fetal outcomes including preeclampsia and gestational hypertension along with preterm birth [32, 33]. It is important to monitor patients with a history of migraine for signs of preeclampsia. Among

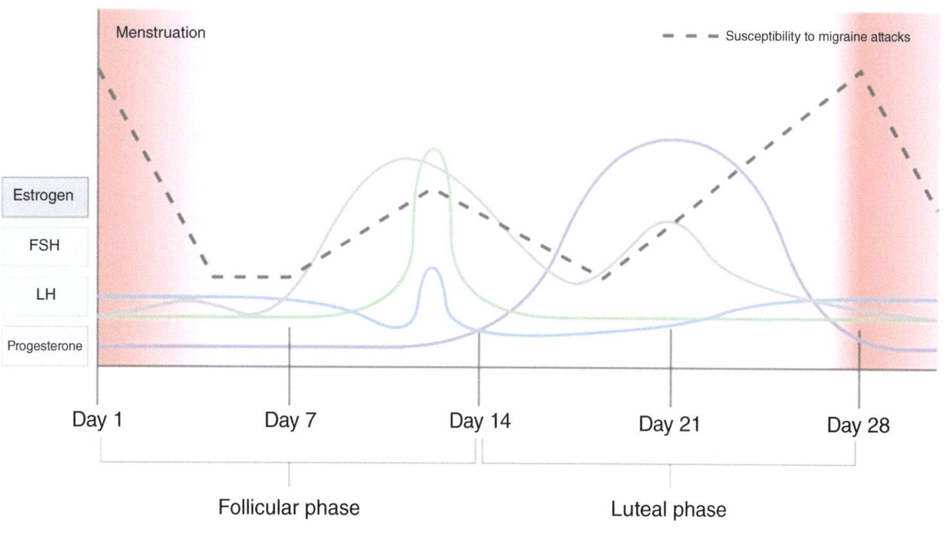

Fig. 32.1 Hormonal fluctuations over the course of the menstrual cycle, in particular the drop in estrogen during the late luteal phase which is thought to be a prominent migraine trigger. (Image is courtesy of Raffaelli et al. [29])

women with multiple risk factors for preeclampsia, low-dose aspirin (81 mg daily), initiated after 12 weeks of gestation, is recommended for preeclampsia prevention. Currently, migraine is not considered a risk factor warranting aspirin use for preeclampsia prevention [34].

Diagnostic considerations for postpartum headaches can be distinct and may warrant further investigation in some instances. In a small retrospective study of 63 postpartum women who presented to the emergency room with headaches, the majority were diagnosed with a secondary headache. Secondary headache etiologies in this study included postdural puncture headaches, hypertensive disorders such as preeclampsia, and cerebrovascular disorders such as pituitary apoplexy, venous thrombosis, and reversible cerebral vasoconstriction syndrome [35]. While preeclampsia alone does not necessarily warrant additional workup, the following symptoms in a woman with preeclampsia should prompt further workup—focal neurologic symptoms, altered level of consciousness, or rapid onset of headache.

Perimenopause

The transition to menopause can distinctly impact migraine based on migraine type. For women with migraine without aura, migraine tends to worsen in perimenopause and improve after menopausal transition. For women with migraine with aura, headaches may become a less frequent feature of migraine attacks [36].

Treatment Considerations

Hormonal epochs in an individual's life can inform migraine treatment considerations. Wellness and biobehavioral strategies serve as an invaluable foundation for migraine treatment. Noninvasive neurostimulation and neuromodulation devices offer a promising new treatment strategy for migraine during pregnancy and lactation. In addition, some patients may require pharmacologic treatments, and we will review important treatment considerations over distinct hormonal epochs in a woman's life.

Menstrually Associated Migraine

Treatment options for menstrual migraine can include standard-of-care migraine rescue (e.g., triptans, NSAIDs, ergotamine, dopamine antagonists, gepants) and prophylactic treatments (e.g., antidepressants, antiepileptics, antihypertensives, anti-CGRP monoclonal antibodies, gepants, onabotulinumtoxinA for chronic migraine). Neuromodulatory devices can also be used for migraine prevention and rescue. These strategies are not unique to menstrual migraine but can certainly be employed to help manage migraine attacks whether menstrually associated or not. Data examining these medications specifically in the setting of menstrual migraine is limited; the following treatments have been studied in the setting of treating menstrual migraine—frovatriptan [37, 38], naproxen and mefenamic acid [38], noninvasive vagal nerve stimulation [39], erenumab [40], and ubrogepant.

Some treatment strategies unique to menstrual migraine can be beneficial as they address the specific nature of these attacks. One strategy involves mini-prophylaxis: using a rescue agent in a prophylactic manner for a brief period of time. Mini-prophylaxis is typically started either at the onset of the perimenstrual headache or in the hours prior to menstruation and continued for 3–5 consecutive days. Mini-prophylaxis is not an appropriate treatment strategy for patients with frequent headaches or unpredictable menstruation. It is ideal for patients with migraine attacks concentrated around menstruation and a few other attacks on other days of the month, and for patients in women menstruation is quite predictable. A calendar tracking this information can be very helpful in determining who would most benefit from this strategy. The medications typically used for mini-prophylaxis include NSAIDs, specifically naproxen, and triptans, often frovatriptan, given their long elimination half-lives [41].

Another option for managing menstrual migraine is to counteract the drop in estrogen that occurs in the late luteal phase of the menstrual cycle and is a potent trigger for migraine attacks. This strategy can involve either using supplemental estrogen or continuous hormonal contraception ideally with monophasic low-dose estrogen-containing hormonal contraceptives or with systemic progestin-only contraceptives that suppress ovulation (injectable progestins, implantable progestins, or daily progestin-only pills). Estrogen supplementation alone is not recommended, given that headaches may be simply delayed until after estrogen withdrawal [42].

Prior to initiating treatment with estrogen-containing hormonal contraceptives, it is critical to assess for the presence of aura, a history of smoking, or hypercoagulable disorder. The data clearly shows that migraine, specifically the subtype of migraine with aura, is a risk factor for stroke. The overall absolute risk is low, but compared to women who do not have migraine, there is about a twofold increased risk of stroke, mostly seen in young premenopausal women who do not otherwise have other traditional stroke risk factors. There is also increasing data regarding the risk of other cardiovascular events in migraine as well. Adding exogenous estrogen can further increase this risk for stroke. The data for this is based on older studies where the estrogen component was high and not in line with the oral contraceptives available today. Due to this conflicting data, there are different recommendations regarding the use of

Table 32.1 Recommendations for use of estrogen-containing hormonal contraception in people with migraine

Organization	Migraine without aura	Migraine with aura	General recommendation
WHO	<35 years: advantages generally outweigh risks ≥35 years: risks generally outweigh advantages	Unacceptable health risks (method not to be used)	If new migraine without aura develops while using an estrogen-containing method, recommendations escalate. <35 years: risks generally outweigh advantages; ≥35 years: unacceptable health risks (method not to be used)
CDC MEC	Advantages generally outweigh risks	Unacceptable health risks (method not to be used)	
IHS	Acceptable	Individualized approach	Avoid with smoking and other risk factors like hypertension

WHO, World Health Organization Medical Eligibility Criteria for Contraceptive Use, 5th edition, 2015; CDC MEC: Center for Disease Control and Prevention US Medical Eligibility Criteria for Contraceptive Use, 2016; IHS, International Headache Society [43]

exogenous estrogen in women who have migraine. Migraine without aura is not considered a contraindication, but both the World Health Organization and United States Center for Disease Control Medical Eligibility Criteria consider the use of exogenous estrogen an "unacceptable health risk" for migraine with aura [44, 45]. The American Headache Society recommends an individualized approach to the use of contraceptives in migraine with aura [46]. See Table 32.1 for further clarification around guidelines for hormonal contraceptives in the setting of migraine.

Transgender Health, Hormone Therapy, and Migraine

Hranilovich et al.'s excellent narrative review of headaches in transgender and gender-diverse patients highlights multiple critical treatment considerations among transgender and gender-diverse patients. One area of focus includes specific medications that can be feminizing and/or masculinizing and/or increase the risk for drug-drug interactions. Antiepileptic drugs, in particular, have the potential to influence estrogen levels, and dose adjustments or alternatives may need to be considered [28].

Pregnancy and Lactation

In light of their quite favorable safety profile, behavioral strategies for managing migraine are strongly recommended for women during preconception and pregnancy. These can include optimizing lifestyle factors such as maintaining regular sleep, exercise, and eating schedules, along with mind-body therapy and body-based practices. Mind-body therapies with the greatest evidence for efficacy in migraine treatment include biofeedback, cognitive behavioral therapy, and relaxation. Body-based practices such as acupuncture, physical therapy, and yoga can also be helpful in managing migraine. It is important to note that specific acupuncture points can induce labor, and these sites should be avoided during acupuncture treatments [47, 48]. Although these authors recommend behavioral strategies as first-line treatment for migraine, at times, medication or neuromodulatory devices may be appropriate to manage migraine during pregnancy.

Given that 50% of pregnancies are unplanned [49], discussions around medication safety during pregnancy should be emphasized whenever a medication is prescribed for a woman of childbearing age, along with counseling on the importance of using effective modes of contraception for those patients who do not desire a pregnancy. A recent study also suggested that among women with migraine with patterns of migraine medication use suggesting increased severity of migraine, the risk for spontaneous abortion was higher, highlighting the importance of developing a safe plan for managing migraine throughout pregnancy [50]. Preconception counseling plays an important role in helping women of childbearing age prepare for a pregnancy. Following a preconception counseling appointment(s), women of childbearing age should understand how pregnancy can influence migraine and how migraine can impact pregnancy outcomes, and have an individualized plan for preventing and managing migraine preconception and during pregnancy. Ideally, counseling would take place months in advance of conception to allow time to review and modify treatment strategies.

There is a paucity of rigorous clinical trials evaluating the safety and efficacy of treatments during specific hormonal epochs of a woman's life. In particular, the treatment of migraine during pregnancy and lactation presents a great challenge for clinicians. Recommendations are, for a large part, based on animal models with at times poor extrapolation to humans, or based on retrospective studies which have their own limitations, namely recall and reporting bias along with misattribution of causality, or extrapolated from use of the same medication in pregnancy for an indication other than headache [51]. Long-term risks to the child after maternal exposure are difficult to ascertain and fraught with confounders. With the elimination of the former Food and Drug

Administration (FDA) letter categorization system for safety of treatments during pregnancy, providers have greater flexibility in informed decision making. The replacement categorization system—Pregnancy and Lactation Labeling (PLLR) is still being phased in.

While the patient is trying to conceive, wherever possible, medication restrictions should be limited. One strategy to optimize for minimal migraine treatment restrictions is to ONLY limit migraine rescue medications during the second half of the menstrual cycle, after ovulation. For the first half of the menstrual cycle, the patient should be able to take most rescue medications with the exception of limiting NSAIDs, as these can potentially interfere with embryo implantation.

Some medications traditionally used for migraine prophylaxis are contraindicated in the setting of pregnancy and should be discontinued prior to trying to conceive. With prophylactic medications, it is important to determine whether prophylaxis is necessary for the patient, as some patients may no longer need prophylaxis at the time of trying to conceive. For those patients who continue prophylaxis, it is important to consider the need for prophylaxis throughout pregnancy as migraine tends to improve in pregnancy and prophylaxis may not be necessary through the duration of the pregnancy. Some medications should be stopped prior to conception due to their teratogenic potential; the elimination half-life of the medication should inform the timing for medication discontinuation. Oral medications such as topiramate, valproic acid, candesartan, and lisinopril can be stopped within a few days of trying to conceive. These specific medications should not be prescribed for women of reproductive age without effective contraception.

It is currently recommended to discontinue anti-CGRP monoclonal antibodies 5–6 months prior to trying to conceive. Despite some reassuring registry data with reports of a limited number of pregnant patients who were on anti-CGRP monoclonal antibodies that did not demonstrate adverse maternal or fetal events [21, 52], concerns remain regarding the safety of this class of medications in pregnancy. The recommendation to discontinue anti-CGRP monoclonal antibodies prior to pregnancy stems from data demonstrating CGRP's roles in fetal development and how abnormal levels may factor into an increased risk for preeclampsia. Monoclonal antibodies are IgGs that also readily cross the placenta [53, 54].

In terms of onabotulinumtoxinA, like many other medications in pregnancy, the safety of onabotulinumtoxinA, injected according to the PREEMPT protocol for chronic migraine prophylaxis, is uncertain during pregnancy. While the molecule is large and is unlikely to cross the placenta, there is a paucity of data proving its safety in pregnancy. Due to a lack of sufficient safety data, many clinicians do not feel comfortable offering onabotulinumtoxinA treatment during pregnancy. Given its long elimination half-life, it is important to discuss discontinuing both CGRP monoclonal antibodies and onbotulinumtoxinA months in advance of conception.

Tables 32.2 and 32.3 highlight the relative safety and efficacy of acute (Table 32.2) and preventive (Table 32.3) treatments for migraines during pregnancy. Behavioral and nonpharmacologic strategies are the preferred first-line treatments for migraine in pregnancy. When needed, rescue migraine treatments to consider for use in pregnancy include acetaminophen, metoclopramide, caffeine, diphenhydramine, occipital nerve blocks with lidocaine, and sumatrip-

Table 32.2 This table highlights the relative safety of migraine acute treatment strategies for migraine during pregnancy

	Safety recommendations	Comments
First line		
Behavioral treatments (cognitive behavioral therapy) Relaxation therapy (biofeedback)	Consider as first line	While the safety data for these strategies in pregnancy is limited, expert consensus suggest that these strategies are relatively safe in pregnancy
Second line		
Acetaminophen (A)	Consider as first line	Saldanha et al.'s systematic review concluded that acetaminophen might be associated with adverse fetal and child events. Poorly powered and potentially biased studies raised the concern for an increased risk of adverse neurodevelopmental outcomes among the offspring of women taking acetaminophen during pregnancy. In light of these studies, there was a call to action to further study the potential impact of acetaminophen [55]. ACOG's response to this call to action was to release a statement reiterating the lack of clear evidence proving a direct relationship between acetaminophen intake during pregnancy and neurodevelopmental disorders in offspring. Acetaminophen should be used as needed
Metoclopramide (B)	Consider as first line	Given its relative efficacy and favorable pregnancy safety profile, metoclopramide may be considered as a first-line migraine rescue medication. According to Saldanha's systematic review, metoclopramide may not be associated with adverse fetal or child effects [56]

(continued)

Table 32.2 (continued)

	Safety recommendations	Comments
Caffeine	Consider as first line	Caffeine can serve as an effective migraine rescue medication, according to ACOG, but amounts should be limited to less than 200 mg/24 hours [56, 57]
Diphenhydramine	Consider as first line	According to Saldanha et al.'s systematic review, diphenhydramine in combination with metoclopramide was shown to be more effective in treating migraine acutely than codeine. It is reasonable to add diphenhydramine as adjunct therapy with metoclopramide for patients during pregnancy as this is a relatively safe medication to use in pregnancy
Nerve blocks	Consider as first line	Occipital nerve blocks should be done with lidocaine and without corticosteroids during pregnancy
Nonsteroidal anti-inflammatory drugs (NSAID) (A)	Balance risks and benefits (only between 12 and 20 weeks)	Avoid NSAIDs during first and third trimesters. Use of NSAIDs in the first trimester may increase the risk of miscarriage, and use during the third trimester may increase the risk for premature closure of the ductus arteriosus
Triptans (A)	Balance risks and benefits	Dudman et al.'s systematic review and meta-analysis conclude that triptans do not increase the risk for adverse maternal events [58]. Saldanha et al.'s systematic review similarly concluded that it may not be associated with adverse fetal or child effects. Among triptans, sumatriptan is preferred during pregnancy as it's less likely to traverse the placenta [59]
Neuromodulatory devices (external trigeminal nerve stimulation (e-TNS), single-pulse transcranial magnetic stimulation (sTMS), noninvasive vagal nerve stimulation, remote electrical neuromodulation (REN), and external combined occipital and trigeminal stimulation (e-COT-n8))	Balance risks and benefits	Devices are not FDA cleared for use in pregnancy and are considered off-label when used during pregnancy. Despite the lack of safety data, expert consensus suggests that devices are relatively safe in pregnancy
Avoid		
Butalbital (C)	Not recommended in pregnancy	Butalbital can readily increase the risk for medication-overuse headache along with increasing the risk for adverse fetal outcomes when used in excess
Opiates (C)	Not recommended in pregnancy	Opiates can readily increase the risk for medication overuse headache along with an increased risk for physical dependence and withdrawal in neonates when used in excess
Ergot alkaloid-containing products (A)	Not recommended in pregnancy	Ergot alkaloid-containing products cause smooth muscle contractions and may stimulate spontaneous abortion or preterm labor
Gepants (ubrogepant, rimegepant)	Not recommended in pregnancy at this time	Gepants such as ubrogepant and rimegepant are well established as effective in treating migraine. Safety data in pregnancy have not been established yet

Saldanha et al.'s systematic review served as a critical source of information, albeit based on limited data, for this table [56]. Included for many medications listed below is a letter adjacent to the medication indicating the American Headache Society (AHS) level of evidence for efficacy in treating migraine. (A) indicates a medication that is established as effective for acute treatment of migraine. (B) indicates medications probably effective for acute treatment of migraine. (C) indicates medications possibly effective for acute treatment of migraine [60]

tan. Of the established first-line preventive treatments for migraine, propranolol is widely used during pregnancy. Other prophylactic options with slightly more favorable pregnancy safety profiles, such as verapamil and cyproheptadine, have less robust efficacy data in preventing migraine.

For further information regarding the relative safety and efficacy of migraine treatments, below are some very helpful resources. The United States Department of Health and Human Services Agency for Healthcare Research and Quality conducted a systematic review of treatments for headaches during pregnancy [56] that is an important source of data when considering migraine treatment options for pregnant patients, albeit based on limited data. The American College of Obstetrics and Gynecology Committee on Clinical Practice Guidelines-Obstetrics also published guidelines on migraine management during pregnancy in 2022. These guidelines can serve as a helpful resource to explore medication safety for pregnant and lactating patients [57]. In addition, Melissa Rayhill's review of Headache in Pregnancy and Lactation is also a helpful source of information on medication safety and efficacy in pregnancy [64].

Table 32.3 This table highlights the relative safety of migraine prophylactic treatment strategies for migraine during pregnancy

	Safety recommendations	Comments
First line		
Propranolol (A)	Consider as first line	Established as effective in preventing migraine and relatively safe in pregnancy. Propranolol should be discontinued prior to labor to avoid reduced uterine contractions and fetal bradycardia. Monitor infants for bradycardia, hypotension, and hypoglycemia
Verapamil (U), amlodipine	Consider as first line	While verapamil and amlodipine are considered relatively safe in pregnancy, data for efficacy in migraine prevention is lacking
Cyproheptadine (C)	Consider as first line	While cyproheptadine is considered relatively safe in pregnancy, data for efficacy in migraine prevention is lacking
Second line		
Antidepressants—amitriptyline (B), nortriptyline	Balance risks and benefits	Tricyclic antidepressants, in particular amitriptyline, which has been most commonly studied in migraine treatment trials, are probably effective in preventing migraine. According to Saldanha et al., tricyclic antidepressants may be associated with adverse fetal effects [56]
Magnesium (B)	Balance risks and benefits	Prolonged IV Mg sulfate exposure during pregnancy was associated with fetal skeletal abnormalities. Given oral magnesium's low bioavailability, doses below 350 mg per day are not thought to compete with calcium in developing bone
Coenzyme Q10 (C)	Balance risks and benefits	One small study of coenzyme Q10 use in pregnancy did not demonstrate increased adverse maternal or fetal outcomes. Coenzyme Q10 is possibly efficacious in preventing migraine
Memantine	Balance risks and benefits	While memantine is not known to cause adverse maternal or fetal effects, data for its efficacy in treating migraine is limited
OnbotulinumtoxinA (A)	Balance risks and benefits	Established as effective in treating migraine although data regarding safety in pregnancy is limited
Avoid		
Butterbur (A)	Not recommended in pregnancy	Preparations may contain pyrrolizidine alkaloids (PA), which are toxic to the liver. It should not be recommended in pregnancy as it could cause congenital malformations
Feverfew (B)	Not recommended in pregnancy	Feverfew can cause uterine contractions and spontaneous abortion
Venlafaxine (B)	Balance risks and benefits	In a case control study of 30 K mothers of infants with birth defects, venlafaxine was found to have the highest proportion of elevated odds ratio with specific birth defects [61]
Topiramate (A)	Not recommended in pregnancy	Not safe in pregnancy, use during the first trimester can increase the risk for cleft lip or palate
Valproic acid (A)	Not recommended in pregnancy	Not safe in pregnancy, use during pregnancy can increase the risk for neural tube defects and impair cognition in children
Candesartan (C)	Not recommended in pregnancy	Not safe in pregnancy
Lisinopril	Not recommended in pregnancy	Not safe in pregnancy
CGRP antagonists (erenumab, fremanezumab, galcanezumab, eptinezumab, rimegepant, atogepant)	Not recommended in pregnancy at this time	While limited data does not demonstrate increased maternal or fetal risks with use of these medications during pregnancy, expert consensus suggest that this class of medications should be avoided during pregnancy due to CGRPs role in pregnancy. These are established as effective in preventing migraine

Saldanha et al.'s systematic review served as a critical source of information, albeit based on limited data, for this table [56]. Included for many medications listed below is a letter adjacent to the medication indicating the American Headache Society (AHS) level of evidence for efficacy in preventing migraine. (A) indicates a medication that is established as effective for preventing migraine. (B) indicates medications are probably effective for preventing migraine. (C) indicates medications possibly effective for preventing migraine. (U) indicates conflicting or inadequate evidence [62, 63]

Lactation

The decision to breastfeed is a deeply personal one dependent on many factors, both maternal and fetal. Patients should be informed regarding the manner in which lactation can influence migraine along with the relative safety of migraine treatment strategies while lactating. Treatment considerations during lactation are distinct from those during pregnancy and preparing patients for this transition is important. While the fourth trimester or postpartum phase is characterized by many potential migraine triggers including poor sleep and stress, lactation can delay the recurrence of migraine [23]. Breastfeeding is also not known to adversely impact migraine.

Medication safety during lactation depends on a number of factors including the maternal plasma concentration, the molecular weight and protein binding of the medication along with the medication half-life, bioavailability, and the baby's age [51]. The Relative Infant Dose (RID) is a measure of the amount of medication excreted in breastmilk, and an

RID less than 10% is considered acceptable. Lactating patients have multiple options including continuing to breastfeed and take needed medications, delaying feeding to allow for drug clearance, and pumping and discarding milk [26]. Clinicians also have multiple resources that can help when evaluating whether a medication is appropriate to take postpartum including the National Library of Medicine Drugs and Lactation (LactMed®) database [65], Thomas Hale's "Medications and Mother's Milk" [23, 66].

Among triptans, sumatriptan has the least excretion into breastmilk and is favored over other triptans during lactation [67]. Among NSAIDs, ibuprofen is preferred because of its relatively shorter elimination half-life. Some medications can also influence the volume of milk production, and it is important to warn patients of this potential; for instance, metoclopramide may increase milk production, whereas diphenhydramine may decrease milk production. Medications contraindicated during breastfeeding include ergotamine, aspirin, atenolol, and venlafaxine. To date, there is no available data on the safety of lasmiditan use during lactation.

Perimenopause

During perimenopause, women with a history of migraine, in particular migraine without aura, experience an increased frequency of headaches, vasomotor symptoms, mood disturbances, sleep disturbances, and increased morbidity [41]. Natural menopause is associated with a lower incidence of migraine compared with surgical menopause [68]. Because of the abrupt reduction in estrogen associated with surgical menopause, bilateral oophorectomy can temporarily increase the incidence of migraine in premenopausal people. Nonhormonal treatment options can be appropriate for the management of migraine during perimenopause, and selective serotonin reuptake inhibitors and selective norepinephrine reuptake inhibitors, in particular, can help with both migraine and vasomotor symptoms of perimenopause [69]. When managing menopausal symptoms, menopausal hormonal therapy is sometimes used and may impact migraine. Based on limited data, transdermal estrogen is preferred to oral estrogen among women with migraine, and continuous combined regimens are better tolerated among women with migraine than cyclical regimens. Reduction of estrogen dose or discontinuation of menopausal hormonal therapy should be considered for women who develop aura or experience an increase in aura [70].

Conclusion

Migraine is predominantly a disorder experienced by women. Reproductive hormones play a critical role in influencing migraine frequency, severity, medication response, and comorbidities. Greater research is needed to identify better-targeted migraine treatments that address the increased disability experienced by women during specific hormonal epochs.

Teaching Points

1. Sex-based factors such as hormonal fluctuations play an important role in influencing migraine incidence and degree of burden.
2. Distinct hormonal milieus can influence migraine differently, resulting in an increased prevalence of migraine among women compared to men after menarche, an improvement for many during pregnancy, and worsening perimenopause.
3. Treatment considerations during specific hormonal epochs can be distinct and should be carefully considered.
4. Preconception counseling is important for patients of childbearing age.

Case

A 35-year-old woman with a history of chronic migraine without aura has experienced a significant reduction in her headache intensity and frequency on monthly erenumab. She presents to the clinic with plans to start trying to conceive in the next year. She inquires whether she can continue erenumab through pregnancy and if not, what she can take to prevent her headaches.

Case Discussion

Despite one small study of 94 cases of pregnant women exposed to erenumab, galcanezumab, and fremanezumab demonstrating reassuring pregnancy safety data, we would advise discontinuation of CGRP blocking treatments prior to conception. This recommendation is rooted in data regarding CGRP's role in fetal development and abnormal levels potentially playing a role in preeclampsia. Gepants can be discontinued days in advance of trying to conceive. However, in light of their long elimination half-lives, CGRP monoclonal antibodies should be discontinued 5–6 months in advance of trying to conceive. It will be important to develop a new migraine action plan for our patient, including discussion of new prophylactic options to help her during the transition off of erenumab. Given her successful migraine response to erenumab, it is reasonable to consider using a gepant to help transition her off of erenumab. Atogepant or rimegepant (dosed every other day) could be used as a prophylactic agent and discontinued for a short time period before conception. Other prophylactic options should be considered once she is trying to conceive.

Questions and Answers

1. Compared to men, women with migraine tend to experience which of the following?
   A. Greater disability from migraine attacks.
   B. Longer lasting migraine attacks.
   C. More frequent migraine attacks.
   D. Increased frequency of accompanying symptoms such as nausea.
   E. Decreased responsiveness to treatments.
   F. Increased risk of transformation from episodic to chronic migraine.
   G. All of the above.

The correct answer is G. Compared to men, women with migraine experience greater disability from migraine attacks with increased duration, frequency, and accompanying symptoms, along with decreased responsiveness to treatments.

2. A 28-year-old woman with a history of migraine without aura currently takes ubrogepant as her migraine rescue medication. She is planning to try to conceive and asks what is the next best step?
   A. Order an MRI of the brain.
   B. Reassure her that it is safe to continue taking ubrogepant as a migraine rescue medication during pregnancy.
   C. Advise her to stop ubrogepant and start fioricet prior to trying to conceive.
   D. Advise her to stop ubrogepant and instead try acetaminophen or metoclopramide for migraine.

The correct answer is D. At this time, we recommend avoiding calcitonin gene-related peptide (CGRP) blocking medications such as ubrogepant during pregnancy as CGRP is known to have a role in fetal development and abnormal levels may play a role in preeclampsia.

References

1. Buse DC, et al. Sex differences in the prevalence, symptoms, and associated features of migraine, probable migraine and other severe headache: results of the American Migraine Prevalence and Prevention (AMPP) Study. Headache. 2013;53:1278–99.
2. GBD 2016 Headache Collaborators. Global, regional, and national burden of migraine and tension-type headache, 1990–2016: a systematic analysis for the Global Burden of Disease Study 2016. Lancet Neurol. 2018;17:954–76.
3. LiptonRB,StewartWF,DiamondS,DiamondML,ReedM.Prevalence and burden of migraine in the united states: data from the American Migraine Study II. Headache J Head Face Pain. 2001;41:646–57. https://doi.org/10.1046/j.1526-4610.2001.041007646.x.
4. Steiner TJ, et al. Migraine remains second among the world's causes of disability, and first among young women: findings from GBD2019. J Headache Pain. 2020;21:137. https://doi.org/10.1186/s10194-020-01208-0.
5. Estave PM, et al. Learning the full impact of migraine through patient voices: a qualitative study. Headache. 2021;61:1004–20.
6. Labastida-Ramírez A, Rubio-Beltrán E, Villalón CM, MaassenVanDenBrink A. Gender aspects of CGRP in migraine. Cephalalgia. 2019;39:435–44.
7. Amir B-Y, et al. Headaches in women undergoing in vitro fertilization and embryo-transfer treatment. Headache. 2005;45:215–9.
8. Martin VT, et al. Perimenopause and menopause are associated with high frequency headache in women with migraine: results of the American Migraine Prevalence and Prevention Study. Headache. 2016;56:292–305.
9. Victor TW, Hu X, Campbell JC, Buse DC, Lipton RB. Migraine prevalence by age and sex in the United States: a life-span study. Cephalalgia. 2010;30:1065–72.
10. Gazerani P, Cairns BE. Sex-specific pharmacotherapy for migraine: a narrative review. Front Neurosci. 2020;14:222.
11. Burch RC, Buse DC, Lipton RB. Migraine. Neurol Clin. 2019;37:631–49. https://doi.org/10.1016/j.ncl.2019.06.001.
12. Tietjen GE, et al. Endometriosis is associated with prevalence of comorbid conditions in migraine. Headache. 2007;47:1069–78.
13. Allais G, et al. Premenstrual syndrome and migraine. Neurol Sci. 2012;33(Suppl 1):S111–5.
14. Glintborg D, Rubin KH, Nybo M, Abrahamsen B, Andersen M. Morbidity and medicine prescriptions in a nationwide Danish population of patients diagnosed with polycystic ovary syndrome. Eur J Endocrinol. 2015;172:627–38. https://doi.org/10.1530/eje-14-1108.
15. Borsook D, et al. Sex and the migraine brain. Neurobiol Dis. 2014;68:200–14.
16. Allais G, et al. Gender-related differences in migraine. Neurol Sci. 2020;41:429–36.
17. Reddy N, Schneeberger S, Schoenbrunner A, Desai M, Janis J. The complex relationship between estrogen and migraines: a scoping review. Syst Rev. 10(1):72. https://doi.org/10.1186/s13643-021-01618-4.
18. Nappi RE, et al. Role of Estrogens in Menstrual Migraine. Cells. 2022;11
19. Warfvinge K, et al. Estrogen receptors α, β and GPER in the CNS and trigeminal system – molecular and functional aspects. J Headache Pain. 2020;21:131.
20. Bharadwaj VN, et al. A new hypothesis linking oxytocin to menstrual migraine. Headache. 2021;61:1051–9.
21. Krause DN, Warfvinge K, Haanes KA, Edvinsson L. Hormonal influences in migraine – interactions of oestrogen, oxytocin and CGRP. Nat Rev Neurol. 2021;17:621–33. https://doi.org/10.1038/s41582-021-00544-2.
22. van Casteren DS, et al. Comparing perimenstrual and non-perimenstrual migraine attacks using an e-diary. Neurology. 2021;97:e1661–71.
23. Sances G, et al. Course of migraine during pregnancy and postpartum: a prospective study. Cephalalgia. 2003;23:197–205.
24. Allais G, Chiarle G, Sinigaglia S, Mana O, Benedetto C. Migraine during pregnancy and in the puerperium. Neurol Sci. 2019;40:81–91. https://doi.org/10.1007/s10072-019-03792-9.
25. Serva WAD, et al. Course of migraine during pregnancy among migraine sufferers before pregnancy. Arq Neuropsiquiatr. 2011;69:613–9.
26. Wells RE, Turner DP, Lee M, Bishop L, Strauss L. Managing migraine during pregnancy and lactation. Curr Neurol Neurosci Rep. 2016;16:40.
27. Ripa P, et al. Migraine in menopausal women: a systematic review. Int J Women's Health. 2015;7:773–82.
28. Hranilovich JA, Kaiser EA, Pace A, Barber M, Ziplow J. Headache in transgender and gender-diverse patients: a narrative review. Headache. 2021;61:1040–50.
29. Raffaelli B, Do TP, Chaudhry BA, Ashina M, Amin FM, Ashina H. Menstrual migraine is caused by estrogen withdrawal: revisit-

ing the evidence. J Headache Pain. 2023;24(1):131. https://doi.org/10.1186/s10194-023-01664-4.
30. Robbins MS, Farmakidis C, Dayal AK, Lipton RB. Acute headache diagnosis in pregnant women: a hospital-based study. Neurology. 2015;85:1024–30.
31. Feske SK, Singhal AB. Cerebrovascular disorders complicating pregnancy. Continuum. 2014;20:80–99.
32. Miller EC, et al. Migraine and adverse pregnancy outcomes: the Nulliparous Pregnancy Outcomes Study: monitoring mothers-to-be. Am J Obstet Gynecol. 2022;227:535–6.
33. Aukes AM, Yurtsever FN, Boutin A, Visser MC, de Groot CJM. Associations between migraine and adverse pregnancy outcomes: systematic review and meta-analysis. Obstet Gynecol Surv. 2019;74:738–48.
34. Liu X, Gong Y. The potential protective role of aspirin against migraine in pregnant women. Med Sci Monit. 2020;26:e923959.
35. Vgontzas A, Robbins MS. A hospital based retrospective study of acute postpartum headache. Headache. 2018;58:845–51.
36. Bernstein C, O'Neal MA. Migraine and menopause – a narrative review. Menopause. 2020;28:96–101.
37. Lichten EM. Menstrual migraine and treatment options: review. Headache. 2018;58:145–6.
38. Allais G, et al. Efficacy of frovatriptan versus other triptans in the acute treatment of menstrual migraine: pooled analysis of three double-blind, randomized, crossover, multicenter studies. Neurol Sci. 2012;33(Suppl 1):S65–9.
39. Grazzi L, et al. Non-invasive Vagus Nerve Stimulation (nVNS) as mini-prophylaxis for menstrual/menstrually related migraine: an open-label study. J Headache Pain. 2016;17:91.
40. Pavlovic JM, et al. Efficacy and safety of erenumab in women with a history of menstrual migraine. J Headache Pain. 2020;21:95.
41. Pavlović JM. Headache in Women. Continuum. 2021;27:686–702.
42. Sacco S, et al. Effect of exogenous estrogens and progestogens on the course of migraine during reproductive age: a consensus statement by the European Headache Federation (EHF) and the European Society of Contraception and Reproductive Health (ESCRH). J Headache Pain. 2018;19:76.
43. Bousser MG, Conard J, Kittner S, de Lignières B, MacGregor EA, Massiou H, et al. Recommendations on the risk of ischaemic stroke associated with use of combined oral contraceptives and hormone replacement therapy in women with migraine. The International Headache Society Task Force on Combined Oral Contraceptives & Hormone Replacement Therapy. Cephalalgia. 2000;20:155–56. https://doi.org/10.1046/j.1468-2982.2000.00035.x.
44. Classifications for Combined Hormonal Contraceptives. https://www.cdc.gov/reproductivehealth/contraception/mmwr/mec/appendixD.html#mec_neurologic. 2020.
45. World Health Organization. Medical eligibility criteria for contraceptive use, 5th ed, 2015. https://iris.who.int/bitstream/handle/10665/181468/9789241549158_eng.pdf?sequence=9
46. Sheikh HU, Pavlovic J, Loder E, Burch R. Risk of stroke associated with use of estrogen containing contraceptives in women with migraine: a systematic review. Headache J Head Face Pain. 2018;58:5–21. https://doi.org/10.1111/head.13229.
47. Holdridge A, Donnelly M, Kuruvilla DE. Integrative, interventional, and non-invasive approaches for the treatment for migraine during pregnancy. Curr Pain Headache Rep. 2022;26:323–30.
48. Riggins N, Ehrlich A. The use of behavioral modalities for headache during pregnancy and breastfeeding. Curr Pain Headache Rep. 2021;25:66.
49. Sawhill IV, Guyot K. Preventing unplanned pregnancy: lessons from the states. Brookings. http://www.brookings.edu/research/preventing-unplanned-pregnancy-lessons-from-the-states/; 2019.
50. Crowe HM, et al. Pre-pregnancy migraine diagnosis, medication use, and spontaneous abortion: a prospective cohort study. J Headache Pain. 2022;23:162.
51. Parikh SK, Delbono MV, Silberstein SD. Managing migraine in pregnancy and breastfeeding. Prog Brain Res. 2020;255:275–309.
52. Noseda R, Bedussi F, Gobbi C, Zecca C, Ceschi A. Safety profile of erenumab, galcanezumab and fremanezumab in pregnancy and lactation: analysis of the WHO pharmacovigilance database. Cephalalgia. 2021;41:789–98.
53. Sandoe CH, Lay C. Secondary headaches during pregnancy: when to worry. Curr Neurol Neurosci Rep. 2019;19:27.
54. Yallampalli C, Chauhan M, Sathishkumar K. Calcitonin gene-related family peptides in vascular adaptations, uteroplacental circulation, and fetal growth. Curr Vasc Pharmacol. 2013;11:641–54.
55. Bauer AZ, et al. Paracetamol use during pregnancy – a call for precautionary action. Nat Rev Endocrinol. 2021;17:757–66. https://doi.org/10.1038/s41574-021-00553-7.
56. Saldanha IJ, et al. Management of primary headaches during pregnancy, postpartum, and breastfeeding: a systematic review. Headache. 2021;61:11–43.
57. ACOG Committee on Clinical Practice Guidelines–Obstetrics. Headaches in pregnancy and postpartum: ACOG clinical practice guideline no. 3. Obstet Gynecol. 2022;139:944–72.
58. Dudman DC, et al. A systematic review and meta-analyses on the prevalence of pregnancy outcomes in migraine treated patients: a contribution from the IMI2 ConcePTION project. J Neurol. 2022;269:742–9.
59. Calhoun AH. Migraine treatment in pregnancy and lactation. Curr Pain Headache Rep. 2017;21:46.
60. Marmura MJ, Silberstein SD, Schwedt TJ. The acute treatment of migraine in adults: the American Headache Society evidence assessment of migraine pharmacotherapies. Headache. 2015;55:3–20.
61. Anderson KN, et al. Maternal use of specific antidepressant medications during early pregnancy and the risk of selected birth defects. JAMA Psychiatry. 2020;77:1246–55.
62. Tfelt-Hansen PC. Evidence-based guideline update: pharmacologic treatment for episodic migraine prevention in adults: report of the Quality Standards subcommittee of the American Academy of Neurology and the American Headache Society. Neurology. 2013;80:869–70.
63. Silberstein SD, et al. Evidence-based guideline update: Pharmacologic treatment for episodic migraine prevention in adults: Table 1. Neurology. 2012;78:1337–45. https://doi.org/10.1212/wnl.0b013e3182535d20.
64. Rayhill M. Headache in pregnancy and lactation. Continuum. 2022;28:72–92.
65. Drugs and Lactation Database (LactMed). (2006).
66. Hale TW, Hilary E, Rowe P. Medications and mothers' milk 2017. Springer; 2016.
67. Amundsen S, et al. Transfer of triptans into human breast milk and estimation of infant drug exposure through breastfeeding. Basic Clin Pharmacol Toxicol. 2021;128:795–804.
68. Characteristics of headache at menopause. A clinico-epidemiologic study. Maturitas. 1993;17:31–7.
69. Arumugam M, Parthasarathy V. Increased incidence of migraine in women correlates with obstetrics and gynaecological surgical procedures. Int J Surg. 2015;22:105–9.
70. MacGregor EA, Anne MacGregor E. Menstrual and perimenopausal migraine: a narrative review. Maturitas. 2020;142:24–30. https://doi.org/10.1016/j.maturitas.2020.07.005.

Migraine in Older Adults

33

Tissa Wijeratne and Chanith Wijeratne

Introduction

Neurological disorders are the leading cause of disability adjusted life years (DALYs) and second leading cause of death globally [1, 2]. The five largest contributors of neurological DALYs in 2016 were stroke (42.2%), migraine (16.3%), dementia (10.4%), meningitis (7.9%), and epilepsy (5%). Approximately 70% of this heavy burden affects low-to-middle-income countries [1]. Migraine remains second among the world's causes of disability (and first among young women) as per the GBD (2019 iteration) [3, 4].

During the last three decades, the total number of deaths and people with disabilities related to neurological disorders have skyrocketed, particularly in low-to-middle-income countries. These figures are only expected to rise further as the COVID-19 pandemic continues to unfold globally [5]. It is worth noting that concomitant diagnosis of COVID-19 in patients with neurological disorders is associated with greater mortality and morbidity [5]. This is a reminder of the importance of neuroinflammation in neurological disorders [6, 7]. Neuroinflammation additionally has a key role in the pathophysiology of migraine, which is a complex neuro-glio-vascular disorder [8, 9].

All these complexities coupled with increased life expectancy worldwide make migraine in older adults an important global public health problem today. This is likely to become an even greater personal and public health problem over the next three to four decades [10]. Despite its significance as a common and debilitating neurological disorder, migraine continues to be neglected and underdiagnosed throughout the world [11–18].

Questions

1. Annual prevalence of migraine in older adults is
   A. 3%
   B. 30%
   C. 10%
   D. 35%
   E. 50%
2. Which of the following statements is true?
   A. Photophobia is common among migraine in older adults
   B. One-year prevalence of migraine in older adults is 30%
   C. Nausea is not reported in migraine in older adults
   D. Bilateral headache is commonly reported in migraine in older adults
   E. Autonomic symptoms are uncommon in migraine in older adults

Migraine Across the Lifespan, Including Later Life

Migraine is generally regarded as a brain disorder that affects young people, though it may be present at any age. Migraine typically begins during early childhood, peaking at puberty [19–23]. Migraine is classically most active between the third and fourth decades of life [24, 25]. The occurrence of a first episode of migraine in the sixth, seventh, and eighth decades of some patients is however well reported [26–29], although the majority of older adults with chronic migraine will have noted the onset of migraine before fifty years of age [27–30].

Migraine is the second most common headache disorder in older adults after tension-type headaches (TTHs), with a

T. Wijeratne (✉)
Department of Neurology, St Albans, VIC, Australia

Sunshine Hospital, Western Health, St Albans, VIC, Australia

Australian Institute of Migraine, Melbourne, VIC, Australia

C. Wijeratne
Australian Institute of Migraine, Melbourne, VIC, Australia

Monash Medical School, Clayton, VIC, Australia

Migraine Foundation Australia, Keilor East, VIC, Australia

T. S. Monteith et al. (eds.), *Comprehensive Migraine Management*, https://doi.org/10.1007/978-3-031-86923-5_33

one-year prevalence of 10% [10, 19, 20, 22, 31]. It is important to note that the population of older adults and disabled patients is noted to have a high burden of migraine [5, 20], with almost one in five members of this cohort bearing a high disease burden [24, 25, 32]. Headache accounts for 14.9% of female patient and 6.1% of male patient general practitioner visits in Australia [33]. Globally, the tenth most common symptom in elderly women is headache [34]. Prevalence of chronic headache among older adults ranges from 5 to 24.4%—note that this occurs more commonly in women, as per a series of publications [30, 35–37].

Migraine Symptoms in Older Adults

Notably, the clinical phenotype of migraine appears to change with age [38]. Photophobia, phonophobia, nausea, and vomiting associated with migraine are reduced, while autonomic symptoms such as bilateral tearing, rhinorrhea, and neck pain may be increased [30, 39]. Wober-Bingol C et al. reported these differences in clinical features in a cross-sectional study of 260 consecutive patients with an age range of 3–69 years [17] [29]. Physical activity-related worsening headache decreased with age [29]. The duration of headache, unilateral pain, light sensitivity, and noise sensitivity all increased with age among females [29]. Interestingly, the percentage of males with migraine tends to decrease from childhood to adulthood [29].

Martins et al. noticed increased autonomic symptoms such as tachycardia, facial flushing, sweating, dry mouth, and reduced sensory sensitivities as migraine tends to occur among older adults [24]. Kelman reported the increased occurrence of neck pain among acute attacks of migraine in older adults [28]. Straub et al. reviewed the pathophysiological changes of migraine across life, linking the different compartments of the brain (hypothalamus, brainstem, components of the autonomic nervous system) to explain the different clinical phenotypes of migraine [40].

The Impact of Comorbidities

Physiological changes of aging, comorbid disorders, and consequent polypharmacy make managing migraine in older adults particularly challenging [10, 32]. Many of these patients are likely to be on long-term therapy for hypertension, ischemic heart disease, diabetes, mood disorders, and/or dyslipidemia [10]. The prevalence of chronic pain among the elderly is also high (estimated at 25–85%) [41]. It is not surprising to see the 30% prevalence of medication overuse headache (MOH) in this cohort [11, 34, 42].

It is worth noting that the female predominance of migraine tends to decrease after menopause [28, 35, 43]. Islamoska et al. argue for the hypothesis that migraine is a midlife risk factor for dementia in later life [43]. Another study reviewed headaches among seniors above the age of 65 years with mild to moderate cognitive impairment (severe cognitive impairment or dementia patients were excluded from the study) [44]. 13.8% of all patients (1237 patients, with a mean age of 75.6 years and with equal representation of men and women) were suffering from probable migraine [44].

Diagnosing Migraine and Other Causes of Headache in Older Adults

Migraine in older adults is more likely to be underdiagnosed, undertreated, and mismanaged.

Alternatively, readers should make a note that certain primary headache disorders such as hypnic headache and primary cough headache are more common among older adults. The prevalence and incidence of primary headache syndromes appear to decrease with age. The majority of older adults suffering from chronic migraine have had the onset of migraine before they were fifty years of age [27–29]. It is well known that the secondary headache syndromes increase in incidence among older adults with sinister differential diagnoses such as neoplasms, postherpetic neuralgia, intracranial hemorrhage, giant cell arteritis, and cervicogenic headaches with sinister pathobiology complicating the clinical picture at times [45, 46].

Late-Life Migraine Accompaniments

One of the reasons behind the misdiagnosis of migraine among older adults is the less classical presentation of symptoms. A Brazilian cohort study of migraine in older adults further confirmed this issue, showing patients may display bilateral headaches with an otherwise featureless presentation to the clinic [30]. Migraine in older adults may also present with aura phase [34]. Some older adult patients may present with shorter attacks of migraine [44].

Late-life migraine accompaniments (LLMA) or migraine without aura is well reported among older adults [47–49]. The late C. M. Fisher reported LLMA in 1980 in a cohort of 120 patients with "unexplained TIA" and a normal comprehensive vascular workup suggesting LLMA [48]. One in six of these patients [25] had paresthesia, while 18 of them had changes in vision and speech. A further 14 had vision changes, speech changes, and paresthesia during the episode. Seven had brain stem involvement and vision involvement. A further one in six of these patients, 25 were patients with an old stroke reproducing the old stroke deficit again. Fisher proposed the term "Late-Life Migraine Accompaniments" to refer to the occurrence of two or more similar episodes in the setting of normal vascular and brain imaging coupled with the presence of migraine-like scintillations. LLMA is thus an important differential diagnosis in the setting of acute stroke diagnosis [47–49].

LLMA tends to generate spreading visual, speech, and sensory disturbances that can present as acute events at times, rarely lasting more than sixty minutes [50]. These symptoms can occur before, during, or after an acute attack of migraine. Fisher reported over 300 cases of LLMA with a comprehensive analysis of clinical phenotypes of LLMA—including his own symptoms—over 27 years with a detailed manuscript [47–49].

C.M. Fisher's criteria for LLMA are as follows:

1. Presence of visual symptoms.
2. A march of paresthesia.
3. Gradual buildup of symptoms (expansion or migration of the symptoms including scintillating display).
4. The serial progression of one type of accompaniment to the other (e.g., visual to paresthesia).
5. The occurrence of two or more identical spells of symptoms.
6. Headache (50% of patients).
7. Slightly longer duration than TIA (majority of TIA lasts less than 15 minutes despite the 24-hour definition by the WHO while LLMA typically lasts up 25 minutes (less than an hour generally).
8. Benign clinical course.
9. Patients between 50 and 60 years of age group may have a flurry of occurrence of LLMA.
10. No evidence of cerebral vascular thrombo-embolism or prothrombotic status.
11. Normal brain and vascular imaging.
12. No evidence of atherosclerosis.

Additional observations from his detailed case studies are summarized below.

Ten patients from his case series were noted to have intermittent horizontal or vertical diplopia lasting from a few seconds to a few minutes. Half of the patients with sensory symptoms experienced numbness of the tongue. Specific focal numbness such as one toe, one finger, tip of the tongue, the chin on one side, or a small patch in the face appears to be more suggestive of LLMA. A few patients reported triggers such as stress or telephone ringing, while some patients described a presyncope experience. A few patients described a sudden, severe pain in the head as if they were struck with a sledgehammer. Some patients experienced a sound in their ear or head or transient tinnitus. Some patients were quite certain that the numbness in their finger or hand lasted only for a second or few seconds. Cerebral amyloid angiopathy (CAA) and amyloid spells are an important differential diagnosis to consider [51]. MRI brain with SWI sequences is most helpful to sort out these two clinical conundrums.

Treatment Considerations

Headache is known to interfere significantly with quality of life by limiting domestic day-to-day activities as well as leisure activities/community activities, thus having a very high burden of disability in older adults [44].

Drug interactions must be considered in the case of migraine in older adults at all times. The 2019 update to the Beer criteria reported that one of the largest relative increases in opioid use was in older adults [52]. Use of simple analgesics such as acetaminophen and nonsteroidal anti-inflammatory drugs should prompt primary care physicians to keep a close eye on renal and liver functions (with special added attention to the function of the gastrointestinal system and cardiovascular system) among older adults with migraine. The prescriber must be cautious with the use of triptans and ergot-based medications due to the vascular effects of these medications on older adults with migraine. Neuroleptics and antiemetics can be used—albeit with caution—among older adults with migraine.

The clinical goal of the management of an acute attack continues to be achieving a sustained pain-free response (both two-hour pain freedom and twenty-four hour pain freedom) [53]. Adverse effects must be monitored cautiously. Novel therapeutic agents such as the one ditan, lasmiditan, and three available calcitonin gene-related peptide (CGRP) receptor antagonists, rimegepant, ubrogepant, and zavegepant, provide promise as nonvasoconstrictor options in the acute management of migraine among older adults [54]. In addition, lifestyle modifications and behavioral interventions, including Life's Ten [55], are of paramount importance in older adults (daily walking, sleep hygiene, mindfulness, etc.) [56, 57].

Of the nonspecific preventive agents, topiramate should be monitored due to the potential for cognitive side effects and weight loss. Tricyclic antidepressants may induce sedation and cardiac conduction abnormalities. Antihypertensive medications may worsen orthostatic hypotension. Beta-blockers should be used with caution to avoid heart block. Candesartan probably has the least adverse effects in this cohort of patients. While sodium valproate is a useful preventative agent, the tremor and gastrointestinal side effects can be bothersome for some patients. CGRP-blocking agents can be safely used in migraine among older adults as per the clinical indications. OnabotulinumtoxinA, neuromodulation therapies, and nerve blocks can be used as appropriate as per the clinical setting.

Conclusion

The prevalence of migraine among older adults has risen over the years. The added differential diagnoses, associated medical conditions and comorbidities, age-specific pharmacodynamic and pharmacokinetic properties, and drug-drug interactions create additional challenges for the physician and the patient. Older adults with migraine must be included in ongoing clinical trials. A careful workup and proper management should help us reduce disability and improve quality of life among older adults with migraine.

Teaching Points

1. Migraine is one of the most common primary headache disorders with significant disability among older adults.
2. Given the aging population in the world, migraine in older adults is an important public health problem.
3. Migraine in older adults can present with unique and different clinical symptoms than in young people.
4. Clinical differentiation, assessment, investigation, and treatment of important secondary headache disorders are particularly important among older adults.
5. Consider the unique comorbidities and drug interactions that are different and common among older adults.

Case

A 79-year-old woman had a four-year history of headaches. She never had headaches as a young person. Headaches were intermittent, occurring 2–3 hours daily. Headaches were associated with sensitivity to light and noise. She denied symptoms suggestive of a visual aura. At times, headaches recurred at nighttime, once or twice per night, with a washed out, drained experience for several days afterward. History included ischemic heart disease, previous right basal ganglia lacunar infarct, controlled hypertension, osteoarthritis, and chronic, mild renal impairment.

Her visual acuity was 20/20, corrected; optic discs showed grade two hypertensive changes. Both temporal arteries were palpable with no tenderness. The rest of the cranial nerves were normal.

She had a good range of neck movements. Assessment of her upper and lower limbs showed normal tone, power, coordination, reflexes and sensory examination for pinprick, touch, joint position sense, and vibration in all four limbs. Her gait was normal.

Her blood pressure in the office was 140/90 mmHg.

Initial investigations revealed elevated creatinine, normal sodium, and potassium. ESR was 11, and CRP was 3. MRI/MRA/MRV brain revealed nonspecific T2 changes considered age-appropriate. On further questioning, she was noted to take Ibuprofen 400–800 mg on most days, more than twenty days per month, for the last four years.

Case Discussion

Based on the clinical features, she was diagnosed with migraine without aura, medication-overuse headaches, and chronic migraine. There were no red flags to suggest a secondary headache disorder.

She was introduced to the concept of SEEDS (Sleep, exercise, healthy diet and fluid intake, diary, and stress management program). She was introduced to magnesium and vitamin B2 daily. Her blood pressure medications were changed to Candesartan tablet daily. She was educated on medication overuse headaches, and acute interventions for headaches with analgesics were restricted to less than two days per week. She underwent a gentle neck physiotherapy program over the next eight weeks.

She had a 50% reduction in headaches within the next three months. Her renal functions improved. She no longer consumes over-the-counter analgesics and is aware of sustained pain-free response and triptan usage.

Questions and Answers

1. Annual prevalence of migraine in older adults is.
   A. 3%
   B. 30%
   C. 10%
   D. 35%
   E. 50%.

The correct answer is C. Migraine has a 10% prevalence in older adults on an annual basis and is the second most common headache disorder after tension headache in older adults (Ref. [10])

2. Which of the following statements is true?
   A. Photophobia is common among migraine in older adults.
   B. One-year prevalence of migraine in older adults is 30%.

C. Nausea is not reported in migraine in older adults.
D. Bilateral headache is commonly reported in migraine in older adults.
E. Autonomic symptoms are uncommon in migraine in older adults.

The correct answer is D. Published work shows that older adults can have different migraine symptomatology. Migraine in elderly is more often bilateral. Migraine in older adults can present without sensitivity to light and sound. Migraine in elderly is noted to be associated with less cranial autonomic symptoms (Ref. [32])

References

1. Steiner TJ, Stovner LJ, Vos T, Jensen R, Katsarava Z. Migraine is first cause of disability in under 50s: will health politicians now take notice? J Headache Pain. 2018;19(1):17.
2. Steiner TJ, Stovner LJ, Jensen R, Uluduz D, Katsarava Z. on behalf of Lifting The Burden: the Global Campaign against H. Migraine remains second among the world's causes of disability, and first among young women: findings from GBD2019. J Headache Pain. 2020;21(1):137.
3. Stovner LJ, Hagen K, Linde M, Steiner TJ. The global prevalence of headache: an update, with analysis of the influences of methodological factors on prevalence estimates. J Headache Pain. 2022;23(1):34.
4. Feigin VL, Vos T, Alahdab F, Amit AML, Bärnighausen TW, Beghi E, et al. Burden of neurological disorders across the US from 1990–2017: a global burden of disease study. JAMA Neurol. 2021;78(2):165–76.
5. Salter A, Fox RJ, Newsome SD, Halper J, Li DKB, Kanellis P, et al. Outcomes and risk factors associated with SARS-CoV-2 infection in a north american registry of patients with multiple sclerosis. JAMA Neurol. 2021;78:699.
6. Wijeratne T, Wijeratne C. Clinical utility of serial systemic immune inflammation indices (SSIIi) in the context of post covid-19 neurological syndrome (PCNS). J Neurol Sci. 2021;423:117356.
7. Wijeratne T, Gillard Crewther S, Sales C, Karimi L. COVID-19 pathophysiology predicts that ischemic stroke occurrence is an expectation, not an exception – a systematic review. Front Neurol. 2021;11(1759)
8. Kursun O, Yemisci M, van den Maagdenberg AMJM, Karatas H. Migraine and neuroinflammation: the inflammasome perspective. J Headache Pain. 2021;22(1):55.
9. Wijeratne T, Murphy MJ, Wijeratne C, Martelletti P, Karimi L, Apostolopoulos V, et al. Serial systemic immune inflammation indices: markers of acute migraine events or indicators of persistent inflammatory status? J Headache Pain. 2025;26(1):7.
10. Wijeratne T, Tang HM, Crewther D, Crewther S. Prevalence of migraine in the elderly: a narrated review. Neuroepidemiology. 2019;52(1–2):104–10. https://doi.org/10.1159/000494758.
11. Wijeratne T, Jenkins B, Stark RJ, Sun-Edelstein C. Assessing and managing medication overuse headache in Australian clinical practice. BMJ Neurol Open. 2023;5(1):e000418.
12. Global age-sex-specific mortality. life expectancy, and population estimates in 204 countries and territories and 811 subnational locations, 1950–2021, and the impact of the COVID-19 pandemic: a comprehensive demographic analysis for the Global Burden of Disease Study 2021. Lancet. 2024;403(10440):1989–2056.
13. Wijeratne T, Dodick D, Grisold W, Carroll W. World brain Day 2019; migraine – the painful truth. Eur J Neurol. 2019;26(11):e92–e3.
14. Wijeratne T, Grisold W, Dodick D, Carroll W. World brain day 2019: migraine, the painful truth. Lancet Neurol. 2019;18(10):914.
15. Stark RJ, Ravishankar K, Siow HC, Lee KS, Pepperle R, Wang SJ. Chronic migraine and chronic daily headache in the Asia-Pacific region: a systematic review. Cephalalgia. 2013;33(4):266–83.
16. Genc D, Vaičienė-Magistris N, Zaborskis A, Şaşmaz T, Tunç AY, Uluduz D, et al. The burden attributable to headache disorders in children and adolescents in Lithuania: estimates from a national schools-based study. J Headache Pain. 2021;22(1):24.
17. Wober-Bingol C, Wober C, Karwautz A, Auterith A, Serim M, Zebenholzer K, et al. Clinical features of migraine: a cross-sectional study in patients aged three to sixty-nine. Cephalalgia. 2004;24(1):12–7.
18. Wöber-Bingöl Ç, Wöber C, Uluduz D, Uygunoğlu U, Aslan TS, Kernmayer M, et al. The global burden of headache in children and adolescents – developing a questionnaire and methodology for a global study. J Headache Pain. 2014;15(1):86.
19. Haan J, Hollander J, Ferrari MD. Migraine in the elderly: a review. Cephalalgia Int J Headache. 2007;27(2):97–106.
20. Eller M, Goadsby PJ. Migraine: a brain state amenable to therapy. Med J Aust. 2020;212(1):32–9.
21. Lipton RB, Fanning KM, Buse DC, Martin VT, Hohaia LB, Adams AM, et al. Migraine progression in subgroups of migraine based on comorbidities: Results of the CaMEO Study. Neurology. 2019;93(24):e2224–e36.
22. Goadsby PJ, Lipton RB, Ferrari MD. Migraine – current understanding and treatment. N Engl J Med. 2002;346(4):257–70.
23. Goadsby PJ. Migraine: diagnosis and management. Intern Med J. 2003;33(9–10):436–42.
24. Burch RC, Loder S, Loder E, Smitherman TA. The prevalence and burden of migraine and severe headache in the United States: updated statistics from government health surveillance studies. Headache. 2015;55(1):21–34.
25. Burch R, Rizzoli P, Loder E. The prevalence and impact of migraine and severe headache in the United States: figures and trends from government health studies. Headache. 2018;58(4):496–505.
26. Stewart WF, Lipton RB, Celentano DD, Reed ML. Prevalence of migraine headache in the United States. Relation to age, income, race, and other sociodemographic factors. JAMA. 1992;267(1):64–9.
27. Lisotto C, Mainardi F, Maggioni F, Zanchin G. Headache in Sturge-Weber syndrome: a case report and review of the literature. Cephalalgia. 2004;24(11):1001–4.
28. Lisotto C, Mainardi F, Maggioni F, Dainese F, Zanchin G. Headache in the elderly: a clinical study. J Headache Pain. 2004;5(1):36–41.
29. Lisotto C, Mainardi F, Maggioni F, Zanchin G. Episodic hypnic headache? Cephalalgia. 2004;24(8):681–5.
30. Martins KM, Bordini CA, Bigal ME, Speciali JG. Migraine in the elderly: a comparison with migraine in young adults. Headache. 2006;46(2):312–6.
31. Prencipe M, Casini AR, Ferretti C, Santini M, Pezzella F, Scaldaferri N, et al. Prevalence of headache in an elderly population: attack frequency, disability, and use of medication. J Neurol Neurosurg Psychiatry. 2001;70(3):377–81.
32. Riggins N, Ehrlich A. Episodic migraine and older adults. Curr Pain Headache Rep. 2022;26(4):331–5. https://doi.org/10.1007/s11916-022-01029-7.
33. Stark RJ, Valenti L, Miller GC. Management of migraine in Australian general practice. Med J Aust. 2007;187(3):142–6.
34. Sharma TL. Common primary and secondary causes of headache in the elderly. Headache. 2018;58(3):479–84.
35. Robblee J, Singh RH. Headache in the older population: causes, diagnoses, and treatments. Curr Pain Headache Rep. 2020;24(7):34.
36. Linn J, Schwarz F, Reinisch V, Straube A. Ophthalmoplegic migraine with paresis of the sixth nerve: a neurovascular compression syndrome? Cephalalgia. 2008;28(6):667–70.

37. Camarda R, Monastero R. Prevalence of primary headaches in Italian elderly: preliminary data from the Zabut Aging Project. Neurol Sci Off J Italian Neurol Soc Italian Soci Clin Neurophysiol. 2003;24(Suppl 2):S122–4.
38. Starling AJ. Diagnosis and management of headache in older adults. Mayo Clin Proc. 2018;93(2):252–62.
39. Kelman L. Migraine changes with age: IMPACT on migraine classification. Headache. 2006;46(7):1161–71.
40. Straube A, Andreou A. Primary headaches during lifespan. J Headache Pain. 2019;20(1):35.
41. Stompór M, Grodzicki T, Stompór T, Wordliczek J, Dubiel M, Kurowska I. Prevalence of chronic pain, particularly with neuropathic component, and its effect on overall functioning of elderly patients. Med Sci Monit Int Med J Exp Clin Res. 2019;25:2695–701.
42. de Rijk P, Resseguier N, Donnet A. Headache characteristics and clinical features of elderly migraine patients. Headache. 2018;58(4):525–33.
43. Islamoska S, Hansen ÅM, Wang H-X, Garde AH, Andersen PK, Garde E, et al. Mid- to late-life migraine diagnoses and risk of dementia: a national register-based follow-up study. J Headache Pain. 2020;21(1):98.
44. Feleppa M, Fucci S, Bigal ME. Primary headaches in an elderly population seeking medical care for cognitive decline. Headache. 2017;57(2):209–16.
45. Schankin CJ, Ferrari U, Reinisch VM, Birnbaum T, Goldbrunner R, Straube A. Characteristics of brain tumour-associated headache. Cephalalgia. 2007;27(8):904–11.
46. Reinisch VM, Schankin CJ, Felbinger J, Sostak P, Straube A. Headache in the elderly. Schmerz. 2008;22(Suppl 1):22–30.
47. Fisher CM. Late-life (migrainous) scintillating zigzags without headache: one person's 27-year experience. Headache. 1999;39(6):391–7.
48. Fisher CM. Late-life migraine accompaniments as a cause of unexplained transient ischemic attacks. Can J Neurol Sci. 1980;7(1):9–17.
49. Fisher CM. Late-life migraine accompaniments – further experience. Stroke. 1986;17(5):1033–42.
50. Headache Classification Committee of the International Headache Society (IHS) The international classification of headache disorders, 3rd edn. Cephalalgia. 2018;38(1):1–211.
51. Caetano A, Pinto M, Calado S, Viana-Baptista M. Amyloid spells and high blood pressure: imminent danger? Case Rep Neurol. 2015;7(1):39–43.
52. American Geriatrics Society 2019. Updated AGS beers criteria® for potentially inappropriate medication use in older adults. J Am Geriatr Soc. 2019;67(4):674–94.
53. VanderPluym JH, Halker Singh RB, Urtecho M, Morrow AS, Nayfeh T, Torres Roldan VD, et al. Acute treatments for episodic migraine in adults: a systematic review and meta-analysis. JAMA. 2021;325(23):2357–69.
54. Johnston K, Popoff E, Deighton A, Dabirvaziri P, Harris L, Thiry A, et al. Comparative efficacy and safety of rimegepant, ubrogepant, and lasmiditan for acute treatment of migraine: a network meta-analysis. Expert Rev Pharmacoecon Outcomes Res. 2022;22(1):155–66.
55. Wijeratne T, Wijeratne C. Unveiling the migraine chronicles 2024. ISBN 9780646898025. Australia: AIM.
56. Buse DC, Fanning KM, Reed ML, Murray S, Dumas PK, Adams AM, et al. Life with migraine: effects on relationships, career, and finances from the Chronic Migraine Epidemiology and Outcomes (CaMEO) study. Headache J Head Face Pain. 2019;59(8):1286–99.
57. Pérez-Muñoz A, Buse DC, Andrasik F. Behavioral interventions for migraine. Neurol Clin. 2019;37(4):789–813.

Vestibular Migraine

34

Danielle Gillard and Jeffrey D. Sharon

Introduction

Dizziness and vertigo are two of the most common chief complaints in medicine, across a variety of settings including the emergency room and outpatient clinics [1, 2]. According to the Barany Society, vertigo is the illusory sensation of movement, whereas dizziness is "disturbed or impaired spatial orientation without a false or distorted sense of motion" [3]. It is important to separate this from presyncope and other feelings of lightheadedness or malaise (e.g., the feeling of hypoglycemia) to avoid diagnostic errors. A thoughtful approach, relying on a detailed history and physical exam, is required for precise diagnosis.

Migraine, a common and complex neurological disorder, is intertwined with dizziness and vertigo in several ways. First, vestibular migraine (VM) is now recognized as a distinct manifestation of migraine, characterized by vestibular symptoms, frequently without headache. Second, there is an association between benign paroxysmal vertigo of childhood and future migraine development. In this disorder, children typically aged 2–8 experience episodic vertigo lasting seconds to minutes [4]. Third, a personal history of migraine is a risk factor for the development of several other vestibular disorders, including BPPV (benign paroxysmal positional vertigo), Meniere's disease, and bilateral vestibular loss [5–7]. Finally, many of those with migraine, even without vertigo, do suffer from high rates of motion sensitivity, and sensitivity to busy visual scenes.

VM is one of the most common causes of dizziness and vertigo in the world. It is more common than other better-known causes of vertigo, such as Meniere's disease. Recent years have seen increased attention from relevant practitioners, including otolaryngologists, neurologists, researchers, audiologists, and physical therapists. In this chapter, we will provide a detailed overview of vestibular migraine.

Questions

1. Which of the following is NOT consistent with a diagnosis of vestibular migraine per Barany Society criteria?
   A. Episodic vertigo lasting hours
   B. Unilateral tinnitus, aural pressure, and hearing loss during vertigo episodes
   C. A prior history of migraine with aura
   D. Photophobia and phonophobia during vertigo episodes
   E. A lifetime total of 17 vertigo episodes
2. A "catch-up saccade" seen during horizontal head impulse testing to the left is most consistent with which diagnosis?
   A. BPPV
   B. Vestibular migraine
   C. Unilateral vestibular hypofunction
   D. Meniere's disease
   E. Superior semicircular canal dehiscence

Epidemiology

VM has an estimated prevalence of between 1% and 2.7% of the adult population [8, 9]. It can present as the initial migraine manifestation or in individuals already diagnosed with a classic migraine syndrome [10, 11]. Based on the 2008 National Health Interview Survey data [8], 11.9% of the US population reported dizziness over the prior year and 23% of those individuals met the case definition for VM. VM is more likely to present between the third and sixth decade of life, and has a female predominance [10, 12]. Sex hormones likely play a role in pathophysiology, with one study showing estradiol levels were negatively correlated with vestibular migraine frequency and severity in post-menopausal women [13, 14]. A majority of patients with VM have had to miss work or school due to dizziness. They also have a higher rate of falls than the general population and individuals with

D. Gillard · J. D. Sharon (✉)
Division of Otology, Neurotology, and Lateral Skull Base Surgery, Department of Otolaryngology-Head and Neck Surgery, University of California, San Francisco, CA, USA

T. S. Monteith et al. (eds.), *Comprehensive Migraine Management*, https://doi.org/10.1007/978-3-031-86923-5_34

non-VM causes of dizziness. Underdiagnosis in this population is common.

Pathophysiology

The pathophysiology of VM is not fully understood but is thought to include the trigeminovascular system, sensory hypersensitivity including to motion, and reciprocal connections between structures involved in trigeminal nociceptive inputs and the vestibular nuclei in the brainstem [15]. The trigeminovascular system is thought to be important for the clinical manifestations of VM. Inflammatory peptides released by this system, especially CGRP (Calcitonin Gene-Related Peptide) may affect inner ear structures. CGRP has been detected in the vestibular system of multiple animal models as well as the human vestibular system [16–20]. CGRP-positive neurons have been located centrally near the vestibular nuclei that project directly to vestibular end organs, the vestibular nucleus, and vestibular cerebellum [20–23]. Expression is also seen in the peripheral vestibular organs where it is co-expressed with choline acetyltransferase. CGRP knockout mice have perturbations of the cochleovestibular system including reductions in sound-evoked activity in the cochlear nerve [24], reduced vestibulo-ocular reflex (VOR) gain, with no effect in VOR phase [25] reduced otolith activation timing and impaired balance [26]. Therefore, one working theory is that activation of the trigeminovascular system during an acute migrainous attack leads to release of peptides like CGRP in the central and peripheral vestibular systems, causing the vestibular symptoms seen in VM. In addition, CGRP and CGRP receptor expression are prominent in the cerebellum [27].

However, patients with VM often report vertigo and motion-sensitivity symptoms between acute migraine attacks. It is thought that patients with VM have lower thresholds for sensory stimuli, including motion. Different tests of multisensory information have shown abnormalities in VM patients [28]. On subjective visual vertical testing, patients with VM make more errors than healthy controls with their head tilted 20 degrees [29] and have lower perceptual thresholds during low frequency roll tilt testing [30], suggesting they have abnormal sensory integration for spatial orientation processing. Functional imaging studies support this theory, with alterations seen in the primary vestibular cortex, multisensory processing areas, and thalamic circuitry [31].

Presentation

It is important to note that postural and balance impairment is common in migraine with and without aura, not necessarily meeting criteria for vestibular migraine.

The most common presenting symptom of VM is vertigo [32], but patients often describe a variety of other symptoms during attacks including nausea, headache, light and sound sensitivity, tinnitus, and aural pressure. An acute episode can last from minutes to days. Between attacks, VM patients may be asymptomatic; however, it is common for patients to report motion sensitivity or sensitivity to certain visual stimuli such as patterns, motion, large amounts of visual information, or certain lighting. They have a higher reported rate of motion sickness than the general population [33].

VM patients can have nystagmus during an acute episode. However, presentation is not consistent across patients and there is not one pattern that is diagnostic for VM. One study of VM has shown that patients had a variety of types of nystagmus including spontaneous nystagmus or positional nystagmus which did not extinguish with time [34]. This is an important distinction between nystagmus in VM and BPPV, as BPPV nystagmus is also positional, but will extinguish with repeat provocation. Like subjective vertigo symptoms, nystagmus can also be seen between acute attacks. On testing, nystagmus has been reported for 60% of VM patients interictally, including gaze-evoked nystagmus with saccadic smooth pursuit, horizontal or vertical spontaneous nystagmus, and central positional nystagmus [11]. However, results are inconsistent across studies.

Lastly, patients can also present with a variety of other otologic symptoms during an acute attack. Patients have reported pulsatile and non-pulsatile tinnitus, aural fullness, subjective hearing loss, neck stiffness, facial numbness, and facial pressure [35]. Patients with VM also report cognitive dysfunction. They have an increased frequency of everyday cognitive slips as measured by the cognitive fails questionnaire compared to individuals with Meniere's disease or BPPV [36–38].

An acute vestibular migraine episode can be triggered by stress, certain food or drink, skipped meals, bright light, allergy, changes in barometric pressure, loud sounds, busy visual scenes, and hormonal changes such as menopause in women [39]. In our center, about half of patients with VM have a positive family history of migraine. Furthermore, almost half of the patients have a comorbid diagnosis of depression or anxiety. It is important to note that VM significantly reduces patient quality of life. Patients are more likely to miss work or school or fall due to their diagnosis [8].

Figure 34.1 shows vertigo triggers, associated symptoms, episode length, episode frequency, and secondary vestibular diagnoses for a cohort of 51 VM patients in the author's practice.

Diagnostic Criteria

Lempert and Neuhauser described the first diagnostic criteria for VM in 2001 based on four basic criteria [40–42]: (1) recurrent vestibular symptoms, (2) migraine based on the

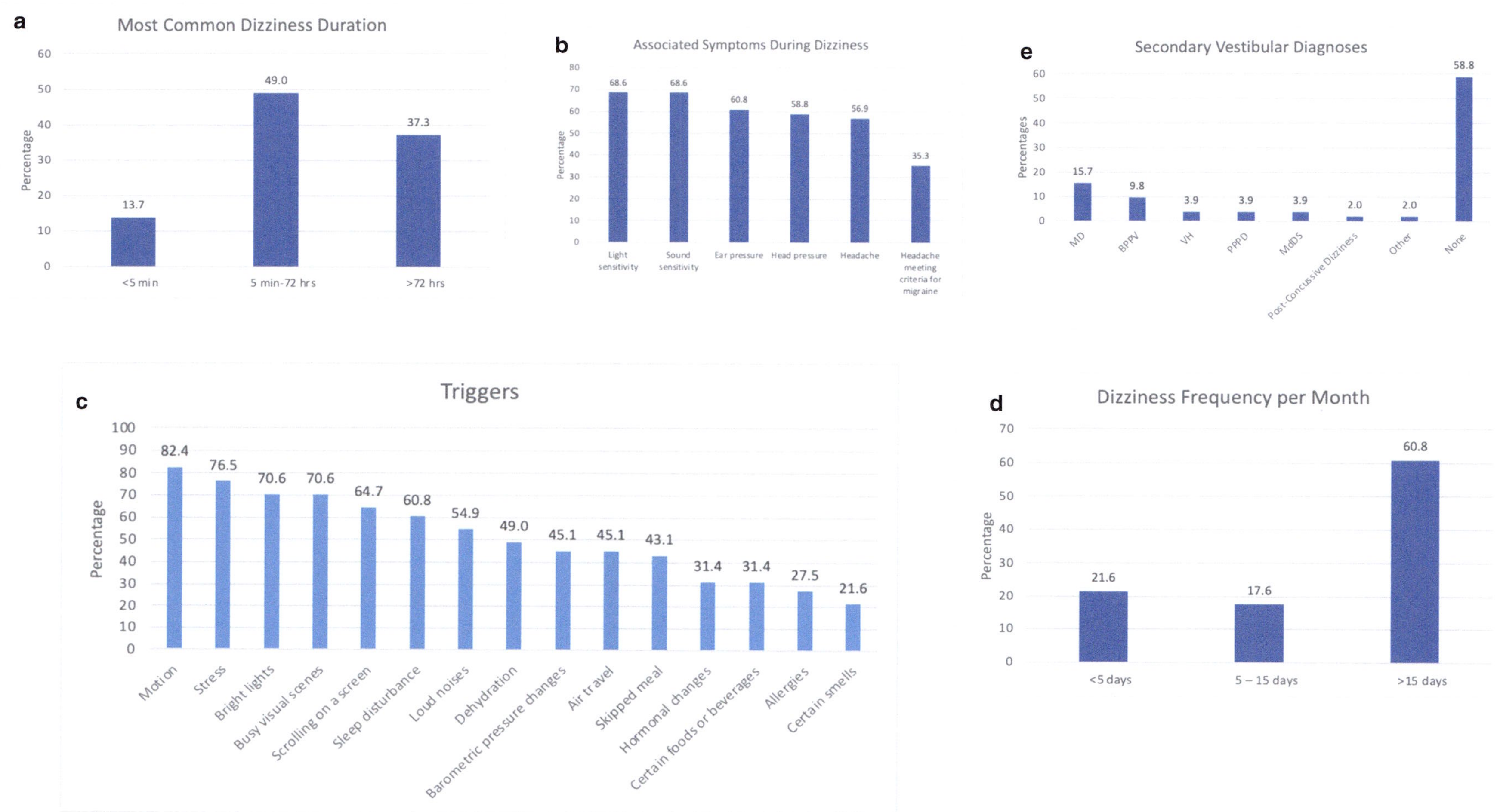

Fig. 34.1 Clinical characteristics of vestibular migraine. Unpublished from a UCSF study of 51 subjects with VM. (**a**) Most common triggers of VM. (**b**) Associated symptoms during dizziness. (**c**) Dizziness duration. (**d**) Dizziness frequency per month. (**e**) Secondary vestibular diagnoses

Table 34.1 Barany Society criteria for the diagnosis of vestibular migraine

A. Vestibular Migraine
(a) At least 5 episodes with vestibular symptoms
(i) Severity: Moderate–severe
(ii) Timing: 5 min–72 h
(b) History of migraine +/− aura according to ICHD-3
(c) ≥1 of the following migraine features occurring with at least 50% of vestibular episodes
(i) Headache
1. Unilateral, pulsating, moderate–severe pain, aggravated by physical activity
(ii) Photophobia, phonophobia
(iii) Visual aura
(d) Not better accounted for by ICHD-3 diagnosis
B. Probable Vestibular Migraine
(a) At least 5 episodes with vestibular symptoms
(i) Severity: Moderate–severe
(ii) Timing: 5 min–72 h
(b) Has either (b) or (c) from above criteria but NOT both
(c) Not better accounted for by ICHD-3 diagnosis

Diagnostic criteria for vestibular migraine and probable vestibular migraine from the Barany Society criteria (Lempert et al. [43])

International Headache Society (IHS) criteria, (3) migraine symptoms such as headache, photophobia, phonophobia, or auras, during vertigo attacks, and (4) other possible causes have been ruled out.

The Barany Society criteria are now more commonly used by practitioners (Table 34.1). This criteria breaks VM down to VM or probable VM. VM is defined as at least five episodes of vestibular symptoms with migrainous features with a personal history of migraine. Probable VM does not require a history of diagnosis of migraine or classical migraine symptoms during vestibular attacks. A description of vestibular migraine can be found in the appendix of the International Classification of Headache Disorders (ICHD-3) [44].

Work-Up

Vestibular migraine is a clinical diagnosis and imaging and laboratory testing is usually normal in these individuals. Appropriate clinical history includes thorough review of vertigo characteristics including timing of episodes, triggers, associated symptoms, stroke risk factors, family history of migraine and history of otologic or neurologic surgery. Episodes triggered by certain foods, pressure changes, visual stimuli, etc., are more indicative of VM, while positional triggers are more consistent with BPPV and Meniere's is often unprovoked. Physical exam should include a complete cranial nerve exam, otoscopy, cerebellar examination, and a vestibular exam. Provocative vestibular testing can help rule out alternative diagnoses such as BPPV. In BPPV, the Dix-Hallpike test provokes a characteristic upbeating nystagmus with a rotational component that beats towards the lower (geotropic) ear. Abnormal head impulse testing, which assesses the vestibulo-ocular-reflex, is indicative of vestibular hypofunction (Fig. 34.2). Abnormal smooth pursuit, inaccurate saccades, and ataxia point to an alternate cerebellar cause of vertigo.

Audiometry can be useful for ruling out other related vertiginous illnesses including vestibular schwannoma, Meniere's disease, and labyrinthitis in which patients also present with sensorineural hearing loss in addition to vertigo. Formal vestibular testing, including videonystagmography, rotational chair testing, video head impulse testing, or vestibular evoked myogenic potentials, has not shown consistent results that are diagnostic for VM. In a study that compared VM patients to patients with other causes of dizziness, there was no significant difference in the majority of neuro-otological tests [45].

There are two major validated surveys that can be used to evaluate symptoms and handicap in patients with VM. The Dizziness Handicap Inventory (DHI) is a validated survey for use in vestibular disorders. More recently, a VM-specific survey tool has been developed, the Vestibular Migraine Patient Assessment Tool and Handicap Inventory (VM-PATHI) [46]. The VM-PATHI is freely available at the University of California San Francisco (USCF) Balance and Falls Website (https://ohns.ucsf.edu/balance-falls/vestibular-migraine). The final validated survey contains 25 symptom-based questions that cover the following domains: cognition, emotional disturbance, disequilibrium, anxiety, motion sensitivity, and headache equivalents (Fig. 34.3).

Differential Diagnosis

VM can be difficult to diagnose, as symptoms may overlap with many other common causes of vertigo and in many patients more than one vestibular disorder can co-exist. Important syndromes on the differential for VM include BPPV, Meniere's disease, superior canal dehiscence syndrome (SCDS), vestibular paroxysmia, mal de debarquement syndrome (MdDS), persistent postural perceptual dizziness (PPPD), vestibular neuritis, bilateral vestibular hypofunction, brainstem aura, post-concussive syndrome, vertebrobasilar TIA or stroke, vertebral artery dissection, orthostatic hypotension, peripheral neuropathy, multiple sclerosis, seizures, and cerebellopontine angle tumors. A proposed approach for a chief complaint of dizziness can be seen in Fig. 34.4. Several vestibular disorders with significant overlap with VM are highlighted below.

VM and BPPV can both present with positional vertigo and nystagmus and patients with both disorders often report disequilibrium and dizziness in between clinical attacks. In BPPV, acute vertiginous episodes generally last less than a minute, while VM vertigo attacks, although variable in duration, tend to last longer on the order of hours to days. Nystagmus in posterior canal BPPV is classically torsional and upbeating, short latency, self-limited, and provoked by the Dix-Hallpike maneuver. On the other hand, the nystag-

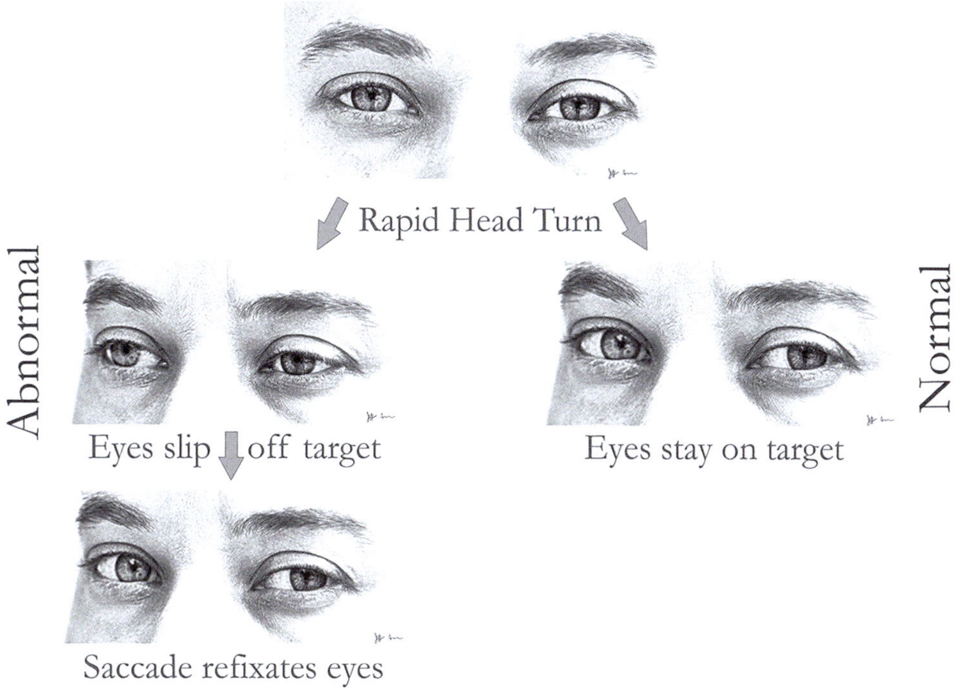

Fig. 34.2 The head impulse test. This is a bedside test of the vestibular system. The test involves a quick head rotation (the impulse) while the patient fixates on a target (typically the examiner's nose). Before performing the test, the practitioner should inquire about neck issues, motion sensitivity, and explain the test in detail. It is best to do the impulse first in "slow motion," to help explain it to the patient. Note that a small rotation is all that is required (5–10 degrees), but that speed is essential (over 150 degrees/second). The figure shows the two possible outcomes. A normal head impulse test indicates a normal vestibulo-ocular reflex for the canal being tested. A normal VOR is far too quick to be seen, so it appears that the eyes just stay fixed on the target. In the abnormal test, the VOR is deficient, and cannot sense the head rotation. Therefore, eyes move with the head, resulting in gaze slippage off target. This is followed by a quick "catch up saccade," in the direction opposite the head turn, which realigns gaze on target. In acute and uncompensated losses, this saccade typically occurs at 200–300 milliseconds, and is therefore visible

Fig. 34.3 VM-PATHI Questionnaire FACTORS. Principal component analysis of VM-PATHI data showed six natural groupings within the data set [46]

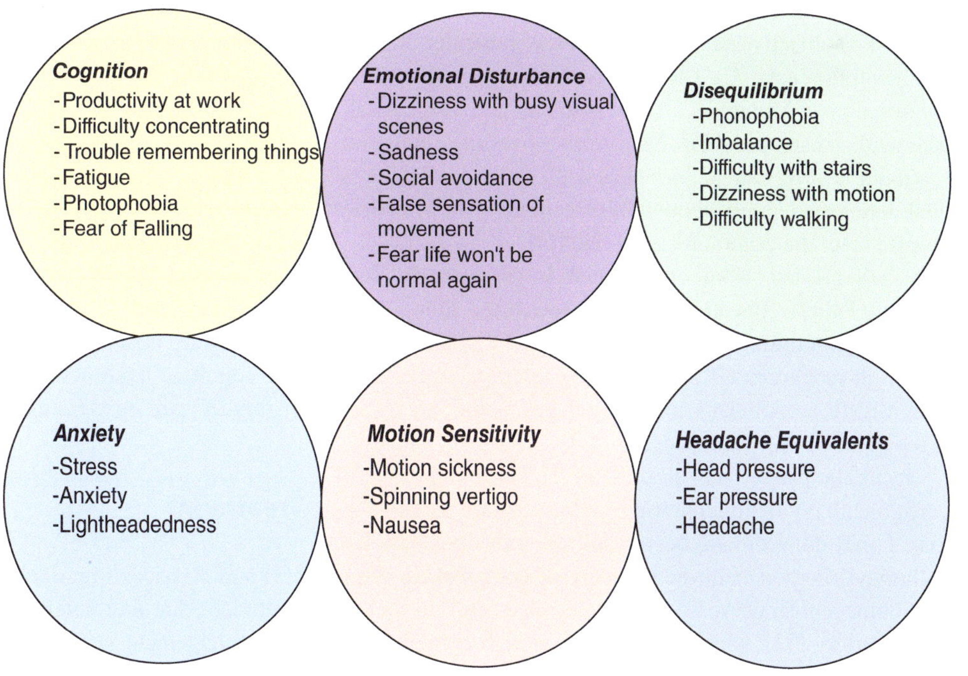

mus seen in VM is variable and can be horizontal, vertical, or torsional [47]. It is often low velocity, low intensity, provoked by head movements, long lasting, and does not fatigue [47]. It is important to note that patients with migraine have an increased risk of BPPV, so both diagnoses can co-exist in one patient [48, 49].

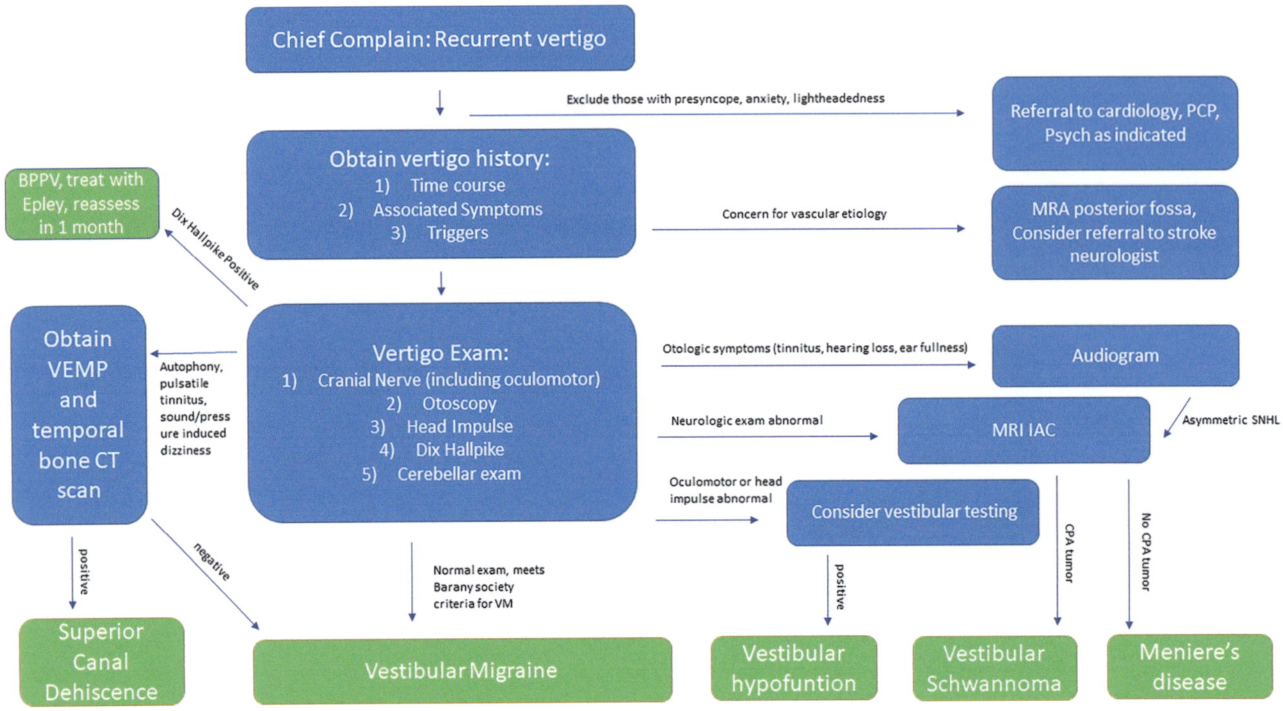

Fig. 34.4 Diagnostic approach to the patient with migraine and recurrent vertigo

VM and Meniere's disease both present with acute attacks of vertigo with longer duration of symptoms. Additionally, both disorders have otologic complaints in addition to vertigo such as tinnitus, aural fullness, and subjective hearing loss. Audiometry in Meniere's disease shows unilateral fluctuating hearing loss, while VM is less likely to have hearing loss on audiometry. Recent studies have shown that VM can progress to objective hearing loss, but it is generally bilateral and low frequency [50]. The most common vestibular testing abnormality in Meniere's disease is unilateral caloric weakness with preserved video head impulse testing. However, vestibular testing can be normal as well. Again, incidence of dual diagnosis is high; about half of patients with Meniere's disease meet the criteria for migraine [6].

SCDS presents with vertigo that is triggered by loud noises (Tulio's phenomenon) or pressure, along with autophony and pulsatile tinnitus (Henneber's sign) [35, 51, 52]. High-resolution CT imaging of the temporal bone, along with VEMP (vestibular evoked myogenic potential) testing is indicated for suspected cases.

Vestibular paroxysmia presents with recurrent episodes of vertigo with no identifiable trigger. Episodes are usually less than 1 min duration and occur multiple times per day. The pathophysiology is believed to be due to compression of the vestibulocochlear nerve by a loop of the anterior inferior cerebellar artery [53], which can be seen on high-resolution T2 MRI.

MdDS is similar to VM in that it can present with chronic dizziness or imbalance and patients report aural fullness, hyperacusis, cognitive disturbance, and visual disturbances [53–56].

PPPD presents with chronic dizziness that is exacerbated by upright posture, motion, or exposure to moving and complex visual stimuli [57]. There is currently overlap between PPPD and vestibular migraine, creating diagnostic confusion. What seems to be clear, though, is that both migraine and central maladaptation including overweighting of visual information (the pathophysiology of PPPD) are frequently seen with chronic vestibular disorders.

Brainstem aura is another migraine subtype that presents with vertigo; however, acute attacks include typical aura (visual and/or sensory and/or speech/language symptoms) and other brainstem symptoms such as ataxia, dysarthria, diplopia, and altered mental status.

Post-concussive syndrome can present identically to VM with vertigo, headache, hypersensitivity to light and sound, and cognitive dysfunction. However, these patients have a history of prior head trauma [57, 58].

Treatment

VM and classical migraine are treated with the same general approach. The first level of treatment consists of conservative management strategies such as stress, reduction, sleep hygiene, treating underlying anxiety, avoiding dietary triggers, stabilizing hormonal fluctuations, and avoiding visual triggers. One study found that 14% of VM patients reported symptomatic improvement after caffeine cessation alone [59].

In addition to conservative management to prevent attacks, symptomatic management of acute attacks is an important part of the initial approach to the treatment of VM. Antiemetics (ondansetron, promethazine, etc.) and vestibular suppressants (meclizine, benzodiazepines, etc.) are important classes of medication to treat acute symptoms. Vestibular specialists are divided as to whether or not they find benzodiazepines helpful for VM. Benzodiazepines are vestibular suppressants, so many (including the authors) feel that long term or daily use can be counterproductive. In addition, physical addiction is a real risk with chronic usage. On the other hand, for select patients who experience discrete episodes of vertigo, and are willing to use the medication responsibly, benzodiazepines can offer powerful symptomatic relief.

Vestibular physical therapy is an important adjuvant treatment for VM [60]. Therapy can restore balance, reduce fall risk, improve motion sensitivity through habituation exercises, and address maladaptive learned behaviors.

Alter failure of conservative management, the next step in therapy is the addition of a prophylactic medication. Tricyclic antidepressants (e.g., nortriptyline), mixed reuptake inhibitors (e.g., venlafaxine), antiepileptics (e.g., topiramate), beta-blockers (e.g., propranolol), and calcium channel blockers (e.g., verapamil) are used to decrease frequency and severity of attacks in VM [61]. Initial choice of medication class is based on comorbidities, medication interactions, and side effect profile (Table 34.2). Some patients can also respond to a combination of multiple prophylactic medications if a single medication does not bring symptoms to manageable levels.

It is unclear if the current approach, which mirrors the paradigm for treatment of classical migraine, is consistently effective for treating VM. In a 2002 retrospective review of this stepwise approach, 16% of patients improved with dietary changes, 66% had significant improvement with medications, and 29% had partial improvement with medications (all patients were started on a tricyclic antidepressant and then a second prophylactic agent was added if symptoms did not have significant improvement) [8, 62]. In another retrospective chart review of the stepwise approach, 15% of patients improved with caffeine cessation while 47% improved with the addition medication (nortriptyline) [59].

There are not many prospective randomized controlled trials of prophylactic medications in VM. A 2013 study comparing betahistidine to paracetamol with or without flunarizine, patients treated with flunarizine had better vertigo control. However, there was no difference in headache symptoms between groups [63]. A 2015 study comparing venlafaxine to propranolol showed both groups had similar, significant improvement in symptoms [63, 64]. It is important to note that neither study has a placebo arm and only the 2015 study measured outcomes with a validated survey tool. Finally, a large German multicenter study of metoprolol (PROVEMIG) was stopped early due to difficulties with patient recruitment. At the end of the study, 114 subjects (54 placebo, 60 metoprolol) were analyzed, and no difference in vertigo rates were seen.

Investigation of abortive therapies is an active area of research for the treatment of VM. Triptans are a promising drug class that have been the subject of a variety of studies. In a randomized, placebo controlled trial, zolmitriptan did not significantly improve symptoms [63–65]. In a survey study, sumatriptan showed benefit with both vertigo and migraine

Table 34.2 Commonly used oral vestibular migraine prophylactic agents (disclaimer—table is incomplete, consult a drug compendia for full information)

Medication	Side effects	Contraindications	Monitoring	Also helpful for
Nortriptyline	Weight gain, sedation, dry mouth	Recent myocardial infarction, MAOI use, Sjogren's	None routinely, but consider EKG (QT prolongation), BMP (SIADH), or psych eval (worsening depression/suicidality) as indicated	Insomnia, anxiety, depression
Topiramate	Tingling in hands/feet, cognitive changes, fatigue, weight loss	H/o kidney stones, acid/base disorders, kidney failure, glaucoma. May worsen balance	BMP annually and with dose changes, annual ophtho exam	Weight loss, seizures
Propranolol	Low BP, worsened depression	Cardiac disease, asthma, diabetes, hypotension	EKG, BP	Anxiety, tremor, HTN
Verapamil	Low BP	Hypotension, cardiac disease	EKG, BP	HTN
Venlafaxine	Nighttime sweating, elevated BP, weight loss, sexual dysfunction	MAOI use	CMP/lipids annually, suicidality	Anxiety, depression, weight loss
Flunarizine[a]	Weight gain, tremor, sedation, parkinsonism	Depression, hepatic impairment, extrapyramidal disorders, hypotension, cardiac arrhythmia	Weight/mood	Weak anti-epileptic drug

Abbreviations: *HTN* hypertension, *BP* blood pressure, *MAOI* monoamine oxidase inhibitor
[a]Flunarizine is not FDA approved in the United States

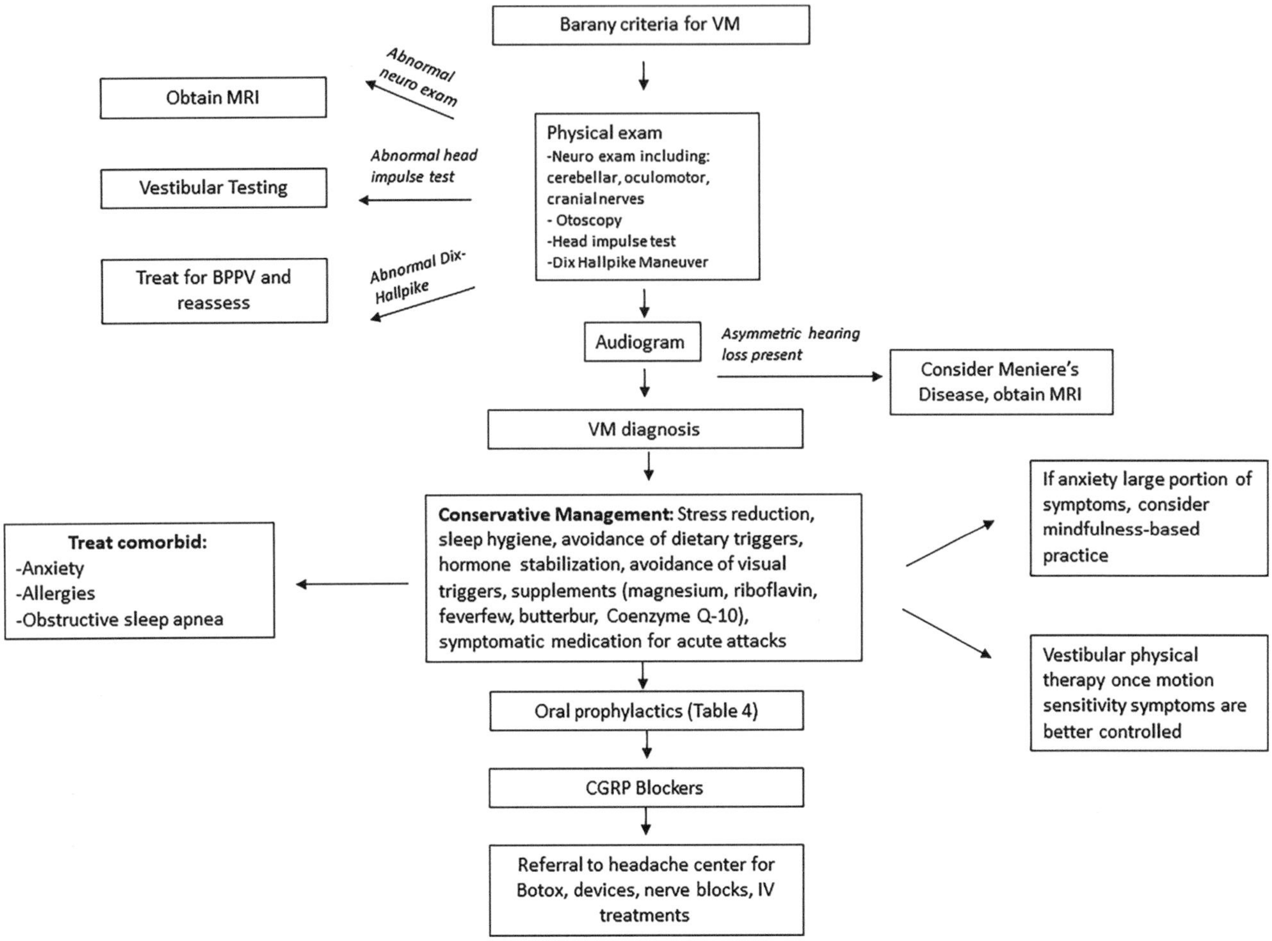

Fig. 34.5 Algorithm for treatment of vestibular migraine. VM Vestibular migraine, CGRP calcitonin-gene-related peptide

symptoms [66]. Almotriptan showed improvement but only in a retrospective study [66, 67]. Rizatriptan decreased motion sickness in VM patients but not in patients with classical migraine [68]. There are also case reports that IV methylprednisolone has efficacy in severe VM [69]. The INVESTMENT study was a double blinded, placebo-controlled trial of galcanezumab for vestibular migraine [70]. Outcomes included the DHI, VM-PATHI, and the count of Definitive Dizzy Days (DDDs). Participants were texted every day asking about dizziness over the prior 24 hours, which was rated as none, mild, moderate, or severe. Days with moderate or severe dizziness were counted as a DDDs. Those randomized to galcanezumab had 5.7 fewer DDDs in the third month of treatment, compared with placebo ($p = 0.026$). They also had a better reduction in DHI scores after 3 months of treatment compared with placebo (–22.0 versus –8.3, $p = 0.018$), and a better reduction in VM-PATHI scores (–14.7 versus –5.1, $p = 0.04$). Overall, there are not enough significantly powered, placebo controlled, randomized clinical trials to determine if current VM treatments are effective [71]. Common prophylactic medications used in the author's practice are detailed in Table 34.2. The treatment paradigm used in the author's clinical practice can be seen in Fig. 34.5.

Conclusion

VM is a common cause of dizziness in the general population. Its presentation can overlap with a variety of other vestibular disorders and it is often under-diagnosed. However, there are clear published diagnostic criteria and validated patient-reported outcome measures that clinicians can use to identify these patients. VM is treatable with non-pharmacological options and classic migraine medications, but there is a lack of high-level evidence to support the currently used treatment paradigm. More work is needed to elucidate the pathophysiology and determine novel therapies for the treatment of this common and debilitating disorder [72]. *See Teaching Points for VM treatment.*

Teaching Points

1. Vestibular migraine is incredibly common. All patients with dizziness should be asked about: personal history of migraine, family history of migraine, and migrainous symptoms during attacks.
2. Patients will not volunteer information about photophobia or phonophobia during attacks—this has to be specifically inquired about.
3. Medication sensitivities are very common with VM. Use low doses of medications to start, taper on and off, and counsel appropriately.
4. Treatment of anxiety, stress, sleep disorders, and allergies may be helpful.
5. Audiometry is helpful in distinguishing Meniere's disease from VM.
6. Adequate time should be set aside for patient counselling about diagnosis and treatment options.
7. Vestibular testing is likely to worsen symptoms, therefore consider using it judiciously when a concurrent issue is suspected.
8. Minor brain white matter abnormalities are very commonly seen on FLAIR or T2 MRI sequences, reassurance to patients can be very helpful regarding those findings, which frequently cause alarm.
9. Periodic follow-up is usually necessary while finding a specific medication regimen that works for a particular patient.
10. Not all patients require pharmacologic intervention.
11. Anxiety is a frequent co-morbidity in this population. We find it most helpful to consider a disease modifier that also requires treatment. Blaming anxiety for dizziness tends to be clinically counterproductive. We find that dizziness and anxiety often make each other worse.
12. Similar to migraine headache (and despite published criteria), there are likely episodic and chronic forms of vestibular migraine.
13. Many symptoms are shared between superior canal dehiscence and vestibular migraine, consider working up for superior canal in select cases, especially when objective findings are present (weber to one ear, negative bone conduction thresholds, etc.).

Case

A 38-year-old woman presents with vertigo. She reports attacks with hours of vertigo, feeling like the world is moving and rocking. On further questioning, light and sound sensitivity are present during those episodes, as well as a moderately severe headache. She does not have a personal history of migraine, but there is a strong family history. She has always been prone to carsickness. In addition, she notes that when she rolls over in bed, she will experience spinning vertigo. On exam, you perform a right Dix Hallpike, which shows upbeating, geotropic rotatory nystagmus consistent with right posterior canal BPPV (benign paroxysmal positional vertigo).

Case Discussion

Vestibular disorders can overlap, and are not mutually exclusive. This patient has a clinical history consistent with both BPPV and vestibular migraine. Her exam confirmed BPPV. The best approach is to treat the BPPV with an Epley maneuver, and then reassess her in 2–4 weeks. It is likely that she also has vestibular migraine, and by eliminating the contribution of BPPV, you will get a clearer picture of symptom burden due to VM. BPPV can take several particle repositioning maneuvers to totally clear, but almost all cases are responsive to treatment.

Questions and Answers

1. Which of the following is NOT consistent with a diagnosis of vestibular migraine per Barany Society criteria?
   A. Episodic vertigo lasting hours
   B. Unilateral tinnitus, aural pressure, and hearing loss during vertigo episodes
   C. A prior history of migraine with aura
   D. Photophobia and phonophobia during vertigo episodes
   E. A lifetime total of 17 vertigo episodes

The correct answer is B. The Barany Society has created diagnostic criteria for many vestibular diseases, and they are quite helpful for both clinical practice and research.

The clinical criteria include all the about except for "b." While tinnitus, aural pressure, and even subjective hearing loss can accompany vestibular migraine episodes, it is uncommon to have all three, and typically it would be bilateral if present. Unilateral tinnitus, aural pressure, and hearing loss accompanying a vertigo episode are more typical of Meniere's disease. Note that tinnitus is a common complaint in those with vestibular migraine. Unilateral hearing loss, documented on audiometry, is not considered a feature of vestibular migraine.

2. A "catch-up saccade" seen during horizontal head impulse testing to the left is most consistent with which diagnosis?
   A. BPPV
   B. Vestibular migraine
   C. Unilateral vestibular hypofunction
   D. Meniere's disease
   E. Superior semicircular canal dehiscence

The correct answer is C. The head impulse test assesses the vestibulo-ocular reflex (VOR). The purpose of the VOR is to keep objects of interest—visual targets—foveated during head and body movements. Whenever the head is quickly rotated, an intact VOR works with the stimulated semicircular canal sensing the rotation, which is then relayed to oculomotor neurons in the brainstem, which in turn cause the eyes to quickly rotate opposite to the direction of the head turn. If they fail to do so, then eyes (and the fovea) will slip off target as the head moves, followed by a corrective saccade (aka catch-up saccade) to return gaze to the visual target. Therefore, in the case above, there is a unilateral vestibular hypofunction affecting the left horizontal canal.

References

1. Kroenke K, Mangelsdorff AD. Common symptoms in ambulatory care: incidence, evaluation, therapy, and outcome. Am J Med. 1989;86(3):262–6.
2. Tehrani S, Ali S, Coughlan D, Hsieh YH, Mantokoudis G, Korley FK, Kerber KA, Frick KD, Newman-Toker DE. Rising annual costs of dizziness presentations to US emergency departments. Acad Emerg Med. 2013;20(7):689–96.
3. Bisdorff AR, Staab JP, Newman-Toker DE. Overview of the international classification of vestibular disorders. Neurol Clin. 2015;33(3):541–50. vii
4. Basser LS. Benign paroxysmal vertigo of childhood: a variety of vestibular neuronitis. Brain J Neurol. 1964;87(March):141–52.
5. Lucieer F, Vonk P, Guinand N, Stokroos R, Kingma H, van de Berg R. Bilateral vestibular Hypofunction: insights in etiologies, clinical subtypes, and diagnostics. Front Neurol. 2016;7(March):26.
6. Radtke A, Lempert T, Gresty MA, Brookes GB, Bronstein AM, Neuhauser H. Migraine and Ménière's disease: is there a link? Neurology. 2002;59(11):1700–4.
7. Uneri A. Migraine and benign paroxysmal positional vertigo: an outcome study of 476 patients. Ear Nose Throat J. 2004;83(12):814–5.
8. Formeister EJ, Rizk HG, Kohn MA, Sharon JD. The epidemiology of vestibular migraine: a population-based survey study. Otol Neurotol. 2018;39(8):1037–44.
9. Lempert T, Neuhauser H. Epidemiology of vertigo, migraine and vestibular migraine. J Neurol. 2009;256(3):333–8.
10. Colombo B, Teggi R, NIVE Project. Vestibular migraine: who is the patient? Neurol Sci. 2017;38(Suppl 1):107–10.
11. Dieterich M, Brandt T. Episodic vertigo related to migraine (90 cases): vestibular migraine? J Neurol. 1999;246(10):883–92.
12. Neuhauser H, Leopold M, von Brevern M, Arnold G, Lempert T. The interrelations of migraine, vertigo, and migrainous vertigo. Neurology. 2001;56(4):436–41.
13. Mucci V, Hamid M, Jacquemyn Y, Browne CJ. Influence of sex hormones on vestibular disorders. Curr Opin Neurol. 2022;35(1):135–41.
14. Tang B, Xiaojun Y, Jiang W, Zhang C, Zhan T, He Y. Clinical significance of serum sex hormones in postmenopausal women with vestibular migraine: potential role of estradiol. J Int Med Res. 2021;49(5):3000605211016379.
15. Espinosa-Sanchez JM, Lopez-Escamez JA. New insights into pathophysiology of vestibular migraine. Front Neurol. 2015;6:12. https://doi.org/10.3389/fneur.2015.00012. PMID: 25705201; PMCID: PMC4319397.
16. Popper P, Ishiyama A, Lopez I, Wackym PA. Calcitonin gene-related peptide and choline acetyltransferase colocalization in the human vestibular periphery. Audiol Neurootol. 2002;7(5):298–302.
17. Tanaka M, Takeda N, Senba E, Tohyama M, Kubo T, Matsunaga T. Localization of calcitonin gene-related peptide in the vestibular end-organs in the rat: an immunohistochemical study. Brain Res. 1988;447(1):175–7.
18. Tanaka. Localization, origin and fine structure of calcitonin gene-related peptide-containing fibers in the vestibular end-organs of the rat. Brain Res. 1989;504(1):31–5.
19. Usami S, Matsubara A, Shinkawa H, Matsunaga T, Kanzaki J. Neuroactive substances in the human vestibular end organs. Acta Otolaryngol Suppl. 1995;520(Pt 1):160–3.
20. Wackym PA, Popper P, Micevych PE. Distribution of calcitonin gene-related peptide mRNA and immunoreactivity in the rat central and peripheral vestibular system. Acta Otolaryngol. 1993;113(5):601–8.
21. Lysakowski A, Goldberg JM. Morphophysiology of the vestibular periphery. In: The vestibular system. New York: Springer; 2004. https://doi.org/10.1007/0-387-21567-0_3.
22. Ohno K, Takeda N, Tanaka-Tsuji M, Matsunaga T. Calcitonin gene-related peptide in the efferent system of the inner ear. A review. Acta Otolaryngol Suppl. 1993;501:16–20.
23. Xiaocheng W, Zhaohui S, Ka B, Junhui X, Lei Z, Feng X, Guoqing Y, Lining F, Zuoming Z. The expression of calcitonin gene-related peptide and acetylcholine in the vestibular-related nucleus population of wild-type mice and retinal degeneration fast mice after rotary stimulation. J Mol Neurosci. 2013;51(2):514–21.
24. Maison SF, Emeson RB, Adams JC, Luebke AE, Charles Liberman M. Loss of alpha CGRP reduces sound-evoked activity in the cochlear nerve. J Neurophysiol. 2003;90(5):2941–9.
25. Luebke AE, Holt JC, Jordan PM, Wong YS, Caldwell JS, Cullen KE. Loss of α-calcitonin gene-related peptide (αCGRP) reduces the efficacy of the Vestibulo-ocular reflex (VOR). J Neurosci Off J Soc Neurosci. 2014;34(31):10453–8.
26. Jones SM, Vijayakumar S, Dow SA, Holt JC, Jordan PM, Luebke AE. Loss of α-calcitonin gene-related peptide (αCGRP) reduces

otolith activation timing dynamics and impairs balance. Front Mol Neurosci. 2018;11(August):289.
27. Eftekhari S, Salvatore CA, Gaspar RC, Roberts R, O'Malley S, Zeng Z, Edvinsson L. Localization of CGRP receptor components, CGRP, and receptor binding sites in human and rhesus cerebellar cortex. Cerebellum. 2013;12(6):937–49.
28. Zhe X, Chen L, Zhang D, Tang M, Gao J, Ai K, Liu W, Lei X, Zhang X. Cortical areas associated with multisensory integration showing altered morphology and functional connectivity in relation to reduced life quality in vestibular migraine. Front Hum Neurosci. 2021;15:717130. https://doi.org/10.3389/fnhum.2021.717130.
29. Winnick A, Sadeghpour S, Otero-Millan J, Chang T-P, Kheradmand A. Errors of upright perception in patients with vestibular migraine. Front Neurol. 2018;9(October):892.
30. King S, Priesol AJ, Davidi SE, Merfeld DM, Ehtemam F, Lewis RF. Self-motion perception is sensitized in vestibular migraine: pathophysiologic and clinical implications. Sci Rep. 2019;9(1):14323.
31. Chen Z, Xiao L, Liu H, Zhang Q, Wang Q, Lv Y, Zhai Y, et al. Altered thalamo-cortical functional connectivity in patients with vestibular migraine: a resting-state fMRI study. Neuroradiology. 2021;64(1):119–27. https://doi.org/10.1007/s00234-021-02777-w.
32. Bisdorff A. Vestibular symptoms and history taking. Handb Clin Neurol. 2016;137:83–90.
33. Cutrer FM, Baloh RW. Migraine-associated dizziness. Headache. 1992;32(6):300–4.
34. Young AS, Lechner C, Bradshaw AP, MacDougall HG, Black DA, Michael Halmagyi G, Welgampola MS. Capturing acute vertigo: a vestibular event monitor. Neurology. 2019;92(24):e2743–53.
35. Weinreich HM, Carey JP. Prevalence of pulsatile tinnitus among patients with migraine. Otol Neurotol. 2016;37(3):244–7.
36. Chari DA, Liu Y-H, Chung JJ, Rauch SD. Subjective cognitive symptoms and dizziness handicap inventory (DHI) performance in patients with vestibular migraine and Menière's disease. Otol Neurotol. 2021;42(6):883–9. https://doi.org/10.1097/MAO.0000000000003081.
37. Liu YF, Locklear TD, Sharon JD, Lacroix E, Nguyen SA, Rizk HG. Quantification of cognitive dysfunction in dizzy patients using the neuropsychological vertigo inventory. Otol Neurotol. 2019;40(7):e723–31.
38. Rizk HG, Sharon JD, Lee JA, Thomas C, Nguyen SA, Meyer TA. Cross-sectional analysis of cognitive dysfunction in patients with vestibular disorders. Ear Hear. 2020;41(4):1020–7.
39. Zhang Y, Kong Q, Chen J, Li L, Wang D, Zhou J. International classification of headache disorders 3rd edition beta-based field testing of vestibular migraine in China: demographic, clinical characteristics, audiometric findings and diagnosis statues. Cephalalgia. 2016;36(3):240–8.
40. Huang T-C, Wang S-J, Kheradmand A. Vestibular migraine: an update on current understanding and future directions. Cephalalgia. 2020;40(1):107–21.
41. Lempert T, Neuhauser H. Vertigo as a symptom of migraine. Med Klin. 2001;96(8):475–9.
42. Schwedt TJ. Chronic migraine. BMJ. 2014;348(March):g1416.
43. Lempert T, Olesen J, Furman J, Waterston J, Seemungal B, Carey J, Bisdorff A, Versino M, Evers S, Newman-Toker D. Vestibular migraine: diagnostic criteria. J Vestib Res Equilib Orientat. 2012;22(4):167–72.
44. Headache Classification Committee of the International Headache Society (IHS). The international classification of headache disorders. 3rd ed. Cephalalgia; 2018. https://doi.org/10.1177/0333102417738202.
45. Vitkovic J, Paine M, Rance G. Neuro-otological findings in patients with migraine- and nonmigraine-related dizziness. Audiol Neurootol. 2008;13(2):113–22.
46. Sharon JD, Krauter R, Kirk L, Pasquesi L, Allen IE, Formeister EJ, Michael RL, Levin M. Development and validation of VM-PATHI: vestibular migraine patient assessment tool and handicap inventory. Otol Neurotol. 2020;41(4):e494–500.
47. Polensek SH, Tusa RJ. Nystagmus during attacks of vestibular migraine: an aid in diagnosis. Audiol Neurootol. 2010;15(4):241–6.
48. Chu C-H, Liu C-J, Lin L-Y, Chen T-J, Wang S-J. Migraine is associated with an increased risk for benign paroxysmal positional vertigo: a nationwide population-based study. J Headache Pain. 2015;16(July):62.
49. Eggers SDZ, Neff BA, Shepard NT, Staab JP. Comorbidities in vestibular migraine. J Vestib Res Equilib Orientat. 2014;24(5–6):387–95.
50. Radtke A, von Brevern M, Neuhauser H, Hottenrott T, Lempert T. Vestibular migraine: long-term follow-up of clinical symptoms and vestibulo-cochlear findings. Neurology. 2012;79(15):1607–14.
51. Bi WL, Brewster R, Poe D, Vernick D, Lee DJ, Eduardo Corrales C, Dunn IF. Superior semicircular canal dehiscence syndrome. J Neurosurg. 2017;127(6):1268–76.
52. Mau C, Kamal N, Badeti S, Reddy R, Ying Y-LM, Jyung RW, Liu JK. Superior semicircular canal dehiscence: diagnosis and management. J Clin Neurosci. 2018;48(February):58–65.
53. Brandt T, Strupp M, Dieterich M. Vestibular paroxysmia: a treatable neurovascular cross-compression syndrome. J Neurol. 2016;263(Suppl 1):S90–6.
54. Cha Y-H, Brodsky J, Ishiyama G, Sabatti C, Baloh RW. Clinical features and associated syndromes of mal de debarquement. J Neurol. 2008;255(7):1038–44.
55. Ghavami Y, Haidar YM, Ziai KN, Moshtaghi O, Bhatt J, Lin HW, Djalilian HR. Management of mal de debarquement syndrome as vestibular migraines. Laryngoscope. 2017;127(7):1670–5.
56. Ombergen V, Van Angelique V, Rompaey LK, Maes PH, de Heyning V, Wuyts FL. Mal de debarquement syndrome: a systematic review. J Neurol. 2016;263(5):843–54.
57. Staab JP, Eckhardt-Henn A, Horii A, Jacob R, Strupp M, Brandt T, Bronstein A. Diagnostic criteria for persistent postural-perceptual dizziness (PPPD): consensus document of the Committee for the Classification of Vestibular Disorders of the Bárány Society. J Vestib Res Equilib Orientat. 2017;27(4):191–208.
58. Chae R, Barber J, Temkin NR, Sharon JD. Dizziness following traumatic brain injury: a TRACH-TBI study; n.d.
59. Mikulec AA, Faraji F, Kinsella LJ. Evaluation of the efficacy of caffeine cessation, nortriptyline, and topiramate therapy in vestibular migraine and complex dizziness of unknown etiology. Am J Otolaryngol. 2012;33(1):121–7.
60. Vitkovic J, Winoto A, Rance G, Dowell R, Paine M. Vestibular rehabilitation outcomes in patients with and without vestibular migraine. J Neurol. 2013;260(12):3039–48.
61. Loder E, Burch R, Rizzoli P. The 2012 AHS/AAN guidelines for prevention of episodic migraine: a summary and comparison with other recent clinical practice guidelines. J Headache Pain. 2012;52(6):930–45. https://doi.org/10.1111/j.1526-4610.2012.02185.x.
62. Reploeg MD, Goebel JA. Migraine-associated dizziness: patient characteristics and management options. Otol Neurotol. 2002;23(3):364–71.
63. Lepcha A, Amalanathan S, Augustine AM, Tyagi AK, Balraj A. Flunarizine in the prophylaxis of migrainous vertigo: a

randomized controlled trial. Eur Arch Otorhinolaryngol. 2014;271(11):2931–6.
64. Salviz M, Yuce T, Acar H, Karatas A, Murat Acikalin R. Propranolol and venlafaxine for vestibular migraine prophylaxis: a randomized controlled trial. Laryngoscope. 2016;126(1):169–74.
65. Neuhauser H, Radtke A, von Brevern M, Lempert T. Zolmitriptan for treatment of migrainous vertigo: a pilot randomized placebo-controlled trial. Neurology. 2003;60(5):882–3.
66. Bikhazi P, Jackson C, Ruckenstein MJ. Efficacy of antimigrainous therapy in the treatment of migraine-associated dizziness. Am J Otol. 1997;18(3):350–4.
67. Cassano D, Pizza V, Busillo V. P074. Almotriptan in the acute treatment of vestibular migraine: a retrospective study. J Headache Pain. 2015;16(Suppl 1):A114.
68. Marcus DA, Furman JM. Prevention of motion sickness with rizatriptan: a double-blind, placebo-controlled pilot study. Med Sci Monit. 2006;12(1):PI1–7.
69. Prakash S, Shah ND. Migrainous vertigo responsive to intravenous methylprednisolone: case reports. Headache. 2009;49(8):1235–9.
70. Sharon JD, Krauter R, Chae R, Gardi A, Hum M, Allen I, Levin M. A placebo controlled, randomized clinical trial of galcanezumab for vestibular migraine: The INVESTMENT study. Headache. 2024 Nov–Dec;64(10):1264–72. https://doi.org/10.1111/head.14835. Epub 2024 Sep 30. PMID: 39344988.
71. Fernández M, Miguel JS, Birdi GJ, Irving LM, Kivekäs I, Strupp M. Pharmacological agents for the prevention of vestibular migraine. Cochrane Database Syst Rev. 2015;6(June):CD010600.
72. Mallampalli MP, Rizk HG, Kheradmand A, Beh SC, Abouzari M, Bassett AM, Buskirk J, et al. Care gaps and recommendations in vestibular migraine: an expert panel summit. Front Neurol. 2022;12:812678. https://doi.org/10.3389/fneur.2021.812678.

Post-traumatic Headache and Migraine

35

Angelica Ahrens and Alan G. Finkel

Introduction

Post traumatic headache (PTH) is classified according to the intensity of the traumatic brain injury (TBI), i.e., mild, moderate, or severe. Based upon the natural history, it is either acute or persistent with the latter defined as greater than three months of pattern change or de novo headache. The onset must occur in seven days, though some have challenged that rule. Persistent Post Traumatic Headache (pPTH) is diagnosed at three months from injury or coming to awareness of the headache since other injuries or treatments may mitigate the awareness of the condition [1]. It is by consensus that many use the term "migraine" or migraine phenotype or type to describe pPTH since an individual attack could meet criteria for either migraine with [2] or without aura [3], though an additional consensus about terminology demands that the designation of PTH must be included, i.e., pPTH with migraine (pheno)type. Thus, migraine-type pPTH after mTBI/concussion is somewhat controversial but is now a focus of intense preclinical and clinical research seeking to understand the presentation and substrates for pathobiology and treatment.

Migraine is a disease of the brain that results in headache in most but not all. Besides the growing understanding of premonitory symptoms and their anatomical basis and the translational importance of aura, changes in sensory processing, e.g., phobias and positive experiences, vestibular, cognitive function, and autonomic changes are included in the spectrum of experiences that associate with a migraine attack. The disability associated with those attacks is well known as pain and other associated symptoms worsen with activity, rendering a migraine attack the seventh most disabling condition according to the World Health Organization (WHO) [4]. The substrates for many of the experiences during an attack are also being identified at the gross, cellular, and submicroscopic levels where targets for treatment are being identified and drugs developed with new successes. Preclinical models verify the human experiences of sensory changes, i.e., conditioned place preference and light aversion [5] to mimic allodynia/pain sensitization and photophobia, respectively. The mainstays of non-human preclinical research, such as cortical spreading depression (CSD) [6, 7], are being studied and used in modeling PTH, both acute and persistent; and calcitonin gene-related peptide (CGRP) and its associated receptors are not only targets for treatment of migraine [8] but also tools in our understanding of the mechanism of headaches following concussion. Taken together, the disease of migraine affects the brain, the head including the face, and the neck, and insights coming from migraine research are now contributing evidence for possible analogy when pPTH has migraine phenotype attacks or phenomenology.

A. Ahrens
Department of Microbiology and Cell Science, College of Agricultural and Life Sciences, University of Florida, Gainesville, FL, USA

A. G. Finkel (✉)
Department of Psychiatry, UNC School of Medicine, Chapel Hill, NC, USA

Carolina Headache Institute, Durham, NC, USA

Questions

1. A significant clinical predictor of persistent headache after concussion is:
   A. A prior history of tension-type headache.
   B. Being a male athlete.
   C. Female gender.
   D. Prior orthopedic injuries.
   E. College education.
2. The treatment of post traumatic headache should:
   A. Always include triptans.
   B. Use hyperbaric oxygen.
   C. Wait for resolution at least 3 months before initiating monoclonal antibodies to CGRP.
   D. Include an assessment of the needs for multidisciplinary care including cognitive and behavioral therapies.
   E. Start with Onabotulinum toxin A injections in areas of nummular pain.

T. S. Monteith et al. (eds.), *Comprehensive Migraine Management*, https://doi.org/10.1007/978-3-031-86923-5_35

The Natural History of pPTH and Diagnosis Type

The prevalence of concussion is not known precisely, likely due to under-reporting, though the Center for Disease Control and Prevention (CDC) estimates that 2.8 million Americans are injured yearly with 166 people dying from TBI-related injuries [9, 10]. A survey of 3009 Americans reported a 23% incidence of lifetime-concussion, with 29% still demonstrating persistent symptoms and effects and as many as nearly 80% stating they had some treatment during the course [11]. Emergency room records are likely to either over or underdiagnose concussion or code incorrectly. Nevertheless, once injured, persistent symptoms, especially PTH, do occur and the rates in real time are being elucidated (Fig. 35.1). A report following patients with moderate to severe TBI due to motor vehicle accident showed that as late as two years from injury, new cases could be seen [12]. Epidemiologic and clinical studies describe the prevalence and diagnosis types with some insight into what our expectations might be after an initial encounter.

The prevalence of PTH changes with time from injury and published reports may vary because of difference in study design and populations. At 1 and 3 months, the 30.4% and 15.35% still had headaches [13] with 30–33% still not fully recovered [14, 15]. At 6 months, as many as one-third had not fully recovered [16]; in another study at one year, three quarters of patients demonstrated worsening or chronic with only 12% completely resolved. At 60 months, 35% of patients having several headaches weekly and 58–62% reporting migraine [13]. Finally, at eleven-year follow-up, 54% of Veterans with a deployment-related TBI reported severe or disabling headache at least two days a week and 44% had "chronic daily headache" [17].

Prognosis for complete recovery appears to be dependent upon premorbid, peri- and post-injury characteristics, and clinical markers [18, 19]. Female gender [20], pre-injury headache and psychiatric comorbidities [18, 21], age, work status, pre-existing headache, and, occurring within 30 days of injury predict headache at 1 year [22]. Acute factors including PTH severity, stiffness in the neck [23], pain modulation, post-traumatic amnesia (PTA), and fatigue [7] and symptoms in arms or hands, dizziness, or unsteadiness [22] also contribute to negative outcomes. In the immediate period, conditional pain modulation at 1 and 2 weeks post-injury [20] and depression and pain catastrophizing scores from 1 week to 4 months [20]. Long term persistence of PTH is predicted by those same psychiatric comorbidities, employment status [22, 24], high levels of catastrophizing and lower recovery expectations [21].

Close interview of patients with PTH often reveals subtle differences in description and phenomenology. Phenotypes not studied or rarely considered in prediction literature include site of injury/nummular pattern, occipital nerve block responses suggesting occipital neuralgia type [25], and trigeminal autonomic cephalalgias [26]. Continuous headache is not uncommon, with descriptions with clinical samples showing as high as 75% of patient describing in detail [27]. We showed that continuous headache, but not primary headache phenotypic diagnosis, was a major determinant of outcomes [28].

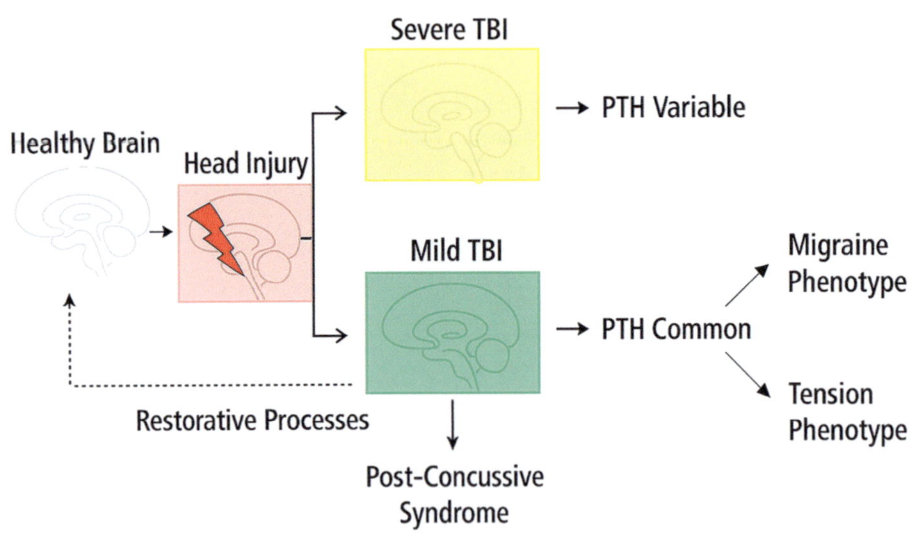

Fig. 35.1 Traumatic brain injury and posttraumatic headache. Mild traumatic brain injury, or concussion, is generally transient due to the brain's restorative process. However, posttraumatic headache is common and a subset of individuals have persistent symptoms including posttraumatic headache. Less is known about the relationship between severe traumatic brain injury and posttraumatic *headache*, because survivors may be either too sick or disabled to report headaches or sensory processing difficulties. A history of repetitive head and neck injuries, premorbid conditions such as migraine and genetic susceptibilities are risk factors of persistence. (Adapted from Monteith TS, Borsook D. Insights and advances in post-traumatic headache: research considerations. Curr Neurol Neurosci Rep. 2014;14(2):428)

With the knowledge that most patients will still express migraine phenotype, it then becomes imperative to be able to predict who amongst those with mTBI are going to persist with ongoing headache since early intervention studies must account for the natural remission of headache after injury [16]. Historically, routine follow-up for TBI is rare, with only <10% of neurotrauma centers scheduling a routine follow-up after discharge from the ED, and a modest 54% after hospital admission [29]. Standardized follow-up is urgently required, with support from the literature implicating the potential value in early indicators of pPTH such as those described.

How Is pPTH Like Migraine?

Preclinical models of migraine are well established. They include CSD to interrogate the connections between brain activation as in aura, and the cascade of events leading to headache and associated features of the migraine attack. Considering open and closed skull, percussion, blast, or weight drop models of different types, there are as many different concerns for confounds, such as craniotomy, fixed and unfixed heads, intact or interrupted dura, and directionality of impact and neck motion, most recently modeled in a weight drop free-fall model, with results suggesting analogy to migraine [30].

Preclinical models of concussion have identified several important occurrences at time of injury, some of which are particularly relevant to our understanding of possible migraine-like headache in humans [29]. When used in preclinical models of PTH and pPTH, CSD is implicated in both anatomical and behavioral changes [30, 31]. Another translational area of research in PTH is CGRP and its family of receptors. Released at the time of injury, "migraine-like" behavioral changes occur within a short time including preference and aversion [30]. These biobehavioral studies have shown dramatic lowering of thresholds to neuronal firing and expansion of receptive fields, which align with findings in non-traumatic models of migraine, including the long-term changes. One study showed that after a period of recovery on measures of migraine-like behaviors and changes in physiology, stress will cause a return of post traumatic "migraine" brought on by stress [32], a known trigger to non-traumatic migraine.

Where Is the Lesion?

The core principle of all neurosciences is the localization of lesions in the nervous system. Whether clinically evident, macroscopic, or molecular, changes in function of the nervous system result in disease. For migraine, we are getting closer to understanding some of the "lesions" including trigeminovascular activation during headache, and central nervous system changes including a possible generator in the hypothalamus [33]. At the anatomical level, imaging changes with chronic migraine [34] and medication overuse [35] may represent surrogates or biomarkers of diagnosis. Where are we with pPTH?

Both structural and functional changes [36] have been reported [37], including gross anatomical loss of cortical thickness [38], cerebrovascular reactivity when compared to healthy controls, and decreases in grey matter even when compared to those with a history of concussion but without pPTH [39]. At the macroscopic level, tract changes in major cortical areas of white matter [40], differences in connectivity [41, 42] between patients with migraine and pPTH, and changes in hypothalamic function [43] have been observed. Recent studies of acute PTH show changes in iron deposition in multiple brain areas in patients acutely concussed and describing PTH, with a dose effect in areas known to be involved with pain processing and recognition [44]. Translating this into the clinic, Chong et al. showed that clinical symptoms may correlate with imaging changes [45], offering a potential for biomarkers to distinguish between chronic migraine, pPTH and those with non-migrainous headaches including those with prior concussion .

What Makes pPTH Different from Migraine?

Migraine Without Aura in pPTH Headache diagnosis is based upon an agreed upon group of symptoms and characteristics, most specifically in primary headaches. Using a 4-point scale (none-mild-moderate-severe), migraine is defined by discrete attacks lasting 4–72 hours with and without aura. Aura is less common than headache without aura and is recognized as the sine qua non of migraine presentation and research.

Migraine with Aura in pPTH Migraine with aura is more prevalent than expected in pPTH [28]. Couch showed that in people with Chronic Daily Headache-Type pPTH, migraine with aura was seen in 41%. In another epidemiologic study of returning soldiers, migraine with aura was found to be the most common phenotype of pPTH in Veterans [46]. Other studies of pPTH describe aura at a higher percentage than expected, with 6% in our clinic-based study [27]; and in the non-clinical study of Mitte in the same population, aura was the most potent predictor of headache in patients with pPTH as well as "definite visual aura," second only to continuous or daily headache [47].

Continuous Headache In chronic migraine, it is accepted that headache-free days occur. In the clinic, non-traumatic continuous headache is seen but poorly recognized and described, often as chronic tension type, though the patients likely have pain grades that are moderate to severe. However, a substantial number of people with pPTH have continuous headaches.

In one of the earliest studies of population-based PTH, continuous headache was present in 19% after head and or neck injury, but 15% of patients with chronic daily headache without injury described continuous pain [48]. In one study, 8% of injured soldiers members reported continuous headache [47]. In the clinic, 75% reported continuous headache, and this was the major determinant of leaving service for medical reasons [27]. In Veterans, all those with TBI had some headache, with migraine-like headache in half of those, and 44% reported "chronic daily headache." In a study of headache burden in Veterans who sustained a deployment-related TBI, 54.5% reported 8+ severe headache days per month, with >75% reporting 10+ total headache days per month, compared to only 20% of matched Veteran controls. Chronic daily headache was observed in 43.6% of TBI Veterans, frequent headache in 32.7% and none reported not having a headache, with 89% migraine prevalence [17].

Separating continuous from extremely frequent or daily may require more detailed interviews than studies of populations could access. In those that do, a wide range of reported constant pain is observed. In addition, patients with continuous headaches may describe episodes of migraine-like pain [27]. Determining research endpoints may be confounded if continuous headaches are not recognized, especially for those whose headaches are not migraine-type-like cluster or nummular site of injury pain [49, 50]?

Treatment

The extant dogma for treating pPTH is to use a primary headache phenotype and apply known therapies. The same would be true of other phenotypes of pPTH, though less common and well studied. Since there are no completed high-quality treatment trials or approvals, the original reports using standard of care migraine drugs has shown some utility. In a military-based clinic study of patients with mTBI-related pPTH, 70–75% of service members responded to triptans [51, 52]. Acutely used occipital nerve blocks were effective in treating pediatric emergency room patients but showed no changes in long-term outcomes [25]. Valproate [53], topiramate and amitriptyline [52], and gabapentin [54] were reported to show some benefits in lesser quality, clinic-based studies, and onabotulinumtoxin A appeared beneficial in clinic-based studies [55, 56], including in our 65 patient report based upon global evaluations of change in soldiers [49]. A controlled study in Veterans showed statistically significant treatment effect in 40 subjects [57].

Using the most recent advances in migraine treatment, drugs that target CGRP and its receptor is an attractive consideration for treatment of PTH. For migraine and chronic migraine(590), erenumab, a CGRP receptor blocking antibody, was shown to be effective in a consecutive patient study that included reductions in headache days and headache impact [58, 59]. Important preclinical studies have demonstrated a role for CGRP in both acute and pPTH models [32]. The recent finding in mice of the loss of diffuse noxious inhibitory controls after mTBI may have great relevance in humans with more regular or even continuous pain. This change in state was prevented by pretreatment with one of the CGRP ligand blocking antibodies [60]. Most recently, fremanezumab, an antibody to the ligand CGRP, was shown to have probable effectiveness, but it did not meet the endpoint of improvement in headache days as defined by moderate severity, compared to placebo [61]. Issues of completing trials may hinge upon the reality that patients with mTBI may have cognitive and memory problems, making primary study protocols such as diary completion difficult. In one trial, this was the reason for early discontinuation. Of the non-pharmacologic treatments that were studied, hyperbaric oxygen did not change the course of pPTH or PTSD [62], nor did pulsed electromagnetic stimulation [63]. Transcranial magnetic stimulation (TMS) shows some relief for acute migraine [64], although likely compounded by reduction in mental health symptoms such as depression, for which this treatment has FDA approval, but effects on chronic migraine are not significant [64]. Moreover, improvements in headache intensity were observed in pPTH at one-week post-intervention but not at four weeks [65]. Some nonpharmacologic treatments for acute PTH in sports have been successful [66] and multidisciplinary treatments [67] and lifestyle modification combined with cognitive behavioral therapy and biofeedback showed dramatic changes in refractory pPTH [68].

Conclusion

Migraine and pPTH are both disabling and occur in individuals with other bothersome symptoms of sensory processing and cognitive changes such as brain fog. Differences in these phenotypes, though, justify the ongoing debates and discussions about etiology and pathobiology. The instant of impact may associate with changes of brain states including CSD and release of CGRP, which could link the injury to a migrainous pathway [69]. Translating preclinical studies to human neuroscience and treatment is still in the initial stages, although there are promising developments in predictive outcome models and biomarker discovery in preclinical models as well as open label studies in humans. Improving outcomes will depend on the strength of those models, and the education necessary to move science onto the playing field, the battlefield, and into the clinic.

Teaching Points

1. Post Traumatic Headache when lasting more than 3 months is persistent and requires additional considerations for evaluation and management. The intensity of service for acute persistent PTH should follow usual guidelines for head injury. For persistent PTH, additional knowledge and specialty training may be necessary.
2. After concussion, the majority of people will recover, but it is likely that a *one-third* of people could have ongoing symptoms for years.
3. Education about the consequences of injury and expected symptoms at the initial point of contact can reduce long term and persistent problems.
4. Persistent post concussive symptoms may complicate improvement for headache since oculo-motor, vestibular, central balance, sleep, and personality changes including mood disorders may occur.
5. Most important: when assessing the patient with a long time since the injury, make sure to assess premorbid factors both personal and biopsychosocial ecologic and medical; factors at the time of injury including the intensity of symptoms and type of injury; and factors that have been impacting since the injury.
6. Treating persistent PTH requires patience, but using medications and other resources to treat the kind of symptoms including headache diagnostic type, i.e., migraine, can mitigate symptoms significantly and improve patient quality of life where cure is not possible.

Case

A 18-year-old senior in high school is finishing her season 3 weeks ago when in cheerleading practice she fell from the top of the "graduation pyramid" striking her head on the floor of the high school lobby where they regularly practice. She has had a continuous headache and nausea since with light sensitivity and feeling off balance. According to the mother, she was not an easy baby and in elementary school had periodic absences for abdominal pain and nausea. She otherwise reported no regular headaches other than "dehydration" and with her menses. She had one prior head injury at 15 when she met head on head with another soccer player, recalling that she only remembers parts of the second period. Her examination is normal. 31-year-old woman with history of episodic migraine presents with increased headache frequency, including 6 debilitating migraine days per month. Following a recent promotion and increased stress, she spends more time in video conferences, a migraine trigger for her. She asks for management suggestions.

Case Discussion

This typical youth athlete has complications known to occur in her sport, sex, and age group. At the evaluation done in the first month if symptoms persist, the importance of prior history becomes essential. In her case, the prior concussion and probable migraine, e.g., childhood precursors of migraine (colic and abdominal symptoms possibly abdominal migraine) and with a normal examination, imaging is not indicated. Careful observation over the next few weeks is essential without a long-term intervention as many athletes will return to baseline within 30 days. If she remains symptomatic, more detailed history and family history will help; and treatment should be aimed at the type of headache, possibly migraine type, that she describes. The clinician should refer to specialists, if necessary, since concurrent symptoms can complicate recovery from PTH and may require more comprehensive concussion evaluation.

Questions and Answers

1. A significant clinical predictor of persistent headache after concussion is:
   A. A prior history of tension-type headache.
   B. Being a male athlete.
   C. Female gender.
   D. Prior orthopedic injuries.
   E. College education.

The correct answer is C. Sex has been found to be a predictor of persistent Post Traumatic Headache where females appear to have more frequent, severe, and migraine-type characteristics. Possible explanations have included anatomical differences in upper body, neck, etc., as well as baseline differences in migraine prevalence prior to injury, sometimes undiagnosed.

2. The treatment of post traumatic headache should:
   A. Always include triptans.
   B. Use hyperbaric oxygen.
   C. Wait for resolution at least 3 months before initiating monoclonal antibodies to CGRP.
   D. Include an assessment of the needs for multidisciplinary care including cognitive and behavioral therapies.
   E. Start with Onabotulinum toxin A injections in areas of nummular pain.

The correct answer is D. The evidence for triptans, though clinically apparent, is from studies of clinic populations including service members that may not represent the other groups including non-athlete civilians. Assessing risks is still important in choice of both acute treatments and preventives. Hyperbaric oxygen has not been shown to be effective and monoclonal antibodies have not been studied though clinic series have suggested efficacy for reduction of headache days. Onabotulinum toxin A has been used in nummular headaches, but post traumatic site of injury pain has not. Multidisciplinary care is one of the only evidence-based treatments thus far shown to be effective with durable effects.

References

1. Headache Classification Committee of the International Headache Society (IHS) The International Classification of Headache Disorders, 3rd edition. Cephalalgia. 2018;38(1):1–211.
2. Hanas JS, Hocker JRS, Lerner MR, Couch JR. Distinguishing and phenotype monitoring of traumatic brain injury and post-concussion syndrome including chronic migraine in serum of Iraq and Afghanistan war veterans. PLoS One. 2019;14(4):e0215762.
3. Theeler BJ, Erickson JC. Mild head trauma and chronic headaches in returning US soldiers. Headache. 2009 Apr;49(4):529–34.
4. GBD 2015 Neurological Disorders Collaborator Group. Global, regional, and national burden of neurological disorders during 1990–2015: a systematic analysis for the Global Burden of Disease Study 2015. Lancet Neurol. 2017;16(11):877–97.
5. De Felice M, Eyde N, Dodick D, Dussor GO, Ossipov MH, Fields HL, et al. Capturing the aversive state of cephalic pain preclinically. Ann Neurol. 2013;74(2):257–65.
6. Noseda R, Burstein R. Migraine pathophysiology: anatomy of the trigeminovascular pathway and associated neurological symptoms, cortical spreading depression, sensitization, and modulation of pain. Pain. 2013;154(Suppl 1):S44–53.
7. Bomyea J, Lang AJ, Delano-Wood L, Jak A, Hanson KL, Sorg S, et al. Neuropsychiatric predictors of post-injury headache after mild-moderate traumatic brain injury in veterans. Headache J Head Face Pain. 2016;56(4):699–710.
8. Edvinsson L. The Trigeminovascular pathway: role of CGRP and CGRP receptors in migraine. Headache. 2017;57(Suppl 2):47–55.
9. Brain Injury Facts & Statistics | Brain Injury Alliance of Connecticut [Internet]. [cited 2021 Oct 24]. Available from: http://www.biact.org/understanding-brain-injury/brain-injury-facts-statistics
10. Get the Facts About TBI | Concussion | Traumatic Brain Injury | CDC Injury Center [Internet]. 2021 [cited 2021 Nov 13]. Available from: https://www.cdc.gov/traumaticbraininjury/get_the_facts.html
11. Hensley S. Poll: Nearly 1 In 4 Americans Reports Having Had A Concussion. NPR [Internet]. 2016 May 31 [cited 2021 Nov 12]; Available from: https://www.npr.org/sections/health-shots/2016/05/31/479750268/poll-nearly-1-in-4-americans-report-having-had-a-concussion
12. Walker WC, Seel RT, Curtiss G, Warden DL. Headache after moderate and severe traumatic brain injury: a longitudinal analysis. Arch Phys Med Rehabil. 2005;86(9):1793–800.
13. Stacey A, Lucas S, Dikmen S, Temkin N, Bell KR, Brown A, et al. Natural history of headache five years after traumatic brain injury. J Neurotrauma. 2017;34(8):1558–64.
14. Sawyer K, Bell KR, Ehde DM, Temkin N, Dikmen S, Williams RM, et al. Longitudinal study of headache trajectories in the year after mild traumatic brain injury: relation to posttraumatic stress disorder symptoms. Arch Phys Med Rehabil. 2015;96(11):2000–6.
15. de Kruijk JR, Leffers P, Menheere P, Meerhoff S, Rutten J, Twijnstra A. Prediction of post-traumatic complaints after mild traumatic brain injury: early symptoms and biochemical markers. J Neurol Neurosurg Psychiatry. 2002;73(6):727–32.
16. Cnossen MC, van der Naalt J, Spikman JM, Nieboer D, Yue JK, Winkler EA, et al. Prediction of persistent post-concussion symptoms after mild traumatic brain injury. J Neurotrauma. 2018;35(22):2691–8.
17. Couch JR, Stewart KE. Headache prevalence at 4–11 years after deployment-related traumatic brain injury in veterans of Iraq and Afghanistan wars and comparison to controls: a matched case-controlled study. Headache J Head Face Pain. 2016;56(6):1004–21.
18. Lingsma HF, Yue JK, Maas AIR, Steyerberg EW, Manley GT, Cooper SR, et al. Outcome prediction after mild and complicated mild traumatic brain injury: external validation of existing models and identification of new predictors using the TRACK-TBI pilot study. J Neurotrauma. 2015;32(2):83–94.
19. Jacobs B, Beems T, Stulemeijer M, van Vugt AB, van der Vliet TM, Borm GF, et al. Outcome prediction in mild traumatic brain injury: age and clinical variables are stronger predictors than CT abnormalities. J Neurotrauma. 2010;27(4):655–68.
20. Guty E, Arnett P. Post-concussion symptom factors and neuropsychological outcomes in collegiate athletes. J Int Neuropsychol Soc JINS. 2018;24(7):684–92.
21. Yue JK, Cnossen MC, Winkler EA, Deng H, Phelps RRL, Coss NA, et al. Pre-injury comorbidities are associated with functional impairment and post-concussive symptoms at 3- and 6-months after mild traumatic brain injury: a TRACK-TBI study. Front Neurol. 2019;10:343.
22. Varner C, Thompson C, de Wit K, Borgundvaag B, Houston R, McLeod S. Predictors of persistent concussion symptoms in adults with acute mild traumatic brain injury presenting to the emergency department. CJEM. 2021;23(3):365–73.
23. Faux S, Sheedy J, Delaney R, Riopelle R. Emergency department prediction of post-concussive syndrome following mild traumatic brain injury--an international cross-validation study. Brain Inj. 2011;25(1):14–22.
24. Lucas S, Hoffman JM, Bell KR, Dikmen S. A prospective study of prevalence and characterization of headache following mild traumatic brain injury. Cephalalgia Int J Headache. 2014;34(2):93–102.
25. Larsen EL, Ashina H, Iljazi A, Al-Khazali HM, Seem K, Ashina M, et al. Acute and preventive pharmacological treatment of

post-traumatic headache: a systematic review. J Headache Pain. 2019;20(1):98.
26. Grangeon L, O'Connor E, Chan C-K, Akijian L, Pham Ngoc TM, Matharu MS. New insights in post-traumatic headache with cluster headache phenotype: a cohort study. J Neurol Neurosurg Psychiatry. 2020;91(6):572–9.
27. Finkel AG, Yerry JA, Klaric JS, Ivins BJ, Scher A, Choi YS. Headache in military service members with a history of mild traumatic brain injury: a cohort study of diagnosis and classification. Cephalalgia. 2017;37(6):548–59.
28. Finkel AG, Ivins BJ, Yerry JA, Klaric JS, Scher A, Sammy CY. Which matters more? A retrospective cohort study of headache characteristics and diagnosis type in soldiers with mTBI/concussion. Headache. 2017;57(5):719–28.
29. Bree D, Levy D. Strides toward better understanding of post-traumatic headache pathophysiology using animal models. Curr Pain Headache Rep. 2018;22(10):67.
30. Bree D, Levy D. Development of CGRP-dependent pain and headache related behaviours in a rat model of concussion: implications for mechanisms of post-traumatic headache. Cephalalgia. 2018;38(2):246–58.
31. Pacheco JM, Hines-Lanham A, Stratton C, Mehos CJ, McCurdy KE, Pinkowski NJ, et al. Spreading Depolarizations occur in mild traumatic brain injuries and are associated with Postinjury behavior. eNeuro. 2019;6(6):ENEURO.0070-19.2019.
32. Navratilova E, Rau J, Oyarzo J, Tien J, Mackenzie K, Stratton J, et al. CGRP-dependent and independent mechanisms of acute and persistent post-traumatic headache following mild traumatic brain injury in mice. Cephalalgia. 2019;39(14):1762–75.
33. Schulte LH, May A. Of generators, networks and migraine attacks. Curr Opin Neurol. 2017;30(3):241–5.
34. Schwedt TJ, Chong CD, Wu T, Gaw N, Fu Y, Li J. Accurate classification of chronic migraine via brain magnetic resonance imaging. Headache. 2015;55(6):762–77.
35. Mehnert J, Hebestreit J, May A. Cortical and subcortical alterations in medication overuse headache. Front Neurol. 2018;9:499.
36. Ofoghi Z, Dewey D, Barlow KM. A systematic review of structural and functional imaging correlates of headache or pain after mild traumatic brain injury. J Neurotrauma. 2020;37(7):907–23.
37. Schwedt TJ. Structural and functional brain alterations in post-traumatic headache attributed to mild traumatic brain injury: a narrative review. Front Neurol. 2019;10:615.
38. Chong CD, Berisha V, Chiang C-C, Ross K, Schwedt TJ. Less cortical thickness in patients with persistent post-traumatic headache compared with healthy controls: an MRI study. Headache. 2018;58(1):53–61.
39. Burrowes SAB, Rhodes CS, Meeker TJ, Greenspan JD, Gullapalli RP, Seminowicz DA. Decreased grey matter volume in mTBI patients with post-traumatic headache compared to headache-free mTBI patients and healthy controls: a longitudinal MRI study. Brain Imaging Behav. 2020;14(5):1651–9.
40. Chong CD, Peplinski J, Berisha V, Ross K, Schwedt TJ. Differences in fibertract profiles between patients with migraine and those with persistent post-traumatic headache. Cephalalgia. 2019;39(9):1121–33.
41. Dumkrieger G, Chong CD, Ross K, Berisha V, Schwedt TJ. Static and dynamic functional connectivity differences between migraine and persistent post-traumatic headache: a resting-state magnetic resonance imaging study. Cephalalgia. 2019;39(11):1366–81.
42. Maleki N, Finkel A, Cai G, Ross A, Moore RD, Feng X, et al. Post-traumatic headache and mild traumatic brain injury: brain networks and connectivity. Curr Pain Headache Rep. 2021;25(3):20.
43. Lu L, Li F, Wang P, Chen H, Chen Y-C, Yin X. Altered hypothalamic functional connectivity in post-traumatic headache after mild traumatic brain injury. J Headache Pain. 2020;21(1):93.
44. Nikolova S, Schwedt TJ, Li J, Wu T, Dumkrieger GM, Ross KB, et al. T2* reduction in patients with acute post-traumatic headache. Cephalalgia. 2021;42(4-5):357–65.
45. Chong CD, Berisha V, Ross K, Kahn M, Dumkrieger G, Schwedt TJ. Distinguishing persistent post-traumatic headache from migraine: classification based on clinical symptoms and brain structural MRI data. Cephalalgia. 2021;41(8):943–55.
46. Couch JR, Stewart KE. Headache prevalence at 4-11 years after deployment-related traumatic brain injury in veterans of Iraq and Afghanistan wars and comparison to controls: a matched case-controlled study. Headache. 2016 Jun;56(6):1004–21.
47. Metti A, Schwab K, Finkel A, Pazdan R, Brenner L, Cole W, et al. Posttraumatic vs nontraumatic headaches: a phenotypic analysis in a military population. Neurology. 2020;94(11):e1137–46.
48. Couch JR, Lipton RB, Stewart WF, Scher AI. Head or neck injury increases the risk of chronic daily headache: a population-based study. Neurology. 2007;69(11):1169–77.
49. Yerry JA, Kuehn D, Finkel AG. Onabotulinum toxin a for the treatment of headache in service members with a history of mild traumatic brain injury: a cohort study. Headache. 2015;55(3):395–406.
50. Cuadrado ML, López-Ruiz P, Guerrero ÁL. Nummular headache: an update and future prospects. Expert Rev Neurother. 2018;18(1):9–19.
51. Scott BR, Uomoto JM, Barry ES. Impact of pre-existing migraine and other co-morbid or co-occurring conditions on presentation and clinical course following deployment-related concussion. Headache. 2020;60(3):526–41.
52. Erickson JC. Treatment outcomes of chronic post-traumatic headaches after mild head trauma in US soldiers: an observational study. Headache. 2011;51(6):932–44.
53. Packard RC. Treatment of chronic daily posttraumatic headache with divalproex sodium. Headache. 2000;40(9):736–9.
54. Cushman DM, Borowski L, Hansen C, Hendrick J, Bushman T, Teramoto M. Gabapentin and tricyclics in the treatment of post-concussive headache, a retrospective cohort study. Headache. 2019;59(3):371–82.
55. Jia C, Lucchese S, Zhang F, Govindarajan R. The role of Onabotulinum toxin type A in the management of chronic non-migraine headaches. Front Neurol. 2019;10:1009.
56. Ferguson LP, Abdukalikov R, Shbeeb D, Gray TK. Shot in the dark: three patients successfully treated with onabotulinum-toxin A injections for relief of post-traumatic chronic headaches and dystonia induced by gunshot wounds. BMJ Case Rep. 2020;13(12):e236433.
57. Zirovich MD, Pangarkar SS, Manh C, Chen L, Vangala S, Elashoff DA, et al. Botulinum toxin type a for the treatment of post-traumatic headache: a randomized, placebo-controlled, cross-over study. Mil Med. 2021;186(5–6):493–9.
58. VanderEnde J, Bateman EA, MacKenzie HM, Sequeira K. Use of CGRP receptor blocker erenumab in the management of post-traumatic headache: a case series of 5 women. Brain Inj. 2020;34(10):1431–4.
59. Ashina H, Iljazi A, Al-Khazali HM, Eigenbrodt AK, Larsen EL, Andersen AM, et al. Efficacy, tolerability, and safety of erenumab for the preventive treatment of persistent post-traumatic headache attributed to mild traumatic brain injury: an open-label study. J Headache Pain. 2020;21(1):62.
60. Kopruszinski CM, Turnes JM, Swiokla J, Weinstein TJ, Schwedt TJ, Dodick DW, et al. CGRP monoclonal antibody prevents the loss

of diffuse noxious inhibitory controls (DNIC) in a mouse model of post-traumatic headache. Cephalalgia. 2021;41(6):749–59.

61. Teva Branded Pharmaceutical Products R&D, Inc. A Phase 2, Multicenter, Randomized, Proof-of-Concept, Double-Blind, Placebo-Controlled, Parallel-Group Study, Including an Open-Label Period, Evaluating the Efficacy and Safety of 1 Subcutaneous Dose Regimen of Fremanezumab for the Treatment of Posttraumatic Headache (PTH) [Internet]. clinicaltrials.gov; 2021 Apr [cited 2021 Oct 24]. Report No.: results/NCT03347188. Available from: https://clinicaltrials.gov/ct2/show/results/NCT03347188
62. Skipper LD, Churchill S, Wilson SH, Deru K, Labutta RJ, Hart BB. Hyperbaric oxygen for persistent post-concussive symptoms: long-term follow-up. Undersea Hyperb Med. 2016;43(5):601–13.
63. Nelson DV, Esty ML. Neurotherapy for chronic headache following traumatic brain injury. Mil Med Res. 2015;2:22.
64. Lan L, Zhang X, Li X, Rong X, Peng Y. The efficacy of transcranial magnetic stimulation on migraine: a meta-analysis of randomized controlled trails. J Headache Pain. 2017;18(1):86.
65. Leung A, Metzger-Smith V, He Y, Cordero J, Ehlert B, Song D, et al. Left dorsolateral prefrontal cortex rTMS in alleviating MTBI related headaches and depressive symptoms. Neuromodulation. 2018;21(4):390–401.
66. Leddy J, Baker JG, Haider MN, Hinds A, Willer B. A physiological approach to prolonged recovery from sport-related concussion. J Athl Train. 2017;52(3):299–308.
67. Janak JC, Cooper DB, Bowles AO, Alamgir AH, Cooper SP, Gabriel KP, et al. Completion of multidisciplinary treatment for persistent Postconcussive symptoms is associated with reduced symptom burden. J Head Trauma Rehabil. 2017;32(1):1–15.
68. Baker VB, Eliasen KM, Hack NK. Lifestyle modifications as therapy for medication refractory post-traumatic headache (PTHA) in the military population of Okinawa. J Headache Pain. 2018;19(1):113.
69. Benemei S, Labastida-Ramírez A, Abramova E, Brunelli N, Caronna E, Diana P, et al. Persistent post-traumatic headache: a migrainous loop or not? The preclinical evidence. J Headache Pain. 2020;21(1):90.

Part VII

The Practice of Headache Medicine

Structured Headache Centers: Establishing Excellence in Migraine Care

36

Teshamae S. Monteith and Gisela M. Terwindt

Introduction

Migraine is a chronic neurovascular disorder that affects one billion people worldwide [1]. The World Health Organization (WHO) ranks migraine fourth among all causes of years lived with disability (YLDs), for all ages and genders, among all countries and across all income levels (GBD2021) [2]. However, migraine ranks 2nd in young adults ages 15–49. Migraine attacks are characterized by moderate to severe headaches, gastrointestinal symptoms, and perceptual disturbances. Migraine attacks result in functional impairment in 75% of patients and is costly to society [3]. For example, one study of healthcare resource utilization and costs in the United States estimated that individuals with migraine had a total annual mean direct and indirect costs that were $8924 higher than matched individuals without migraine [4]. In addition, nearly 30% of individuals with migraine experience reduced school and work productivity [5]. To this extent, migraine is one of the most common reasons individuals seek care in primary care settings, neurology consultations, and emergency room departments [6, 7]. The debilitating nature of migraine results in high costs due in part to healthcare expenditure, work absenteeism and presenteeism, often less recognized [8]. Taken together, there are major socioeconomic consequences as migraine is associated with high direct and indirect costs, lack of insurance/underinsurance, unemployment, poverty, and food insecurity [9–11]. Although primary care physicians manage most patients with primary headaches, headache centers and high-quality specialized programs are needed to effectively and efficiently diagnose and treat primary and secondary headache disorders requiring further evaluation and management.

A Center of Excellence is defined as a specialized and concentrated hub of dedicated individuals managed from a common point or within a network to drive excellence, innovation, and continuous improvement. In healthcare, the term implies access and healthcare delivery innovation among highly skilled and knowledge professionals [12]. There are several key foundations of Centers of Excellence, which include organizational structure and leadership, quality service, specialized expertise, innovation and research, accreditation and set standards, as well as collaboration and partnership [13]. A fundamental focus is to provide leadership, promotion of best practices, support and education, and research and development (Table 36.1). Critical to the success includes centralization of resources and expertise, increasing efficiency, and reducing costs. There is a need for specialized headache centers although systems of care may differ by region and country (Fig. 36.1). In this chapter, we focus on the concept of Headache Centers of Excellence although formal criteria have not been fully established. The mission, infrastructure, and proposed standards for specialized centers are also discussed [14].

T. S. Monteith (✉)
Department of Neurology, Headache Division,
University of Miami, Miller School of Medicine, Miami, FL, USA

G. M. Terwindt
Department of Neurology, Leiden University Medical Center,
Leiden, The Netherlands

T. S. Monteith et al. (eds.), *Comprehensive Migraine Management*, https://doi.org/10.1007/978-3-031-86923-5_36

Table 36.1 Criteria for center of excellence: implications for migraine

1. *Specialized medical services*:
Provide specialized medical services for migraine diagnosis and management and apply guidelines-based treatments and procedures
2. *Clinical excellence*:
Focus on achieving high standards of clinical excellence and best practices in patient care, treatment, and medical interventions.
3. *Research and innovation*:
Conduct medical research to advance knowledge and innovation in migraine science, delivery, and treatment through clinical trials. This may involve developing new treatment protocols, medical technologies, or pharmaceuticals.
4. *Training and education*:
Serve as a training and education hub for healthcare professionals, including physicians, nurses, and allied health professionals. This can involve residency programs, continuing education, and skill development.
5. *Quality improvement*:
Implement quality improvement initiatives to enhance patient safety, reduce medical errors, and improve overall healthcare quality.
6. *Collaboration and networking*:
Facilitate collaboration and networking among healthcare professionals, researchers, and institutions. This can lead to the exchange of knowledge and best practices among key stakeholders (i.e. emergency room physicians, ophthalmology, radiology, gynecology)
7. *Patient outcomes and experience*:
Focus on improving patient outcomes (i.e. patient-reported outcome measures) and experiences by adopting evidence-based practices, patient-centered care models, and personalized medicine approaches.
8. *Disease management*:
Specialize in the management and treatment of migraine and comorbidities contributing to advancements in disease prevention, diagnosis, and treatment.
9. *Technology integration*:
Incorporate cutting-edge medical technologies (i.e. E-diary, telemedicine) and innovations to enhance diagnostic capabilities, treatment options, and overall healthcare delivery.
10. *Multidisciplinary approach*:
Adopt a multidisciplinary approach to healthcare, bringing together experts from various medical fields to address complex presentations and refractory disorders.
11. *Public health initiatives*:
Engage in public health initiatives and advocacy, such as community outreach programs, health education, and preventive care, and policy to improve the overall health of the population.
12. *Cost efficiency and effectiveness*:
Strive for cost efficiency and effectiveness in healthcare delivery, optimizing resource utilization and providing value-based care for migraine.
13. *Regulatory compliance*:
Adhere to and often surpass regulatory standards and guidelines to ensure patient safety and maintain high ethical standards

This Chart was Created with ChatGPT 3.5 modified search results for medical center of excellence on November 24, 2023. https://chat.openai.com/c/4ec2485a-59f0-48be-94e6-cba046f51cb7

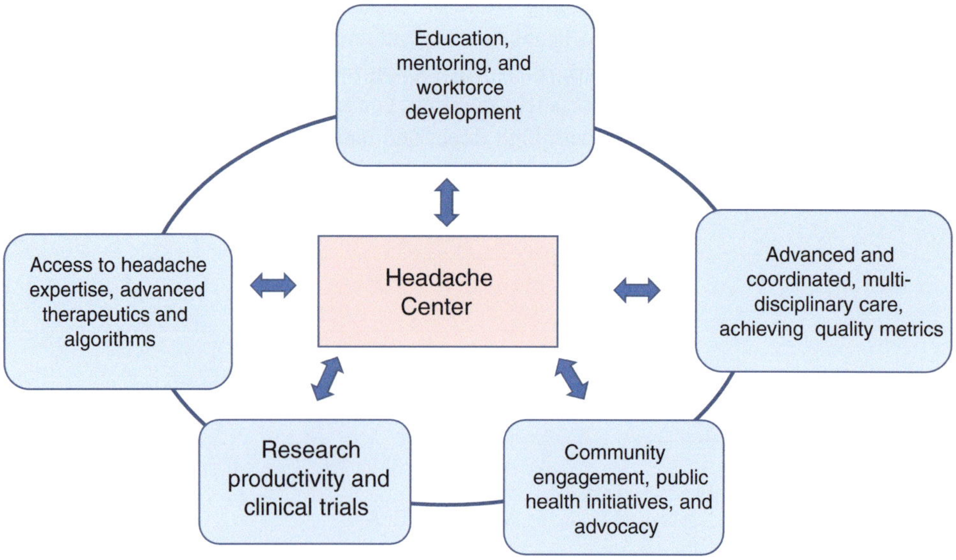

Fig. 36.1 Components of structured headache centers (Model for Centers of Excellence)

Questions

1. To achieve excellence in clinical migraine care, essential components of a structured headache center should include which of the following:
   A. Advanced imaging techniques for the diagnosis of migraine
   B. Coordination of care
   C. Expertise in migraine surgery
   D. Expedited access for migraine with aura
2. Which of the following may explain the potential cost effectiveness of headache centers?
   A. Protocols are avoided so that treatment is personalized.
   B. Patient education modules encourage emergency department visits for severe attacks.
   C. Evidenced-based treatments are initiated early to reduce disability.
   D. The availability of genetic tests may predict migraine progression.

Barriers to Care and Access Considerations

Clinically, migraine is often under-diagnosed, under-managed, and under-treated [15]. To address this issue, the Institute of Medicine (IOM) framework of six aims for healthcare quality that may be applied to migraine when considered system-based levels of care [16]. They include considerations on effectiveness, safety, efficiency, timeliness, equity, and patient/family-centeredness. According to a group of experts from the Global Campaign against Headache, European Federation, and Lifting the Burden, good quality care includes 30 indicators that include adequate referrals and ultimately evaluation of outcomes [17, 18]. Quality measures are important as a study by Buse et al. showed that there are barriers to migraine care including consultation, failure to receive correct diagnosis, not receiving acute and preventive treatment, and lack of management of medication overuse [15]. Despite excessive prior neuroimaging, treatment for individuals with migraine referred to specialty centers remain with low use of preventive therapies, migraine-specific therapies such as triptans or with inappropriate uses of benzodiazepines and opiates [19, 20]. Although quality is less in primary care, wait times are delayed for specialty centers; innovation is greatly needed to improve health delivery.

The burden of migraine in patients with prior preventive medication failures is particularly concerning [21]. A guideline put forth includes definitions for resistant and refractory migraine [22]. In a survey from the European Headache Federation, specialty respondents in headache centers reported very frequently seeing resistant and refractory migraine (75% and 46%, respectively) and had high levels of confidence in providing care (63% and 39%, respectively) for these groups. In the study, there was an overall low rate of referrals for resistant and refractory migraine to specialized centers although general attitudes were that headache centers were best for management. However, the authors raise attention that there are no uniform criteria for escalation to headache centers. Some guidance is available for the management of migraine and other headache disorders in primary care [23]. In this guidance, suggested recommendations for referral include diagnostic uncertainty, suspicion of secondary headache where investigations are not available, and certain primary headache disorders including trigeminal autonomic cephalalgias, and trigeminal neuralgia. In addition, certain clinical presentations of migraine such as chronic migraine, hemiplegic migraine, presence of brainstem symptoms, prolonged aura, or new-onset aura without headache in a person 50 or older without a prior history of migraine, the presence of medication failures and comorbidities are also important reasons for referrals.

If leveraged, structured headache programs may meet many healthcare goals across systems of care. The emergency room continues to have excessive levels of non-urgent visits for migraine; severe headache and prolonged aura are common risk factors as compared to outpatients [24]. Rapid referrals from emergency rooms to headache specialty care, ideally within the same hospital system for sharing of records, may reduce return to the emergency room and result in cost savings [25].

Access to Specialized Interventions and Emerging Therapeutics

Headache medicine programs focus on providing outpatient, inpatient, and clinical research areas in headache medicine, with the goals of establishing excellence through evidence-based treatment of migraine [26]. In terms of standardization, clinical protocols can be implemented to improve treatment efficiency and safety during care of status migrainosus, refractory chronic migraine, and medication overuse headache [27]. Treatment is provided by clinicians, nurses and physician assistants, psychologists, and other providers working closely together. Efficiency is improved by dedicated and trained administrative assistants that understand administrative needs of patients with migraine. This will help to improve access, facilitate authorizations allowing for access to the newest therapeutics, and for essential communications with patients, insurers, caregivers, and referring providers.

In addition, protocols should be established to facilitate patient volumes and safety. For example, a survey of U.S. headache programs found that 68% of the respondents provided outpatient infusion services typically using 3 medications and availability 5 days per week [28]. However, lack of staffing was identified as the most common barrier. Qualified specialists perform common procedures such as neurotoxin injections, FDA approved for chronic migraine in the United States since 2010. In addition, trigger points, peripheral nerve, and sphenopalatine ganglion blocks are performed by headache neurologist or interventionalist. While a few centers offer surgical interventions such as decompressive surgeries, these procedures are considered experimental and should not be offered for management of migraine outside of randomized controlled trials [29]. Although evidenced-based neuromodulation devices for migraine are non-invasive, knowledge of the appropriate indications and administration, as well as efficacy and safety are important for improving adherence, patient satisfaction, and optimal outcomes.

Optimizing Migraine Outcomes

Optimizing migraine outcomes requires adhering to evidence-based guidelines, while considering disability, costs, and tolerability. Careful and routine assessments are needed to optimize migraine; for chronic migraine alone, switching among oral migraine preventive medications is common, and persistence of use at 6 and 12 months is reported low [30]. This suggests significant unmet needs and opportunities to improve patient satisfaction. Clinical guidance from the American Headache Society and the European Headache Federation is available to integrate newer therapies that are associated with increased cost [31, 32]. For example, guidance on treatment with neuromodulation and migraine-specific calcitonin gene-related peptide inhibitors, both small-molecule receptor antagonists and monoclonal antibodies to the ligand or receptor are available for personalized medicine. Standardized headache questionnaires and validated tools are also useful (Table 36.2), as poor treatment outcomes have been linked to low dosing, early discontinuation, and poor tolerability [33].

As new treatment has emerged, the American Academy of Neurology and the American Headache Society organized a work group consisting of headache care team members to develop an evidenced-based headache quality measurement set [34]. Initial high-priority topics included documentation of migraine frequency, counseling, regarding modifiable lifestyle and chronification factors, as well as treatment with acute and preventive therapies. While not a part of the measurement set, there are several validated instruments that can be used for to evaluate acute treatment response and reduction in disability (Table 36.2). However, there are no widely accepted instruments, and some are associated with costs. Electronic medical records for migraine should incorporate fields for headache quality measures [35]. Structured headache forms on initial and follow-up visit can improve efficiency and help communicate prior use of acute and preventive therapies, including safety and efficacy. To evaluate clinical responses and the need for adjustments, clinical trial endpoints should be used during clinical encounters

Table 36.2 Validated instruments for migraine assessments (Recommended by the American Headache Society [26])

Acute therapies	
The Migraine Treatment Optimization Questionnaire (mTOQ) [85]	Assesses treatment efficacy based on 4 aspects of response to acute treatment (very poor, poor, moderate, and maximum treatment efficacy)
Migraine Assessment of Current Therapy (Migraine-ACT) [86]	Assessment tool to identify patients with suboptimal response to acute migraine treatment
Patient Perception of Migraine Questionnaire (PPMQ-R) [87]	Satisfaction measure for acute migraine treatment
Functional Impairment Scale (FIS) [88]	A 4-point scale, single global item, addressing functional status and intensity of impairment during daily activities
Preventive therapies	
Patient Global Impression of Change Scale (PGIC)	A 7-point scale characterizing a patient's self-rating of overall improvement
Migraine Functional Impact Questionnaire (MFIQ) [89]	A 26-item self-administered instrument for the assessment of the impact of migraine: on physical functioning, usual activities, social functioning, and emotional functioning over the past 7 days
Migraine-Specific Quality of Life questionnaire version 2.1 (MSQ v2.1) [90]	A 14-item instrument that measures the impact of migraine over the past 4 weeks: role function-restrictive, role function-preventive, and emotional function
Migraine Physical Function Impact Diary (MPFID) [91]	A 13-item self-administered instrument that assesses the impact of migraine on everyday activities and physical impairment in the past 24 hours
Headache Impact Test (HIT-6) [92]	A six-item evaluation on the impact of headache on the ability to function on the job, at school, at home, and in social situations.
Migraine Disability Assessment (MIDAS) [93]	A 6-item questionnaire used to assess impact of headache on life; work/school, household work, and social activities
Work Productivity and Activity Impairment (WPAI) [94]	A 6-item tool that assess migraine-related disability related to work, both absenteeism and presenteeism
Generic measures of HRQoL	Generic measures of perceived health and impact on quality of life

Collection of Instruments based on the American Headache Society Consensus Statement [26]

such as mean migraine days, individual 50% and 75% responder rates for prescribed preventive treatment, and sustained pain freedom, 2-hour pain relief, and pain freedom for acute attacks [36, 37]. For value-based care, the International Headache Society published a position statement on health technology assessments of acute and preventive interventions, to assess value from different perspectives, ranging from providers, patients and caregivers, healthcare systems, insurers, employers, to society [38]. A wholistic migraine care plan is ultimately needed, which is patient-centered.

Digital Tools: Telemedicine and E-Diaries

Telemedicine utilizes technology such as video conferencing, remote monitoring, and smartphone apps to remotely provide healthcare services, including headache care. This approach improves access to care for those who face barriers, reduces costs, and enhances efficiency. Patients with migraine are ideal candidates for telemedicine since regular physical examinations are not always necessary. Monitoring of treatment can take place through collection of diary data combined with patient-reported outcomes. A validated and easy-to-use daily headache diary is essential for reliable data collection, and the Leiden Headache Center E-diary is a validated algorithm for determining migraine characteristics and monitoring treatment [39–41]. The Leiden Headache E-tools include validated screening and extensive questionnaires, and a daily E-headache diary, all available in one application that can be downloaded on a smartphone. These tools have proved helpful during the COVID-19 pandemic for the continuation of migraine care through telephone and video consultations [42].

We identified a group of 1009 patients at the Leiden Headache Center with migraine that were followed from April 2022 until March 2023 and used the E-headache diary imbedded in the newly developed Patient Journey App (42.9% Android users and 57.1% Apple users). Of these 1009 patients, 55 (5%) were excluded due to a follow-up time of less than 2 weeks, leaving a representative group of 954 patients to which a one-time patient satisfaction questionnaire was sent. The response rate for this one-time patient satisfaction questionnaire was 56%. Patients rated their satisfaction with the E-diary with an over the E-diary, with 84.4% of patients reporting that the amount of push notifications was adequate.

Video consultations are increasingly used for remote medical care, especially when in-person visits are not feasible. At the Leiden Headache Center, the majority of patients and healthcare providers considered video consults a good replacement for physical visits [43]. Thus, both patients and healthcare providers value video consultation, which is in line with previous research that describes telemedicine as a valuable alternative for headache patients with high patient satisfaction [44]. In headache care, the most critical aspect of a consultation is the headache history, which can be obtained accurately through telemedicine [45]. Patients can track their symptoms and share them during video consultations. Some guidelines are available for providing a second opinion through telemedicine [46], although formal guidelines are lacking. In certain clinical scenarios with indications of secondary headache, we do recommend performing a physical neurological assessment during an in-person consultation. For widespread implementation, systems must be in place to assure health equity, reduce disparities, and improve access to care with the use of digital health applications [47].

Multidisciplinary Care

Headache Centers are multidisciplinary programs that are experienced in the care of complex or refractory headache conditions and utilize a collaborative approach to management [48]. Multidisciplinary care models are efficient and effective approaches for management of chronic pain, including migraine and associated comorbidities [49]. In addition, integrated and coordinated care services between specialists and primary care are essential for continuity of care. However, communication barriers between general practitioners, specialists and patients, lack of education and follow through of the care plan may negatively impact outcomes. To facilitate care, simple migraine screening tools, linkage protocols, and online education may improve outcomes [50, 51].

In one study, multidisciplinary care was associated with a reduction in headache frequency, medication overuse, and work absenteeism [52]. In another study of a headache center of excellence group model approach, headache outcomes, healthcare utilization, and patient and provider satisfaction were evaluated prospectively [53]. After an educational session with a neurologist and nurse practitioner followed by a coordinated care plan by a nurse practitioner, statistically significant improvements were seen in the Migraine-Specific Questionnaire and the Short Form-36 measurements at 8 weeks and for 6 months after completion of the program. During the study period, there was a 92% subjective improvement, a reduction in emergency room and primary care visits, and high levels of patient satisfaction. Taken together, this study demonstrated the value of multidisciplinary teams for individualized patient care.

Structured headache programs can provide expert encounters with treatment complexities. This includes pregnancy and lactation, metabolic and nutritional disorders, hormonal dysfunction, sleep disorders, cardiovascular disease, evaluation of genetic syndromes such as hemiplegic migraine, cerebral autosomal dominant arteriopathy with subcortical infarcts and leukoencephalopathy (CADASIL), and Ehlers-Danlos Syndrome. Access to neuroradiologists and other diagnosticians are needed to evaluate secondary disorders such as idiopathic intracranial hypertension, low-pressure headache syndromes, peripheral causes of vertigo, and autonomic dysfunction. In addition, migraine is associated with a several medical and psychological comorbidities, which may complicate care and increase risks of progression. For example, several studies have shown the emergence of comorbidity profiles or clusters of natural chronic migraine phenotypes [54, 55]. In one study of individuals receiving care at a headache center, it was estimated that almost 50% suspected to have migraine, either episodic or chronic, also had insomnia and may benefit from cognitive behavioral therapy [56]. Behavioral therapies are underutilized for headache management, but evaluations by psychologists for migraine increase use of cognitive behavioral therapies, which may be associated with several societal and cultural factors [57, 58]. As another example, Headache Centers of Excellence designations by Veterans Health Administration allows for the specialized care needs and research priorities in enriched populations carrying higher rates of migraine, in addition to comorbid pain disorders, traumatic brain injuries, and psychiatric comorbidities. The center designation facilities investigate to meet the clinical needs, such as a recent study suggesting that multimodalities should be encouraged including complimentary and integrative medicine [59]. Implementation of behavioral interventions might be particularly relevant in the care of headache patients with medication overuse headache (MOH). A recent trial suggested modest benefit of behavioral intervention by a headache nurse during withdrawal therapy for medication overuse headache, to reduce acute medication use during and shortly after intervention, but extension seems warranted for a prolonged effect [60].

Migraine Education and Specialization

Headache education is an important component of Headache Centers of Excellence, as there is a serious deficiency in the number of headache specialists available to support population demands [61]. In a summary to address the headache specialty shortage, Huang et al. describe exposure to a headache center during residency training as one of the top 3 most commonly cited reasons for developing interest in headache medicine [62]. In reality, exposure to formal headache education is low. It is the lowest of all neurologic subspecialty topics, occurring in 4–6% of all grand round lectures, and with estimates of just 3 hours during undergraduate medical education [63, 64]. Ongoing continuing medical education programs for headache specialists, neurologists, primary care providers, and advanced nurse practitioners can be facilitated best on local needs in addition to prominent national and international efforts.

At headache centers, rigorous educational programs should be leveraged to develop many more qualified headache specialists. This includes clinical fellowship programs and a Master's degrees in Headache Medicine, based on standardized curriculums. High-quality educational strategies include case-based learning, hands on as well as procedural workshops, and exposures to inpatient units and outpatient care. Long distance learning can be supported with newer virtual platforms, as well as mentoring, limiting geographic boundaries. International clinical collaborations are useful to improve headache education and can be organized through formalized international scholar exchange programs [65].

Advances in Scientific Research

Migraine shows familial occurrence, with complex inheritance and a combination of genetic and environmental factors together conferring disease susceptibility [66]. The influence of genetics on migraine has been widely acknowledged for a considerable period. Notably, various monogenic migraine syndromes underscore this genetic connection, wherein migraine serves as a central symptom or is part of a broader array of symptoms. In the case of common migraine forms, such as those with or without aura, extensive genome-wide association studies (GWAS) have significantly broadened our understanding of the genetic factors involved [67]. These studies highlight the importance of both neuronal and vascular pathways in the manifestation of migraines. Analyzing the genetic makeup of prevalent migraine subtypes contributes to our understanding of the relationships between different subtypes and their links to concurrent disorders. While currently limited in its applicability for diagnosis or personalized treatments, the landscape may evolve with emerging genetic studies focusing on neuropharmacology (pharmacogenetics) [66]. In contrast, the clinical significance of identifying monogenic migraine syndromes and comprehending their underlying genetic architecture has been firmly established for quite some time.

The International Headache Genetics Consortium is a multinational research collaboration that collects diagnostic and genetic information for genome wide association studies, to inform future therapeutics [70].

Research programs at headache centers range from translational to clinical-oriented research, case studies, quality care service, and public health research. A study investigating migraine research trends from 2010–2019 was conducted using scientometric methods and found key topics which included causes and pathophysiological mechanisms, migraine genes, diagnostic criteria, epidemiology, preventive drugs, and other treatments [68]. In a collaboration with NIH and the American Headache Society, eight headache research priorities were established through working groups, which will help drive research for the next decade [69]. Structured headache centers will play a critical role in research workforce development and migraine-specific research.

Team science, defined as a collaborative effort utilizing the strengths and expertise of different fields, can be successfully applied to investigate migraine. Cohesiveness among different interdisciplinary research created by the Centers of Excellence may strengthen funding potential, as well as collaboration between patient care and research activities. Administrative and scientific core reduce redundancy and improve efficiency through a centralized process. The foundation of team science includes capacity to develop a shared vision, open communication, trust, accountability, and conflict resolution. The NIH's National Cancer Institute developed a Team Science Toolkit, with insights that can be applied to headache research [70]. A major part of the mission of the headache center is the training and mentoring of the next generation of scientists [71]. Due to the COVID19 pandemic, there has been a rise in the use of virtual platforms for mentoring and thesis or dissertation defense, which may continue years to come.

Headache centers participate in multi-centered, randomized clinical trials to assure accurate diagnoses and adequate recruitment of subjects with migraine, as well as representative samples that may be more difficult to treat. To guide clinical trials, the International Headache Society has published several clinical trial guidelines for migraine, including for investigation of therapeutics for acute migraine attacks and preventive therapies of episodic and chronic migraine [72–74]. Patient input is necessary to assure research studies and clinical outreach are patient-centric [75]. Patient collaboration should occur in every step of the research process, including informed consent and study design.

Real world and registries studies are a useful way to capture real-world responses and adverse events to newer agents, with varying demographics and comorbidities that may have been excluded in clinical trials. In addition, the American Registry for Migraine Research, or ARMR, collects patient data and biospecimens to understand the cause, characteristics, and management of migraine [76]. The NIH Common Data Elements Repository provides structured human and machine-readable definitions of data elements for migraine [77]. At headache centers, databases powered by searchable headache intakes are useful for clinic-based studies and the development of hypotheses-driven aims, and for prospective studies [78]. In addition, patient registries may be useful to improve in the recruitment of clinical trials. Moreover, headache specialty clinics may contribute to the validation of the International Classification of Headache Disorders system, through field testing, such as the call to validate the proposed vestibular migraine diagnose and others [79].

Community Engagement and Patient Education

Headache centers are principal settings for patient advocacy, education, and community engagement [80]. To increase awareness and reduce stigma and disability, the rapid acceleration of digital platforms may improve the accessibility to support and education globally. In addition, education programs for patients on waitlists may reduce emergency department visits, analgesic overuse, and disability [81]. Partnership with patient advocacy groups and community representatives may result in more patient-centric services and higher rates of satisfaction. Support groups can organize within headache centers and may be supplemented by online platforms such as those hosted by the American Migraine Foundation or Miles for Migraine, to name a few.

Conclusion

Migraine is a leading cause of disability, suffering, and socioeconomic loss. Yet, this is an exciting time practice headache medicine, with novel advances and greater opportunities for migraine education and research collaboration. Structured headache programs provide high-quality care to reduce the burden of migraine and other headache disorders. Universal outcome measures are available for headache treatments and health care systems, factoring time loss during migraine attacks and disability [82]. The societal gains of headache centers go beyond utilization of evidenced-based treatment to reduce disability, but also include gains from training providers, investments from scientific advancements, and public education. The business of a headache center, including financial benchmarks and center goals should be clearly outlined with regional and national support to strengthen referral base, infrastructure, and ultimately improve outcomes for the lives of those with migraine [48]. As seen in an evaluation of European regions, analytic models are available to link direct and indirect costs with health outcomes and allow for comparisons in cost-effectiveness structured headache services [83]. Overall, specialized headache programs are cost-effective, and reduce healthcare utilization, disability, and costs [84]. Partnerships with federal funding agencies, local health institutions, and academic headache societies are needed to accelerate scientific discovery on a large scale, which may be supported regionally, nationally, or internationally.

Teaching Points

1. Structured headache centers aim to provide excellence in migraine care through several main features: expertise in migraine care, access to multidisciplinary specialties, protocols based on clinical guidelines, and the use of clinical measures, including those necessary to assess quality care delivery.
2. While barriers to migraine care occur on every level, systems that implement policies to improve access and parameters for referral, digital tools, and coordination of care may optimize care delivery, including the diagnosis and treatment.
3. Structured headache centers should include education and research productivity, in addition to involvement in public health initiatives and community engagement; participation may vary based on preferences.

Questions and Answers

1. To achieve excellence in clinical migraine care, essential components of a structured headache center should include which of the following:
   A. Advanced imaging techniques for the diagnosis of migraine
   B. Coordination of care
   C. Expertise in migraine surgery
   D. Expedited access for migraine with aura

The correct answer is B. A defining feature of a structured headache center is the ability to provide high-quality treatment and coordination of services including multidisciplinary referrals. Migraine surgery is not a recognized evidence-based intervention for migraine and is therefore not a recommended service of structured headache center. Advances in imaging techniques such as functional MRI and diffusion tensor imaging (DTI) may be useful for research purposes, but do not play a role in the diagnosis of migraine. Migraine with aura may be common among people seeking care; however, uncomplicated migraine with aura is not an indication for expedited referrals and can be managed without subspecialists. However, most patients with refractory headache disorders, including chronic migraine, are best managed at structured headache centers.

2. Which of the following may explain the potential cost effectiveness of headache centers?
   A. Protocols are avoided so that treatment is personalized.
   B. Patient education modules encourage emergency department visits for severe attacks.
   C. Evidenced-based treatments are initiated early to reduce disability.
   D. The availability of genetic tests may predict migraine progression.

The correct answer is C. Structured headache programs have increased efficiency as a consequence of multiple clinical protocols available to provide care for patients in a systematic way (i.e. infusions, neurotoxin injections, rescue plans, and status migrainosus protocols). Protocols may also be in place for establishing support for work disability or other aspects of patient care. Patient education is designed to improve migraine outcomes and reduce healthcare utilization such as due to frequent emergency department visits. Migraine guidelines and consensus statements are closely followed to improve outcomes and provide the highest standard of care. Outcomes can be captured by quality measures and with validated clinical instruments. At this time, genetic testing is not available to provide migraine progression or prognosis.

References

1. Collaborators GBDH. Global, regional, and national burden of migraine and tension-type headache, 1990–2016: a systematic analysis for the Global Burden of Disease Study 2016. Lancet Neurol. 2018;17(11):954–76.
2. Steiner TJ, Husoy A, Stovner LJ. GBD2021: headache disorders and global lost health – a focus on children, and a view forward. J Headache Pain. 2024;25(1):91.
3. Clarke CE, MacMillan L, Sondhi S, Wells NE. Economic and social impact of migraine. QJM. 1996;89(1):77–84.
4. Bonafede M, Sapra S, Shah N, Tepper S, Cappell K, Desai P. Direct and indirect healthcare resource utilization and costs among migraine patients in the United States. Headache. 2018;58(5):700–14.
5. Lipton RB, Bigal ME, Diamond M, Freitag F, Reed ML, Stewart WF, et al. Migraine prevalence, disease burden, and the need for preventive therapy. Neurology. 2007;68(5):343–9.
6. Latinovic R, Gulliford M, Ridsdale L. Headache and migraine in primary care: consultation, prescription, and referral rates in a large population. J Neurol Neurosurg Psychiatry. 2006;77(3):385–7.
7. Gibbs TS, Fleischer AB Jr, Feldman SR, Sam MC, O'Donovan CA. Health care utilization in patients with migraine: demographics and patterns of care in the ambulatory setting. Headache. 2003;43(4):330–5.
8. Shimizu T, Sakai F, Miyake H, Sone T, Sato M, Tanabe S, et al. Disability, quality of life, productivity impairment and employer costs of migraine in the workplace. J Headache Pain. 2021;22(1):29.
9. Messali A, Sanderson JC, Blumenfeld AM, Goadsby PJ, Buse DC, Varon SF, et al. Direct and indirect costs of chronic and episodic migraine in the United States: a web-based survey. Headache. 2016;56(2):306–22.
10. Nagata JM, Weiser SD, Gooding HC, Garber AK, Bibbins-Domingo K, Palar K. Association between food insecurity and migraine among US young adults. JAMA Neurol. 2019;76(9):1121–2.
11. Burch R, Rizzoli P, Loder E. The prevalence and impact of migraine and severe headache in the United States: updated age, sex, and socioeconomic-specific estimates from government health surveys. Headache. 2021;61(1):60–8.

12. Farmer P. The major infectious diseases in the world--to treat or not to treat? N Engl J Med. 2001;345(3):208–10.
13. Manyazewal T, Woldeamanuel Y, Oppenheim C, Hailu A, Giday M, Medhin G, Belete A, Yimer G, Collins A, Makonnen E, Fekadu A. Conceptualising centres of excellence: a scoping review of global evidence. BMJ Open. 2022;12(2):e050419.
14. Steiner TJ, Gobel H, Jensen R, Lampl C, Paemeleire K, Linde M, et al. Headache service quality: the role of specialized headache centres within structured headache services, and suggested standards and criteria as centres of excellence. J Headache Pain. 2019;20(1):24.
15. Buse DC, Armand CE, Charleston L, Reed ML, Fanning KM, Adams AM, et al. Barriers to care in episodic and chronic migraine: results from the chronic migraine epidemiology and outcomes study. Headache. 2021;61(4):628–41.
16. Improvement IoMIPMA. Performance measurement: accelerating improvement. Washington, DC: National Academy Press; 2005.
17. Lenz B, Katsarava Z, Gil-Gouveia R, Karelis G, Kaynarkaya B, Meksa L, et al. Headache service quality evaluation: implementation of quality indicators in primary care in Europe. J Headache Pain. 2021;22(1):33.
18. Peters M, Jenkinson C, Perera S, Loder E, Jensen R, Katsarava Z, et al. Quality in the provision of headache care. 2: defining quality and its indicators. J Headache Pain. 2012;13(6):449–57.
19. Fejes E, Feher G, Gurdan Z, Gombos K, Koltai K, Pusch G, et al. Characteristics of patients referred to a specialized headache clinic. Sci Rep. 2020;10(1):1146.
20. Fischer M, Frank F, Wille G, Klien S, Lackner P, Broessner G. Triptans for acute migraine headache: current experience with triptan use and prescription habits in a tertiary care headache outpatient clinic: an observational study. Headache. 2016;56(6):952–60.
21. Pozo-Rosich P, Lucas C, Watson DPB, Gaul C, Ramsden E, Ritter S, et al. Burden of migraine in patients with preventive treatment failure attending European headache specialist centers: real-world evidence from the BECOME study. Pain Ther. 2021;10(2):1691–708.
22. Sacco S, Braschinsky M, Ducros A, Lampl C, Little P, van den Brink AM, et al. European headache federation consensus on the definition of resistant and refractory migraine : developed with the endorsement of the European Migraine & Headache Alliance (EMHA). J Headache Pain. 2020;21(1):76.
23. Steiner TJ, Jensen R, Katsarava Z, Linde M, MacGregor EA, Osipova V, et al. Aids to management of headache disorders in primary care (2nd edition): on behalf of the European Headache Federation and Lifting The Burden: the Global Campaign against Headache. J Headache Pain. 2019;20(1):57.
24. Vigano A, Savastano E, Petolicchio B, Toscano M, De Sanctis R, Maestrini I, et al. A study of clinical features and risk factors of self-referring emergency department headache patients: a comparison with headache center outpatients. Eur Neurol. 2020;83(1):34–40.
25. Negro A, Spuntarelli V, Sciattella P, Martelletti P. Rapid referral for headache management from emergency department to headache centre: four years data. J Headache Pain. 2020;21(1):25.
26. Ailani J, Burch RC, Robbins MS, Board of Directors of the American Headache Society. The American Headache Society Consensus Statement: update on integrating new migraine treatments into clinical practice. Headache. 2021;61:1021.
27. Diener HC, Gaul C, Jensen R, Gobel H, Heinze A, Silberstein SD. Integrated headache care. Cephalalgia. 2011;31(9):1039–47.
28. Strauss LD, Yugrakh MS, Kaplan KE, Minen MT, Ahs Emergency Department IRSIG. Headache infusion centers: a survey on treatments provided, infusion center operations, and barriers to developing new infusion centers. Headache. 2021;61(9):1364–75.
29. Mathew PG. A critical re-evaluation of migraine trigger site decompression surgery. Headache. 2014;54(7):1231–3.
30. Hepp Z, Dodick DW, Varon SF, Chia J, Matthew N, Gillard P, et al. Persistence and switching patterns of oral migraine prophylactic medications among patients with chronic migraine: a retrospective claims analysis. Cephalalgia. 2017;37(5):470–85.
31. Burch RC, Ailani J, Robbins MS. The American Headache Society Consensus Statement: update on integrating new migraine treatments into clinical practice. Headache. 2022;62(1):111–2.
32. Sacco S, Bendtsen L, Ashina M, Reuter U, Terwindt G, Mitsikostas DD, et al. European headache federation guideline on the use of monoclonal antibodies acting on the calcitonin gene related peptide or its receptor for migraine prevention. J Headache Pain. 2019;20(1):6.
33. Sharon R, Rayhill M, Viknevich J, Charleston L, Mathew PG. An analysis of UCNS certified headache center patient intake forms. Headache. 2016;56(3):519–27.
34. Robbins MS, Victorio MCC, Bailey M, Cook C, Garza I, Huff JS, et al. Quality improvement in neurology: headache quality measurement set. Headache. 2021;61(1):219–26.
35. Marmura MJ, Nahas SJ. What might the ideal electronic medical record for migraine headache look like? Curr Pain Headache Rep. 2010;14(3):233–7.
36. Houts CR, McGinley JS, Nishida TK, Buse DC, Wirth RJ, Dodick DW, et al. Systematic review of outcomes and endpoints in acute migraine clinical trials. Headache. 2021;61(2):263–75.
37. McGinley JS, Houts CR, Nishida TK, Buse DC, Lipton RB, Goadsby PJ, et al. Systematic review of outcomes and endpoints in preventive migraine clinical trials. Headache. 2021;61(2):253–62.
38. Diener HC, Ashina M, Durand-Zaleski I, Kurth T, Lanteri-Minet M, Lipton RB, et al. Health technology assessment for the acute and preventive treatment of migraine: a position statement of the International Headache Society. Cephalalgia. 2021;41(3):279–93.
39. van Casteren DS, Verhagen IE, de Boer I, de Vries Lentsch S, Fronczek R, van Zwet EW, et al. E-diary use in clinical headache practice: a prospective observational study. Cephalalgia. 2021;41(11–12):1161–71.
40. Verhagen IE, Spaink HA, van der Arend BW, van Casteren DS, MaassenVanDenBrink A, Terwindt GM. Validation of diagnostic ICHD-3 criteria for menstrual migraine. Cephalalgia. 2022;42(11–12):1184–93.
41. van der Arend BWH, Verhagen IE, van Leeuwen M, van der Arend M, van Casteren DS, Terwindt GM. Defining migraine days, based on longitudinal E-diary data. Cephalalgia. 2023;43(5):3331024231166625.
42. Verhagen IE, van Casteren DS, de Vries Lentsch S, Terwindt GM. Effect of lockdown during COVID-19 on migraine: a longitudinal cohort study. Cephalalgia. 2021;41(7):865–70.
43. van der Arend BWH, Holwerda LJ, Verhagen IE, van Casteren DS, Timmers T, Terwindt GM. Practical experience with the use of electronic headache diaries and video consultations in migraine care from a longitudinal cohort study. Telemed e-Health. 2024;30:2696–703.
44. Clausen TC, Greve NK, Muller KI, Kristoffersen ES, Schytz HW. Telemedicine in headache care: a systematic review. Cephalalgia. 2022;42(13):1397–408.
45. Spina E, Tedeschi G, Russo A, Trojsi F, Iodice R, Tozza S, et al. Telemedicine application to headache: a critical review. Neurol Sci. 2022;43(6):3795–801.
46. Pereira-Monteiro J, Wysocka-Bakowska MM, Katsarava Z, Antonaci F, European HF. Guidelines for telematic second opinion consultation on headaches in Europe: on behalf of the European Headache Federation (EHF). J Headache Pain. 2010;11(4):345–8.
47. Gordon Perue GL, Fox-Rosellini SE, Sur NB, Marulanda-Londono E, Margolesky J, Tornes L, et al. Development of an equity, diversity, inclusion, and anti-racism pledge as the foundation for action in an Academic Department of Neurology. Neurology. 2021;97:729.
48. Minen MT, Wells RE, Gautreaux JR, Szperka CL, Rayhill M, Orlova Y, et al. Responding to the needs of early career physi-

cians and fellows in headache medicine: career planning, getting involved, and considerations in building a headache center. Headache. 2020;60(7):1453–62.
49. Gaul C, Liesering-Latta E, Schafer B, Fritsche G, Holle D. Integrated multidisciplinary care of headache disorders: a narrative review. Cephalalgia. 2016;36(12):1181–91.
50. La Pegna GB, Brighina F, Saporito V, Aloisio A, Morreale C, D'Agati A. Continuity of healthcare for headache patients: a problem of communication between headache specialists and general practitioners. J Headache Pain. 2005;6(4):310–1.
51. Ashina M, Katsarava Z, Do TP, Buse DC, Pozo-Rosich P, Ozge A, et al. Migraine: epidemiology and systems of care. Lancet. 2021;397(10283):1485–95.
52. Zeeberg P, Olesen J, Jensen R. Efficacy of multidisciplinary treatment in a tertiary referral headache centre. Cephalalgia. 2005;25(12):1159–67.
53. Blumenfeld A, Tischio M. Center of excellence for headache care: group model at Kaiser Permanente. Headache. 2003;43(5):431–40.
54. Woldeamanuel YW, Sanjanwala BM, Peretz AM, Cowan RP. Exploring natural clusters of chronic migraine phenotypes: a cross-sectional clinical study. Sci Rep. 2020;10(1):2804.
55. Lipton RB, Fanning KM, Buse DC, Martin VT, Reed ML, Manack Adams A, et al. Identifying natural subgroups of migraine based on comorbidity and concomitant condition profiles: results of the Chronic Migraine Epidemiology and Outcomes (CaMEO) study. Headache. 2018;58(7):933–47.
56. Begasse de Dhaem O, Seng E, Minen MT. Screening for insomnia: an observational study examining sleep disturbances, headache characteristics, and psychiatric symptoms in patients visiting a headache center. Pain Med. 2018;19(5):1067–76.
57. Langenbahn D, Matsuzawa Y, Lee YSC, Fraser F, Penzien DB, Simon NM, et al. Underuse of behavioral treatments for headache: a narrative review examining societal and cultural factors. J Gen Intern Med. 2021;36(10):3103–12.
58. Minen MT, Azarchi S, Sobolev R, Shallcross A, Halpern A, Berk T, et al. Factors related to migraine patients' decisions to initiate behavioral migraine treatment following a headache specialist's recommendation: a prospective observational study. Pain Med. 2018;19(11):2274–82.
59. Kuruvilla DE, Lindsey H, Grinberg AS, Goldman RE, Riley S, Baird S, et al. Complementary and integrative medicine perspectives among veteran patients and VHA healthcare providers for the treatment of headache disorders: a qualitative study. BMC Complement Med Ther. 2022;22(1):22.
60. Pijpers JA, Kies DA, van Zwet EW, Rosendaal FR, Terwindt GM. Behavioural intervention in medication overuse headache: a concealed double-blind randomized controlled trial. Eur J Neurol. 2022;29(5):1496–504.
61. Begasse de Dhaem O, Burch R, Rosen N, Shubin Stein K, Loder E, Shapiro RE. Workforce gap analysis in the field of headache medicine in the United States. Headache. 2020;60(2):478–81.
62. Huang H, Minen MT. Eleven reasons people decide to choose headache medicine: there may be a headache medicine provider shortage but there are ways to foster interest. Headache. 2020;60(8):1846–52.
63. Gallagher RM, Alam R, Shah S, Mueller L, Rogers JJ. Headache in medical education: medical schools, neurology and family practice residencies. Headache. 2005;45(7):866–73.
64. Vollbracht S, Masters-Israilov A. The unmet need of headache medicine grand rounds education in neurology. Headache. 2021;61(7):988–9.
65. Rizzoli PB, Lauria Pinter G, Grazzi L. International clinical collaboration in headache medicine: the international visiting scholars program. Headache. 2019;59(3):446–9.
66. de Boer I, van den Maagdenberg A, Terwindt GM. Advance in genetics of migraine. Curr Opin Neurol. 2019;32(3):413–21.
67. Hautakangas H, Winsvold BS, Ruotsalainen SE, Bjornsdottir G, Harder AVE, Kogelman LJA, et al. Genome-wide analysis of 102,084 migraine cases identifies 123 risk loci and subtype-specific risk alleles. Nat Genet. 2022;54(2):152–60.
68. Lu T, Li J, Li J, Li M, Feng L, Li X, et al. The global trends of migraine research from 2010 to 2019: a scientometric study. Ann Palliat Med. 2021;10(5):5767–79.
69. Stroke NIoNDa. Headache research priorities. 2023. Available from: https://ninds.ideascalegov.com/c/campaigns/1263/about.
70. Institute NIoHNC. Team Science Toolkit. 2018.
71. Minen MT, Monteith T, Strauss LD, Starling A. New investigator and trainee task force survey on the recruitment and retention of headache specialists. Headache. 2015;55(8):1092–101.
72. Tassorelli C, Diener HC, Dodick DW, Silberstein SD, Lipton RB, Ashina M, et al. Guidelines of the International Headache Society for controlled trials of preventive treatment of chronic migraine in adults. Cephalalgia. 2018;38(5):815–32.
73. Diener HC, Tassorelli C, Dodick DW, Silberstein SD, Lipton RB, Ashina M, et al. Guidelines of the International Headache Society for controlled trials of preventive treatment of migraine attacks in episodic migraine in adults. Cephalalgia. 2020;40(10):1026–44.
74. Alpuente A, Tassorelli C, Diener HC, Silberstein SD, Pozo-Rosich P. Have the IHS guidelines for controlled trials of acute treatment of migraine attacks been followed? Laying the ground for the 4th edition. Cephalalgia. 2020;40(8):778–87.
75. Sharma NS. Patient centric approach for clinical trials: current trend and new opportunities. Perspect Clin Res. 2015;6(3):134–8.
76. Schwedt TJ, Digre K, Tepper SJ, Spare NM, Ailani J, Birlea M, et al. The American Registry for Migraine Research: research methods and baseline data for an initial patient cohort. Headache. 2020;60(2):337–47.
77. https://www.commondataelements.ninds.nih.gov/headache
78. Marmura MJ, Hopkins M, Andrel J, Young WB, Biondi DM, Rupnow MF, et al. Electronic medical records as a research tool: evaluating topiramate use at a headache center. Headache. 2010;50(5):769–78.
79. Groezinger M, Huppert D, Strobl R, Grill E. Development and validation of a classification algorithm to diagnose and differentiate spontaneous episodic vertigo syndromes: results from the DizzyReg patient registry. J Neurol. 2020;267(Suppl 1):160–7.
80. Monteith TS. Advocacy for migraine relief: strategic planning to eliminate the burden. Curr Pain Headache Rep. 2022;26(8):567–74.
81. Lagman-Bartolome AM, Lawler V, Lay C. Headache education active-waiting directive: a program to enhance well-being during long referral wait times. Headache. 2018;58(1):109–17.
82. Steiner TJ, Linde M, Schnell-Inderst P. A universal outcome measure for headache treatments, care-delivery systems and economic analysis. J Headache Pain. 2021;22(1):63.
83. Tinelli M, Leonardi M, Paemeleire K, Mitsikostas D, de la Torre ER, Steiner TJ, et al. Structured headache services as the solution to the ill-health burden of headache. 2. Modelling effectiveness and cost-effectiveness of implementation in Europe: methodology. J Headache Pain. 2021;22(1):99.
84. Freitag FG, Lyss H, Nissan GR. Migraine disability, healthcare utilization, and expenditures following treatment in a tertiary headache center. Baylor Univ Med Cent Proc. 2013;26(4):363–7.
85. Lipton RB, Kolodner K, Bigal ME, Valade D, Lainez MJ, Pascual J, et al. Validity and reliability of the Migraine-Treatment Optimization Questionnaire. Cephalalgia. 2009;29(7):751–9.
86. Dowson AJ, D'Amico D, Tepper SJ, Baos V, Baudet F, Kilminster S. Identifying patients who require a change in their current acute migraine treatment: the Migraine Assessment of Current Therapy (Migraine-ACT) questionnaire. Neurol Sci. 2004;25(Suppl 3):S276–8.

87. Kimel M, Hsieh R, McCormack J, Burch SP, Revicki DA. Validation of the revised Patient Perception of Migraine Questionnaire (PPMQ-R): measuring satisfaction with acute migraine treatment in clinical trials. Cephalalgia. 2008;28(5):510–23.
88. Silberstein SD, Cady RK, Sheftell FD, Almas M, Parsons B, Albert KS. Efficacy of eletriptan in migraine-related functional impairment: functional and work productivity outcomes. Headache. 2007;47(5):673–82.
89. Hareendran A, Skalicky A, Mannix S, Lavoie S, Desai P, Bayliss M, et al. Development of a new tool for evaluating the benefit of preventive treatments for migraine on functional outcomes – the Migraine Functional Impact Questionnaire (MFIQ). Headache. 2018;58(10):1612–28.
90. Martin BC, Pathak DS, Sharfman MI, Adelman JU, Taylor F, Kwong WJ, et al. Validity and reliability of the migraine-specific quality of life questionnaire (MSQ Version 2.1). Headache. 2000;40(3):204–15.
91. Kawata AK, Hsieh R, Bender R, Shaffer S, Revicki DA, Bayliss M, et al. Psychometric evaluation of a novel instrument assessing the impact of migraine on physical functioning: the migraine physical function impact diary. Headache. 2017;57(9):1385–98.
92. Pryse-Phillips W. Evaluating migraine disability: the headache impact test instrument in context. Can J Neurol Sci. 2002;29(Suppl 2):S11–5.
93. Stewart WF, Lipton RB, Kolodner K, Liberman J, Sawyer J. Reliability of the migraine disability assessment score in a population-based sample of headache sufferers. Cephalalgia. 1999;19(2):107–14; discussion 74.
94. Reilly MC, Zbrozek AS, Dukes EM. The validity and reproducibility of a work productivity and activity impairment instrument. Pharmacoeconomics. 1993;4(5):353–65.

Underserved Populations, Reducing Health Disparities, and Improving Equity

37

Charles Flippen II

Introduction

Treatment of primary headache disorders, not unlike other chronic conditions, have multiple axes of disparate care [1, 2]. The optimal, just (and equitable) care for patients with headache disorders requires access to primary care providers with basic knowledge of the diagnosis and management of primary headache disorders. Ideally, patients would have access to referral networks to general neurological or headache medicine subspecialty expertise to provide an accurate diagnosis and treatment plan. Meeting those minimal requirements has challenged all migraine sufferers. Only 26.3% of adult patients with episodic migraine and less than 5% of adult chronic migraine patients receive appropriate care with regards to acute and preventive treatments [3, 4]. The structure of care disparity in headache medicine involves social determinants of health (SDH) (race, socioeconomic stability/status, social location, education) along with access to well-trained providers with the resources (medications, procedures, behavioral medicine) to provide quality care (Fig. 37.1).

Questions

1. How does lower socioeconomic status impact migraine prevalence?
   A. It reduces the likelihood of experiencing migraine.
   B. It has no significant effect on migraine prevalence.
   C. It predicts worse health outcomes associated with migraine.
   D. It decreases the risk of transitioning from episodic to chronic migraine.
2. Which of the following is NOT a core tenet of intersectionality?
   A. Personal experiences are complex, with high variation within an identity categorization.
   B. Human beings exist in the simultaneously overlapping margins of multiple identities.
   C. Intersectionality focuses solely on individual identity without considering broader social contexts.
   D. Intersectionality centers on the experiences of historically marginalized individuals and groups.

C. Flippen II (✉)
Department of Neurology, David Geffen School of Medicine at UCLA, Los Angeles, CA, USA

T. S. Monteith et al. (eds.), *Comprehensive Migraine Management*, https://doi.org/10.1007/978-3-031-86923-5_37

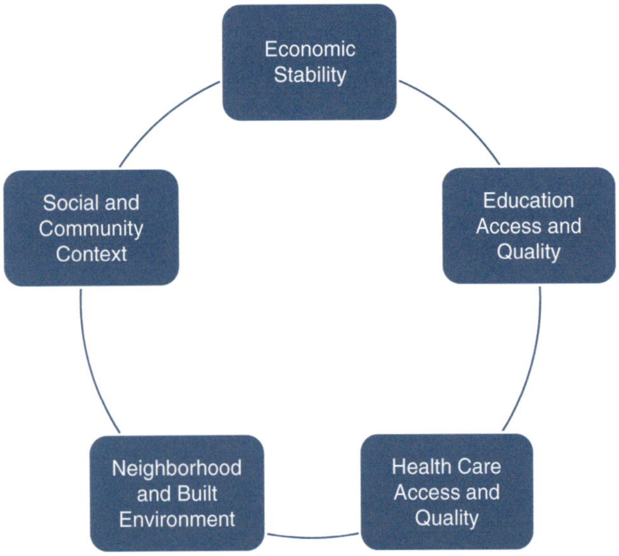
Economic Stability
Education Access and Quality
Health Care Access and Quality
Neighborhood and Built Environment
Social and Community Context

Fig. 37.1 Social determinants of health are thought to have major impacts on health and well-being, including chronic diseases such as migraine. (https://odphp.health.gov/healthypeople)

Disparity Factors and Social Determinants of Health

Race/Ethnicity

Race as a social construct has influenced both the consignment of patients to lower status within other social determinants of health as well as provider reaction to and treatment of non-White patients. Most of the literature on the influence of race on diagnosis and treatment of migraine is from the study of Black migraine sufferers [5]. Although migraine and severe headache prevalence is similar among groups (White 15.5%; Black 15%; Hispanic 14.9%) in the United States, diagnosis rates are lower for Black (25% less) and Hispanic (50% less) than for White patients. Black patients with headache were 4.8 times less likely than White patients presenting with a complaint of headache to receive CT of head in the emergency department (ED) setting in evaluation for headache etiology [6]. While ED imaging is not an indicator of appropriate or care quality, it could be inferred to be a marker of increased provider concern in not wanting to "miss something".

Socioeconomic Factors

Lower socioeconomic status is a known predictor of worse health outcomes with migraine prevalence directly associated with annual household income [6, 7] The effect of low-income status may compound the disparity encumbered by a patient who have additional factors known to promote healthcare disparities. Most of the headache literature on the impact of income and insurance status comes from the migraine population that has the most robust epidemiological studies and data. There is a 60% higher rate of migraine in lower annual income patient groups (<$10,000) compared to patients from higher (>$30,000) income groups [6]. The prevalence of migraine is highest in those with the lowest incomes, below the poverty line and those uninsured (17%) or those with Medicaid (26%) when compared to migraine patients with private insurance (15%) [4].

Low income and uninsured patients are less likely to receive migraine-specific acute treatments [7]. The absence of effective acute treatments is associated with progression to and increased risk of chronic migraine [8].

Social Location

Migraine disproportionately affects people in low-social locations, people experiencing intersecting, mutually constitutive disadvantages that creates susceptibility to poor outcomes, at the same time alienating them from protective factors [9]. This places migraine within the social causation hypothesis that theorizes the likelihood of a disorder and severity once initiated are increased by occupying a low social location and the subsequent higher stress and associated exogenous factors, such as food insecurity, personal safety, access to healthcare, and employment [9]. Adversities in childhood, such as physical and sexual abuse, as well as witnessing domestic violence, are significantly correlated with migraine in men and women in adulthood [10, 11]. Food insecurity is reported twice as frequently by people with migraine [12].

Education

Education level appears to impact the migraine population by virtue of those episodic sufferers who transition to chronic migraine usually due to abortive medication overuse (MOH). At least two-thirds of people with MOH have migraine as their primary headache disorder [13]. The sociodemographic profile of the MOH population with chronic migraine is characterized by a higher proportion of women, a lower education level, and a higher level of unemployment as compared to those with episodic migraine [14]. Low socioeconomic status defined by education and occupation has been found to be associated with increased risk of frequent and chronic headache [15].

The social determinants of health are key to the disparities seen in migraine care through influence on self-management choices [16], access [17], and type of care received [18] that directly correlates to health outcomes [16, 17]. They must be factored into the care of the underserved.

Intersectionality and Care Delivery

Intersectionality, the premise that social disadvantages and marginalization are a function of multiple interacting factors and not on any one single or separable group identity (e.g., racial and social class categorizations) [19, 20]. Intersectionality provides a multidisciplinary, theoretical framework for examining and understanding identity and experiences of oppression [21]. It includes the following core tenets:

1. Human beings exist in the simultaneously overlapping margins of multiple identities [22, 23].
2. Personal experiences are complex, with high variation within an identity categorization (e.g., racial variation within socioeconomic class) [24].
3. Intersectionality centers on the experiences of individuals and groups who historically have been ignored, marginalized, and underserved [22, 25] and urges a vision of equity that draws on the unique histories and experiences of those who have been marginalized [24].

Taking an intersectional approach to care has been proposed by Befus et al. [24] The use of a trauma and violence-informed paradigm whereby the clinician creates an emotionally and physically safe care environment to mitigate the known health effects of past trauma and violence. This approach is based on six principles: safety, trustworthiness, peer support, collaboration, empowerment and cultural, historical, and gender issues [26, 27]. This approach to care may be applied across the provider and system levels [28]. Examples of how this approach may be implemented at the provider level includes examination of personal experiences, assumptions, and power and how these affect interactions with patients and clinical decision-making [29], and recognition of trauma as a risk factor for physical and behavioral outcomes [30].

Paired with the acknowledgement of trauma and violence as a clinical factor, social determinants must influence the clinical encounter by use of clinical tools such as the PRAPARE instrument (Protocol for Responding to and Assessing Patients' Assets, Risks, and Experiences) [31]. It allows providers to collect data to better understand and act on patients' social determinants of health, engage patients to optimize care accounting for social determinants (can your patient enact the care plan you formulated?), diversify treatment options, including evidence-based behavioral and non-pharmacological approaches. Use of equity-oriented engagement around lifestyle modifications that gives guidance in consideration to social determinants of health when making care recommendations [32].

Provider/Organization Factors

The provision of equitable headache medicine care to underserved populations in many communities falls to safety net health care systems. As defined by the Institute of Medicine (IOM), these systems are "providers that organize and deliver a significant level of healthcare and other needed services to uninsured, Medicaid and other vulnerable patients." [33] These systems are by legal obligation, under funding agreements and/or mission, obligated to provide healthcare to individuals regardless of insurance or resource status. These systems have been the stop gap in the US healthcare system to provide access to uninsured/underinsured populations in the absence of a universal program to ensure access to healthcare services. The commentary by Waitzkin [34] provides a historical overview of the US safety net system that is instructive in understanding the current state of these systems.

Patient access to these systems are through three conduits: hospital-based primary care and specialty clinics, the Emergency Department, and community-based primary care clinics. Prior work has identified 3 crucial steps for adequate medical care for migraine: (1) appropriate medical consultation; (2) an accurate diagnosis; and (3) an effective treatment regimen [39]. The challenges to delivering headache care in this setting involves 3 key factors; (1) the limited number of providers coupled with the number of available appointments exacerbate a baseline access issue, (2) medication formularies with regard to both acute and preventive headache medications are restricted (only 2 triptans, oral preventives are available but limited availability to novel medications), (3) there are few accommodations for procedures, mechanisms for provision of neuromodulation devices or reliable access to Behavioral Health support (limited referrals, poor communication channels to community clinics). These factors result in delayed diagnoses, much more intractable conditions once patients are diagnosed and few options once patients have tried the available medications. Another factor may be the lack of limits on prescribing non-migraine-specific abortive medications, may lead to more frequent use as an entry for patients to medication overuse. High rates of comorbid conditions (particularly the high prevalence of uncontrolled vascular risk factors) contraindicate many abortive medication options.

Potential Provider/Organizational Remedies

Attempts to improve the three factors for effective migraine treatment combines a mix of technology and resource reallocation. Electronic consultation systems where advice is given to primary care providers (mostly APPs) on patient evaluation and treatment to lessen the need for limited specialty appointments. A standing set of expected practices for common neurological complaints including headache could be made available online for additional guidance. Refinement of the dialogue processes to prompt provision of key clinical data by referring providers to allow meaningful communication within the platform is needed. Ongoing efforts to educate our primary care colleagues in basics of headache diagnosis and initial management through seminars and potential online offerings are being developed.

Regarding physical space, several DHS facilities have undergone significant upgrades and replacement of the main DHS hospital in recent years. It is also hoped that the physician (neurologists/headache medicine specialists)/APP staff would increase at a proportional rate to the physical space since current workforce levels are not matched to current patient volume data. Telemedicine has been introduced, spurred by the COVID-19 pandemic but only by telephone conversations.

Formulary issues are framed by a limited budget and resource competition with other disease processes (chemotherapies comprise a significant budget demand on many public systems). The process for formulary additions is cumbersome. Attempts to streamline those processes should be considered.

The systems must engage with community partner pain management physicians to provide some procedural services though this approach is not optimal due to limited capacity and communication. Until capacity is created within safety net systems, these collaborations are neccessary for provision of comprehensive care. Behavioral services may occur primarily through neuropsychology to identify the presence of DSM-5, Axis 1 diagnoses, somatoform tendencies, and/or challenging personality traits. Though not ideal in that psychopharmacological care may be delayed, non-Axis 2 issues may be identified and considered when constructing a care plan.

The care of the underserved migraine patient must not only acknowledge the role of social determinants of health along with the impact of violence and trauma, but consideration of those factors must also be actively incorporated in the clinical care plan if equitable outcomes are to be achieved.

Global Issues

The Global Burden of Disease Study performed by the Institute for Health Metrics and Evaluation, a longitudinal observational epidemiological study of disease burden and Lifting the Burden (LtB), a UK NGO with an official collaboration with the WHO, focused on improving headache healthcare worldwide, have identified the need and with LtB, strategies for improving headache healthcare. Addressing headache medicine care disparities in underserved/underresourced communities in non-US countries can involve several approaches. Here are some examples of how these disparities might be addressed (Table 37.1).

Table 37.1 Global and regional solutions for headache medicine

Increase Access to Healthcare	One of the primary steps is to improve access to healthcare services in underserved communities. LtB suggests a 3-tiered approach with (a) the bulk of care given by primary, community-based providers, (b) special interest headache providers, and (c) headache specialty hospital-based centers [40]
Community Education and Awareness	Raising awareness about headaches, their causes, and available treatment options is crucial. Community education programs can be organized to provide information on the different types of headaches, triggers, and lifestyle modifications that may help alleviate symptoms. By increasing knowledge about headache disorders, individuals in underserved communities can make informed decisions about seeking appropriate care.
Training Healthcare Providers	Enhancing the knowledge and skills of healthcare providers working in underserved communities is essential. Medical professionals should receive training on headache management, diagnosis, and appropriate prescription of medication. This can help ensure that individuals with headaches receive accurate diagnoses and appropriate treatment options.
Improving Medication Availability	Ensuring a steady supply of headache medications is vital. Efforts should be made to make essential headache medicines readily available in local pharmacies and healthcare facilities. This may involve collaborations between pharmaceutical companies, government agencies, and non-governmental organizations (NGOs) to improve distribution networks and affordability.
Telemedicine and Telehealth Services	In areas where access to healthcare is limited, telemedicine and telehealth services can play a significant role. Utilizing digital platforms, individuals can consult with healthcare providers remotely, allowing them to receive medical advice, prescriptions, and follow-up care without the need for physical travel. This approach can bridge the gap between underserved communities and healthcare professionals.
Collaboration with NGOs and International Organizations	NGOs and international organizations focused on healthcare can provide support by initiating programs specifically targeting headache care in underserved communities. These organizations can offer funding, resources, and expertise to improve healthcare infrastructure, develop educational materials, and train local healthcare providers.
Research and Data Collection	Conducting research studies and collecting data on headache prevalence, impact, and treatment outcomes in underserved communities is crucial for understanding the scope of the problem and designing effective interventions. Such data can help guide policymakers, healthcare providers, and organizations in developing evidence-based strategies to address the disparities.

Conclusion

Healthcare equity and initiatives to reduce disparities in headache medicine are important imperatives both nationally and globally. It is important to note that the specific strategies employed may vary depending on the country, cultural factors, and available resources. Tailoring interventions to the unique needs of each community is essential for addressing headache medicine care disparities effectively [40, 41]. Effective care of patients with migraine includes consideration of the impact of social determinants of health and barriers at the system level. The recognition of these factors alone will not improve care, but active partnering between the provider and patient is the essential first step to mitigate SDH effects. Potential solutions have been suggested to mitigate the effect of race/ethnicity, socioeconomic standing, education, and social location were discussed to improve the opportunity to provide culturally sensitive care. Further research in this area is greatly needed, in addition to partnerships with federal/governmental agencies, academic and hospital systems, and the public.

It is important to note that the specific strategies employed may vary depending on the country, cultural factors, and available resources. Tailoring interventions to the unique needs of each community is essential for addressing headache medicine care disparities effectively [40, 41].

Teaching Points

1. Headache care of the underserved is disparate.
2. Recognition of social determinants of health and traumas—violence is essential to delivery of equitable care.
3. The role of unconscious bias.
4. Use of evidence-based scales can aid clinicians in data collection and acting on a patient's social determinants of health.
5. Safety net health systems must assess their processes and practices to eliminate barriers to the provision of access, up-to-date therapies, and behavioral medicine resources.
6. Telemedicine and other digital technologies may increase equity by increasing access but should be monitored for the potential of increasing inequities for individuals with technological challenges such as broad band connectivity barriers.

Case Study: As an Example, We May Look at the Los Angeles County Safety Net System

Los Angeles County is the largest county in the United States with a population of approximately 10 million people. It is one of the most racially and ethnically diverse counties in the United States. About 7 million non-White residents account for nearly three quarters of the population. It is home to more than one million undocumented immigrants [35]. The demographic breakdown of the population includes nearly half (48.6%) of LA county residents identifying themselves as Latinos, 15.4% as Asian, and 9% as African American. Eleven percent of the population under the age of 65 years lack health insurance [36]. The Los Angeles County Department of Health Services (LAC-DHS) safety net health system, the second largest of its kind in the United States serves over 800,000 patients annually; most are non-White, uninsured, or underinsured [37]. It has been established that access to and outcomes from care are generally worse in county hospital systems than in private hospitals [38].

A 39-year-old Hispanic woman presented with headache in the setting of working two jobs, caring for her mother and two teenaged daughters. She has one day off weekly and as a domestic worker with no sick time. She has limited public insurance and medication benefits. She has used mostly simple analgesics and NSAIDs for abortive therapy and had trials of propranolol and amitriptyline for prevention (former was ineffective, later limited by side effects). Her nurse practitioner sought help via electronic consultation from the neurology service, although a specific diagnosis of chronic migraine was given, it had yet to be recorded in her record. Due to a limited formulary for her health plan, many suggested options were not available.

The patient was interviewed via telephonic interpreter in Spanish. It was determined she was surprisingly not in medication overuse, needed both improved (effective) abortive and preventive therapy. Challenges included lifestyle changes (improved/adequate sleep in the context of two jobs); having follow-up at reasonable intervals; access to specific migraine medications; need to refer to the one center in the system with botulinum toxin injections for migraine prevention or to contracted provider outside of health system EHR.

Considering her intersectional characteristics: Mexican heritage, female, Spanish-speaking, cisgender, able-bodied and episodically disabled, low-middle income, secondary education; the following were done to address some of the systemic challenges:

- Plan to use telephone follow-up appointments with Spanish interpreting services (due to lack of cameras on system computers, conventional video telehealth not an option at that time)
- Provide Spanish language patient education materials on migraine treatment and prevention to better understand condition
- Write a letter to her employers that she may intermittently need time off or altered work hours until her condition has improved (6 months).
- Trial of formulary triptan for abortive therapy
- While awaiting the botulinum toxin injection appointment (6 months), use of a drug maker patient assistance program allowed a trial of CGRP monoclonal antibody for prevention.
- Schedule a meeting with the social worker to review her eligibility for a different public insurer option with broader pharmacy options.

Questions and Answers

1. How does lower socioeconomic status impact migraine prevalence?
   A. It reduces the likelihood of experiencing migraine.
   B. It has no significant effect on migraine prevalence.
   C. It predicts worse health outcomes associated with migraine.
   D. It decreases the risk of transitioning from episodic to chronic migraine.

The correct answer is C. *It predicts worse health outcomes associated with migraine*. There is a 60% higher rate of migraine in lower annual income patient groups (<$10,000) compared to patients from higher (>$30,000) income groups [6]. Low income and uninsured patients are less likely to receive migraine-specific acute treatments [7]. The absence of effective acute treatments is associated with progression to and increased risk of chronic migraine [8].

2. Which of the following is NOT a core tenet of intersectionality?
   A. Personal experiences are complex, with high variation within an identity categorization.
   B. Human beings exist in the simultaneously overlapping margins of multiple identities.
   C. Intersectionality focuses solely on individual identity without considering broader social contexts.
   D. Intersectionality centers on the experiences of historically marginalized individuals and groups.

The correct answer is C. Intersectionality focuses solely on individual identity without considering broader social contexts. Intersectionality is a theoretical framework that emphasizes the presence and interaction of multiple identity and social factors that influence disease course and care [24]. For a given patient, recognition of a single identity factor to the exclusion of others (e.g. Black woman who is also lesbian), would potentially create blind spots to communications, care collaboration, and trust.

References

1. Kiarashi J, et al. Factors associated with, and mitigation strategies for, health care disparities faced by patients with headache disorders. Neurology. 2021;97:280–9. https://n.neurology.org/content/97/6/280. Accessed 16 Oct 2021
2. Saadi A, et al. Racial disparities in neurologic healthcare access and utilization in the United States. Neurology. 2017;88(24):2268–75. https://n.neurology.org/. Accessed 16 Oct 2021
3. Lipton RB, Buse DC, Serrano D, Holland S, Reed ML. Examination of unmet needs among persons with episodic migraine: results of the American Migraine Prevalence and Prevention (AMPP) Study. Headache. 2013;53(8):1300–11.
4. Dodick DW, Loder EW, Manack Adams A, et al. Assessing barriers to chronic migraine consultation, diagnosis, and treatment: results from the Chronic Migraine Epidemiology and Outcomes (CaMEO) study. Headache. 2016;56(5):821–34.
5. Burch R, Rizzoli P, Loder E. The prevalence and impact of migraine and severe headache in the United States: figures and trends from government health studies. Headache. 2018;58(4):496–505.
6. Stewart W, Lipton R, Celentano D, Reed M. Prevalence of migraine headache in the United Stats: relation to age, income, race, and other sociodemographic factors. JAMA. 1992;267(1):64–9.
7. Wu J, Noxon V, Lu ZK. Patterns of use and health expenses associated with triptans among adults with migraine. Clin J Pain. 2015;31(8):673–9.
8. Lipton RB, Fanning KM, Serrano D, Reed MI, Cady R, Buse DC. Ineffective acute treatment of episodic migraine is associated with new-onset chronic migraine. Neurology. 2015;84(7):688–95.
9. Charleston L IV, et al. Migraine care challenges and strategies in US uninsured and underinsured adults: a narrative review, part 1. Headache. 2018;58(4):506–11.
10. Brennenstuhl S, Fuller-Thomson E. The painful legacy of childhood violence: migraine headaches among adult survivors of adverse childhood experiences. Headache. 2015;55(7):973–83.
11. Anda R, Tietjen G, Schulman E, Felitti V, Croft J. Adverse childhood experiences and frequent headaches in adults. Headache. 2010;50(9):1473–81.

12. Dooley JM, Gordon KE, Kuhle S. Food insecurity and migraine in Canada. Cephalalgia. 2016;36(10):936–42.
13. Diener HC, Dalhof CGH. Headache associated with chronic use of substances. In: Olesen J, Tfelt-Hansen P, Welch KMA, editors. The headaches. 2nd ed. Philadelphia: Lippincott, Williams and Wilkins; 1999. p. 671–878.
14. Ferrari A, Leone S, Vergoni AV, Bertolini A, Sances G, Coccia CPR. Similarities and differences between chronic migraine and episodic migraine. Headache. 2007;47:65–72.
15. Scher AI, Stewart WF, Liberman J, Lipton RB. Prevalence of frequent headache in a population sample. Headache. 1998;38:497–506.
16. Ahnquist J, Wamala SP, Lindstrom M. Social determinants of health—a question of social or economic capital? Interaction effects of socioeconomic factors on health outcomes. Soc Sci Med. 2012;74(6):930–9.
17. Marmot M, Freil S, Bell R, Houweling TA, Taylor S. Closing the gap in a generation: health equity through action on the social determinants of health. Lancet. 2008;372(9650):1661–9.
18. Lipton RB, Serrano D, Holland S, Fanning KM, Reed ML, Buse DC. Barriers to the diagnosis and treatment of migraine: effects of sex, income, and headache features. Headache. 2013;53(1):81–92.
19. Stewart WF, Roy J, Lipton RB. Migraine prevalence, socioeconomic status, and social causation. Neurology. 2013;81(11): 948–55.
20. Dill BT, Zinn MB. Theorizing difference from multiracial feminism. In: race, gender and class. Routledge; 2016. p. 76–82.
21. McCall L. The complexity of intersectionality. Signs J Women Cult Soc. 2005;30(3):1771–800.
22. Nash JC. Re-thinking intersectionality. Fem Rev. 2008;89(1):1–15. 1. Delgado R. Rodrigo's reconsideration: intersectionality and the future of critical race theory. Iowa Law Rev 2011;96(4):1247–88
23. Delgado R. Rodrigo's reconsideration: intersectionality and the future of critical race theory. Iowa Law Rev. 2011;96(4):1247–88.
24. Befus DR, Irby MB, Coeytaux RR, Penzien DB. A critical exploration of migraine as a health disparity: the imperative of an equity-oriented, intersectional approach. Curr Pain Headache Rep. 2018;22:79.
25. Matsuda MJ, et al. Words that wound. Boulder: Westview; 1993.
26. Leitch L. Action steps using ACEs and trauma-informed care: a resilience model. Health Justice. 2017;5(1):5.
27. Substance Abuse and Mental Health Services Administration. Trauma-informed approach and trauma-specific interventions. 2015 [cited 2022 March 7]; Available from: https://www.samhsa.gov/nctic/trauma-interventions
28. EQUIP Health Care. Trauma-and-violence-informed care (TVIC): a tool for health and social service organizations and providers. 2017 [cited 2022 March 7]; Available from: http://www.equiphealthcare.ca/
29. Browne AJ, et al. EQUIP healthcare: an overview of a multicomponent intervention to enhance equity-oriented care in primary health care settings. Int J Equity Health. 2015;14(1):152.
30. Norman RE, Byambaa M, De R, Butchart A, Scott J, Vos T. The long-term health consequences of child physical abuse, emotional abuse, and neglect: a systematic review and meta-analysis. PLoS Med. 2012;9(11):e1001349.
31. National Association of Community Health Centers. PRAPARE 2018 [cited 2022 March 2]; Available from: http://www.nachc.org/research-and-data/prapare/
32. Walker RJ, Gebregziabher M, Martin-Harris B, Egede LE. Independent effects of socioeconomic and psychological social determinants of health on self-care and outcomes in type 2 diabetes. Gen Hosp Psychiatry. 2014;36(6):662–8.
33. Institute of Medicine. America's Health Care Safety Net: Intact but Endangered. Washington, D.C.: The National Academies Press; 2000.
34. Waitzkin H. Commentary—the history and contradictions of the health care safety net. Health Serv Res. 2005;40(3):941–52. PubMed. Accessed 16 October 2021
35. Migration Policy Institute. Profile of Unauthorized Population: Los Angeles County, CA. Migration Policy, 2020, www.migrationpolicy.org/data/unauthorized-immigrant-population/county/6037. Accessed 16 Oct 2021.
36. US Bureau of Census. Los Angeles County Quick Facts. https//www.census.gov/quickfacts/fact/table/losangelescountycalifornia,losangelescitycalifornia,US/PST045219, 2019. Accessed 16 Oct 2021. https://www.census.gov/quickfacts/fact/table/losangelescountycalifornia/LFE041223.
37. Los Angeles County Department of Health Services. DHS annual report 2018–2019. Available at: https://file.lacounty.gov/SDSInter/dhs/1066922_2018-19MHLAAnnualReportFINAL.pdf. Accessed 16 Oct 2021.
38. Baker CL, Messmer PL, Gyurko CC, et.al. Hospital ownership, performance, and outcomes: assessing the state-of-the-science. J Nurs Adm 2000; 30:227–240.
39. Lipton RB, Amatniek JC, Ferrari MD, Gross M. Migraine: Identifying and removing barriers to care. Neurology. 1994;44(Suppl. 4):S63–8.
40. Steiner TJ. Lifting the burden: the global campaign against headache. Lancet Neurol. 2004;3:204–5.
41. Lifting the Burden: The Global Campaign Against Headache, on locality and national fronts. https://www.l-t-b.org/go/on_locality_national_fronts. Accessed 5 June 2023.

Coding, Telehealth, and Management Basics for the Headache Practice

38

Brad Klein

Introduction

The management of a headache practice continues to become more complex, similarly to evolving science and clinical care. As the discipline of headache grows, diagnostic criteria are honed [1] and the classification of headache diseases improves [2]. The impact of language, gender, culture, race, ethnicity, and care disparities is also better understood and thus incorporated into care management. Lastly, due to the technological breakthroughs in hardware, software, and broadband access, and the need to rapidly adapt in the setting of Coronavirus Disease 2019 (COVID-19), telehealth was catalyzed on a global scale [3]. Nonetheless, a financially viable model remains critical to provide headache care.

Financing a practice may be embedded within diverse delivery systems unique to a particular country or region. For instance, the US model is largely based on fee for service, with increasing inertia towards value-based care. In other countries, such as Denmark, care is publicly financed, offering largely free primary, specialist, hospital, mental health, preventive, and long-term care services [4]. In this chapter, we will review aspects of the administrative foundation needed to provide excellence in clinical care. Much of this chapter provides an updated understanding of the application of telehealth in headache care, followed by a deeper appreciation of some of the associated legal, coding, and billing issues that impact care in the United States.

B. Klein (✉)
Abington Neurological Associates, Abington, PA, USA

Abington Headache Center, Jefferson Abington Hospital, Abington, PA, USA

Thomas Jefferson University, Philadelphia, PA, USA

Questions

1. Which of the following statements regarding telehealth is NOT true according to the text?
   A. Telehealth encompasses various electronic and telecommunication technologies.
   B. It allows for improved access to expert neurological evaluation.
   C. Telemedicine has been shown to have inferior clinical outcomes compared to in-person visits.
   D. Telehealth reduces travel time and associated costs for patients and care partners
2. In the United States, what is the recommended approach for billing telehealth services based on the text?
   A. Use HCPCS Level I codes only.
   B. Bill using ICD codes exclusively.
   C. Utilize both ICD and CPT® codes for accurate billing.
   D. Billing is not necessary for telehealth services in the United States

An Overview of Headache Service Administration

There is an old maxim in medical care: success is based on the "three A's": affability, ability, and availability. By prioritizing these traits in the practice, clinicians help deliver on their patients' expectations. Affability may be defined as having a friendly and good-natured manner. When new patients call the office due to a headache, many may be unsure if they are suffering a tension headache, migraine, tumor, or other life-threatening disease. For the patient, a headache can be frightening. Thus, when patients call the office for the appointment, invariably the office staff will answer the phone. Professionalism, sincerity, and compassion by the staff can help put the patient at ease and set the

T. S. Monteith et al. (eds.), *Comprehensive Migraine Management*, https://doi.org/10.1007/978-3-031-86923-5_38

tone for what the patient can expect when meeting the provider. A defined script can aid the conversation, while also ensuring consistent messaging. Office space also can impact perceptions: a clean and quiet waiting room, with dim lighting, a space to sit, and an efficient front desk or user friendly digital application check-in process will convey a very different message than a bright, unkempt, and disorganized staff. Office locations with a good cellular signal and/or Wi-Fi access is an expectation by most all patients.

Access to Headache Care Providers

Availability can be difficult for a headache specialist as there remain few providers within the United States, or globally, to address the demand. As a result, the provider needs to develop access strategies. This may include hiring and training another physician, advanced practice provider, or nurse whereby each person's scope of practice is maximized. It could also mean improving efficiencies such as a medical assistant or scribe that can help shrink provider time per visit to see more patients. For instance, patients can fill out paperwork ahead of a visit and a medical assistant can collate and collect missing information into the chart. Patients may also be able to enter information via patient portals ahead of the visit. Providers can also offer written educational material for patients instead of verbally communicating information as part of counseling. Another approach is to have emergency or urgent referral slots available, or "frozen." If someone truly needs help, they can be fit in to these open appointments. Slots not filled within a reasonable period can then be opened, or "thawed," for patients on the wait list. A standard within practice management is to track the number of business days until the 3rd next available appointment. If the number of days is excessive, the demand is not being met.

The third A, Ability, references the clinical knowledge needed to care for headache patients, which is covered in the other chapters of this book.

Telehealth

Telehealth is the broad term referring to various electronic and telecommunication technologies to deliver virtual medical, health, and education services. Within this collection are four modalities: synchronous or two-way, real-time interactive audio and video, and often colloquially referred to as telemedicine; mobile health, ranging from targeted text messages promoting healthy behavior to wide-scale alerts about disease outbreaks; remote patient monitoring, whereby data is transferred to providers in a different location; and exchange of medical information through electronic communication via store-and-forward, or asynchronous exchange, where transmission of medical information, such as digital images, documents, and pre-recorded videos is completed through communication such as secure email, patient portal, or secure file exchange [5].

The benefits of telehealth are copious, including improved access to expert neurological evaluation; enhanced comfort, convenience, and safety, particularly for patients with limited mobility or need for home medical support equipment; reduced travel time and associated costs; decreased time away from work or other essential activities for patients and care partners; reduced caregiver stress; increased care partner and provider participation during a visit; better assessment of social determinants of health, including the patient's home environment; early intervention prior to a scheduled office visit, based on remote monitoring of disease progression and treatment efficacy; and protection of patient and providers from infectious disease exposure and reducing use of personal protective equipment in times of contagious pandemics [6]. Further, studies suggest telemedicine for headache care may result in noninferior clinical outcomes to in-person visits [7, 8] as well as high patient satisfaction [9, 10].

Despite the myriad of benefits for patients, there are challenges providers must consider in providing telehealth, including the feeling of connectedness, assessing body language, and mitigating accidental distractions and interruptions on either end of the camera. In both telehealth and in-person, the provider must relate to the patient's concerns and needs, help them understand their diagnoses, and develop a sound treatment plan. As most providers have electronic medical records, it remains paramount that the desk is set up such that the provider can maximize eye contact when recording their history either in-person or by telemedicine.

Clinical Considerations

Taking a comprehensive history is a critical component to understand a patient's headache disorder and screening for red flags is paramount [11]. An intake form may help expedite relevant questions, provide a broader understanding of the patient, and make the visits more efficient [12].

History taking via telehealth may provide a unique understanding of the patient not available during an in-person visit, such as seeing and hearing the patient's home life. As part of the examination, patients may record and report their own vitals, and much of the general neurological examination is within reach by telemedicine for headache [13, 14] (Table 38.1)

There are limitations to the telemedicine examination. Auscultation and fundoscopic examinations are difficult to perform without specialized equipment. Other assessments may be limited as well. This may include the inability for

Table 38.1 Example of a telemedicine examination for headache [15]

Vital signs:	The patient can use home equipment, if available, to check blood pressure, pulse, and weight.
Environment features:	Assess for evidence of photophobia (i.e. dark room/sunglasses), or phonophobia (i.e. irritation due to loud noise in the background).
General features:	Assess for head deformities, visualization of temporal arteries, and posture, including evidence of dystonia.
Mental status	Orientation: State name, date, and home address.
	Language, recent and remote memory: Ask a question about recent events. Assess fluency of speech, naming, repetition, and ability to follow commands. Administer 3-word registration and recall.
	Attention: Count backward from 100 by 7's or spell WORLD backwards.
Cranial nerves	Pupils: Have the patient hold the camera close to their eyes. Observe for symmetry then reaction to light by having the patient cover and uncover each eye independently.
	Eye movements: Look in the nine cardinal positions of gaze with brief pause at each position. For fixation, have the patient look at the camera and rotate the head from side to side. Assess for nystagmus.
	Saccades: Alternate gaze between upper right and left corner of screen, and then just above and below the screen.
	Facial strength: Lift eyebrows, squeeze eyes shut, show teeth, and purse the lips, observing for any asymmetry or ptosis.
	Facial sensation: Ask the patient to compare light touch to the face, ask if it feels unusual, particularly uncomfortable or painful, to assess for allodynia.
	Speech: Comment on dysarthria or dysphonia.
	Hearing: Evaluate grossly and document that it is intact to voice or with patient's own fingers using bilateral finger rubs.
	Palate: If appropriate lighting and quality video, look into their mouths to assess uvula. Of note, the provider may also be able to assess Mallampati score (for sleep apnea [16]), mouth span, jaw clicking, and teeth for evidence of grinding down.
	Neck rotation and flexion: Turn head right and left, attempting to touch their chin to their shoulders bilateral. Assess degree of rotation. Then shrug shoulders.
	Tongue: Observe the tongue at rest for bulk and fasciculations, then stick out tongue and move side to side.
Motor exam	Assess muscle bulk in upper and lower limbs.
	Observe for abnormal movements in the limbs including tremors or other dyskinetic movements.
	Assess for pronator drift, barrel rolling, and fine finger movements.
	As a basic assessment of symmetric antigravity power, have the patient move through a full range of motion in both upper and lower limbs, this could include squats.
Sensory	Ask the patient to compare light touch (or cold using ice) on the index fingers of both hands and the top of the big toes. A safety pin can be used to assess pinprick if needed. Romberg testing may be performed with the assistance of a bystander to ensure the patient does not fall.
Coordination	Rapid-alternating, finger-to-nose (or finger-to-object), and heel-to-shin movements.
	Bradykinesia testing with finger tapping and opening/closing fist.
Gait	Observe gait, including heel walk and toe walk.

the patient and/or friend, family, neighbor, etc., to fully understand and comply with instructions given through a screen and speaker. Further, the clinician will be limited in the assessment of several aspects of the examination, such as assessing the temporomandibular joint, motor strength and reflexes, and looking for subtle sensory deficits. The use of telemedicine to accurately evaluate and manage of the patient must be weighed carefully based on the patient, the technology available, the history, and limitations of the telemedicine modality.

As the telemedicine experience is different from an in-person visit for both the patient and provider, it is important the provider adapts to maximize an authentic engagement, such as ensuring appropriate lighting and audio, minimizing background noise, avoiding glare due to shiny surfaces, framing oneself in the picture, and nonverbal cue management [17].

Additional barriers may limit the value of telehealth and require alternative engagement strategies to support people with disabilities, older individuals, uninsured and underinsured, those who may have limited language or digital proficiency, and lack of adequate hardware and broadband access. Specific provider and staff training may be needed, including communication tactics to recognize different cultures, provide material that is accessible in different formats and in multiple languages, and developing an educational awareness campaign within the community of services offered. Post-visit surveys are invaluable to improve service, reduce barriers to care, and make patients more comfortable before, during, and after a virtual visit.

Legal Considerations for Telehealth

Within the United States, there are multiple legal concerns in performing telehealth visits, and each state may have unique laws and regulations [18]. Informed consent may be required either verbally or written with respect to the patient's commercial payer or state's Medicaid programs. Providers must also understand specific rules related to compliance of telehealth visits consistent with the Health Insurance Portability and Accountability Act of 1996 (HIPAA) to ensure the confidentiality of patients' personal health information. Failure to comply may result in penalties imposed by the U.S. Department of Health and Human Services Office for Civil Rights. While federal rules were loosened during the public health emergency of COVID-19, under Sec. 13410(e) of the HITECH Act [19], State Attorney Generals are still permitted to obtain civil money penalties on behalf of state residents for HIPAA violations.

Providers may deliver telehealth services across state lines, though contingent on rules set by state and federal policies. Malpractice coverage also varies by policy and may or may not cover telehealth. Further, a policy may not cover telehealth in more than one state or even in counties within the state outside of where the practitioner is located for in-person visits. Prior to telehealth implementation, the provider must reach out to their malpractice insurer and determine what is and is not covered by the carrier.

Billing Considerations for Telehealth

Billing for telehealth services, similar to clinical care, must first be considered in terms of the contract signed by the provider's employer. If reimbursements are documented as guaranteed for specific services, the provider should expect appropriate payments. Outside of this agreement, the provider not only needs to maintain a master fee schedule that tracks contracted payments of each payer, but also potentially the agreed upon payments of different products within a payer, and understand policies that may impact payments such as collecting coinsurance, deductibles, or copays. The provider must also be aware if a service offered by the provider is, or is no longer, deemed a covered service. Of note, it is standard practice for practices to collect all copays, coinsurance, and deductibles at the time of the visit. If by telehealth, the office may be able to collect by credit or debit services ahead of the visit.

During the COVID-19 public health emergency, section 1135 of the Social Security Act allowed the Health and Human Services (HHS) secretary to temporarily waive or modify certain Medicare, Medicaid, and Children's Health Insurance Program (CHIP) policies. Along with the Coronavirus Preparedness and Response Supplemental Appropriations Act, passed in 2020, Centers for Medicare and Medicaid Services (CMS)' flexibilities allowed broadened access to Medicare telehealth services on a temporary and emergency basis. Amongst many flexibilities, this allowed physicians and other healthcare professionals licensed in one state to be reimbursed for services in another state in which they were not licensed. Specifically, services could be rendered at an originating site outside of the state they were licensed. The originating site refers to where the Medicare beneficiary (the patient) is located, while the distant site refers to the location of the eligible healthcare provider. However, each state also has the authority to approve of such arrangements, regardless of emergency, and allow interstate waivers. Thus, providers must also understand current laws relevant to the state where the originating site is located. During COVID-19, the Center for Connected Health Policy was an important resource for providers to monitor such activity [20]. Nonetheless, certain states have developed or are developing interstate medical licensure compacts to help expedite health care services across state lines [21].

Coding Basics

Published by the World Health Organization, the International Statistical Classification of Diseases and Related Health Problems (ICD) defines the diseases, disorders, injuries, and other related health conditions. These codes are listed in a comprehensive, hierarchical fashion. ICD provides coding for diseases, signs and symptoms, abnormal findings, complaints, social circumstances, and external causes of injury or diseases and is the accepted classification globally [22].

Within the United States, providers also use the Healthcare Common Procedure Coding System (HCPCS), also known as "hicks-picks," as a standardized code system for medical providers to submit healthcare claims to Medicare and other payers. HCPCS comprises two medical code sets, HCPCS Level I and HCPCS Level II. HCPCS Level I consist of the Current Procedural Terminology (CPT®) code set, used to submit medical claims to payers for procedures and services performed by physicians, nonphysician practitioners, hospitals, laboratories, and outpatient facilities. This includes evaluation and management (E/M) and procedures such as botulinum toxin injections, nerve blocks. CPT® is updated annually by the American Medical Association and it is a valuable reference for a practice [23]. CMS may also develop temporary codes separate from CPT®. These include G-codes.

HCPCS) Level II is the national procedure code set for healthcare practitioners, providers, and medical equipment suppliers when filing health plan claims for medical devices, supplies, medications, transportation services, and other items and services. This would include J codes that identify medications used, such as botulinum toxin, eptinezumab, or anesthetics for nerve blocks. Thus, for a patient visit in-person or by telehealth, providers in the United States will code both an ICD and CPT®. It is critical that the provider also understands that certain CPT® codes can only be applied to certain ICD codes. For instance, in order to bill CPT® 64615, the procedure for botulinum toxin administration for chronic migraine, one must use a chronic migraine ICD code. If the practice buys and bills botulinum toxin for this procedure, the visit will also include a HCPCS Level II code: J0585 to inform the payer that the claim includes a request for payment of the procedure in addition to the medication.

Effective as of January 1, 2021, the American Medical Association's Current Procedural Terminology (CPT®) code set revised the Evaluation and Management (E/M) office visit CPT® code (99201-99215) descriptors and documentation standards that directly address the continuing problem of administrative burden for physicians in nearly every specialty for the first time since 1997. Major changes included: eliminating history and physical as elements for code selection, allow qualified providers to choose whether their documentation is based on Medical Decision Making (MDM) or Total Time, modifications to the criteria for MDM, deletion of CPT® code 99201, and the creation of a shorter prolonged services code.

Coding

To ensure accurate billing in the United States, headache providers should understand E/M at a minimum, including how to code by either medical decision-making or by time. As of this writing, synchronous audio and video, or telemedicine, follows the same rules as outlined for evaluation and management codes. If using medical decision management in the outpatient clinic, the provider will base their level of coding based on the highest levels of coding relevant to two of three categories: First, the "Number and Complexity of Problems Addressed" considers the disease, syndrome, injury, symptom, sign, finding, or complaint. The second: "Amount and/or Complexity of Data to be Reviewed and Analyzed" includes 3 subcategories: review of tests & documents, or independent historian history; independent interpretation of tests; and discussion of management or test interpretation. The third comprises the "Risk of Complications and/or Morbidity or Mortality of Patient Management." [24]

If the amount of time invested during a telemedicine visit is significant (including time spent by the provider in preparation of the visit, time spent with the patient during the visit, and time spent in chart completion, calls, etc., throughout the day of the visit), then the provider may choose to bill by time instead of MDM, and document the total time spent (Table 38.2). However, reaching a level 4 visit by MDM may not require 30 minutes of total time if the provider documents a diagnosis of migraine (presuming it is a chronic illness with exacerbation) and requires prescription drug management.

Providers should only code ICDs when they provided (documented) care management services for the particular ICD. Thus, if the provider manages migraine without aura, and addressed muscle spasms during the visit (and documented the management), the provider codes both diagnoses. If only one issue is managed (with documentation), only the one ICD is coded. Of note, the provider can code a diagnosis without a change in management, but must document that they considered management. For instance, the provider does not have to prescribe a drug during the visit, but documents a consideration of a medication prescription, explaining that no changes should be made to the medication dosing or no refill was necessary.

As per AMA guidelines, if the total time exceeds 60 minutes for a new patient or 40 minutes for a follow-up patient, and the coding is based on total time, providers can add on a unit of the prolonged service code 99417 for every additional 15 minutes (Table 38.3). At the time of this writing, this code applies to commercial payers, but not Medicare. Instead, with different criteria, Medicare accepts HCPCS G2212.

Procedures may support the management of headache disorders (Table 38.4). Unfortunately, payer policies change with time, and procedures that may have been covered may no longer be covered, and vice versa. It is thus imperative that the provider is aware of current payer policies before providing such services. To mitigate financial harm to the

Table 38.2 Ambulatory evaluation and management coding by time:

New Patient Visit	Typical Time (minutes)	Established Patient Visit	Typical Time (minutes)
99202	15–29	99212	10–19
99203	30–44	99213	20–29
99204	45–59	99214	30–39
99205	60–74	99215	40–54

Table 38.3 Prolonged service codes

CPT®	Time	CPT®	Time
99205	60–74	99215	40–54
99417	75–89	99417	55–69
+99417x 2	90–104	+99417x 2	70–84
+99417x3	105–119	+99417x3	85–99

Table 38.4 Common procedure codes in headache medicine

CPT®	Procedure[a]
20552	Injection of trigger points, 1–2 muscles
20553	Injection of trigger points, 3 muscles or more
62270	Lumbar Puncture
64400	Injection of anesthetic agent and/or steroid, trigeminal nerve (i.e. ophthalmic, maxillary, mandibular)
64405	Injection of anesthetic agent and/or steroid, greater occipital nerve
64505	Injection of anesthetic agent, sphenopalatine ganglion
64615	Chemodenervation of muscles (i.e. for chronic migraine)
64616	Chemodenervation of muscles (i.e. for cervical dystonia)

[a]Procedures involving injections may also require J codes for billing purposes.

Table 38.5 Telephone codes

Telephone Codes	Time
99441	5–10 minutes
99442	11–20 minutes
99443	21–30 minutes

Table 38.6 Online digital E/M codes

Online digital E/M codes, such as secure email and patient portal communications	Time
99421	5–10 minutes
99422	11–20 minutes
99423	21–30 minutes

practice, financial policies should be transparent and all patients should sign a waiver recognizing their financial responsibility for services rendered. Depending on applicable laws, waivers may need to be resigned periodically, such as an annual basis. Lastly, the practice should also re-affirm the patient's current insurance is up to date during appointment registration to mitigate additional risks that a procedure is no longer covered when they arrive for their service.

Telephone Services and Digital Communication

Telephone E/M services may be reimbursable by payors. However, their rate may not equal patient E/M visits, or be paid (CPT® 99441-99443; Table 38.4). Telephone visits can be provided by a qualified provider, but not originating from a related E/M service provided within the previous 7 days nor leading to an E/M service or procedure within the next 24 hours or soonest available appointment. Patients must initiate the request for this service as well. Further, the provider must verify with the payer if there is an expectation to collect a copay, coinsurance, or deductible when billing for this service (Table 38.5).

Virtual check-in (HCPCS G2012) was designed to provide a brief communication by a technology-based service, including audio-only real-time telephone interactions, that last 5–10 minutes in medical discussion. Other billable communications by technology include HCPCS G2010, whereby established patients can submit recorded video and/or images for the provider's review. Of note, the provider cannot submit for billing of G2012 or G2010 if they originate from a related E/M service provided within the previous 7 days nor leading to an E/M service or procedure within the next 24 hours or soonest available appointment.

Billing by providers for online digital E/M or e-visits (CPT® 99421-99423; Table 38.6 may be a submittable claim to a payer as well. These are patient-initiated requests for evaluation and are billed based on cumulative time spent by the qualified provider (not including clinical staff) within 7 days. That is, the provider must track and document the time spent in communication with a patient. Examples of services are secure communications through email and the patient portal. Online digital E/M or e-visits cannot be reported on a day when the qualified health care professional reports E/M services or bills for remote monitoring, chronic care management, transitional care management, care plan oversight, or supervision of the patient in a home, domiciliary or rest home for the same communication(s).

Remote Monitoring

Remote monitoring, involving asynchronous transmission of information, can be used for established patients (CPT® 99453-99455; Table 38.7). Examples include weight, blood pressure, pulse oximetry, and respiratory flow rate.

Table 38.7 Remote monitoring

Remote monitoring of physiologic parameter(s) codes	Description
99453	initial; set-up and patient education on use of equipment
99454	initial; device(s) supply with daily recording(s) or programmed alert(s) transmission, each 30 days
99455	Remote physiologic monitoring treatment management services, 20 minutes or more of clinical staff, physician, or other qualified health professional time in a calendar month requiring interactive communication with the patient/caregiver during the month

Table 38.8 Interprofessional consultation codes

Interprofessional consultation codes			
Verbal and written report	Time	Written report only	Time
99446	5–10 minutes	99451	for consulting physician
99447	11–20 minutes		
99448	21–30 minutes		
99449	> 31 minutes	99452	treating/requesting physician or other qualified health care provider

Interprofessional Consultations

Interprofessional consultations are consults provided without seeing the patient in person. This may be to minimize exposure to patients with communicable disease, when advice is needed but a consulting provider is unable to provide a visit in a timely manner, or for other team-based care approaches. There are 2 sets of codes that may be considered in this situation: a verbal and written report or for a written report only (CPT® 99446-99449 or 99451-99452; Table 38.8). In either case, these codes require patient consent because copays may also be charged to the patient if not waived by payor policy. These codes cannot be used if the consultation leads to a transfer of care within 14 days or the soonest available appointment date. More than 50% of the time cannot be spent in data review, and the codes should not be reported more than once within a 7-day interval. The codes should only be reported by the consultative physician, although the treating/requesting physician can also bill with CPT® 99452 if the service takes 30 minutes or longer.

Modifiers and Place of Service

Modifiers are used when additional information may be beneficial to the payor or provider in order to have a claim paid in a timely manner. These codes are also used as a shorthand to explain specific details about a patient encounter. Place of service (POS) codes are used on professional claims to specify the entity where service(s) were rendered to inform payors.

With respect to telehealth, 4 modifiers are typically considered, depending on the payor and service.

1. GT, meaning "via interactive audio and video telecommunications systems"
2. 95, meaning "synchronous telemedicine service rendered via a real-time interactive audio and video telecommunications system"
3. GQ, meaning "via an asynchronous telecommunications system." This is for the federal telemedicine demonstration project conducted in Alaska or Hawaii
4. G0 (G Zero), meaning "telehealth services furnished for purposes of diagnosis, evaluation, or treatment of symptoms of an acute stroke."

Medicare discontinued modifier GT in 2017 when POS-02 (telehealth) was introduced. However, private payors may still use this modifier. Modifier 95 should not be used with in-person visits, virtual visits (G2012), or digital evaluations (99421-99423), although payors may vary in their approach to how telehealth claims are coded.

Conclusion

A common expression in academic centers is "no margin, no mission". Without operational success, one cannot provide excellence in care. Understanding the basics of coding and payment are thus critical components to the success of the organization. While also part of the fabric of healthcare, telehealth is relatively "young" in medicine and it will continue to evolve as clinicians and patients learn to master it while government and payers understand its implications in medical economics and health policy. It is in the provider's interest to not only continue growing their knowledge in the science of headache, but the larger world around them, recognizing how rules, regulations, policies, revenues, and expenses will continue to impact care.

> **Teaching Point**
> As an experiment, try calling your own practice to see how your staff interacts with you as a patient. That is, can you reach a live person in your office, and if so, how did the staff make you feel? Was the scheduling process reasonable?

Common Migraine-Related ICD10 Codes [25]

- G43 Migraine
  - G43.0 Migraine without aura
    - G43.00 Migraine without aura, not intractable
      - G43.001 ...... with status migrainosus
      - G43.009 ...... without status migrainosus
    - G43.01 Migraine without aura, intractable
      - G43.011 ...... with status migrainosus
      - G43.019 ...... without status migrainosus
  - G43.1 Migraine with aura
    - G43.10 Migraine with aura, not intractable
      - G43.101 ...... with status migrainosus
      - G43.109 ...... without status migrainosus
    - G43.11 Migraine with aura, intractable
      - G43.111 ...... with status migrainosus
      - G43.119 ...... without status migrainosus
  - G43.4 Hemiplegic migraine
    - G43.40 Hemiplegic migraine, not intractable
      - G43.401 ...... with status migrainosus
      - G43.409 ...... without status migrainosus
    - G43.41 Hemiplegic migraine, intractable
      - G43.411 ...... with status migrainosus
      - G43.419 ...... without status migrainosus
  - G43.5 Persistent migraine aura without cerebral infarction
    - G43.50 Persistent migraine aura without cerebral infarction, not intractable
      - G43.501 ...... with status migrainosus
      - G43.509 ...... without status migrainosus
    - G43.51 Persistent migraine aura without cerebral infarction, intractable
      - G43.511 ...... with status migrainosus
      - G43.519 ...... without status migrainosus
  - G43.6 Persistent migraine aura with cerebral infarction
    - G43.60 Persistent migraine aura with cerebral infarction, not intractable
      - G43.601 ...... with status migrainosus
      - G43.609 ...... without status migrainosus
    - G43.61 Persistent migraine aura with cerebral infarction, intractable
      - G43.611 ...... with status migrainosus
      - G43.619 ...... without status migrainosus
  - G43.7 Chronic migraine without aura
    - G43.70 Chronic migraine without aura, not intractable
      - G43.701 ...... with status migrainosus
      - G43.709 ...... without status migrainosus
    - G43.71 Chronic migraine without aura, intractable
      - G43.711 ...... with status migrainosus
      - G43.719 ...... without status migrainosus
  - G43.A Cyclical vomiting
    - G43.A0 ...... in migraine, not intractable
    - G43.A1 ...... in migraine, intractable
  - G43.B Ophthalmoplegic migraine
    - G43.B0 ...... not intractable
    - G43.B1 ...... intractable
  - G43.C Periodic headache syndromes in child or adult
    - G43.C0 ...... not intractable
    - G43.C1 ...... intractable
  - G43.D Abdominal migraine
    - G43.D0 ...... not intractable
    - G43.D1 ...... intractable
  - G43.8 Other migraine
    - G43.80 Other migraine, not intractable
      - G43.801 ...... with status migrainosus
      - G43.809 ...... without status migrainosus
    - G43.81 Other migraine, intractable
      - G43.811 ...... with status migrainosus
      - G43.819 ...... without status migrainosus
    - G43.82 Menstrual migraine, not intractable
      - G43.821 ...... with status migrainosus
      - G43.829 ...... without status migrainosus
    - G43.83 Menstrual migraine, intractable
      - G43.831 ...... with status migrainosus
      - G43.839 ...... without status migrainosus
  - G43.9 Migraine, unspecified
    - G43.90 Migraine, unspecified, not intractable
      - G43.901 ...... with status migrainosus
      - G43.909 ...... without status migrainosus
    - G43.91 Migraine, unspecified, intractable
      - G43.911 ...... with status migrainosus
      - G43.919 ...... without status migrainosus

Questions and Answers

1. Which of the following statements regarding telehealth is NOT true according to the text?
   A. Telehealth encompasses various electronic and telecommunication technologies.
   B. It allows for improved access to expert neurological evaluation.
   C. Telemedicine has been shown to have inferior clinical outcomes compared to in-person visits.

D. Telehealth reduces travel time and associated costs for patients and care partners.

The correct answer is C. Telemedicine has been shown to have inferior clinical outcomes compared to in-person visits. Current literature continues to demonstrate telemedicine is not inferior to in-person visits, particularly in patients with established neurological disorders. However, capabilities to perform a comprehensive neurological examination may be limited despite audio and video capabilities. This may include the inability to perform an ophthalmological examination, assessment of muscle trigger points, as well as appreciation of muscle strength, reflexes, and subtleties in sensory deficits.

2. In the United States, what is the recommended approach for billing telehealth services based on the text?
   A. Use HCPCS Level I codes only.
   B. Bill using ICD codes exclusively.
   C. Utilize both ICD and CPT® codes for accurate billing.
   D. Billing is not necessary for telehealth services in the United States

The correct answer is C. Utilize both ICD and CPT® codes for accurate billing. The International Statistical Classification of Diseases and Related Health Problems (ICD) defines the diseases, disorders, injuries, and other related health conditions. In other words, ICD clarifies why the provider "did" something. Current Procedural Terminology (CPT®) code set, which falls under Healthcare Common Procedure Coding System (HCPCS) level I, is necessary to clarify what procedures and services were performed. In other words, CPT® clarifies what the provider did. To ensure the CPT® must also be connected to an appropriate ICD to ensure payment. For instance, connecting CPT® 64615 with an ICD for insomnia may result in denied payment as botulinum toxin administration (chemodenervation) is not indicated for insomnia.

References

1. https://ichd-3.org. Last accessed August 11 2021.
2. https://www.who.int/standards/classifications/classification-of-diseases. Last accessed August 11 2021.
3. Klein BC, Busis NA. COVID-19 is catalyzing the adoption of teleneurology. Neurology. 2020;94(21):903–4. https://doi.org/10.1212/WNL.0000000000009494.
4. https://www.commonwealthfund.org/international-health-policy-center/countries/denmark. Last accessed August 11 2021.
5. Center for Connected Health Policy. https://www.cchpca.org. Last accessed March 21 2020.
6. Hatcher-Martin JM, Busis NA, Cohen BH, Wolf RA, Jones EC, Anderson ER, Fritz JV, Shook SJ, Bove RM. American Academy of Neurology Telehealth Position Statement. Neurology. 2021; https://doi.org/10.1212/WNL.0000000000012185.
7. Friedman DI, Rajan B, Seidmann A. A randomized trial of telemedicine for migraine management. Cephalalgia. 2019;39:1577–85. https://orcid.org/0000-0001-7802-7172
8. Hatcher-Martin JM, Adams JL, Anderson ER, Bove R, Burrus TM, Chehrenama M, Dolan O'Brien M, Eliashiv DS, Erten-Lyons D, Giesser BS, Moo LR, Narayanaswami P, Rossi MA, Soni M, Tariq N, Tsao JW, Vargas BB, Vota SA, Wessels SR, Planalp H, Govindarajan R. Telemedicine in neurology: Telemedicine Work Group of the American Academy of Neurology update. Neurology. 2020;94(1):30–8. https://doi.org/10.1212/WNL.0000000000008708. Epub 2019 Dec 4. PMID: 31801829.
9. Müller KI, Alstadhaug KB, Bekkelund SI. Headache patients' satisfaction with telemedicine: a 12-month follow-up randomized non-inferiority trial. Eur J Neurol. 2017;24:807–15.
10. Chiang C-C, Halker SR, Lalvani N, Shubin SK, Henscheid LD, Lay C, Dodick DW, Newman LC. Patient experience of telemedicine for headache care during the COVID-19 pandemic: an American Migraine Foundation survey study. Headache. 2021;61:734–9. https://doi.org/10.1111/head.14110.
11. Do TP, Remmers A, Schytz HW, et al. Red and orange flags for secondary headaches in clinical practice: SNNOOP10 list. Neurology. 2019;92(3):134–44. https://doi.org/10.1212/WNL.0000000000006697.
12. Sharon R, Rayhill M, Viknevich J, Charleston L 4th, Mathew PG. An analysis of UCNS certified headache center patient intake forms. Headache. 2016;56(3):519–27. https://doi.org/10.1111/head.12739. Epub 2016 Feb 15. PMID: 26875592.
13. https://americanheadachesociety.org/news/telemedicine-neurologic-examination/ Last accessed August 7 2021.
14. Al Hussona M, Maher M, Chan D, et al. The virtual neurologic exam: instructional videos and guidance for the COVID-19 era. Can J Neurol Sci. 2020;47(5):598–603. https://doi.org/10.1017/cjn.2020.96.
15. Al Hussona M, Maher M, Chan D, Micieli JA, Jain JD, Khosravani H, Izenberg A, Kassardjian CD, Mitchell SB. The virtual neurologic exam: instructional videos and guidance for the COVID-19 era. Can J Neurol Sci. 2020;47(5):–598–603. https://doi.org/10.1017/cjn.2020.96. Epub 2020 May 21. PMID: 32434626; PMCID: PMC7347716.
16. Yurcheshen ME, Pigeon W, Marcus CZ, et al. Interrater reliability between in-person and telemedicine evaluations in obstructive sleep apnea. J Clin Sleep Med. 2021;17(7):1435–40.
17. https://www.youtube.com/watch?v=IpF9gW9OZQQ. Last accessed August 7 2021.
18. https://www.cchpca.org/all-telehealth-policies/ Last accessed August 8 2021.
19. https://www.govinfo.gov/content/pkg/FR-2010-07-14/pdf/2010-16718.pdf. Last accessed August 7 2021.
20. https://www.cchpca.org/topic/cross-state-licensing-covid-19/ Last accessed August 8 2021.
21. https://www.imlcc.org Last accessed August 8 2021.
22. https://www.who.int/standards/classifications/classification-of-diseases. Last accessed August 8 2021.
23. American Medical Association. 2020 CPT. Professional ed. Chicago: American Medical Association; 2019.
24. https://www.ama-assn.org/system/files/2019-06/cpt-revised-mdm-grid.pdf Last accessed August 8 2021.
25. https://www.who.int/standards/classifications/classification-of-diseases/list-of-official-icd-10-updates. Last accessed September 5 2022.

Migraine Advocacy

39

William B. Young, Ellen Gibson Depoy, Brittany Heckel, and Marianna Vinokur

Introduction

At its core, advocacy involves intervention on behalf of "vulnerable" people in need although more recent advocacy movements discuss and teach self-advocacy. Historians postulate that advocacy evolved in bureaucratic societies for the benefit of individual citizens. The role of an ombudsman was created in Sweden in 1809 to protect individual rights against the excess of bureaucracy. In the early twentieth century, nurses' code of ethics promoted the rights of patients, which nurses then and now "advocate for" [1]. Modern patient advocacy can be traced back to the 1950s cancer advocacy movement, the March of Dimes, and the precursor to Planned Parenthood. Patient advocacy evolved further in the 1960s and 1970s from self-help organizations. The HIV/AIDS movement of the 1980s crystallized the concept of the grassroots movement with disease reframing, social justice, and competition for resources at its core [2]. In the 1990s, the Food and Drug Administration (FDA) evolved the Patient Representative Program, which solicits the involvement of patients through committees and panels [2]. The number of disease-related non-profits evolved from under 500 in 1991 to close to 1200 in 2003 [3].

In the USA, migraine disease advocacy was spearheaded by physicians through the organized recognition of headache disorders as a legitimate area of medical study began. American Association for the Study of Headache (AASH), the precursor to the American Headache Society (AHS), was established in 1959. Modern disease advocacy for migraine headaches could have started in Britain with the Migraine Trust, founded in 1965 as a largely patient-driven organization. In the USA, modern patient advocacy can be traced back to the separation of the National Headache Foundation (NHF) from the AASH in 1970. The NHF assumed a leadership position in patient education and support. Eventually, the AHS began to view patient education as part of its mission as well. A fledgling patient-driven advocacy movement evolved in the early 1990s, surprisingly housed under an organization of rare diseases. The patient-led advocacy movement has evolved, and multiple organizations with headache patient constituencies or mixed physician–patient constituencies are now in operation, housed under the Coalition of Headache and Migraine Patients (CHAMP), which began operations in 2017. Cluster headache organizations evolved as OUCH (USA) in 1998, OUCH (UK) in 2001, and Cluster Busters (USA) soon after. Cluster Busters' position was more patient centric than migraine's, taking the approach that the medical world was not adequately studying or developing new treatments for the most painful disease in the world and that patients would take matters into their own hands including use and research on psychedelics and oxygen.

In the USA, disease advocacy is a critical predictor of the resources allocated to that disease [3]. Patient advocacy, and to a lesser extent physician advocacy, has fundamentally changed public attitudes toward diseases such as AIDS, breast cancer, autism, epilepsy, and other chronic illnesses. It is hard to compare diseases in terms of sympathy, respect, or acceptability. One of the only quantifiable domains with available data, National Institutes of Health (NIH) funding, has come to stand in for overall disease respectability and sympathy.

The table below illustrates the burden of illness measured in disability-adjusted life years (DALYs) as a percent of total US DALYs, the relative size of the advocacy movement measured by the number of advocacy organizations, the budget of the largest patient organization, and the amount of funding from NIH (Table 39.1).

W. B. Young (✉) · E. G. Depoy · B. Heckel · M. Vinokur
Jefferson Headache Center, Jefferson University, Philadelphia, PA, USA

T. S. Monteith et al. (eds.), *Comprehensive Migraine Management*, https://doi.org/10.1007/978-3-031-86923-5_39

The size of the migraine advocacy movement is miniscule compared to other diseases of comparable and lesser disease burden. Also, NIH funding is negligible compared to other diseases with comparable or lesser disease burden. The calculations in Table 39.1 confirm Best's observation that advocacy size is a better predictor of NIH funding than disease burden [3]. In addition, the underfunding of migraine and other headache disorders could only occur to a stigmatized disease.

Questions

1. Three types of stigma we discussed are:
   A. Personal stigma, public and institutional stigma
   B. Self-stigma, public stigma, and institutional stigma
   C. Self-stigma, public stigma, and structural stigma
   D. Individual stigma, group stigma, and structural stigma
2. The most persistent issue for migraine advocacy organizations in the USA has been:
   A. Creating a new institute of headache medicine at NIH
   B. Addressing the underfunding of headache research by NIH
   C. New legislation demanding employers offer accommodations for people with migraine
   D. Creating a CMS "blue book" listing for migraine

Table 39.1 Comparison of disability (DALYS); strength of advocacy movement in numbers as nonprofits and income. Compared to NIH funding and disability and advocacy strength adjusted NIH funding

	Disability-adjusted life years (DALYs; % US total DALYs)	Number of advocacy organizations (2021)	Income of largest patient advocacy group	NIH funding (2021 est) in millions of dollars ($)	NIH funding millions $/1% of DALYs	NIH funding/million advocacy $ of largest patient organization
Migraine	1.86	31	$1,345,000 (Miles for Migraine, 2019)	25	15.1	19.2
Multiple sclerosis	0.19	133	$196,890,000 (National MS Society)	109	573.7	0.5
Epilepsy	0.30	176	$28,595,000 Epilepsy Foundation of America	185	617	6.5
Parkinson's disease	0.44	291	161,693,000 (Michael J. Fox Foundation for Parkinson's research)	218	495	5.1
Alzheimer's disease	1.83	293	$389,665,878 (Alzheimer's Association)	2240	1224	5.7
Autism spectrum	0.17	1477	$37,893,000 (Anderson Center for Autism)	305	1794	8.2
Nonneurological diseases						
Arthritis	2.01	56	$73,080,000 (Arthritis Foundation Inc.)	413	205	5.6
Chronic kidney disease	1.64	140	$43,218,000 (National Kidney Foundation)	660	402	15.2

1. https://vizhub.healthdata.org/gbd-compare/
2. https://projects.propublica.org/nonprofits/search?utf8=%E2%9C%93&q=&state%5Bid%5D=&ntee%5Bid%5D=&c_cod+e%5Bid%5D=
3. https://report.nih.gov/funding/categorical-spending#/

Table 39.2 Types of stigma with examples for migraine

Type of stigma	Definition	Migraine-specific examples
Public = enacted	Stereotypes, prejudice, and discrimination	"It's just a headache" from a parent, teacher, or a friend "I get migraine, and I can do that"—bullying
Structural	Shame, low self-esteem, and lack of engagement in treatment	Not seeking a diagnosis or treatment Negative self-talk
Self-stigma = internalized	Prejudice and discrimination by policies, laws, and constitutional practice	Lack of accommodations—at school with low funding, access to medication, making up tests, or lack of a quiet environment for learning

What Is Stigma?

There are several types of stigmas that impact migraine (Table 39.2). Stigma was defined by Goffman in 1963 as an "attribute that is deeply discrediting" (Goffman, 1963). He further notes that persons who are stigmatized are "disqualified from full social acceptance and tainted or discounted." Stigma has two components: (1) the individual is devalued and viewed negatively because of a characteristic or disease, poisoned identity; (2) the individual is sanctioned for that condition. This sanctioning can have many forms including direct punishment by limiting access to various resources.

Stigma can manifest very differently across various conditions. The stigma of having a skin disease differs from the stigma of depression or being LGBTQ. The burden of having a visible, stigmatized condition differs qualitatively from an invisible condition. Since Goffman, alternative or elaborated definitions have varied considerably. Research on stigma is clearly unique and multidisciplinary, including contributions by psychologists, sociologists, anthropologists, political scientists, and mental health experts. Stigma has been widely studied across many disease states, for example, HIV and epilepsy. Despite this, only limited work has been done in migraine, and none in other headache diseases.

History of Migraine Stigma

Historian Katherine Foxhall traced the origins of migraine stigma attached [4]. Societal understanding of migraine began with the coining of hemicrania by Galen, a Roman Empire era physician who treated migraine as a disease of real pain [4]. The term emerged as magryne in the works of sixteenth-century Scottish poet William Dunbar, who described not only the head pain, but also the associated debilitating symptoms and postdrome of migraine [4]. A 1642 recipe book detailed a range of treatments for mild-to-severe forms of megrim [4]. In the sixteenth and seventeenth centuries, society legitimized migraine with its accompanying symptoms, as well as an appreciation as a disease afflicting both men and women [4]. However, in the eighteenth and nineteenth centuries, migraine became discredited by being associated with "ladies of fashion," "young female martyrs," and "mothers in the lower classes of life" [4].

The questioning of migraine as an actual disease started with the scientific revolution. This evolves as previous theories of unseen bodily humors and malaise transform into the tangible and objective evidence of visible anatomy and pathology. This transformation in public and medical thought may be one reason an invisible disease such as pain or migraine lost its credibility as a legitimate medical disease. This stigma, seeded in the objective lack of migraine manifestations, still plays a role in social understanding of migraine and availability of economic and political resources, as well as in how people with migraine themselves view and treat the disease. The "gendering" of migraine is also stigmatizing and an ongoing practice. An estimated 6% of American men have migraine [5]. Despite the prevalence of migraine among men outweighing the prevalence of many other diseases, such as prostate disease or diabetes, migraine is still regarded as a "women's disease" [6]. Pharmaceutical marketing exacerbates this stigma: a female subject is up to four times more likely to portray a person with migraine on a pharmaceutical website [6]. Gendered metaphors appealing to women, such as comparing a treatment to a "spa" experience and gendered messages through visual narratives of women as caretakers, further enhance this notion [6]. This stigma misconstrues migraine as a disease of women, which perpetuates misdiagnosis and delay in medical care for men with migraine.

Stigma in Migraine

Kempner studied migraine as having a "legitimacy deficit" with experience by both providers and patients [6]. Migraine stigma has been studied from the perspective of the stigmatized subject, the stigmatizer in the community, and messaging in advertisements and films about migraine. Over the last decade, the discussion of migraine stigma, as well as advocacy, has increased. It is not clear at a population level whether this movement has led to more NIH or other research funding, more accommodations and better work conditions for persons with migraine, or more sympathy and understanding from friends and family.

Shapiro found a link between disability and stigma. Upon using a large panel of test-takers, there was more desire for social distance for persons who missed more days of work due to migraine. Other features of stigmatizers include maleness and being non-white [7] . Moreover, it showed that persons who knew more people with migraine were greater stigmatizers. This finding is not completely understood, but it could suggest that people know of an individual's migraine because of their work-related disability (it is otherwise hidden) and that work-related disability negatively colors attitudes not just to the known individual with migraine but to all other persons with migraine.

Young studied migraine stigma in a clinic population of highly impacted patients, comparing them with epilepsy patients from a specialty clinic [8]. Patients with migraine were subdivided into patients with chronic and episodic migraine. Persons with episodic migraine experienced similar levels of stigma compared to persons with epilepsy—and persons with chronic migraine experienced more stigma than individuals in the other groups. In these cohorts, patients with chronic migraine experienced more disability than those with epilepsy, while epilepsy and episodic migraine were similar. Disability had the strongest correlation with stigma scores; thus, patients with chronic migraine experienced more stigma than either patients with epilepsy or episodic migraine. Once disability was accounted for, chronic migraine and epilepsy had similar stigma scores, which was more than episodic migraine [8]. This may be because chronic migraine is less familiar and viewed as an aberrant brain like epilepsy, not like episodic migraine, which is viewed as more normal.

Similar findings were seen in a smaller Spanish study. Stigma was greater in patients who were unemployed, divorced, and who had migraine with aura [9]. In a Turkish study, the stigma was greater in epilepsy [9]. The instrument used to measure stigma in the US and Italian studies differed from the one in the Turkish study, so it is unclear if the differences arise from study characteristics or represent differences in cultural attitudes across countries. Seng evaluated the extent to which stigma contributes to migraine-related disability and quality of life beyond migraine and psychiatric symptoms, and pain conditions. In 121 clinic-based subjects, stigma (using the Stigma Scale for Chronic Illnesses 8-item version or SSCI-8) was correlated with disability, migraine-related quality of life, allodynia, pain catastrophizing, and psychiatric symptoms. Stigma was associated with higher headache frequency, anxiety, depression, and quality of life sub scores. The SSCI-8 contributed significantly beyond migraine symptoms to measures of emotional function and disability. Consistent with current models, these findings suggest that migraine-related stigma reduction may improve quality of life and possibly function [10].

Shapiro examined stigma in a web-based population study of 59,004 subjects with migraine. Stigma was measured with a newly developed stigma instrument, the Migraine-Related Stigma scale (MiRs). MiRs had two factors: secondary gain and minimizing burden. Even patients with low-frequency migraine (0–3 headache days per month) experienced migraine-related stigma often or very often 25% percent of the time. Subjects with high-frequency headache (15 or more headache days a month) experienced stigma often or very often 47% of the time. Three measures of disease impact were correlated with MiRs across all headache frequencies. These findings are consistent with the notion that disease-related disabling symptoms cause stigma, although the causal direction between stigma and measures of disease impact is not proven [11].

Best analyzed 4.5 million news articles to create new measures of stigma across 107 health conditions. This allowed for the comparison of public stigma across these conditions. Among ten neurological conditions, migraine disease was the most stigmatized. Migraine ranked 18 of 107. The conditions that were more stigmatized were mental health disorders, addictions, and several of the sexually transmitted diseases. Conditions that were less stigmatized than this measure included obesity, fibromyalgia, and chronic fatigue syndrome [3].

In a survey of neurologists in an academic medical center with a strong headache medicine program, half reported that they believe that there is a stigma against patients with migraine among healthcare professionals [12]. Almost 82% of respondents reported that they view treating patients with migraine as challenging, whereas 67% of respondents reported that they feel patients with migraine drain them emotionally. These findings need to be confirmed and explored. Do the stigmatizing physicians recognize the stigma in themselves and others? And how does this awareness determine how much a physician is a stigmatizer?

Types of Stigma

Public Stigma

Public stigma is characterized by labeling and stigmatizing stereotypes [13]. Jokes about migraine and use of headache or migraine as a metaphor for something annoying but unimportant. Negative labels for persons with migraine are: whiney, malignant, pill-popping, hypochondriacs, weak willed, lazy, and incapable of handling stress [6]. These perceptions are shared with diseases that are invisible spectrum disorders like depression and other pain disorders [13]. Patients with migraine often live with insensitive or insulting statements made by others that blame or belittle them. Developing strategies to reduce these "micro-aggressions" or change the attitudes that underlie them has become a central pillar of the advocacy movement.

Table 39.3 Suggested language guide simplified from Migraine Australia Language guide [37]

Migraine language quick guide	This quick guide contains the most important points from our migraine language guide. If you can change the language you use to talk about migraine on these five points, you will help reduce the stigma for everyone living with migraine!
1: Say migraine attack or episode, not "a migraine"	Migraine is a life-long medical condition. The term migraine attack is more accurate to describe the symptoms we experience. Migraine episode is also acceptable.
2: Say migraine, not "migraines"	The term migraines (i.e., with an "s") suggests that migraine comes and goes, when this is not the case. The way migraine affects people can change from one day to another and between attacks, but the condition is always there. Migraine disorder is also acceptable.
3: Say "people living with migraine," not "migraine sufferers"	Migraine can be awful and people with migraine suffer from the *symptoms* of migraine attacks. The term "migraine sufferer" is not helpful as it focuses on the disorder instead of the person.
4: Don't call your headache a migraine, or migraine a headache	The "just a headache" myth is the leading cause of migraine stigma. Headache is a common symptom, but some people living with migraine do not experience headache at all! Other types of headache, no matter how severe, are not migraine.
5: Don't call anything else migraine	Please try not to use the word migraine unless you are actually talking about migraine. The term migraine should not be used to describe something else. It also should not be used in casual conversation, for example, do not say things like "I'm getting a migraine just thinking about that."

The language used about migraine is a form of public stigma and can make a difference in how patients are treated by the medical community and be influenced by the public at large (Table 39.3). Studies conducted in substance use disorders, another stigmatized disease, demonstrate that using terms such as being a "substance abuser" contrasted with "having substance use disorder," results in substantially different provider attitudes toward otherwise identical patients [14, 15]. The migraine patient community has endorsed a set of recommendations that they believe are less stigmatizing. One notable difference between the Australian and the US language guide is that the word "migraineur" is discouraged by the US version and not mentioned by the Australian version [16]. In general, a person's first language is endorsed by the medical community. The patient community sometimes endorses the term "migraineur" or other labels of a person with a chronic illness because they feel their disease is indeed a defining feature of their identity. Most providers feel that they should use person's first language, accepting self-labeling only after an individual has chosen this language. In the USA, CHAMP identified the term "medication overuse" as stigmatizing, suggesting "medication adaption headache" as more appropriate and precise [17].

Structural Stigma

Structural stigma is prejudice and discrimination by policies, laws, or real practice. Like public stigma, this can be a feature of the general culture so pervasive that it is unnoticed by anyone embedded in that culture.

We have already demonstrated the pervasive underfunding of migraine research by NIH. This has been a persistent problem since funding of migraine and headache have been tracked by NIH. Congress has issued 17 report language statements since 2009 urging NIH to increase programmatic funding specifically for migraine and headache disorders, yet NIH has not significantly increased migraine funding relative to other disease [18]. The NIH's funding curve for headache diseases has remained relatively flat, even in the face of enormous funding increases for pain research in the face of the opioid crisis [19].

Disability (Supplemental Security Income, Social Security Disability Insurance) for chronic illness is hard to obtain in general. This difficulty is particularly acute for migraine and other headache diseases. Patients with migraine apply for federal disability benefits at a rate that is disproportionately small relative to their populations burden of disability (0.3% of disability claims versus 5.6% of US YLDs (Years Lived with Disability), an 18.6 fold lower rate of application); and yet, their applications are far less likely to be initially approved by the Social Security claims process [19]. The absence of "blue book" (Social Security Administration Listing of Impairments) listing for migraine and other headache diseases has persisted despite advocacy efforts to change this [19]. This is astounding since migraine is the number two source of YLDs worldwide [20].

The Alliance for Headache Disorders Advocacy (AHDA) is a coalition of patient and physician organizations that lobbies for policy changes to improve the lives of patients with headache diseases. Over the 15 years of its existence, the AHDA has gone to congress with a specific task for legislation or regulation changes. Some of these efforts are listed in Table 39.4. The AHDA also meets with Federal agencies, disability lawyer organizations, and device manufacturers to envision and work toward policies beneficial to people with headache disorders. It has worked with other stakeholders toward migraine and headache screening standards in women's health clinics and in primary care for both men and women.

Self-Stigma (Internalized Stigma)

After a lifetime of exposure to public and structural stigma, persons with chronic disease incorporate these negative attitudes toward their own self-perception [21]. One study [8] showed an extremely tight correlation between public

Table 39.4 Policies addressed by the Alliance for Headache Disorders Advocacy

Policy Areas of Advocacy by AHDA
Increase National Institutes of Health (NIH) funding for migraine research
Adding migraine and headache as categories of NIH expenditure
Fair review of NIH by experienced reviewer
Request for Proposal (RFP) for headache related grants
Correlating NIH expenditure with disease burden
Improving pay-line for headache related grants
Increasing headache research funding through the Congressionally Directed Medical Research Program (CDMRP)
Increasing headache research funding as part of efforts to find alternatives to opioid use
Increasing headache fellowship funding to provide expertise in the fight against opioid substance disorder
Improving headache care for veterans
Establishing Veterans Administration (VA) centers of excellence
Increasing numbers of established centers
Establish Indian Health Service (HIS) centers of excellence
Medicare coverage of oxygen for cluster headache
Adding Headache Disorders to the Social Security Administration listing of impairments

(enacted) and internalized stigma. Both stigmas are encountered in migraine and epilepsy, thus confirming the model [21] in which the conversion of public to internalized stigma is nearly inevitable. Internalized self-stigma has a profound effect on the quality of life and mental health of those who experience pain. Psychological disorders due to perceived discrimination are associated with worsened chronic pain. These align with a robust literature on internalized stigma's effect on health [22–24]. Internalized stigma has a corrosive effect on patients with chronic pain, as demonstrated by racial discrimination's effect on pain in the National Survey of Midlife Development in the United States (MIDUS) study [23], and in migraine disease [10].

Advocacy Efforts

A number of strategies to reduce stigma and improve understanding of headache diseases and access to resources could be adopted. It is clear that the problem of stigma and under-resourcing is pervasive and requires concerted efforts across multiple domains. History demonstrates that well-meaning interventions can be counterproductive, so new endeavors should be carefully considered. Advocacy efforts can be grouped into three broad categories: education, contact, and protest [25].

Education

Public education about a disease serves the public good while legitimizing a condition. Currently, mental health diseases—depression and substance use disorders—receive the bulk of attention. In recent years, the American Migraine Foundation (AMF) has had a public awareness campaign with billboards over Times Square; CHAMP and Miles for Migraine have a pilot campaign to educate about migraine and to normalize receiving care. Curated patient educational materials are provided by most advocacy organizations. The Migraine World Summit educates patients from around the world with a yearly multiday virtual symposium on a variety of topics, reaching tens of thousands of persons with migraine each year. Advertising for headache treatments can frame how migraine is viewed. Some negative examples of this are: companies persist in using the term "migraines"; fail to show the spectrum of disease severity; and give the impression that migraine should be universally successfully treatable [26]. Physician education should be seen as a kind of advocacy, given the paucity of headache providers and the poor state of education on headache disease at all levels including medical school [27–30]. Physician education has been at the core of the AHS mission since its inception, and it is also at the core of the mission of The International Headache Society, NHF, and Association of Migraine Disorders (AMD). CHAMP, a patient organization, has created a neutral list of provider educational opportunities in the USA, highlighting its view of the importance of physician training for the headache community [16].

Contact Strategies

Contact strategies are among the most effective advocacy and anti-stigma strategies based on the results from the mental health and anti-stigma campaign [25, 31]. Contact strategies encourage patients to identify themselves as persons with migraine or other headache diseases, view themselves as educators of the community, and access accommodations. It takes courage for people to self-identify as someone with a stigmatized disease, particularly with migraine, because there may be a potential impact on professional and personal relationships. Advocacy groups, such as Miles for Migraine, are training future advocates for success in those actions. These include the interaction between individuals of the general population and with the stigmatized disease, as well as between patients. Grassroots contact has twice as much impact as population-based contact [32]. In-person support groups and walk-runs can be important activities to reduce stigma.

Protest

Protest efforts speak out against injustices and discrimination caused by stigma. These strategies are notably successful in HIV advocacy, changing "politically correct" representations and speech. There is a possibility of backfire

Table 39.5 Coalition for Headache and Migraine. Patients (CHAMP) declaration of rights

CHAMP Declaration of Rights for People with Headache Diseases (Shortened)
We, the people with headache, migraine and cluster disease, deserve respect and empathy for the serious and sometimes debilitating medical conditions with which we live. We will not be disempowered, minimized or stigmatized by society....
Recommendations For All People
1. *Honor and believe* the struggle of people living with headache, migraine and cluster disease to cope with their pain and many other symptoms
2. *Educate and work* to correct the culture that penalizes people with severe headache, migraine and cluster disease
3. *Learn* about these diseases and understand the systemic nature of them
Recommendations For People With Headache Diseases
1. When you can, *reject the stigma* of headache, migraine and cluster in yourself, and confront it in others. This takes work and time to understand the messages we have received about living with a chronic disease.
2. When you can, *be visible* as a person with headache, migraine or cluster disease.
3. And when you can, *participate in awareness and advocacy* efforts. Seek out policymakers and advocate for understanding, research and treatment.
Rights Of People With Headache Diseases
1. *Live a life of dignity*, despite whatever limitations may be caused by our disease.
2. *Not be blamed or dismissed* for having a headache disease when all we want is effective treatment.
3. Gain access to quality medical treatment and social service provision not limited by external forces, financial or otherwise.
Advance robust scientific research that addresses the impact of headache disease and chronic pain on people living these diseases, their caregivers and families and society.

despite the accomplishments, due to forced suppression of stereotypes showing an increase in stereotypes arising [26]. With this in mind, protest approaches to migraine stigma should proceed with caution. CHAMP made an effort in this direction with its declaration of rights, which has a tone of protest (Table 39.5).

Advocacy Targets and Methods

Recently, a review of migraine expert action plans and online resources was evaluated to develop and identify high-yield advocacy goals that could improve the lives of patients with migraine. Six domains of action were identified: stigma and awareness, public health, access to care, research, social determinants of health, and workforce education. For each domain, specific goals were identified for 37 directions that advocacy efforts could have a profitable take (Table 39.6) [24]. The work of advocating is overdue, enormous, and will require the engagement of patients, physicians, scientists, and others.

Table 39.6 Procedure for developing an advocacy strategy from the Bill and Melinda Gates Foundation

Strategic Planning for Migraine Advocacy					
Stigma and awareness	Public health	Access to care	Research	Social determinants of health	Education and workforce
Educate patient and public on migraine diagnosis, prevention and treatment Educate to reduce disease progression Reframe with language choice and messaging Increase awareness of diversity including BIPOC and LGBQT communities Reduce stigma of migraine and associated comorbidities Eliminate migraine stereotypes and bias Form coalitions with advocacy groups	Improve CDC reporting Track indirect and direct costs Target opiate epidemic by preventing inappropriate use of opiates and increasing education of migraine specific treatments and prevention Address headache disorders linked to the COVID-19 Pandemic and Long-COVID Expand access to migraine care for veterans with migraine and posttraumatic headache	Improve clinical access and quality Eliminate arbitrary limits on personalized medicine Address rising costs Reform prior authorization and eliminate step care Eliminate non-medical switching Support widespread of telemedicine adoption Assure transitions from pediatric to adult clinics Improve access to affordable behavioral health services	Fund translational studies including biomarker programs Fund accelerated therapeutic development Increase health disparities and inequities research Develop coordinated multidisciplinary centers and networks Increase recruitment and retention of underrepresented minorities in trials and as investigators Engage patients and stakeholders for patient centered outcomes	Support policies resulting in affordable care Accommodations and workplace outreach Reduce discrimination Increase collaborations with social workers and other allied services Increase studies that identify the impact of social determinants of health and interventions for migraine Address the impact of environmental factors and structural barriers that may be linked to migraine	Increase headache education in residency and medical schools Train more headache specialists Increase continuing medical education opportunities for front line providers Increase diversity and inclusion efforts Incorporate advocacy training as a part of professional development Reduce burnout Support global collaborations for shared resources

Reprinted by permission from Current Pain and Headache Reports. Monteith [38]

Structural Advocacy

Regulations and policies skew against patients with headache disorders and the doctors who treat them. To combat these unfair policies, including the National Institutes of Health (NIH) underfunding migraine research, the lack of insurance coverage of oxygen for patients with cluster headaches, the lack of a category for migraine in the Social Security bluebook for headache disorders, and the absence of headache centers in the Veterans' Administrative system, the Alliance for Headache Disorders Advocacy (AHDA) have lobbied Congress since 2007 (Table 39.4) [19]. In a joint effort to improve access to newly developed drugs, both patients and physicians participate in the Institute for Clinical and Economic Review process that assigns a value to newly developed drugs. The patient community (The Danielle Byron Henry Foundation and CHAMP) has spearheaded migraine screening in schools by requiring a mandatory program teaching about migraine in the school curriculum [33]. A coalition of physicians and patients is currently pushing for migraine screening in women's health. Physician and patient groups continue to advocate for accommodations and screening at work.

Physician and Healthcare Professional Impact

People with migraine need access to medical professionals to receive a prompt diagnosis and to help to manage the stigmatizing landscape of their diagnosis. One way to do this is to change the emphasis and tone of trigger management, which is clearly given too great a role in patient care. Public stigma blames patients for exposing themselves to triggers, which are viewed as a "cause of migraine," which they are not. Emphasizing the management of "triggers" and medication "overuse" (as opposed to medication adaptation headache) harkens to stigma experiences by those with substance use disorder, creating an atmosphere in which patients blame themselves each time they have a migraine attack.

Healthcare professionals must teach the normality of migraine-related disability. Teaching empowerment and self-determination in patient counseling is a successful approach against stigma for healthcare professionals. Patients with a severe primary headache disorder can manage their diseases to be able to continue to work, while making them aware of how to secure workplace accommodations through the Americans with Disabilities Act. The use of terms like "discrimination" may help patients understand the nature of the

Table 39.7 A migraine-specific advocacy agenda

Phase 1		Phase 2		Phase 3	
Build consensus		Focus efforts		Achieve change	
Step 1	*Understand the landscape*	Step 4	*Know the decision-maker*	Step 7	*Present the case*
Step 2	*Decide who to involve*	Step 5	*Determine the ask*	Step 8	*Monitor the plan*
Step 3	*Set a SMART objective*	Step 6	*Create a work plan*	Step 9	*Capture results*

stigmatizing world in which they are functioning. Healthcare professionals can help reframe the patient's disease with the use of non-stigmatizing language [34].

International Headache Advocacy

In Europe, Canada, Australia, and South America, headache societies and patient advocacy organizations evolved in a similar manner to the USA. In 2017 [35], the first Global Patient Advocacy Summit was convened, bringing together patients, patient advocates, patient advocacy organizations, healthcare professionals, pharmaceutical manufacturers, scientists, and regulatory agencies. The parties agreed on the need to challenge pervasive stigma and assure access to competent, evidence-based treatment by providers with adequate training. In 2019 [36], the group reconvened and chose to focus on the education of employees and employers to support programs about migraine and reduce the burden of illness and workplace productivity. This strategy is logical, given the observation (in the USA) that stigma is strongly correlated with workplace disability.

Developing Advocacy Strategies

Advocacy is encouraged in many fields of medicine. The Bill & Melinda Gates Institute for Population and Reproductive Health pioneered Specific, Measurable, Attainable, Relevant, and Time-bound (SMART) advocacy as an effective structure to achieve changes toward advocacy goals. While initially developed for family planning, it is designed to be adapted for any health issue. SMART stands for Specific, Measurable, Attainable, Relevant, and Time-bound. It focuses on decision makers who have the power to act on requests of well-prepared advocates. It envisions three phases to a successful advocacy plan, each with three steps, for a nine-step process to achieving change. The process is thus broken down into manageable steps (Table 39.7). SMART advocacy builds consensus from the start. Training materials for the development of a successful SMART advocacy plan are available at https://www.gatesinstitute.org/sites/default/files/SMART%20Advocacy%20Brief%20English%20Final.pdf.

Conclusion

Advocacy for migraine and other headache diseases has been accelerating over the last 30 years, but it remains tiny compared to other diseases of similar or lesser burden. In the competition for resources, headache remains far behind less burdensome diseases, as manifested by the anemic NIH funding of migraine and other headache disorders. The most important cause of this under-advocacy and under-resourcing is stigma. Migraine is depicted as a disorder of weak and whiney women and is strongly linked in the individual to the disability that it causes. Migraine stigma exists in three domains: public, structural, and self-stigma. Different advocacy strategies should be used to reduce each type of stigma. We review past and current advocacy targets and suggested areas of future advocacy. We provide a list of some notable US and international advocacy organizations.

Teaching Points

1. The size of the migraine advocacy movement is miniscule compared to other diseases of comparable and lesser disease burden.
2. This stigma, seeded in the objective lack of migraine manifestations, still plays a role in the social understanding of migraine and the availability of economic and political resources.
3. After a lifetime of exposure to public and structural stigma, persons with chronic disease incorporate these negative attitudes toward their own self-perception.
4. For effective migraine advocacy, six domains of action have been identified: stigma and awareness, public health, access to care, research, social determinants of health, and workforce education.
5. Teaching empowerment and self-determination in patient counseling is a successful approach against stigma for healthcare professionals.

Important Advocacy Organizations for Physicians and Patients

ABRACES

https://abraces.me

The Associação Brasileira de Cefaleia em Salvas e Enxaqueca (Brazilian Association for Cluster Headache and Migraine) is a cluster headache and migraine advocacy association aimed at improving patients' quality of life through lifestyle change approaches, mental health support, raising awareness, promoting disease education, and fighting for disability rights. Their very successful campaign for cluster headache awareness reached 44 million people (famous artists joined). Currently, efforts are focused on public policies for headache disorders.

Alliance for Headache Disorders Advocacy

http://allianceforheadacheadvocacy.org/what-we-can-do/

The alliance is a group of nonprofits focused on fighting for policy changes to benefit persons with headache disorders, including migraine disease.

AMCEMIG (Mexico)

https://amcemig.com/ is an association that addresses the educational, academic, and research needs of Mexico's neurologists and health professionals. It provides the neurological community and health professionals with scientific information and carries out various activities through congresses that spread knowledge for better care of patients. It educates the population through forums, congresses, courses, publications, and conferences on headache and migraine problems.

American Migraine Foundation

https://americanmigrainefoundation.org/migraine-stories/

The American Migraine Foundation provides education, support, and resources for persons with migraine. Its mission is to advance migraine research, promote patient advocacy, and expand access to care for patients worldwide.

Association of Migraine Disorders

www.migrainedisorders.org/get-involved

The Association of Migraine Disorders (AMD) is devoted to improving the understanding of migraine disease. Because migraine is a full-body condition with a broad spectrum of symptoms, AMD incorporates the experience of many medical specialties in managing this disease.

CHAMP (Coalition for Headache & Migraine Patients)

https://headachemigraine.org

The Coalition for Headache and Migraine Patients (CHAMP) brings together organizations and leaders in this disease area to enhance communication, coordination, and collaboration to help people more effectively wherever they are on their patient journey. CHAMP is working to identify and address the unmet needs of those with headache, migraine, and cluster diseases.

Chronic Migraine Awareness

https://chronicmigraineawareness.org/

Chronic Migraine Awareness upholds a mission to be the voice of the chronic migraine community by offering support, information, and education to empower individuals to advocate for their own health.

Cluster Busters

https://clusterbusters.org/

Cluster Busters supports research for better treatments and a cure while advocating to improve the lives of those struggling with cluster headaches. Their purpose is to help its members find solutions to problems that exist as a result of cluster headaches, including supporting research. Cluster Busters was born out of the discovery that psychedelics may be valuable in the management of cluster headaches, and the need to help patients navigate this tricky scientific and legal environment. It provides general information and support to help persons with cluster headaches.

The European Migraine Headache Alliance

https://www.emhalliance.org/

The European Migraine & Headache is a nonprofit umbrella organization that includes over 33 patient associations for migraine, cluster headache, trigeminal neuralgia, and other headache diseases, across Europe. EMHA speaks on behalf of and to advocate for the rights and needs of the 138 million people in Europe living with headache disorders. It works closely with organizations such as the European Headache Federation (EHF).

Miles for Migraine

www.milesformigraine.org

Miles for Migraine creates live, patient-participatory events that reduce the burden of isolation and stigma for people with migraine and headache diseases, and their caregivers. It builds community by bringing people together at fun walk/runs and through educational and support programs. It is building local advocacy movements in 24 cities with fellowship training programs. Funds raised support fellowship training programs and research in the community.

The Migraine World Summit

www.migraineworldsummit.com

The Migraine World Summit is the largest patient event in the world for those with chronic headache and migraine disease while bringing together tens of thousands of people to learn from world-leading doctors, experts, and specialists.

National Headache Foundation

https://headaches.org/

National Headache Foundation is the oldest and largest foundation for patients with headache disorders. It supports programs for headache awareness, advocacy, education, and research.

US Pain Foundation

www.uspainfoundation.org/get-involved

The US Pain Foundation is the leading advocacy organization for people with pain. It empowers, educates, connects, and advocates for individuals living with chronic illness that causes pain, as well as their caregivers and clinicians, through multiple programs and services.

Migraine & Headache Australia

https://www.headacheaustralia.org.au

Migraine & Headache Australia is the only organization in Australia that has supported more than 5 million Australians affected by headaches and migraine for over 20 years. Its mission is to fund headache research, provide trustworthy information for patients, and advocate and support the patient community.

Migraine Association of Ireland

http://migraine.ie/

The Migraine Association of Ireland is Ireland's only patient charity providing support, education, information, and reassurance to people with migraine and other headache disorders. They provide free educational courses on self-management and understanding migraine for people with migraine, and certified health professional courses for General Pratictioners and other healthcare professionals; lobby and advocate on behalf of people with migraine to access new treatments and to ensure they have access treatments.

Migraine Canada

https://migrainecanada.org/

Migraine Canada is a nationally registered charity organization dedicated to improving the lives of all Canadians living with migraine and other headache disorders. Its mission is to improve the lives of Canadians with migraine and other headache disorders through awareness, support, education, advocacy, and research.

Migraine Foundation Aotearoa New Zealand

https://www.migrainefoundation.org.nz/

Migraine Foundation Aotearoa New Zealand is the only not-for-profit, incorporated society in New Zealand supporting people living with migraine. They provide a collective voice for people in New Zealand living with this invisible and disabling condition with the goal of raising awareness and supporting people living with migraine in New Zealand.

The Migraine Trust

https://migrainetrust.org/

The Migraine is the only UK migraine charity providing information and support, campaigning for awareness and change, and funding and promoting research. Their goals are: encouraging new research and treatment; ensuring an accurate, timely diagnosis and access to the best possible information, care, and treatment; ensuring people with headache disorders have the same legal protections as other disabled people; and building an active and supportive community of people affected by migraine.

OUCH, UK

https://ouchuk.org

The Organization for Understanding Cluster Headache (OUCH, UK) exists to raise awareness of cluster headaches within the medical profession and the general public and to offer support and guidance to people with migraine and their families. OUCH is a member of Headache UK, an umbrella organization of headache charities. They link patients to educational materials, research, and work for accommodations and disability rights.

The International Headache Society-Global Patient Advocacy Coalition (IHS-GPAC)

https://ihs-gpac.org/

IHS-GPAC works in collaboration with patients, patient advocacy organizations, healthcare providers, and headache, pain and neurology associations worldwide to improve the lives of those affected by migraine, cluster, and other diseases that cause severe head pain. Recent focus has been on workplace and school initiatives. Produced Vancouver documents advocating for reducing stigma, workplace initiatives, and access to care.

Questions and Answers

1. Three types of stigma relevant to migraine are:
   A. Personal stigma, public and institutional stigma.
   B. Self-stigma, public stigma and institutional stigma.

C. Self-stigma, public stigma and structural stigma.
D. Individual stigma, group stigma, and structural stigma.

The correct answer is B. In this article, we discussed stigma according to the categories listed in answer B. While other, often overlapping categorizations of stigma have been used, we believe this research consensus terminology serves the headache community best.

2. The most persistent issue for migraine advocacy organizations in the USA has been:
   A. Creating a new institute of headache medicine at NIH.
   B. Addressing the underfunding of headache research by NIH.
   C. New legislation demanding employers offer accommodations for people with migraine.
   D. Creating a CMS "blue book" listing for migraine.

The correct answer is B. AHDA has gone to Congress and had 17 report language statements that should have resulted increased NIH funding for headache diseases, but this has not substantially happened. Congress has not been asked to create a new institute for headache diseases. Various advocacy organizations have programs to educated employers and employees about appropriate accommodations and rights under the ADA—these pro grams need expansion, but the rights exist under the ADA. The AHDA has only had one Congressional ask related to CMS recognizing migraine as a disability.

References

1. Dahnke MD. The role of the American Nurses Association code in ethical decision making. Holist Nurs Pract. 2009;23(2):112–9.
2. Gonzalez AR. Patient advocacy history, evolution and impact on health. Juniper Online J Public Health. 2018;3(3):1.
3. Best RK. Disease politics and medical research funding: three ways advocacy shapes policy. Am Sociol Rev. 2012;77(5):780–803.
4. Foxhall K. Migraine: a history. Johns Hopkins University Press; 2019.
5. Lipton RB, Scher A, Kolodner K, Liberman J, Steiner T, Stewart W. Migraine in the United States: epidemiology and patterns of health care use. Neurology. 2002;58(6):885–94.
6. Kempner J. Not tonight. Not tonight. University of Chicago Press; 2014.
7. Shapiro R, Araujo A, Nicholson R, Reed M, Buse D, Ashina S, et al., editors. Stigmatizing attitudes about migraine by people without migraine: results of the OVERCOME study. Headache. Hoboken: Wiley; 2019.
8. Young WB, Park JE, Tian IX, Kempner J. The stigma of migraine. PLoS One. 2013;8(1):e54074.
9. Aydemir N, Özkara Ç, Ünsal P, Canbeyli R. A comparative study of health related quality of life, psychological well-being, impact of illness and stigma in epilepsy and migraine. Seizure. 2011;20(9):679–85.
10. Seng EKSR, Buse DC, Robbins MS, Lipton RB, Parker A. Headache: the Journal of Head and Face Pain. American Headache Society 64th Annual scientific meeting June 9–12, 2022; 2022. p. 99–100.
11. Shapiro RENR, Seng EK, Buse DC, Reed ML, Zagar AJ, et al. Headache: the Journal of Head and Face Pain. Denver, Colorado: American Headache Society 64th Annual scientific meeting June 9–12, 2022; 2022. p. 34–5.
12. Zubair AS, Sico JJ, Kuruvilla DE. Presence of stigma in the treatment of patients with migraine among neurologists. Pain Med. 2021;22:2135.
13. Parikh SK, Young WB. Migraine: stigma in society. Curr Pain Headache Rep. 2019;23(1):1–6.
14. Kelly JF, Dow SJ, Westerhoff C. Does our choice of substance-related terms influence perceptions of treatment need? An empirical investigation with two commonly used terms. J Drug Issues. 2010;40(4):805–18.
15. Kelly JF, Westerhoff CM. Does it matter how we refer to individuals with substance-related conditions? A randomized study of two commonly used terms. Int J Drug Policy. 2010;21(3):202–7.
16. CHAMP. HeadEd: Headache & Migraine Education for Healthcare Providers 2022. Available from: https://headachemigraine.org/headed/.
17. Solomon M, Nahas SJ, Segal JZ, Young WB. Medication adaptation headache. London: SAGE Publications Sage UK; 2011. p. 515–7.
18. Australia, M. Language guide, n.d.. Retrieved February 2, 2024, from https://assets.nationbuilder.com/migraineaus/pages/408/attachments/original/1657878609/Migraine_Australia_-_Language_Guide_-_2022_v1.pdf?1657878609.
19. Allianceforheadacheadvocacy.org. 2022 Headache on the Hill | Alliance for Headache Advocacy 2022. Available from: https://allianceforheadacheadvocacy.org/headache-on-the-hill/2022-headache-on-the-hill/.
20. Shapiro RE. What will it take to move the needle for headache disorders? An advocacy perspective. Headache. 2020;60(9):2059–77.
21. Murray JL, C. Global burden of 369 diseases and injuries in 204 countries and territories, 1990–2019: a systematic analysis for the Global Burden of Disease Study 2019. Lancet. 2020;396(10258):1204–22.
22. Rao D, Choi SW, Victorson D, Bode R, Peterman A, Heinemann A, et al. Measuring stigma across neurological conditions: the development of the stigma scale for chronic illness (SSCI). Qual Life Res. 2009;18(5):585–95.
23. Nichols VP, Ellard DR, Griffiths FE, Kamal A, Underwood M, Taylor SJ. The lived experience of chronic headache: a systematic review and synthesis of the qualitative literature. BMJ Open. 2017;7(12):e019929.
24. Brown TT, Partanen J, Chuong L, Villaverde V, Griffin AC, Mendelson A. Discrimination hurts: the effect of discrimination on the development of chronic pain. Soc Sci Med. 2018;204:1–8.
25. Livingston JD, Boyd JE. Correlates and consequences of internalized stigma for people living with mental illness: a systematic review and meta-analysis. Soc Sci Med. 2010;71(12):2150–61.
26. Corrigan PW, River LP, Lundin RK, Penn DL, Uphoff-Wasowski K, Campion J, et al. Three strategies for changing attributions about severe mental illness. Schizophr Bull. 2001;27(2):187–95.
27. Parikh SK, Kempner J, Young WB. Stigma and migraine: developing effective interventions. Curr Pain Headache Rep. 2021;25(11):1–10.
28. Finkel A. American academic headache specialists in neurology: practice characteristics and culture. Cephalalgia. 2004;24(7):522–7.
29. Kommineni M, Finkel AG. Teaching headache in America: survey of neurology chairs and residency directors. Headache. 2005;45(7):862–5.

30. Minen MT, Monteith T, Strauss LD, Starling A. New investigator and trainee task force survey on the recruitment and retention of headache specialists. Headache. 2015;55(8):1092–101.
31. Pace A, Orr SL, Rosen NL, Safdieh JE, Cruz GB, Sprouse-Blum AS. The current state of headache medicine education in the United States and Canada: an observational, survey-based study of neurology clerkship directors and curriculum deans. Headache. 2021;61(6):854–62.
32. Corrigan PW, Morris SB, Michaels PJ, Rafacz JD, Rüsch N. Challenging the public stigma of mental illness: a meta-analysis of outcome studies. Psychiatr Serv. 2012;63(10):963–73.
33. Corrigan PW, Fong MW. Competing perspectives on erasing the stigma of illness: what says the dodo bird? Soc Sci Med. 2014;103:110–7.
34. Utahpta.org. Migraine at school, Utah PSA, 2022.
35. Arca KN, Starling AJ. Advocacy in headache medicine: tips at the bedside, the institutional level, and beyond. Curr Neurol Neurosci Rep. 2020;20(11):52.
36. Dodick D, Edvinsson L, Makino T, Grisold W, Sakai F, Jensen R, et al. Vancouver declaration on global headache patient advocacy 2018. Cephalalgia. 2018;38(13):1899–909.
37. Dodick DW, Ashina M, Sakai F, Grisold W, Miyake H, Henscheid-Lorenz D, et al. Vancouver declaration II on global headache patient advocacy 2019. Cephalalgia. 2020;40(10):1017–25.
38. Monteith TS. Advocacy for migraine relief: strategic planning to eliminate the burden. Curr Pain Headache Rep. 2022:1–8. https://doi.org/10.1007/s11916-022-01059-1. Epub ahead of print.

Teaching the World About Migraine: A Narrative Review

40

Henrik W. Schytz and R. Allan Purdy

Learning is lifelong.

Sir William Osler, 1874.

Introduction

Teaching can be hard work, and of course, teaching neurology has its own special requirements. Teaching about migraine and other headache disorders can be very challenging, but all teaching can be rewarding. In the past three decades, the knowledge about headache and migraine, in particular, has expanded in an exponential manner [6, 7]. It has become an area of neurology specialization that deals with primary and secondary headaches and has fallen under the rubric of "Headache Medicine."

Headache, of course, is a cardinal symptom of various neurological diseases and as such deserves a lot of study and interest to ensure the diagnostician understands what needs to be known to practice medicine dealing with any type of headache complaint [3, 10]. Neurologists see many patients with headaches, and migraine is the most common headache seen by neurologists in the USA [11], for example. Around the world, about 1 billion people have migraine [4, 10, 11], and the prevalence of migraine is no less than 19% for women and 10% for men [1]. However, despite migraine being highly frequent, medical schools and neurologists in training are often only presented with headache and migraine as a very limited part of the curriculum [25–27]. Insufficient headache education may also result in diagnostic failure and inappropriate treatment of headache patients [28]. As an example, a recent study from Norway showed that only half of the participating general practitioners were aware that different types of acute headache medication can lead to a very frequent secondary headache: medication-overuse headache (MOH) [29]. The initial need to separate secondary headache diseases from primary headache disorders remains the most important thing that physicians need to know. Thus, even though only a relatively small percentage of cases are secondary headache etiologies [2], it should be a matter of attention as some secondary headaches are preventable and treatable but may lead to disability or may even be life-threatening if not properly diagnosed and treated. In fact, about 18% of patients presenting with headaches to tertiary care centers could have an underlying secondary cause [2].

H. W. Schytz
Danish Headache Center, Department of Neurology, Copenhagen University Hospital – Rigshospitalet, Copenhagen, Denmark

Department of Clinical Medicine, Faculty of Health and Medical Sciences, University of Copenhagen, Copenhagen, Denmark

R. A. Purdy (✉)
Medicine (Neurology), Dalhousie University, Halifax, NS, Canada

Process of Knowledge Acquisition

The new knowledge about migraine and other headaches disorders, along with advanced technology, has helped make the diagnosis of headache disorders easier, especially imaging of the nervous system [4, 11]. What has also changed most dramatically is the knowledge about migraine. Migraine has been studied for centuries, but effective therapies have eluded caregivers. With the advent of the triptans over 30 years ago [7, 8, 14], the field has changed in a positive way. Now, three decades later, the advent of new calcitonin gene-related peptide monoclonal antibodies, and gepants in particular [9, 10, 14], as well as other treatments, has started a new cycle of effective therapies.

So, specialists in migraine and other headaches are now found around the world, but it is also necessary to spread this knowledge to other specialists, such as generalists in neurology and primary care physicians, to ensure the newer knowledge is applied in clinical practice at every level. This is not an easy task without major guideposts along the way. Learning what is required to become a headache practitioner takes time. However, the increase in research, treatments, and clinical care directed toward headaches in recent decades has created a golden opportunity, mainly because of migraine, the most common primary headache disorder, to advance the field.

T. S. Monteith et al. (eds.), *Comprehensive Migraine Management*, https://doi.org/10.1007/978-3-031-86923-5_40

Migraine is more than a headache and is among the most common neurological diseases [1]. It is the focus of much study and disability for people with migraine [1]. Migraine may be understood as a neurological disorder, which in a sense highjacks the normal pain and other brain pathways and structures to produce its plethora of symptomatology. Other diseases like stroke and tumors do the same thing, and thus, many mimic migraine or vice versa when presented to diagnosticians on a regular basis [15]. This is key to understanding the field, and as indicated, most headaches presenting to neurologists are migraine [11].

Relationship to Current Knowledge

This book has excellent content. It shows the amazing understanding and underpinnings of the clinical and scientific progress of the field of headache medicine as it relates to migraine. The authors behind this book know a lot, and their chapters reflect that. However, there are many around the world who need to be taught more about the new science, clinical changes in therapies, and opportunities. How is this best accomplished?

In this chapter, there are some hints of what has worked. In essence, teaching involves both an engaging teacher and an interested student, connected to an interesting topic such as migraine or neurology. If the student also possesses "insatiable curiosity," then the mixture works, magic occurs, and learning can take place. If knowledge acquisition can be constructed around a clinical case, it becomes even more contextual for the learner [16]. In the past three decades, it has been possible to make this happen on a wide scale regarding migraine and other headache disorders around the world.

Opportunities arose when major national headache societies took on increasing continuing medical education (CME) and continuing professional development (CPD) about headaches. They produced the content and course material to train doctors. This expanded into regional and local groups. Residency training followed in some countries and resident programs; however, to reach medical students has proven more difficult, but help is on the way. Primary care physicians see a lot of patients with migraine, so they need to know a lot about headaches to practice medicine. They must know about migraine.

Role of Multiple Groups, Societies, and Journals

A specific course for neurology residents has been taking place in Canada since 1998, and another recently began in the USA. There have been local attempts in the past in the USA, and later in the USA and Canada, directed to medical school teaching of headache with curriculum development in the past [22, 23]; additionally, international meetings of headache fellows occur in North America by way of the International Headache Academy (IHA in USA; iHead in Europe), both of which have proven extremely successful in creating and mentoring a future cadre of headache clinicians and researchers. Journals on headache continue to evolve including *Headache and Facial Pain* from the American Headache Society (AHS), Cephalalgia and now Cephalalgia Reports from the International Headache Society (IHS) and the *Journal of Headache and Pain* from the European Headache Federation (EHF).

Many other journals around the world are directed to headache medicine and the basic science of headache, migraine, and other headache disorders. It is a truly remarkable explosion in knowledge. Residency programs are starting to incorporate headache into their curricula, Grand Rounds and elective and clinical rotations, and clinical fellowships are plentiful. In Europe, for example, at the Danish Headache Center and University of Copenhagen in Denmark, there has been an accredited Master of Headache Disorders program since 2016, which has been highly successful. At the Sapienza University in Rome, Italy, a highly successful master's program in headache medicine has existed for more than 19 years, endorsed by the European Headache Federation (EHF). At the University of Kiel in Germany, a master of migraine and headache medicine has just been launched.

Role of the International Headache Society with Other Societies and Teaching Methods

Another leap in the field to help with training physicians and other healthcare providers came about with the ongoing evolution of the IHS and its biennial Congresses (IHC), rotating in many countries for 20 Congresses, which include science, clinical information, and many teaching courses about migraine and headache. The IHS with the latest International Classification of Headache Disorders, currently in its third iteration [5], provided fertile soil for meetings and gatherings, and the evolution of clinical knowledge in practice, the science of migraine, and other headache disorders. Evidence-based medicine became an important cornerstone of clinical trials, as did primary basic and clinical research. New journals evolved and progressed, and in the latter part of the twentieth century and into the twenty-first century, online learning modules, including seminars, courses, and podcasts, have been disseminating knowledge about headaches and migraine.

Patient societies have formed, as have advocacy groups worldwide which further defined and were highlighted by the IHS Global Patient Advocacy Coalition by way of the

Vancouver Declaration [12, 13]. It is hard to escape the new growth in migraine knowledge and other headache disorders with respect to diagnosis, investigations, and treatments.

Notwithstanding the above, all teaching about migraine and other headache disorders begins with the patient or person with a headache and the diagnostician, usually in a room conversing and talking about their headache. This process is time consuming and repetitive, which is both the magic of the process and the potential Achilles' heel. New algorithmic approaches, machine learning [20], and artificial intelligence [19] have helped, and in certain circumstances are better, but nothing will replace this need to get the correct diagnosis from the start and apply it individually in each case, as every person is unique in practice and life.

The IHS through its Education Committee has created learning opportunities in the field. There are regular courses that are either supported or endorsed by IHS at other society meetings, and speakers from the membership attending or being involved with in-person meetings and recently online teaching. A Visiting Professor Programme has evolved [VP Programme IHS]; the definition of a Visiting Professor from the IHS website is *Visiting Professors is an initiative of the IHS Education committee with the aim to send headache specialists as representatives of IHS to attend regional meetings, or teach at a headache centre, in countries that might need or want increased headache education and motivation and where, without financial support, attendance of an international specialist would not be possible*. This placed emphasis outside the European and North American corridor, where major efforts for headache education prevailed, yet did not exclude countries with well-developed local, regional, and even national headache societies of their own. The VPs have travelled to several countries to help with the teaching and conveyance of new knowledge on migraine backed by the latest clinical and basic science findings. Recent VPs have gone to Nepal, Iran, Kyrgyzstan, and Mexico, for example. A new VP Plus Programme was developed to allow VPs to be sent to countries and stay a while to mentor clinicians and researchers. Programs for clinical and research fellowships are awarded annually, as are short-stay programs. The importance of mentorship in headache education has also been acknowledged by the Junior Group of the IHS by organizing a yearly virtual mentoring program to promote global collaborations, mentorship, and support to aspiring headache specialists.

A Core Curriculum has been produced and recently updated by the Education Committee with translated versions into Spanish, Italian, French, Turkish, Brazilian Portuguese, Japanese, Korean, Chinese, Chinese Traditional, Russian, and Arabic. The IHS homepage (https://www.ihs-headache.org) is now available in English, Spanish, Chinese, and Russian. It also contains many short videos on various headache topics (with Spanish and Chinese subtitles), podcasts, previous webinars, and recorded lectures from the IHC and other conferences around the world. In addition, several e-learning modules on primary and secondary headaches are in development for IHS members, which will be accredited by the European Accreditation Council for Continuing Medical Education online courses. Other major national and regional headache societies have also put learning material online.

IHS has supported Headache Master Schools in many areas around the world: Sao Paulo, Brazil, 2011; Tokyo, Japan, 2013; Mumbai, India, 2014; Beijing, China, 2015; Sydney, Australia, 2018; and Bogota, Colombia, 2019, in cooperation with local/regional headache societies, and individuals who helped facilitate the programs and Master's courses. One of us (RAP) personally attended four of the schools. These evolved from IHS supporting local, national, or regional societal requests for support and the subsequent detailed processes needed to create good educational offerings and have visiting faculty to work with local faculty to enhance the learning. Currently, there are 54 Affiliate Headache Societies listed in relation to IHS, which look to the Society for guidance in teaching. Core knowledge is conveyed by prior reading, testing sometimes, and at the usual 3–4 days meeting with plenary sessions of focused lectures, and lots of interactive sessions to include small and large group teaching, debates, and other learning tools. The feedback thus far has been very good, and the outcomes remain sustainable as many places continue with annual headache meetings with elements of the Masters School experience, being part of the programs.

The usual plan for a Masters School was as follows:

1. Pretest of prior knowledge
2. Course
   (a) Didactic Core Lectures
   (b) Small or large group sessions with cases
   (c) Other interactive sessions with debates and/or facilitated by experts in the field, using local and visiting faculty
3. Posttest of gained knowledge
4. Follow-up in 6 months to see how they did

Having attended four of these courses, one of us (RAP) had first-hand experience in the outcomes. Focused plenary sessions were excellent and welcome. Large group sessions dealt with many areas of the migraine and headache in general. Small group sessions were based on cases and followed generally the principles of Case Based Learning (CBL). There were groups of eight to ten or and even more in some large groups, and they brought cases or used the tutors' cases, which involved lots of interaction and learning, along with an approach to migraine and other headache disorders. Informal discussion of migraine and other aspects of the field occurred during nutrition breaks, common meals, and social events. Anecdotally, such informal learning is highly valuable and approaches the concept of an "unconference" [24]. A lot of time and effort is given to make the meeting more interactive and less didactic using fewer lectures. In the last Master's School in Colombia, a video link was done over an hour or more so the course organizers could show the IHS Education Chair (RAP at the time) the venue, lecture room, and breakout rooms to ensure that a lot of effort had been put into getting this right space and atmosphere for the attendees.

The European Headache Federation has played a role to take on teaching on the continent, while in North America the AHS has led the way in creating meetings and courses on headaches. The Migraine Trust in the United Kingdom has held successful meetings for decades. South American, Asian, and Australian/New Zealand Headache Societies are evolving rapidly. Recent endeavors in Africa are also beginning to grow, as are efforts in Russia and the Middle East. Many other individual countries, including India, have now evolved teaching courses on migraine and other headache disorders. Regional centers for teaching about migraine and other headaches exist in most countries. It is really phenomenal to share knowledge of headache around the world.

During the pandemic, there was a concern that all of this effort and teaching about migraine may be impacted; however, in reality, it might just have increased for everybody. Virtual meetings now regularly have visiting speakers from all around the world doing live synchronous sessions and not infrequently video talks, which allow for time differences to be respected, and subsequent online and on-time demand follow-up on the presentations. Asynchronous learning occurred in the past with a diverse group around the world interacting with a tutor, and now webinars and podcasts make the interactions personalized and interactive. Nevertheless, a lot of experience indicates that in-person meetings have great value for the attendees, in developing relationships and knowledge. Hybrid models might help facilitate change which is what is happening with large international headache symposia and congresses. It looks like these might point the way to involvement of many areas around the world in the future.

In the end, however, we go back to that triangle of the student and teacher interacting with a case, a live patient or person with a headache, or a topic in the field of headaches. This is where the teaching takes place, and where there has been a tremendous opportunity to change what we do. As each person who has been taught and that learning continues to be taught to others, we are developing the underpinnings of our field worldwide.

In terms of teaching, the method that appears to attract the most attention and works best for learners is Case Based Learning (CBL). Problem Based Learning (PBL) [21] preceded CBL as an educational technique in the past decades where the onus was on the learner to do the work and the tutor acted to guide them along in the process. CBL then became more efficient than PBL and allowed the focus to come to the learner with some direction from the tutor. Although the outcome of a direct lecture-based curriculum with PBL has been studied [17, 18], without a major difference in the learning, the PBL method showed that the participants enjoyed it more and were more active in the learning process [17, 18]. Questions over tutor variability came up in general curricula, but in the field of migraine and headache, this was generally avoided due to the fact that most teachers were neurologists.

It is important not to dismiss lectures as they can provide expert transfer of knowledge, condensed over years of learning combined with recent knowledge. However, lectures are best limited, and cases are the international communication of physicians while learning. In many countries, despite significant language and other barriers to learning, cases have stood out as the way to communicate medical knowledge, and by and large, the process appears to have worked.

Conclusion

Many people around the world played an important role in making this process a success. In each country, there were a few leaders who helped set the stage for the educational courses. There are just too many to mention in this overview article. In many national societies, people worked to make this learning invaluable and to reach multiple levels of learners, with great success. Many faculty travelled to various parts of the world, with the sole purpose of making migraine and headache medicine viable and part of the broader goal to teach the world about migraine.

Migraine, we believe, and this book clearly makes the point, is unique in the medical disorders. Generally, when a migraine attack affects the brain, it presents as an episodic disorder that produces a remarkable symptomatology. After the migraine attack, the brain returns to a normal or resting state of less excitability. We do this teaching to help people with migraine, but they and many among us who have experienced the perturbations of a migraine attack, get back something special in return from this remarkable neurological disorder—migraine teaches us how the brain works and migraine is the ultimate teacher of headache.

Teaching Points

- Teaching migraine requires a broad and comprehensive approach including: expert knowledge of migraine, clinical and scientific, by way of lectures, debates, focused discussion, case-based and other interactive sessions to give context to the learning.
- Teaching about migraine is best done while teaching about other primary headache disorders and secondary headaches to reflect the broad reach of headaches in medicine, with recognition that migraine is the most common headache disorder seen by physicians.
- Creating teaching sessions on headaches is best facilitated by local, regional, and national headache societies, first supported by international symposia and congresses.
- The International Headache Society is positioned to help with creating and fostering high-level knowledge in all aspects of headache medicine around the world. Online options for programming support and teaching resources are outlined on their site at: https://www.ihs-headache.org.

Acknowledgments We would like to mention three people who helped this along around the world. Professors Alan Rapoport, Vincenzo Guidetti, and Carlos Bordini had an idea about a Master School for IHS, and all brought it to fruition. Professor Alan Rapoport developed the Visiting Professor Programme. They all worked hard with many others to make this work by facilitating change and serving as tutors and guides with other local and visiting faculty to bring the world of migraine to the world. They should be thanked for their vision around the world.

The authors would also like to thank Carol Taylor of the International Headache Society for looking at this manuscript and making useful suggestions. Without her considerable talent and help, a lot of the process of teaching migraine around the world would not have been possible.

Disclosure HS is the current Chair of the Education Committee of the International Headache Society and RAP is the past Chair. Both of us have a long-time interest in migraine and other headache disorders, and a particular interest in medical education and teaching as it applies to the emerging field of Headache Medicine.

References

1. GBD 2016 Headache Collaborators. Global, regional, and national burden of migraine and tension-type headache, 1990-2016: a systematic analysis for the Global Burden of Disease Study 2016. Lancet Neurol. 2018;17(11):954–976. https://doi.org/10.1016/S1474-4422(18)30322-3.
2. Do TP, Remmers A, Schytz HW, et al. Red and orange flags for secondary headaches in clinical practice: SNNOOP10 list. Neurology. 2019;92(3):134–44. https://doi.org/10.1212/WNL.0000000000006697.
3. Dodick DW. Pearls: headache. Semin Neurol. 2010;30(1):74–81. https://doi.org/10.1055/s-0029-1245000.
4. Dodick DW. Diagnosing secondary and primary headache disorders. Continuum (Minneap Minn). 2021;27(3):572–85. https://doi.org/10.1212/CON.0000000000000980. PMID: 34048392.
5. Headache Classification Committee of the International Headache Society (IHS) The International Classification of Headache Disorders, 3rd edition. Cephalalgia. 2018;38(1):1–211. https://doi.org/10.1177/0333102417738202.
6. Charles A. The pathophysiology of migraine: implications for clinical management. Lancet Neurol. 2018;17(2):174–82. https://doi.org/10.1016/S1474-4422(17)30435-0. Epub 2017 Dec 8. PMID: 29229375.
7. Goadsby PJ, Holland PR, Martins-Oliveira M, Hoffmann J, Schankin C, Akerman S. Pathophysiology of Migraine: a disorder of sensory processing. Physiol Rev. 2017;97(2):553–622. https://doi.org/10.1152/physrev.00034.2015. PMID: 28179394; PMCID: PMC5539409.
8. Loder E. Triptan therapy in migraine. N Engl J Med. 2010;363(1):63–70. https://doi.org/10.1056/NEJMct0910887. PMID: 20592298.
9. Chan C, Goadsby PJ. Recent advances in pharmacotherapy for Episodic Migraine. CNS Drugs. 2019;33(11):1053–71. https://doi.org/10.1007/s40263-019-00665-9. PMID: 31556018.
10. Dodick DW. Migraine. Lancet. 2018;391(10127):1315–30. https://doi.org/10.1016/S0140-6736(18)30478-1. Epub 2018 Mar 6. PMID: 29523342.
11. Evans RW. Migraine and other primary headaches. Neurol Clin. 2019;37(4):xiii–xiv. https://doi.org/10.1016/j.ncl.2019.07.011. Epub 2019 Aug 21. PMID: 31563238.
12. Dodick DW, Edvinsson L, Makino T, Grisold W, Sakai F, Jensen R, Balch A, Ruiz de la Torre E, Henscheid-Lorenz D, Craven A, Messoud A, on behalf of the International Headache Society Global Patient Advocacy Coalition. Vancouver declaration on global headache patient advocacy 2018. Cephalalgia. 2018;38(13):1899–909. https://doi.org/10.1177/0333102418781644. PMID: 29882695.
13. Dodick DW, Ashina M, Sakai F, Grisold W, Miyake H, Henscheid-Lorenz D, Craven A, de la Ruiz Torre E, Koh R, Reznik N, Bance L, Leroux E, Edvinsson L, International Headache Society Global Patient Advocacy Coalition. Vancouver declaration II on global headache patient advocacy 2019. Cephalalgia. 2020;40(10):1017–25. https://doi.org/10.1177/0333102420921162. Epub 2020 Apr 28. PMID: 32345038.
14. Migraine AM. N Engl J Med. 2020;383(19):1866–76. https://doi.org/10.1056/NEJMra1915327. PMID: 33211930.
15. Angus-Leppan H. Migraine: mimics, borderlands and chameleons. Pract Neurol. 2013;13(5):308–18. https://doi.org/10.1136/practneurol-2012-000502. Epub 2013 Aug 1. PMID: 23906594.
16. Kassirer JP. Teaching clinical reasoning: case-based and coached. Acad Med. 2010;85(7):1118–24. https://doi.org/10.1097/acm.0b013e3181d5dd0d. PMID: 20603909.
17. Doucet MD, Purdy RA, Kaufman DM, Langille DB. Comparison of problem-based learning and lecture format in continuing medical education on headache diagnosis and management. Med Educ. 1998;32(6):590–6. https://doi.org/10.1046/j.1365--2923.1998.00277.x. PMID: 10211248.
18. Sargeant JM, Purdy RA, Allen MJ, Nadkarni S, Watton L, O'Brien P. Evaluation of a CME problem-based learning internet discussion. Acad Med. 2000;75(10 Suppl):S50–2. https://doi.org/10.1097/00001888-200010001-00016. PMID: 11031172.
19. Pedersen M, Verspoor K, Jenkinson M, Law M, Abbott DF, Jackson GD. Artificial intelligence for clinical decision support in neurology. Brain Commun. 2020;2(2):fcaa096. https://doi.org/10.1093/braincomms/fcaa096. PMID: 33134913; PMCID: PMC7585692.

20. Kwon J, Lee H, Cho S, Chung CS, Lee MJ, Park H. Machine learning-based automated classification of headache disorders using patient-reported questionnaires. Sci Rep. 2020;10(1):14062. https://doi.org/10.1038/s41598-020-70992-1. PMID: 32820214; PMCID: PMC7441379.
21. Barrows H, Tamblyn R, Gliva G, Baxter D, Murray J, Dunne P. Design and evaluation of problem-based learning units in neurology. Trans Am Neurol Assoc. 1979;104:236–8. PMID: 553419.
22. Young WB, Rosen N, Sheftell F. Square one: headache education for the medical student. Headache. 2007;47(3):351–4. https://doi.org/10.1111/j.1526-4610.2007.00726.x. PMID: 17371351.
23. Pace A, Orr SL, Rosen NL, Safdieh JE, Cruz GB, Sprouse-Blum AS. The current state of headache medicine education in the United States and Canada: an observational, survey-based study of neurology clerkship directors and curriculum deans. Headache. 2021;61(6):854–62. https://doi.org/10.1111/head.14134. Epub 2021 Jun 29. PMID: 34184273.
24. Budd A, Dinkel H, Corpas M, Fuller JC, Rubinat L, Devos DP, Khoueiry PH, Förstner KU, Georgatos F, Rowland F, Sharan M, Binder JX, Grace T, Traphagen K, Gristwood A, Wood NT. Ten simple rules for organizing an unconference. PLoS Comput Biol. 2015;11(1):e1003905. https://doi.org/10.1371/journal.pcbi.1003905. PMID: 25633715; PMCID: PMC4310607
25. Ong JJY, Chan YC. Medical undergraduate survey on headache education in Singapore: knowledge, perceptions, and assessment of unmet needs. Headache. 2017;57(6):967–78. https://doi.org/10.1111/head.13110.
26. Kristoffersen ES, Faiz KW, Winsvold BS. Neurology residents' knowledge of the management of headache. Cephalalgia. 2019;39(11):1396–406. https://doi.org/10.1177/0333102419847973.
27. World Health Organization. Atlas of headache disorders and resources in the world, 2011.
28. Gallagher RM, Alam R, Shah S, Mueller L, Rogers JJ. Headache in medical education: medical schools, neurology and family practice residencies. Headache. 2005;45(7):866–73. https://doi.org/10.1111/j.1526-4610.2005.05155.x.
29. Kristoffersen ES, Faiz KW, Hansen JM, Tronvik EA, Frich JC, Lundqvist C, Winsvold BS. The management and clinical knowledge of headache disorders among general practitioners in Norway: a questionnaire survey. J Headache Pain. 2021;22(1):136. https://doi.org/10.1186/s10194-021-01350-3.

Correction to: Migraine, Psychiatric Disorders and Psychopharmacology

Michelle Bravo, Maria Adelaida Rueda-Lara,
and Noah Rosen

Correction to:
Chapter 11 in: T. S. Monteith et al. (eds.), *Comprehensive Migraine Management*,
https://doi.org/10.1007/978-3-031-86923-5_11

This title has been published recently. Table 11.11 in Chapter 11 was published incorrectly and has now been corrected with the updated table.

Table 11.11 Neuroleptics

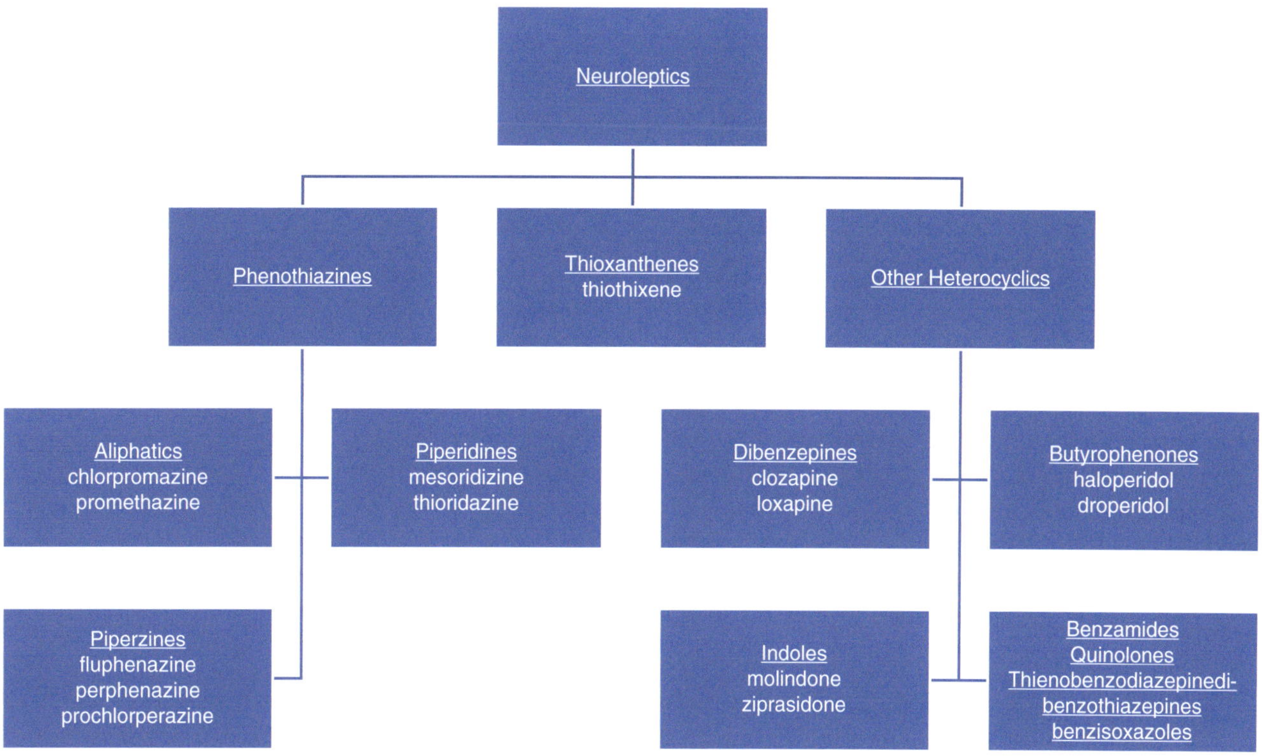

The updated version of this chapter can be found at
https://doi.org/10.1007/978-3-031-86923-5_11

T. S. Monteith et al. (eds.), *Comprehensive Migraine Management*, https://doi.org/10.1007/978-3-031-86923-5_41

Index

T. S. Monteith et al. (eds.), *Comprehensive Migraine Management*, https://doi.org/10.1007/978-3-031-86923-5

Q

R

S

MIX
Papier aus verantwortungsvollen Quellen
Paper from responsible sources
FSC® C105338

If you have any concerns about our products,
you can contact us on
ProductSafety@springernature.com

In case Publisher is established outside the EU,
the EU authorized representative is:
Springer Nature Customer Service Center GmbH
Europaplatz 3, 69115 Heidelberg, Germany

Printed by Libri Plureos GmbH
in Hamburg, Germany